Nursing Outcomes Classification (NOC)

Measurement of Health Outcomes

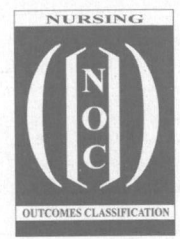

EDITORS

Sue Moorhead, RN, PhD, FAAN
Elizabeth Swanson, PhD, RN
Marion Johnson, PhD, RN

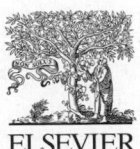

ELSEVIER

3251 Riverport Lane
St. Louis, Missouri 63043

NURSING OUTCOMES CLASSIFICATION (NOC), SEVENTH EDITION ISBN: 978-0-323-88252-1

Notices

International Standard Book Number: 978-0-323-88252-1

Senior Content Strategist: Sandra Clark
Senior Content Development Specialist: Kathleen Nahm
Publishing Services Manager: Deena Burgess
Project Manager: Anne Collett
Design Direction: Margaret Reid

Printed in India

Last digit is the print number: 9 8 7 6 5 4 3 2

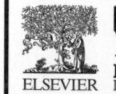

Working together
to grow libraries in
developing countries

www.elsevier.com • www.bookaid.org

The editors of this edition of NOC would like to
dedicate this book to the memory of our colleague,

Dr. Meridean L. Maas

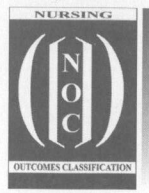

About the Editors

Dr. Sue Moorhead RN, PhD, FAAN received her undergraduate degree from the University of Maryland through the Walter Reed Army Institute of Nursing (WRAIN) at Walter Reed Army Medical Center in Washington, DC and received her commission as a 1st Lieutenant in the Army Nurse Corps after receiving her BSN in 1972. After graduation, she was stationed at the community hospital at Fort Belvoir, Virginia working on a medical surgical unit. She served on active duty for 7 years before returning to Iowa. As a member of the Army Reserves, she served as the chief nurse at the 73rd Combat Support Hospital in Cedar Rapids, Iowa and the chief nurse of the 830th Station Hospital in Des Moines, Iowa. She retired from the Army Nurse Corps as a Colonel after 27 years of active and reserve service in 1997. Her clinical experiences were primarily in medical surgical nursing and renal dialysis. She received her Master's degree in nursing focused on adult health in 1982 and her Doctoral degree in nursing focused on nursing administration in 1993 from the University of Iowa. During her PhD program, she worked for over 3 years as a research assistant on the Nursing Interventions Classification team and as a new faculty member started working with Marion Johnson and Meridean Maas on classifying nursing-sensitive patient outcomes. She has been a faculty member at the University of Iowa for more than 30 years. Dr. Moorhead's teaching focused primarily on leadership, nursing administration, and nursing process, and the use of standardized nursing terminologies. She served for 5 years as the director of the PhD program and for 16 years as the Director of the Center for Nursing Classification and Clinical Effectiveness (CNC). Her research focuses on the development and implementation of standardized nursing terminologies and effectiveness research. She has served as the lead editor of the Nursing Outcomes Classification (NOC) since the third edition. She has published 11 books and over 100 articles and book chapters. In her last years as a faculty member, she primarily mentored doctoral students from Iowa and other international universities. She is a fellow of the Center for Nursing Classification and Clinical Effectiveness, NANDA International, and the American Academy of Nursing. She retired from the University of Iowa in 2021 but remains active in her role with NOC and the CNC and mentors young scholars interested in using nursing terminologies.

Dr. Elizabeth (Liz) Swanson PhD, RN completed her BSN degree at The University of Iowa (UI) College of Nursing, her MA in medical-surgical nursing from the UI College of Nursing and her PhD in Student Development and Personnel from the UI College of Education. Her career at the University of Iowa has included various positions: staff nurse, faculty member, investigator, collegiate administrator, and a stint in central administration. Dr. Swanson's initial exposure to the Nursing Outcomes Classification (NOC), was as a focus group leader in the interest area of caregivers and caregiving. This work produced numerous caregiver outcomes, which are still prominent in the editions. Through her many positions within the University of Iowa, she has consistently been involved in advancing the financial stability of the units in which she worked. Her fund-raising efforts generated numerous opportunities for nursing students and faculty members to acquire support for educational, research, and programmatic initiatives through the completion of a major campaign. Dr. Swanson is the author of 78 journal articles and book chapters. In addition, she has edited with colleagues' 10 books including three NOC editions and three linkage editions. She and her colleagues released the sixth edition of Nursing Outcomes Classification (NOC) in 2018 and now this seventh edition. In addition, she is a part of a work group defining the value of the discipline of nursing. Dr. Swanson is a member of NANDA-International and associated with ACENDIO. She has also had the opportunity to provide nursing process content and impact the view of nursing education in Russia. She serves as a manuscript reviewer for *Applied Nursing Research, Journal of Nursing Scholarship, Midwest Nursing Research Journal, Scandinavian Journal of Caring Sciences, Geriatric Nursing, and the American Journal of Nursing.* She is currently an Associate Professor Emeritus from the University of Iowa, College of Nursing.

Dr. Marion Johnson, PhD, RN received her education at the College of St. Teresa in Winona, Minnesota (BSN); Case-Western Reserve, Cleveland (MSN), and The University of Iowa (PhD). The emphasis of her undergraduate and Master's degree was nursing. Her doctoral work focused on administration and the development of research skills. Immediately after receiving her BSN, Dr. Johnson spent 1 year working as a staff nurse at St. Mary's Hospital in Rochester, Minnesota before going to graduate school. She also worked as a staff nurse at a community hospital in Cleveland while in school. She moved to Iowa City in 1968 to take a position at University of Iowa Hospitals as a Clinical Specialist in the Neuroscience division. During her 6 years at University Hospitals, she held positions as a Clinical Director and as a research assistant on a lung cancer study with an oncologist and a pulmonary surgeon. It was during this time that she recognized the need to identify patient outcomes influenced by nursing to quantify nursing's contribution to patient care. After receiving her MSN, Dr. Johnson taught for 2 years at Case-Western Reserve school of nursing and for 13 years at South Dakota State University as an Assistant Professor and later an Acting Head of the nursing program. Dr. Johnson assumed an Assistant Professor position at the College of Nursing at The University of Iowa in 1980 and retired as a Full Professor in 2001. It was during these years that she received a num-

ber of small grants to study outcomes of nursing care and two large grants from NIH, National Institute of Nursing Research to continue this work. In addition, she served as Project Director on a grant to implement a Family Nurse Practitioner Program at the College and was an Assistant Director on two grants to expand the graduate program in Nursing Administration. During her professional career, Dr. Johnson was an active member of six nursing organizations focused on nursing practice, education, and research. She served on of a number of committees for these organizations and for the college and university. Dr. Johnson taught clinical courses in the undergraduate program and graduate courses in the nursing administration program at Iowa. She served terms as director of the nursing administration area and of the graduate programs. She has three children and as many women do, she juggled work and childcare during her career. She considers her major contribution to nursing the work reflected in the series of books titled, *Nursing Outcomes Classification*.

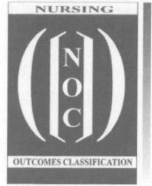

Recognition List, Seventh Edition

We want to thank the following individuals who have shared their knowledge and expertise by reviewing or developing outcomes. The editors deeply appreciate and value their contributions to the development of nursing-sensitive outcomes.

Elenice Valentim Carmona, PhD, MSN, RN, Associate Professor, School of Nursing, Universidade Estadual de Campinas (UNICAMP), São Paulo, Brazil.

Sena Chae, PhD, RN, Assistant Professor, University of Iowa, College of Nursing, Iowa City, IA, USA.

Mary F. Clarke, PhD, RN-BC, NE-BC, Vice President of Nursing Excellence, HealthLinx, Columbus, OH, USA.

Natany da Costa Ferreira Oberfrank, PhD, RN, Assistant Professor, College of Nursing, University of Iowa, Iowa City, IA, USA.

Erica Davisson Watkinson, PhD, RN-BC, Lecturer, University of Iowa, College of Nursing; Staff Nurse, University of Iowa Hospitals and Clinics, Iowa City, IA, USA.

Miriam de Abreu Almeida, PhD, RN, Professor, School of Nursing, Universidade Federal do Rio Grande do Sul (UFRGS), Porto Alegre, RS, Brazil.

Amália de Fátima Lucena, PhD, RN, Associate Professor, School of Nursing, Universidade Federal do Rio Grande do Sul (UFRGS), Porto Alegre, RS, Brazil. Coordinator of the Nursing Process Committee, Hospital de Clínicas de Porto Alegre, Porto Alegre, RS, Brazil.

Karina de Oliveira Azzolin, PhD, RN. Associate Professor, School of Nursing, Universidade Federal do Rio Grande do Sul (UFRGS), Porto Alegre, RS, Brazil.

Fernanda de Souza Freitas Abbud, RN, Ob/Gyn NP, Master's student, School of Nursing, Universidade Estadual de Campinas (UNICAMP),), São Paulo, SP, Brazil

Ana Railka de Souza Oliveira-Kumakura, Assistant Professor, School of Nursing, Universidade Estadual de Campinas (UNICAMP), São Paulo, SP, Brazil.

Suellen Cristina Dias Emidio, PhD, Assistant Professor, Universidade Federal do Tocantins (UFT), Nursing Department, Palmas, TO, Brazil.

Murilo dos Santos Graeff, MSN, RN, Doctoral student, School of Nursing, Universidade Federal do Rio Grande do Sul (UFRGS), Porto Alegre, RS, Brazil.

Isabel Cristina Echer, PhD, RN. Associate Professor, School of Nursing, Universidade Federal do Rio Grande do Sul (UFRGS), Porto Alegre, RS, Brazil.

Maria Lindell Joseph, Clinical Professor, PhD, RN, FAAN, FAONL, College of Nursing, University of Iowa, Iowa City, IA, USA.

Antonieta Keiko Kakuda Shimo, RN, PhD, Ob/Gyn NP, Professor, School of Nursing, Universidade Estadual de Campinas (UNICAMP), School of Nursing, São Paulo, SP, Brazil.

Rosana Pinheiro Lunelli, MSc, RN, Nursing Professor, Centro Universitário da Serra Gaúcha (FSG), -Caxias do Sul, RS, Brazil; Doctoral student in Nursing, School of Nursing, Universidade Federal do Rio Grande do Sul (UFRGS), Porto Alegre, RS, Brazil.

Vanessa Monteiro Mantovani, PhD, MSc, RN, Social Projects Nurse, Hospital Moinhos de Vento, Porto Alegre, RS, Brazil.

Intansari Nurjannah, PhD, M.NSc., S.Kp., RN, Associate Professor, Department of Mental Health and Community Nursing, Faculty of Medicine, Public Health and Nursing, Universitas Gadjah Mada, Yogyakarta, Indonesia.

Eneida Rejane Rabelo-Silva, PhD, RN, Professor, School of Nursing, Universidade Federal do Rio Grande do Sul (UFRGS), Porto Alegre, RS, Brazil; Cardiology Division, Hospital de Clínicas de Porto Alegre, Porto Alegre, RS, Brazil.

Rejane Reich, PhD, RN, Cardiology Division, Hospital de Clínicas de Porto Alegre, Porto Alegre, RS, Brazil.

Dawn E. Sugarman, PhD, Assistant Professor, Department of Psychiatry, Harvard Medical School; Research Psychologist, Alcohol, Drug, and Addiction Clinical and Health Services Research Program, McLean Hospital, Belmont, MA, USA.

Preface

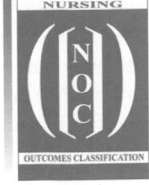

This edition of *Nursing Outcomes Classification (NOC)* represents over 30 years of work by the NOC team to develop nursing terminology focused on patient, family, and community outcomes at the Center for Nursing Classification and Clinical Effectiveness located at the University of Iowa, College of Nursing. The classification standardizes nursing outcome concepts, definitions, indicators, and measurement scales for use in practice, education, and research. Each outcome includes a label name, a definition, a set of indicators that describe specific states, perceptions, or behaviors related to the outcome, a five-point Likert measurement scale(s), and selected references used in the development of the outcome. The outcomes assist nurses and other health care providers to evaluate and quantify the status of the patient, caregiver, family, or community.

The classification focuses on the measurement of outcomes across a variety of specialties and settings with outcomes for use with patients, families, and communities. Nurses incorporating NOC into their practice can quantify the change in patient status after nursing interventions and consistently monitor the patients' progress toward the desired outcome status. Feedback from educators, researchers, and clinicians using the outcome measures has been positive, and their suggestions have helped to improve the classification over the years. NOC is included in many of the nursing textbooks currently in use. It has been licensed for use in vendor products such as care planning, documentation, and staffing software.

The need for nursing to define patient outcomes that are responsive to nursing care has continued to increase since the first edition of this book was published. The growth of managed care, the emphasis on cost containment and safety, and the need for evidence-based practice continues to bring concerns about the effectiveness of nursing interventions and health care quality to the attention of nurses, consumers, health care organizations, payers, and policy makers. Being the largest group of health professionals, nursing plays a key role in the delivery of safe, cost-effective care in every health care setting; therefore it is imperative that nursing data are included in the evaluation of health care effectiveness. The COVID-19 pandemic has only served to reinforce the importance of delivering outcome-based care. The increasing uptick in the number of natural disasters and health emergencies like COVID-19 demonstrates the importance of having an educated, competent, and skilled nursing work force to respond to these calamities. COVID-19, as well as the environmental disasters, have heightened the presence of an ineffective and inefficient health care system. Of note, is the major impact this lack of effectiveness has on persons of color with preexisting health conditions, persons who are economically disadvantaged, and persons with limited access to health professionals. It is critical nurses respond to these circumstances in the years to come. We have attempted to respond to this call by developing new outcomes to respond to the future threats selected populations may experience. Examples of new outcomes that have been developed are *Community Pandemic Readiness*, *Community Pandemic Recovery*, *Community Pandemic Response*, *Family Risk Control: Household Food Insecurity*, *Knowledge: Community Health Resources*, *Risk Control: Food Insecurity*, and *Risk Control: Housing Insecurity*.

The NOC completes the nursing process elements of the Nursing Minimum Data Set (NMDS). NOC is a companion language to the Nursing Interventions Classification (NIC) interventions and the NANDA-I nursing diagnoses. Standardized nursing terminologies are required to assure that the nursing elements identified in the NMDS are included in electronic databases. They also facilitate the study and teaching of diagnostic reasoning and the development of midrange theory as linkages between patient characteristics, nursing diagnoses, nursing interventions, and nursing-sensitive outcomes are tested.

This edition contains 612 outcomes and includes 82 new outcomes. A complete list of new outcomes and changes in previously published outcomes can be found in Appendix A. We have revised the label of the domain Perceived Health to Health and Life Quality with the addition of two new classes: Health Status and Health Supporting Life Skills. Part 1 describes the current classification, addresses frequently asked questions, and highlights new features. A model of how diagnoses, outcomes, and interventions can be used for building nursing knowledge and supporting clinical reasoning is included in this edition as well as resources to support the use of NOC by educators, clinicians, and researchers.

The editors of this book want to thank the many nurses who have contributed to the development of NOC. The team has worked diligently to continue to expand

and evaluate the NOC outcomes. Many individuals have shared their knowledge and work with us or have agreed to review an outcome related to their specialty. Without them, this seventh edition would not be possible. NOC has been translated into 12 languages, allowing adoption to be expanded to nurses around the globe. We value the use of NOC in these countries and welcome their suggestions and feedback as they measure outcomes with the patients they serve.

Sue Moorhead and Liz Swanson

Strengths of the Nursing Outcomes Classification

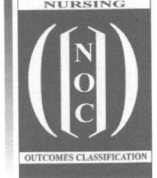

Comprehensive. The Nursing Outcomes Classification (NOC) contains outcomes for individuals, caregivers, families, and communities that can be used with all clinical specialties in care settings across the continuum of care. Although there are still outcomes to develop, the outcomes in this seventh edition are useful for the entire scope of nursing practice and can be used by other health care providers. It also reflects on new global health challenges facing individuals, families, and communities and health care professionals.

Research-based. The research, conducted by a large team of University of Iowa, College of Nursing faculty and students in conjunction with clinicians from a variety of settings, began in 1991. Both qualitative and quantitative strategies were used to develop the classification. Methods included content analysis, concept analysis, survey of experts, similarity analysis, hierarchical clustering analysis, multidimensional scaling, and clinical field site testing. The outcomes were evaluated for inter-rater reliability, validity, and usefulness in 10 clinical sites representing the care continuum. Research continues to validate the content and measurement scales thanks to the efforts of our students and colleagues, both nationally and internationally. This edition provides a comprehensive summary of research focused on NOC.

Developed inductively and deductively. Sources of data for the initial development of outcomes and indicators were nursing textbooks, care plan guides, nursing clinical information systems, standards of practice, and research instruments. Research team focus groups reviewed outcomes in eight broad categories that were drawn from the Medical Outcomes Study and nursing literature. Based on a review of the literature, outcomes were grouped in broad categories and refined through concept analysis. This was the foundation for the development of the NOC taxonomy and this process is still used today to develop new outcomes.

Grounded in clinical practice and research. Developed initially from nursing texts, care plan guides, and clinical information systems, the outcomes were reviewed by clinical experts, and many were tested in clinical field sites. Feedback from clinicians and educators is solicited through a defined feedback process. Beginning work on core NOC outcomes for specialty practice was first included in the third edition. This grounding in clinical practice continues with this edition as numerous outcomes were developed by clinical experts and forwarded to the authors. To be useful, the classification must be updated and refined to meet the needs of practicing nurses and support the scope of practice for nurses globally. The updating in this edition included the addition of several specialty groups not previously included.

Has an easy-to-use organizing structure. The taxonomy has five levels: domains, classes, outcomes, indicators, and measurement scales. All five levels have been coded for use in practice. New outcomes are added to the taxonomy as the classification is further developed. This structure aids nurses in identifying outcomes for use in clinical practice and provides a framework for teaching NOC to students in educational settings. The taxonomy has been an important part of the development of this classification of outcomes. A major review of the taxonomy for this edition was conducted and revisions were made to improve its fit with the classes and outcomes in the classification.

Outcomes can be shared by all disciplines. Although the NOC emphasizes outcomes that are responsive to nursing interventions, the outcomes describe patient, caregiver, family, or community states at a conceptual level. Thus, the NOC provides a classification of patient outcomes that are influenced by all health care disciplines. Use of the outcomes by all members of the interdisciplinary team provides standardization yet allows the selection of indicators that are most responsive to each discipline. Research in clinical setting across the care continuum demonstrated that the outcomes and indicators were useful to interdisciplinary teams in practice.

Optimizes information used for the evaluation of nursing effectiveness. The outcomes and indicators are variable concepts. They allow for measurement of the patient, caregiver, family, or community outcome at any point on a continuum from most negative to most positive and at different points in time. Rather than the limited information of whether a goal is met or unmet, NOC outcomes can be used to monitor the extent of progress, or lack of progress, throughout an episode of care and across different care settings. Change in outcome ratings can be reported and documented as a result of nursing interventions instituted across time and care settings.

Funded by extramural grants. The initial NOC research received 9 years of peer-reviewed grant funding: 1 year from Sigma Theta Tau International and 8 years from the National Institute of Nursing Research (NINR).

Tested in clinical field sites. Testing of the NOC has been conducted in a variety of clinical field sites, including tertiary care hospitals, intermediate care hospitals, a nursing home, home health care settings, nurse-managed clinics, and through a parish nursing organization. The field tests have provided important information about the clinical usefulness of the outcomes and indicators; linkages between nursing diagnoses, interventions, and outcomes; and the process of implementing the outcomes in clinical nursing information systems.

Dissemination emphasized. Information about the classification, its development, and its use is available in this book published by Elsevier every 5 to 6 years and in numerous journal articles, book chapters, and dissertations. The NOC is described on the University of Iowa College of Nursing website (https://nursing.uiowa.edu/center-for-nursing-classification-and-clinical-effectiveness). The NOC work has been disseminated in numerous national and international presentations. Although developed in the United States, nurses in other countries are finding the classification useful. Translations are available for the following languages: Chinese, Dutch, French, German, Indonesian, Italian, Japanese, Korean, Norwegian, Portuguese, Spanish, and Taiwanese. The English editions and the translations are listed in Appendix B.

Linked to other nursing languages. Linkages have been developed by the NIC and NOC editors and other scholars to assist nurses with the use of the classifications and to facilitate use in clinical information systems. Linkages among NANDA diagnoses, NOC outcomes, and NIC interventions are available in the book NANDA, NIC, and NOC linkage: Nursing Diagnoses, Interventions and Outcomes, published by Elsevier in 2012.

Included in initiatives for the electronic clinical record. All outcomes in the sixth edition of NOC have been included in SNOMED Clinical Terms, a reference terminology for use in clinical information systems. NOC has been registered with Health Level 7, a U.S. standards organization dedicated to simplifying the exchange, management, and integration of clinical and administrative data in health records. A growing number of vendors have licensed NOC for inclusion in their software focused on the nursing component of an electronic clinical record.

Developed as companion to the NIC. Experience with the NIC at Iowa has aided the NOC research. Both classifications are comprehensive, research-based, and reflect current clinical nursing practice. They are both housed in the Center for Nursing Classification and Clinical Effectiveness.

Recipient of national recognition. NOC is recognized by the American Nurses Association (ANA), included in the Metathesaurus for a Unified Medical Language at the National Library of Medicine, included in the CINAHL index, and listed as one of the languages that met the standards set by the ANA's Nursing Information and Data Set Evaluation Center (NIDSEC).

Validation of the outcomes and indicators. Because of the conceptual based development of the outcomes and indicators, validation work of NOC is being conducted within the United States and internationally. This work is being reviewed by the research team and used to address the revision and review of published outcomes. Since the last edition, many validation studies focused on NOC have been published. A summary of validation studies is included in this edition.

Structure for continued development and refinement. The classification continues to be evaluated, developed, and refined by the NOC research team. Continued refinement will be facilitated through the Center for Nursing Classification and Clinical Effectiveness, the College of Nursing, and the University of Iowa. A $1 million endowment is being raised to ensure a solid financial foundation for supporting further development of both NIC and NOC. Revenue from the book sales and licensing are used to support the staff and work of the Center for Nursing Classification and Clinical Effectiveness.

Definition of Terms

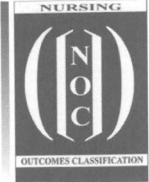

Nursing-Sensitive Patient Outcome

An individual, family, or community state, behavior, or perception that is measured along a continuum in response to a nursing intervention(s). Each outcome has an associated group of indicators that are used to determine patient status in relation to the outcome. To be measured, the outcome requires identification of a series of more specific indicators.

Outcome Indicator

A more concrete individual, family, or community state, behavior, or perception that serves as a cue for measuring an outcome. Nursing-sensitive patient outcome indicators characterize a patient, family, or community state at the concrete level. Some examples of indicators include "describes strategies to maximize health," "maintains usual family routines," or "intake of adequate fluid."

Measure

A five-point Likert type scale that quantifies a patient outcome or indicator status on a continuum from least to most desirable and provides a rating at a point in time. Measurement will reflect a continuum, such as 1 = Severely compromised; 2 = Substantially compromised; 3 = Moderately compromised; 4 = Mildly compromised; 5 = Not compromised.

Change Score

The difference between a baseline rating of the outcome and the postintervention rating(s) of the outcome. This change score can be positive (the outcome rating increased), negative (the outcome rating decreased), or there can be no change (the outcome rating stayed the same).

This change in rating score represents the outcome achieved following a health care intervention(s).

NOC Taxonomy

A systematic organization of outcomes into groups or categories based on similarities, dissimilarities, and relationships among the outcomes. The NOC taxonomy structure has five levels: domains, classes, outcomes, indicators, and measures.

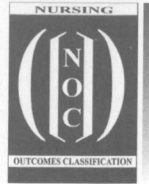

Acknowledgments

Continual development of the Nursing Outcomes Classification (NOC) and this publication would not have been possible without the work and support of numerous individuals and organizations. We are indebted to the many individuals who have supported our work and encouraged us along the way. We would like to acknowledge and thank the following individuals and organizations for their efforts:

- *Sigma Theta Tau International* for a 1-year grant (1992–1993) and the Office of Nursing Research, University of Iowa, for seed grants (1992–1993). These grants partially funded the pilot work and beginning development of the NOC.
- *The National Institute of Nursing Research, National Institutes of Health*, for a 4-year grant (1993–1997) to continue the development of the classification, construct the taxonomy, and field test the outcomes and for a 4-year continuation grant (1998–2001) entitled "Evaluation of Nursing-Sensitive Patient Outcome Measures" to pilot the outcomes and evaluate the measurement scales in clinical sites.
- The *College of Nursing* at the *University of Iowa* for support of this work by *past Deans Geraldene Felton, Melanie Dreher,* and *Rita Frantz, and Interim Deans Martha Craft-Rosenberg* and *Thad Wilson.* Thank you to our current *Dean Julie Zerwic* for her support as well. This support for the Center for Nursing Classification and Effectiveness since it was founded in 1995 has been instrumental in the continuing development and refinement of both NIC and NOC and our work on linkages among diagnoses, interventions, and outcomes.
- The *Director of the Center for Nursing Classification and Effectiveness Karen Dunn-Lopez* for continuing to acknowledge the contribution of this work to the nursing profession.
- The *team members, clinicians, educators, fellows, and students* who have devoted hours of work to develop, review, and refine the outcomes, associated indicators, and measurement scales that appear in NOC.
- The *NANDA International* organization for its partnership that enables the NOC team to link our languages to support the nursing profession. We also appreciate the organization's efforts through The Margery Gordon program to advance nursing diagnoses at the same time, preparing global scholars to advance nursing knowledge.
- *The National Library of Medicine* for including since the sixth edition, NOC terms in SNOMED Clinical Terms (SNOMED-CT). In addition, we acknowledge that NOC has been registered with Health Level 7, a U.S. standards organization dedicated to quality data within the health care records.
- *Nurses from a variety of nursing specialty organizations* who shared their expertise by completing validation surveys and core surveys to further this effort. In addition, interacting with us to improve the usability of the outcomes in clinical practice.
- The many *patients and their families* who were willing to participate in our research and complete both outcome ratings and criterion tool measures as we tested our outcomes in clinical settings.
- *Contributors to our endowment fund* to support the efforts of the Center for Nursing Classification and Clinical Effectiveness.
- The great staff we work with at Elsevier, *Sandra Clark* and *Bonita Allen,* for their diligent work on our behalf.
- The many nurses who have been named *Fellows* of the Center for Nursing Classifications and Clinical Effectiveness.
- Our very competent staff member, *Noriko Abe,* who manages the data and many details of this classification to make this edition possible.

Contents

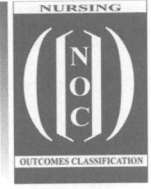

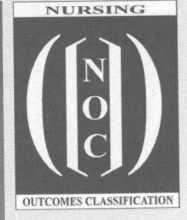

Overview and Use of Nursing Outcomes Classification (NOC)

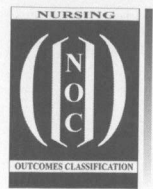

Overview and Use of Nursing Outcomes Classification (NOC)

OVERVIEW OF THE CLASSIFICATION
What is the Nursing Outcomes Classification (NOC)?

This book presents standardized terminology for outcomes for use by nurses across specialties and practice settings to capture changes in status after intervention. Each outcome represents a concept that can be used to measure the state of a patient, caregiver, family, or community before and after intervention. In some clinical situations, outcomes from a variety of these perspectives may be used for a patient situation. The outcomes have been developed for use by nurses, but other disciplines may find them helpful for evaluating the effectiveness of the interventions they provide independently or in collaboration with nurses. Each outcome has a definition, a measurement scale(s), a list of associated indicators for the concept, and supporting content references. For this edition, we expanded the number of references for most new and revised outcomes because more literature is available to support our work. The outcomes are organized in a taxonomy that facilitates the identification of outcomes for use in practice, education, and research. The three levels of the taxonomy, domains, classes, and outcomes help nurses and other care providers quickly identify outcomes useful for their practice. The current classification contains 612 outcomes including 82 new outcomes developed after the publication of the sixth edition in 2018.[218] This edition of NOC includes the *revision* or *review* of over 400 outcomes from prior editions.

Significance of NOC

Measuring the health outcomes of clinical care is a standard of professional practice across all health disciplines in today's health care environment, and it has global implications. Identifying patient outcomes responsive to nursing care is critical work for nurses who are facing the challenges of implementing electronic health records. In addition, there are continued efforts to engage patients in shared decision-making. This is an important goal for nurses and other health care providers as patients use a variety of media and website sources to learn about their health condition and possible treatment options. Other advantages of using outcomes are important to the discipline of nursing. Key is the continued focus of all health professionals and

government officials to control cost, improve safety, and enhance the effectiveness of care in an ever-changing health care system. Evidence-based practice has become an essential requirement for nurses to provide care that reflects current professional nursing practice. It is also vital for nurses to measure outcomes and capture changes in the status of patients over time, as this demonstrates the impact of the profession of nursing. In the past, nurses used outcomes primarily from physician practice to assess impact. Today, the existence of the NOC enables nurses to conduct ratings of progress in patients through the documentation of nursing-based outcomes. Many nurses believe that the use of standardized nursing terminologies can transform practice.[57,105,149,161,183,188,242] The ability to measure the effectiveness of nursing's role in health care has become even more important in the last years with the occurrence of the pandemic and other disasters.

Why is an Outcome Classification Needed?

The NOC includes patient, caregiver, family, and community outcomes that are responsive to nursing interventions. The outcomes in NOC are not intended to be unique to nursing. Most, if not all, patient outcomes are influenced by multiple health care providers, by environmental factors, and by other patient, caregiver, family, and community characteristics; however, it is critically important for nurses to measure the effects of their interventions on patient outcomes. The NOC provides a set of indicators for each outcome that is sensitive to nursing interventions. When used with interdisciplinary teams, different indicators may be the focus of interventions for other disciplines involved in the care of the patient. Without discipline-specific indicators for shared outcomes, it is impossible to monitor the accountability of each discipline for its contribution to outcome improvement or deterioration. To ensure that the contributions of nursing interventions to patient outcomes are not credited to other health care providers, standardized nursing data elements must be included in clinical electronic databases. Large data sets that include these data along with other salient system, patient, caregiver, family, or community characteristics, including provider characteristics, are necessary to isolate the independent effects of nursing interventions on patient outcomes. With the publication of this seventh edition, NOC remains the only comprehensive classification of outcomes available for health care providers across settings.

Identifying patient outcomes responsive to nursing care is critical work for nurses who face the challenge of implementing electronic health records. Efforts to engage patients and families in shared decision-making are growing, and this is an important goal for nurses and other health care providers as patients use the web to learn about their health conditions and possible treatment options. Key to this is the continued focus of health professionals and government officials on cost, safety, and effectiveness of care in the changing health care system in the United States and internationally. Evidence-based practice has become an essential requirement for nurses to provide care that reflects current professional nursing practice. Efforts by nurses to measure outcomes and capture changes in the status of patients over time provide a way to improve the quality of patient care and add to the knowledge base of nursing.

Historical Overview of the Development of NOC

Initially, NOC was developed to be used with nursing diagnoses and nursing interventions as an important part of using the nursing process, care planning, and documentation. Our initial work focused on the development of nursing-sensitive patient outcomes to enable nurses to measure the effects of the interventions they provide to patients, families, and communities. The focus of the early research of the NOC team was testing the reliability, validity, and sensitivity of the NOC outcomes and measurement scales.[22,87,141,144–146,148,154,157,193–195,280] Reed[270] examined the characteristics of patients and settings related to the choice of indicators by nurses providing care using NOC to see differences in use across the continuum of care. Box 1.1 summarizes the criteria we established in the original research

Criteria for Evaluating Nursing Sensitivity

A nursing intervention produces a positive outcome.
A nursing intervention influences a positive outcome.
A nursing intervention is implemented with the intent of producing or influencing the outcome.
A nursing intervention produces improvement or maintenance of the outcome.
A nursing intervention prevents deterioration or occurrence of a negative outcome.
The nursing intervention occurs before observation of the outcome.
The interventions that produce or influence the outcome are within the scope of practice of nursing.

to meet the standard for an outcome to be considered nurse sensitive. These criteria have served us well and continue to be relevant as we develop new nursing-sensitive patient outcomes for use by nurses.

Many factors in nursing and the health care environment stimulated the need for an outcomes classification in nursing to be developed over the last 30 years. The creation of NOC provides terminology for the outcome identification and evaluation steps of the nursing process and nursing content for the outcomes element of the Nursing Minimum Data Set[322,323] published by Werley and colleagues.[323] NOC can also be used as a key component of the Outcome-Present State Test Model for clinical reasoning developed by Pesut and Herman[258,259] and the application of this framework in nursing education[326] and advanced practice.[167] In addition, the documentation of outcomes has been encouraged by the work of NANDA International (NANDA-I) as it developed patient problems as nursing diagnoses, and the early work of the Nursing Interventions Classification (NIC) team.[136,198] As nursing terminology was developed, several nurse leaders in language development identified the issues that needed to be addressed that contributed to the development of outcomes for nursing as a profession.[192,198] In addition, the development of computerized information systems in health care created the capacity to generate large uniform databases and encouraged efforts supporting meaningful use of health care data.[104,156,158,159,285,318] The emphasis on demonstrating health care effectiveness and evidence-based practice[74,152,153,211,216,316,330] also supported the development of NOC. The definition and classification of clinically useful nursing-sensitive patient outcomes, however, was not realized until the first edition of NOC edited by Marion Johnson and Meridean Maas was published in 1997.[137] Expanded editions were published in 2000,[138] 2004,[212] 2008,[214] 2013,[215] and 2018.[218] A detailed timeline of the development of NOC is available in Appendix D.

The NOC is globally significant because standardized terminologies for computerized nursing diagnoses, interventions, and outcomes are needed for the study of linkages among these patient phenomena using actual patient data. Further, the standardized nursing terminologies represent concepts that describe basic phenomena the nursing discipline is accountable for as part of clinical practice. In addition, the linkages among the concepts of diagnoses, outcomes, and interventions represent an important stage of nursing theory development as the relationship between nursing diagnoses, outcomes, and interventions are identified for patient populations treated by nurses. Nurse researchers from around the world have contributed to the refinement of NOC with publications in English from Brazil, China, Greece, Iceland, Indonesia, Israel, Italy, Nigeria, Portugal, Spain, South Korea, Switzerland, and Turkey.

Who Should Use NOC?

Nurses working in any clinical setting across the care continuum can use NOC. Nurses working in specialty areas identify nursing outcomes important to their practice area such as advanced practice,[60,108,154,158] cancer,[304,313,314] community,[8,125–127] gerontology,[5,14,29,128,129,180] hemodialysis,[75] home care,[15,16,157,289,303] hospice/palliative care,[38,140,187,200,267,275] intensive care,[56,86,87,206,219] long-term care,[61,62,73,110] medical/surgical,[6,19,67,82,112,113,115,202,232,243,244,252,276,292,317] obstetrics,[90,91,327] neurology,[99,133,134,173,177] orthopedics,[68,201,274] parish nursing,[40,41,89] pediatrics,[1,26,50,72,192,287] peri-operative nursing,[30,81,264] psychiatry,[93,139,263,308] rehabilitation,[9,145,286] and school nursing.[51,52,189,328] Another group who can use nursing-sensitive patient outcomes in support of patients are family caregivers.[301,306] The use of the knowledge and self-management outcomes by patients and family caregivers has added a new dimension to our work and offered another perspective to outcome development efforts. More recently, the knowledge outcomes have been used to evaluate the knowledge base of practicing nurses caring for patients with clinical conditions.[35] The list of ways NOC is being used to support quality care and enhance nursing practice continues to expand.

As knowledge of NOC has expanded within health care organizations and across the globe, interest in using outcomes by other health care providers has greatly increased. Some of the disciplines that want to include measurement of clinical outcomes in their practice are nutritionists, physical therapists, occupational therapists, speech pathologists,[284] respiratory therapists, social workers, and pastoral care providers.[41] Using NOC in clinical practice is also of interest to nurse managers and nurse executives who want to have data to describe the quality of care provided by their organization.[149] Zugcic and colleagues[331] have linked patient satisfaction to the use of NOC outcomes, an important focus of organizations today. Anderson and colleagues[11] describe how to use bibliometrics to select nursing terminologies for use in practice and Scherb and Weydt[288] use NIC and NOC to describe the complexity of nurse work environments. For nurse managers or executives trying to decide how to use NOC in their organization, Moorhead[208] describes 10 paths for using nursing terminologies in clinical practice.

BASIC COMPONENTS OF NOC
Definition of a Nursing-Sensitive Patient Outcome

A nursing-sensitive patient outcome is an individual, family, or community state, behavior, or perception that is measured along a continuum in response to a nursing intervention(s). The outcomes are variable concepts that can be measured by nurses, other health care providers,

caregivers, or patients using a 5-point measurement scale(s). The outcomes are stated as concepts that reflect a patient, caregiver, family, or community state, behavior, or perception rather than as expected goals. Key terms and definitions used in the development of NOC outcomes are listed in Box 1.2. Each outcome has an associated group of indicators that are used to determine patient status in relation to the outcome. Outcome indicators are defined as a more concrete individual, family, or community state, behavior, or perception that serves as a cue for measuring an outcome. The definitions and indicators acknowledge that nurses, family caregivers, and patients provide outcome data, and that both the patient and family caregiver are the focus of outcomes for individuals. Some outcomes can be measured only by the patient, some only by the nurse, and some by the patient (or family) and the nurse or other health provider. This is an important consideration when nurses use NOC outcomes in their clinical practice. The outcomes that are based on the patient's perception of the outcome must be measured by the patient. Examples of this type of outcome are *Pain Level*, *Nausea & Vomiting Severity*, and *Suffering Severity*. Examples of outcomes that are measured by the nurse or other health professional are *Respiratory Function*, *Blood Loss Severity*, *Wound Healing: Secondary Intention*, and *Kidney Function*. It is important that the nurse is aware of the importance of perspective (whose viewpoint is needed) and the primary focus or priority of care for a patient when selecting outcomes.[207]

Most patient outcomes, including those traditionally used to evaluate physician care, are not influenced by any one discipline alone. For nursing to monitor and improve its practice, it is important to identify the outcomes that are responsive to nursing care. If the care provider is a nurse, the term *nursing-sensitive* patient outcomes is used. The more abstract and global the outcome, the more likely its achievement will be the result of interventions from several health care disciplines. Specific disciplines will have more influence on certain intermediate outcomes than others. For example, at various times nursing, medicine, and physical therapy may have the most impact on the outcome *Mobility* (0208), although all interventions provided by health professionals impact the outcome. Another example is *Respiratory Function* (0415) that may be shared among medicine, nursing, and respiratory therapy. Specific indicators of an outcome are more likely to be sensitive to the interventions of a single discipline; therefore it is essential to identify the indicators that are most sensitive to nursing interventions. This enables nurses to document the effects of their interventions and to be held individually and collectively accountable for care delivered to patients. In this book, we do not always use the term nurse-sensitive patient outcomes but simply call them patient outcomes or outcomes for simplicity.

Box 1.2

Definitions of Selected Terms Used in NOC

Ability

Power or capacity to perform actions.

Adaptation

The action or process of changing or adjusting.

Adherence

To hold fast to a selected action to improve health.

Adolescence

The period in a child's life from 12 years through 17 years.

Adulthood

A period in the human lifespan in which full physical and intellectual maturity have been attained.

Appropriate

Suitable to meet requirements, demands, or needs.

Assistive Device

Any tool or apparatus that helps an individual do something that he/she might not otherwise be able to do.

Avoids

Withdrawing from something; to keep away from.

Behavior

The observable or reported response of an individual, family, or community to its environment.

Caregiver

A family member, significant other, friend, or other person who cares for or acts on behalf of the patient.

Care Recipient

The person, such as patient, caregiver (specify), parent (specify), family (specify), or community (specify), receiving services from a professional.

Change in Rating Score

The difference between a baseline rating of the outcome and the post-intervention rating(s) of the outcome. This change score can be positive (the outcome rating increased), negative (the outcome rating decreased) or there can be no change (the outcome rating stayed the same). This change in rating score represents the outcome achieved following a health care intervention(s).

Child

Overall term for childhood from 1 year through 17 years old.

Childcare Provider

Family caregiver or an individual who is paid to provide childcare.

Clinical Condition

A medical, nursing diagnosis or patient state that may be associated with multiple diagnoses or that is undiagnosed.

Chronic Disease

A human health condition or illness that is persistent and long-lasting in its effects on the individual usually lasting for more than 3 months.

Classification

A process of classifying something according to shared qualities or characteristics.

Community

An interactive population with relationships that emerge as members develop and use, in common, some agencies and institutions.

Confidence

Belief that one can act to achieve a desired goal.

Conservation

The act of trying to protect or preserve something or limiting how much of a resource you use.

Convey

To express a thought, feeling, or idea so that it is understood.

Core Outcomes

A concise set of outcomes that capture the essence of an area of specialty practice.

Data Source

Documentation of where data are obtained from, such as the patient, family member, caregiver, direct observation by health care provider, clinical record, or other sources.

Decreased

Lesser in size, degree, or amount.

Disease

A specific pathological process defined by a set of signs and symptoms that affects a body part or the whole body where the etiology, pathology, and prognosis may be known or unknown.

Discharge

The action of arranging for someone to leave a hospital or other health care facility.

Domain

The highest-level abstraction in the NOC taxonomy.

Early Childhood

The period in a child's life from 1 year through 5 years (includes Toddler and Preschool).

Effective

Producing desired health-related results.

Electronic Health Record

An electronic version of a patient's medical history that is maintained by an organization or provider over time and may in-

Box 1.2—cont'd

Definitions of Selected Terms Used in NOC

clude all important administrative clinical data relevant to the person's care.

Established Adulthood

Period in an adult's life from 30 to 44 years old.

Equilibrium

A state or situation in which opposing forces or influences are balanced.

Family

Two or more people who are related biologically, legally, or by choice that has a societal expectation to socialize, enculturate, and care for its members.

Function

Special action or physiologic property of an organ or other part of the body to perform its specific work.

Functioning

To carry out a set of actions in the expression or performance of a role.

Health

A state of physical, psychological, social, and spiritual functioning.

Health Professionals

Individuals with advanced education and licensure that are reimbursed for providing health care services.

Health Providers

Professional and assistive personnel who are reimbursed for providing health care services.

Home

A place of residence where an individual lives permanently or for a length of time as a member of a family or household.

Hospitalization

A situation where a patient is admitted to a hospital for evaluation or treatment.

Inappropriate

Not suitable for meeting requirements, demands, or needs.

Increased

Greater in amount, degree, or size.

Infant

The term used for a baby from birth to first birthday.

Late Adulthood

Period in an adult's life from 65 years and older.

Level

A position on a real or imaginary scale of amount, quantity, extent, or quality.

Linkages

The existence or forming of a connection between two or more concepts.

Literacy

Competence or knowledge in a specified area.

Knowledge

The accumulation of facts, information, and skills acquired by a person through experience or education.

Measure

A five-point Likert-type scale that quantifies a patient outcome or indicator status on a continuum from least-to-most desirable and provides a rating at a point in time.

Medication

A substance used for the treatment of a health condition.

Mental

Total emotional and intellectual response.

Middle Adulthood

Period in an adult's life from 45 years through 64 years.

Middle Childhood

The period in a child's life from 6 years through 11 years.

Newborn

The term used for a baby the first 28 days of life.

NOC Taxonomy

A systematic organization of outcomes into groups or categories based upon similarities, dissimilarities, and relationships among the outcomes. The NOC taxonomy structure has five levels: domains, classes, outcomes, indicators, and measures.

Non-Parenteral Medication

A substance used to treat a clinical condition administered as oral medications (pills, capsules, syrups), topical medications (ointments, patches like nitro), or suppositories (vaginal and rectal).

Normalization

The process of bringing or returning something to a normal condition or state.

Nursing-Sensitive Outcome

An individual, family, or community state, behavior, or perception that is measured along a continuum in response to a nursing intervention(s). Each outcome has an associated group of indicators that are used to determine patient status in relation to the outcome.

Obtains

To gain or attain by planned effort or action.

Outcome Indicator

A more concrete individual, family, or community state, behavior, or perception that serves as a cue for measuring an outcome.

Box 1.2—cont'd

Definitions of Selected Terms Used in NOC

Pandemic

An epidemic occurring worldwide, or over a very wide area, crossing international boundaries and usually affecting many people.

Parent

Mother, father, or individual assuming the childrearing role.

Participation

The act of joining with others in doing something.

Perception

A conscious mental thought or an image or sensation from a sensory stimulus.

Personal Actions

Actions taken by the individual, caregiver, significant other, or family member.

Preterm Infant

A term used for babies born alive before 37 weeks of pregnancy are completed.

Prevention

Actions taken by an individual to stop something from happening.

Population

A collection of individuals who have one or more personal (e.g., gender, age, illness) or environmental (e.g., country, worksite) characteristics in common.

Preschool

The term used for a child from 3 years through 5 years.

Protection

Actions taken by an individual to prevents someone or something from suffering harm or injury.

Readiness

A state or condition of being fully prepared for something.

Recommended

Presented as worthy of confidence, acceptance, or use.

Recovery

The process of getting something back that was lost or almost destroyed.

Reference Person

A healthy person of the same age and gender used for comparison when rating an outcome or indicator.

Refrains

Keeps oneself from following a passing impulse.

Response

A reaction to a question, experience, or some other type of stimulus.

Reputable

Recognized as positive by health providers or experts in the field.

Resilience

The ability to become strong, healthy, or successful again after a negative event or experience.

Resources

Source of supply, support, or information.

Risk Control

Personal actions to understand and avoid, limit or control identified health risks.

Satisfaction

A happy or pleased feeling because of something that you did or something that happened to you.

School-Age Child

The term used for a child from 6 years through 17 years.

Self-Care Behavior

Decisions and actions that an individual can take to cope with a health problem or to improve their health.

Self-Control

The ability to control oneself, one's emotions and desires or the expression of them in one's behavior, especially in demanding situations.

Self-Management

The personal application of behavior-change tactics that produces a desired change in behavior including self-control and self-monitoring skills that an individual can do without supervision.

Severity

The degree of something undesirable.

Status

State of health of the focus of the outcome. This may be at the individual, family, or community level or a function of a system or state of the body.

Stability

A state or quality of being stable, or without change.

Syndrome

A group of symptoms, which consistently occur together, or a condition characterized by a set of associated symptoms.

Toddler

The term used for a child from 1 year through 2 years.

Well-Being

Extent of positive perception of one's own health status.

Young Adulthood

Period in an adult's life from 21 years through 29 years.

Sensitivity of the Outcomes

Each concept represents a patient, caregiver, family, or community state that is sensitive in varying degrees to nursing interventions. Originally, the research team assessed sensitivity to nursing interventions by: (1) selecting the concepts from outcomes in nursing literature and clinical information systems, (2) determining that the outcomes have been used to measure the effects of nursing interventions, and (3) surveying expert nurses about the importance of the outcomes as measures of the effects of nursing interventions. The ultimate test of sensitivity will be the widespread selection and use of outcomes in practice and research with careful analyses that isolate the effects of interventions on patient outcomes. Because the outcomes have been developed for use in all settings where nurses provide care, some of the outcome indicators may be more applicable in one setting than another. For example, blood values and other diagnostic results used as indicators may be pertinent in an intensive or acute care setting, but they may be less useful in a home or nursing home setting. Community-level outcomes are more likely to be used in community health settings or in the evaluation of community actions.

Identification of the Recipient of Care

Patient outcomes focus on the care recipient, although this traditional use of the term *patient* is too limiting. *Patient* traditionally is defined as an individual recipient of care; however, family caregivers and significant others often are involved substantially with patients or may be recipients of care themselves. The term *patient* is used in many of the outcomes even though the care recipient may be called *client, consumer,* or *resident* in some settings. The first two editions of NOC used the term *patient* consistently. When the satisfaction outcomes were added to the third edition, the term *patient satisfaction* was considered by the team to be too limiting, so the term *client satisfaction* is used to describe these outcomes. The issue has continued to evolve in nursing, with some health care organizations using the term *consumer* to refer to their patients. Regardless of what word is used to describe these individuals, the research team decided to use individuals as the focal unit for the development of NOC, with family caregivers included as an individual to facilitate assessing the impact of nursing on individual family members. The recipient of care can also be the family as a unit of care, or the community. In this edition, 88% of the outcomes are developed for use at the individual level. Thus, recipient of care can address the individual and/or the family member/caregiver.

Taxonomy and Levels of Abstraction

The NOC contains health outcomes presented at four general levels of abstraction with measurement procedures at the

Table 1.1	LEVELS OF ABSTRACTION IN TAXONOMY
Level of Abstraction	**Level in Taxonomy**
Most Abstract	Nursing-Sensitive Outcome Domain
High Middle Level Abstraction	Nursing-Sensitive Outcome Classes
Middle Level Abstraction	Nursing-Sensitive Outcome
Low Level Abstraction	Nursing-Sensitive Outcome Indicators
Empirical Level	Measurement of Outcomes

empirical level (Table 1.1). The highest levels of abstraction, outcome domains and classes were derived from the results of hierarchical clustering and qualitative strategies used in the development of the taxonomy. The least level of abstraction contains the indicator statements for each of the outcome labels. While the outcomes are the middle level of abstraction, and in some unique instances, indicators are more abstract. The global outcomes are developed as more specific, less abstract outcomes. The levels of the taxonomy, domains, classes, and outcomes help nurses and other care providers quickly identify outcomes useful for their practice.

How to Choose Outcomes

Selecting health outcomes for a specific patient or group of patients is one step in the nurse's clinical decision-making process. The use of standardized terms and measures to evaluate outcomes does not decrease the nurse's responsibility to make an informed assessment and engage in clinical reasoning. Selected factors are paramount in the nurse's choice of health outcomes. These factors include the type of health problem, the nursing or medical diagnoses, patient characteristics, available resources, patient preferences, and treatment potential.

Health concerns identified for the patient can be categorized as: (1) problems for referral addressed primarily by other health professionals, (2) interdisciplinary problems addressed collaboratively with other providers, and (3) nursing diagnoses for which nurses have primary responsibility. These categories were clarified by the early work of the Iowa Intervention Project.[136] When the health concern falls in the first category, the primary accountability for identifying the desired outcome resides with the responsible health provider. When the health concern falls in the second category, nurses and other responsible providers should work together to identity the outcomes for the patient or patient population. When the health concern is a nursing diagnosis, nurses should assume primary responsibility for identifying patient outcomes related to the identified nursing diagnosis and include the patient in the decision-making process as much as possible. When selecting the appropriate outcomes using the nursing diagnoses, consideration needs to be given to the definition of the nursing diagnoses, the defining characteristics, related factors for each diagnosis, and the associated conditions.[131] If the nursing diagnosis is a risk diagnosis, consideration should be given to the listed risk factors. When the outcome selection is based on the medical diagnosis or a clinical condition, nurses should consider the signs and symptoms of the medical diagnosis or clinical condition, as well as causative and other related factors.

Another key component of the health care provider's decisions should be prioritization of the identified problems and associated outcomes. This is especially true when caring for older individuals with serious illness challenges such as cancer or dementia. Patients making complex treatment decisions commonly choose treatments based on remaining independent and extending life.[98] All individuals have a unique journey through their care and what matters to them should be considered by nurses and other health care providers when setting priorities[123] and selecting care facilities.[234]

Several additional factors are especially important in the selection of the health outcomes. Patient characteristics to consider include demographic factors, psychological and cognitive processes, illness and health-related factors, prior health challenges, and personal health beliefs or values. Education level is important when selecting outcomes related to knowledge and participation in health care decisions by the patient and family. Psychological and cognitive variables such as depression or anxiety and processes such as concentration, memory, information processing ability, and decision-making can influence the response of the patient to illness, the ability to learn, and motivation. It is critical that knowledge outcomes should not be selected for the patient who does not have the ability to recall the information or the ability to process information. When this situation arises, family members or significant others can be involved in the care situation and help with decision-making with the patient. Additional factors that impact outcome selection include severity of the illness, functional status, and the ability to perform activities of daily living and instrumental living. Financial concerns may also impact outcome selection.

There are numerous resources available to patients and their caregivers (family or professional). These can be financial, social, family, and health resources that influence lifestyle, living situation, and access to health care. These resources have a major impact positively or negatively on the outcomes and even in some cases, have the potential to limit the outcomes selected. Social factors include social support, social relationships, and the availability of others to assist the patient as needed. Preferences are influenced by the patient's personal perceptions of health, desired health goals, prior illness experiences, and preferences in relation to treatment, religious, and cultural beliefs. If patients believe their health is satisfactory, they may be less inclined to accept outcomes aimed at measuring improvements in overall health. Patients and their health professionals should collaborate on selecting outcomes and participating in how much change in the outcome they want to achieve. This impacts the decision focused on setting a target rating. While this is a collaborative process, nurses can assist patients in identifying realistic outcome scores. Treatment potential is also an important consideration, and the nurse needs to determine whether an intervention exists to achieve the desired outcome. In addition, it is important to determine whether the nursing personnel have the skills and are available to implement the designated intervention. Once the nurse and patient identify the relevant health outcomes, the initial evaluation of the patient's state, behavior or perception is conducted using the outcomes and indicators.

How Outcomes are Stated

Because outcomes and indicators are conceptualized as variable patient, caregiver, family, or community states, behaviors, or perceptions, they are given labels representing concepts that can be measured along a continuum as negative or positive states. Whenever possible, we avoid labels that describe an undesirable state; however, because of the common use of some concepts in practice or difficulty identifying an anonym, some outcomes do describe an undesirable state. Examples are *Infection Severity, Discomfort Level, Fear Level, Lymphedema Severity,* and *Pain Level.* These types of outcomes are used frequently by nurses to help recipients of care validate the severity of the symptoms they experience. From the recipients' point of view, these symptoms are their perceptions of the extent to which they are experiencing the indicators present in the outcome. Conceptualization of the outcomes as variable states allows for the measurement of negative or positive changes, as well as no change in the recipients' status after nursing interventions.

Some outcomes are more concrete than others. A colon is used within the outcome to depict this idea. An example of a general outcome is *Nutritional Status* (1004); more specific outcomes are *Nutritional Status: Food & Fluid Intake* (1008) or *Nutritional Status: Nutrient Intake* (1009). Box 1.3 summarizes the basic rules for developing the nursing-sensitive outcomes for this classification. These rules were established early in the development of NOC and have provided a sound foundation for outcome development requiring very few revisions. Examples of developing a new outcome that describe this process are available for direct and indirect caregiving outcomes,[290] *Hyperactivity Level* (0915),[43,321] *Personal Autonomy* (1614),[44] and more recently *Tissue Injury Severity: Percutaneous Procedure Integrity* (1109).[272]

Box 1.3

Rules for Standardization of Nursing-Sensitive Outcomes

Outcomes labels should be concise (stated in five words or less).

Outcome labels should be stated in non-evaluative terms rather than as decreased, increased, or improved.

Outcome labels should use common nursing terms as much as possible.

Outcomes should not describe a nurse behavior or intervention.

Outcome labels should not be stated as a nursing diagnosis.

Outcomes should describe a state, behavior, or perception.

Outcome labels should be inherently variable and can be measured and quantified.

Outcome labels should be conceptualized and stated at a middle level of abstraction.

Outcomes may be developed using one or two measurement scales.

Definitions for outcomes should be defined consistently with the measurement scale.

Wording of indicators should be standardized for outcomes using the same measurement scale.

Colons should be used to make broader concept labels more specific (e.g., Nutritional Status: Nutrient Intake, Self-Care Behavior: Bathing).

Use of Reference Person

To measure the outcomes, we advocate that health professionals use a "reference person" for comparison to the patient they are caring for. The reference person is defined as a *healthy* person of the same age and gender. For example, the health professional compares a 60-year-old male patient to a *healthy* 60-year-old male, implying the professional uses clinical cases of other patients in the same age group in their practice for comparison. This is a crucial step in ensuring that the measurement of outcomes is comparable across populations and settings. When a patient has a chronic condition, such as arthritis, and the health professional may be providing care to improve the patient's mobility, the comparison is not to a 60-year-old man with arthritis but a *healthy* man of the same age. This comparison sets the bar or benchmark to aim for a healthy rating of a "5" on the measurement scale with this particular care situation. Thus, the rating of "5" reflects the best state possible for the patients in the health professionals' practice. Although there are conditions that present in patients, which do not allow for the rating of a "5" on a relevant outcome. This is especially true for populations of patients with serious conditions, such as renal failure or congestive heart failure. In these situations, the health professional and the patient may attempt to achieve a "5", but in practice the highest rating the patient may be able to achieve is a "3". Because all health professionals are

working to benchmark outcomes to support their effectiveness, this is an important requirement for measuring health outcomes for their patients. The use of a "reference family" and "reference community" is more difficult to define and would need to include cultural and social elements within the definition to function as a conceptual comparison at the family and community levels.

Use of Measurement Scales

A five-point Likert type scale is used with all the outcomes and the indicators providing an adequate number of options to demonstrate variability in the state, behavior, or perception described by the outcome. For example, the outcome *Cognition* is measured on a five-point scale from "never demonstrated" (1) to "consistently demonstrated" (5) and *Rest* is measured on a five-point scale from "severely compromised" (1) to "not compromised" (5). The most frequently used scales in the classification are associated with behaviors (demonstrated scale) and the knowledge of the patient (knowledge scale). The measurement scales are standardized, so a rating of "5" is always the best possible score, and the rating of "1" is the worst possible score. Each scale provides the anchors for the scores from "1" to "5." There is an option to rate an indicator as "not applicable" for the patient by selecting the NA column. This scale structure does not demand the degree of precision required for a 10-point format but has been successful in capturing incremental changes for short acute care hospitalizations. It is critical the scales are sensitive enough to capture minor changes in patient's status after a nursing intervention. The overall outcome score should be determined by considering the importance of each indicator to the outcome.

The indicator ratings provide the nurse with important pieces of information. First, these ratings provide the nurse with the evidence to assist in determining the patient's overall rating on the outcome. The evaluation of the indicator ratings also gives the nurse clues as to appropriate nursing interventions particularly if key indicators have lower ratings (i.e., 1 to 2). Indicators currently are not weighed to provide a mean or summated rating. It is recommended that nurses and other health professionals use both the range of scores on the indicators (i.e., 1 to 5) and the frequency of scores indicator ratings as an aid in arriving at the overall outcome rating. In general, ratings of important indicators on the scale as "1" and "2" means the patient has a "1" or "2" rating on the overall outcome. For example, a patient has indicator ratings of "1"s and "2"s on all the indicators of the outcome *Activity Tolerance*. This evaluation would suggest that *Activity Tolerance* be rated as "severely compromised" because several indicators are rated as severely compromised. Data from another patient may present a different situation. In this patient scenario, the selected indicators range from "severely compromised" on a single indicator, of *ability to speak with physical activity,* while the remaining indicators are rated as "mildly compromised" and "not compromised." Because there is only one indicator that is rated as "severely compromised" and not consistent with the other indicator ratings, the nurse may want to determine whether the "severely compromised" rating is correct. Specifically, does this patient rating on this indicator occur only with intense activity or is it with minimal activity? If the patient is having difficulty only with intense activity, the nurse may rate the patient as "mildly compromised" on the outcome instead of "severely compromised." If this is a new symptom and it occurs with minimal activity, the nurse may adjust the indicator and the outcome rating to "moderately compromised." Novice nurses find rating outcomes more challenging because they do not have the experience of caring for large numbers of patients with a specific problem. Expert nurses can share their experience with these nurses and help them to see examples of patients with scores from 1 to 5 on a measurement scale for the outcome they have chosen. Nurses should use their expertise to determine an overall score for the outcomes. We know some indicators are more important than others to the overall score. Because of this, we do not recommend totaling the scores of the indicators and dividing by the number to arrive at an average indicator score. Organizations may choose to record indicator scores for each outcome, but in most situations the overall outcome score is adequate for determining the changes in patient status.

When to Measure an Outcome

The timing to measure the patient status against the chosen outcomes is critical. At a minimum, the outcomes selected should be rated and documented when: (1) the patient or family is admitted to a care setting or makes an initial visit to a nurse for care; (2) the patient or family is discharged, transferred, or referred to another setting or clinician for care; or (3) there is a significant change in the status of the patient. It is important to time the outcome measure to the patient response and being sensitive to the length of time the intervention may take to have an impact. Some patients may respond very quickly to the interventions and other respond over a longer time period. In addition, some interventions may require assessment over additional time periods to reflect the true impact of the nursing care. For example, if the intervention is *Progressive Muscle Relaxation,* the nurse may need to evaluate the patient over an extended period of time to assess the impact of the intervention on the outcome of *Comfort Status: Physical* because of the degree of learning that is required by the patient with this therapy. While assessing the outcome *Pain Level,* it may require a shorter interval of time to measure the intervention *Medication Administration.* One problem is selecting the time for measurement close enough to the implementation

of the intervention to be assured the change is the result of the intervention, but enough time for all the measurement to detect change in the outcome. In other words, the time intervals for measurement of outcomes will vary based on the characteristics of the concept. Other conditions impact the intervals of measurement of the outcomes. Currently, nurses determine the intervals for measurement and documentation of change in the outcome based on their clinical judgment or by organizational polices as to when effects of the intervention are assessed. If the nurse and/or the interdisciplinary health care team is using the classification, they should consult with one another to determine the measurement time frames for the family and community outcomes.

As previously mentioned, measurement and documentation of the outcomes is conducted at various times. An essential time for measuring the outcome is when the patient or family is discharged, transferred, or referred to another setting or clinician for care. This measurement and documentation are a key component to the continuity of care individuals and/or their family members receive when they experience different care settings. In the current resource-constrained health care environment, substantial emphasis is being placed on continuity of care to reduce costs for individuals and their families and increase efficiencies within the health care system. Further, networks that include providers and settings across the continuum of care are being developed to optimize care in the most cost-efficient environment. The effort to reduce costs has prompted a corresponding emphasis on outcomes and the acknowledgement that outcomes need to be evaluated across different care settings. NOC provides a standardized terminology for health outcomes that can be measured across the continuum of care, providing essential information to nurses, other health professionals, and administrators to achieve consistent care for patients and reduce system inefficiencies.

Setting a Target Rating

The target rating is used within this system to replace the goal statement. It is our contention that very rarely do nurses set goals for the patients that cannot be achieved. But a target rating is set to determine the expected effect or impact of the selected nursing intervention. The initial rating is determined at and the target rating in discussion with the patient is set. As you recall, the scales for the outcomes are numbered from 1 to 5. In general, the numbers of the scale to work toward improvement is the target rating. For the patient with an outcome rating of "2," the target rating to show improvement could be a "3 or 4" based on the intervention and the time frame of the episode of care. Sometimes a target rating in the plan of care is designated to maintain the current rating of the outcome. This is particularly relevant to patients in long-term care or those with severe illness or advanced cancer.

The patient and the family should be involved with setting the target rating as part of the care planning process. It is critical the nursing interventions selected be acceptable to the patient. At times because of a change in the patient status, the target rating may be adjusted. Nurses should be aware of whether there is a change in the target rating. If there is no change in the rating of the outcome after implementation of a selected intervention, other interventions need to be considered. Nurses need to have a minimum of two outcome ratings to adequately determine whether change has occurred and to what degree of change has occurred after an intervention.

Using Change Scores for Outcome Evaluation

By measuring the outcome before the intervention, the nurse establishes a baseline overall outcome score on the selected outcome and then needs to rate the outcome after the intervention is implemented. This allows nurses to follow changes in patient status or identify whether the outcome is being maintained at the same level or changing over time and across settings. For example, if a patient is rated a "2" before the intervention and a "4" after the intervention, then the change score is a +2. Hopefully the "4" was the target rating the nurse and the patient agreed on. The **true outcome** is the **change** seen in the overall outcome rating after the nursing intervention. This change score can be positive (the outcome rating increased), negative (the outcome rating decreased), or there can be no changes (the outcome rating stayed the same). In some patients' situations a change score of zero is the best outcome because of the patient's status. This degree of evaluation reinforces the relevance of the change scores. Examples of change scores reported in research are published for older adults with heart failure,[251,282] patients with pneumonia,[282] and cancer patients.[313]

FREQUENTLY ASKED QUESTIONS

Initial work on the NOC identified conceptual questions that have formed the foundation for this outcome work. The original research team reviewed the extensive literature on patient outcomes, information systems, taxonomic classification science, effectiveness research, and relevant qualitative and quantitative methods to address these issues. Team members reviewed multiple sources of patient outcomes used by nurses (textbooks, nursing information systems, critical pathways and care plans, outcome studies, standards of practice, conceptual frameworks, and outcome classifications) to identify the types of outcomes needed to capture changes in patient status after a nursing intervention. Because nurses wanted to use standardized outcomes rather than goals in their practice, many of these initial issues and other key questions needed to be answered. Some questions have remained relevant as nurses and health care organizations have learned about NOC. The most frequently asked

questions about the classification and its use are included here and brief answers are provided for each question.

What is the Difference Between the Terms Standardized Nursing Languages and Standardized Nursing Terminologies?

When classification work first developed in nursing, most of the literature used the phrase *standardized nursing languages*. As the nursing classifications became more popular and translations of NANDA-I diagnoses and NIC interventions were being done, the word "language" was used to describe Spanish or Portuguese versions of these classifications. We prefer using *standardized nursing terminologies* because it better describes what we create when we develop an outcome. We are not creating a new language but are standardizing and defining the words we prefer to use in nursing. In some specialties, for example informatics, the word "nomenclature" is also used. In a thesaurus, these three terms languages, terminology, and nomenclature, are listed as synonyms.

How are Outcomes Different From Nursing Diagnoses?

NOC outcomes describe a variable state, behavior, or perception. The overall outcome rating at a specific time can be at any point on a negative-to-positive continuum. The outcomes can be used with problem-focused diagnoses, health promotion diagnoses, risk diagnoses, or syndromes. Nursing diagnoses, in contrast, generally describe states that are in some way less positive than what is desired. Nursing diagnoses describe problem-focused and risk diagnoses that the nurse plans to resolve through nursing interventions. More recently, nursing diagnoses focused on wellness have been developed. The relationship between these diagnoses and outcomes needs further discussion and evaluation as the NOC and NANDA-I classifications evolve. Some research has been published that compare nursing diagnoses and related outcomes.[76]

Why are the Outcomes not Stated as Goals?

The outcomes are developed as variable concepts for several reasons. First, NOC outcomes measure the response of the patient, caregiver, family, or community to nursing interventions and can be documented and monitored over time and across settings and compared. A goal statement developed specifically for each patient does not allow for this cross-comparison among populations of patients. Second, variable outcomes yield more information than just whether a goal is met. For clinical and research purposes, either/or type data provide extremely limited information and constrain nurses' abilities to adequately evaluate the effectiveness of the interventions they provide. If goals are not met, it is important to know whether any progress was made or to what extent the outcome status deteriorated, if at all. Third, with the current short length of stays in acute care settings, it has become important to be able to document even slight improvements in outcome scores at discharge. Goal statements for short time frames become meaningless for monitoring progress over time. NOC outcomes can be used to state a goal for a patient, family, or community, but this should be in addition to the measurement of the outcome at baseline and over time. Fourth, in many cases, the goal of nursing care may be to maintain a patient at a particular outcome rating when an improvement in status is not possible. For example, the goal for a patient with self-care issues may be to maintain the outcome status at a "3" for the outcome *Self-Care Behavior: Bathing*. It may not be realistic to expect all patients to regain the ability to bathe themselves because of a progressive decline in their functional abilities. Finally, a major strength of using outcomes rather than goals is that an *overall change score* can be determined after nursing care is provided. This overall change score is not possible with goals and is important for evaluating the effectiveness of nursing treatments and comparing outcomes for specific patient populations over time. In addition, it truly measures the impact of the nursing care provided.

Why is Standardization of Outcomes Recommended When We Consider Each Patient, Caregiver, Family, or Community as Unique?

Standardizing the terminology used to describe outcomes in no way interferes with assessing the unique response of each patient, caregiver, family, or community/population. Use of NOC enables nurses to measure an outcome state for an individual, caregiver, family, and community, and provides more information for monitoring progress. Specific, quantified targets can be set for each outcome, and the extent that the target ratings are or are not met can be documented over time and compared across settings. In other words, using nursing standardized terminologies for nursing diagnoses, interventions, and outcomes can increase the ability of nurses to identify and document the nursing diagnoses that are unique for each patient, prescribe interventions that are tailored for the patient, and document outcomes in response to the interventions across time and care settings. Recipients of care can be actively engaged in determining priority problems, desired interventions, and timeframes for evaluating the care provided.

Why are There So Many Different Measurement Scales?

Although we have tried to limit the number of measurement scales used in the classification, there are currently outcomes with one or two scales used in the 612 outcomes in this edition. Because the outcomes focus on states, behaviors, or perceptions, it is not surprising that different measurement scales are needed to fit the focus of the outcome. After a careful review of field-testing results in 10 clinical settings, an effort was made to solve some of the problems encountered

by nurses using NOC in practice. In the third edition, the measurement scales for each outcome and the corresponding outcome definition were carefully reviewed and resulted in a reduction in the number of scales and a standard format for definitions based on the specific measurement scale. The evaluation of the anchors for each of the scales resulted in modifications, and some outcomes had a change in measurement scale. A more detailed description of this review is available in the third edition. Table 1.2 identifies the primary measurement scales with anchors, a definition of the focus of each scale. Table 1.3 provides examples of the outcomes using one scale, the classes in the taxonomy that use that scale, and the number of outcomes using the scale. Appendix C provides a complete list of all outcomes using one scale.

Why do Some Outcomes Have Two Scales?

An issue identified from the testing of the NOC in clinical sites was that some indicators were difficult to use because they contained double negatives to fit the measurement scale. Nurses felt the negative indicators were important to document because they focused on symptoms indicating complications of the patient's condition and were frequently monitored by nurses in practice. As a solution to this problem, a second scale for measuring the negative states was added to 72 outcomes in the third edition. This was an important revision to the classification because it allowed for better documentation of complications associated with the outcome. A second problem that made the indicators difficult to use was the wording of indicators as "free of" (e.g., "free of bleeding"). A second scale allowed the nurse to rate the severity of bleeding experienced by the patient, rather than whether bleeding was present or absent in the outcome *Oral Health*. This use of the second scale provided better data and more information on a change in the status of the patient. In this edition, we have tried to reduce the number of outcomes using two scales. Table 1.4 lists examples of the outcomes using two scales in combination, the classes in the taxonomy that use each combined scale, and the total number of outcomes for each scale. Appendix C contains a complete list of all outcomes using combined scales.

What Revisions Were Made to the Measurement Scales?

We made several changes to the list of scales used in NOC for this edition. As we reviewed and revised outcomes, we decided to eliminate the adequate scale as an option for several reasons. First, there were only 20 outcomes that used this scale. These included several outcomes focused on breastfeeding, caregivers, and community outcomes. We felt that describing patient's behavior as "not adequate" was awkward and not supportive of nurses trying to increase their engagement with patients and families during their care. Most of the outcomes that used the adequate scale were moved to the demonstrated

Table 1.2	MEASUREMENT SCALES WITH CODES AND DEFINITIONS

01 Compromised Scale
Definition: Extent of impairment of health or well-being

Severely Compromised	Substantially Compromised	Moderately Compromised	Mildly Compromised	Not Compromised

02 Deviation Scale
Definition: Extent of departure from an established norm or standard

Severe Deviation from Normal Range	Substantial Deviation from Normal Range	Moderate Deviation from Normal Range	Mild Deviation from Normal Range	No Deviation from Normal Range

07 Occurrence Scale
Definition: Number of occurrences

10 and over	7–9	4–6	1–3	None

09 Range Scale
Definition: Range over which an entity extends

None	Limited	Moderate	Substantial	Extensive

11 Positive Scale
Definition: Frequency of an affirmative and accepting perception or characteristics

Never Positive	Rarely Positive	Sometimes Positive	Often Positive	Consistently Positive

12 Strength Scale
Definition: Extent of intensity

Very Weak	Weak	Moderate	Strong	Very Strong

13 Demonstrated Scale
Definition: Frequency of making clear by report or behavior

Never Demonstrated	Rarely Demonstrated	Sometimes Demonstrated	Often Demonstrated	Consistently Demonstrated

14 Severity Scale
Definition: Extent of a negative or adverse state or response

Severe	Substantial	Moderate	Mild	None

17 Excellence Scale
Definition: Extent of proximity to a desired state

Poor	Fair	Good	Very Good	Excellent

18 Satisfaction Scale
Definition: Extent of perception of positive expectations

Not at All Satisfied	Somewhat Satisfied	Moderately Satisfied	Very Satisfied	Completely Satisfied

19 Reversed Demonstration Scale
Definition: Frequency of making clear by report or behavior

Consistently Demonstrated	Often Demonstrated	Sometimes Demonstrated	Rarely Demonstrated	Never Demonstrated

20 Knowledge Scale
Definition: Extent of cognitive information that is understood

No Knowledge	Limited Knowledge	Moderate Knowledge	Substantial Knowledge	Extensive Knowledge

Table 1.3	EXAMPLES OF OUTCOMES USING ONE MEASUREMENT SCALE

Compromised Scale (01)
Used in Classes: Digestion & Nutrition, Energy Maintenance, Family Member Health Status, Fluid & Electrolytes, Growth & Development, Health Status, Immune Status, Mobility, Neurocognitive, Perceived Health & Life Situation, Sensory Function, Symptom Status

Selected Examples:

Activity Tolerance	Personal Health Status
Appetite	Sensory Function
Caregiver Physical Health Status	Spiritual Health

Deviation Scale (02)
Used in Classes: Cardiopulmonary, Digestion & Nutrition, Fluid & Electrolytes, Growth & Development, Metabolic Regulation, Mobility, Therapeutic Response

Selected Examples:

Blood Glucose Control	Newborn Adaptation
Electrolyte Balance	Nutritional Status
Joint Movement	Vital Signs

Occurrence Scale (07)
Used in Class: Safety

Selected Examples:

Elopement Occurrence	Falls Occurrence

Range Scale (09)
Used in Classes: Family Member Health Status

Selected Examples:

Abuse Cessation	Neglect Cessation

Positive Scale (11)
Used in Class: Psychological Well-Being

Selected Examples:

Body Image	Self-Esteem

Strength Scale (12)
Used in Class: Health Beliefs

Selected Examples:

Health Beliefs	Health Orientation

Demonstrated Scale (13)
Used in Classes: Digestion & Nutrition, Energy Maintenance, Family Caregiver Performance, Family Member Health Status, Family Well-Being, Growth, & Development, Health Behavior, Health Management, Health Status, Health Supporting Life Skills, Mobility, Neurocognitive, Parenting, Psychological Well-Being, Psychosocial Adaptation, Risk Control, Safety, Self-Care, Self-Control, Social Interaction

Selected Examples:

Adaptation to Physical Disability	Participation in Health Care Decisions
Cardiac Rehabilitation Participation	Patient Engagement Behavior
Parent-Infant Attachment	Seizure Self-Control

Severity Scale (14)
Used in Classes: Cardiopulmonary, Energy Maintenance, Family Caregiver Performance, Fluid & Electrolytes, Immune Response, Mobility, Neurocognitive, Psychological Well-Being, Symptom Status, Tissue Integrity, Therapeutic Response

Continued

Table 1.3	EXAMPLES OF OUTCOMES USING ONE MEASUREMENT SCALE—cont'd

Selected Examples:

Anxiety Level	Hyponatremia Severity
Blood Loss Severity	Nausea & Vomiting Severity
Fear Level	Seizure Severity

Excellence Scale (17)
Used in Classes: Community Health Protection, Community Well-Being, Safety

Selected Examples:

Community Competence	Community Risk Control: Lead Exposure
Community Health Screening Effectiveness	Community Risk Control: Obesity
Community Health Status	Community Risk Control: Suicide

Satisfaction Scale (18)
Used in Classes: Family Member Health Status, Perceived Health & Life Situation, Satisfaction with Care

Selected Examples:

Caregiver Well-Being	Client Satisfaction: Physical Care
Client Satisfaction	Personal Well-Being
Client Satisfaction: Access to Care	Quality of Life

Reversed Demonstrated Scale (19)
Used in Class: Safety

Selected Example:
Elopement Propensity Risk

Knowledge Scale (20)
Used in Classes: Knowledge Health Condition, Knowledge Health Promotion

Selected Examples:

Knowledge: Acute Illness Management	Knowledge: Cancer Management
Knowledge: Dementia Management	Knowledge: Fall Management
Knowledge: Healthy Diet	Knowledge: Infection Management
Knowledge: Personal Safety	Knowledge: Time Management

Note: Scale code is in parenthesis.

scale and the indicators were structured using verbs. Three community outcomes (*Community Disaster Readiness*, *Community Disaster Response*, and *Community Grief Response*) were changed to the poor to excellent scale to be consistent with the other community outcomes.

A second change we made as we revised outcomes was to try to eliminate the second measurement scale when possible. In some cases, for this edition, the disruptive effects of a concept were separated from the original outcome and became a new outcome. In the previous edition, we had 95 outcomes that used a combination of two scales. For this edition, we reduced the number to 77. A third change in the measurement scales for this edition was that two combined scales were eliminated based on these revisions. The combined scales of *severe to none* with the *severely compromised* scale, which had five outcomes and the *severe to none* scale used with the *severe to no deviation,* which had one outcome (*Pain Level*) were eliminated.

Why is it Necessary to use the Outcome Labels When the Indicators may be More Useful?

Along with medicine, the nursing profession is a key member of the interdisciplinary health care team. The profession's contribution to interdisciplinary outcomes must be documented, and the effectiveness of nursing interventions must be evaluated. Large, standardized databases contain outcomes, such as those provided by NOC, but likely not discipline-specific indicators in all cases because of space limitations. It is therefore essential that the nursing profession uses standardized outcomes that are included in large databases so that the profession's contributions to outcomes can be used to determine nursing effectiveness and influence health policy. The concepts used for outcome labels represent a higher level of abstraction that better captures the status of the patient.

Table 1.4	EXAMPLES OF OUTCOMES USING COMBINATION MEASUREMENT SCALE

Compromised Scale and Severity Scale (21)

Used in Classes: Cardiopulmonary, Digestion & Nutrition, Elimination, Energy Maintenance, Family Member Health Status, Family Well-Being, Health Status, Metabolic Regulation, Mobility, Neurocognitive, Perceived Health & Life Skills, Sensory Function, Therapeutic Response, Tissue Integrity

Selected Examples:

Bowel Elimination	Neurological Function
Caregiver Emotional Health Status	Oral Health
	Thermoregulation
Family Health Status	

Deviation Scale and Severity Scale (22)

Used in Classes: Cardiopulmonary, Fluid & Electrolytes, Therapeutic Response

Selected Examples:

Blood Coagulation	Respiratory Function
Electrolyte & Acid/Base Balance	Surgical Recovery: Convalescence
	Tissue Perfusion: Abdominal Organs
Post-Procedure Recovery	

Range Scale & Reversed Range Scale (23)

Used in Classes: Tissue Integrity

Selected Examples:

Bone Healing	Wound Healing: Primary Intention
Burn Recovery	

Demonstrated Scale and Reversed Demonstrated Scale (24)

Used in Classes: Elimination, Energy Maintenance, Family Member Health Status, Psychosocial Adaptation, Psychological Well-Being, Safety, Self-Control

Selected Examples:

Bowel Continence	Psychomotor Energy
Eating Disorder Self-Control	Relocation Adaptation
	Successful Aging

Note: Scale code is in parenthesis.

How are Outcomes Used in Standardized Care Plans?

NOC outcomes are extremely useful in care plans because they allow quantification of the patient state, behavior, or perception that is expected to occur at specific points in time for an episode of care. Major advantages of their use are: (1) the ability to evaluate the effectiveness of nursing treatments, (2) the ability to monitor variance from the expected time frames for a specific patient, and (3) the ability to compare the achievement of specific patient populations across settings and providers. Use of standardized outcomes greatly facilitates the development of large databases of clinical information across settings and providers, rather than the more limited, unique databases that result when setting- or provider-specific outcomes are used in care planning. Care plans can be developed by experts in the care of specific populations and shared with less experienced nurses to ensure quality care is provided to all patients.

Why is it Important to Measure Outcomes Across Different Care Settings?

Continuity of care has always an important value for the nursing profession, yet communication among various settings and nurse providers is often limited and routinely constrained. A major obstacle is the lack of standardized nursing terminologies to describe the problems that nurses treat; the interventions used; and the resulting individual, family, or community outcomes. The inability to optimize continuity of care is costly to patients, families, and the health care system. In the current resource-constrained health care environment, substantial emphasis is placed on continuity of care to reduce costs. This issue has become even more important during the challenges presented by the global pandemic focused on SARS-CoV-2 (COVID-19). A trend is the creation or merger of health care networks into larger entities that include providers and settings across the continuum of care to enhance continuity and optimize care in a more cost-efficient environment. The effort to reduce costs has prompted a corresponding emphasis on outcomes and clinical effectiveness. The NOC provides a standardized terminology for outcomes that can be measured across the entire continuum of care, providing essential information that health care providers need to achieve care continuity and to evaluate the cost-effectiveness of care across different settings.

What are Core Outcomes?

We define core outcomes as a set of outcomes that capture the essence of a specialty area of practice. Nurses that are experts in a specialty area or are credentialed in that specialty would be very familiar with the outcomes described as core to their practice. The list represents outcomes that would be commonly used on a daily or weekly basis to serve patients in need of specialty care. Areas of expertise vary greatly between nursing specialties because of the difference in scope of practice. For example, nurses working in dermatology have a shorter list of core outcomes than nurses working in medical surgical units or critical care. Health care organizations can identify core outcomes for their organization as a whole and for specific units. This information is especially useful when evaluating staff competencies. The core outcomes for nursing specialties are also useful for assisting nurses to identify core outcomes for specialty care. Part 5 of this edition addresses core outcomes for 51 nursing specialties and describes the historical development of the core outcome lists.

How do I Identify Outcomes for use in my Practice?

With 612 outcomes in the seventh edition of NOC, this task may seem difficult at first. The scope of the classification is to identify all outcomes needed by nurses to evaluate the effectiveness of nursing interventions. Most nurses will focus on a limited set of outcomes based on their specialty and practice setting. Beginning efforts to identify core outcomes for specialty practice have supported the belief that nurses can identify a list of outcomes they use daily with their patients. The easiest way to identify outcomes for use in clinical practice is to review the NOC Taxonomy where similar outcomes are grouped under key concepts in nursing. A second method is to use linkages of outcome to common patient problems or nursing diagnoses addressed in your practice. A third way is to review the list of core outcomes of a nursing specialty discussed in the previous question. It is especially important that specialty practice is adequately reflected in this classification.

Why are There so Many Knowledge and Self-Management Outcomes?

We have developed knowledge and self-management outcomes for several reasons. The knowledge outcomes provide a list of the information needed for patients to maintain their health or to learn about a health condition that they are being treated for as part of their care. Nurses can use the indicators to assess the patient's knowledge and create a teaching plan based on the areas the patient needs to learn about. The indicators, in general, are focused on symptoms, treatment options, required medications, and how to manage the health condition. In addition, family caregivers or parents can also make use of the knowledge outcomes to prepare for a caregiver role. The self-management outcomes are based on the knowledge outcomes and measure the behaviors the patient needs to demonstrate to manage their health or a health condition. As more and more patients are treated as outpatients, these outcomes have become important tools for patients and families to use to address diagnosed health conditions. Part Four of this book provides linkages of all knowledge outcomes with behavior outcomes in NOC using the classes in the taxonomy focused on *Knowledge Health Conditions* and *Knowledge Health Promotion*. The linkages of knowledge and behavior outcomes are important to identify whether teaching interventions and increased patient knowledge lead to enhanced engagement, motivation, and improved health.

When is a New Outcome Developed and how is it Done?

Outcomes are developed throughout the months between the publication dates. As we have numerous colleagues around the world working to develop outcomes for their practice and they routinely submit their work for the editors' review. In addition, the team responds to changes in practice, education, or research and reviews literature to assess whether there is enough conceptual depth to develop the proposed outcome (i.e., definition and indicators). Once it is decided by the editors, the idea has the required conceptual depth, a member of the team extensively reviews current literature to develop a definition, outcome label, indicators and selects a scale consistent with the outcome definition. References are also identified, which support the selection of the outcome. Upon completion of this work, the designated team member presents the proposed outcome for extensive review by the team. The elements of the outcomes are fully discussed, and revisions made as appropriate. Once the editors sign off on the proposed outcome, it is formatted for publication. As will be discussed in the section "Global Model of Nursing Caring", we attempt in developing new outcomes to respond to the demands of nursing care as they surface within health care. For example, in response to the pandemic, we published several articles for health professionals during this challenging time. These articles focused on the unique care demands and needs of individuals, families, and communities experiencing COVID-19. The aims of these papers were to present linkages between the NANDA-I, NIC, and NOC terminologies as guides for nurses to create care plans focused on problems related to COVID-19 and assist to provide the needed care.[217,307,319] Some of the new outcomes included in this edition of NOC to assist health professionals to evaluate the impact of the care during severe crisis situations are *Community Pandemic Readiness, Community Pandemic Recovery, Community Pandemic Response*, and *Knowledge: Community Health Resources*. Another challenge facing the profession is the focus on the social determinants of health.[231] We have tried to respond to this call by developing new outcomes in response to circumstances that contribute to poorer health outcomes within the United States and abroad. Some examples of these new outcomes are *Family Risk Control: Household Food Insecurity, Risk Control: Food Insecurity*, and *Risk Control: Housing Insecurity*. As the readers will note, we use several approaches to identify content for new outcomes.

How Frequently are Outcomes Reviewed and Revised?

The outcomes are reviewed and/or revised every 4 to 6 years based on the publication deadline. Prior to publication, the major focus of the team is on the review of outcomes, not reviewed since the last publication. If the review suggests changes in any elements of the outcome (i.e., label, definition, indicators, scale), revisions are made after an extensive literature review. In addition, references are updated to reflect the latest literature.

Although this timeline is based on book publication submission, editors with intense regularity review current literature to identify trends and relevant content to enhance the comprehensiveness of the classification. For example, for this edition we reviewed *Knowledge: Breastfeeding* (1800) and found a research study published in 2017 that used the indicators to develop a questionnaire for parents to evaluate their knowledge of breastfeeding.[248] We added this reference to the content references so that others interested in using this outcome could review the publication. This work includes updating previous published outcomes and the development of new outcomes for the next publication. Over the recent years, the editors have reviewed many publications about the NOC. We want to thank the authors of these publications as well as persons associated with *The International Journal of Nursing Knowledge* for being the main vehicle of dissemination for these works. These excellent resources of validation studies, conceptual reviews of outcomes, and linkage work enable the team of editors to examine the classification based on the work of these scholars and users of NOC. Thank you to all of you who are contributing to the refinement of the classification.

How are new Outcomes Added to the Taxonomy?

The editors follow a detailed method of review when new outcomes are added to the taxonomy. The definitions of each of the domains are reviewed and the appropriate domain is selected. With the identification of the domain, all definitions of the classes within that domain are reviewed to establish the best fit for the new outcome within the respective class. In addition, the outcomes within the class are reviewed by label name to confirm the consistency between those outcomes with the new outcome to be placed. If we still question the placement of the new outcome in the chosen class, we will review the definitions and indicators of the individual outcomes already assigned to the class to ensure the appropriate fit. Once these reviews are complete, outcome(s) are placed and coded within the taxonomy.

What Translations of NOC are Available?

Translations of the NOC are available in Chinese (simplified and traditional), Dutch, French, German, Indonesian, Italian, Japanese, Korean, Norwegian, Portuguese, and Spanish. In most cases, the translation into another language is published about a year after the publication in English. Translation rights are granted by our publisher and require a forward and back translation and the involvement of a nurse fluent in both English and the chosen language. Translations are important because they facilitate the use of NOC across cultures and make research feasible because of

the coding structure of NOC. A more detailed list of publications can be found in Appendix B. Some translations of NOC have been published as part of a research project such as the translation and validation of NOC into Icelandic for use in acute care.[121]

How are NOC Outcome Terms Added to the Systematized Nomenclature of Medical Terms

The current process of adding new terms to Systematized Nomenclature of Medical Terms (SNOMED-CT) is done by dedicated nurses working at the Library of Medicine. The definition of a new outcome is compared to terms currently in SNOMED-CT and if the NOC outcome is a new term, it is added to the list of terms. SNOMED-CT only contains the label name and does not provide definitions, indicators, or measurement scales used in NOC. An example of the process developed for this is available in the literature.[179] In addition, there is a published scoping review on nursing's current status on implementing SNOMED-CT in practice[164] and a literature review for 2013 to 2020.[54]

Is a License Required to use NOC?

A license is required to use NOC if it is used in an electronic information system or if you use more than a few outcomes in a product for commercial gain. The use of NOC in an electronic system requires a license because significant portions of the book will be available to multiple users. Fees for the use of NOC in an organization's electronic system depend on the number of users in most cases. If the user purchases a software product that uses NOC, the license fees often will be included as part of the product cost. In addition, a license is required if a sizable portion of the classification is used in a book or products using portions of the book are being sold. Many requests are consistent with fair use and do not require fees. Fees are not required if the organization uses the outcomes in a paper format; however, the organization should purchase enough books that they do not have to make multiple copies of the classification. Fees are generally not required for schools of nursing that want to use NOC in educational products for their own students; however, if the school is using a significant portion of NOC, it is expected that students will have the books to use with the products produced by the schools. Fees are generally not required for research using NOC, and fees for use in other publication will depend on the number of outcomes used. Elsevier holds the copyright on NOC. Details of how to contact Elsevier are located on the inside cover.

RESOURCES TO SUPPORT AND ENHANCE THE USE OF NOC

The last section of Part I is focused on providing the reader with resources that could be helpful for nurses implementing, teaching, or conducting research focused on nursing terminologies and NOC. A brief overview of each topic is provided with an emphasis on identifying helpful resources to support nurses interested in using nursing terminologies. The section includes an overview of related terminologies, strategies for teaching and implementing NOC and standardized nursing terminologies, references for care planning and documentation, models of clinical decision-making, the nursing process, Nursing Diagnoses, Nursing Interventions, and Nursing Outcomes (NNN) linkages, and global health as well as useful summaries of outcome validation research, linkage research, and integrative, scoping, and systematic reviews focused on nursing terminologies.

Companion Nursing Terminologies

Although NOC can be used with any nursing terminology, medical diagnosis, or mental health classification, its use with NANDA-I and NIC are the most common. Two publications compare the frequency of publications focused on different terminologies. The first by Anderson and colleagues[11] identified that use of NNN nursing terminologies had strongest pattern of publications and potential for sustainability. Those are both excellent reasons to choose to use NNN terminologies. The second publication by Tastan and colleagues[309] found evidence supporting the successful integration of NNN in electronic health records.

NANDA International Diagnoses Classification

The NANDA International (NANDA-I) Organization develops and maintains a classification of nursing diagnoses that describe clinical judgements made by nurses focused on the human response of an individual, caregiver, family, group, or community to a health condition, life process, or susceptibility to that response.[131] Nursing diagnoses may be problem-focused, health promotion, risk diagnoses, or syndromes made up of a cluster of nursing diagnoses. Each diagnosis has a label name, definition, defining characteristics, risk factors, related factors, at risk populations, and associated conditions depending on the type of diagnosis. The current NANDA-I taxonomy has 13 domains, 47 classes, and 267 nursing diagnoses in the 12th edition.[131] NANDA-I publishes a new edition every 2 years, so it is important to have a current edition. The work of NANDA-I has been translated into 20 languages and is frequently linked with nursing interventions and outcomes. Members of the NIC and NOC research teams have a long history as members of NANDA-I.

A conference focused on combining the three taxonomies of NANDA-I, NOC, and NIC was held and reported in 2003.[92] One of the challenges was trying to combine the classes from the three terminologies that were at various levels of abstraction. Another issue focused on the fact that two of the classifications were focused on patients, caregivers, families, and communities, while NIC addresses the actions of nurses. Researchers have also examined the correspondence of NANDA-I nursing diagnoses to NOC outcomes. For example, Johnson and Maas reported their findings on the correspondence of problem-focused nursing diagnoses to the NOC indicators in the sixth edition of NOC[218] and de Carvalho and colleagues did a similar comparison of NANDA-I terms and NOC outcomes in 2018.[76]

Nursing Interventions Classification

The Nursing Interventions Classification (NIC),[320] now in its eighth edition, contains treatments that nurses perform in their care of patients, families, and communities. The focus of this classification is on nurse behavior, rather than the patient. It provides standardized terminology for both nurse-initiated and physician-initiated nursing treatments. Each NIC intervention has a label name, definition, a set of activities that a nurse does to carry out the intervention, and a concise list of references used to support the intervention. The coded interventions are classified into a taxonomic structure with domains, classes, and interventions. The interventions are used in documentation and can be used for reimbursement. The classification was designed to support implementation of the Nursing Minimum Data Set. The use of NIC to plan and document care facilitates the collection of large databases that allow nurses to study the effectiveness and cost of nursing treatments. NIC is frequently used with NANDA-I nursing diagnoses and NOC outcomes in practice and education. NIC is a valuable resource for nurses wanting to describe the treatments they provide and document their practice using an electronic health record. The classification also offers performance time frames and educational level suggestions for all interventions.

Educational Strategies for Teaching NNN and Implementation of NNN

One of the first steps in using nursing terminologies is to teach students, staff nurses, nurse practitioners, and faculty members how to use the terminologies. The models discussed in a later section may be useful when considering your approach to educating nurses in practice or educational settings. In addition to using a clinical reasoning model, nurse educators have used a variety of methods to improve their NNN teaching strategies. Early in the implementation of NNN into curriculum, Denehy[88] discussed this topic using three approaches: teaching undergraduate students, graduate students, and faculty. Her suggestions are still relevant today. Based on the experience level of the nurse, different approaches are important to consider. Teaching students new to nursing is sometimes easier than teaching experienced nurses who learned nursing from a system or medical model approach. Several authors have described how to use NNN in baccalaureate education[39,100,170,255,296] that will be helpful in thinking about teaching students. More recently, teaching approaches have adopted web-based approaches[18] and software programs to teach NNN.[107]

Case studies have been an important teaching method to provide clinical scenarios for students to learn care planning and documentation skills. Many examples of case studies are available in the literature and include case studies focused on stroke patients,[34] patients with urinary incontinence and psychosocial problems,[37] patients with diabetes,[102] teen parenting,[45] an oncology patient using Roger's theory of Unitary Human Beings,[95] a patient with schizophrenia,[166] and a patient with COVID-19.[10] We have also had success having beginning nursing students write a case study about a family member with a health concern during their first course focused on the nursing process. This allows the students to practice a patient interview with someone they already have a relationship with and to begin to "think" like a nurse. When teaching about outcomes, it is important that nurses and students practice doing an initial evaluation of the selected outcome, establish a target rating, measure indicators of the outcome and determine an overall outcome score. This process then allows the nurse or student to calculate a changed score and see the impact of the intervention. When using a case study, this can be built into the scenario and allow the nurse to see the longitudinal effects of the intervention provided and the improvement in the patient's problems. Box 1.4 provides a list of recommended publications focused on educational strategies for teaching NNN.[150,171,184,186,315]

Examples of Using NOC and NNN in Care Planning and Documentation

Interest in using NOC in clinical settings is frequently associated with the need for developing nursing care plans and documenting the interventions provided to patients and families. Evaluation of the status change of the patient after intervention is a major part of completing the steps of the nursing process. Box 1.5 provides publications focused on care planning and documentation of care.[7,33,65,106,122,155,229,236,246,247,266,297,310] Keenan and colleagues[162] provide an overview of care planning and documentation in nursing that highlights the importance of having the ability to collect these data electronically. What is interesting about this list of publications is the international interest in this topic. For example, three publications focus on care planning and documentation in Nigeria.[2,4,242] There are also publications from Brazil,[256] China,[132] Greece,[254] Indonesia,[124] Italy,[8] Spain,[257] and South Korea.[176,253] There are also three books that provide linkages of NOC and NIC to NANDA-I nursing diagnoses based on prior editions.[142,143,147]

To help evaluate the quality of nursing documentation, Müller-Staub and colleagues[226,228,230] developed a literature-based audit instrument for nursing documentation called the

Q-DIO. The strength of this instrument is its ability to measure the quality of nursing diagnoses, interventions, and outcomes documented in clinical practice and set criteria for documentation in electronic health records. Additional publications report the results of testing the psychometric properties of the Q-DIO[227,293] and validation of the instrument for use in Brazil and the United States.[178] This tool is an important contribution to improving the documentation of care by nurses.

Examples and Strategies for Implementation of NOC and NNN

Examples of implementing specific NOC outcomes with patient populations and typical application of nursing terminologies in clinical settings can be found in the literature. Box 1.6 provides a list of publications focused on using NOC in clinical settings.[21,27,42,46,58,66,94,130,165,209,213,224,235,240,265,311] It is common to find examples of evaluating the use of a NOC outcome for a specific care need of patients. For example, the research by Monteiro Mantovani and colleagues[204,205] evaluated two NOC outcomes, *Smoking Cessation Behavior* (1625) and *Substance Withdrawal Severity* (2108) with patients in a smoking cessation program in Brazil. Johnson and colleagues[140] identified outcomes for patients at the end of life experiencing anticipatory grieving using electronic data health care data. Burkhart and colleagues[41] used NOC to communicate outcomes of providing spiritual care in an electronic health record. Two publications highlight adaptations of NOC used in China with stroke patients.[132,133] Most of the evaluation articles focused on using NOC in China are published in Chinese research journals making it difficult for us to include publications on the use of standardized nursing terminologies in practice by nurses in China. These are examples of nurses and other disciplines using NOC to evaluate interventions provided to specific types of patient situations. Other publications highlighted in Box 1.6 are more general examples of implementation projects. Some focus on a specific area of practice, while others discuss nurses' attitudes to implementation of nursing terminologies including the advantages or barriers experienced during the transition in care processes created by adoption of nursing standardized terminologies. Researchers are beginning to investigate strategies to improve interface prototypes for nurses using electronic health records.[302]

Models that Support the use of NOC in Practice and Education

This section highlights a variety of models we have found especially useful in our work supporting teaching, implementation, and research focused on NOC and the use of standardized nursing terminologies. In her most recent publication, Flanagan[103] writes of the benefits to nursing for using these paths to facilitate the development

Box 1.4

Education Strategies for Teaching NNN

Basit, G., & Korkmaz, F. (2021). The effect of web-based nursing process teaching on senior nursing students' care planning skills. *International Journal of Nursing Knowledge, 32*(1), 4–19.

Brito-Brito, P. R., Fernandez-Gutierrez, D. A., & Smith, H. M. (2016). Case study: Community nursing care plan for a man with functional and psychosocial problems following a stroke. *International Journal of Nursing Knowledge, 27*(3), 170–174.

Brito-Brito, P. R., Oter-Quintana, C., Martín-García, Á., Alcolea-Cosín, M. T., Martín-Iglesias, S., & Fernández-Gutiérrez, D. Á. (2014). Case Study: Community nursing care plan for an elderly patient with urinary incontinence and social interaction problems after prostatectomy. *International Journal of Nursing Knowledge, 25*(1), 62–65.

Bros, I., & Serra, M. (2006). Application of the NANDA, NOC and NIC standardised languages to a geriatric nursing undergraduate course. *Gerokomos, 17*(3), 140–143.

Cardaci, R. (2011). A case study of teen parenting. *International Journal of Nursing Terminologies & Classifications, 22*(1), 40–43.

Denehy, J. (1998). Integrating Nursing Outcomes Classification in nursing education. *Journal of Nursing Care Quality, 12*(5), 73–84.

Farren, A. T. (2009). An oncology case study demonstrating the use of Rogers's Science of Unitary Human Beings and standardized nursing languages. *International Journal of Nursing Terminologies & Classifications, 20*(1), 34–39.

Finesilver, C., & Metzler, D. (2003). Use of NANDA, NIC, and NOC in a baccalaureate curriculum. *International Journal of Nursing Terminologies & Classifications, 14*(Suppl. 4), 34–35.

Frigstad, V., & von Krogh, G. (2006). Training nursing students in NANDA, NIC, and NOC terminology using a software program. *International Journal of Nursing Terminologies & Classifications, 17*(1), 70–71.

Gloskey, D., Kravutske, M. E., & Zugcic, M. (2006). Do you need to educate RNs on how to document using the Nursing Outcome Classification? *International Journal of Nursing Terminologies & Classifications, 17*(1), 34–35.

Karaca, T., & Aslan, S. (2018). Effect of 'nursing terminologies and classifications' course on nursing students' perception of nursing diagnosis. *Nurse Education Today, 67*, 114–117.

Kumar, C. P. (2007). Application of Orem's Self-Care Deficit Theory and standardized nursing languages in a case study of a woman with diabetes. *International Journal of Nursing Terminologies & Classifications, 18*(3), 103–110.

Lunney, M. (2006a). Helping nurses use NANDA, NOC, and NIC: Novice to expert. *Nurse Educator, 31*(1), 40–46.

Lunney, M. (2006b). Staff development. Helping nurses use NANDA, NOC, and NIC: Novice to expert. JONA: *The Journal of Nursing Administration, 36*(3), 118–125.

Pehler, S., & Bodenbender, K. (2003). Concept maps as a tool for learning standardized languages. *International Journal of Nursing Terminologies & Classifications, 14*(Suppl. 4), 39.

Smith, K. J., & Craft-Rosenberg, M. (2010). Using NANDA, NIC, and NOC in an undergraduate nursing practicum. *Nurse Educator, 35*(4), 162–166.

Van De Castle, B. (2003). Comparisons of NANDA/NIC/NOC linkages between nursing experts and nursing students. *International Journal of Nursing Terminologies & Classifications, 14*(Suppl. 4), 40.

---

of nursing knowledge. It is the intent of the team with these applications to address gaps in the outcome classification as well as make useful suggestions from the comprehensiveness of our work to augment the theoretical frameworks chosen. In some of the comparisons, the researchers also included all the nursing terminologies in the examinations.

Nursing Process Model

Since the development of NOC, the nursing process has expanded to six phases: assessment, diagnosis, outcome identification, planning, implementation, and evaluation.[218] The addition of a new phase devoted to outcome identification has placed the selection of a nursing outcome before the selection of an intervention and care planning. This is an important addition to the nursing process because it forces the nurse to consider the preferred outcome early in the planning of care. After implementation of the care plan and interventions, the nurse can evaluate the effectiveness of the care provided by calculating a change score using NOC. The

nurse can use NOC to evaluate care for groups of patients on a unit, for an organization, or across settings. Fig. 1.1 depicts the six phases of the nursing process and the use of NANDA-I, NOC, and NIC in the planning of care.

Pesut and Herman[259] described six nursing process generations in their book *Clinical Reasoning: The Art & Science of Critical & Creative Thinking.* The first three generations of the nursing process are described as *Problems to process* (1950–1970), *Diagnosis and reasoning* (1970–1990), and *Outcome specification and testing* (1990–2010). These generations closely align with the development of the classifications of nursing diagnoses, interventions, and outcomes in nursing. According to their predicted generation categories, today we are in the fourth generation of the nursing process focused on *Knowledge building* (2010–2025). The next two generations of the nursing process are *Models of Care Archetypes* (2025–2035) and *Predictive Care* (2035–2050). Research is critical to having the knowledge base in nursing to support the development of models of care and predictive care criteria for the future. These nursing process genera-

Box 1.5

Care Planning and Documentation Using NNN

Adubi, I. O., Olaogun, A. A., Adejumo, P.O. (2018). Effect of standardized nursing language continuing education programme on nurses' documentation of care at University College Hospital, Ibadan. *Nursing Open, 5*, 37–44.

Adereti, C. S., & Olaogun, A. A. (2019). Use of electronic and paper-based standardized nursing care plans to improve nurses' documentation quality in a Nigerian teaching hospital. *International Journal of Nursing Knowledge, 30*(4), 219–227.

Albers, C., Gloskey, D., Pahl, J., Kravutske, M. E, & Zugcic, M. (2006). Methods of educating RNs to use the NOCs in their documentation. *International Journal of Nursing Terminologies & Classifications, 17*(1), 92–93.

Aleandri, M., Scalorbi, S., & Pirazzini, M. C. (2022). Electronic nursing care plans through the use of NANDA, NOC and NIC taxonomies in community setting: A descriptive study in northern Italy. *International Journal of Nursing Knowledge, 33*, 72–80.

Brier, J. (2006). NANDA/NIC/NOC care plans enhance communication among caregivers and improve measurable outcomes for patients and staff. *International Journal of Nursing Terminologies & Classifications, 17*(1), 61.

D'Agostino, F., Barbaranelli, C., Paans, W., Belsito, R., Juarez Vela, R., Alvaro, R., et al. (2017). Psychometric evaluation of the D-Catch, an instrument to measure the accuracy of nursing documentation. *International Journal of Nursing Knowledge, 28*(3), 145–152.

Frederick, J., & Watters, M. (2003). Integrating nursing acuity, NANDA, NIC, and NOC into an automated nursing documentation system. *International Journal of Nursing Terminologies & Classifications, 14*(Suppl. 4), 26.

García-Garcés, L., & Bellver Capella, V. (2021). Advance-care planning implementation through the nursing process. *Nursing Science Quarterly, 34*(4), 440–447.

González Aguña, A., Fernández Batalla, M., Díaz-Tendero Rodríguez, J., Sarrión Bravo, J. A., Gonzalo de Diego, B., & Santamaría García, J. M. (2021). Validation of a manual of care plans for people hospitalized with COVID-19. *Nursing Open, 8*, 3495–3515.

Hajewski, C., Maupin, J. M., Rapp, D. A., Sitterding, M., & Pappas, J. (1998). Implementation and evaluation of Nursing Interventions Classification and Nursing Outcomes Classification in a patient education plan. *Journal of Nursing Care Quality, 12*(5), 30–40.

Hariyati, R. T. S., Yani, A., Eryando, T., Hasibuan, Z., & Milanti, A. (2016). The effectiveness and efficiency of nursing care documentation using the SIMPRO Model. *International Journal of Nursing Knowledge, 27*(3), 136–142.

Hou, S., Li, B., Luo, Y., & Shang, S. (2019). Creation and location-specific revision of a core nursing outcomes evaluation system based on Nursing Outcomes Classification for stroke inpatients in China. *International Journal of Nursing Knowledge, 30*(3), 154–161.

Keenan, G. M., Falan, S., Heath, C., & Treder, M. (2003). Establishing competency in the use of North American Nursing Diagnosis Association, Nursing Outcomes Classification, and Nursing Interventions Classification terminology. *Journal of Nursing Measurement, 11*(2), 183–198.

Keenan, G. M., Yakel, E., Tschannen, D., & Mandeville, M. (2008). Documentation and the nurse care planning process. Patient safety and quality: An evidence-based handbook for nurses. In R. G. Hughes. (Ed.), *Patient safety and quality: An evidence-based handbook for nurses.* Agency for Healthcare Research and Quality.

Lee, E., & Noh, H. K. (2016). The effects of a web-based nursing process documentation program on stress and anxiety of nursing students in South Korea. *International Journal of Nursing Knowledge, 27*(1), 35–42.

Müller-Staub, M., Needham, I., Odenbreit, M., Lavin, M. A., & van Achterberg, T. (2007). Improved quality of nursing documentation: Results of a nursing diagnoses, interventions, and outcomes implementation study. *International Journal of Nursing Terminologies & Classifications, 18*(1), 5–17.

Odutayo, P. O., Olaogun, A. A. E., Oluwatosin, A. O., & Ogunfowokan, A. A. (2013). Impact of an educational program on the use of standardized nursing languages for nursing documentation among public health nurses in Nigeria. *International Journal of Nursing Knowledge, 24*(2), 108–112.

Paans, W., & Müller, S. M. (2015). Patients' care needs: Documentation analysis in general hospitals. *International Journal of Nursing Knowledge, 26*(4), 178–186.

Paans, W., Sermeus, W., Nieweg, R. M. B., & van der Schans, C. P. (2010). D-Catch instrument: Development and psychometric testing of a measurement instrument for nursing documentation in hospitals. *Journal of Advanced Nursing, 66*(6), 1388–1400.

Park, H., & Lee, E. (2015). Incorporating standardized nursing languages into an electronic nursing documentation system in Korea: A pilot study. *International Journal of Nursing Knowledge, 26*(1), 35–42.

Patiraki, E., Katsaragakis, S., Dreliozi, A., & Prezerakos, P. (2017). Nursing care plans based on NANDA, Nursing Interventions Classification, and Nursing Outcomes Classification: The investigation of the effectiveness of an educational intervention in Greece. *International Journal of Nursing Knowledge, 28*(2), 88–93.

Peres, H., Cruz, D., Tellez, M., de Cássia Gengo e Silva, R., Ortiz, D., Diogo, R., & Ortiz, D. R. (2016). Implementation of improvements in an electronic documentation nursing process system structured on NANDA-I, NOC and NIC (NNN) classification. *Studies in Health Technology & Informatics, 225*, 1082–1083.

Pérez Rivas, F. J., Martín, I. S., Pacheco del Cerro, J. L., Minguet Arenas, C., García López, M., & Beamud Lagos, M. (2016). Effectiveness of nursing process use in primary care. *International Journal of Nursing Knowledge, 27*(1), 43–48.

Prophet, C. M., & Delaney, C. W. (1998). Nursing Outcomes Classification: Implications for nursing information systems and the computer-based patient record. *Journal of Nursing Care Quality, 12*(5), 21–29.

Roecklein, N. (2012). Using standardized nursing languages in end-of-life care plans. *International Journal of Nursing Knowledge, 23*(3), 183–185.

Smith, K., Smith, V., Krugman, M., & Oman, K. (2005). Evaluating the impact of computerized clinical documentation. *CIN: Computers, Informatics, Nursing, 23*(3), 132–138.

Thoroddsen, A., Ehnfors, M., & Ehrenberg, A. (2011). Content and completeness of care plans after implementation of standardized nursing terminologies and computerized records. *CIN: Computers, Informatics, Nursing, 29*(10), 599–607.

Wuryanto, E., Rahayu, G. R., Emilia, O., Harsono, & Octavia, A. P. R. (2017). Application of an outcome present test-peer learning model to improve clinical reasoning of nursing students in the intensive care unit. *Annals of Tropical Medicine & Public Health, 10*(3), 657–663.

Box 1.6

Implementation of NOC and Nursing Terminologies

Behrenbeck, J. G. (2003). Nursing-sensitive outcome implementation and reliability testing in a tertiary care setting. *International Journal of Nursing Terminologies & Classifications, 14*(Suppl. 4), 12.

Behrenbeck, J. G., Timm, J. A., Griebenow, L. K., & Demmer, K. A. (2005). Nursing-sensitive outcome reliability testing in a tertiary care setting. *International Journal of Nursing Terminologies & Classifications, 16*(1), 14–20.

Bernhart-Just, A., Hillewerth, K., Holzer-Pruss, C., Paprotny, M., & Heinrich, H. Z. (2009). The electronic use of the NANDA-, NOC- and NIC-classifications and implications for nursing practice. *Pflege, 22*(6), 443–454.

Bernhart-Just, A., Lassen, B., & Schwendimann, R. (2010). Representing the nursing process with nursing terminologies in electronic medical record systems: A Swiss approach. *CIN: Computers, Informatics, Nursing, 28*(6), 345–352.

Bjornsdottir, G., & Thorhallsdottir, I. (2003). An internet-based survey of Icelandic nurses on their use of and attitudes toward NANDA, NIC, and NOC. *International Journal of Nursing Terminologies & Classifications, 14*(S4), 32–33.

Burkhart, L., Coglianese, M., Kaelin, J., Moorhead, S., & Joyce, C. (2021). Communicating spiritual care in the electronic health record. *CIN: Computers, Informatics, Nursing, 39*(10), 538–546.

Cachón Pérez, J. M., Alvarez-López, C., & Palacios-Ceña, D. (2012). The meaning of standardized language NANDA-NIC-NOC to intensive care nurses in Madrid: A phenomenological approach. *Enfermería Intensiva, 23*(2), 68–76.

Carrington, J. M. (2012). The usefulness of nursing languages to communicate a clinical event. *CIN: Computers, Informatics, Nursing, 30*(2), 82–8; quiz 89.

Clancy, T. R., Delaney, C. W., Morrison, B., & Gunn, J. K. (2006). The benefits of standardized nursing languages in complex adaptive systems such as hospitals. *JONA: The Journal of Nursing Administration, 36*(9), 426–434.

Clarke, M. (1998). Implementation of nursing standardized languages: NANDA, NIC & NOC. *Online Journal of Nursing Informatics, 2*(2).

Conrad, D., Hanson, P. A., Hasenau, S. M., & Stocker-Schneider, J. (2012). Identifying the barriers to use of standardized nursing language in the electronic health record by the ambulatory care nurse practitioner. *Journal of the American Academy of Nurse Practitioners, 24*(7), 443–451.

D'Agostino, F., Zeffiro, V., Vellone, E., Ausili, D., Belsito, R., Leto, A., et al. (2020). Cross-mapping of nursing care terms recorded in Italian hospitals into the standardized NNN terminology. *International Journal of Nursing Knowledge, 31*(1), 4–13.

Daly, J. M., Maas, M., & Buckwalter, K. (1995). Use of standardized nursing diagnoses and interventions in long-term care. *Journal of Gerontological Nursing, 8*, 29–36.

Demmer, K. A., McKane, C., Griebenow, L., Behrenbeck, J., & Timm, J. (2004). Nursing-sensitive outcome implementation and reliability testing in two cardiac surgery intensive care units. *Online Journal of Nursing Informatics, 8*(3), 6.

Eun, K., & Hyang-Sook, S. (2013). Construction and application of nursing information system using NANDA-NOC-NIC linkage in medical-surgical nursing units. *Korean Journal of Adult Nursing, 25*(4), 365–376.

Finesilver, C. (2003). Use of standardized language in neuroscience nursing. *International Journal of Nursing Terminologies & Classifications, 14*(Suppl. 4), 52.

Frederick, J., Scherb, C. A., Smith-Foreman, K., Wit, T. S., Quiram, J., Wagenaar, J., et al. (2001). Speaking a common language: Standardized nursing languages have increased the visibility of nursing practice at three facilities. *AJN: American Journal of Nursing, 101*(3), 2400-TT.

Hajewski, C., Maupin, J. M., Rapp, D. A., Sitterding, M., & Pappas, J. (1998). Implementation and evaluation of Nursing Interventions Classification and Nursing Outcomes Classification in a patient education plan. *Journal of Nursing Care Quality, 12*(5), 30–40.

Hendrix, S. E. (2009). An experience with implementation of NIC and NOC in a clinical information system. *CIN: Computers, Informatics, Nursing, 27*(1), 7–11.

Johnson, J., Lodhi, M. K., Cheema, U., Stifter, J., Dunn-Lopez, K., Yingwei Yao, et al. (2017). Outcomes for end-of-life patients with anticipatory grieving: Insights from practice with standardized nursing terminologies within an interoperable internet-based electronic health record. *Journal of Hospice & Palliative Nursing, 19*(3), 223–231.

Johnson, M., & Maas, M. (1998). Implementing the Nursing Outcomes Classification in a practice setting. *Outcomes Management for Nursing Practice, 2*(3), 99–104.

Klehr, J., Hafner, J., Spelz, L. M., Steen, S., & Weaver, K. (2009). Implementation of standardized nomenclature in the electronic medical record. *International Journal of Nursing Terminologies & Classifications, 20*(4), 169–180.

Kravutske, M, E., Zugcic, M., Gloskey, D., & Reed, D. (2006). Initial results from using NOCs in an acute care setting. *International Journal of Nursing Terminologies & Classifications, 17*(1), 93.

Lundberg, C., Brokel, J. M., Bulechek, G. M, Butcher, H. K., Martin, K. S., et al. (2008). Selecting a standardized terminology for the electronic health record that reveals the impact of nursing on patient care. *Online Journal of Nursing Informatics, 12*(2), 19.

Maas, M. L., Reed, D., Reeder, K. M., Kerr, P., Specht, J., Johnson, M., et al. (2002). Nursing outcomes classification: A preliminary report of field testing. *Outcomes Management, 6*(3), 112–119.

Moorhead, S., Clarke, M., Willits, M., Tomsha, K. A. (1998). Nursing Outcomes Classification implementation projects across the care continuum. *Journal of Nursing Care Quality, 12*(5), 52–63.

Moorhead, S., Johnson, M., Maas, M., & Reed, D. (2003). Testing the Nursing Outcomes Classification in three clinical units in a community hospital. *Journal of Nursing Measurement, 11*(2), 171–181.

Müller-Staub M. (2009). Study to the implementation of NANDA-1 nursing diagnosis, interventions and nursing sensitive patient outcomes. *Pflegewissenschaft, 11*(12), 688–696

O'Connor, N. A., Hameister, A. D., & Kershaw, T. (2000). Applications of standardized nursing language to describe

Continued

Box 1.6—cont'd

Implementation of NOC and Nursing Terminologies

adult nurse practitioner practice. *International Journal of Nursing Knowledge, 11*, 109–120.

Olatubi, M. I., Oyediran, O. O., Faremi, F. A., & Salau, O. R. (2019). Knowledge, perception, and utilization of standardized nursing language (SNL) (NNN) among nurses in three selected hospitals in Ondo State, Nigeria. *International Journal of Nursing Knowledge, 30*(1), 43–48.

Powelson, S., & Leiby, K. (2003), Implementation of standardized nursing language at a university. *International Journal of Nursing Terminologies & Classifications, 14*(Suppl. 4), 60.

Timm, J. A., & Behrenbeck, J. G. (1998). Implementing the Nursing Outcomes Classification in a clinical information system in a tertiary care setting. *Journal of Nursing Care Quality, 12*(5), 64–72.

von Krogh, G., Dale, C., & Naden, D. (2005). A framework for integrating NANDA, NIC, and NOC terminology in electronic patient records. *Journal of Nursing Scholarship, 37*(3), 275–281.

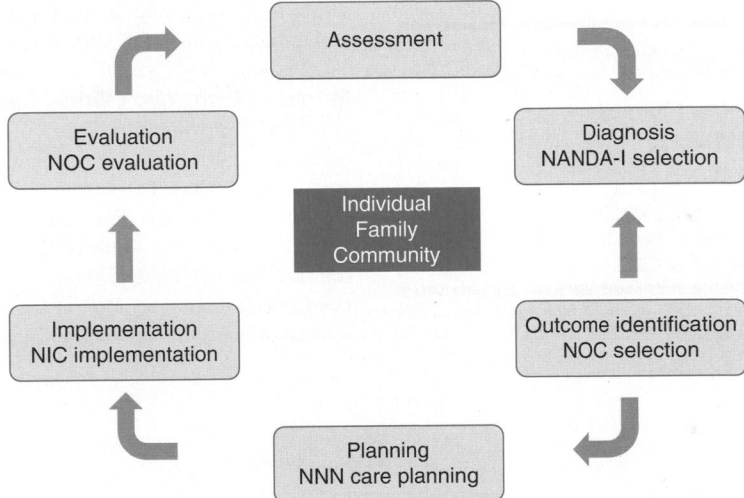

Fig. 1.1 Use of NNN in six phases of the nursing process. *NANDA-I,* the North American Nursing Diagnosis Association; *NIC,* Nursing Interventions Classification; *NNN,* nursing diagnosis, nursing outcomes, and nursing interventions; *NOC,* Nursing Outcomes Classification. (© *2014 Center for Nursing Classification & Clinical Effectiveness*)

tions predicted by Pesut and Herman[259] are another example of the development and evolution of the nursing process and can be found in Box 1.7.

Nursing research continues to support the evolution of the nursing process to support clinical practice, decision-making, and knowledge generation. The nursing process has been used to structure electronic care planning systems for nursing by nurses in Switzerland[28] and in the United States by Keenan and colleagues[160] as the HANDS research project to collect standardized nursing data.

Model of Linkages of NNN

The first NNN model published in 1996 by the Iowa Intervention Project[136] combined the use of NNN focusing on nursing knowledge and clinical decision-making as a framework for nurses to choose diagnoses, interventions, and outcomes for a patient. At the time, the original model was created, the North American Nursing Diagnosis Association (now NANDA-I) had a published classification of nursing problems, and the Iowa Intervention Project was in the second edition of NIC.[136] The outcomes component of the model was just a placeholder for the development of a classification of nursing outcomes. The addition of outcomes was considered an important next step for classification efforts for nursing.

The description of the generations of the nursing process discussed in the previous section, impacted our current work and a revision of a model depicting the linkages among diagnoses, interventions, and outcomes was developed in 2012 to describe the relationship of nursing diagnoses, outcomes, and nursing interventions to clinical reasoning and knowledge development. The revised model is shown in Fig. 1.2. Several revisions were made to the original model published by the Nursing Interventions Project.[136] First, the term *clinical decision-making* was replaced with the term *clinical reasoning* to better depict the concepts in use. Second, the placement of the outcomes moved to the middle of the model to reflect the changes in the phases of the nursing process and the addition of an outcome identification step. Third, the interventions content was moved to the far right to follow selection of outcomes in the care planning process.

We added two new areas under the "choice" boxes. Each classification has a list of three components that are impor-

tant to the specific classification. These areas include patient preferences and involvement in the care process and areas of strengths of each type of classification such as diagnostic accuracy, measurement accuracy, and nurse competencies. The final area added corresponds to the building of nursing knowledge to tie back to the *Knowledge* at the top of the model. Here the predictions of Pesut and Herman[259] focusing on the evolution of the nursing process were included to reflect the advancement of the nursing profession to *Models of care* for populations of patients (2025–2035) and the final goal of *Predictive care* based on practice evidence (2035–2050). These examples of changes in the supporting concepts and models in nursing have assisted in the development of a robust outcome classification for use by professional nurses and may be useful frameworks for teaching and implementing NOC and other nursing terminologies.

Model of Reflective Clinical Reasoning

This model provides a new way of thinking about clinical reasoning and the use of nursing diagnoses, interventions, and outcomes. Based on the need to improve critical thinking skills in nursing, Pesut and Herman[258,259] developed a process to support iterative thinking in the model they call the *Outcome-Present State-Test* (OPT) *Model of Reflective Clinical Reasoning*. One of the strengths of this model is that it helps nurses begin thinking about the client's

---

Box 1.7

Nursing Process Generations

Years	Focus of Nursing
1950–1970	Problems to Process
1970–1990	Diagnosis and Reasoning
1990–2010	Outcome Specification & Testing
2010–2025	Knowledge Building
2025–2035	Models of Care Archetypes
2035–2050	Predictive Care

From Pesut, D., & Herman J. (1999). *Clinical reasoning: The art & science of critical & creative thinking.* Delmar.

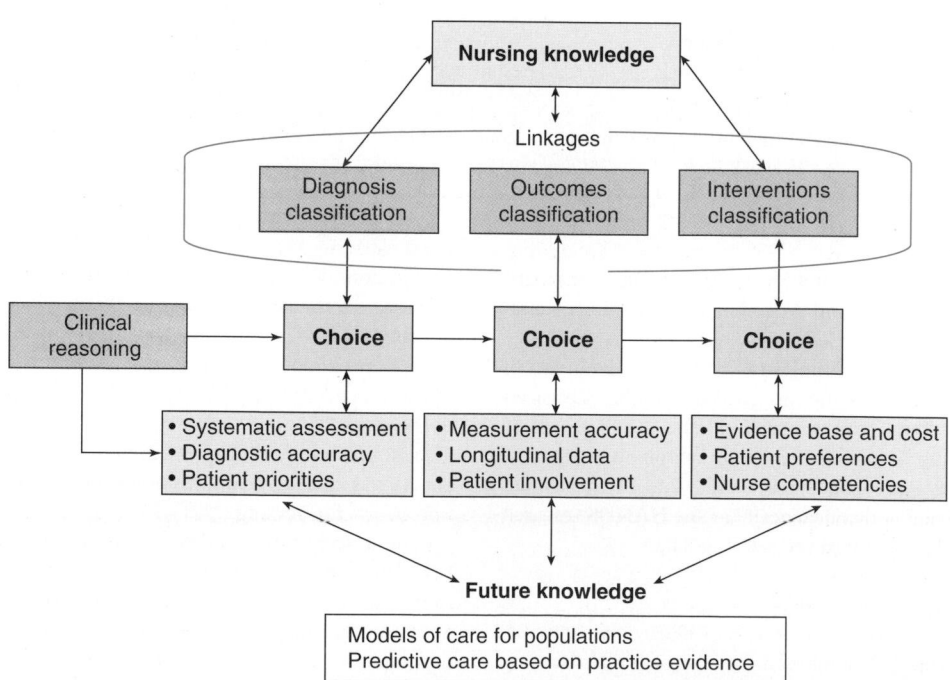

Fig. 1.2 Relationship of nursing classifications to clinical reasoning and knowledge development. (© *2012 Center for Nursing Classification & Clinical Effectiveness*)

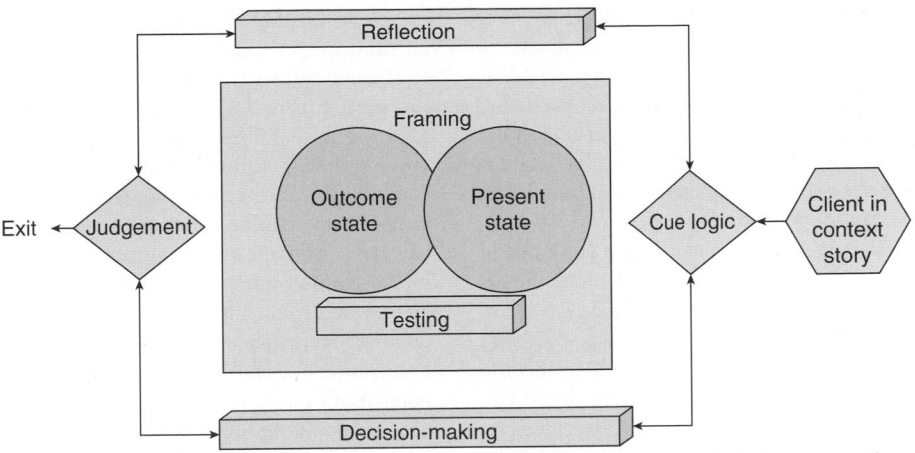

Fig. 1.3 Outcome-present state-test model of clinical reasoning. (*Pesut, D. J. & Herman, J. (1999). Clinical reasoning: The art & science of critical & creative thinking. Delmar.*)

care through listening to the client's story and identifying relevant cues and information in a logical way using what they call "*cue logic.*" The information the nurse gains from the client's story helps determine the frame, outcome state, present state, and test needed to identify if the desired state has been selected. Reflection, a major strategy of the model, and decision-making help the nurse determine the interventions needed to move the individual from the present state to the desired outcome state. The model is presented in Fig. 1.3. The model is unique in that it progresses from right to left ending with the nurse making a judgement. This final judgement about the client's care needs results in the nurse exiting the model, altering the decisions made about the needed nursing care, reformatting the test situation set up in the model, or reframing the client situation. The client participates in the process and helps to determine the priority problem needed to be addressed by the nurse. The model is also based on creating web diagrams of the patient's problems to create visual images of the connections of the problems and determine the keystone issue that will be the focus of care. Pesut and Herman[259] and Kautz and colleagues[151] offer examples of using the model with NANDA-I nursing diagnoses, NIC, and NOC. Kuiper, Pesut, and Arms[169] have applied this model to advanced practice and care coordination. We have found this model an excellent resource to support clinical reasoning and teach nurses how to use NNN in care planning with their patient.

Global Model of Nursing

The global community's expectations of the role of the nurse are expanding, as nurses increase their contact with individuals in their respective communities.[325] Nurses as the largest group of health professionals have the most direct impact on people's health. They also have a critical role in the delivery of safe, cost-effective care in every health care setting in which they practice. The health care system and the profession of nursing has been challenged in the past number of years because of major world events. Although regions of the world experience different health challenges due to varied socioeconomic and geographical conditions; at the same time, there are common health concerns. The increasing uptick in the number of natural disasters and health emergencies like COVID-19 has demonstrated health problems and issues most dramatically, as well as commonalities across the world.

COVID-19 as well as the environmental disasters have heightened the presence of ineffective and inefficient health care systems. With this being our seventh edition of Nursing Outcomes Classification initiated in 1994, the authors could not have envisioned the world would be experiencing the challenges of a pandemic and the shortage of nursing professionals and hospital beds worldwide. We strongly believe that as professionals, we need to respond to the current health issues facing the populations we serve as well as be resources to the members of the health care system. In response to this pandemic, the NIC and NOC teams developed linkages between NANDA-I, NOC, and NIC to guide nurses in caring for these complex patients.[217,307,319] We hope these publications can be used as references worldwide to guide nurses in the care of COVID-19 patients.

Not only is the profession of nursing facing natural and pandemic challenges but there are other critical situations involving the social determinants of health that dramatically impact the health outcomes of selected populations. This phenomenon is not only in the United States but a major concern of the World Health Organization (WHO).[299,300] Worldwide, the health systems are focused on these nonclinical psychosocial and socioeconomic factors or social determinants of health, because of their interrelationship with quality health outcomes. There is growing evidence of the presence of inequities in both health and access to health care that has further enhanced the world view of the complexities and impact of these important social determinants.[101] The American Academy of Nursing recently published a consensus paper defining the social determinants of health for nursing efforts to achieve health equity that focuses on individual, family, and population levels with an emphasis on health policy.[168] As noted in the publication, *The Future of Nursing 2020-2030: Charting a Path to Achieve Health Equity* published in 2021,[231] there are two key frameworks that explain the interaction between the social determinants and health. These two frameworks are: the model of Social Determinants of Health conceptual framework developed by the WHO's Commission on the Social Determinants of Health,[300] and the Social Determinants of Health and Social Needs Model developed by Castrucci and Auerbach.[47]

In 2010 the WHO's Commission on the Social Determinants of Health developed a framework to explain the complexities between social determinants and their impact on health.[300] This framework divides the determinants into two different sections: structural determinants and intermediary determinants. The structural determinants are defined as inequities and represent the socioeconomic and political context, social class gender, and ethnicity inequities.[300] Whereas the intermediary determinants are defined as material circumstances, psychosocial conditions, and behavioral and biological factors. The authors of the WHO model contend that the inequities created by policies, social class, gender, and ethnicity shape the material circumstances (e.g., working conditions, food availability) and behaviors (e.g., substance abuse) and other psychosocial factors that underlie health.[300] For example, Solar and Irwin (2010) suggest that the lack of education in turn impacts job security, resultant income, and access to health care. While the WHO model explains the relationship between social determinants of health and quality health outcomes, the model presented by Castrucci and Auerbach,[47] focuses on strategies to be used by nurses to improve the individual and population health primarily within the United States. Although in reviewing the suggested strategies, it is clear they can be adapted to countries outside the United States. The categories of strategies are upstream, midstream, and downstream strategies.[47] In each case, nurses can have an impact but at a different component of society. For example, upstream strategies may focus on the larger issues of income disparity or discrimination within the community. Whereas midstream strategies may emphasize individual factors that influence health. Nurses may focus on preventing disease and assisting their clients to meet their social needs.[47] The remaining group of strategies focus on disease treatment and management of chronic disease and nurses and other staff can address these areas in hospitals, clinics, and home settings.

These situations demonstrate the importance of having an educated, competent, and skilled worldwide nurse force to respond to these calamities.[325] Nurses are well prepared to create, partner, or lead the complex initiatives of integrating social and health sectors in support of the health and well-being of disadvantaged individuals, families, and communities. Nurses working with social services professionals across ambulatory-care and public health settings can develop point-of-care interventions to advance care models for outcome-based care for all patients they serve.[231] Nurses are called on to address and implement policies that do affect many persons in the most dramatic ways. It has been noted by health professionals that poor policies like poor health care can undermine the health and well-being of individuals, families, and communities.[101] Nursing like other professions, need to find broader and collaborative solutions to address the increasing complexity of the global issues facing health care.[222]

It is critical nurses respond to these challenges in the years to come since the health care industry worldwide has heightened its focus on the social determinants of health. We have attempted to respond to this call by developing new outcomes to respond to some of these circumstances that contribute to health outcomes within the United States and abroad. Selected new outcomes developed to address these issues are *Community Pandemic Readiness, Community Pandemic Recovery, Community Pandemic Response, Family Risk Control: Household Food Insecurity, Knowledge: Community Health Resources, Risk Control: Food Insecurity,* and *Risk Control: Housing Insecurity.* We hope these new outcomes will provide nurses and other health professionals, the tools they need to identify and evaluate the care for patients, families, and communities to achieve the best health outcomes possible. Fig. 1.4 was initially designed to depict the impact of the pandemic, but it can be renamed as a Global Model of Nursing to address the physiological and psychosocial problems others experience in pandemics, natural disasters, and the nonclinical psychosocial and socioeconomic conditions or social determinants of health select populations in the world face today.

Gordon's Functional Health Patterns

The first opportunity the team had to develop linkages with the NOC was to Gordon's Functional Health Patterns.[117] This work was initially published in the second edition of NOC[138] and reflected the three levels of abstraction presented within the NOC taxonomy. We noted that because of the frequent use of Gordon's Functional Health Patterns within nursing, linkages among the outcomes and the 11 health patterns would assist nurses who routinely used the health patterns as an assessment structure in clinical practice to identify outcomes as well.[215] In addition, these linkages provided another means for identifying relevant outcomes for nurses using

NOC in education and research. The process the team used to develop the linkages was as follows: the outcome was placed under a specific pattern consistent with the pattern name and definition developed by Gordon,[118] and general outcomes as opposed to the actual health status, were placed in the Health Perception-Health Management Pattern. We concluded that 36 of the 490 outcomes of the fifth edition[215] could not be placed in the Functional Health Patterns structure. A complete listing of the NOC outcomes organized by the 11 Gordon Health Patterns can be reviewed in the fifth edition.[215] It also includes the outcomes, which did not fit with the Health Patterns framework. As we concluded, it is critical to develop linkages based on these health patterns. It assists others in learning, improves diagnostic reasoning, helps to identify new outcomes relevant to nursing practice, and emphasizes the impact of nursing interventions due to the focus on outcomes.[215] With the importance of Gordon's work continuing,[111] it is our intent to review the 612 outcomes in this new edition and update and publish the linkages of NOC and Gordon's Functional Health Patterns to support this critical resource for the profession of nursing.

International Classification of Functioning, Disability, and Health

Another project to link the NOC to a framework was the linking of NOC to the International Classification of Functioning, Disability, and Health (ICF) (WHO, 2001).[135,305] Although there is limited use of ICF in the United States, it is used heavily internationally. The team felt that if nursing was going to embrace an interdisciplinary approach, ICF seems appropriate because it incorporates the discipline of nursing. However, given its unfamiliarity within the United States, work needs to be advanced to establish the importance to nursing. We did link parts of the ICF to the NOC,[215] although the results are not available currently for review. The use of this framework is more common in Europe.

Multi-Dimensional Model of Successful Aging

Another project compared the physiological, psychological, and sociological domains of the Multi-Dimensional Model of Successful Aging (MMSA)[329] with the nursing terminologies of NANDA-I, NIC, and NOC to define similarities or gaps across the model and the terminologies.[181] This was a cross-mapping study, which allowed for the comparison of data from various sources. We established rules for the methodologic process, and then compared the similarity of meanings of each MMSA domain with the domains and classes of NNN, considering words that were equal, similar, or have to have the same meaning, and considering opposing concepts when making the comparison with NIC and NOC.[181,182,210] This cross-mapping was completed by seven Brazilian and North American research nurses with knowledge of MMSA and NNN, as well as knowledge and clinical experience with the care of the older adults. All the initial reviews were conducted independently and afterwards, colleagues met virtually to discuss the results and arrive at a consensus. Upon completion of the discussion, it was verified that the NOC and NIC domains could be mapped with similarity to the MMSA domains. In addition, 12 of the 13 NANDA-I domains were mapped to the MMSA domains. A complete

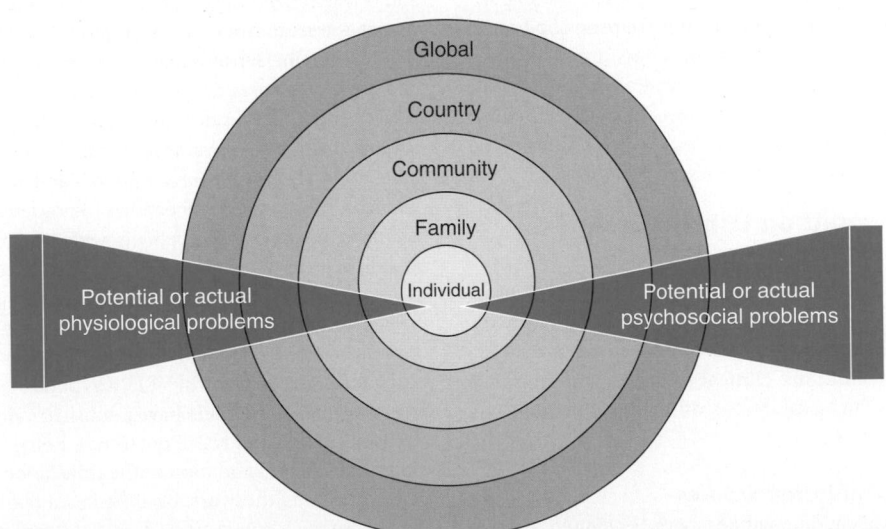

Fig. 1.4 Global Model of Nursing. (© *2022 The Center for Nursing Classification and Clinical Effectiveness*)

discussion of the detailed results has been published by Lucena and colleagues.[181]

Although most NANDA-I domains and all the NIC and NOC domains mapped to the domains of MMSA, several of the classes of NANDA-I, NIC, and NOC did not map to the MMSA. It was basically because of the unique specificity of the respective classes within the terminologies. Some of the examples were NANDA-I class of Growth and Development, NIC classes of Perioperative Care, Childbearing Care, and Childrearing Care, and NOC classes of Parenting and Family Member Health Status.[181] As one can note, these classes were not a match due to the lack of age-appropriate fit with the domains of MMSA. In conclusion, the association of NNN and MMSA promotes understanding of the needs of care in the elderly population. NNN provides the elements of nursing practice, while the MMSA provides the structure for the evaluation of elderly to achieve successful aging and to achieve quality nursing care.[181]

NOC and the Self- and Family Management Framework

A project currently being conducted is the linking of NOC outcomes to the Self and Family Management Framework (SFMF). The SFMF was originally developed by Grey and her colleagues.[119] The most recent version of the framework[120] was used in this project after we made some minor adjustments. The unique contribution of this version is the inclusion of four dimensions: Facilitators & Barriers, Processes, Proximal Outcomes, and Distal Outcomes.[120] The team was drawn to the potential of suggesting outcomes for the framework to perhaps enhance its usability in clinical practice, education, and research. Thus, the purpose of this work is to develop linkages between the components of the revised SFMF to NOC outcomes.[218] To our knowledge, this comparison across this framework and NOC has not been conducted. As the work continues several manuscripts are in process. Hopefully over the next several years, work to apply the NOC to other model and theoretical frameworks can enable us to fully develop a comprehensive taxonomy with appropriate domains, classes, and outcomes to support nurses.

Research Focused on Using Nursing Terminologies

Research focused on NOC has used a variety of approaches including validation studies and clinical validations with specific populations, linkages of NNN for nursing diagnoses, and clinical conditions, clinical validations of proposed linkages of NNN, and evaluations of nursing interventions using NOC outcomes.

NOC Content Validation Studies

Several content validation methods have been used to validate nursing diagnoses and outcomes. Content validation is the process of obtaining expert opinions about the degree to which some attributes represent a concept. The original method developed by Fehring[96] has been used extensively to validate nursing diagnoses and Fehring[96] includes recommendations on how to determine the expertise of nurses included in the validation process. The Fehring method was modified for content validation research with NOC and used in research by the NOC team.[125–127] More recently the Rasch model[31,32,223,324] has become a second methodology used to validate nursing diagnoses.[84,85] The Rasch model has been used to estimate the validity of nursing diagnoses, whether established categorically (present or absent of the attribute) or ordinally (measured by Likert-type scales). This method has potential for content validation studies evaluating NOC outcomes in the future and much of the literature about this method has been published in Brazil. New methods for determining nurse experts have also been published from scholars in Brazil focused on valuing clinical experience higher that nurses' experts from academia[268] and address the need for clear criteria for content experts in validation studies. A new method, the Nurse-Patient Outcome Content Validation Method, has been published that uses patients as experts in validation studies of content focused on living with a chronic disease.[63] Research using this method found that patients with heart failure viewed an indicator focused on depression especially important to living with cardiac problems and the nurses, in contrast, felt it could be eliminated from the outcome.

Several of the first studies focused on content validation of NOC outcomes were conducted as dissertation work of doctoral students working with the Center for Nursing Classification and Clinical Effectiveness at the University of Iowa. For example, research on the validation of outcomes for rural and urban community elders was the first dissertation focused on NOC[125] and a second dissertation focused on describing nursing effectiveness using standardized nursing terminologies and computerized nursing data.[281] Other populations and approaches were the focus of dissertations testing the reliability of selected nursing-sensitive outcomes on organizational, patient, and nurse characteristics,[280] determining linkages of NANDA-I, NOC, and NIC used in nursing care plans for hospitalized patients with congestive heart failure,[250] identifying linkages of nursing diagnoses, interventions, and outcomes used in intensive care units,[206] validation of knowledge and self-management outcomes with patients with cardiovascular disease and diabetes[36,237] and the use of NNN in the care of cancer patients using electronic heath record data.[313] These dissertations helped define methods for validation studies and linkage work for future research focused on NOC.

Since the last edition of NOC was published in 2018, many international researchers have published validation research focused on specific NOC outcomes. Some of these studies have focused on validation of the translation of specific outcomes such as the work by Bellido-Vallejo and colleagues on the Spanish translation of pain outcomes.[23–25,249] Other researchers have focused on the validation of outcomes with Portuguese patients such as the work by Sampaio and colleagues on *Anxiety Level* and *Anxiety Self-Control*[277] and Coelho and colleagues on the outcome *Cognition*.[59] There is also research to validate outcomes on breastfeeding for both the infant and mother[90,91] and self-management outcomes for cardiac patients by Cavalcante and colleagues.[48,49] Many of the publications are in both English and Portuguese in Brazil making the sharing of research results very feasible. Table 1.5 summarizes the validations studies focused on specific outcomes published to date that are available in English.[3,12,13,55,64,69,78,79,83,197,220,238,239,261,269,273,291] We have included these publications on the content references for these outcomes so others can read about their research and results. In some cases, we have modified the outcome based on the published recommendations from the research. In other situations, we hope additional research will be conducted to further clarify the needed revisions. It would be extremely helpful in the future if researchers would share their results, recommendations, and publications with us. We would be delighted to share these publications with others interested in similar methods or patient populations. We are excited to see the quality of validation studies being conducted on NOC outcomes and hope to see more cross-cultural studies in the future.

Research Focused on Linkages of Nursing Diagnoses, Outcomes, and Interventions

The literature review of research focused on linking nursing diagnoses, outcomes, and interventions for populations of patients identified 60 publications. Table 1.6 groups the publications identified into categories based on the population studied.[109,116,172,174,175,190,203] Some of the populations are very specific. For example, there are six publications focused on patients experiencing pain: one publication focused on acute pain,[77] two on chronic pain,[200,271] one on palliative care,[199] and one on perimenstrual pain and discomfort.[163] Some NNN linkage publications are more aligned with an age group of patients such as school age children[185,189,191] or older adults.[5,14,129,180,181,295]

Eleven studies focus on respiratory problems including seven published recently on COVID-19.[10,17,114,115,217,307,319] The literature review identified nine NNN publications on heart disease[26,82,221] and heart failure,[15,16,128,252,283] and nine publications focused on NNN linkages for problems with

Table 1.5 VALIDATION STUDIES OF SPECIFIC NOC OUTCOMES

Nursing Outcome	Validation Study
Anxiety Level (1211) Anxiety Self-Control (1402)	Sampaio, F. M. C., Araújo, O. S. S. L., Sequeira, C. A. da C., Lluch Canut, M. T., & Martins, T. (2018). Evaluation of the psychometric properties of NOC outcomes "Anxiety Level" and "Anxiety Self-Control" in a Portuguese outpatient sample. *International Journal of Nursing Knowledge, 29*(3), 184–191.
Breastfeeding Establishment: Infant (1000) Breastfeeding Establishment: Maternal (1001)	Dias Emidio, S. C., Barbosa Dias, F. de S., Moorhead, S., Deberg, J., de Souza Oliveira-Kumakura, A. R., & Valentim Carmona, E. (2020a). Conceptual and operational definition of nursing outcomes regarding the breastfeeding establishment. *Revista Latino-Americana de Enfermagem (RLAE), 28*, 1–12. Dias Emidio, S. C., Moorhead, S., Oliveira, H. C., Herdman, T. H., Oliveira, K. A. R. de S., & Carmona, E. V. (2020b). Validation of nursing outcomes related to Breastfeeding Establishment. *International Journal of Nursing Knowledge, 31*(2), 134–144.
Caregiver Performance: Direct Care (2205)	Adistya, V. K., Nurjannah, I., & Subekti, H. (2018). The interrater reliability of Nursing Outcome Classification (NOC): "Caregiver Performance: Direct Care." *International Journal of Nursing Knowledge, 29*(3), 192–199. Head, B. J., Maas, M., & Johnson, M. (2003). Validity and community-health-nursing sensitivity of six outcomes for community health nursing with older clients. *Public Health Nursing, 20*(5), 385–398.
Caregiver Physical Health Status (2507)	Head, B. J., Maas, M., & Johnson, M. (2003). Validity and community-health-nursing sensitivity of six outcomes for community health nursing with older clients. *Public Health Nursing, 20*(5), 385–398.
Cognition (0900)	Coelho, J. C. F., Ribeiro, A. R. M., Sampaio, F. M. C., Sequeira, C. A. da C., Lleixà Fortuño, M. del M., & Roldán Merino, J. (2020). Cultural adaptation and psychometric properties assessment of the NOC outcome "Cognition" in a sample of Portuguese adults with mental illness. *International Journal of Nursing Knowledge, 31*(3), 180–187.
Community Competence (2700)	Head, B. J., Aquilino, M. L., Johnson, M., Reed, D., Maas, M., & Moorhead, S. (2004). Content validity and nursing sensitivity of community-level outcomes from the Nursing Outcomes Classification (NOC). *Journal of Nursing Scholarship, 36*(3), 251–259.
Community Health Status (2701)	Head, B. J., Aquilino, M. L., Johnson, M., Reed, D., Maas, M., & Moorhead, S. (2004). Content validity and nursing sensitivity of community-level outcomes from the Nursing Outcomes Classification (NOC). *Journal of Nursing Scholarship, 36*(3), 251–259.
Community Immune Status (2800)	Head, B. J., Aquilino, M. L., Johnson, M., Reed, D., Maas, M., & Moorhead, S. (2004). Content validity and nursing sensitivity of community-level outcomes from the Nursing Outcomes Classification (NOC). *Journal of Nursing Scholarship, 36*(3), 251–259.

Continued

Table 1.5	Studies of Specific NOC Outcomes—cont'd
Community Risk Control: Chronic Disease (2801)	Head, B. J., Aquilino, M. L., Johnson, M., Reed, D., Maas, M., & Moorhead, S. (2004). Content validity and nursing sensitivity of community-level outcomes from the Nursing Outcomes Classification (NOC). *Journal of Nursing Scholarship, 36*(3), 251–259.
Community Risk Control: Communicable Disease (2802)	Head, B. J., Aquilino, M. L., Johnson, M., Reed, D., Maas, M., & Moorhead, S. (2004). Content validity and nursing sensitivity of community-level outcomes from the Nursing Outcomes Classification (NOC). *Journal of Nursing Scholarship, 36*(3), 251–259.
Community Risk Control: Lead Exposure (2803)	Head, B. J., Aquilino, M. L., Johnson, M., Reed, D., Maas, M., & Moorhead, S. (2004). Content validity and nursing sensitivity of community-level outcomes from the Nursing Outcomes Classification (NOC). *Journal of Nursing Scholarship, 36*(3), 251–259.
Dignified Life Closure (1307)	Puente, F. D., Palma, A. E., Sánchez, G. M. R., Hueso, M. C., Esteban, B. A. A., Montoya, J. R. (2020). Development of a scale based on Nursing Outcome Classification "Dignified Life Closure" (1307) to assess end-of-life dignity of patients in care homes for the elderly. *International Journal of Nursing Knowledge, 31*(1), 44–49.
Fall Prevention Behavior (1909)	Araújo, J. N. M., Nunes de Lima Fernandes, A. P., Silva, A. B., Moura, L. A., Ferreira, M. A. Jr., Vitor, A. F. (2018). Clinical validation of Fall Prevention Behavior in a hospital environment. *Revista Brasileira de Enfermagem, 71*(4), 1841–1849. Araújo, J. N. M., Nunes de Lima Fernandes, A. P., Moura, L. A., Palhano dos Santos, M. M., Ferreira Júnior. M, A., Fortes Vitor, A. (2017). Validation of nursing outcome content Fall Prevention Behavior in a hospital environment. *Rev Rene, 18*(3), 337–344. de Sousa Costa, A. G., Leite de Araujo, T., Frota Cavalcante, T., Oliveira Lopes, M. V., de Souza Oliveira-Kumakura, A. R., & Chaves Costa, F. B. (2017). Clinical validation of the nursing outcome Fall Prevention Behavior in people with stroke. *Applied Nursing Research, 33*, 67–71.
Health Seeking Behavior (1603)	Macnee, C. L., Edwards, J., Kaplan, A., Reed, S., Bradford, S., Walls, J., & Schaller-Ayers, J. M. (2006). Evaluation of NOC standardized outcome of "health seeking behavior" in nurse-managed clinics. *Journal of Nursing Care Quality, 21*(3), 242–247.
Knowledge: Cardiac Disease	Rodrigues de Alvarenga, S., de Souza Carneiro, C., Batista Santos, V., & Lopes Moreira, R. S. (2015). Instructional instrument of the NOC outcomes: Control knowledge of cardiac disease for patients with heart failure. *Revista Eletronica de Enfermagem, 17*(4), 1–10.
Knowledge: Diabetes Management (1820)	Oh, H., & Moorhead, S. (2019). Validation of the knowledge and self-management Nursing Outcomes Classification for adults with diabetes. *CIN: Computers, Informatics, Nursing, 37*(4), 222–228.
Knowledge: Fall Prevention (1828)	de Freitas Luzia, M., Argenta, C., de Abreu Almeida, M., & de Fátima Lucena, A. (2018). Conceptual definitions of indicators for the nursing outcome "Knowledge: Fall Prevention." *Revista Brasileira de Enfermagem, 71*(2), 431–439. de Freitas Luzia, M., Vidor, I. D., da Silva, A. C. F. E., & de Fátima Lucena, A. (2020). Fall prevention in hospitalized patients: Evaluation through the Nursing Outcomes Classification/NOC. *Applied Nursing Research, 54*, 151273.
Knowledge: Health Behavior (1805)	Head, B. J., Maas, M., & Johnson, M. (2003). Validity and community-health-nursing sensitivity of six outcomes for community health nursing with older clients. *Public Health Nursing, 20*(5), 385–398.
Knowledge: Heart Failure Management (1835)	da Costa Ferreira, N., Takao Lopes, C., Moorhead, S., Gengo e Silva Butcher, R. de C. (2021). Content validation of the nursing outcome Knowledge Heart Failure Management: Brazilian nurses' opinions. *International Journal of Nursing Knowledge, 32*(3), 206–214.
Knowledge: Hypertension Management (1873)	Oh, H., & Moorhead, S. (2020). Validation of the knowledge and self-management Nursing Outcomes Classification outcomes for adults with hypertension and lipid disorder. *Online Journal of Nursing Informatics, 24*(2), 1.
Knowledge: Lipid Disorder Management (1858)	Oh, H., & Moorhead, S. (2020). Validation of the knowledge and self-management Nursing Outcomes Classification outcomes for adults with hypertension and lipid disorder. *Online Journal of Nursing Informatics, 24*(2), 1.
Mobility (0208)	Moreira, R. P., de Araujo, T. L., Cavalcante, T. F., Guedes, N. G., Costa, A. G. d. S. & Lopes, M. V. d. O. (2013), Validation of the mobility nursing outcome in stroke survivors. *International Journal of Nursing Knowledge, 24*(3), 157–162. da Silva, M. B., de Almeida, M. A., Panato, B. P., de Siqueira, A. P. O., da Silva, M. P., & Reisderfer, L. (2015). Clinical applicability of nursing outcomes in the evolution of orthopedic patients with impaired physical mobility. *Revista Latino-Americana de Enfermagem, 23*, 51–58.
Pain: Adverse Psychological Response (1306)	Bellido-Vallejo, J. C., & Pancorbo-Hidalgo, P. L. (2020), Psychometric evaluation of the nursing outcome "Pain: Adverse Psychological Response" in patients with chronic pain. *International Journal of Nursing Knowledge, 31*(3), 164–172.

Table 1.5   STUDIES OF SPECIFIC NOC OUTCOMES—cont'd

Pain Control (1605)	Bellido-Vallejo, J. C., & Pancorbo-Hidalgo, P. L. (2017). Cultural adaptation and psychometric evaluation of the Spanish version of the nursing outcome "Pain Control" in primary care patients with chronic pain. *Pain Management Nursing, 18*(5), 337–350.
Pain: Disruptive Effects (2101)	Pancorbo-Hidalgo, P. L., & Bellido-Vallejo, J. C. (2019). Clinical validation of the nursing outcome "Pain: Disruptive Effects" in people with chronic pain in Spain. *Journal of Nursing Measurement, 27*(3), 384–400.
Pain Level (2102)	Bellido-Vallejo, J. C., Rodríguez, T. M. C., López, M. I. M., & Pancorbo-Hidalgo, P. L. (2016). Psychometric testing of the Spanish version of the Pain Level outcome scale in hospitalized patients with acute pain. *International Journal of Nursing Knowledge, 27*(1), 10–16.
Risk Control (1902)	Peters, R. M. (2000). Using NOC outcome of risk control in prevention, early detection, and control of hypertension: Nursing Outcomes Classification system. *Outcomes Management for Nursing Practice, 4*(1), 39–45.
Self-Care Behavior: Activities of Daily Living (ADL) (0300)	Head, B. J., Maas, M., & Johnson, M. (2003). Validity and community-health-nursing sensitivity of six outcomes for community health nursing with older clients. *Public Health Nursing, 20*(5), 385–398.
Self Care: Instrumental Activities of Daily Living (IADL) (0306)	Head, B. J., Maas, M., & Johnson, M. (2003). Validity and community-health-nursing sensitivity of six outcomes for community health nursing with older clients. *Public Health Nursing, 20*(5), 385–398.
Self-Management: Cardiac Disease (1617)	Cavalcante, A. M, Lopes, C. T., Swanson, E., Moorhead, S. A., Bachion, M. M., Barros, A. L. (2020). Validation of definitions of the indicators for Nursing Outcomes Classification outcomes: Self-Management cardiac disease. *Acta Paulista de Enfermagem, 33*(1), 1–9. Cavalcante, A. M. R. Z., Lopes, C. T., Brunori, E. F. R., Swanson, E., Moorhead, S. A., Bachion, M. M., & de Barros, A. L. B. L. (2018). Self-care behaviors in heart failure. *International Journal of Nursing Knowledge, 29*(3), 146–155.
Self-Management: Diabetes (1619)	Oh, H., & Moorhead, S. (2019). Validation of the knowledge and self-management Nursing Outcomes Classification for adults with diabetes. *CIN: Computers, Informatics, Nursing, 37*(4), 222–228.
Self-Management: Hypertension (3107)	Oh, H., & Moorhead, S. (2020). Validation of the knowledge and self-management Nursing Outcomes Classification outcomes for adults with hypertension and lipid disorder. *Online Journal of Nursing Informatics, 24*(2), 1.
Self-Management: Lipid Disorder (3109)	Oh, H., & Moorhead, S. (2020). Validation of the knowledge and self-management Nursing Outcomes Classification outcomes for adults with hypertension and lipid disorder. *Online Journal of Nursing Informatics, 24*(2), 1.
Substance Addiction Consequences (1407)	Seabra, P. R. C., Amendoeira, J. J. P., Sá, L. O., & Capelas, M. L. V. (2018). Clinical validation of the Portuguese version of "Substance Addiction Consequences" derived from the Nursing Outcomes Classification. *Issues in Mental Health Nursing, 39*(9), 779–785.
Swallowing Status (1010)	de Souza Oliveira-Kumakura, A. R., Alonso, J. B., & Campos de Carvalho, E. (2019). Psychometric assessment of the nursing outcome Swallowing Status: Rasch model approach. *International Journal of Nursing Knowledge, 30*(4), 197–202. Railka de Souza Oliveira, A., Leite de Araujo, T., Campos de Carvalho, E., Gabrielle de Sousa Costa, A., Frota Cavalcante, T., & Veníícios de Oliveira Lopes, M. (2015). Construction and validation of indicators and respective definitions for the nursing outcome Swallowing status. *Revista Latino-Americana de Enfermagem (RLAE), 23*(3), 450–457.
Tissue Integrity: Skin & Mucous Membranes (1101)	Chantal Magalhães da Silva, N., de Souza Oliveira, K. A. R., Moorhead, S., Pace, A. E., & Carvalho, E. (2017). Clinical validation of the indicators and definitions of the nursing outcome "Tissue Integrity: Skin and Mucous Membranes" in people with Diabetes Mellitus. *International Journal of Nursing Knowledge, 28*(4), 165–170. da Silva, M. B., Barreto, L. N. M., Panato, B. P., Engelman, B., Figueiredo, M. S., Rodríguez, A. A. L., & Almeida, M. de A. (2019). Clinical indicators for evaluation of outcomes of impaired tissue integrity in orthopedic patients: Consensus study. *International Journal of Nursing Knowledge, 30*(2), 81–86.
Wound Healing: Primary Intention (1102)	da Silva, M. B., Barreto, L. N. M., Panato, B. P., Engelman, B., Figueiredo, M. S., Rodríguez, A. A. L., & Almeida, M. de A. (2019). Clinical indicators for evaluation of outcomes of impaired tissue integrity in orthopedic patients: Consensus study. *International Journal of Nursing Knowledge, 30*(2), 81–86. Menna Barreto, L. N., Silva, M., Engelman, B., Figueiredo, M. S., Rodríguez-Acelas, A. L., Cañon-Montañez, W., & Almeida, M. A. (2019). Evaluation of Surgical Wound Healing in Orthopedic Patients with Impaired Tissue Integrity According to Nursing Outcomes Classification. *International Journal of Nursing Knowledge, 30*(4), 228–233. Seyhan Ak, E., Kilinc Akman, E., & Gencbas, D. (2021). Evaluation of wound healing in patients with hip prosthesis according to nursing outcome classification. *International Journal of Nursing Knowledge, 33*(3), 185–195.

tissue integrity. These publications focused on venous ulcers,[20,279] pressure ulcers, or risk of pressure ulcers,[201,233,278]or wound healing.[201,241,262,294] It is good to see research focused on linkages for mental health issues identified four publications, but more studies are needed. What is surprising is that there are only two publications identifying NNN linkages for patients with cancer[304,313] and no NNN linkage publications for patients with diabetes or children from birth to 5 years old. These populations need to be included in linkage research by nurses in the future and more clinical validation studies of NNN linkages are needed.

Integrative, Scoping, and Systematic Reviews focused on Nursing Terminologies

Several types of reviews were found in the literature related to nursing terminologies. These include integrative, scoping, and systematic reviews. For example, in a recent publication, da Silva and colleagues[71] explored the use of integrative reviews to generate or test nursing theories. Several published reviews examined the use and impact of standardized nursing terminologies on nursing practice. For example, a systematic review was conducted with a focus on the impact of nursing diagnoses, interventions, and outcomes on practice by Müller-Staub and colleagues[225] (2007) and a literature review by Törnvall and Jansson.[312] Chae and colleagues[53] conducted an integrative review focused on the effectiveness of nursing interventions using standardized nursing terminologies and Zhang and colleagues[330] examined the effectiveness of nursing terminologies for nursing practice and improved health care outcomes. Fennelly and colleagues[97] conducted an extensive scoping review focused on the use of standardized nursing terminologies in clinical practice. Box 1.8 contains a reference list of all the reviews related to the use of nursing terminologies identified.[70,80,196,245] The box also includes some helpful articles on integrative reviews[298] and scoping reviews[260] that would support further research on the impact of nursing terminologies on practice.

Refinement of the Classification: Ongoing and Future Development

The seventh edition of NOC represents the completion of more than 30 years of research to develop and test a classification and taxonomy of nursing-sensitive patient

| Table 1.6 | RESEARCH FOCUSED ON NURSING OUTCOME LINKAGES TO NURSING DIAGNOSES, CLINICAL CONDITIONS, AND/OR NURSING INTERVENTIONS |

Patients with Heart Problems

Ahern, C. K. (2003). Applying standardized nursing language to three cardiac and pulmonary rehabilitation programs in a rural setting. *International Journal of Nursing Terminologies & Classifications, 14*(Suppl. 4), 32.

Alessandra, Z., Silla, A., & Marilisa, C. (2011). A retrospective study of nursing diagnoses, outcomes, and interventions for patients admitted to a cardiology rehabilitation unit. *International Journal of Nursing Terminologies & Classifications, 22*(4), 148–156.

Azzolin, K., de Souza, E. N., Ruschel, K. B., Mussi, C. M., de Lucena, A. F, Rabelo, E. R. (2012). Consensus on nursing diagnoses, interventions and outcomes for home care of patients with heart failure. *Revista Gaucha de Enfermagem, 33*(4), 56–63.

Azzolin, K., Mussi, C. M., Ruschel, K. B., de Souza, E. N., de Fátima Lucena, A., & Rabelo-Silva, E. R. (2013). Effectiveness of nursing interventions in heart failure patients in home care using NANDA-I, NIC, and NOC. *Applied Nursing Research, 26*(4), 239–244.

Beltrão, B. A., da Silva, V. M., de Araujo, T. L., & Lopes, M. V. de O. (2011). Clinical indicators of Ineffective Breathing Pattern in children with congenital heart diseases. *International Journal of Nursing Terminologies & Classifications, 22*(1), 4–12.

de Lima Lopes, J., de Barros, A. L. B. L., & Marlene Michel, J. L. (2009). A pilot study to validate the priority Nursing Interventions Classification interventions and Nursing Outcomes Classification outcomes for the nursing diagnosis "excess fluid volume" in cardiac patients. *International Journal of Nursing Terminologies & Classifications, 20*(2), 76–88.

Head, B. J., Scherb, C. A., Maas, M. L., Swanson, E. A., Moorhead, S., Reed, D., Conley, D. M., & Kozel, M. (2011). Nursing clinical documentation data retrieval for hospitalized older adults with heart failure: Part 2. *International Journal of Nursing Terminologies & Classifications, 22*(2), 68–76.

Moreira, R. P., Guerra, F. V. G., Ferreira, G. O., Cavalcante, T. F., Felício, J. F., Ferreira, L. C. C., & Guedes, N. G. (2021). Effects of the nursing intervention Fall Prevention in older adults with arterial hypertension using NANDA-I, NIC and NOC. *International Journal of Nursing Knowledge, 33*(2), 147–161.

Park, H. (2014). Identifying core NANDA-I nursing diagnoses, NIC interventions, NOC outcomes, and NNN linkages for heart failure. *International Journal of Nursing Knowledge, 25*(1), 30–38.

Rodrigues de Alvarenga, S., de Souza Carneiro, C., Batista Santos, V., & Lopes Moreira, R. S. (2015). Instructional instrument of the NOC outcomes: Control knowledge of cardiac disease for patients with heart failure. *Revista Eletronica de Enfermagem, 17*(4), 1–10.

Scherb, C. A., Head, B. J., Maas, M. L., Swanson, E. A., Moorhead, S., Reed, D., Conley, D. M., & Kozel, M. (2011). Most frequent nursing diagnoses, nursing interventions, and nursing-sensitive patient outcomes of hospitalized older adults with heart failure: Part 1. *International Journal of Nursing Terminologies & Classifications, 22*(1), 13–22.

Van Horn, E. R., & Kautz, D. D. (2010). NNN language and evidence-based practice guidelines for acute cardiac care: Retaining the essence of nursing. *Dimensions of Critical Care Nursing, 29*(2), 69–72.

Table 1.6	RESEARCH FOCUSED ON NURSING OUTCOME LINKAGES TO NURSING DIAGNOSES, CLINICAL CONDITIONS, AND/OR NURSING INTERVENTIONS—cont'd

Patients Experiencing Pain

de Fátima Lucena, A., Holsbach, I., Pruinelli, L., Serdotte Freitas Cardoso, A., & Schroeder Mello, B. (2013). Brazilian validation of the nursing outcomes for acute pain. *International Journal of Nursing Knowledge, 24*(1), 54–58.

Killeen, M. B. (2003). Use of NANDA, NIC, and NOC as a framework for cyclic perimenstrual pain and discomfort. *International Journal of Nursing Terminologies & Classifications, 14*(Suppl. 4), 19–20.

Mello, B. S., Almeida, M. A., Pruinelli, L., & Lucena, A. F. (2019). Nursing outcomes for pain assessment of patients undergoing palliative care. Reben-Revista Brasileira de Enfermagem, *72*, 64–72.

Mello, B. S., Massutti, T. M., Longaray, V. K., Trevisan, D. F., & de Fátima Lucena, A. (2016). Applicability of the Nursing Outcomes Classification (NOC) to the evaluation of cancer patients with acute or chronic pain in palliative care. *Applied Nursing Research, 29*, 12–18.

Régis, C. C., Santos, C. T., Einhardt, R. S., Lucena, A. F. (2020). Chronic pain evaluated by the Nursing Outcomes Classification. *Revista de Enfermagem UFPE, 14*, e243932.

School Age Children

Lunney, M. (2006). NANDA diagnoses, NIC interventions, and NOC outcomes used in an electronic health record with elementary school children. *Journal of School Nursing, 22*(2), 94–101.

Lunney, M., & Parker, L. (2003). Effects of using NANDA, NIC, and NOC on health outcomes of school children: A pilot study. *International Journal of Nursing Terminologies & Classifications, 14*(Suppl. 4), 21.

Lunney, M., Parker, L., Fiore, L., Cavendish, R., & Pulcini, J. (2004). Feasibility of studying the effects of using NANDA, NIC, and NOC on nurses' power and children's outcomes. *CIN: Computers, Informatics, Nursing, 22*(6), 316–325.

Older Patients

Aguilar, L. V., & Pancorbo-Hidalgo, P. L. (2011). Nursing diagnoses, outcomes and interventions identified in multimorbidity aged patients after discharge. *Gerokomos, 22*(4), 152–161.

Argenta, C., Zanatta, E. A., Adamy, E. K., Lucena, A. F. (2022). Nursing outcomes and interventions associated with the nursing diagnoses: Risk for or actual frail elderly syndrome. *International Journal of Nursing*, Advance online publication.

Head, B. J., Scherb, C. A., Reed, D., Conley, D. M., Weinberg, B., Kozel, M., Gillette, S., Clarke, M., & Moorhead, S. (2011). Nursing diagnoses, interventions, and patient outcomes for hospitalized older adults with pneumonia. *Research in Gerontological Nursing, 4*(2), 95–105.

Lee, E. (2019). Use of the Nursing Outcomes Classification for falls and fall prevention by nurses in South Korea. *International Journal of Nursing Knowledge, 30*(1), 28–33.

Lucena, A. de F., Argenta, C., Almeida, M. de A., Moorhead, S., & Swanson, E. (2019). Validation of nursing outcomes and interventions to older adults' care with risk or frail elderly syndrome: Proposal of linkages among NOC, NIC, and NANDA-I to clinical practice. *International Journal of Nursing Knowledge, 30*(3), 147–153.

Lucena, A. de F., Argenta, C., Luzia, M. F., Almeida, M. A., Barreto, L. N. M., Swanson, E. (2020). Multidimensional model of successful aging and nursing terminologies: Similarities for use in the clinical practice. *Revista Gaúcha de Enfermagem, 41*, e20190148.

Shin, J. H., Choi, G. Y., & Lee, J. (2021). Identifying frequently used NANDA-I nursing diagnoses, NOC outcomes, NIC interventions, and NNN linkages for nursing home residents in Korea. *International Journal of Environmental Research and Public Health, 18*(21), 11505.

Patients with Neurological Problems/Spinal Cord Injury

Hughes, R. (2003). The use of NANDA, NIC, and NOC in the identification and measurement of problems, interventions, and outcomes in spinal cord injury. *International Journal of Nursing Terminologies & Classifications, 14*, 18–19.

Lee, E. (2006b). Analysis of Nursing Outcomes Classification (NOC) used in neurosurgical units in Korea. *International Journal of Nursing Terminologies & Classifications, 17*(1), 73–74.

Lee, E., Park, H., Whyte, J., Kim, Y., & Park, S. Y. (2014). Identifying core nursing sensitive outcomes associated with the most frequently used North American Nursing Diagnosis Association-International nursing diagnoses for patients with cerebrovascular disease in Korea. *International Journal of Nursing Practice, 20*(6), 636–645.

Lunney, M., Mcguire, M., Endozo, N., & Mclutsh-Waddy, D. (2010). Consensus validation study identifies relevant nursing diagnoses, nursing interventions, and health outcomes for people with traumatic brain injuries. *Rehabilitation Nursing, 35*(4), 161–166.

Continued

Table 1.6	RESEARCH FOCUSED ON NURSING OUTCOME LINKAGES TO NURSING DIAGNOSES, CLINICAL CONDITIONS, AND/OR NURSING INTERVENTIONS—cont'd

Patients with Tissue Integrity Problems

Bavaresco, T., Pires, A. U. B., Moraes, V. M., Osmarin, V. M., Silveira, D. T., & Lucena, A. de F. (2018). Low-level laser therapy for treatment of venous ulcers evaluated with the Nursing Outcome Classification: Study protocol for a randomized controlled trial. *Trials, 19*(1), 372.

Menna Barreto, L. N., da Silva, M. B., Engelman, B., Figueiredo, M. S., Rodríguez-Acelas, A. L., Cañon-Montañez, W., & de Abreu Almeida, M. (2019). Evaluation of surgical wound healing in orthopedic patients with impaired tissue integrity according to Nursing Outcomes Classification. *International Journal of Nursing Knowledge, 30*(4), 228–233.

Menna Barreto, L. N., Swanson, E. A., & de Abreu Almeida, M. (2016). Nursing outcomes for the diagnosis impaired tissue integrity (00044) in adults with pressure ulcer. *International Journal of Nursing Knowledge, 27*(2), 104–110.

Nunes Caldini, L., Alves Silva, R., Alencar Melo, G. A., Fernandes Pereira, F. G., Marques Frota, N., & Áfio Caetano, J. (2017). Nursing interventions and outcomes for pressure ulcer risk in critically ill patients. *Rev Rene, 18*(5), 598–605.

Oliveira, M.C., Flores, F. S., Barbosa, F. M.; Fujii, C. D. C., Rabelo-Silva, E. R., Lucena A.F., (2021). Evaluation of percutaneous renal biopsy complications based on outcomes and indicators of the Nursing Outcomes Classification. *Revista Latino-Americana de Enfermagem, 29*, e3415.

Pezzi, M. V., Rabelo, S. E. R., Paganin, A., & Souza, E. N. (2016). Nursing interventions and outcomes for the diagnosis of Impaired Tissue Integrity in patients after cardiac catheterization: Survey. *International Journal of Nursing Knowledge, 27*(4), 215–219.

Santos, C. T., Barbosa, F. M., Almeida, T., Silva, A. C. F. E., Einhardt, R. S., Lucena, A. F. (2021). Indicators of Nursing Outcomes Classification for evaluation of patients with pressure injury: Expert consensus. *Escola Anna Nery. Revista de Enfermagem, 25*, e20200155.

Santos, F. A. A. S., de Melo, R. P., & de Oliveira Lopes, M. V. (2010). Characterization of health status with regard to tissue integrity and tissue perfusion in patients with venous ulcers according to the Nursing Outcomes Classification. *Journal of Vascular Nursing, 28*(1), 14–20.

Seyhan Ak, E., Kilinc Akman, E., & Gencbas, D. (2021). Evaluation of wound healing in patients with hip prosthesis according to nursing outcome classification. *International Journal of Nursing Knowledge, 33*(3), 185–195.

Patients with Mental Health Problems

Escalada-Hernández, P., Muñoz-Hermoso, P., González-Fraile, E., Santos, B., González-Vargas, J. A., Feria-Raposo, I., Girón-García, J. L., & García-Manso, M. (2015). A retrospective study of nursing diagnoses, outcomes, and interventions for patients with mental disorders. *Applied Nursing Research, 28*(2), 92–98.

Jennewein, C. (2006). Development/implementation of NNN-language care plans in an electronic medical record for a behavioral health population. *International Journal of Nursing Terminologies & Classifications, 17*(1), 72.

Pires, A. U. B., Lucena, A. F., Behenck, A., Heldt, E. (2020). Results of the Nursing Outcomes Classification/NOC for patients with obsessive-compulsive disorder. *Revista Brasileira de Enfermagem, 73*, 1.

Taghavi Larijani, T., Saatchi, B. (2019). Training of NANDA-I nursing diagnoses (NDs), Nursing Interventions Classification (NIC) and Nursing Outcomes Classification (NOC) in psychiatric wards: A randomized controlled trial. *Nursing Open, 6*, 612–619.

Patients Admitted to Intensive Care Unit or Medical Surgical Units

Garutti Rodrigues, F., Andrade dos Santos, F., & Bottura Leite de Barros, A. L. (2006). NIC interventions and NOC outcomes in patients with activity intolerance. *International Journal of Nursing Terminologies & Classifications, 17*(1), 79.

Gengo e Silva, R. de C., dos Santos Diogo, R. C., da Cruz, D. de A. L. M., Ortiz, D., Ortiz, D., Peres, H. H. C., & Moorhead, S. (2018). Linkages of nursing diagnoses, outcomes, and interventions performed by nurses caring for medical and surgical patients using a decision support system. *International Journal of Nursing Knowledge, 29*(4), 269–275.

Lee, E., & Choi, S. (2011). Identification of nursing diagnosis-outcome-intervention (NANDA-NOC-NIC) linkages in surgical nursing unit. *Korean Journal of Adult Nursing, 23*(2), 180–188.

Moon, M. (2011). Relationship of nursing diagnoses, nursing outcomes, and nursing interventions for patient care in intensive care units (Publication No. 3526851) [Doctoral dissertation, University of Iowa]. ProQuest Dissertations and Theses Global.

Noh, H. K., & Lee, E. (2015). Relationships among NANDA-I diagnoses, Nursing Outcomes Classification, and nursing interventions classification by nursing students for patients in medical-surgical units in Korea. *International Journal of Nursing Knowledge, 26*(1), 43–51.

Patients with Cancer

Su, M.-S., So, H., & An, M. (2014). Identification of major nursing diagnosis, nursing outcomes, and nursing interventions (NNN) linkage for cancer patients undergoing chemotherapy. *Korean Journal of Adult Nursing, 26*(4), 413–423.

Tseng, H. C. (2012). Use of standardized nursing terminologies in electronic health records for oncology care: The impact of NANDA-I, NOC, and NIC (Publication No. 3638443) [Doctoral dissertation, University of Iowa]. ProQuest Dissertations and Theses Global.

Tseng, H., & Moorhead, S. (2014). The use of standardized terminology to represent nursing knowledge: Nursing interventions relevant to safety for patients with cancer. *Studies in Health Technology & Informatics, 201*, 298–303.

Continued

Table 1.6	RESEARCH FOCUSED ON NURSING OUTCOME LINKAGES TO NURSING DIAGNOSES, CLINICAL CONDITIONS, AND/OR NURSING INTERVENTIONS—cont'd

Patients with Urinary Problems

Gencbas, D., Bebis, H., & Cicek, H. (2018). Evaluation of the efficiency of the nursing care plan applied using NANDA, NOC, and NIC linkages to elderly women with incontinence living in a nursing home: A randomized controlled study. *International Journal of Nursing Knowledge, 29*(4), 217–226.

Patients with Respiratory Problems or COVID-19

Ahern, C. K. (2003). Applying standardized nursing language to three cardiac and pulmonary rehabilitation programs in a rural setting. *International Journal of Nursing Terminologies & Classifications, 14*(Suppl. 4), 32.

Allande-Cussó, R., Fernández-Garcia, E., Barrientos-Trigo, S., Rapela-Sánchez-Campa, M. A., & Porcel-Gálvez, A. M. (2021). Implementing holistic care in isolated patients during COVID-19 Pandemic: A case study using Nursing Outcomes (NOC) and Interventions (NIC) Classifications. *Holistic Nursing Practice, 35*(6), 326–331.

Barros, A. L. B. L., Silva, V. M., Santana, R. F., Cavalcante, A. M. R. Z., Vitor, A. F., Lucena, A. F., et al. (2020). Brazilian Nursing Process Research Network contributions for assistance in the COVID-19 pandemic. *Revista Brasileira de Enfermagem, 73*(S2), e20200798.

da Silva, L. F. M., Pascoal, L. M., Nunes, S. F. L., de Sousa Freire, V. E. C., de Araújo Almeida, A. G., Gontijo, P. V. C. & Neto, M. S. (2019). Ineffective airway clearance in surgical patients: Evaluation of nursing interventions and outcomes. *International Journal of Nursing Knowledge, 30*(4), 251–256.

da Silva, V. M., de Oliveira Lopes, M. V., de Araujo, T. L., Beltrao, B. A., Monteiro, F. P. M., Cavalcante, T. F., Moreira, R. P., & Santos, F. A. A. S. (2011). Operational definitions of outcome indicators related to ineffective breathing patterns in children with congenital heart disease. *Heart & Lung, 40*(3), e70–e77.

Gomes, G. L. L., de Oliveira F. M. R. L., Leal, N. P. da R., Guimarães, K. S. L., Silva, D. F. da, Barbosa, K. T. F. et al. (2021). Nursing diagnoses/outcomes and interventions for patients with COVID-19: A retrospective documentary study. *Online Brazilian Journal of Nursing,* Supplement *20*, 16–27.

González Aguña, A., Fernández Batalla, M., Díaz-Tendero Rodríguez, J., Sarrión Bravo, J. A., Gonzalo de Diego, B., & Santamaría García, J. M. (2021). Validation of a manual of care plans for people hospitalized with COVID-19. *Nursing Open, 8*, 3495–3515.

Head, B. J., Scherb, C. A., Reed, D., Conley, D. M., Weinberg, B., Kozel, M., Gillette, S., Clarke, M., & Moorhead, S. (2011). Nursing diagnoses, interventions, and patient outcomes for hospitalized older adults with pneumonia. *Research in Gerontological Nursing, 4*(2), 95–105.

Lee, E. (2006a). Analysis of nursing diagnoses and outcomes used in a respiratory unit in Korea. *International Journal of Nursing Terminologies & Classifications, 17*(1), 42.

Moorhead, S., Macieira, T. G. R., Lopez, K. D., Mantovani, V. M., Swanson, E., Wagner, C., & Abe, N. (2021). NANDA-I, NOC, and NIC linkages to SARS-Cov-2 (COVID-19): Part 1. Community response. *International Journal of Nursing Knowledge, 32*(1), 59–67.

Swanson, E., Mantovani, V. M., Wagner, C., Moorhead, S., Lopez, K. D., Macieira, T. G. R., & Abe, N. (2021). NANDA-I, NOC, and NIC linkages to SARS-CoV-2 (COVID-19): Part 2. Individual response. *International Journal of Nursing Knowledge, 32*(1), 68–83.

Wagner, C. M., Swanson, E., Moorhead, S., Mantovani, V. M., Dunn-Lopez, K., Macieira, T.G.R., Abe, N., & Breitenstein, S. (2022). NANDA-I, NOC, and NIC linkages to SARS-CoV-2 (COVID-19): Part 3. Family response. *International Journal of Nursing Knowledge, 33*(1), 5–17.

Patients with Nutritional Problems

Monteiro Mantovani, V., Moorhead, S., & Abe, N. (2020). NANDA-I, NOC, and NIC linkages for nutritional problems. *International Journal of Nursing Knowledge, 31*(4), 246–252.

Maternity Patients

Yang, M. J., Kim, H. Y., Ko, E., & Kim, H. K. (2019). Identification of nursing diagnosis–outcome–intervention linkages for inpatients in the obstetrics department nursing unit in South Korea. *International Journal of Nursing Knowledge, 30*(1), 12–20.

outcomes. The classification contains 612 outcomes designed for measuring the impact of nursing interventions on individual, caregiver, family, and community outcomes. The seventh edition provides nurses with 82 new outcomes, 337 revised, and eight reviewed outcomes. Ten outcomes were retired based on the review process. This edition provides the reader with the most comprehensive review of the classification ever completed. Nine new community outcomes and four new family outcomes were added based on needs identified by the global pandemic. Five new risk control outcomes were created to address health challenges. The number of outcomes developed for use with teaching interventions continues to increase with each edition. This edition added eight new knowledge outcomes and five new

Box 1.8

Integrative, Scoping, and Systematic Research Reviews Focused on Use of NNN Nursing Terminologies

Chae, S., Oh, H., & Moorhead, S. (2020). Effectiveness of nursing interventions using standardized nursing terminologies: An integrative review. *Western Journal of Nursing Research, 42*(11), 963–973.

da Silva, N. C. M., de Souza Oliveira, A. R., & de Carvalho, E.C. (2015). Knowledge produced from the outcomes of the "Nursing Outcomes Classification - NOC": Integrative review. *Revista Gaucha de Enfermagem, 36*(4),104–111.

da Silva, R. N., Brandão, M. A. G., & Ferreira, M. de A. (2020). Integrative review as a method to generate or to test nursing theory. *Nursing Science Quarterly, 33*(3), 258–263.

de Groot, K., Triemstra, M., Paans, W., & Francke, A. L. (2019). Quality criteria, instruments, and requirements for nursing documentation: A systematic review of systematic reviews. *Journal of Advanced Nursing, 75*(7), 1379–1393.

de Souza Oliveira-Kumakura, A. R., Caldeira, S., Prado Simão, T., Camargo, F. F. A., de Almeida Lopes Monteiro da Cruz, D., & Campos de Carvalho, E. (2018). The contribution of the Rasch Model to the clinical validation of nursing diagnoses: Integrative literature review. *International Journal of Nursing Knowledge, 29*(2), 89–96.

Fennelly, O., Grogan, L., Reed, A., & Hardiker, N. R. (2021). Use of standardized terminologies in clinical practice: A scoping review. *International Journal of Medical Informatics, 149,* 104431.

Gengo e Silva Butcher, R. de C., & Jones, D. A. (2021). An integrative review of comprehensive nursing assessment tools developed based on Gordon's Eleven Functional Health Patterns. *International Journal of Nursing Knowledge, 32*(4), 294–307.

Kim, J., Macieira, T., Meyer, S. L., Ansell Maggie, M., Bjarnadottir Raga, R. I., Smith, M. B., et al. (2020). Towards implementing SNOMED CT in nursing practice: A scoping review. *International Journal of Medical Informatics, 134,* 104035.

Macieira, T. G. R., Chianca, T. C. M., Smith, M. B., Yao, Y., Bian, J., Wilkie, D. J., et al. (2019). Secondary use of standardized nursing care data for advancing nursing science and practice: A systematic review. *Journal of the American Medical Informatics Association, 26*(11), 1401–1411.

Müller-Staub, M, Lavin, M. A., Needham, I., & van Achterberg, T. (2007). Pflegediagnosen, -interventionen und -ergebnisse—Anwendung und Auswirkungen auf die Pflegepraxis: eine systematische Literaturübersicht [Nursing diagnoses, interventions, and outcomes -- application and impact on nursing practice: A systematic literature review]. *Pflege, 20*(6), 352–371.

Othman, E. H., Shatnawi, F., Alrajabi, O., & Alshraideh, J. A. (2020). Reporting nursing interventions classification and Nursing Outcomes Classification in nursing research: A systematic review. *International Journal of Nursing Knowledge, 31*(1), 19–36.

Peters, M. D. J., Marnie, C. Colquhoun, H., Garritty, C. M., Hempel, S., Horsley, T., et al. (2021). Scoping reviews: Reinforcing and advancing the methodology and application. *Systematic Reviews, 10*(1), 263.

Soares, C. B., Komura Hoga, L. A., Peduzzi, M., Sangaleti, C., Yonekura, T., & Delage Silva, D. R. A. (2014). Integrative review: Concepts and methods used in nursing. *Revista Da Escola de Enfermagem Da USP, 48*(2), 329–339.

Tastan, S., Linch, G. C. F., Keenan, G. M., Stifter, J., McKinney, D., Fahey, L., et al. (2014). Evidence for the existing American Nurses Association-recognized standardized nursing terminologies: A systematic review. *International Journal of Nursing Studies, 51*(8), 1160–1170.

Törnvall, E., & Jansson, I. (2017). Preliminary evidence for the usefulness of standardized nursing terminologies in different fields of application: A literature review. *International Journal of Nursing Knowledge, 28*(2), 109–119.

Zhang, T., Wu, X., Peng, G., Zhang, Q., Chen, L., Cai, Z., & Ou, H. (2021). Effectiveness of standardized nursing terminologies for nursing practice and healthcare outcomes: A systematic review. *International Journal of Nursing Knowledge, 32*(4), 220–228.

self-management outcomes. The entire class of client satisfaction outcomes were revised, and three new outcomes were added. We want to thank the many nurses who helped us accomplish this updated edition of NOC. The names of nurses who participated in this review are listed in the front part of the book in the recognition list. The guidelines for submitting new or revised outcomes are in Appendix E.

SUMMARY

This chapter provides an overview of the current outcome classification, defining important components of an outcome and its use. Frequently asked questions about NOC are discussed. For this edition, we have added a new section focused on resources to complement the use of NOC and standardized nursing terminologies in education, practice, and research. This resource section highlights the many nurses who support the use of NOC and are dedicated to increasing the knowledge base of nursing. As the work to maintain NOC continues, we need to find better ways to identify published research related to the outcomes in the classification. We hope anyone who publishes research using NOC will share their work with us. A classification of nursing-sensitive patient, family, and community outcomes will never be complete, but will continue to expand to meet the demands of nursing practice. Readers and users of the classification are encouraged to provide feedback to the editors of NOC.

Even after 30 years of work, the contributions of nurses remain invisible in most cases. The nursing research completed to date are often conducted in a single health care system and electronic health records are not well developed for nursing. The use of NOC in a well-developed nursing system can provide data so that contributions made by the nursing profession to health care are documented and made visible. Use of NOC over the last decade has demonstrated that nurses can make dramatic improvements in outcomes in a short time period. With shorter lengths of stay in acute care institutions, it is critical that nurses choose interventions that are effective in improving patient outcomes. Nurses also need to identify ineffective or poorly timed interventions in current practice. Nurses need to identify outcomes that are essential to basic care delivery and determine the key outcomes for specialty practice. Organizations beyond acute care hospitals should use outcomes in evaluating nursing care because the ability to evaluate NOC outcomes across settings is one of its strengths.

Classification work of this kind is essential to the future of the nursing profession. All nurses can join in the effort to include nursing terminologies in clinical information systems so that comparable nursing data are available in large local, national, and international data sets. We invite our colleagues to assist with further testing of the psychometric integrity and clinical usefulness of the NOC outcomes. Over 60 journals have published manuscripts related to NOC and use of NNN based on our review for this edition. Research published by nurse scientists, clinicians, and graduate students and shared with the NOC research team impacts the nursing profession and benefits the patients who nurses serve. Armed with data that demonstrates nursing effectiveness and impact on health care, nurses can influence health policy to optimally benefit the individuals, families, and communities to whom they provide care. Today nurses across the world are working together to improve nursing care using standardized nursing terminologies. Morley and Cunningham[222] worked with other European countries to improve education across borders. Their research concludes that "only by growing international champions" through funded and well constituted projects can a genuine impact on the global health and educational needs in nursing be met. The lessons they learned can also be applied to nurses working with standardized nursing terminologies.

References

1. Abreu Almeida, M., Silva, M. B., Panato, B. P., Oliveira Siqueira, A. P., & Laurent, M. D. C. R. (2013). Nursing outcomes for Brazilian pediatric patients hospitalized with deficient diversional activity. *International Journal of Nursing Knowledge*, *24*(2), 85–92. https://doi.org/10.1111/j.2047-3095.2013.01233.x

2. Adereti, C. S., & Olaogun, A. A. (2019). Use of electronic and paper-based standardized nursing care plans to improve nurses' documentation quality in a Nigerian teaching hospital. *International Journal of Nursing Knowledge*, *30*(4), 219–227. https://doi.org/10.1111/2047-3095.12232

3. Adistya, V. K., Nurjannah, I., & Subekti, H. (2018). The interrater reliability of Nursing Outcome Classification (NOC): "Caregiver Performance: Direct Care".

International Journal of Nursing Knowledge, *29*(3), 192–199. https://doi.org/10.1111/2047-3095.12164

4. Adubi, I. O., Olaogun, A. A., & Adejumo, P. O. (2018). Effect of standardized nursing language continuing education programme on nurses' documentation of care at University College Hospital, Ibadan. *Nursing Open*, *5*, 37–44. https://doi.org/10.1002/nop2.108

5. Aguilar, L. V., & Pancorbo-Hidalgo, P. L. (2011). Nursing diagnoses, outcomes and interventions identified in multimorbidity aged patients after discharge. *Gerokomos*, *22*(4), 152–161.

6. Ahern, C. K. (2003). Applying standardized nursing language to three cardiac and pulmonary rehabilitation programs in a rural setting. *International Journal of Nursing Terminologies & Classifications*, *14*(Suppl. 4), 32. https://doi.org/10.1111/j.1744-618x.2003.032_1.x

7. Albers, C., Gloskey, D., Pahl, J., Kravutske, M. E., & Zugcic, M. (2006). Methods of educating RNs to use the NOCs in their documentation. *International Journal of Nursing Terminologies & Classifications*, *17*(1), 92–93. https://doi.org/10.1002/mc.22044

8. Aleandri, M., Scalorbi, S., & Pirazzini, M. C. (2022). Electronic nursing care plans through the use of NANDA, NOC and NIC taxonomies in community setting: A descriptive study in northern Italy. *International Journal of Nursing Knowledge*, *33*(1), 72–80. https://doi.org/10.1111/2047-3095.12326

9. Alessandra, Z., Silla, A., & Marilisa, C. (2011). A retrospective study of nursing diagnoses, outcomes, and interventions for patients admitted to a cardiology rehabilitation unit. *International Journal of Nursing Terminologies & Classifications*, *22*(4), 148–156. https://doi.org/10.1111/j.1744-618X.2011.01184.x

10. Allande-Cussó, R., Fernândez-Garcia, E., Barrientos-Trigo, S., Rapela-Sânchez-Campa, M. A., & Porcel-Gâlvez, A. M. (2021). Implementing holistic care in isolated patients during COVID-19 Pandemic: A case study using Nursing Outcomes (NOC) and Interventions (NIC) Classifications. *Holistic Nursing Practice*, *35*(6), 326–331. https://doi.org/10.1097/HNP.0000000000000479

11. Anderson, C. A., Keenan, G., & Jones, J. (2009). Using bibliometrics to support your selection of a nursing terminology set. *CIN: Computers, Informatics, Nursing*, *27*(2), 82–90. https://doi.org/10.1097/ncn.0b013e3181972a24

12. Araújo, J. N. M., Nunes de Lima Fernandes, A. P., Moura, L. A., Palhano dos Santos, M. M., Ferreira, M. A., Jr., & Fortes Vitor, A. (2017). Validation of nursing outcome content Fall Prevention Behavior in a hospital environment. *Rev Rene*, *18*(3), 337–344. https://doi.org/10.15253/2175-6783.2017000300008

13. Araújo, J. N. M., Nunes de Lima Fernandes, A. P., Silva, A. B., Moura, L. A., Ferreira, M. A., Jr., & Vitor, A. F. (2018). Clinical validation of Fall Prevention Behavior in a hospital environment. *Revista Brasileira de Enfermagem*, *71*(4), 1841–1849. https://doi.org/10.1590/0034-7167-2017-0212

14. Argenta, C., Zanatta, E. A., Adamy, E. K., & Lucena, A. F. (2022). Nursing outcomes and interventions associated with the nursing diagnoses: Risk for or actual frail elderly syndrome. *International Journal of Nursing Knowledge*, Advance online publication. https://doi.org/10.1111/2047-3095.12357

15. Azzolin, K., de Souza, E. N., Ruschel, K. B., Mussi, C. M., de Lucena, A. F., & Rabelo, E. R. (2012). Consensus on nursing diagnoses, interventions and outcomes for home care of patients with heart failure. *Revista Gaucha de Enfermagem*, *33*(4), 56–63.

16. Azzolin, K., Mussi, C. M., Ruschel, K. B., de Souza, E. N., de Fátima Lucena, A., & Rabelo-Silva, E. R. (2013). Effectiveness of nursing interventions in heart failure patients in home care using NANDA-I, NIC, and NOC. *Applied Nursing Research*, *26*(4), 239–244. https://doi.org/10.1016/j.apnr.2013.08.003

17. Barros, A. L. B. L., Silva, V. M., Santana, R. F., Cavalcante, A. M. R. Z., Vitor, A. F., Lucena, A. F., et al. (2020). Brazilian Nursing Process Research Network contributions for assistance in the COVID-19 pandemic. *Revista Brasileira de Enfermagem*, *73*(Suppl. 2), e20200798. https://doi.org/10.1590/0034-7167-2020-0798

18. Basit, G., & Korkmaz, F. (2021). The effect of web-based nursing process teaching on senior nursing students' care planning skills. *International Journal of Nursing Knowledge*, *32*(1), 4–19. https://doi.org/10.1111/2047-3095.12283

19. Bavaresco, T., & Lucena, A. F. (2022). Low-laser light therapy in venous ulcer healing: A randomized clinical trial. *Reben-Revista Brasileira De Enfermagem*, *75*, 1–7. https://doi.org/10.1590/0034-7167-2021-0396

20. Bavaresco, T., Pires, A. U. B., Moraes, V. M., Osmarin, V. M., Silveira, D. T., & Lucena, A. de F. (2018). Low-level laser therapy for treatment of venous ulcers evaluated with the Nursing Outcome Classification: Study protocol for a randomized controlled trial. *Trials*, *19*(1), 372. https://doi.org/10.1186/s13063-018-2729-x

21. Behrenbeck, J. G. (2003). Nursing-sensitive outcome implementation and reliability testing in a tertiary care setting. *International Journal of Nursing Terminologies & Classifications*, *14*(Suppl. 4), 12. https://doi.org/10.1111/j.1744-618X.2003.012_1.x

22. Behrenbeck, J. G., Timm, J. A., Griebenow, L. K., & Demmer, K. A. (2005). Nursing-sensitive outcome reliability testing in a tertiary care setting. *International Journal of Nursing Terminologies & Classifications*, *16*(1), 14–20. https://doi.org/10.1111/j.1744-618x.2005.00002.x

23. Bellido-Vallejo, J. C., & Pancorbo-Hidalgo, P. L. (2017). Cultural adaptation and psychometric evaluation of the Spanish version of the nursing outcome "Pain Control" in primary care patients with chronic pain. *Pain Management Nursing*, *18*(5), 337–350. https://doi.org/10.1016/j.pmn.2017.04.001

24. Bellido-Vallejo, J. C., & Pancorbo-Hidalgo, P. L. (2020). Psychometric evaluation of the nursing outcome "Pain: Adverse Psychological Response" in patients with chronic pain. *International Journal of Nursing Knowledge*, *31*(3), 164–172. https://doi.org/10.1111/2047-3095.12267

25. Bellido-Vallejo, J. C., Rodríguez, T. M. C., López, M. I. M., & Pancorbo-Hidalgo, P. L. (2016). Psychometric testing of the Spanish version of the Pain Level outcome scale in hospitalized patients with acute pain. *International Journal of Nursing Knowledge*, *27*(1), 10–16. https://doi.org/10.1111/2047-3095.12070

26. Beltrão, B. A., da Silva, V. M., de Araujo, T. L., & Lopes, M. V. de O. (2011). Clinical indicators of ineffective breathing pattern in children with congenital heart diseases. *International Journal of Nursing Terminologies & Classifications*, *22*(1), 4–12. https://doi.org/10.1111/j.1744-618X.2010.01169.x

27. Bernhart-Just, A., Hillewerth, K., Holzer-Pruss, C., Paprotny, M., & Heinrich, H. Z. (2009). The electronic use of the NANDA-, NOC- and NIC-classifications and implications for nursing practice. *Pflege*, *22*(6), 443–454. https://doi.org/10.1024/1012-5302.22.6.443

28. Bernhart-Just, A., Lassen, B., & Schwendimann, R. (2010). Representing the nursing process with nursing terminologies in electronic medical record systems: A Swiss approach. *CIN: Computers, Informatics, Nursing*, *28*(6), 345–352. https://doi.org/10.1097/NCN.0b013e3181f69bb3

29. Bitencourt, G. R., Alves, L. de A. F., Santana, R. F., & Lopes, M. V. de O. (2016). Agreement between experts regarding assessment of postoperative urinary elimination nursing outcomes in elderly patients. *International Journal of Nursing Knowledge*, *27*(3), 143–148. https://doi.org/10.1111/2047-3095.12094

30. Bjorklund, L. L., Müller, S. M., Cardozo, M. C. E., Souza Bernardes, D., & Rabelo, S. E. R. (2019). Clinical indicators of Nursing Outcomes Classification for patient with risk for perioperative positioning injury: A cohort study. *Journal of Clinical Nursing*, *28*(23/24), 4367–4378. https://doi.org/10.1111/jocn.15019

31. Bond, T. G., & Fox, C. M. (2015). *Applying the Rasch model: Fundamental measurement in the human sciences* (3rd ed.). Routledge.

32. Boone, W. J. (2016). Rasch analysis for instrument development: Why, when, and how? *CBE Life Sciences Education*, *15*(4), rm4. https://doi.org/10.1187/cbe.16-04-0148

33. Brier, J. (2006). NANDA/NIC/NOC care plans enhance communication among caregivers and improve measurable outcomes for patients and staff. *International Journal of Nursing Terminologies & Classifications*, *17*(1), 61

34. Brito-Brito, P. R., Fernandez-Gutierrez, D. A., & Smith, H. M. (2016). Case study: Community nursing care plan for a man with functional and psychosocial problems following a stroke. *International Journal of Nursing Knowledge*, *27*(3), 170–174. https://doi.org/10.1111/2047-3095.12084

35. Brito-Brito, P. R., Fernández-Gutiérrez, D. Á., Martínez-Alberto, C. E., Sáez-Rodríguez, M. J., Núñez-Marrero, J., & García-Hernández, A. M. (2021). Use of the Nursing Outcomes Classification (NOC) to measure perceived knowledge about the control of SARS-CoV-2 infection: The impact of a training programme in primary healthcare professionals. *International Journal of Nursing Knowledge*. Advance online publication. https://doi.org/10.1111/2047-3095.12356

36. Brito-Brito, P. R., Martín, G. Á., Oter-Quintana, C., Paloma, C. O., & Romero, S. J. M. (2020). Development and content validation of a NOC-based instrument for measuring dietary knowledge in patients with diabetes: CoNOCidiet–Diabetes. *International Journal of Nursing Knowledge*, *31*(1), 59–73. https://doi.org/10.1111/2047-3095.12243

37. Brito-Brito, P. R., Oter-Quintana, C., Martín-García, Á., Alcolea-Cosín, M. T., Martín-Iglesias, S., & Fernández-Gutiérrez, D. Á. (2014). Case study: Community nursing care plan for an elderly patient with urinary incontinence and social interaction problems after prostatectomy. *International Journal of Nursing Knowledge*, *25*(1), 62–65. https://doi.org/10.1111/2047-3095.12021

38. Brokel, J. M., & Hoffman, F. (2005). Hospice methods to measure and analyze nursing-sensitive patient outcomes. *Journal of Hospice & Palliative Nursing*, *7*(1), 37–44. https://doi.org/10.1097/00129191-200501000-00013

39. Bros, I., & Serra, M. (2006). Application of the NANDA, NOC and NIC standardised languages to a geriatric nursing undergraduate course. *Gerokomos*, *17*(3), 140–143.

40. Burkhart, L., & Androwich, I. (2009). Measuring spiritual care with informatics. *Advances in Nursing Science*, *32*(3), 200–210. https://doi.org/10.1097/ANS.0b013e3181b0d6a6

41. Burkhart, L., Coglianese, M., Kaelin, J., Moorhead, S., & Joyce, L. (2021). Communicating spiritual care in the electronic health record. *CIN: Computers, Informatics, Nursing*, *39*(10), 538–546. https://doi.org/10.1097/CIN.0000000000000707

42. Cachón Pérez, J. M., Alvarez-López, C., & Palacios-Ceña, D. (2012). The meaning of standardized language NANDA-NIC-NOC intensive care nurses in Madrid: A phenomenological approach. *Enfermería Intensiva*, 23(2), 68–76.

43. Caldwell, C. L., Wasson, D., Anderson, M. A., Brighton, V., & Dixon, L. (2005). Development of the Nursing Outcome (NOC) label: Hyperactivity Level. *Journal of Child & Adolescent Psychiatric Nursing*, 18(3), 95–102. https://doi.org/10.1111/j.1744-6171.2005.00004.x

44. Caldwell, C., Wasson, D., Brighton, V., Dixon, L., & Anderson, M. A. (2003). Personal Autonomy: Development of a NOC label. *International Journal of Nursing Terminologies & Classifications*, 14(Suppl. 4), 12–13. https://doi.org/10.1111/j.1744-618x.2003.012_2.x

45. Cardaci, R. (2011). A case study of teen parenting. *International Journal of Nursing Terminologies & Classifications*, 22(1), 40–43. https://doi.org/10.1111/j.1744-618X.2010.01176.x

46. Carrington, J. M. (2012). The usefulness of nursing languages to communicate a clinical event. *CIN: Computers, Informatics, Nursing*, 30(2), 82–88. https://doi.org/10.1097/NCN.0b013e318224b338

47. Castrucci, B., & Auerbach, J. (2019). January 16). Health affairs: Meeting individual social needs falls short of addressing social determinants of health. *Health Affairs Blog*, 10. https://doi.org/10.1377/hblog20190115.234942

48. Cavalcante, A. M. R. Z., Lopes, C. T., Brunori, E. F. R., Swanson, E., Moorhead, S. A., Bachion, M. M., et al. (2018). Self–care behaviors in heart failure. *International Journal of Nursing Knowledge*, 29(3), 146–155. https://doi.org/10.1111/2047-3095.12170

49. Cavalcante, A. M. R. Z., Lopes, C. T., Swanson, E., Moorhead, S. A., Bachion, M. M., & Barros, A. L. (2020). Validation of definitions of the indicators for Nursing Outcomes Classification outcomes: Self-Management cardiac disease. *Acta Paulista de Enfermagem*, 33(1), 1–9. https://doi.org/10.37689/acta-ape/2020AO0265

50. Cavendish, R. (2003). School nurses' use of NANDA, NIC, and NOC to describe children's abdominal pain. *International Journal of Nursing Terminologies & Classifications*, 14(Suppl. 4), 17–18. https://doi.org/10.1111/j.1744-618X.2003.017_2.x

51. Cavendish, R., Lunney, M., Luise, B. K., & Richardson, K. (2001). The Nursing Outcomes Classification: Its relevance to school nursing. *Journal of School Nursing*, 17(4), 189–197. https://doi.org/10.1177/10598405010170040401

52. Celona, C. A. (2015). Measuring acuity and patient progress for youth with special health care needs in transition care utilizing nursing outcomes. *Journal of Pediatric Nursing*, 30(5), e15–e18. https://doi.org/10.1016/j.pedn.2015.05.005

53. Chae, S., Oh, H., & Moorhead, S. (2020). Effectiveness of nursing interventions using standardized nursing terminologies: An integrative review. *Western Journal of Nursing Research*, 42(11), 963–973. https://doi.org/10.1177/0193945919900488

54. Chang, E., & Mostafa, J. (2021). The use of SNOMED CT, 2013-2020: A literature review. *Journal of the American Medical Informatics Association*, 28(9), 2017–2026. https://doi.org/10.1093/jamia/ocab084

55. Chantal Magalhães da Silva, N., de Souza Oliveira, K. A. R., Moorhead, S., Pace, A. E., & Carvalho, E. (2017). Clinical validation of the indicators and definitions of the nursing outcome "Tissue Integrity: Skin and Mucous Membranes" in people with diabetes mellitus. *International Journal of Nursing Knowledge*, 28(4), 165–170. https://doi.org/10.1111/2047-3095.12150

56. Chianca, T. C. M., de Oliveira Salgado, P., Albuquerque, J. P., Campos, C. C., Tannure, M. C., & Ercole, F. F. (2012). Mapping nursing goals of an intensive care unit to the Nursing Outcomes Classification. *Revista Latino-Americana de Enfermagem*, 20(5), 854–862. https://doi.org/10.1590/S0104-11692012000500006

57. Clancy, T. R., Delaney, C. W., Morrison, B., & Gunn, J. K. (2006). The benefits of standardized nursing languages in complex adaptive systems such as hospitals. *JONA: The Journal of Nursing Administration*, 36(9), 426–434. https://doi.org/10.1097/00005110-200609000-00009

58. Clarke, M. (1998). Implementation of nursing standardized languages: NANDA, NIC & NOC. *Online Journal of Nursing Informatics*, 2(2). https://ojni.org/2_2/index.htm

59. Coelho, J. C. F., Ribeiro, A. R. M., Sampaio, F. M. C., Sequeira, C. A. da C., Lleixà Fortuño, M., del, M., et al. (2020). Cultural adaptation and psychometric properties assessment of the NOC outcome "Cognition" in a sample of Portuguese adults with mental illness. *International Journal of Nursing Knowledge*, 31(3), 180–187. https://doi.org/10.1111/2047-3095.12268

60. Conrad, D., Hanson, P. A., Hasenau, S. M., & Stocker-Schneider, J. (2012). Identifying the barriers to use of standardized nursing language in the electronic health record by the ambulatory care nurse practitioner. *Journal of the American Academy of Nurse Practitioners*, 24(7), 443–451. https://doi.org/10.1111/j.1745-7599.2012.00705.x

61. Cook, E. K. (2012). *Nursing Outcomes Classification: A cross-link to assign nursing home recertification survey severity scores* (Publication No. 3567996) [Doctoral dissertation, University of Iowa]. ProQuest Dissertations and Theses Global.

62. Cox, R. A. (2003). Using NANDA, NIC, and NOC with Levine's conservation principles in a nursing home. *International Journal of Nursing Terminologies & Classifications*, 14(Suppl. 4), 41. https://doi.org/10.1111/j.1744-618x.2003.040_2.x

63. da Costa Ferreira, N., Moorhead, S., & Gengo e Silva Butcher, R. de C. (2021). The nurse–patient outcome content validation method. *International Journal of Nursing Knowledge*, 32(2), 88–95. https://doi.org/10.1111/2047-3095.12298

64. da Costa Ferreira, N., Takáo Lopes, C., Moorhead, S., & Gengo e Silva Butcher, R. de C. (2021). Content validation of the nursing outcome Knowledge Heart Failure Management: Brazilian nurses' opinions. *International Journal of Nursing Knowledge*, 32(3), 206–214. https://doi.org/10.1111/2047-3095.12312

65. D'Agostino, F., Barbaranelli, C., Paans, W., Belsito, R., Juarez Vela, R., Alvaro, R., et al. (2017). Psychometric evaluation of the D-Catch, an instrument to measure the accuracy of nursing documentation. *International Journal of Nursing Knowledge*, 28(3), 145–152. https://doi.org/10.1111/2047-3095.12125

66. D'Agostino, F., Zeffiro, V., Vellone, E., Ausili, D., Belsito, R., Leto, A., et al. (2020). Cross-mapping of nursing care terms recorded in Italian hospitals into the standardized NNN terminology. *International Journal of Nursing Knowledge*, 31(1), 4–13. https://doi.org/10.1111/2047-3095.12200

67. da Silva, L. F. M., Pascoal, L. M., Nunes, S. F. L., de Sousa Freire, V. E. C., de Araújo Almeida, A. G., Gontijo, P. V. C., et al. (2019). Ineffective airway clearance in surgical patients: Evaluation of nursing interventions and outcomes. *International Journal of Nursing Knowledge*, 30(4), 251–256. https://doi.org/10.1111/2047-3095.12242

68. da Silva, M. B., Almeida, M. de A., Panato, B. P., de Siqueira, A. P. O., da Silva, M. P., & Reisderfer, L. (2015). Clinical applicability of nursing outcomes in the evolution of orthopedic patients with impaired physical mobility. *Revista Latino-Americana de Enfermagem, 23*, 51–58. https://doi.org/10.1590/0104-1169.3526.2524

69. da Silva, M. B., Barreto, L. N. M., Panato, B. P., Engelman, B., Figueiredo, M. S., Rodríguez, A. A. L., et al. (2019). Clinical indicators for evaluation of outcomes of impaired tissue integrity in orthopedic patients: Consensus study. *International Journal of Nursing Knowledge, 30*(2), 81–86. https://doi.org/10.1111/2047-3095.12204

70. da Silva, N. C. M., de Souza Oliveira, A. R., & de Carvalho, E. C. (2015). Knowledge produced from the outcomes of the "Nursing Outcomes Classification - NOC": Integrative review. *Revista Gaucha de Enfermagem, 36*(4), 104–111. https://doi.org/10.1590/1983-1447.2015.04.53339

71. da Silva, R. N., Brandão, M. A. G., & Ferreira, M. de A. (2020). Integrative review as a method or to test nursing theory. *Nursing Science Quarterly, 33*(3), 258–263. https://doi.org/10.1177/0894318420920602

72. da Silva, V. M., de Oliveira Lopes, M. V., de Araujo, T. L., Beltrao, B. A., Monteiro, F. P. M., Cavalcante, T. F., et al. (2011). Operational definitions of outcome indicators related to ineffective breathing patterns in children with congenital heart disease. *Heart & Lung, 40*(3), e70–e77. https://doi.org/10.1016/j.hrtlng.2010.12.002

73. Daly, J. M., Maas, M., & Buckwalter, K. (1995). Use of standardized nursing diagnoses and interventions in long-term care. *Journal of Gerontological Nursing, 21*(8), 29–36. https://doi.org/10.3928/0098-9134-19950801-09

74. Daly, J. M., Maas, M. L., & Johnson, M. (1997). Nursing Outcomes Classification: An essential element in data sets for nursing and health care effectiveness. *Computers in Nursing, 15*(Suppl. 2), S82–S86.

75. de Araújo Ferreira, J. K., Costa Pessoa, N. R., Pereira Pôrto, N., Mendes Santos, L. N., de Carvalho Lira, A. L. B., & de Queiroz Frazão, C. M. F. (2018). Knowledge: Disease Process in patients undergoing hemodialysis. *Investigacion & Educacion En Enfermeria, 36*(2), 26–35. https://doi.org/10.17533/udea.iee.v36n2e04

76. de Carvalho, E. C., Eduardo, A. H. A., Romanzini, A., Simão, T. P., Zamarioli, C. M., Garbuio, D. C., et al. (2018). Correspondence between NANDA international nursing diagnoses and outcomes as proposed by the Nursing Outcomes Classification. *International Journal of Nursing Knowledge, 29*(1), 66–78. https://doi.org/10.1111/2047-3095.12135

77. de Fátima Lucena, A., Holsbach, I., Pruinelli, L., Serdotte Freitas Cardoso, A., & Schroeder Mello, B. (2013). Brazilian validation of the nursing outcomes for acute pain. *International Journal of Nursing Knowledge, 24*(1), 54–58. https://doi.org/10.1111/j.2047-3095.2012.01230.x

78. de Freitas Luzia, M., Argenta, C., de Abreu Almeida, M., & de Fátima Lucena, A. (2018). Conceptual definitions of indicators for the nursing outcome "Knowledge: Fall Prevention". *Revista Brasileira de Enfermagem, 71*(2), 431–439. https://doi.org/10.1590/0034-7167-2016-0686

79. de Freitas Luzia, M., Vidor, I. D., da Silva, A. C. F. E., & de Fátima Lucena, A. (2020). Fall prevention in hospitalized patients: Evaluation through the Nursing Outcomes Classification/NOC. *Applied Nursing Research, 54*, 151273. https://doi.org/10.1016/j.apnr.2020.151273

80. de Groot, K., Triemstra, M., Paans, W., & Francke, A. L. (2019). Quality criteria, instruments, and requirements for nursing documentation: A systematic review of systematic reviews. *Journal of Advanced Nursing, 75*(7), 1379–1393. https://doi.org/10.1111/jan.13919

81. de Lima, L. B., e Cardozo, M. C., Bernardes, D. de S., & Rabelo-Silva, E. R. (2019). Nursing outcomes for patients with risk of perioperative positioning injury. *International Journal of Nursing Knowledge, 30*(2), 114–119. https://doi.org/10.1111/2047-3095.12209

82. de Lima Lopes, J., de Barros, A. L. B. L., & Michel, J. L. M. (2009). A pilot study to validate the priority Nursing Interventions Classification interventions and Nursing Outcomes Classification outcomes for the nursing diagnosis "excess fluid volume" in cardiac patients. *International Journal of Nursing Terminologies & Classifications, 20*(2), 76–88. https://doi.org/10.1111/j.1744-618X.2009.01118.x

83. de Sousa Costa, A. G., Leite de Araujo, T., Frota Cavalcante, T., Oliveira Lopes, M. V., de Souza Oliveira-Kumakura, A. R., & Chaves Costa, F. B. (2017). Clinical validation of the nursing outcome Fall Prevention Behavior in people with stroke. *Applied Nursing Research, 33*, 67–71. https://doi.org/10.1016/j.apnr.2016.10.003

84. de Souza Oliveira-Kumakura, A. R., Alonso, J. B., & Campos de Carvalho, E. (2019). Psychometric assessment of the nursing outcome Swallowing Status: Rasch model approach. *International Journal of Nursing Knowledge, 30*(4), 197–202. https://doi.org/10.1111%2F2047-3095.12229

85. de Souza Oliveira-Kumakura, A. R., Caldeira, S., Prado Simão, T., Camargo, F. F. A., de Almeida Lopes Monteiro da Cruz, D., & Campos de Carvalho, E. (2018). The contribution of the Rasch Model to the clinical validation of nursing diagnoses: Integrative literature review. *International Journal of Nursing Knowledge, 29*(2), 89–96. https://doi.org/10.1111/2047-3095.12162

86. Demmer, K. (2003). NOC Implementation and testing in a cardiac surgery ICU. *International Journal of Nursing Terminologies & Classifications, 14*(Suppl. 4), 13–14. https://doi.org/10.1111/j.1744-618X.2003.012_3.x

87. Demmer, K. A., McKane, C., Griebenow, L., Behrenbeck, J., & Timm, J. (2004). Nursing-sensitive outcome implementation and reliability testing in two cardiac surgery intensive care units. *Online Journal of Nursing Informatics, 8*(3), 6.

88. Denehy, J. (1998). Integrating Nursing Outcomes Classification in nursing education. *Journal of Nursing Care Quality, 12*(5), 73–84. https://doi.org/10.1097/00001786-199806000-00011

89. Devesa, A. M., Moreno, I. M., Bermejo Higuera, J. C., & González Serna, J. M. G. (2014). Nursing care and spiritual suffering. *Index de Enfermería, 23*(3), 153–156. https://doi.org/10.4321/S1132-12962014000200008

90. Dias Emidio, S. C., Barbosa Dias, F. de S., Moorhead, S., Deberg, J., de Souza Oliveira-Kumakura, A. R., & Valentim Carmona, E. (2020). Conceptual and operational definition of nursing outcomes regarding the breastfeeding establishment. *Revista Latino-Americana de Enfermagem (RLAE), 28*, 1–12. https://doi.org/10.1590/1518-8345.3007.3259

91. Dias Emidio, S. C., Moorhead, S., Oliveira, H. C., Herdman, T. H., Oliveira, K. A. R. de S., & Carmona, E. V. (2020). Validation of nursing outcomes related to breastfeeding establishment. *International Journal of Nursing Knowledge, 31*(2), 134–144. https://doi.org/10.1111/2047-3095.12256

92. Dochterman, J. C., & Jones, D. A. (2003). *Unifying nursing languages: The harmonization of NANDA. NIC and NOC.* American Nurses Association.

93. Escalada-Hernández, P., Muñoz-Hermoso, P., González-Fraile, E., Santos, B., González-Vargas, J. A., Feria-

Raposo, I., et al. (2015). A retrospective study of nursing diagnoses, outcomes, and interventions for patients with mental disorders. *Applied Nursing Research*, 28(2), 92–98. https://doi.org/10.1016/j.apnr.2014.05.006

94. Eun, K., & Hyang-Sook, S. (2013). Construction and application of nursing information system using NANDA-NOC-NIC linkage in medical-surgical nursing units. *Korean Journal of Adult Nursing*, 25(4), 365–376. https://doi.org/10.7475/kjan.2013.25.4.365

95. Farren, A. T. (2009). An oncology case study demonstrating the use of Rogers's Science of Unitary Human Beings and standardized nursing languages. *International Journal of Nursing Terminologies & Classifications*, 20(1), 34–39. https://doi.org/10.1111/j.1744-618X.2008.01111

96. Fehring, R. J. (1987). Methods to validate nursing diagnoses. *Heart & Lung*, 16(6), 625–629.

97. Fennelly, O., Grogan, L., Reed, A., & Hardiker, N. R. (2021). Use of standardized terminologies in clinical practice: A scoping review. *International Journal of Medical Informatics*, 149, 104431. https://doi.org/10.1016/j.ijmedinf.2021.104431

98. Festen, S., van Twisk, Y. Z., van Munster, B. C., & de Graeff, P. (2021). What matters to you? Health outcome prioritization in treatment decision-making for older patients. *Age & Ageing*, 50(6), 2264–2269. https://doi.org/10.1093/ageing/afab160

99. Finesilver, C. (2003). Use of standardized language in neuroscience nursing. *International Journal of Nursing Terminologies & Classifications*, 14(Suppl. 4), 52. https://doi.org/10.1111/j.1744-618x.2003.051_2x

100. Finesilver, C., & Metzler, D. (2003). Use of NANDA, NIC, and NOC in a baccalaureate curriculum. *International Journal of Nursing Terminologies & Classifications*, 14(Suppl. 4), 34–35. https://doi.org/10.1111/j.1744-618x.2003.032_5.x

101. Fink-Samnick, E. (2021). The social determinants of mental health. Definitions, distinctions, and dimensions for professional case management: Part 1. *Professional Case Management*, 26(3), 121–137. https://doi.org/10.1097/NCM.0000000000000497

102. Fischetti, N. (2008). Using standardized nursing languages: A case study exemplar on management of diabetes mellitus. *International Journal of Nursing Terminologies & Classifications*, 19(4), 163–166. https://doi.org/10.1111/j.1744-618x.2008.00105.x

103. Flanagan, J. (2021). From concepts and systematic reviews: A path to enhancing nursing knowledge development. *International Journal of Nursing Knowledge*, 32(3), 217. https://doi.org/10.1111/2047-3095.12353

104. Flanagan, J., & Weir, H. D. (2016). NANDA-I NIC and NOC, the EHR, and meaningful use. *International Journal of Nursing Knowledge*, 27(4), 183. https://doi.org/10.1111/2047-3095.12156

105. Frederick, J., Scherb, C. A., Smith-Foreman, K., Wit, T. S., Quiram, J., Wagenaar, J., et al. (2001). Speaking a common language: Standardized nursing languages have increased the visibility of nursing practice at three facilities. *AJN: American Journal of Nursing*, 101(3), 2400–TT https://doi.org/10.1097/00000446-200103000-00032

106. Frederick, J., & Watters, M. (2003). Integrating nursing acuity, NANDA, NIC, and NOC into an automated nursing documentation system. *International Journal of Nursing Terminologies & Classifications*, 14(Suppl. 4), 26. https://doi.org/10.1111/j.1744-618x.2003.023_5.x

107. Frigstad, V., & von Krogh, G. (2006). Training nursing students in NANDA, NIC, and NOC terminology using a software program. *International Journal of Nursing Terminologies & Classifications*, 17(1), 70–71. https://doi.org/10.1111/2047-3095.12326

108. García-Garcés, L., & Bellver Capella, V. (2021). Advance-care planning implementation through the nursing process. *Nursing Science Quarterly*, 34(4), 440–447. https://doi.org/10.1177/08943184211031576

109. Garutti Rodrigues, F., Andrade dos Santos, F., & Bottura Leite de Barros, A. L. (2006). NIC interventions and NOC outcomes in patients with activity intolerance. *International Journal of Nursing Terminologies & Classifications*, 17(1), 79. https://doi.org/10.1111/j.1744-618X.2011.01184.x

110. Gencbas, D., Bebis, H., & Cicek, H. (2018). Evaluation of the efficiency of the nursing care plan applied using NANDA, NOC, and NIC linkages to elderly women with incontinence living in a nursing home: A randomized controlled study. *International Journal of Nursing Knowledge*, 29(4), 217–226. https://doi.org/10.1111/2047-3095.12180

111. Gengo e Silva Butcher, R. de C., & Jones, D. A. (2021). An integrative review of comprehensive nursing assessment tools developed based on Gordon's Eleven Functional Health Patterns. *International Journal of Nursing Knowledge*, 32(4), 294–307. https://doi.org/10.1111/2047-3095.12321

112. Gengo e Silva, R. de C., dos Santos Diogo, R. C., da Cruz, D. de A. L. M., Ortiz, D., Ortiz, D., Peres, H. H. C., et al. (2018). Linkages of nursing diagnoses, outcomes, and interventions performed by nurses caring for medical and surgical patients using a decision support system. *International Journal of Nursing Knowledge*, 29(4), 269–275. https://doi.org/10.1111/2047-3095.12185

113. Gloskey, D., Kravutske, M. E., & Zugcic, M. (2006). Do you need to educate RNs on how to document using the Nursing Outcome Classification? *International Journal of Nursing Terminologies & Classifications*, 17(1), 34–35.

114. Gomes, G. L. L., de Oliveira, F. M. R. L., Leal, N. P. da R., Guimarães, K. S. L., Silva, D. F. da, & Barbosa, K. T. F. (2021). Nursing diagnoses/outcomes and interventions for patients with COVID-19: A retrospective documentary study. *Online Brazilian Journal of Nursing*, 20, 16–27. https://doi.org/10.17665/1676-4285.20216512

115. Gómez De Segura Navarro, C., Esain Larrambe, A., Tina Majuelo, P., Guembe Ibañez, I., Fernández Perea, L., & Narvaiza Solis, M. J. (2006). Interrelationship among NANDA, NOC and NIC: A pilot study and an evaluation of a nursing document. *Revista de Enfermeria (Barcelona, Spain)*, 29(7-8), 21–26.

116. González Aguña, A., Fernández Batalla, M., Díaz-Tendero Rodríguez, J., Sarrión Bravo, J. A., Gonzalo de Diego, B., & Santamaría García, J. M. (2021). Validation of a manual of care plans for people hospitalized with COVID-19. *Nursing Open*, 8, 3495–3515. https://doi.org/10.1002/nop2.900

117. Gordon, M. (1994). *Nursing diagnosis: Process and application* (3rd ed.). McGraw-Hill.

118. Gordon, M. (2011). *Manual of nursing diagnosis* (12th ed.). Jones & Bartlett Learning.

119. Grey, M., Knafl, K., & McCorkle, R. (2006). A framework for the study of self- and family management of chronic conditions. *Nursing Outlook*, 54(5), 278–286. https://doi.org/10.1016/j.outlook.2006.06.004

120. Grey, M., Schulman-Green, D., Knafl, K., & Reynolds, N. R. (2015). A revised Self- and Family Management Framework. *Nursing Outlook*, 63(2), 162–170. https://doi.org/10.1016/j.outlook.2014.10.003

121. Gudmundsdottir, E., Delaney, C., Thoroddsen, A., & Karlsson, T. (2004). Translation and validation of the Nursing Outcomes Classification labels and definitions for acute care nursing in Iceland. *Journal of Advanced Nursing*, 46(3), 292–302. https://doi.org/10.1111/j.1365-2648.2004.02989.x

122. Hajewski, C., Maupin, J. M., Rapp, D. A., Sitterding, M., & Pappas, J. (1998). Implementation and evaluation of Nursing Interventions Classification and Nursing Outcomes Classification in a patient education plan. *Journal of Nursing Care Quality, 12*(5), 30–40. https://doi.org/10.1097/00001786-199806000-00007

123. Hansen, F., Berntsen, G. K. R., & Salamonsen, A. (2018). "What matters to you?" A longitudinal qualitative study of Norwegian patients' perspectives on their pathways with colorectal cancer. *International Journal of Qualitative Studies on Health and Wellbeing, 13*(1), 1548240. https://doi.org/10.1080/17482631.2018.1548240

124. Hariyati, R. T. S., Yani, A., Eryando, T., Hasibuan, Z., & Milanti, A. (2016). The effectiveness and efficiency of nursing care documentation using the SIMPRO Model. *International Journal of Nursing Knowledge, 27*(3), 136–142. https://doi.org/10.1111/2047-3095.12086

125. Head, B. J. (1997). *Validation of nursing-sensitive outcomes for rural and urban community elderly* (Publication No. 9819945) [Doctoral dissertation, University of Iowa]. ProQuest Dissertations and Theses Global.

126. Head, B. J., Aquilino, M. L., Johnson, M., Reed, D., Maas, M., & Moorhead, S. (2004). Content validity and nursing sensitivity of community-level outcomes from the Nursing Outcomes Classification (NOC). *Image: Journal of Nursing Scholarship, 36*(3), 251–259. https://doi.org/10.1111/j.1547-5069.2004.04046.x

127. Head, B. J., Maas, M., & Johnson, M. (2003). Validity and community-health-nursing sensitivity of six outcomes for community health nursing with older clients. *Public Health Nursing, 20*(5), 385–398. https://doi.org/10.1046/j.1525-1446.2003.20507.x

128. Head, B. J., Scherb, C. A., Maas, M. L., Swanson, E. A., Moorhead, S., Reed, D., et al. (2011). Nursing clinical documentation data retrieval for hospitalized older adults with heart failure: Part 2. *International Journal of Nursing Terminologies & Classifications, 22*(2), 68–76. https://doi.org/10.1111/j.1744-618X.2010.01177.x

129. Head, B. J., Scherb, C. A., Reed, D., Conley, D. M., Weinberg, B., Kozel, M., et al. (2011). Nursing diagnoses, interventions, and patient outcomes for hospitalized older adults with pneumonia. *Research in Gerontological Nursing, 4*(2), 95–105. https://doi.org/10.3928/19404921-20100601-99

130. Hendrix, S. E. (2009). An experience with implementation of NIC and NOC in a clinical information system. *CIN: Computers, Informatics, Nursing, 27*(1), 7–11. https://doi.org/10.1097/NCN.0b013e31818d498c

131. Herdman, T. H., Kamitsuru, S., & Takáo Lopes, C. (2021). *NANDA International nursing diagnoses: Definitions and classification 2021–2023* (12th ed.). Thieme.

132. Hou, S., Li, B., Luo, Y., & Shang, S. (2019). Creation and location-specific revision of a core nursing outcomes evaluation system based on Nursing Outcomes Classification for stroke inpatients in China. *International Journal of Nursing Knowledge, 30*(3), 154–161. https://doi.org/10.1111/2047-3095.12222

133. Hou, S., Zhang, H., Li, B., Luo, Y., Han, Z., & Shang, S. (2020). Validation and evaluation of the core nursing outcomes evaluation system for inpatients with stroke. *International Journal of Nursing Knowledge, 31*(3), 173–179. https://doi.org/10.1111/2047-3095.12259

134. Hughes, R. (2003). The use of NANDA, NIC, and NOC in the identification and measurement of problems, interventions, and outcomes in spinal cord injury. *International Journal of Nursing Terminologies & Classifications, 14*(Suppl. 4), 18–19. https://doi.org/10.1111/j.1744-618x.2003.017_3.x

135. *International classification of functioning, disability, and health (ICF).* (2001). World Health Organization.

136. Iowa Intervention Project. (1996). *Nursing interventions classification (NIC)* (2nd ed.). Mosby-Year Book.

137. Iowa Outcomes Project, Johnson, M. & Maas, M. (Eds.). (1997). *Nursing outcomes classification (NOC)*. Mosby-Yearbook.

138. Iowa Outcomes Project, Johnson, M., Maas, M. & Moorhead, S. (Eds.). (2000). *Nursing outcomes classification (NOC)* (2nd ed.). Mosby.

139. Jennewein, C. (2006). Development/implementation of NNN-language care plans in an electronic medical record for a behavioral health population. *International Journal of Nursing Terminologies & Classifications, 17*(1), 72.

140. Johnson, J., Lodhi, M. K., Cheema, U., Stifter, J., Dunn Lopez, K., Yingwei, Y., et al. (2017). Outcomes for end-of-life patients with anticipatory grieving: Insights from practice with standardized nursing terminologies within an interoperable internet-based electronic health record. *Journal of Hospice & Palliative Nursing, 19*(3), 223–231. https://doi.org/10.1097/NJH.0000000000000333

141. Johnson, M. (1998). Overview of the Nursing Outcomes Classification (NOC). *Online Journal of Nursing Informatics, 2*(2). https://ojni.org/2_2/index.htm

142. Johnson, M., Bulechek, G., Dochterman, J. M., Maas, M., & Moorhead, S. (Eds.). (2001). *Nursing diagnoses, outcomes, and interventions: NANDA, NOC, & NIC linkages.* Mosby.

143. Johnson, M., Bulechek, G., Dochterman, J. M., Maas, M., Moorhead, S., & Swanson, E. (Eds.). (2006). *NANDA, NOC, & NIC linkages: Nursing diagnoses, outcomes, and interventions* (2nd ed.). Mosby.

144. Johnson, M., & Maas, M. (1994). *Nursing focused patient outcomes:* Challenges for the nineties. In J. McCloskey & H. Grace (Eds.), *Current issues in nursing* (4th ed., pp. 643–649). Mosby.

145. Johnson, M., & Maas, M. (1998). Implementing the Nursing Outcomes Classification in a practice setting. *Outcomes Management for Nursing Practice, 2*(3), 99–104.

146. Johnson, M., & Maas, M. (1998). The Nursing Outcomes Classification. *Journal of Nursing Care Quality, 12*(5), 9–87. https://doi.org/10.1097/00001786-199806000-00005

147. Johnson, M., Moorhead, S., Bulechek, G., Butcher, H., Maas, M., & Swanson, E. (Eds.). (2012). *NOC, and NIC linkages to NANDA-I and clinical conditions: Supporting critical reasoning and quality care* (3rd ed.). Elsevier Mosby.

148. Johnson, M., Moorhead, S., Maas, M., & Reed, D. (2003). Evaluation of the sensitivity and use of the Nursing Outcomes Classification. *Journal of Nursing Measurement, 11*(2), 119–134. https://doi.org/10.1891/jnum.11.2.119.57282

149. Jones, D., Lunney, M., Keenan, G., & Moorhead, S. (2010). Standardized nursing languages essential for the nursing workforce. *Annual Review of Nursing Research, 28*(1), 253–294. https://doi.org/10.1891/0739-6686.28.253

150. Karaca, T., & Aslan, S. (2018). Effect of 'nursing terminologies and classifications' course on nursing students' perception of nursing diagnosis. *Nurse Education Today, 67,* 114–117. https://doi.org/10.1016/j.nedt.2018.05.011

151. Kautz, D. D., Kuiper, R., Pesut, D. J., & Williams, R. L. (2006). Using NANDA, NIC, and NOC (NNN) language for clinical reasoning with the Outcome-Present State-Test (OPT) Model. *International Journal of Nursing Terminologies & Classifications, 17*(3), 129–138. https://doi.org/10.1111/j.1744-618X.2006.00033.x

152. Kautz, D. D., & Van Horn, E. R. (2008). An exemplar of the use of NNN language in developing evidence-based practice guidelines. *International Journal of Nursing Terminologies & Classifications, 19*(1), 14–19. https://doi.org/10.1111/j.1744-618x.2007.00074.x

153. Keenan, G. M., & Aquilino, M. (1998). Standardized nomenclatures: Key to continuity of care, nursing accountability, and nursing effectiveness. *Outcomes Management for Nursing, 2*(2), 81–86.

154. Keenan, G. M., Barkauskas, V., Stocker, J., Johnson, M., Maas, M., Moorhead, S., et al. (2003). Establishing the validity, reliability, and sensitivity of NOC in an adult care nurse practitioner setting. *Outcomes Management, 7*(2), 74–83.

155. Keenan, G. M., Falan, S., Heath, C., & Treder, M. (2003). Establishing competency in the use of North American Nursing Diagnosis Association, Nursing Outcomes Classification, and Nursing Interventions Classification terminology. *Journal of Nursing Measurement, 11*(2), 183–198. https://doi.org/10.1891/jnum.11.2.183.57286

156. Keenan, G. M., Lopez, K. D., Sousa, V. E. C., Stifter, J., Macieira, T. G. R., Yao, Y., et al. (2018). A shovel–ready solution to fill the nursing data gap in the interdisciplinary clinical picture. *International Journal of Nursing Knowledge, 29*(1), 49–58. https://doi.org/10.1111/2047-3095.12168

157. Keenan, G. M., Stocker, J., Barkauskas, V., Johnson, M., Maas, M., Moorhead, S., et al. (2003). Assessing the reliability, validity, and sensitivity of nursing outcomes classification in home care settings. *Journal of Nursing Measurement, 11*(2), 135–155. https://doi.org/10.1891/jnum.11.2.135.57285

158. Keenan, G. M., Stocker, J., Barkauskas, V., Treder, M., & Heath, C. (2003a). Toward collecting a standardized nursing data set across the continuum: Case of adult care nurse practitioner setting. *Outcomes Management, 7*(3), 113–120.

159. Keenan, G. M., Stocker, J., Barkauskas, V., Treder, M., & Heath, C. (2003b). Toward integrating a common nursing data set in home care to facilitate monitoring outcomes across settings. *Journal of Nursing Measurement, 11*(2), 157–169. https://doi.org/10.1891/jnum.11.2.157.57288

160. Keenan, G. M., Stocker, J. R., Geo-Thomas, A. T., Soparkar, N. R., Barkauskas, V. H., & Lee, J. L. (2002). The HANDS project: Studying and refining the automated collection of a cross-setting clinical data set. *CIN: Computers, Informatics, Nursing, 20*(3), 89–100. https://doi.org/10.1097/00024665-200205000-00008

161. Keenan, G. M., Tschannen, D., & Wesley, M. (2008). Standardized nursing terminologies can transform practice. *JONA: The Journal of Nursing Administration, 38*(3), 103–106. https://doi.org/10.1097/01.NNA.0000310728.50913.de

162. Keenan, G. M., Yakel, E., Tschannen, D., & Mandeville, M. (2008). Documentation and the nurse care planning process. In R. G. Hughes (Ed.), *Patient safety and quality: An evidence-based handbook for nurses* (pp. 3-175–3-206). Agency for Healthcare Research and Quality (U.S.).

163. Killeen, M. B. (2003). Use of NANDA, NIC, and NOC as a framework for cyclic perimenstrual pain and discomfort. *International Journal of Nursing Terminologies & Classifications, 14*(S4), 19–20. https://doi.org/10.1111/j.1744-618X.2003.017_5.x

164. Kim, J., Macieira, T., Meyer, S. L., Ansell Maggie, M., Bjarnadottir Raga, R. I., Smith, M. B., et al. (2020). Towards implementing SNOMED CT in nursing practice: A scoping review. *International Journal of Medical Informatics, 134*, 104035. https://doi.org/10.1016/j.ijmedinf.2019.104035

165. Klehr, J., Hafner, J., Spelz, L. M., Steen, S., & Weaver, K. (2009). Implementation of standardized nomenclature

in the electronic medical record. *International Journal of Nursing Terminologies & Classifications, 20*(4), 169–180. https://doi.org/10.1111/j.1744-618X.2009.01132.x

166. Kotowski, A. (2012). Case study: A young male with auditory hallucinations in paranoid schizophrenia. *International Journal of Nursing Knowledge, 23*(1), 41–44. https://doi.org/10.1111/j.2047-3095.2011.01197.x

167. Kravutske, M. E., Zugcic, M., Gloskey, D., & Reed, D. (2006). Initial results from using NOCs in an acute care setting. *International Journal of Nursing Terminologies & Classifications, 17*(1), 93.

168. Kuehnert, P., Fawcett, J., DePriest, K., Chinn, P., Cousin, L., Ervin, N., et al. (2022). Defining the social determinants of health for nursing action to achieve health equity: A consensus paper from the American Academy of Nursing. *Nursing Outlook, 70*(1), 10–27. https://doi.org/10.1016/j.outlook.2021.08.003

169. Kuiper, R., Pesut, D. J., & Arms, T. E. (2016). *Clinical reasoning and care coordination in advance practice nursing.* Springer.

170. Kuiper, R., Pesut, D., & Kautz, D. (2009). Promoting the self-regulation of clinical reasoning skills in nursing students. *Open Nursing, 3,* 76–85. https://doi.org/10.2174/18744346000903010076

171. Kumar, C. P. (2007). Application of Orem's Self-Care Deficit Theory and standardized nursing languages in a case study of a woman with diabetes. *International Journal of Nursing Terminologies & Classifications, 18*(3), 103–110. https://doi.org/10.1111/j.1744-618x.2007.00058.x

172. Lee, E. (2006a). Analysis of nursing diagnoses and outcomes used in a respiratory unit in Korea. *International Journal of Nursing Terminologies & Classifications, 17*(1), 42.

173. Lee, E. (2006b). Analysis of Nursing Outcomes Classification (NOC) used in neurosurgical units in Korea. *International Journal of Nursing Terminologies & Classifications, 17*(1), 73–74.

174. Lee, E. (2019). Use of the Nursing Outcomes Classification for falls and fall prevention by nurses in South Korea. *International Journal of Nursing Knowledge, 30*(1), 28–33. https://doi.org/10.1111/2047-3095.12201

175. Lee, E., & Choi, S. (2011). Identification of nursing diagnosis-outcome-intervention (NANDA-NOC-NIC) linkages in surgical nursing unit. *Korean Journal of Adult Nursing, 23*(2), 180–188.

176. Lee, E., & Noh, H. K. (2016). The effects of a web-based nursing process documentation program on stress and anxiety of nursing students in South Korea. *International Journal of Nursing Knowledge, 27*(1), 35–42. https://doi.org/10.1111/2047-3095.12072

177. Lee, E., Park, H., Whyte, J., Kim, Y., & Park, S. Y. (2014). Identifying core nursing sensitive outcomes associated with the most frequently used North American Nursing Diagnosis Association- International nursing diagnoses for patients with cerebrovascular disease in Korea. *International Journal of Nursing Practice, 20*(6), 636–645. https://doi.org/10.1111/ijn.12224

178. Linch, G. F., da, C., Rabelo-Silva, E. R., Keenan, G. M., Moraes, M. A., Stifter, J., et al. (2015). Validation of the Quality of Diagnoses, Interventions, and Outcomes (Q-DIO) Instrument for use in Brazil and the United States. *International Journal of Nursing Knowledge, 26*(1), 19–25. https://doi.org/10.1111/2047-3095.12030

179. Lu, D., Park, H., Ucharattana, P., Konicek, D., & Delaney, C. (2007). Nursing Outcomes Classification in the systematized nomenclature of medicine clinical terms: A cross-mapping validation. *CIN: Computers, Informatics, Nursing, 25*(3), 159–170. https://doi.org/10.1097/01.NCN.0000270042.22164.21

180. Lucena, A. de F., Argenta, C., Almeida, M. de A., Moorhead, S., & Swanson, E. (2019). Validation of nursing outcomes and interventions to older adults care with risk or frail elderly syndrome: Proposal of linkages among NOC, NIC, and NANDA–I to clinical practice. *International Journal of Nursing Knowledge, 30*(3), 147–153. https://doi.org/10.1111/2047-3095.12225

181. Lucena, A. de F., Argenta, C., Luzia, M. F., Almeida, M. A., Barreto, L. N. M., & Swanson, E. (2020). Multidimensional model of successful aging and nursing terminologies: Similarities for use in the clinical practice. *Revista Gaúcha de Enfermagem, 41*, e20190148. https://doi.org/10.1590/1983-1447.2020.20190148

182. Lucena, A. de F., & Barros, A. L. B. L. (2005). Cross-mapping: An alternative to data analysis in nursing. *Acta Paulista Enfermeria, 18*(1), 82–88. https://doi.org/10.1590/S0103-21002005000100011

183. Lundberg, C., Brokel, J. M., Bulechek, G. M., Butcher, H. K., Martin, K. S., Moorhead, S., et al. (2008). Selecting a standardized terminology for the electronic health record that reveals the impact of nursing on patient care. *Online Journal of Nursing Informatics, 12*(2), 19.

184. Lunney, M. (2006a). Helping nurses use NANDA, NOC, and NIC: Novice to expert. *Nurse Educator, 31*(1), 40–46. https://doi.org/10.1097/00006223-200601000-00011

185. Lunney, M. (2006b). NANDA diagnoses, NIC interventions, and NOC outcomes used in an electronic health record with elementary school children. *Journal of School Nursing, 22*(2), 94–101. https://doi.org/10.1177/105984050602200206

186. Lunney, M. (2006c). Staff development. Helping nurses use NANDA, NOC, and NIC: Novice to expert. *JONA: The Journal of Nursing Administration, 36*(3), 118–125. https://doi.org/10.1097/00005110-200603000-00004

187. Lunney, M., Caffrey, P. M., & Umbro, J. (2013). Participant action research with staff nurses in end-of-life care. *Journal of Hospice & Palliative Nursing, 15*(3), 156–162. https://doi.org/10.1097/NJH.0b013e3182735d48

188. Lunney, M., Delaney, C., Duffy, M., Moorhead, S., & Welton, J. (2005). Technology. Advocating for standardized nursing languages in electronic health records. *JONA: The Journal of Nursing Administration, 35*(1), 1–3. https://doi.org/10.1097/00005110-200501000-00001

189. Lunney, M., & Parker, L. (2003). Effects of using NANDA, NIC, and NOC on health outcomes of school children: A pilot study. *International Journal of Nursing Terminologies & Classifications, 14*(Suppl. 4), 21. https://doi.org/10.1111/j.1744-618x.2003.017_7.x

190. Lunney, M., McGuire, M., Endozo, N., & Mclutsh-Waddy, D. (2010). Consensus validation study identifies relevant nursing diagnoses, nursing interventions, and health outcomes for people with traumatic brain injuries. *Rehabilitation Nursing, 35*(4), 161–166. https://doi.org/10.1002/j.2048-7940.2010.tb00042.x

191. Lunney, M., Parker, L., Fiore, L., Cavendish, R., & Pulcini, J. (2004). Feasibility of studying the effects of using NANDA, NIC, and NOC on nurses' power and children's outcomes. *CIN: Computers, Informatics, Nursing, 22*(6), 316–325. https://doi.org/10.1097/00024665-200411000-00006

192. Maas, M. L., & Delaney, C. (2004). Nursing process outcome linkage research: Issues, current status, and health policy implications. *Medical Care, 42*(2), 11–40. https://doi.org/10.1097/01.mlr.0000109291.44014.cb

193. Maas, M. L., Johnson, M., & Moorhead, S. (1996). Classifying nursing–sensitive patient outcomes. *Image: The Journal of Nursing Scholarship, 28*(4), 295–302. https://doi.org/10.1111/j.1547-5069.1996.tb00377.x

194. Maas, M. L., Johnson, M., Moorhead, S., Reed, D., & Sweeney, S. (2003). Evaluation of the reliability and validity of Nursing Outcomes Classification patient outcomes and measures. *Journal of Nursing Measurement, 11*(2), 97–117. https://doi.org/10.1891/jnum.11.2.97.57284

195. Maas, M. L., Reed, D., Reeder, K. M., Kerr, P., Specht, J., & Johnson, M. (2002). Nursing outcomes classification: A preliminary report of field testing. *Outcomes Management, 6*(3), 112–119.

196. Macieira, T. G. R., Chianca, T. C. M., Smith, M. B., Yao, Y., Bian, J., Wilkie, D. J., et al. (2019). Secondary use of standardized nursing care data for advancing nursing science and practice: A systematic review. *Journal of the American Medical Informatics Association, 26*(11), 1401–1411. https://doi.org/10.1093/jamia/ocz086

197. Macnee, C. L., Edwards, J., Kaplan, A., Reed, S., Bradford, S., Walls, J., et al. (2006). Evaluation of NOC standardized outcome of "health seeking behavior" in nurse-managed clinics. *Journal of Nursing Care Quality, 21*(3), 242–247. https://doi.org/10.1097/00001786-200607000-00009

198. McCloskey, J., & Bulechek, G. (1994). Standardizing the language for nursing treatments: An overview of the issues. *Nursing Outlook, 42*(2), 56–63. https://doi.org/10.1016/s0029-6554(06)80022-9

199. Mello, B. S., Almeida, M. A., Pruinelli, L., & Lucena, A. F. (2019). Nursing outcomes for pain assessment of patients undergoing palliative care. *Reben-Revista Brasileira de Enfermagem, 72*, 64–72. https://doi.org/10.1590/0034-7167-2018-0307

200. Mello, B. S., Massutti, T. M., Longaray, V. K., Trevisan, D. F., & de Fátima Lucena, A. (2016). Applicability of the Nursing Outcomes Classification (NOC) to the evaluation of cancer patients with acute or chronic pain in palliative care. *Applied Nursing Research, 29*, 12–18. https://doi.org/10.1016/j.apnr.2015.04.001

201. Menna Barreto, L. N., da Silva, M. B., Engelman, B., Figueiredo, M. S., Rodríguez-Acelas, A. L., & Cañon-Montañez, W. (2019). Evaluation of surgical wound healing in orthopedic patients with impaired tissue integrity according to Nursing Outcomes Classification. *International Journal of Nursing Knowledge, 30*(4), 228–233. https://doi.org/10.1111/2047-3095.12233

202. Menna Barreto, L. N., Swanson, E. A., & de Abreu Almeida, M. (2016). Nursing outcomes for the diagnosis impaired tissue integrity (00044) in adults with pressure ulcer. *International Journal of Nursing Knowledge, 27*(2), 104–110. https://doi.org/10.1111/2047-3095.12081

203. Monteiro Mantovani, V., Moorhead, S., & Abe, N. (2020). NANDA–I, NOC, and NIC linkages for nutritional problems. *International Journal of Nursing Knowledge, 31*(4), 246–252. https://doi.org/10.1111/2047-3095.12279

204. Monteiro Mantovani, V., Rodríguez Acelas, A. L., Klockner Boaz, S., Cañon, M. W., Lucena, A. de F., & Echer, I. C. (2019). Evaluation of patients in a smoking cessation support group using the Nursing Outcomes Classification. *International Journal of Nursing Knowledge, 30*(3), 125–130. https://doi.org/10.1111/2047-3095.12213

205. Monteiro Mantovani, V., Rodríguez Acelas, A. L., Lucena, A. de F., Abreu Almeida, M., Paz da Silva Heldt, E., Klockner Boaz, S., et al. (2017). Nursing outcomes for the evaluation of patients during smoking cessation. *International Journal of Nursing Knowledge, 28*(4), 204–210. https://doi.org/10.1111/2047-3095.12138

206. Moon, M. (2011). *Relationship of nursing diagnoses, nursing outcomes, and nursing interventions for patient care in intensive care units* (Publication No. 3526851) [Doctoral dissertation, University of Iowa]. ProQuest Dissertations and Theses Global.

207. Moorhead, S. (2006). The importance of perspective and primary focus in choosing and measuring outcomes. *International Journal of Nursing Terminologies & Classifications, 17*(1), 83–84.

208. Moorhead, S. (2019). Ten paths to data-driven care using NIC and NOC. *Nurse Leader, 17*(6), 522–525. https://doi.org/10.1016/j.mnl.2019.09.010

209. Moorhead, S., Clarke, M., Willits, M., & Tomsha, K. A. (1998). Nursing Outcomes Classification implementation projects across the care continuum. *Journal of Nursing Care Quality, 12*(5), 52–63. https://doi.org/10.1097/00001786-199806000-00009

210. Moorhead, S., & Delaney, C. (1997). Mapping nursing intervention data into the Nursing Interventions Classification (NIC): Process and rules. *Nursing Diagnosis, 8*(4), 137–144. https://doi.org/10.1111/j.1744-618X.1997.tb00468.x

211. Moorhead, S., & Johnson, M. (2004). Diagnostic-specific outcomes and nursing effectiveness research. *International Journal of Nursing Terminologies & Classifications, 15*(2), 49–57. https://doi.org/10.1111/j.1744-618x.2004.00049.x

212. Moorhead, S., Johnson, M., & Maas, M. (Eds.). (2004). *Nursing outcomes classification (NOC)* (3rd ed.). Mosby.

213. Moorhead, S., Johnson, M., Maas, M., & Reed, D. (2003). Testing the Nursing Outcomes Classification in three clinical units in a community hospital. *Journal of Nursing Measurement, 11*(2), 171–181. https://doi.org/10.1891/jnum.11.2.171.57287

214. Moorhead, S., Johnson, M., Maas, M., & Swanson, E. (Eds.). (2008). *Nursing outcomes classification (NOC)* (4th ed.). Mosby/Elsevier.

215. Moorhead, S., Johnson, M., Maas, M., & Swanson, E. (Eds.). (2013). *Nursing outcomes classification (NOC): Measurement of health outcomes* (5th ed.). Elsevier.

216. Moorhead, S., Johnson, M., Michel, J., de Barros, A., & Apalategui, M. U. (2004). Diagnostic-specific outcomes and nursing effectiveness research. *International Journal of Nursing Terminologies & Classifications, 15*(2), 49–57. https://doi.org/10.1111/j.1744-618X.2004.00049.x

217. Moorhead, S., Macieira, T. G. R., Lopez, K. D., Mantovani, V. M., Swanson, E., Wagner, C., et al. (2021). NANDA–I, NOC, and NIC linkages to SARS–Cov–2 (COVID–19): Part 1. Community response. *International Journal of Nursing Knowledge, 32*(1), 59–67. https://doi.org/10.1111/2047-3095.12291

218. Moorhead, S., Swanson, E., Johnson, M., & Maas, M. L. (Eds.). (2018). *Nursing outcomes classification (NOC): Measurement of health outcomes* (6th ed.). Elsevier.

219. Morales, J. M., Torres, A., Muñoz, F., León, J., & Miralles, L. (2003). Development of consensus-based clinical guidelines in critical care through standardized nursing language. *International Journal of Nursing Terminologies & Classifications, 14*(Suppl. 4), 54. https://doi.org/10.1111/j.1744-618x.2003.051_7.x

220. Moreira, R. P., de Araujo, T. L., Cavalcante, T. F., Guedes, N. G., Costa, A. G. D. S., & Lopes, M. V. D. O. (2013). Validation of the mobility nursing outcome in stroke survivors. *International Journal of Nursing Knowledge, 24*(3), 157–162. https://doi.org/10.1111/j.2047-3095.2013.01245.x

221. Moreira, R. P., Guerra, F., Ferreira, G. O., Cavalcante, T. F., Felício, J. F., Ferreira, L., et al. (2022). Effects of the nursing intervention fall prevention in older adults with arterial hypertension using NANDA-I, NIC, and NOC. *International Journal of Nursing Knowledge, 33*(2), 147–161. https://doi.org/10.1111/2047-3095.12346

222. Morley, D. A., & Cunningham, S. (2021). Global partnerships in nursing – a qualitative study in lessons for success. *Nurse Education in Practice, 54*, 1–8. https://doi.org/10.1016/j.nepr.2021.103069

223. Müller, M. (2020). Item fit statistics for Rasch analysis: Can we trust them? *Journal of Statistical Distributions and Applications, 7*(5). https://doi.org/10.1186/s40488-020-00108-7

224. Müller-Staub, M. (2009). Study to the implementation of NANDA-I nursing diagnosis, interventions and nursing sensitive patient outcomes. *Pflegewissenschaft, 11*(12), 688–696.

225. Müller-Staub, M., Lavin, M. A., Needham, I., & van Achterberg, T. (2007). Pflegediagnosen, -interventionen und -ergebnisse—Anwendung und Auswirkungen auf die Pflegepraxis: eine systematische Literaturübersicht [Nursing diagnoses, interventions, and outcomes—Application and impact on nursing practice: A systematic literature review]. *Pflege, 20*(6), 352–371. https://doi.org/10.1024/1012-5302.20.6.352

226. Müller-Staub, M., Lunney, M., Lavin, M. A., Needham, I., Odenbreit, M., & van Achterberg, T. (2008). Testing the Q-DIO as an instrument to measure the documented quality of nursing diagnoses, interventions, and outcomes. *International Journal of Nursing Knowledge, 19*(1), 20–27. https://doi.org/10.1111/j.1744-618X.2007.00075.x

227. Müller-Staub, M., Lunney, M., Lavin, M. A., Needham, I., Odenbreit, M., & van Achterberg, T. (2010). Psychometric properties of Q-DIO, an instrument to measure the quality of documented nursing diagnoses, interventions, and outcomes. *Pflege, 23*(2), 119–128. https://doi.org/1012-5302/a000024

228. Müller Staub, M., Lunney, M., Odenbreit, M., Needham, I., Lavin, M. A., & van Achterberg, T. (2009). Development of an instrument to measure the quality of documented nursing diagnoses, interventions and outcomes: The Q-DIO. *Journal of Clinical Nursing, 18*(7), 1027–1037. https://doi.org/10.1111/j.1365-2702.2008.02603.x

229. Müller-Staub, M., Needham, I., Odenbreit, M., Lavin, M. A., & van Achterberg, T. (2007). Improved quality of nursing documentation: Results of a nursing diagnoses, interventions, and outcomes implementation study. *International Journal of Nursing Terminologies & Classifications, 18*(1), 5–17. https://doi.org/10.1111/j.1744-618x.2007.00043.x

230. Müller-Staub, M., Needham, I., Odenbreit, M., Lavin, M. A., & van Achterberg, T. (2008). Quality of nursing diagnoses, interventions and outcomes: Criteria and operationalization of the measurement instrument Q-DIO. *Pflege, 21*(5), 327–338. https://doi.org/10.1024/1012-5302.21.5.327

231. National Academies of Sciences, Engineering, and Medicine. (2021). *The future of nursing 2020-2030: Charting a path to achieve health equity.* The National Academies Press. https://doi.org/10.17226/25982

232. Noh, H. K., & Lee, E. (2015). Relationships among NANDA-I diagnoses, Nursing Outcomes Classification, and Nursing Interventions Classification by nursing students for patients in medical-surgical units in Korea. *International Journal of Nursing Knowledge, 26*(1), 43–51. https://doi.org/10.1111/2047-3095.12044

233. Nunes Caldini, L., Alves Silva, R., Alencar Melo, G. A., Fernandes Pereira, F. G., Marques Frota, N., & Áfio Caetano, J. (2017). Nursing interventions and outcomes for pressure ulcer risk in critically ill patients. *Rev Rene, 18*(5), 598–605. https://doi.org/10.15253/2175-6783.2017000500006

234. Nygaard, A., Halvorsrud, L., Grov, E. K., & Bergland, A. (2022). "What matters to you?"—A qualitative study on the views of nursing home residents with dementia regarding the health care they receive. *Journal of Clinical Nursing, 31*(1/2), 262–274. https://doi.org/10.1111/jocn.15904

235. O'Connor, N. A., Hameister, A. D., & Kershaw, T. (2000). Applications of standardized nursing language to describe adult nurse practitioner practice. *International Journal of Nursing Knowledge, 11*(3), 109–120. https://doi.org/10.1111/j.1744-618X.2000

236. Odutayo, P. O., Olaogun, A. A. E., Oluwatosin, A. O., & Ogunfowokan, A. A. (2013). Impact of an educational program on the use of standardized nursing languages for nursing documentation among public health nurses in Nigeria. *International Journal of Nursing Knowledge, 24*(2), 108–112. https://doi.org/10.1111/j.2047-3095.2013.01239.x

237. Oh, H. (2016). *Validation of nursing-sensitive knowledge and self-management outcomes for adults with cardiovascular diseases and diabetes.* (Publication No. 10143103) [Doctoral dissertation, University of Iowa]. ProQuest Dissertations and Theses Global.

238. Oh, H., & Moorhead, S. (2019). Validation of the knowledge and self-management Nursing Outcomes Classification for adults with diabetes. *CIN: Computers, Informatics, Nursing, 37*(4), 222–228. https://doi.org/10.1097/CIN.0000000000000495

239. Oh, H., & Moorhead, S. (2020). Validation of the knowledge and self-management Nursing Outcomes Classification outcomes for adults with hypertension and lipid disorder. *Online Journal of Nursing Informatics, 24*(2), 1.

240. Olatubi, M. I., Oyediran, O. O., Faremi, F. A., & Salau, O. R. (2019). Knowledge, perception, and utilization of standardized nursing language (SNL) (NNN) among nurses in three selected hospitals in Ondo State, Nigeria. *International Journal of Nursing Knowledge, 30*(1), 43–48. https://doi.org/10.1111/2047-3095.12197

241. Oliveira, M. C., Flores, F. S., Barbosa, F. M., Fujii, C. D. C., Rabelo-Silva, E. R., & Lucena, A. F. (2021). Evaluation of percutaneous renal biopsy complications based on outcomes and indicators of the Nursing Outcomes Classification. *Revista Latino-Americana de Enfermagem, 29*, e3415. https://doi.org/10.1590/1518-8345.3759.3415

242. Oreofe, A. I., & Oyenike, A. M. (2018). Transforming practice through nursing innovative patient centered care: Standardized nursing languages. *International Journal of Caring Sciences, 11*(2), 1319–1322.

243. Osmarin, V. M., Bavaresco, T., Hirakata, V., Lucena, A. F., & Echer, I. C. (2021). Venous ulcer healing treated with conventional therapy and adjuvant laser: Is there a difference? *Revista Brasileira de Enfermagem, 74*, 1–7. https://doi.org/10.1590/0034-7167-2020-1117

244. Osmarin, V. M., Guarilha Boni, F., Bavaresco, T., de Fátima Lucena, A., & Echer, I. C. (2020). Use of the Nursing Outcomes Classification—NOC to assess the knowledge of patients with venous ulcer. *Revista Gaucha de Enfermagem, 41*, 1–7. https://doi.org/10.1590/1983-1447.2020.20190146

245. Othman, E. H., Shatnawi, F., Alrajabi, O., & Alshraideh, J. A. (2020). Reporting nursing interventions classification and Nursing Outcomes Classification in nursing research: A systematic review. *International Journal of Nursing Knowledge, 31*(1), 19–36. https://doi.org/10.1111/2047-3095.12265

246. Paans, W., & Müller, S. M. (2015). Patients' care needs: Documentation analysis in general hospitals. *International Journal of Nursing Knowledge, 26*(4), 178–186. https://doi.org/10.1111/2047-3095.12063

247. Paans, W., Sermeus, W., Nieweg, R. M. B., & van der Schans, C. P. (2010). D-Catch instrument: Development and psychometric testing of a measurement instrument for nursing documentation in hospitals. *Journal of Advanced Nursing, 66*(6), 1388–1400. https://doi.org/10.1111/j.1365-2648.2010.05302.x

248. Paloma, C. O., Romero, S. J. M., Paramio, C. J. C., Pastor, M. S. M., Carmen Sánchez, D. M., Rozadillas, S. E., et al. (2017). Development and psychometric evaluation of a questionnaire based on the Nursing Outcomes Classification to determine the knowledge of parents on breast-feeding: Research protocol. *International Journal of Nursing Knowledge, 28*(2), 100–108. https://doi.org/10.1111/2047-3095.12101

249. Pancorbo-Hidalgo, P. L., & Bellido-Vallejo, J. C. (2019). Clinical validation of the nursing outcome "Pain: Disruptive Effects" in people with chronic pain in Spain. *Journal of Nursing Measurement, 27*(3), 384–400. https://doi.org/10.1891/1061-3749.27.3.384

250. Park, H. (2010). *NANDA-I, NOC, and NIC linkages in nursing care plans for hospitalized patients with Congestive Heart Failure* (Publication No. 3409520) [Doctoral dissertation, University of Iowa]. ProQuest Dissertations and Theses Global.

251. Park, H. (2013). Nursing-sensitive outcome change scores for hospitalized older adults with heart failure: A preliminary descriptive study. *Research in Gerontological Nursing, 6*(4), 234–241. https://doi.org/10.3928/19404921-20130802-01

252. Park, H. (2014). Identifying core NANDA-I nursing diagnoses, NIC interventions, NOC outcomes, and NNN linkages for heart failure. *International Journal of Nursing Knowledge, 25*(1), 30–38. https://doi.org/10.1111/2047-3095.12010

253. Park, H., & Lee, E. (2015). Incorporating standardized nursing languages into an electronic nursing documentation system in Korea: A pilot study. *International Journal of Nursing Knowledge, 26*(1), 35–42. https://doi.org/10.1111/2047-3095.12038

254. Patiraki, E., Katsaragakis, S., Dreliozi, A., & Prezerakos, P. (2017). Nursing care plans based on NANDA, Nursing Interventions Classification, and Nursing Outcomes Classification: The investigation of the effectiveness of an educational intervention in Greece. *International Journal of Nursing Knowledge, 28*(2), 88–93. https://doi.org/10.1111/2047-3095.12120

255. Pehler, S., & Bodenbender, K. (2003). Concept maps as a tool for learning standardized languages. *International Journal of Nursing Terminologies & Classifications, 14*(Suppl. 4), 39. https://doi.org/10.1111/j.1744-618x.2003.32_12.x

256. Peres, H., Cruz, D., Tellez, M., de Cássia Gengo e Silva, R., Ortiz, D., Diogo, R., et al. (2016). Implementation of improvements in an electronic documentation nursing process system structured on NANDA-I, NOC and NIC (NNN) classification. *Studies in Health Technology & Informatics, 225*, 1082–1083. https://doi.org/10.3233/978-1-61499-658-3-1082

257. Pérez Rivas, F. J., Martín, I. S., Pacheco del Cerro, J. L., Minguet Arenas, C., García López, M., & Beamud Lagos, M. (2016). Effectiveness of nursing process use in primary care. *International Journal of Nursing Knowledge, 27*(1), 43–48. https://doi.org/10.1111/2047-3095.12073

258. Pesut, D. J., & Herman, J. (1998). OPT: Transformation of nursing process for contemporary practice: Outcome-Present State-Test. *Nursing Outlook, 46*(1), 29–36. https://doi.org/10.1016/s0029-6554(98)90022-7

259. Pesut, D. J., & Herman, J. (1999). *Clinical reasoning: The art & science of critical & creative thinking.* Delmar.

260. Peters, M. D. J., Marnie, C., Colquhoun, H., Garritty, C. M., Hempel, S., Horsley, T., et al. (2021). Scoping reviews: Reinforcing and advancing the methodology and application. *Systematic Reviews, 10*(1), 263. https://doi.org/10.1186/s13643-021-01821-3

261. Peters, R. M. (2000). Using NOC outcome of risk control in prevention, early detection, and control of hypertension: Nursing Outcomes Classification system. *Outcomes Management for Nursing Practice, 4*(1), 39–45.

262. Pezzi, M. V., Rabelo, S. E. R., Paganin, A., & Souza, E. N. (2016). Nursing interventions and outcomes for the diagnosis of impaired tissue integrity in patients after cardiac catheterization: Survey. *International Journal of Nursing Knowledge, 27*(4), 215–219. https://doi.org/10.1111/2047-3095.12140

263. Pires, A. U. B., Lucena, A. F., Behenck, A., & Heldt, E. (2020). Results of the Nursing Outcomes Classification/NOC for patients with obsessive-compulsive disorder. *Revista Brasileira de Enfermagem, 73*, 1. https://doi.org/10.1590/0034-7167-2018-0209

264. Porcella, A. (2003). Nursing outcomes across a surgical care episode. *International Journal of Nursing Terminologies & Classifications, 14*(Suppl. 4), 15. https://doi.org/10.1111/j.1744-618x.2003.012_5.x

265. Powelson, S., & Leiby, K. (2003). Implementation of standardized nursing language at a university. *International Journal of Nursing Terminologies & Classifications, 14*(Suppl. 4), 60. https://doi.org/10.1111/j.1744-618X.2003.059_3.x

266. Prophet, C. M., & Delaney, C. W. (1998). Nursing Outcomes Classification: Implications for nursing information systems and the computer-based patient record. *Journal of Nursing Care Quality, 12*(5), 21–29. https://doi.org/10.1097/00001786-199806000-00006

267. Puente, F. D., Palma, A. E., Sánchez, G. M. R., Hueso, M. C., Esteban, B. A. A., & Montoya, J. R. (2020). Development of a scale based on Nursing Outcome Classification "Dignified Life Closure" (1307) to assess end–of–life dignity of patients in care homes for the elderly. *International Journal of Nursing Knowledge, 31*(1), 44–49. https://doi.org/10.1111/2047-3095.12264

268. Quatrini Carvalho Passos Guimarães, H. C., Pena, S. B., Lopes, J. de L., Lopes, C. T., & Bottura Leite de Barros, A. L. (2016). Experts for validation studies in nursing: New proposal and selection criteria. *International Journal of Nursing Knowledge, 27*(3), 130–135. https://doi.org/10.1111/2047-3095.12089

269. Railka de Souza Oliveira, A., Leite de Araujo, T., Campos de Carvalho, E., Gabrielle de Sousa Costa, A., Frota Cavalcante, T., & Venícios de Oliveira Lopes, M. (2015). Construction and validation of indicators and respective definitions for the nursing outcome Swallowing Status. *Revista Latino-Americana de Enfermagem (RLAE), 23*(3), 450–457. https://doi.org/10.1590/0104-1169.0377.2575

270. Reed, D. (2006). Characteristics of patients and settings related to the choice of indicators for Nursing Outcome Classification outcomes. *International Journal of Nursing Terminologies & Classifications, 17*(1), 83.

271. Régis, C. C., Santos, C. T., Einhardt, R. S., & Lucena, A. F. (2020). Chronic pain evaluated by the Nursing Outcomes Classification. *Revista de Enfermagem UFPE, 14*, e243932. https://doi.org/10.5205/1981-8963.2020.243932

272. Reich, R., Rabelo-Silva, E. R., Swanson, E., Moorhead, S., & Almeida, M. de A. (2021). Development of a nursing outcome for a percutaneous procedure. *International Journal of Nursing Knowledge, 33*(2), 84–92. https://doi.org/10.1111/2047-3095.12329

273. Rodrigues de Alvarenga, S., de Souza Carneiro, C., Batista Santos, V., & Lopes Moreira, R. S. (2015). Instructional instrument of the NOC outcomes: Control knowledge of cardiac disease for patients with heart failure. *Revista Eletronica de Enfermagem, 17*(4), 1–10. https://doi.org/10.5216/ree.v17i4.26530

274. Rodríguez-Acelas, A. L., Cañon-Montañez, W., Mantovani, V. M., Figueiredo, M. S., Silva, M. B., & Almeida, M. A. (2019). Nursing outcomes for pain assessment after hip arthroplasty. *Revista Cuidarte, 10*(2), 1–9. https://doi.org/10.15649/cuidarte.v10i2.651

275. Roecklein, N. (2012). Using standardized nursing languages in end-of-life care plans. *International Journal of Nursing Knowledge, 23*(3), 183–185. https://doi.org/10.1111/j.2047-3095.2012.01211.x

276. Roman Cereto, M., Campos Rico, A., Viñas Heras, C., Palop, R., Zamudio Sánchez, A., Domingo García, R., et al. (2005). The nursing taxonomies, NANDA, NIC and NOC in hospital practice. *Enfermería Clínica, 15*(3), 163–166.

277. Sampaio, F. M. C., Araújo, O. S. S. L., Sequeira, C. A. da C., Lluch Canut, M. T., & Martins, T. (2018). Evaluation of the psychometric properties of NOC outcomes "Anxiety Level" and "Anxiety Self–Control" in a Portuguese outpatient sample. *International Journal of Nursing Knowledge, 29*(3), 184–191. https://doi.org/10.1111/2047-3095.12169

278. Santos, C. T., Barbosa, F. M., Almeida, T., Silva, A. C. F. E., Einhardt, R. S., & Lucena, A. F. (2021). Indicators of Nursing Outcomes Classification for evaluation of patients with pressure injury: Expert consensus. *Escola Anna Nery. Revista de Enfermagem, 25*, 20200155. https://doi.org/10.1590/2177-9465-ean-2020-0155

279. Santos, F. A. A. S., de Melo, R. P., & de Oliveira Lopes, M. V. (2010). Characterization of health status with regard to tissue integrity and tissue perfusion in patients with venous ulcers according to the Nursing Outcomes Classification. *Journal of Vascular Nursing, 28*(1), 14–20. https://doi.org/10.1016/j.jvn.2009.11.001

280. Sanubol, M. (2005). *Reliability of six outcomes from the Nursing Outcomes Classification (NOC) and the relationships of organizational, patient and nurse characteristics to these outcomes* (Publication No. 3172437) [Doctoral dissertation, University of Iowa]. ProQuest Dissertations and Theses Global.

281. Scherb, C. A. (2001). *Describing nursing effectiveness through standardized nursing languages and computerized clinical data* (Publication No. 3034148) [Doctoral dissertation, University of Iowa]. ProQuest Dissertations and Theses Global.

282. Scherb, C. A., Head, B. J., Hertzog, M., Swanson, E., Reed, D., Maas, M. L., et al. (2013). Evaluation of outcome change scores for patients with pneumonia or heart failure. *Western Journal of Nursing Research, 35*(1), 117–140. https://doi.org/10.1177/0193945911401429

283. Scherb, C. A., Head, B. J., Maas, M. L., Swanson, E. A., Moorhead, S., Reed, D., et al. (2011). Most frequent nursing diagnoses, nursing interventions, and nursing-sensitive patient outcomes of hospitalized older adults with heart failure: Part 1. *International Journal of Nursing Terminologies & Classifications, 22*(1), 13–22. https://doi.org/10.1111/j.1744-618X.2010.01164.x

284. Scherb, C. A., Lehmkuhl, J., & Leasman, E. (2003). The use of standardized nursing language by physical therapy, occupational therapy, and speech pathology in acute care. *International Journal of Nursing Terminologies & Classifications, 14*(Suppl. 4), 44–45. https://doi.org/10.1111/j.1744-618x.2003.040_8.x

285. Scherb, C. A., Maas, M. L., Head, B. J., Johnson, M. R., Kozel, M., Reed, D., et al. (2013). Implications of electronic health record meaningful use legislation for nursing clinical information system development and refinement. *International Journal of Nursing Knowledge, 24*(2), 93–100. https://doi.org/10.1111/j.2047-3095.2013.01235.x

286. Scherb, C. A., Rapp, C. G., Johnson, M., & Maas, M. (1998). The Nursing Outcomes Classification: Validation by rehabilitation nurses. *Rehabilitation Nursing, 23*(4), 174–178, 191 https://doi.org/10.1002/j.2048-7940.1998.tb01776.x

287. Scherb, C. A., Stevens, M. S., & Busman, C. (2007). Outcomes related to dehydration in the pediatric population. *Journal of Pediatric Nursing, 22*(5), 376–382. https://doi.org/10.1016/j.pedn.2006.10.004

288. Scherb, C. A., & Weydt, A. P. (2009). Work complexity assessment, Nursing Interventions Classification, and Nursing Outcomes Classification: Making connections. *Creative Nursing, 15*(1), 16–22. https://doi.org/10.1891/1078-4535.15.1.16

289. Schneider, J. S., Barkauskas, V., & Keenan, G. (2008). Evaluating home health care nursing outcomes with OASIS and NOC. *Journal of Nursing Scholarship, 40*(1), 76–82. https://doi.org/10.1111/j.1547-5069.2007.00209.x

290. Schoenfelder, D. P., Swanson, E. A., Specht, J. K. P., Maas, M., & Johnson, M. (2000). Outcome indicators for direct and indirect caregiving. *Clinical Nursing Research, 9*(1), 47–69. https://doi.org/10.1177/10547730022158438

291. Seabra, P. R. C., Amendoeira, J. J. P., Sá, L. O., & Capelas, M. L. V. (2018). Clinical validation of the Portuguese version of "Substance Addiction Consequences" derived from the Nursing Outcomes Classification. *Issues in Mental Health Nursing, 39*(9), 779–785. https://doi.org/10.1080/01612840.2018.1462870

292. Seganfredo, D. H., & Almeida, M. de A. (2011). Nursing outcomes content validation according to Nursing Outcomes Classification (NOC) for clinical, surgical and critical patients. *Revista Latino-Americana de Enfermagem (RLAE), 19*(1), 34–41. https://doi.org/10.1590/S0104-11692011000100006

293. Šerková, D., & Marečková, J. (2018). Creation and validation of Q-DIO, an instrument for rating the quality of nursing documentation -- literature review. *Central European Journal of Nursing & Midwifery, 9*(1), 799–810. https://doi.org/10.15452/CEJNM.2018.09.0007

294. Seyhan Ak, E., Kilinc Akman, E., & Gencbas, D. (2021). Evaluation of wound healing in patients with hip prosthesis according to nursing outcome classification. *International Journal of Nursing Knowledge, 33*(3), 185–195.

295. Shin, J. H., Choi, G. Y., & Lee, J. (2021). Identifying frequently used NANDA-I nursing diagnoses, NOC outcomes, NIC interventions, and NNN linkages for nursing home residents in Korea. *International Journal of Environmental Research and Public Health, 18*(21), 11505. https://doi.org/10.3390/ijerph182111505

296. Smith, K. J., & Craft-Rosenberg, M. (2010). Using NANDA, NIC, and NOC in an undergraduate nursing practicum. *Nurse Educator, 35*(4), 162–166. https://doi.org/10.1097/NNE.0b013e3181e33953

297. Smith, K., Smith, V., Krugman, M., & Oman, K. (2005). Evaluating the impact of computerized clinical documentation. *CIN: Computers, Informatics, Nursing, 23*(3), 132–138. https://doi.org/10.1097/00024665-200505000-00008

298. Soares, C. B., Komura Hoga, L. A., Peduzzi, M., Sangaleti, C., Yonekura, T., & Delage Silva, D. R. A. (2014). Integrative review: Concepts and methods used in nursing. *Revista Da Escola de Enfermagem Da USP, 48*(2), 329–339. https://doi.org/10.1590/s0080-6234201400002000020

299. Solar, O., & Irwin, A. (2006). Social determinants, political contexts and civil society action: A historical perspective on the Commission on Social Determinants of Health. *Health Promotion Journal of Australia, 17*(3), 180–185. https://doi.org/10.1071/he06180

300. Solar, O., & Irwin, A. (2010). *A conceptual framework for action on the social determinants of health. Social Determinants of Health Discussion Paper 2 (Policy and Practice)*. World Health Organization.

301. Specht, J. (2003). Nursing outcomes for evaluations of caregiver outcomes in a rural Alzheimer demonstration project. *International Journal of Nursing Terminologies & Classifications, 14*(Suppl. 4), 51–51. https://doi.org/j.1744-618X.2003.050_2.x

302. Stifter, J., Sousa, V. E. C., Febretti, A., Dunn Lopez, K., Johnson, A., Yao, Y., et al. (2018). Acceptability of clinical decision support interface prototypes for a nursing electronic health record to facilitate supportive care outcomes. *International Journal of Nursing Knowledge, 29*(4), 242–252. https://doi.org/10.1111/2047-3095.12178

303. Stocker, J. R. (2005). *Evaluating home health care nursing outcomes with OASIS and NOC* (Publication No. 3163939) [Doctoral dissertation, University of Iowa]. ProQuest Dissertations and Theses Global.

304. Su, M.-S., So, H., & An, M. (2014). Identification of major nursing diagnosis, nursing outcomes, and nursing interventions (NNN) linkage for cancer patients undergoing chemotherapy. *Korean Journal of Adult Nursing, 26*(4), 413–423. https://doi.org/10.7475/kjan.2014.26.4.413

305. Swanson, E. A., Moorhead, S., Johnson, M., & Maas, M. (2006). Using the model of mapping nursing outcomes classification (NOC) to the International Classification of Functioning, Disability and Health (ICF) to map NANDA, NIC and NOC. *International Journal of Nursing Terminologies & Classifications, 17*(1), 56–57.

306. Swanson, E., Jensen, D. P., Specht, J., Saylor, D., Johnson, M., & Maas, M. L. (1997). Caregiving: Concept analysis and outcomes. *Scholarly Inquiry for Nursing Practice: An International Journal, 11*(1), 65–76.

307. Swanson, E., Mantovani, V. M., Wagner, C., Moorhead, S., Lopez, K. D., Macieira, T. G. R., et al. (2021). NANDA−I, NOC, and NIC linkages to SARS−CoV−2 (COVID−19): Part 2. Individual response. *International Journal of Nursing Knowledge, 32*(1), 68–83. https://doi.org/10.1111/2047-3095.12307

308. Taghavi Larijani, T., & Saatchi, B. (2019). Training of NANDA-I nursing diagnoses (NDs), Nursing Interventions Classification (NIC) and Nursing Outcomes Classification (NOC), in psychiatric wards: A randomized controlled trial. *Nursing Open, 6*(2), 612–619. https://doi.org/10.1002/nop2.244

309. Tastan, S., Linch, G. C. F., Keenan, G. M., Stifter, J., McKinney, D., Fahey, L., et al. (2014). Evidence for the existing American Nurses Association-recognized standardized nursing terminologies: A systematic review. *International Journal of Nursing Studies, 51*(8), 1160–1170. https://doi.org/10.1016/j.ijnurstu.2013.12.004

310. Thoroddsen, A., Ehnfors, M., & Ehrenberg, A. (2011). Content and completeness of care plans after implementation of standardized nursing terminologies and computerized records. *CIN: Computers, Informatics, Nursing, 29*(10), 599–607. https://doi.org/10.1097/ncn.0b013e3182148c31

311. Timm, J. A., & Behrenbeck, J. G. (1998). Implementing the Nursing Outcomes Classification in a clinical information system in a tertiary care setting. *Journal of Nursing Care Quality, 12*(5), 64–72. https://doi.org/10.1097/00001786-199806000-00010

312. Törnvall, E., & Jansson, I. (2017). Preliminary evidence for the usefulness of standardized nursing terminologies in different fields of application: A literature review.

International Journal of Nursing Knowledge, *28*(2), 109–119. https://doi.org/10.1111/2047-3095.12123

313. Tseng, H. C. (2012). *Use of standardized nursing terminologies in electronic health records for oncology care: The impact of NANDA-I, NOC, and NIC* (Publication No. 3638443) [Doctoral dissertation, University of Iowa]. ProQuest Dissertations and Theses Global.

314. Tseng, H., & Moorhead, S. (2014). The use of standardized terminology to represent nursing knowledge: Nursing interventions relevant to safety for patients with cancer. *Studies in Health Technology & Informatics*, *201*, 298–303. https://doi.org/10.3233/978-1-61499-415-2-298

315. Van De Castle, B. (2003). Comparisons of NANDA/NIC/NOC linkages between nursing experts and nursing students. *International Journal of Nursing Terminologies & Classifications*, *14*(Suppl. 4), 40. https://doi.org/10.1111/j.1744-618x.2003.32_13.x

316. Van Horn, E. R., & Kautz, D. D. (2010). NNN language and evidence-based practice guidelines for acute cardiac care: Retaining the essence of nursing. *Dimensions of Critical Care Nursing*, *29*(2), 69–72. https://doi.org/10.1097/DCC.0b013e3181c92fea

317. Vargas-Escudero, A., Moya-Muñoz, N., Capilla-Díaz, C., Sánchez-Crisol, I., & Hueso-Montoro, C. (2019). Altered body image in stoma patients: Evaluation through classification of nursing outcomes. *Gastrointestinal Nursing*, *17*(Suppl. 5), S24–S30. https://doi.org/10.12968/gasn.2019.17.Sup5.S24

318. von Krogh, G., Dale, C., & Naden, D. (2005). A framework for integrating NANDA, NIC, and NOC terminology in electronic patient records. *Journal of Nursing Scholarship*, *37*(3), 275–281. https://doi.org/10.1111/j.1547-5069.2005.00047.x

319. Wagner, C. M., Swanson, E., Moorhead, S., Mantovani, V. M., Dunn-Lopez, K., Macieira, T. G. R., et al. (2022). NANDA-I, NOC, and NIC linkages to SARS-CoV-2 (COVID-19): Part 3. Family response. *International Journal of Nursing Knowledge*, *33*(1), 5–17. https://doi.org/10.1111/2047-3095.12323

320. Wagner, C., Butcher, H., & Clarke, M. (2024). *Nursing interventions classification (NIC)* (8th ed.). Elsevier.

321. Wasson, D., Dixon, L., Brighton, V., Caldwell, C., & Anderson, M. A. (2003). Hyperactivity Level: Development of a Nursing Outcome Label. *International Journal of Nursing Terminologies & Classifications*, *14*(Supp. 4), 16–16. https://doi.org/10.1111/j.1744-618X.2003.012_7.x

322. Werley, H. H., & Devine, E. C. (1987). The Nursing Minimum Data Set: Status and implications. In K. J. Hanna, M. Reimer, W. C. Mills, & S. Letourneau (Eds.), *Clinical judgment and decision-making: The future of nursing diagnosis* (pp. 540–551). John Wiley.

323. Werley, H. H., & Lang, N. M. (Eds.). (1988). *Identification of the nursing minimum data set*. Springer.

324. Wolfe, E. W., & Smith, E. V. (2007). Instrument development tools and activities for measure validation using Rasch models: Part I and Part II -Instrument development tools. In E. V. Smith, & R. M. Smith (Eds.), *Rasch measurement: Advanced and specialized applications* (pp. 202–290). JAM Press.

325. Wong, F. K. Y., Liu, H., Wang, H., Anderson, D., Seib, C., & Molasiotis, A. (2015). Global nursing issues and development: Analysis of World Health Organization documents. *Journal of Nursing Scholarship*, *47*(6), 574–583. https://doi.org/10.1111/jnu.12174

326. Wuryanto, E., Rahayu, G. R., Emilia, O., Harsono, & Octavia, A. P. R. (2017). Application of an outcome present test-peer learning model to improve clinical reasoning of nursing students in the intensive care unit. *Annals of Tropical Medicine & Public Health*, *10*(3), 657–663. https://doi.org/10.4103/ATMPH.ATMPH_201_17

327. Yang, M. J., Kim, H. Y., Ko, E., & Kim, H. K. (2019). Identification of nursing diagnosis–outcome–intervention linkages for inpatients in the obstetrics department nursing unit in South Korea. *International Journal of Nursing Knowledge*, *30*(1), 12–20. https://doi.org/10.1111/2047-3095.12187

328. Yearous, S. K. G. (2011). *School nursing documentation: Knowledge, attitude, and barriers to using standardized nursing languages and current practices* (Publication No. 3526877) [Doctoral dissertation, University of Iowa]. ProQuest Dissertations and Theses Global.

329. Young, Y., Frick, K. D., & Phelan, E. A. (2009). Can successful aging and chronic illness coexist in the same individual? A multidimensional concept of successful aging. *Journal of the American Medical Directors Association*, *10*(2), 87–92. https://doi.org/10.1016/j.jamda.2008.11.003

330. Zhang, T., Wu, X., Peng, G., Zhang, Q., Chen, L., Cai, Z., et al. (2021). Effectiveness of standardized nursing terminologies for nursing practice and healthcare outcomes: A systematic review. *International Journal of Nursing Knowledge*, *32*(4), 220–228. https://doi.org/10.1111/2047-3095.12315

331. Zugcic, M., Kravutske, M. E., & Gloskey, D. (2006). Relationship between utilization of selected NOCs and patient satisfaction. *International Journal of Nursing Terminologies & Classifications*, *17*(1), 82.

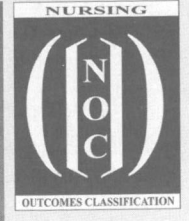

PART TWO

Nursing Outcomes Classification Taxonomy

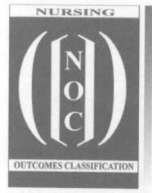

Overview of the NOC Taxonomy

The following section of this book contains the three-level taxonomy for the Nursing Outcomes Classification (NOC). The NOC taxonomy was created to: (1) organize the key concepts in the classification into domains, classes, and outcomes, (2) provide a stable structure for outcome placement over time, (3) allow for the addition of new outcomes, (4) allow for the expansion of classes within the domains, (5) identify missing outcomes needed for future editions, and 6) assist nurses and other health care providers to identify and select outcomes for the nursing diagnoses and clinical conditions they treat for patients, families, and communities. Use of the taxonomy makes identification of possible outcomes for use in practice easier than an alphabetical list of outcomes. The domain and class levels of the taxonomy have become even more important as the classification has grown over time. This edition has a total of 612 outcomes placed in the taxonomy.

HISTORICAL DEVELOPMENT OF THE NOC TAXONOMY

The taxonomic structure was developed during the second phase of the original NOC research and was first distributed in a publication from the Center[1] and then published in an article overviewing the methods in 1998.[5] The NOC taxonomic structure was developed using strategies refined by the Iowa Intervention Project.[2] The goal was to create a three-level taxonomic structure like the one developed for the Nursing Interventions Classification (NIC).[3] This required an inductive approach using qualitative similarity-dissimilarity analysis by many participants sorting outcomes into clusters. Nurse participants identified a concept label they felt captured the essence of the cluster of outcomes. In the first sort, 175 outcomes were grouped in this manner and the participants were asked to create 15 to 25 clusters based on the sorting process. Hierarchical cluster analysis was then applied to combine the results of each participant's individual sort. This process created the class level of the NOC taxonomy, which when finalized created 24 classes: *Energy Maintenance, Growth and Development, Mobility, Self-Care, Cardiopulmonary, Elimination, Fluid and Electrolytes, Immune Response, Metabolic Regulation, Neurocognitive, Nutrition, Tissue Integrity, Psychological Well-Being, Psychological Adaptation, Self-Control, Social Interaction, Health Behavior, Health Beliefs, Health Knowledge, Risk Control and Safety, Health and Life Quality, Symptom Status, Family Caregiver Status,* and *Maltreatment Resolution.* Each outcome is listed in only one class in the taxonomy.

In the second phase of the development of the taxonomy, the 24 classes were sorted by participants to create the top level of the taxonomy using the same methods used to create concept labels for each class. The results of this process identified six domains: *Functional Health, Physiologic Health, Psychosocial Health, Health Knowledge and Behavior, Perceived Health,* and *Family Health.* By the time the first publication was available 197 outcomes had been placed in the taxonomy including several outcomes that were included for the first time in the second edition of NOC. A more detailed description of the process used to create the taxonomy is available elsewhere.[4]

REVISIONS MADE IN THE TAXONOMY SINCE ITS CREATION

The following sections highlight the changes made in the NOC taxonomy by edition. The reader can review a more complete list of new and revised outcomes in the appendix of previous editions. In general, new classes are added to the taxonomy when outcomes are identified that do not fit easily into the current classes in the taxonomy or when a substantial number of outcomes focused on a concept are added to the classification.

Second Edition

The NOC taxonomy was first published within the classification in the second edition[3] in 2000. At that time there were 7 domains, 29 classes, and 260 outcomes. The revisions to the taxonomy for the second edition included five new classes: *Therapeutic Response* and *Sensory Function* in the *Functional Health* domain, *Family Member Health Status* in the *Family Health* domain, and *Community Well-Being* and *Community Health Protection* in the new domain *Community Health. Community Health* was added as a domain to the taxonomy to allow for inclusion of outcomes focused on the community as the recipient of care. This domain contains outcomes that describe the health, well-being, and functioning of a community or population. Like the *Family Health* domain, the focus of care is on a group rather than an individual. In this case, the population might be an entire community, a neighborhood, or a population of patients with the same health concern, for example patients with diabetes. The addition of another domain enlarged the taxonomy to 7 domains, 29 classes, and 260 outcomes. In addition, the definitions for four classes were modified: *Nutrition, Symptom Status, Family Care Status,* and *Family Well-Being.* The class *Maltreatment Resolution* was changed to *Family Well-Being.*

Third Edition

The addition of two new classes to the NOC taxonomy in the third edition[6] resulted in some changes in the placement of outcomes within the taxonomy. A class called *Satisfaction with Care* was added that includes outcomes that describe an individual's perceptions of the quality and adequacy of their health care. Because of this addition to the taxonomy the definition of the class *Health and Life Quality* was modified. Several changes were made in Domain VI, *Family Health*. A second class was added called *Parenting* containing outcomes that describe behaviors of parents that promote growth and development of children. The class *Family Care Status* was renamed *Family Caregiver Performance* to better reflect the outcomes in this class. This enlarged the taxonomy to 7 domains, 31 classes, and 330 outcomes. Overall, the definitions for three classes were modified: *Health Knowledge, Health and Life Quality,* and *Family Well-Being* and one domain *Perceived Health*.

Fourth Edition

The NOC taxonomy in the fourth edition[7] contained 7 domains, 31 classes, and 385 outcomes. In this edition the class *Nutrition* was changed to *Digestion and Nutrition* and the definition was modified to define this broader class. Three other class definitions were modified: *Satisfaction with Care, Family Member Health Status,* and *Family Well-Being*.

Fifth Edition

The taxonomy for the fifth edition of NOC[8] had 7 domains, 32 classes, and 490 outcomes. The class *Health Management* was added to include outcomes that describe the individual's role in the management of an acute or chronic condition. Definition changes to the *Psychologic Well-Being* and *Health Behavior* classes were also made in this edition.

Sixth Edition

The taxonomy of the sixth edition of NOC[9] had 7 domains, 34 classes, and 540 outcomes. We made several modifications in the fourth domain of the NOC Taxonomy, *Health Knowledge and Behavior*. The class *Health Knowledge* was divided into two classes: *Knowledge Health Condition* and *Knowledge Health Promotion*. As we continued to develop outcomes focused on knowledge, we realized that they were easily divided into two groups: one focused on knowledge of health promotion and one focused on knowledge of health conditions. We divided this class into two categories to make it easier to find an outcome. This change allowed for further development of outcomes in these classes. Eleven new knowledge outcomes were added to the sixth edition with all but one focused on knowledge related to a clinical condition.

A second revision of the NOC taxonomy focused on the class *Risk Control & Safety*. We divided this class into *Risk Control* with a separate class for *Safety*. The sixth edition added eight new risk control outcomes. One outcome was reclassified; *Physical Injury Severity* was moved from the Class *Risk Control & Safety* to *Tissue Integrity* because it was a better match for this class.

Seventh Edition

The taxonomy of the seventh edition of NOC has 7 domains, 36 classes, and 612 outcomes. We added a new class to the fourth domain, *Health Knowledge and Behavior*, called *Health Supporting Life Skills* that includes behaviors that enhance health and life quality. We moved several previously published outcomes into this class and added several new outcomes focused on literacy. Major changes were made to the fifth domain. We changed the domain name to *Health & Life Quality*, which was previously a class under this domain and changed the name of that class to *Health Status* to include status health outcomes. The previous domain name, *Perceived Health*, was felt to be to narrow and did not support including actual measurements of health status within the domain. We also added a new class, *Perceived Health & Life Situation*, to this domain, increasing the number of classes from 3 to 4. Seven classes have minor definition changes for this edition. All domains have new outcomes added to the taxonomy. The *Health Knowledge & Behavior Domain* remains the largest with a total of 211 outcomes. Outcomes for the *Family Health* and *Community Health Domains* expanded based on new outcomes to address the impact of the global pandemic.

Table 2.1 summarizes the changes made to the NOC taxonomy from the second through seventh editions. Details of these changes can be found by comparing previous editions of the taxonomy. The expansion of the number of classes in the taxonomy are consistent with the development of new areas of outcomes since the original taxonomy was added to the classification in the second edition. The seven domains have remained stable as the organizing concepts of this outcomes classification.

CODING OF THE CLASSIFICATION

Once the taxonomic structure was created, coding of the NOC became a high priority and was first included in the second edition of the classification. Coding is important because it creates a way to: (1) represent each of the taxonomic elements, (2) facilitate use of NOC in electronic health records or computer systems, (3) create nursing data sets that can be linked with large regional and national health care databases, (4) facilitate client outcome evaluation to improve the quality of patient care, and (5) ease use of NOC outcomes in research using multiple translations. The coding structure for NOC includes the domains, classes, outcomes, indicators of each outcome, the measurement scales, and scale values (see Table 2.2). The actual outcome scores are recorded by users of NOC for a specific client.

| Table 2.1 | | DEVELOPMENT OF THE NOC TAXONOMY ACROSS EDITIONS | | | | | |

NOC Taxonomy	Original[a]	2nd edition	3rd edition	4th edition	5th edition	6th edition	7th edition
Energy Maintenance	4	6	6	7	8	8	7
Growth and Development	18	20	21	24	24	24	30
Mobility	11	12	20	21	22	22	22
Self-Care	11	11	13	13	13	13	14[c]
Functional Health	**44**	**49**	**60**	**65**	**67**	**67**	**73**
Cardiopulmonary	9	11	14	17	23	23	23
Digestion and Nutrition	10	14[c]	14	15[bc]	20	20	20[c]
Elimination	4	4	5	5	5	5	5
Fluid and Electrolytes	3	3	4	4	21	21	22
Immune Response	4	5	7	7	7	7	7
Metabolic Regulation	3	3	4	4	5	6	6[c]
Neurocognitive	15	15	16	19	21	21	22
Sensory Function	-	5	6	6	6	6	7
Therapeutic Response	-	3	4	4	6	6	8[c]
Tissue Integrity	5	6	6	8	8	9	12
Physiologic Health	**53**	**69**	**80**	**89**	**122**	**124**	**132**
Psychological Well-Being	7	9	14	15	17[c]	18	23
Psychosocial Adaptation	7	7	7	8	10	11	15
Self-Control	9	10	10	9	11	12	12
Social Interaction	5	5	5	5	5	5	5
Psychosocial Health	**28**	**31**	**36**	**37**	**43**	**46**	**55**
Health Behavior	10	14	22	32	31[c]	35	36
Health Beliefs	6	6	6	6	6	6	6
Health Knowledge[e]	15	26	30[c]	42	64	-	-
Health Management	-	-	-	-	16	29	35
Knowledge Health Condition	-	-	-	-	-	40	45
Knowledge: Health Promotion	-	-	-	-	-	34	37
Risk Control and Safety[d]	14	19	18	26	34	-	-
Risk Control	-	-	-	-	-	30	35
Safety	-	-	-	-	-	10	11
Health Supporting Life Skills	-	-	-	-	-	-	6
Health Knowledge & Behavior	**45**	**65**	**76**	**106**	**151**	**184**	**211**
Health Status	-	-	-	-	-	-	6
Health and Life Quality[e]	3	5	8[c]	12	13	15	-
Perceived Health & Life Situation	-	-	-	-	-	-	9
Satisfaction with Care	-	-	14	17[c]	17	17	21
Symptom Status	5	6[c]	9	12	18	21	25[c]
Health & Life Quality[e]	**8**	**11**	**31**[b]	**41**	**48**	**53**	**61**

| Table 2.1 | DEVELOPMENT OF THE NOC TAXONOMY ACROSS EDITIONS—cont'd |

NOC Taxonomy	Original[a]	2nd edition	3rd edition	4th edition	5th edition	6th edition	7th edition
Family Caregiver Performance	12	9[c]	8[b]	8	8	9	8
Family Member Health Status	-	13	15	15[c]	15	15	12
Family Well-Being	7	7[bc]	10[c]	9[c]	10	13	18[c]
Parenting	-	-	5	5	10	10	14
Family Health	**19**	**29**	**38**	**37**	**43**	**47**	**52**
Community Health Protection	-	4	5	6	10	13	17[c]
Community Well-Being	-	2	4	4	6	6	11
Community Health	**-**	**6**	**9**	**10**	**16**	**19**	**28**
	6 domains	7 domains	7 domains	7 domains	7 domains	7 domains	7 domains
	24 classes	29 classes	31 classes	31 classes	32 classes	34 classes	36 classes
	197 outcomes	260 outcomes	330 outcomes	385 outcomes	490 outcomes	540 outcomes	612 outcomes

[a]From: Iowa Outcomes Project. (1997). Taxonomy of Nursing Outcomes Classification (NOC).
[b]Change in class name
[c]Change in class definition
[d]Division of class
[e]Change in domain name

| Table 2.2 | CODING STRUCTURE OF NOC |

Domain (1–9)	Class (A–Z) or (AA–ZZ)	Outcome (4 numbers)	Indicator (01–99)	Scale (01–99)	Scale Value (1–5)
#	##	####	##	##	#

Every effort has been made to retain codes used in the previous editions of this classification. With classification work it is important to keep coding of the outcomes consistent across editions. When changes were made in this edition, careful consideration of whether the outcome was a new outcome, or a revision of a previously published outcome had to be made. Any outcome that was just updated or revised retained its original code. In a few cases, revisions resulted in the creation of new outcomes from a previous published outcome in the classification. In this case, the old outcome was retired (along with its code) and the new outcome was given a new code. Codes for any indicator retired from the outcome resulted in the retiring of the code assigned to that indicator. Some minor edits to indicators have been made where the meaning of the indicator phrase did not change. In many outcomes, the indicators were reordered, and the indicators retained their original code, despite changes in placement within the outcome.

The addition of a second scale to some outcomes in the third edition resulted in the need to modify the coding scheme for the scale data. Scales in the second edition were coded with a letter of the alphabet. We now have moved to assigning numbers to each scale or combination of scales. This is a change in the coding schema since the third edition. The coding uses a number to reflect what scale or scale combinations are used for that outcome, and because there are more than nine scales, the codes for the scales require two spaces in the structure. In the second edition, numbers were used for the original set of measurement scales. If a scale was previously attached to a number, we have reinstituted that number as the code for the scale. This means that numbers for scales previously retired have not been used in newer editions. In addition, we have altered the code for the classes to use all capital letters and have used A–Z and have started using double letters such as AA. We have identified that the use of capitals and lower-case letters was confusing in database entries. This also requires two spaces.

This coding structure allows for expansion of the NOC at every level of the taxonomy and creates a unique identifier for each outcome, indicator, and measurement scale. For example, two additional domains can be added to the NOC taxonomy and 19 new classes can be added, each containing up to 99 outcomes. This structure allows for substantial additions to the classifications without changing the coding structure. Since the first draft of the taxonomy was created, new outcomes have been developed and easily placed in the taxonomy. Few changes in the structure have been needed to accomplish this. The next section provides the 612 outcomes in this edition listed in alphabetical order.

The NOC Taxonomy

	Domain I	Domain II	Domain III
Level 1 Domains	**Functional Health** Outcomes that describe the capacity for and performance of basic tasks of life	**Physiologic Health** Outcomes that describe organic functioning	**Psychosocial Health** Outcomes that describe psychological and social functioning
Level 2 Classes	**Energy Maintenance** Outcomes that describe an individual's energy rejuvenation, conservation, and expenditure	**Cardiopulmonary** Outcomes that describe an individual's cardiac, pulmonary, circulatory, or tissue perfusion status	**Psychological Well-Being** Outcomes that describe an individual's emotional health and related self-perception
	Growth & Development Outcomes that describe an individual's physical, emotional, and social maturation	**Digestion & Nutrition** Outcomes that describe an individual's eating, digestion, and nutritional patterns	**Psychosocial Adaptation** Outcomes that describe an individual's psychological and/or social adaptation to altered health or life circumstances
	Mobility Outcomes that describe an individual's physical mobility and the sequelae of restricted movement	**Elimination** Outcomes that describe an individual's waste excretion, elimination patterns, and status	**Self-Control** Outcomes that describe an individual's ability to restrain behavior that may be emotionally or physically harmful to self or others
	Self-Care Outcomes that describe an individual's performance of basic and instrumental activities of daily living	**Fluid & Electrolytes** Outcomes that describe an individual's fluid and electrolyte status	**Social Interaction** Outcomes that describe an individual's relationships with others
		Immune Response Outcomes that describe an individual's physiological reaction to substances that are foreign or interpreted by the body as foreign	
		Metabolic Regulation Outcomes that describe an individual's ability to regulate body metabolism or body functions	
		Neurocognitive Outcomes that describe an individual's neurological and cognitive status	
		Sensory Function Outcomes that describe an individual's perception and use of sensory information	
		Therapeutic Response Outcomes that describe an individual's systemic reaction to a health treatment, agent, or method	
		Tissue Integrity Outcomes that describe the condition and function of an individual's body tissues	

Domain IV	Domain V	Domain VI	Domain VII
Health Knowledge & Behavior Outcomes that describe attitudes, comprehension, and actions with respect to health and illness	**Health & Life Quality** Outcomes that describe an individual's health and perception of health care and life circumstances	**Family Health** Outcomes that describe health status, behavior, or functioning of the family as a whole or a family member	**Community Health** Outcomes that describe the health, well-being, and functioning of a community or population
Health Behavior Outcomes that describe an individual's actions to promote or restore health	**Health Status** Outcomes that describe an individual's overall health	**Family Caregiver Performance** Outcomes that describe the adaptation and performance of a family member caring for a dependent child or adult	**Community Health Protection** Outcomes that describe the community structures, processes, and programs to eliminate or reduce health risks and increase community resistance to health threats
Health Beliefs Outcomes that describe an individual's ideas and perceptions that influence health behavior	**Symptom Status** Outcomes that describe an individual's indications of a disease, injury, disruption, or loss	**Family Member Health Status** Outcomes that describe the physical, psychological, social, and spiritual health of a family member	**Community Well-Being** Outcomes that describe the overall health status and social competence of a community or population
Health Management Outcomes that describe an individual's actions to manage an acute or chronic condition	**Satisfaction with Care** Outcomes that describe an individual's perceptions of the quality and adequacy of health care provided	**Family Well-Being** Outcomes that describe the family environment, overall health status, and social competence of a family as a unit	
Knowledge Health Condition Outcomes that describe an individual's understanding in applying information to manage a health condition	**Perceived Health & Life Situation** Outcomes that describe an individual's perceived health status and related life circumstances	**Parenting** Outcomes that describe behaviors of parents that promote optimum growth and development of a child	
Knowledge Health Promotion Outcomes that describe an individual's understanding in applying information to optimize health			
Risk Control Outcomes that describe an individual's actions to understand, avoid, limit, or control identifiable health threats			
Safety Outcomes that describe an individual's behaviors or status that promotes protection from harm			
Health Supporting Life Skills Outcomes that describe behaviors that enhance an individual's health and life quality or circumstances			

Level 1 Domain	(1) Domain I–Functional Health
	Outcomes that describe the capacity for and performance of basic tasks of life

Level 2 Classes	**A-Energy Maintenance**	**B-Growth & Development**
	Outcomes that describe an individual's energy rejuvenation, conservation, and expenditure	Outcomes that describe an individual's physical, emotional, and social maturation

Level 3 Outcomes	
0005-Activity Tolerance	0120-Child Development: 1 Month
0001-Endurance	0100-Child Development: 2 Months
0002-Energy Conservation	0101-Child Development: 4 Months
0007-Fatigue Level	0102-Child Development: 6 Months
0006-Psychomotor Energy	0125-Child Development: 9 Months
0003-Rest	0103-Child Development: 12 Months
0004-Sleep	0126-Child Development: 18 Months
	0104-Child Development: 2 Years
	0105-Child Development: 3 Years
	0106-Child Development: 4 Years
	0107-Child Development: 5 Years
	0127-Child Development: 6–7 Years
	0128-Child Development: 8–10 Years
	0129-Child Development: Early Adolescence
	0130-Child Development: Late Adolescence
	0131-Child Development: Middle Adolescence
	0127-Development: Established Adulthood
	0121-Development: Late Adulthood
	0122-Development: Middle Adulthood
	0123-Development: Young Adulthood
	0111-Fetal Status: Antepartum
	0112-Fetal Status: Intrapartum
	0110-Growth
	0118-Newborn Adaptation
	0113-Physical Aging
	0114-Physical Maturation: Female
	0115-Physical Maturation: Male
	0116-Play Participation
	0117-Preterm Infant Organization
	0119-Sexual Functioning

C-Mobility

Outcomes that describe an individual's physical mobility and the sequelae of restricted movement

0200-Ambulation
0201-Ambulation: Wheelchair
0202-Balance
0203-Body Positioning: Self-Initiated
0212-Coordinated Movement
0222-Gait
0204-Immobility Consequences: Physiological
0205-Immobility Consequences: Psycho-Cognitive
0206-Joint Movement
0213-Joint Movement: Ankle
0214-Joint Movement: Elbow
0215-Joint Movement: Fingers
0216-Joint Movement: Hip
0217-Joint Movement: Knee
0218-Joint Movement: Neck
0207-Joint Movement: Passive
0219-Joint Movement: Shoulder
0220-Joint Movement: Spine
0221-Joint Movement: Wrist
0208-Mobility
0211-Skeletal Function
0210-Transfer Performance

D-Self-Care

Outcomes that describe an individual's performance of basic and instrumental activities of daily living

0311-Discharge Readiness: Independent Living
0312-Discharge Readiness: Supported Living
0313-Self-Care Behavior
0300-Self-Care Behavior: Activities of Daily Living (ADL)
0301-Self-Care Behavior: Bathing
0302-Self-Care Behavior: Dressing
0303-Self-Care Behavior: Eating
0314-Self-Care Behavior: Feet
0305-Self-Care Behavior: Hygiene
0306-Self-Care Behavior: Instrumental Activities of Daily Living (IADL)
0307-Self-Care Behavior: Non-Parenteral Medication
0308-Self-Care Behavior: Oral Hygiene
0309-Self-Care Behavior: Parenteral Medication
0310-Self-Care Behavior: Toileting

Level 1 *Domain*	**(2) Domain II–Physiologic Health** **Outcomes that describe organic functioning**

Level 2 *Classes*	**E-Cardiopulmonary** Outcomes that describe an individual's cardiac, pulmonary, circulatory, or tissue perfusion status	**K-Digestion & Nutrition** Outcomes that describe an individual's eating, digestion, and nutritional patterns
Level 3 *Outcomes*	0409-Blood Coagulation 0413-Blood Loss Severity 0400-Cardiac Pump Effectiveness 0414-Cardiopulmonary Function 0401-Circulation Status 0411-Mechanical Ventilation Response: Adult 0412-Mechanical Ventilation Weaning Response: Adult 0415-Respiratory Function 0410-Respiratory Function: Airway Patency 0402-Respiratory Function: Gas Exchange 0403-Respiratory Function: Ventilation 0417-Shock Severity: Anaphylactic 0418-Shock Severity: Cardiogenic 0419-Shock Severity: Hypovolemic 0420-Shock Severity: Neurogenic 0421-Shock Severity: Septic 0422-Tissue Perfusion 0404-Tissue Perfusion: Abdominal Organs 0405-Tissue Perfusion: Cardiac 0416-Tissue Perfusion: Cellular 0406-Tissue Perfusion: Cerebral 0407-Tissue Perfusion: Peripheral 0408-Tissue Perfusion: Pulmonary	1014-Appetite 1016-Bottle Feeding Establishment: Infant 1017-Bottle Feeding Performance 1000-Breastfeeding Establishment: Infant 1001-Breastfeeding Establishment: Maternal 1002-Breastfeeding Maintenance 1003-Breastfeeding Weaning 1018-Cup Feeding Establishment: Infant 1019-Cup Feeding Performance 1015-Gastrointestinal Function 1020-Infant Nutritional Status 1004-Nutritional Status 1005-Nutritional Status: Biochemical Measures 1007-Nutritional Status: Energy 1008-Nutritional Status: Food & Fluid Intake 1009-Nutritional Status: Nutrient Intake 1010-Swallowing Status 1011-Swallowing Status: Esophageal Phase 1012-Swallowing Status: Oral Phase 1013-Swallowing Status: Pharyngeal Phase

F-Elimination	**G-Fluid & Electrolytes**	**H-Immune Response**
Outcomes that describe an individual's waste excretion, elimination patterns, and status	Outcomes that describe an individual's fluid and electrolyte status	Outcomes that describe an individual's physiological reaction to substances that are foreign or interpreted by the body as foreign
0500-Bowel Continence 0501-Bowel Elimination 0504-Kidney Function 0502-Urinary Continence 0503-Urinary Elimination	0604-Acute Respiratory Acidosis Severity 0605-Acute Respiratory Alkalosis Severity 0621-Dehydration Severity 0600-Electrolyte & Acid/Base Balance 0606-Electrolyte Balance 0601-Fluid Balance 0603-Fluid Overload Severity 0602-Hydration 0607-Hypercalcemia Severity 0608-Hyperchloremia Severity 0609-Hyperkalemia Severity 0610-Hypermagnesemia Severity 0611-Hypernatremia Severity 0612-Hyperphosphatemia Severity 0613-Hypocalcemia Severity 0614-Hypochloremia Severity 0615-Hypokalemia Severity 0616-Hypomagnesemia Severity 0617-Hyponatremia Severity 0618-Hypophosphatemia Severity 0619-Metabolic Acidosis Severity 0620-Metabolic Alkalosis Severity	0705-Allergic Response: Localized 0706-Allergic Response: Systemic 0700-Blood Product Transfusion Reaction 0707-Immune Hypersensitivity Response 0702-Immune Status 0703-Infection Severity 0708-Infection Severity: Newborn

Level 1 Domain	(2) Domain II–Physiologic Health (Continued)	
Level 2 Classes	**I-Metabolic Regulation** Outcomes that describe an individual's ability to regulate body metabolism or body functions	**J-Neurocognitive** Outcomes that describe an individual's neurological and cognitive status
Level 3 Outcomes	0803-Liver Function 0804-Metabolic Function 0800-Thermoregulation 0801-Thermoregulation: Newborn 0802-Vital Signs 1006-Weight: Body Mass	0919-Abstract Thinking 0921-Attention Deficit Level 0900-Cognition 0901-Cognitive Orientation 0902-Communication 0903-Communication: Expressive 0904-Communication: Receptive 0905-Concentration 0906-Decision-Making 0916-Delirium Level 0920-Dementia Level 0918-Heedfulness of Affected Side 0915-Hyperactivity Level 0907-Information Processing 0908-Memory 0909-Neurological Function 0910-Neurological Function: Autonomic 0911-Neurological Function: Central Motor Control 0912-Neurological Function: Consciousness 0913-Neurological Function: Cranial Sensory/Motor 0917-Neurological Function: Peripheral 0914-Neurological Function: Spinal Sensory/Motor

Y-Sensory Function

Outcomes that describe an individual's perception and use of sensory information

2405-Sensory Function
2401-Sensory Function: Hearing
2402-Sensory Function: Proprioception
2406-Sensory Function: Smell
2400-Sensory Function: Tactile
2407-Sensory Function: Taste
2404-Sensory Function: Vision

AA-Therapeutic Response

Outcomes that describe an individual's systemic reaction to a health treatment, agent, or method

2300-Blood Glucose Control
2306-Hemodialysis: Disruptive Effects
2301-Medication Response
2307-Peritoneal Dialysis: Disruptive Effects
2303-Post-Procedure Recovery
2304-Surgical Recovery: Convalescence
2305-Surgical Recovery: Immediate Post-Operative
2302-Systemic Toxin Clearance: Dialysis

L-Tissue Integrity

Outcomes that describe the condition and function of an individual's body tissues

1104-Bone Healing
1106-Burn Healing
1107-Burn Recovery
1108-Foot Health
1105-Hemodialysis Access
1100-Oral Health
1913-Physical Injury Severity
1101-Tissue Integrity: Skin & Mucous Membranes
1109-Tissue Injury Severity: Percutaneous Procedure
1110-Vocal Function
1102-Wound Healing: Primary Intention
1103-Wound Healing: Secondary Intention

Level 1 *Domain*	**(3) Domain III–Psychosocial Health** **Outcomes that describe psychological and social functioning**

Level 2 *Classes*	**M-Psychological Well-Being** Outcomes that describe an individual's emotional health and related self-perception	**N-Psychosocial Adaptation** Outcomes that describe an individual's psychological and/or social adaptation to altered health or life circumstances
Level 3 *Outcomes*	1214-Agitation Level 1211-Anxiety Level 1200-Body Image 1208-Depression Level 1210-Fear Level 1218-Fear Level: Adolescent 1219-Fear Level: Middle Childhood 1220-Fear Level: Preschooler 1221-Gender Identity 1222-Hoarding Behavior Severity 1201-Hope 1203-Loneliness Severity 1204-Mood Equilibrium 1209-Motivation 1217-Panic Level 1202-Personal Identity 1215-Self-Awareness 1205-Self-Esteem 1207-Sexual Identity 1216-Social Anxiety Level 1223-Social Identity 1212-Stress Level 1206-Will to Live	1300-Acceptance: Health Status 1315-Adaptation to Hospitalization: Adolescent 1314-Adaptation to Hospitalization: Middle Childhood 1313-Adaptation to Hospitalization: Preschooler 1308-Adaptation to Physical Disability 1312-Childhood Bullying Recovery 1302-Coping 1307-Dignified Life Closure 1304-Grief Resolution 1310-Guilt Resolution 1316-Parent Adaptation to Infant Hospitalization 1317-Parent Adaptation to Toddler Hospitalization 1309-Personal Resilience 1305-Psychosocial Adjustment: Life Change 1311-Relocation Adaptation

O-Self-Control

Outcomes that describe an individual's ability to restrain behavior that may be emotionally or physically harmful to self or others

1400-Abusive Behavior Self-Restraint
1401-Aggression Self-Restraint
1410-Anger Self-Restraint
1402-Anxiety Self-Control
1409-Depression Self-Control
1403-Distorted Thought Self-Control
1411-Eating Disorder Self-Control
1404-Fear Self-Control
1405-Impulse Self-Control
1412-Panic Self-Control
1414-Self-Harm Restraint
1408-Suicide Self-Restraint

P-Social Interaction

Outcomes that describe an individual's relationships with others

1500-Parent-Infant Attachment
1501-Role Performance
1502-Social Interaction Skills
1503-Social Involvement
1504-Social Support

Level 1 Domain	(4) Domain IV–Health Knowledge & Behavior Outcomes that describe attitudes, comprehension, and actions with respect to health and illness	
Level 2 Classes	**Q-Health Behavior** Outcomes that describe an individual's actions to promote or restore health	**R-Health Beliefs** Outcomes that describe an individual's ideas and perceptions that influence health behavior
Level 3 Outcomes	1600-Adherence Behavior 1640-Adherence Behavior: Clinical Condition 1621-Adherence Behavior: Healthy Diet 1632-Adherence Behavior: Prescribed Activity 1622-Adherence Behavior: Prescribed Diet 1623-Adherence Behavior: Prescribed Medication 1629-Alcohol Abuse Cessation Behavior 1616-Body Mechanics Performance 1636-Cardiac Rehabilitation Participation 1630-Drug Abuse Cessation Behavior 1633-Exercise Participation 1641-Group Therapy Participation 1602-Health Promoting Behavior 1603-Health Seeking Behavior 1610-Hearing Compensation Behavior 1413-Hoarding Cessation Behavior 1604-Leisure Participation 1637-Musculoskeletal Rehabilitation Participation 1618-Nausea & Vomiting Control 1605-Pain Control 1606-Participation in Health Care Decisions 1638-Patient Engagement Behavior 1614-Personal Autonomy 1634-Personal Health Screening Behavior 1624-Postpartum Maternal Health Behavior 1607-Prenatal Health Behavior 1620-Seizure Self-Control 1613-Self-Direction of Care 1639-Self-Direction of Instrumental Activities of Daily Living 1642-Sleep Enhancement Behavior 1625-Smoking Cessation Behavior 1608-Symptom Control 1611-Vision Compensation Behavior 1626-Weight Gain Behavior 1627-Weight Loss Behavior 1628-Weight Maintenance Behavior	1700-Health Beliefs 1701-Health Beliefs: Perceived Ability to Perform 1702-Health Beliefs: Perceived Control 1703-Health Beliefs: Perceived Resources 1704-Health Beliefs: Perceived Threat 1705-Health Orientation

FF-Health Management

Outcomes that describe an individual's actions to manage an acute or chronic condition

3100-Self-Management: Acute Illness
3101-Self-Management: Anticoagulation Therapy
3112-Self-Management: Arthritis
0704-Self-Management: Asthma
3113-Self-Management: Autism Spectrum Disorder
3114-Self-Management: Cancer
1617-Self-Management: Cardiac Disease
3115-Self-Management: Celiac Disease
3116-Self-Management: Chronic Anemia
3102-Self-Management: Chronic Disease
3103-Self-Management: Chronic Obstructive Pulmonary Disease
3104-Self-Management: Coronary Artery Disease
1619-Self-Management: Diabetes
3105-Self-Management: Dysrhythmia
3106-Self-Management: Heart Failure
3117-Self-Management: Human Immunodeficiency Virus
3107-Self-Management: Hypertension
3118-Self-Management: Infection
3119-Self-Management: Inflammatory Bowel Disease
3108-Self-Management: Kidney Disease
3125-Self-Management: Kidney Failure
3120-Self-Management: Known Allergy
3109-Self-Management: Lipid Disorder
3126-Self-Management: Liver Disease
3121-Self-Management: Lymphedema
1631-Self-Management: Multiple Sclerosis
3110-Self-Management: Osteoporosis
1615-Self-Management: Ostomy
3127-Self-Management: Parkinson Disease
3111-Self-Management: Peripheral Artery Disease
3122-Self-Management: Pneumonia
3123-Self-Management: Stroke
3128-Self-Management: Treatment Procedure
3129-Self-Management: Treatment Regimen
3124-Self-Management: Wound

Level 1 *Domain*	**(4) Domain IV–Health Knowledge & Behavior (Continued)**
Level 2 *Classes*	**GG- Knowledge Health Condition** Outcomes that describe an individual's understanding in applying information to manage a health condition	**S-Knowledge Health Promotion** Outcomes that describe an individual's understanding in applying information to optimize health
Level 3 *Outcomes*	1844-Knowledge: Acute Illness Management 3200-Knowledge: Allergy Management 1845-Knowledge: Anticoagulation Therapy Management 1868-Knowledge: Anxiety Management 1831-Knowledge: Arthritis Management 1832-Knowledge: Asthma Management 1869-Knowledge: Attention Deficit Hyperactivity Disorder (ADHD) Management 3201-Knowledge: Autism Spectrum Disorder Management 1833-Knowledge: Cancer Management 1830-Knowledge: Cardiac Disease Management 3202-Knowledge: Cardiac Rehabilitation 3203-Knowledge: Celiac Disease Management 3204-Knowledge: Chronic Anemia Management 1847-Knowledge: Chronic Disease Management 1848-Knowledge: Chronic Obstructive Pulmonary Disease Management 1849-Knowledge: Coronary Artery Disease Management 1851-Knowledge: Dementia Management 1836-Knowledge: Depression Management 1820-Knowledge: Diabetes Management 1803-Knowledge: Disease Management 1852-Knowledge: Dysrhythmia Management 1853-Knowledge: Eating Disorder Management 3205-Knowledge: Epilepsy Management 1835-Knowledge: Heart Failure Management 3206-Knowledge: Human Immunodeficiency Virus Management 1837-Knowledge: Hypertension Management 1842-Knowledge: Infection Management 1856-Knowledge: Inflammatory Bowel Disease Management 1857-Knowledge: Kidney Disease Management 1872-Knowledge: Kidney Failure Management 1858-Knowledge: Lipid Disorder Management 1873-Knowledge: Liver Disease Management 3207-Knowledge: Lymphedema Management 1838-Knowledge: Multiple Sclerosis Management 3208-Knowledge: Musculoskeletal Rehabilitation 1859-Knowledge: Osteoporosis Management 1874-Knowledge: Parkinson Disease Management 1860-Knowledge: Peripheral Artery Disease Management 1861-Knowledge: Pneumonia Management 1811-Knowledge: Prescribed Activity 1802-Knowledge: Prescribed Diet 1863-Knowledge: Stroke Management 1814-Knowledge: Treatment Procedure 1813-Knowledge: Treatment Regimen 3209-Knowledge: Wound Management	1827-Knowledge: Body Mechanics 1846-Knowledge: Bottle Feeding 1800-Knowledge: Breastfeeding 1834-Knowledge: Cancer Threat Reduction 1801-Knowledge: Child Physical Safety 1870-Knowledge: Community Health Resources 1821-Knowledge: Conception Prevention 1850-Knowledge: Cup Feeding 1867-Knowledge: Diagnostic & Therapeutic Procedures 1804-Knowledge: Energy Conservation 1828-Knowledge: Fall Prevention 1816-Knowledge: Fertility Promotion 1871-Knowledge: Foot Care 1805-Knowledge: Health Behavior 1806-Knowledge: Health Resources 1854-Knowledge: Healthy Diet 1855-Knowledge: Healthy Lifestyle 1819-Knowledge: Infant Care 1817-Knowledge: Labor & Delivery 1808-Knowledge: Medication 1829-Knowledge: Ostomy Care 1843-Knowledge: Pain Management 1826-Knowledge: Parenting 1809-Knowledge: Personal Safety 1818-Knowledge: Postpartum Maternal Health 1822-Knowledge: Preconception Maternal Health 1810-Knowledge: Pregnancy 1839-Knowledge: Pregnancy & Postpartum Sexual Function 1840-Knowledge: Preterm Infant Care 1875-Knowledge: School Age Child Psychosocial Safety 1815-Knowledge: Sexual Function 1862-Knowledge: Stress Management 1864-Knowledge: Stroke Threat Reduction 1812-Knowledge: Substance Use Control 1865-Knowledge: Thrombus Threat Reduction 1866-Knowledge: Time Management 1841-Knowledge: Weight Management

T-Risk Control	**HH-Safety**	**II-Health Supporting Life Skills**
Outcomes that describe an individual's actions to understand, avoid, limit, or control identifiable health threats	Outcomes that describe an individual's behaviors or status that promotes protection from harm	Outcomes that describe behaviors that enhance an individual's health and life quality or circumstances
1902-Risk Control	1919-Elopement Occurrence	2040-Digital Literacy Behavior
1903-Risk Control: Alcohol Use	1920-Elopement Propensity Risk	2014-Financial Literacy Behavior
1935-Risk Control: Aspiration	1909-Fall Prevention Behavior	2041-Health Insurance Literacy Behavior
1917-Risk Control: Cancer	1912-Falls Occurrence	2015-Health Literacy Behavior
1914-Risk Control: Cardiovascular Disease	1900-Immunization Behavior	2013-Lifestyle Balance
1936-Risk Control: Child Bullying	1911-Personal Safety Behavior	1635-Personal Time Management
1937-Risk Control: Dehydration	1921-Pre-Procedure Readiness	
1904-Risk Control: Drug Use	1934-Safe Health Care Environment	
1927-Risk Control: Dry Eye	1910-Safe Home Environment	
1938-Risk Control: Environmental Hazards	1947-Safe Home Environment: Nursery	
1939-Risk Control: Falls	1926-Safe Wandering	
1943-Risk Control: Food Insecurity		
1915-Risk Control: Hearing Impairment		
1944-Risk Control: Housing Insecurity		
1928-Risk Control: Hypertension		
1922-Risk Control: Hyperthermia		
1933-Risk Control: Hypotension		
1923-Risk Control: Hypothermia		
1940-Risk Control: Infant Allergies		
1924-Risk Control: Infectious Process		
1929-Risk Control: Lipid Disorder		
1941-Risk Control: Obesity		
1930-Risk Control: Osteoporosis		
1945-Risk Control: Prediabetes		
1942-Risk Control: Pressure Injury		
1946-Risk Control: Problematic Internet Use		
1905-Risk Control: Sexually Transmitted Diseases (STDs)		
1931-Risk Control: Stroke		
1925-Risk Control: Sun Exposure		
1932-Risk Control: Thrombus		
1906-Risk Control: Tobacco Use		
1907-Risk Control: Unintended Pregnancy		
1916-Risk Control: Visual Impairment		
1948-Risk Control: Voice Disorder		
1908-Risk Detection		

Level 1
Domain

(5) Domain V–Health & Life Quality

Outcomes that describe an individual's health and perception of health care and life circumstances

Level 2
Classes

JJ-Health Status	V-Symptom Status
Outcomes that describe an individual's overall health	Outcomes that describe an individual's indications of a disease, injury, disruption, or loss

Level 3
Outcomes

2509-Maternal Status: Antepartum	2515-Abuse: Disruptive Effects
2510-Maternal Status: Intrapartum	2116-Chemotherapy: Disruptive Physical Effects
2511-Maternal Status: Postpartum	2109-Discomfort Level
2006-Personal Health Status	2110-Dry Eye Severity
2004-Physical Fitness	0008-Fatigue: Disruptive Effects
2005-Student Health Status	2111-Hyperglycemia Severity
	2112-Hypertension Severity
	2113-Hypoglycemia Severity
	2114-Hypotension Severity
	2117-Lymphedema Severity
	2106-Nausea & Vomiting: Disruptive Effects
	2107-Nausea & Vomiting Severity
	2516-Neglect: Disruptive Effects
	1306-Pain: Adverse Psychological Response
	2101-Pain: Disruptive Effects
	2102-Pain Level
	2104-Perimenopause Symptom Severity
	2115-Peripheral Artery Disease Severity
	2105-Premenstrual Syndrome (PMS) Severity
	2118-Seizure Severity
	2119-Sleep Disruption Severity
	1407-Substance Addiction Consequences
	2108-Substance Withdrawal Severity
	2003-Suffering Severity
	2103-Symptom Severity

EE-Satisfaction with Care	**U-Perceived Health & Life Situation**
Outcomes that describe an individual's perceptions of the quality and adequacy of health care provided	Outcomes that describe an individual's perceived health status and related life circumstances

3014-Client Satisfaction	2008-Comfort Status
3000-Client Satisfaction: Access to Care Resources	2009-Comfort Status: Environment
3017-Client Satisfaction: Acute Care Transition Process	2010-Comfort Status: Physical
3001-Client Satisfaction: Caring	2011-Comfort Status: Psychospiritual
3015-Client Satisfaction: Case Management	2012-Comfort Status: Sociocultural
3002-Client Satisfaction: Communication	2002-Personal Well-Being
3003-Client Satisfaction: Continuity of Care	2000-Quality of Life
3004-Client Satisfaction: Cultural Needs Fulfillment	2001-Spiritual Health
3018-Client Satisfaction: Discharge Process	2016-Successful Aging
3005-Client Satisfaction: Functional Assistance	
3019-Client Satisfaction: Labor & Delivery	
3016-Client Satisfaction: Pain Management	
3006-Client Satisfaction: Physical Care	
3007-Client Satisfaction: Physical Environment	
3008-Client Satisfaction: Protection of Rights	
3009-Client Satisfaction: Psychological Care	
3010-Client Satisfaction: Safety	
3011-Client Satisfaction: Symptom Control	
3012-Client Satisfaction: Teaching	
3013-Client Satisfaction: Technical Aspects of Care	
3020-Client Satisfaction: Telehealth Services	

Level 1 Domain	(6) Domain VI–Family Health **Outcomes that describe health status, behavior, or functioning of the family as a whole or of an individual as a family member**	
Level 2 Classes	**W-Family Caregiver Performance** Outcomes that describe the adaptation and performance of a family member caring for a dependent child or adult	**Z-Family Member Health Status** Outcomes that describe the physical, psychological, and social health of a family member
Level 3 Outcomes	2200-Caregiver Adaptation to Patient Institutionalization 2202-Caregiver Home Care Readiness 2203-Caregiver Lifestyle Disruption 2204-Caregiver-Patient Relationship 2205-Caregiver Performance: Direct Care 2206-Caregiver Performance: Indirect Care 2210-Caregiver Role Endurance 2208-Caregiver Stressors	2500-Abuse Cessation 2501-Abuse Protection 2514-Abuse Recovery 2502-Abuse Recovery: Emotional 2503-Abuse Recovery: Financial 2504-Abuse Recovery: Physical 2505-Abuse Recovery: Sexual 2506-Caregiver Emotional Health Status 2507-Caregiver Physical Health Status 2508-Caregiver Well-Being 2513-Neglect Cessation 2512-Neglect Recovery

X-Family Well-Being	**DD-Parenting**
Outcomes that describe the family environment, family health status, family behaviors, and social competence of a family as a unit	Outcomes that describe behaviors of parents that promote optimum growth and development of a child

X-Family Well-Being	DD-Parenting
2600-Family Coping	2211-Parenting Performance
2602-Family Functioning	2903-Parenting Performance: Adolescent
2606-Family Health Status	2902-Parenting Performance: Adolescent Physical Safety
2603-Family Integrity	2908-Parenting Performance: Attention Deficit Hyperactivity Disorder
2604-Family Normalization	2909-Parenting Performance: Early Childhood Psychosocial Safety
2613-Family Normalization: Autism Spectrum Disorder	2901-Parenting Performance: Early/Middle Childhood Physical Safety
2611-Family Normalization: Dementia	2904-Parenting Performance: Infant
2605-Family Participation in Professional Care	2910-Parenting Performance: Infant Physical Safety
2212-Family Performance: Dementia Care	2911-Parenting Performance: Infant Psychosocial Safety
2608-Family Resilience	2905-Parenting Performance: Middle Childhood
2612-Family Risk Control: Bullying	2906-Parenting Performance: Preschooler
2614-Family Risk Control: Elopement	2912-Parenting Performance: School Age Child Psychosocial Safety
2620-Family Risk Control: Household Food Insecurity	2907-Parenting Performance: Toddler
2610-Family Risk Control: Obesity	2913-Parenting Performance: Toddler Physical Safety
2615-Family Risk Control: Violence	
2601-Family Social Climate	
2630-Family Social Network Support	
2609-Family Support During Treatment	

Level 1 *Domain*	**(7) Domain VII–Community Health** **Outcomes that describe the health, well-being, and functioning of a community or population**
Level 2 *Classes*	**CC-Community Health Protection** Outcomes that describe the community structures, processes, and programs to eliminate or reduce health risks and increase community resistance to health threats
Level 3 *Outcomes*	2804-Community Disaster Readiness 2806-Community Disaster Response 2703-Community Grief Response 2807-Community Health Screening Effectiveness 2799-Community Immunity Effectiveness 2707-Community Pandemic Readiness 2709-Community Pandemic Response 2808-Community Program Effectiveness 2811-Community Risk Control: Bullying 2801-Community Risk Control: Chronic Disease 2802-Community Risk Control: Communicable Disease 2812-Community Risk Control: Environmental Hazards 2803-Community Risk Control: Lead Exposure 2809-Community Risk Control: Obesity 2813-Community Risk Control: Suicide 2810-Community Risk Control: Unhealthy Cultural Traditions 2805-Community Risk Control: Violence

BB-Community Well-Being

Outcomes that describe the overall health status
and social competence of a community or population

2700-Community Competence
2705-Community Disaster Recovery
2706-Community Grief Recovery
2701-Community Health Status
2800-Community Immune Status
2796-Community Immune Status: Adult
2797-Community Immune Status: School Age Child
2798-Community Immune Status: Young Child
2709-Community Pandemic Recovery
2704-Community Resilience
2702-Community Violence Level

References

1. Iowa Outcomes Project. (1997). *Taxonomy of nursing outcomes classification (NOC)*. IA: Iowa City.
2. Iowa Intervention Project. (1993). The NIC taxonomy structure. *IMAGE: Journal of Nursing Scholarship, 25*(3), 187–192.
3. Iowa Intervention Project. (1996). In J. C. McCloskey, & G. M. Bulechek (Eds.), *Nursing interventions classification (NIC)* (2nd ed.). Mosby.
4. Iowa Outcomes Project. (2000). In M. Johnson, M. Maas, & S. Moorhead (Eds.), *Nursing outcomes classification (NOC)* (2nd ed.). Mosby.
5. Moorhead, S., Head, B., Johnson, M., & Maas, M. (1998). The nursing outcomes taxonomy: Development and coding. *Journal of Nursing Care Quality, 12*(6), 56–63.
6. Moorhead, S., Johnson, M., & Maas, M. (Eds.). (2004). *Nursing outcomes classification (NOC)* (3rd ed.). Mosby.
7. Moorhead, S., Johnson, M., Maas, M., & Swanson, E. (Eds.). (2008). *Nursing outcomes classification (NOC)* (4th ed.). Mosby/Elsevier.
8. Moorhead, S., Johnson, M., Maas, M., & Swanson, E. (Eds.). (2013). *Nursing outcomes classification (NOC): Measurement of health outcomes* (5th ed.). Elsevier.
9. Moorhead, S., Swanson, E., Johnson, M., & Maas, M. (Eds.). (2018). *Nursing outcomes classification (NOC): Measurement of health outcomes* (6th ed.). Elsevier.

PART THREE

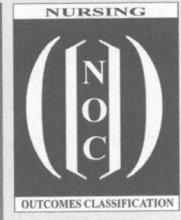

Outcomes

OVERVIEW

Part three contains 612 outcomes listed in alphabetical order in the seventh edition. Each outcome has an outcome label, definition, list of indicators, measurement scale(s), and content references. In addition, the code for each outcome is listed in the upper right corner. The indicators for the outcomes are configured with the first four numbers representing the outcome code and the last two numbers assigned to a specific indicator. This allows for 99 potential indicators for each outcome. For previously published outcomes, the indicators may not be in numerical order because as the outcomes are revised, some indicators may have been eliminated and others may have been shifted within the outcome, so they are presented in a logical order. Each outcome includes a space to record the outcome target rating that the patient and nurse set as a goal. Two options are available: maintain at a specific score (3, for example) or increase to a higher score than the patient is currently rated. Ideally, the nurse or patient depending on the outcomes provides an overall rating based on the review of the indicators for the outcome. This rating can be circled on the top rating scale. At the bottom of each outcome, there is a summary line that provides the domain and class of the outcome within the taxonomy and information about when it was first added to the classification. Following the original date of the outcome, are the years the outcome was revised or reviewed for outcomes included in more than one edition. A change in the outcome content is considered a *revision* when the definition, scale, or indicators are modified. As part of the revision process new content references are added based on a review of the literature. In most cases, the literature review is primarily based on articles published in English. For this edition, we were able to include research focused on validation of specific Nursing Outcomes Classification (NOC) outcomes.

In the case of outcomes that are in the reviewed category, no changes were made to the definition, scale, or indicators. This indicates that a search of the literature did not reveal any modifications were needed in the outcome label, definition, or list of indictors. When an outcome is reviewed, references for that outcome are evaluated and new references are added. For both revised and reviewed outcomes, we retain references that are considered foundational to the development of the outcome. If the class changes for an outcome, this is not considered a revision to the outcome but is reflected as a revision of the NOC taxonomy.

Some new, reviewed, or revised outcomes also include references for other measurement tools for the concept. They are identified with the symbol "+" before the reference. Many of these measurement tools were used when we did the original validation of the measurement scales. Details

of this research can be found in the third edition of Nursing Outcomes Classification (NOC) (Moorhead, et al., 2008). When a new outcome is developed, measurement scales focused on the concept are included in the content references.

For this edition we revised 371 outcomes by adding new content, reviewed 28 previously published outcomes without making content changes to the outcome, and retired 10 outcomes. In addition, 37 outcomes had label name changes, 87 outcomes had definition changes, and 63 had scale modifications. Most of the outcomes that were retired were revised as a new outcome and made more specific than the previous version. For example, the development outcomes focused on adults were organized into three age groups in the previous edition (*Development: Young Adulthood, Development: Middle Adulthood,* and *Development Late Adulthood*) and the literature review we conducted now uses four adult age groups, so these outcomes were modified to reflect this change in the theoretical literature. Most outcomes are revised during this process but some outcomes, especially those that are physiological in nature tend to remain stable over time.

The extensive revisions we did for this edition resulted in more label name changes than in the past. Here are some examples. We added the term "*behavior*" to the outcomes focused on self-care. These outcomes use the demonstrated scale to measure the indicators and we wanted to reinforce that these outcomes were not focused on the *ability* to perform the indicators but on the *action* of doing self-care. For example, *Self-Care: Bathing* became *Self-Care Behavior: Bathing.* A second example is we eliminated the use of the concept "compliance" in this edition to better fit the use of the concept in current literature. We chose to retain the concept "adherence" and modified the compliance outcomes to fit within this concept. *Compliance Behavior* (1601) was retired from the seventh edition and the outcomes *Compliance Behavior: Prescribed Activity* became *Adherence Behavior: Prescribed Activity* retaining the original code (1622). Two other compliance outcomes were modified in this way. Current literature uses the term compliance to refer to nurses' behavior, rather than that of the patient. A third example is we split the outcome *Sensory Function: Taste & Smell* into two outcomes: *Sensory Function: Smell* and *Sensory Function: Taste*. With loss of taste as a common symptom of SARS-CoV-2 (COVID-19), we felt measuring these concepts together was not helpful.

Appendix A contains a complete summary of the new, revised, reviewed, and retired outcomes for this edition. This includes outcomes with label name changes, definition changes, and scale changes. We believe this information is important for organizations and users who want to update their electronic health records and care planning systems.

Abstract Thinking   0919   A

Definition: Ability to recognize multiple meanings and patterns of concepts and generalize to new meanings, ideas, or contexts

OUTCOME TARGET RATING: Maintain at_____ Increase to_____

		Never Demonstrated	Rarely Demonstrated	Sometimes Demonstrated	Often Demonstrated	Consistently Demonstrated	
OUTCOME OVERALL RATING		1	2	3	4	5	
Indicators:							
091916	Identifies multiple meanings of a concept	1	2	3	4	5	NA
091917	Identifies separate components of a concept	1	2	3	4	5	NA
091918	Uses concrete thinking	1	2	3	4	5	NA
091919	Uses critical thinking	1	2	3	4	5	NA
091920	Uses creative thinking	1	2	3	4	5	NA
091921	Compares unfamiliar experiences to familiar ones	1	2	3	4	5	NA
091922	Uses memories to retrieve patterns of similar situations	1	2	3	4	5	NA
091923	Uses memories to assist in solving problems	1	2	3	4	5	NA
091924	Uses visual representations to accelerate understanding of concepts and relationships	1	2	3	4	5	NA
091925	Identifies missing concepts in abstract patterns	1	2	3	4	5	NA
091926	Uses previously understood concept relationships in judgments	1	2	3	4	5	NA
091927	Uses cues to identify new contexts	1	2	3	4	5	NA
091928	Uses complex problem-solving	1	2	3	4	5	NA
091929	Applies concepts to new contexts	1	2	3	4	5	NA
091930	Describes the thought process	1	2	3	4	5	NA
091931	Draws reasonable assertions or conclusions from inferences	1	2	3	4	5	NA
091932	Uses imagery as an abstract form of visual input	1	2	3	4	5	NA

Domain-Physiologic Health (II)   ***Class**-Neurocognitive (J)*   5th edition 2013; revised 2024

OUTCOME CONTENT REFERENCES:

Katz, S. J., & Byrne, S. (2019). Cognitive bridging: Using strategic communication to connect abstract goals with the means to achieve them. *Health Communication, 34*(4), 484–499. https://www.doi.org/10.1080/10410236.2018.1428848

Potter, P. A., Perry, A. G., Stockert, P. A., & Hall, A. M. (2021). *Fundamentals of nursing* (10th ed.). Elsevier.

Williams, P. (2020). *Basic geriatric nursing* (7th ed.). Elsevier.

Zebehazy, K. T., Weber, R. C., Murphy, M., & Ghani, A. (2020). Divergent thinking: The performance of students with visual impairments on abstract and scenario-based tasks and their correlates. *Journal of Visual Impairment & Blindness, 114*(4), 301–314. https://www.doi.org/10.1177/0145-482X20940101

Abuse Cessation 2500

Definition: Evidence that the victim is no longer hurt or exploited

OUTCOME TARGET RATING: Maintain at_____ Increase to_____

OUTCOME OVERALL RATING		None 1	Limited 2	Moderate 3	Substantial 4	Extensive 5	
Indicators:							
250002	Evidence that physical abuse has ceased	1	2	3	4	5	NA
250003	Evidence that emotional abuse has ceased	1	2	3	4	5	NA
250004	Evidence that sexual abuse has ceased	1	2	3	4	5	NA
250006	Evidence that financial exploitation has ceased	1	2	3	4	5	NA

Domain-Family Health (VI)   **Class**-Family Member Health Status (Z)   *1st edition 1997; revised 2004; reviewed 2018*

OUTCOME CONTENT REFERENCES:

Bhilwar, M., Upadhyay, R. P., Rajavel, S., Singh, S. K., Vasudevan, K., & Chinnakali, P. (2015). Childhood experiences of physical, emotional and sexual abuse among college students in South India. *Journal of Tropical Pediatrics, 61*(5), 329–338. https://doi.org/10.1093/tropej/fmv037

Cowen, P. S. (1991). *The Iowa crisis nursery project as a factor in the prevention of child abuse.* Dissertation Abstracts International, *52*(8-A) (UMI No. 9136912).

Gassoumis, Z., Navarro, A., & Wilber, K. H. (2015). Protecting victims of elder financial exploitation: The role of an elder abuse forensic center in referring victims for conservatorship. *Aging & Mental Health, 19*(9), 790–798. https://doi.org/10.1080/13607863.2014.962011

Nanda, M. M., Reichert, E., Jones, U. J., & Flannery-Schroeder, E. (2016). Childhood maltreatment and symptoms of social anxiety: Exploring the role of emotional abuse, neglect, and cumulative trauma. *Journal of Child & Adolescent Trauma, 9*(3), 201–207. https://doi.org/10.1007/s40653-015-0070-z

+Postmus, J. L., Stylianou, A. M., & McMahon, S. (2016). The Abusive Behavior Inventory- revisited. *Journal of Interpersonal Violence, 31*(17), 2867–2888. https://doi.org/10.1177/0886260515581882

+Shepard, M., & Campbell, J. A. (1992). The Abusive Behavior Inventory: A measure of psychological and physical abuse. *Journal of Interpersonal Violence, 7*(3), 291–305.

Wang, J. J., Lin, J. N., & Lee, F. P. (2006). Psychologically abusive behaviors by those caring for the elderly in a domestic context. *Geriatric Nursing, 27*(5), 284–291. https://doi.org/10.1016/j.gerinurse.2006.08.016

Abuse: Disruptive Effects 2515

Definition: Severity of observed or reported disruptive effects due to experiences of emotional, physical, sexual abuse, and financial exploitation

OUTCOME TARGET RATING: Maintain at_____ Increase to_____

OUTCOME OVERALL RATING		Severe 1	Substantial 2	Moderate 3	Mild 4	None 5	
Indicators:							
251501	Anxiety	1	2	3	4	5	NA
251502	Anger	1	2	3	4	5	NA
251503	Impaired mental health	1	2	3	4	5	NA
251504	Depression	1	2	3	4	5	NA
251505	Fear	1	2	3	4	5	NA
251506	Panic	1	2	3	4	5	NA
251507	Hopelessness	1	2	3	4	5	NA
251508	Neurotic behaviors	1	2	3	4	5	NA
251509	Antisocial behaviors	1	2	3	4	5	NA
251510	Trauma-induced psychoneurotic behaviors	1	2	3	4	5	NA
251511	Malnutrition	1	2	3	4	5	NA
251512	Alcohol consumption	1	2	3	4	5	NA
251513	Substance abuse of opioids	1	2	3	4	5	NA
251514	Substance abuse of cocaine	1	2	3	4	5	NA
251515	Smoking	1	2	3	4	5	NA
251516	Impaired physical health	1	2	3	4	5	NA

Abuse: Disruptive Effects—cont'd

		Severe	Substantial	Moderate	Mild	None	
251517	Bodily complaints (somatic)	1	2	3	4	5	NA
251518	Sleep disruptions	1	2	3	4	5	NA
251519	Food insecurity	1	2	3	4	5	NA
251520	Housing instability	1	2	3	4	5	NA
251521	Financial hardship	1	2	3	4	5	NA
251522	Delinquency	1	2	3	4	5	NA
251523	Criminal behaviors	1	2	3	4	5	NA
251524	Communication ability delay	1	2	3	4	5	NA
251525	Developmental delay	1	2	3	4	5	NA
251526	Self-injurious behaviors	1	2	3	4	5	NA
251527	Suicide ideation	1	2	3	4	5	NA
251528	Suicide attempts	1	2	3	4	5	NA
251529	Injurious behaviors toward others	1	2	3	4	5	NA
251530	Need of restraining order	1	2	3	4	5	NA
251531	Intimate partner violence	1	2	3	4	5	NA
251532	Venerable victim to abuse	1	2	3	4	5	NA
251533	Neglectful parenting	1	2	3	4	5	NA
251534	Violence based parenting	1	2	3	4	5	NA
251535	Sexual difficulties	1	2	3	4	5	NA
251536	Isolation	1	2	3	4	5	NA
251537	Hopelessness	1	2	3	4	5	NA

Domain-Health & Life Quality (V)   *Class*-Symptom Status (V)   7th edition 2024

OUTCOME CONTENT REFERENCES:

Carr, A. (2018). Couple therapy, family therapy and systemic interventions for adult-focused problems. *Journal of Family Therapy, 41*(4), 492–536. https://doi.org/10.1111/1467-6427.12225

Carr, A. (2019). Family therapy and systemic interventions for child-focused problems: The current evidence base. *Journal of Family Therapy, 41*(2), 153–213. https://doi.org/10.1111/1467-6427.12226

Crowder, J., Burnett, C., Laughon, K., & Dreisbach, C. (2019). Elder abuse in American Indian communities: An integrative review. *Journal of Forensic Nursing, 15*(4), 250–258. https://doi.org/10.1097/JFN.0000000000000259

Cui, N., & Liu, J. (2020). Physical abuse, emotional abuse, and neglect and childhood behavior problems: A meta-analysis of studies in mainland China. *Trauma, Violence, & Abuse, 21*(1), 206–224. https://doi.org/10.1177/1524838018757750

Digman, C. (2020). Lost voices part 2: Modifying psychological therapies for two young men with complex learning disabilities following alleged sexual and physical abuse: A case study in trauma recovery. *British Journal of Learning Disabilities, 49*(2), 205–216. https://doi.org/10.1111/bld.12370

Lange, B. C., Condon, E. M., & Gardner, F. (2019). A systematic review of the association between the childhood sexual abuse experiences of mothers and the abuse status of their children: Protection strategies, intergenerational transmission, and reactions to the abuse of their children. *Social Science & Medicine, 233*, 113–137. https://doi.org/10.1016/j.socscimed.2019.05.004

Lansford, J. E., Godwin, J., McMahon, R. J., Crowley, M., Pettit, G. S., Bates, J. E., Cole, J. D., & Dodge, K. A. (2021). Early physical abuse and adult outcomes. *Pediatrics, 147*(1), e20200873. https://doi.org/10.1542/peds.2020-0873

McCarthy, A., Cyr, M., Fernet, M., & Hébert, M. (2019). Maternal emotional support following the disclosure of child sexual abuse: A qualitative study. *Journal of Child Sexual Abuse, 28*(3), 259–279. https://doi.org/10.1080/10538712.2018.1534919

Makaroun, L. K., Bachrach, R. L., & Rosland, A. M. (2020). Elder abuse in the time of COVID-19: Increased risks for older adults and their caregivers. *The American Journal of Geriatric Psychiatry, 28*(8), 8756–880. https://doi.org/10.1016/j.jagp.2020.05.017

Palmer, C. J., Williams, Y., & Harrington, A. (2019). Repairing the effects of childhood trauma: The long and winding road. *Journal of Psychiatric and Mental Health Nursing. 27*(3), 205–210. https://doi.org/10.1111/jpm.12581

Schuster, I., & Tomaszewska, P. (2021). Pathways from child sexual and physical abuse to sexual and physical intimate partner violence victimization through attitudes toward intimate partner violence. *Journal of Family Violence, 36*(4), 443–453. https://doi.org/10.1007/s10896-020-00180-2

Sierau, S., Warmingham, J., White, L. O., Klein, A. M., & von Klitzing, K. (2020). Childhood emotional and conduct problems in childhood and adolescence differentially associated with intergenerational maltreatment continuity and parental internalizing symptoms. *Journal of Abnormal Child Psychology, 48*(1), 29–42. https://doi.org/10.1007/s10802-019-00575-w

Thulin, J., Kjellgren, C., & Nilsson, D. (2019). Children's experiences with an intervention aimed to prevent further physical abuse. *Child & Family Social Work, 24*(1), 17–24. https://doi.org/10.1111/cfs.12476

Widom, C. S. (2017). Long term impact of childhood abuse and neglect on crime and violence. *Clinical Psychology: Science and Practice, 24*(2), 186–202. https://doi.org/10.1111/cpsp.12194

Wilson, P. R., Thorpe, R. J. Jr., Sharps, P., & Laughon, K. (2021). The relationship between housing instability and intimate partner violence: A retrospective study. *Public Health Nursing, 38*(1), 32–39. https://doi.org/10.1111/phn.12819

Yoon, S., Cummings, S., Nugent, W., & Forrest-Bank, S. (2020). Protective factors against suicidal ideation among community-dwelling older adults with experience of spousal physical abuse: Focusing on direct and indirect protections. *Aging & Mental Health, 24*(11), 1854–1863. https://doi.org/10.1080/13607863.2019.1636208

A

Abuse Protection

2501

Definition: Protection of self and/or dependent others from abuse

OUTCOME TARGET RATING: Maintain at_____ Increase to_____

OUTCOME OVERALL RATING	Never Demonstrated 1	Rarely Demonstrated 2	Sometimes Demonstrated 3	Often Demonstrated 4	Consistently Demonstrated 5	
Indicators:						
250117 Prepares to leave situation	1	2	3	4	5	NA
250118 Provides safe residence	1	2	3	4	5	NA
250119 Reports plan for avoiding abuse	1	2	3	4	5	NA
250120 Implements plan to avoid abuse	1	2	3	4	5	NA
250121 Reports plan for haven	1	2	3	4	5	NA
250122 Provides safety of self	1	2	3	4	5	NA
250123 Provides safety of children	1	2	3	4	5	NA
250124 Reports having mental plan to disconnect from abuser	1	2	3	4	5	NA
250125 Limits contact with abuser	1	2	3	4	5	NA
250126 Maintains self-advocacy	1	2	3	4	5	NA
250127 Facilitates access to counseling for abused person	1	2	3	4	5	NA
250128 Plans to withdraw when relationship is unsafe	1	2	3	4	5	NA
250129 Reports severance of relationship with abuser	1	2	3	4	5	NA
250130 Provides safety of dependent adult	1	2	3	4	5	NA
250131 Uses restraining order	1	2	3	4	5	NA
250132 Uses resources for social support	1	2	3	4	5	NA
250133 Uses formal help-seeking strategies	1	2	3	4	5	NA
250134 Uses coping strategies	1	2	3	4	5	NA
250135 Receives support from a confidant	1	2	3	4	5	NA

Domain-*Family Health (VI)*   **Class**-*Family Member Health Status (Z)*   *1st edition 1997; revised 2004, 2008, 2024*

OUTCOME CONTENT REFERENCES:

Bermea, A. M., Khaw, L., Hardesty, J. L., Rosenbloom, L., & Salerno, C. (2020). Mental and active preparation: Examining variations in women's processes of preparing to leave abusive relationships. *Journal of Interpersonal Violence, 35*(3-4), 988–1011. https://doi.org/10.1177/0886260517692332

Kennedy, C., & Will, J. (2021). Interventions for preventing abuse in the elderly. *International Journal of Nursing Practice, 27*, e12870, 1–3. https://doi.org/10.1111/ijn.12870

Weisz, A., & Schell, M. (2020). Responding to intimate partner violence: Urban women's decisions about getting personal protection orders when other resources are scare. *Violence Against Women, 26*(1), 243–261. https://doi.org/10.1177/1077801219854537

Yoon, S., Cummings, S., Nugent, W. R., & Forrest-Bank, S. (2020). Protective factors against suicidal ideation among community-dwelling older adults with experience of spousal physical abuse: Focusing on direct and indirect protections. *Aging & Mental Health, 24*(11), 1854–1863. https://doi.org/10.1080/13607863.2019.1636208

Abuse Recovery   2514

Definition: Personal actions to promote healing of physical or psychological abuse that may include sexual or financial exploitation

OUTCOME TARGET RATING: Maintain at_____ Increase to_____

		Never Demonstrated	Rarely Demonstrated	Sometimes Demonstrated	Often Demonstrated	Consistently Demonstrated	
OUTCOME OVERALL RATING		1	2	3	4	5	
Indicators:							
251411	Seeks medical treatment for injuries	1	2	3	4	5	NA
251412	Recognizes characteristics of abusive relationship(s)	1	2	3	4	5	NA
251413	Reports healing of psychological injuries	1	2	3	4	5	NA
251414	Reports healing of physical injuries	1	2	3	4	5	NA
251416	Controls personal finances following financial exploitation	1	2	3	4	5	NA
251417	Controls legal matters following financial exploitation	1	2	3	4	5	NA
251418	Exhibits self-esteem	1	2	3	4	5	NA
251419	Expressed feelings of empowerment	1	2	3	4	5	NA
251420	Establishes interpersonal relationships	1	2	3	4	5	NA
251421	Maintains positive interpersonal relationships	1	2	3	4	5	NA
251422	Avoids contact with abuser	1	2	3	4	5	NA
251423	Keeps appointments with health professional	1	2	3	4	5	NA

Domain-Family Health (VI)   **Class**-Family Member Health Status (Z)   *3rd edition 2004; revised 2008, 2024*

OUTCOME CONTENT REFERENCES:

Carr, A. (2018). Couple therapy, family therapy and systemic interventions for adult-focused problems. *Journal of Family Therapy 40*(4), 492–536. https://doi.org/10.1111/1467-6427.12225

Carr, A. (2019). Family therapy and systemic interventions for child-focused problems: The current evidence base. *Journal of Family Therapy, 41*(2), 153–213. https://doi.org/10.1111/1467-6427.12226

Cui, N., & Liu, J. (2020). Physical abuse, emotional abuse, and neglect and childhood behavior problems: A meta-analysis of studies in mainland China. *Trauma, Violence, & Abuse, 21*(1), 206–224. https://doi.org/10.1177/1524838018757750

Lansford, J. E., Godwin, J., McMahon, R. J., Crowley, M., Pettit, G. S., Bates, J. E., Cole, J. D., & Dodge, K. A. (2021). Early physical abuse and adult outcomes. *Pediatrics, 147*(1), e20200873. https://doi.org/10.1542/peds.2020-0873

Lee, K., Tang, W., Jones, S., Xu, L., & Cong, Z. (2021). The money smart for older adults' program: A qualitative study of the participants' financial well-being. *Journal of Gerontological Social Work, 64*(2), 120–134. https://doi.org/10.1080/01634372.2020.1814477

Lichtenberg, P. A, Gross, E., & Ficker, L. J. (2020). Quantifying risk of financial incapacity and financial exploitation in community-dwelling older adults: Utility of a scoring system for the Lichtenberg Financial Decision-Making Rating Scale. *Clinical Gerontologist, 36*(2), 132–146. https://doi.org/10.1080/07317115.2018.1485812

Russo, A., Reginelli, A., Pignatiello, M., Cioce, F., Mazzei, G., Fabozzi, O., Parlato, V., Cappabianca, S., & Giovine, S. (2018). Imaging of violence against the elderly and the women. *Seminars in Ultrasound, CT, and MRI, 40*, 18–24. https://doi.org/10.1053/j.sult.2018.10.004

Salimath, G., & Raddi, S. A. (2020). Correlation between physical abuse and depression among school going adolescents (10–16 years of age) - A school-based study. *Online Journal of Health and Allied Sciences, 19*(2), 1–5.

Wilson, P. R., Thorpe, R. J. Jr., Sharps, P., & Laughon, K. (2019). The relationship between housing instability and intimate partner violence: A retrospective study. *Public Health Nursing, 38*, 32–39. https://doi.org/10.1111/phn.12819

Yoon, S., Cummings, S., Nugent, W. R., & Forrest-Bank, S. (2020). Protective factors against suicidal ideation among community-dwelling older adults with experience of spousal physical abuse: Focusing on direct and indirect protections. *Aging & Mental Health, 24*(11), 1854–1863. https://doi.org/10.1080/13607863.2019.1636208

A

Abuse Recovery: Emotional 2502

Definition: Personal actions to heal from psychological injuries due to abuse

OUTCOME TARGET RATING: Maintain at_____ Increase to_____

OUTCOME OVERALL RATING		Never Demonstrated	Rarely Demonstrated	Sometimes Demonstrated	Often Demonstrated	Consistently Demonstrated	
		1	2	3	4	5	
Indicators:							
250224	Expresses self-confidence	1	2	3	4	5	NA
250225	Exhibits self-esteem	1	2	3	4	5	NA
250226	Exhibits self-sufficiency	1	2	3	4	5	NA
250227	Uses anxiety management strategies	1	2	3	4	5	NA
250228	Uses problem-solving strategies	1	2	3	4	5	NA
250229	Uses coping strategies	1	2	3	4	5	NA
250230	Exhibits affect appropriate for situation	1	2	3	4	5	NA
250231	Controls impulses	1	2	3	4	5	NA
250232	Advocates for self	1	2	3	4	5	NA
250233	Trusts others	1	2	3	4	5	NA
250234	Expresses feelings of independence	1	2	3	4	5	NA
250235	Expresses feelings of empowerment	1	2	3	4	5	NA
250236	Recognizes characteristics of abusive relationships	1	2	3	4	5	NA
250237	Expresses insight into abusive relationship	1	2	3	4	5	NA
250238	Resolves feelings about abuse	1	2	3	4	5	NA
250239	Resolves guilt	1	2	3	4	5	NA
250240	Interacts socially with others	1	2	3	4	5	NA
250241	Maintains positive interpersonal relationships	1	2	3	4	5	NA
250242	Adjusts to change in living arrangements	1	2	3	4	5	NA
250243	Avoids contact with abuser	1	2	3	4	5	NA

Domain-Family Health (VI)   **Class**-Family Member Health Status (Z)   *1st edition 1997; revised 2004, 2013, 2024*

OUTCOME CONTENT REFERENCES:

Carr, A. (2018). Couple therapy, family therapy and systemic interventions for adult-focused problems. *Journal of Family Therapy, 40*(4), 492–536. https://doi.org/10.1111/1467-6427.12225

Carr, A. (2019). Family therapy and systemic interventions for child-focused problems: The current evidence base. *Journal of Family Therapy, 41*(2), 153–213. https://doi.org/10.1111/1467-6427.12226

Cui, N., & Liu, J. (2020). Physical abuse, emotional abuse, and neglect and childhood behavior problems: A meta-analysis of studies in mainland China. *Trauma, Violence, & Abuse, 21*(1), 206–224. https://doi.org/10.1177/1524838018757750

Digman, C. (2020). Lost voices part 2: Modifying psychological therapies for two young men with complex learning disabilities following alleged sexual and physical abuse: A case study in trauma recovery. *British Journal of Learning Disability, 49*(2), 205–216. https://doi.org/10.1111/bld.12370

Palmer, C. J., Williams, Y., & Harrington, A. (2019). Explaining the effects of childhood trauma: The long and winding road. *Journal of Psychiatric and Mental Health Nursing, 27*(2), 205–210. https://doi.org/10.1111/jpm.12581

Sierau, S., Warmingham, J., White, L. O., Klein, A. M., & von Klitzing, K. (2020). Childhood emotional and conduct problems in childhood and adolescence differentially associated with intergenerational maltreatment continuity and parental internalizing symptoms. *Journal of Abnormal Child Psychology, 48*(1), 29–42. https://doi.org/10.1007/s10802-019-00575-w

Widom, C. S. (2017). Long-term impact of childhood abuse and neglect on crime and violence. *Clinical Psychology: Science and Practice. 24*(2), 186–202. https://doi.org/10.1111/cpsp.12194

Abuse Recovery: Financial

2503

Definition: Personal actions to control investments, money, property, or legal matters following financial exploitation

OUTCOME TARGET RATING: Maintain at_____ Increase to_____

		Never Demonstrated	Rarely Demonstrated	Sometimes Demonstrated	Often Demonstrated	Consistently Demonstrated	
OUTCOME OVERALL RATING		1	2	3	4	5	
Indicators:							
250317	Exhibits financial independence	1	2	3	4	5	NA
250318	Expresses ability to pay bills	1	2	3	4	5	NA
250319	Develops financial literacy	1	2	3	4	5	NA
250320	Controls personal possessions	1	2	3	4	5	NA
250321	Manages personal finances	1	2	3	4	5	NA
250322	Balances personal bank account	1	2	3	4	5	NA
250323	Controls withdrawal of money from account(s)	1	2	3	4	5	NA
250324	Controls social security and pension income	1	2	3	4	5	NA
250325	Controls earned income	1	2	3	4	5	NA
250326	Controls court-ordered benefits	1	2	3	4	5	NA
250327	Protects financial resources	1	2	3	4	5	NA
250328	Protects personal identity	1	2	3	4	5	NA
250329	Monitors financial resources	1	2	3	4	5	NA
250330	Makes informed financial decisions	1	2	3	4	5	NA
250331	Explains legal matters	1	2	3	4	5	NA
250332	Controls legal matters	1	2	3	4	5	NA
250333	Exercises legal rights	1	2	3	4	5	NA
250334	Participates in financial planning	1	2	3	4	5	NA
250335	Acknowledges investment risks	1	2	3	4	5	NA
250336	Acknowledges importance of financial well-being	1	2	3	4	5	NA

Domain-Family Health (VI)   *Class*-Family Member Health Status (Z)   *1st edition 1997; revised 2004, 2008, 2013, 2024*

OUTCOME CONTENT REFERENCES:

Acierno, R., Hernandez-Tejada, M. A., Anetzberger, G. J., Loew, D., & Muzzy, W. (2017). The national elder mistreatment study: An 8-year longitudinal study of outcomes. *Journal of Elder Abuse & Neglect, 29*(4), 254–269. https://doi.org/10.1080/08946566.2017.1365031

Coluccia, A., Pozza, A., Ferretti, F., Carabellese, E., Masti, A., & Gualtieri, G. (2020). Online romance scams: Relational dynamics and psychological characteristics of the victims and scammers. A scoping review. *Clinical Practice and Epidemiology in Mental Health, 16*, 24–35. https://doi.org/10.2174/1745017902016010024

Lee, K., Tang, W., Jones, S., Xu, L., & Cong, Z. (2021). The money smart for older adults' program: A qualitative study of the participants' financial well-being. *Journal of Gerontological Social Work, 64*(2), 120–134. https://doi.org/10.1080/01634372.2020.1814477

+Lictenberg, P. A., Gross, E., & Ficker, L. J. (2020). Quantifying risk of financial incapacity and financial exploitation in community-dwelling older adults: Utility of a scoring system for the Lichtenberg Financial Decision-Making Rating Scale. *Clinical Gerontologist, 36*(2), 132–146. https://doi.org/10.1080/073171115.2018.1485812

Nguyen, A. L., Mosqueda, L., Windisch, N., Weissberger, G., Axelrod, J., & Han, S. D. (2021). Perceived types, causes, and consequences of financial exploitation: Narratives from older adults. *The Journal of Gerontology: Series B, 76*(5), 996–1004. https://doi.org/10.1093/geronb/gbab01

Santos, A. M. R., Nolêto, R. D. S., Rodrigues, R. A. P., Andrade, E. M. L. R., Bonfim, E. G., & Rodrigues, T. S. (2019). Economic-financial and patrimonial elder abuse: A documentary study. *Revista da Escola de Enfermagem da USP, 53*, e03417. https://doi.org/10.1590/S1980-220X20170438003417

A

Abuse Recovery: Physical 2504

Definition: Personal actions to heal physical injuries due to abuse

OUTCOME TARGET RATING: Maintain at_____ Increase to_____

OUTCOME OVERALL RATING	Never Demonstrated	Rarely Demonstrated	Sometimes Demonstrated	Often Demonstrated	Consistently Demonstrated	
	1	2	3	4	5	
Indicators:						
250412 Seeks medical treatment for injuries	1	2	3	4	5	NA
250413 Implements treatment plan	1	2	3	4	5	NA
250414 Exhibits expected response to treatment	1	2	3	4	5	NA
250415 Uses therapeutic health care as needed	1	2	3	4	5	NA
250416 Keep appointments with health professional	1	2	3	4	5	NA
250417 Reports healing of physical injuries	1	2	3	4	5	NA
250418 Uses preventive health care services	1	2	3	4	5	NA
250419 Avoids contact with abuser	1	2	3	4	5	NA

Domain-Family Health (VI)   **Class**-Family Member Health Status (Z)   *1st edition 1997; revised 2004, 2008, 2024*

OUTCOME CONTENT REFERENCES:

Cui, N., & Liu, J. (2020). Physical abuse, emotional abuse, and neglect and childhood behavior problems: A meta-analysis of studies in mainland China. *Trauma, Violence, & Abuse, 21*(1), 206–224. https://doi.org/10.1177/1524838018757750

Lansford, J. E., Godwin, J., McMahon, R. J., Crowley, M., Pettit, G. S., Bates, J. E., Cole, J. D., & Dodge, K. A. (2021). Early physical abuse and adult outcomes. *Pediatrics, 147*(1), e20200873. https://doi.org/10.1542/peds.2020-0873

Salimath, G., & Raddi, S. A. (2020). Correlation between physical abuse and depression among school going adolescents (10–16 years of age)—A school-based study. *Online Journal of Health and Allied Sciences, 19*(2), 1–5.

Wilson, P. R., Thorpe, R. J. Jr., Sharps, P., & Laughon, K. (2019). The relationship between housing instability and intimate partner violence: A retrospective study. *Public Health Nursing, 38*(1), 32–39. https://doi.org/10.1111/phn.12819

Yoon, S., Cummings, S., Nugent, W. R., & Forrest-Bank, S. (2020). Protective factors against suicidal ideation among community-dwelling older adults with experience of spousal physical abuse: Focusing on direct and indirect protections. *Aging & Mental Health, 24*(11), 1854–1863. https://doi.org/10.1080/13607863.2019.1636208

Abuse Recovery: Sexual 2505

Definition: Personal actions to heal physical and psychological injuries due to sexual abuse or exploitation

OUTCOME TARGET RATING: Maintain at_____ Increase to_____

OUTCOME OVERALL RATING	Never Demonstrated	Rarely Demonstrated	Sometimes Demonstrated	Often Demonstrated	Consistently Demonstrated	
	1	2	3	4	5	
Indicators:						
250528 Acknowledges right to disclose abusive situation	1	2	3	4	5	NA
250529 Expresses right to have been protected from abuse	1	2	3	4	5	NA
250530 Willingness to accept support	1	2	3	4	5	NA
250531 Seeks medical treatment for injuries	1	2	3	4	5	NA
250532 Exhibits emotional stability	1	2	3	4	5	NA
250533 Trusts others	1	2	3	4	5	NA
250534 Uses strategies to control anger in non-destructive ways	1	2	3	4	5	NA
250535 Advocates for self	1	2	3	4	5	NA
250536 Expresses self-compassion	1	2	3	4	5	NA

Abuse Recovery: Sexual—cont'd

		Never Demonstrated	Rarely Demonstrated	Sometimes Demonstrated	Often Demonstrated	Consistently Demonstrated	
250537	Expresses self-worth	1	2	3	4	5	NA
250538	Exhibits feelings of empowerment	1	2	3	4	5	NA
250539	Expresses hope	1	2	3	4	5	NA
250540	Maintains behaviors within social norms	1	2	3	4	5	NA
250541	Expresses affection toward others	1	2	3	4	5	NA
250542	Expresses comfort with gender identity	1	2	3	4	5	NA
250543	Expresses comfort with sexual orientation	1	2	3	4	5	NA
250544	Verbalizes accurate information about sexual functioning	1	2	3	4	5	NA
250545	Resolves feelings about abuse	1	2	3	4	5	NA
250546	Resolves guilt	1	2	3	4	5	NA
250547	Reports healing of physical injuries	1	2	3	4	5	NA
250548	Keeps appointment with health professional	1	2	3	4	5	NA
250549	Avoids contact with abuser	1	2	3	4	5	NA

Domain-Family Health (VI)   **Class**-Family Member Health Status (Z)   *1st edition 1997; revised 2004, 2013, 2024*

OUTCOME CONTENT REFERENCES:

Alix, S., Cossette, L., Cyr, M., Frappier, J. Y., Caron, P. O., & Hébert, M. (2020). Self-blame, shame, avoidance, and suicidal ideation in sexually abused adolescent girls: A longitudinal study. *Journal of Child Sexual Abuse, 29*(4), 432–447. https://doi.org/10.1080/10538712.2019.1678543

Carr, A. (2018). Couple therapy, family therapy and systemic interventions for adult-focused problems. *Journal of Family Therapy, 40*(4), 492–536. https://doi.org/10.1111/1467-6427.12225

Digman, C. (2020). Lost voices part 2: Modifying psychological therapies for two young men with complex learning disabilities following alleged sexual and physical abuse: A case study in trauma recovery. *British Journal of Learning Disabilities, 49*(2), 205–216. https://doi.org/10.1111/bld.12370

Gueta, K., Cohen-Leibovich, Y., & Tonel, N. (2021). "Even crap can be fertilizer": The experience of volunteering at sexual assault crisis center for women survivors of sexual assault. *Feminism & Psychology, 31*(20), 270–290. https://doi.org/10.1177/0959353520955141

Karlsson, M. E., Zielinski, M. J., & Bridges, A. J. (2020). Replicating outcomes of survivors healing from abuse: Recovery through Exposure (SHARE): A brief exposure-based group treatment for incarcerated survivors of sexual violence. *Psychological Trauma: Theory, Research, Practice, and Policy, 12*(3), 300–305. https://doi.org/10.1037/tra0000504

Kirkner, A., Relyea, M., & Ullman, S. E. (2019). Predicting the effects of sexual assault research participation: Reactions, perceived insight, and help-seeking. *Journal of Interpersonal Violence, 34*(17), 3592–3713. https://doi.org/10.1177/0886260516670882

MacGinley, M., Breckenridge, J., & Mowll, J. (2019). A scoping review of adult survivors' experience of shame following sexual abuse in childhood. *Health & Social Care in the Community, 27*(5), 1135–1146. https://doi.org/10.1111/hsc.12771

McLean, L., Bambling, M., & Steindl, S. R. (2021). Perspectives on self-compassion form adult female survivors of sexual abused and the counselors who work with them. *Journal of Interpersonal Violence, 36*(9-10), NP4564–NP4587. https://doi.org/10.1177/0886260518793975

Palmer, C. J., Williams, Y., & Harrington, A. (2019). Explaining the effects of childhood trauma: The long and winding road. *Journal of Psychiatric Mental Health Nursing. 27*(1), 205–210. https://doi.org/10.1111/jpm.12581

Salimath, G., & Raddi, S. A. (2020). Correlation between physical abuse and depression among school going adolescents (10–16 years of age) - A school-based study. *Online Journal of Health and Allied Sciences, 19*(2), 1–5.

Sierau, S., Warmingham, J., White, L. O., Klein, A. M., & von Klitzing, K. (2020). Childhood emotional and conduct problems in childhood and adolescence differentially associated with intergenerational maltreatment continuity and parental internalizing symptoms. *Journal of Abnormal Child Psychology, 48,* 29–42. https://doi.org/10.1007/s10802-019-00575-w

Widom, C. S. (2017). Long term impact of childhood abuse and neglect on crime and violence. *Clinical Psychology: Science and Practice. 24*(2), 186–202. https://doi.org/10.1111/cpsp.12194

Yoon, S., Cummings, S., Nugent, W. R., & Forrest-Bank, S. (2020). Protective factors against suicidal ideation among community-dwelling older adults with experience of spousal physical abuse: Focusing on direct and indirect protections. *Aging & Mental Health, 24*(11), 1854–1863. https://doi.org/10.1080/13607863.2019.1636208

A

Abusive Behavior Self-Restraint 1400

Definition: Personal actions to refrain from emotional, physical, sexual, and financial abusive and neglectful behaviors towards others

OUTCOME TARGET RATING: Maintain at_____ Increase to_____

	Never Demonstrated	Rarely Demonstrated	Sometimes Demonstrated	Often Demonstrated	Consistently Demonstrated	
OUTCOME OVERALL RATING	1	2	3	4	5	
Indicators:						
140029 Obtains needed mental health treatment	1	2	3	4	5	NA
140030 Obtains needed physical health treatment	1	2	3	4	5	NA
140020 Participates in required treatment regimens	1	2	3	4	5	NA
140031 Uses substance abuse services	1	2	3	4	5	NA
140007 Identifies factors contributing to abusive behavior	1	2	3	4	5	NA
140006 Discusses the abusive behavior	1	2	3	4	5	NA
140032 Uses strategies to deal with frustrations	1	2	3	4	5	NA
140033 Uses strategies to deal with conflicts	1	2	3	4	5	NA
140034 Uses strategies to deal with anxiety	1	2	3	4	5	NA
140035 Uses strategies for anger management	1	2	3	4	5	NA
140036 Uses strategies to control aggression	1	2	3	4	5	NA
140037 Uses strategies to control impulses	1	2	3	4	5	NA
140005 Uses alternative coping mechanisms for stress	1	2	3	4	5	NA
140038 Identifies basic needs of significant others	1	2	3	4	5	NA
140039 Participates in providing basic needs to significant others	1	2	3	4	5	NA
140040 Participates in child-rearing classes	1	2	3	4	5	NA
140018 Uses correct role behaviors	1	2	3	4	5	NA
140041 Adapts positive attitudes toward child-rearing	1	2	3	4	5	NA
140024 Uses appropriate caregiving techniques	1	2	3	4	5	NA
140013 States expectations congruent with developmental level	1	2	3	4	5	NA
140042 Uses strategies to cope with disabilities of others	1	2	3	4	5	NA
140023 Uses personal support system	1	2	3	4	5	NA
140025 Refrains from physically abusive behavior	1	2	3	4	5	NA
140026 Refrains from emotionally abusive behavior	1	2	3	4	5	NA
140027 Refrains from sexually abusive behavior	1	2	3	4	5	NA
140043 Refrains from financial abusive behavior	1	2	3	4	5	NA
140028 Refrains from neglect of dependent's basic needs	1	2	3	4	5	NA
140008 Expresses feelings about victim	1	2	3	4	5	NA
140016 Expresses empathy for victim	1	2	3	4	5	NA

A

Abusive Behavior Self-Restraint—cont'd

	Never Demonstrated	Rarely Demonstrated	Sometimes Demonstrated	Often Demonstrated	Consistently Demonstrated	
140011 Uses nurturing behavior toward victim	1	2	3	4	5	NA
140044 Recognizes when to contact health professionals for assistance	1	2	3	4	5	NA
140009 Identifies available community resources	1	2	3	4	5	NA

Domain-Psychosocial Health (III)   **Class**-Self-Control (O)   *1st edition 1997; revised 2000, 2004, 2008, 2013, 2024*

OUTCOME CONTENT REFERENCES:

Ellis, A. E., Simiola, V., Mackintosh, M. A., Schlaudt, V. A., & Cook, J. A. (2020). Perceived helpfulness and engagement in mental health treatment: A study of male survivors of sexual abuse. *Psychology of Men & Masculinities, 21*(4), 632–642. https://doi.org/10.1037/men0000313

Gülirmak, K., & Orak, O. S. (2021). Effectiveness of web-based distance education for parents in the prevention of emotional neglect and abuse: A randomized controlled study. *Perspectives in Psychiatric Care, 57*(2), 573–582. https://doi.org/10.1111/ppc.12580

Hefti, S., Pérez, T., Fürstenau, U., Rhiner, B., Swenson, C. C., & Schmid, M. (2020). Multisystemic therapy for child abuse and neglect: Do parents show improvement in parental mental health problems and parental stress? *Journal of Marital and Family Therapy, 46*(1), 95–109. https://doi.org/10.1111/jmft.12367

Iob, E., Steptoe, A., & Fancourt, D. (2020). Abuse, self-harm and suicidal ideation in the UK during the COVID-19 pandemic. *The British Journal of Psychiatry, 217*(4), 543–546. https://doi.org/10.1192/bjp.2020.130

Johnson, E. J. (2020). An exploratory study on the prevention of school children for violence and abuse. *Journal of Human Behavior in the Social Environment, 30*(4), 399–409. https://doi.org/10.1080/10911359.2019.1688220

Palusci, V. J., & Ilardi, M. (2020). Risk factors and services to reduce child sexual abuse recurrence. *Child Maltreatment, 25*(1), 106–116. https://doi.org/10.1177/1077559519848489

Reitan, T. (2019). Substance abuse during pregnancy: A 5-year follow-up of mothers and children. *Drugs: Education, Preventions and Policy, 26*(3), 219–228. https://doi.org/10.1080/09687637.2018.1432568

Thulin, J., Kjellgren, C., & Nilsson, D. (2018). Children's experiences with an intervention aimed to prevent further physical abuse. *Child & Family Social Work, 24*(1), 17–24. https://doi.org/10.1111/cfs.12476

Acceptance: Health Status   1300

Definition: Personal actions to reconcile significant changes in health circumstances

OUTCOME TARGET RATING: Maintain at_____ Increase to_____

	Never Demonstrated	Rarely Demonstrated	Sometimes Demonstrated	Often Demonstrated	Consistently Demonstrated	
OUTCOME OVERALL RATING	1	2	3	4	5	
Indicators:						
130002 Relinquishes previous concept of personal health	1	2	3	4	5	NA
130008 Recognizes reality of health situation	1	2	3	4	5	NA
130022 Reports reduced anxiety	1	2	3	4	5	NA
130020 Reports positive self-regard	1	2	3	4	5	NA
130023 Reports sense of control in health situation	1	2	3	4	5	NA
130016 Maintains relationships	1	2	3	4	5	NA
130024 Seeks social support as needed	1	2	3	4	5	NA
130007 Reports decreased need to verbalize feelings about health	1	2	3	4	5	NA
130017 Adjusts to change in health status	1	2	3	4	5	NA
130021 Expresses inner peace	1	2	3	4	5	NA
130018 Exhibits resilience	1	2	3	4	5	NA
130009 Pursues information about health	1	2	3	4	5	NA

Continued

A

Acceptance: Health Status—cont'd

		Never Demonstrated	Rarely Demonstrated	Sometimes Demonstrated	Often Demonstrated	Consistently Demonstrated	
130010	Copes with health situation	1	2	3	4	5	NA
130011	Makes decisions about health	1	2	3	4	5	NA
130025	Reports importance of health-related quality of life	1	2	3	4	5	NA
130012	Clarifies personal values	1	2	3	4	5	NA
130019	Clarifies life priorities	1	2	3	4	5	NA
130013	Reports sense of life being worth living	1	2	3	4	5	NA
130026	Reports use of self-care strategies to maintain current health status	1	2	3	4	5	NA
130014	Performs self-care tasks	1	2	3	4	5	NA

Domain-Psychosocial Health (III)   **Class**-Psychosocial Adaptation (N)   1st edition 1997; revised 2000, 2004, 2008, 2013, 2024

OUTCOME CONTENT REFERENCES:

Bellagamba, G., Descamps, A., Cypowyj, C., Eisinger, F., Villa, A., & Lehucher-Michel, M. P. (2021). Cancer survivors' efforts to facilitate return to work. *Psychology, Health & Medicine, 26*(7), 845–852. https://doi.org/10.1080/13548506.2020.1795212

Dattilo, T. M., Roberts, C. M., Fisher, R. S., Traino, K. A., Edwards, C. S., Pepper-Davis, M., Chaney, J. M., & Mullins, L. L. (2021). The role of avoidance coping and illness uncertainty in the relationship between transition readiness and health anxiety. *Journal of Pediatric Nursing, 59*(1), 125–130. https://doi.org/10.1016/j.pedn.2021.04.006

Liu, Y., Wei, M., Guo, L., Guo, Y., Zhu, Y., & He, Y. (2020). Association between illness perception and health behavior among stroke patients: The mediation effect of coping style. *Journal of Advanced Nursing, 77*(5), 2307–2318. https://doi.org/10.1111/jan.14761

Nair, D., Bonnet, K., Wild, M. G., Umeukeje, E. M., Fissell, R. B., Faulkner, M. L., Bahri, N.S., Bruce, M. A., Schlundt, D. G, Wallston, K. A., & Cavanaugh, K. L. (2021). Psychological adaptation to serious illness: A qualitative study of culturally diverse patients with advanced chronic kidney disease. *Journal of Pain and Symptom Management, 61*(1), 32–41. https://doi.org/10.1016/j.jpainsymman.2020.07.014

Ogawa, T., Saito, N., Fukuzawa, K., Kiuchi, K., Takami, M., Hayashi, M., Tanioka, R., Ota, M., Komoriya, K., Miyawaki, I., & Hirata, K. (2021). Device nurse intervention facilities the patients' adaptation to cardiac shock devices in the remote monitoring era. *Pacing Clinical Electrophysiology, 44*(11), 1874–1883. https://doi.org/10.1111/pace.14348

Patra, S., & Unisa, S. (2021). Addressing reproductive health knowledge, infertility and coping strategies among rural women in India. *Journal of Biosocial Science, 53*(4), 557–565. https://doi.org/10.1017/S0021932020000371

Ruile, S., Meisinger, C., Burkhardt, K., Heier, M., Thilo, C., & Kirchberger, I. (2021). Effort-reward imbalance at work and overcommitment in patients with acute myocardial infarction (AMI): Associations with return to work 6 months after AMI. *Journal of Occupational Rehabilitation, 31*, 532–542. https://doi.org/10.1007/s10926-020-09942-7

Activity Tolerance   0005

Definition: Physiologic response to energy-consuming movements with daily activities

OUTCOME TARGET RATING: Maintain at_____ Increase to_____

		Severely Compromised	Substantially Compromised	Moderately Compromised	Mildly Compromised	Not Compromised	
OUTCOME OVERALL RATING		1	2	3	4	5	
Indicators:							
000501	Oxygen saturation with activity	1	2	3	4	5	NA
000502	Pulse rate with activity	1	2	3	4	5	NA
000503	Respiratory rate with activity	1	2	3	4	5	NA
000508	Ease of breathing with activity	1	2	3	4	5	NA
000504	Systolic blood pressure with activity	1	2	3	4	5	NA
000505	Diastolic blood pressure with activity	1	2	3	4	5	NA
000506	Electrocardiogram findings	1	2	3	4	5	NA
000507	Skin color	1	2	3	4	5	NA
000509	Walking pace	1	2	3	4	5	NA
000510	Walking distance	1	2	3	4	5	NA
000519	Walking tolerance	1	2	3	4	5	NA

Activity Tolerance—cont'd

		Severely Compromised	Substantially Compromised	Moderately Compromised	Mildly Compromised	Not Compromised	
000511	Stair climbing tolerance	1	2	3	4	5	NA
000520	Coordination of movement	1	2	3	4	5	NA
000521	Hand strength	1	2	3	4	5	NA
000516	Upper body strength	1	2	3	4	5	NA
000517	Lower body strength	1	2	3	4	5	NA
000518	Ease of performing activities of daily living	1	2	3	4	5	NA
000522	Ease of performing instrumental activities of daily living	1	2	3	4	5	NA
000514	Ability to speak during physical activity	1	2	3	4	5	NA

Domain-Functional Health (I)   **Class**-Energy Maintenance (A)   2nd edition 2000; revised 2004, 2018

OUTCOME CONTENT REFERENCES:

Arikan, H., Yatar, I., Calik-Kutukcu, E., Aribas, Z., Saglam, M., Vardar-Yagli, N., Savci, S., Inal-Ince, D., Ozcelik, U., & Kiper, N. (2015). A comparison of respiratory and peripheral muscle strength, functional exercise capacity, activities of daily living and physical fitness in patients with cystic fibrosis and healthy subjects. *Research in Developmental Disabilities, 45–46*, 147–156. https://doi.org/10.1016/j.ridd.2015.07.020

Cho, M. H. (2016). Preliminary reliability of the five-item physical activity questionnaire. *The Journal of Physical Therapy Science, 28*(12), 3393–3397. https://doi.org/10.2174/1745017902016010024

Harcombe, H., Samaranayaka, A., & Derrett, S. (2016). Predictors of reduce frequency of physical activity 3 months after injury: Findings from the prospective outcomes of injury study. *Physical Therapy, 96*(12), 1885–1895. https://doi.org/10.2522/ptj.20160038

Kunkel, D., Fitton, C., Burnett, M., & Ashburn, A. (2015). Physical inactivity post-stroke: A 3-year longitudinal study. *Disability and Rehabilitation, 37*(4), 304–310. https://doi.org/10.3109/09638288.2014.918190

Mungovan, S. F., Singh, P., Gass, G., Smart, N. A., & Hirschhorn A. D. (2017). Effect of physical activity in the first five days after cardiac surgery. *Journal of Rehabilitation Medicine, 49*(1), 71–77. https://doi.org/10.2340/16501977-2165

Taylor, N. F., Peiris, C. L., Kennedy, G., & Shields, N. (2016). Walking tolerance of patients recovering from hip fracture: A phase I trial. *Disability and Rehabilitation, 38*(19), 1900–1908. https://doi.org/10.3109/09638288.2015.1107776

Acute Respiratory Acidosis Severity

0604

Definition: Severity of signs and symptoms of decreased blood pH and increased partial arterial carbon dioxide pressure due to hypoventilation and retention of carbon dioxide

OUTCOME TARGET RATING: Maintain at_____ Increase to_____

		Severe	Substantial	Moderate	Mild	None	
OUTCOME OVERALL RATING		1	2	3	4	5	
Indicators:							
060401	Decrease in blood plasma pH	1	2	3	4	5	NA
060402	Increase in serum hydrogen ions	1	2	3	4	5	NA
060403	Increase in serum partial arterial carbon dioxide pressure ($PaCO_2$)	1	2	3	4	5	NA
060404	Decrease in serum partial arterial oxygen pressure (PaO_2)	1	2	3	4	5	NA
060405	Hypoxia	1	2	3	4	5	NA
060406	Increased apical heart rate	1	2	3	4	5	NA
060407	Arrhythmias	1	2	3	4	5	NA
060408	Increased respiratory rate	1	2	3	4	5	NA
060409	Increased blood pressure	1	2	3	4	5	NA
060410	Muscle twitching	1	2	3	4	5	NA
060411	Drowsiness	1	2	3	4	5	NA
060412	Decreased level of consciousness	1	2	3	4	5	NA

Continued

Acute Respiratory Acidosis Severity—cont'd

		Severe	Substantial	Moderate	Mild	None	
060413	Confusion	1	2	3	4	5	NA
060414	Slowed verbal response	1	2	3	4	5	NA
060415	Dizziness	1	2	3	4	5	NA
060416	Dilated conjunctival blood vessels	1	2	3	4	5	NA
060419	Blurred vision	1	2	3	4	5	NA
060417	Headache	1	2	3	4	5	NA
060420	Restlessness	1	2	3	4	5	NA
060418	Diaphoresis	1	2	3	4	5	NA
060421	Nasal flaring	1	2	3	4	5	NA

Domain-Physiologic Health (II)   **Class**-Fluid & Electrolytes (G)   5th edition 2013; revised 2024

OUTCOME CONTENT REFERENCES:
Appel, S. J., & Downs, C. A. (2007). Steady a disturbed equilibrium. *Nursing Critical Care, 2*(4), 45–53.
Clancy, J., & McVicar, A. (2007). Intermediate and long-term regulation of acid-base homeostasis. *British Journal of Nursing, 16*(17), 1076–1079.
Huether, S. E., McCance, K. L., & Brashers, V.L. (2020). *Understanding pathophysiology* (7th ed.). Elsevier.
Isenhour, J. L., & Slovis, C. M. (2008). Arterial blood gas analysis: A 3-step approach to acid-base disorders. *The Journal of Respiratory Diseases, 29*(2), 74–82.
Kraut, J. A., & Madeas, N. E. (2001). Approach to patients with acid-base disorders. *Respiratory Care, 46*(4), 392–402.
Lian, J. X. (2010). Interpreting and using the arterial blood gas analysis. *Nursing Critical Care, 5*(3), 26–36.
Lynch, F. (2009). Arterial blood gas analysis: Implications for nursing. *Paediatric Nursing, 21*(1), 41–44.
Porth, C. M. (2019). *Essentials of pathophysiology* (6th ed.). Lippincott Williams & Wilkins.
Ruholl, L. (2006). Arterial blood gases: Analysis and nursing responses. *MEDSURG Nursing, 15*(6), 343–351.
Zorrilla-Riveiro, J. G., Arnau-Bartés, A., Rafat-Sellarés, R., García-Pérez, D., Mas-Serra, A., & Fernández-Fernández, R. (2017). Nasal flaring as a clinical sign of respiratory acidosis in patients with dyspnea. *American Journal of Emergency Medicine, 35*(4), 548–553. https://doi.org/10.1016/j.ajem.2016.12.008

Acute Respiratory Alkalosis Severity

0605

Definition: Severity of signs and symptoms of increased blood pH and decreased partial arterial carbon dioxide pressure due to hyperventilation and increased elimination of carbon dioxide

OUTCOME TARGET RATING: Maintain at_____ Increase to_____

		Severe	Substantial	Moderate	Mild	None	
OUTCOME OVERALL RATING		1	2	3	4	5	
Indicators:							
060501	Increase in blood plasma pH	1	2	3	4	5	NA
060502	Decrease in serum hydrogen ions	1	2	3	4	5	NA
060503	Decrease in serum bicarbonate	1	2	3	4	5	NA
060504	Decrease in partial pressure of carbon dioxide in arterial blood ($PaCO_2$)	1	2	3	4	5	NA
060505	Decrease in partial pressure of oxygen in arterial blood (PaO_2)	1	2	3	4	5	NA
060506	Decrease in serum potassium	1	2	3	4	5	NA
060507	Decrease in ionized serum calcium	1	2	3	4	5	NA
060508	Decrease in serum phosphate	1	2	3	4	5	NA
060509	Increased apical heart rate	1	2	3	4	5	NA
060510	Arrhythmias	1	2	3	4	5	NA
060511	Heart palpitations	1	2	3	4	5	NA
060512	Increased respiratory rate	1	2	3	4	5	NA
060513	Increased respiratory depth	1	2	3	4	5	NA
060514	Tinnitus	1	2	3	4	5	NA
060515	Dizziness	1	2	3	4	5	NA
060516	Lightheadedness	1	2	3	4	5	NA

Acute Respiratory Alkalosis Severity—cont'd

		Severe	Substantial	Moderate	Mild	None	
060522	Confusion	1	2	3	4	5	NA
060517	Decreased level of consciousness	1	2	3	4	5	NA
060519	Hyperactive reflexes	1	2	3	4	5	NA
060520	Hypertonic muscles	1	2	3	4	5	NA
060521	Paresthesias	1	2	3	4	5	NA

Domain-Physiologic Health (II)   **Class**-Fluid & Electrolytes (G)   5th edition 2013; revised 2024

OUTCOME CONTENT REFERENCES:

Appel, S. J., & Downs, C. A. (2007). Steady a disturbed equilibrium. *Nursing Critical Care, 2*(4), 45–53.

Clancy, J., & McVicar, A. (2007). Intermediate and long-term regulation of acid-base homeostasis. *British Journal of Nursing, 16*(17), 1076–1079.

Foster, G. T., Vaziri, N. D., & Sassoon, C. S. (2001). Respiratory alkalosis. *Respiratory Care, 46*(4), 384–391.

Huether, S. E., McCance, K. L., & Brashers, V. L. (2020). *Understanding pathophysiology* (7th ed.). Elsevier.

Isenhour, J. L., & Slovis, C. M. (2008). Arterial blood gas analysis: A 3-step approach to acid-base disorders. *The Journal of Respiratory Diseases, 29*(2), 74–82.

Kraut, J. A., & Madeas, N. E. (2001). Approach to patients with acid-base disorders. *Respiratory Care, 46*(4), 392–402.

Lian, J. X. (2010). Interpreting and using the arterial blood gas analysis. *Nursing Critical Care, 5*(3), 26–36.

Larkin, B. G., & Zimmanck, R. J. (2015). Interpreting arterial blood gases successfully. *AORN Journal, 102*(4), 343–357.
https://doi.org/10.1016/j.aorn.2015.08.002

Lynch, F. (2009). Arterial blood gas analysis: Implications for nursing. *Paediatric Nursing, 21*(1), 41–44.

Ruholl, L. (2006). Arterial blood gases: Analysis and nursing responses. *MEDSURG Nursing, 15*(6), 343–351.

Adaptation to Hospitalization: Adolescent   **1315**

Definition: Adaptive response of a child from 12 through 17 years of age to hospitalization

OUTCOME TARGET RATING: Maintain at_____ Increase to_____

		Never Demonstrated	Rarely Demonstrated	Sometimes Demonstrated	Often Demonstrated	Consistently Demonstrated	
OUTCOME OVERALL RATING		1	2	3	4	5	
Indicators:							
131501	Communicates with parents	1	2	3	4	5	NA
131502	Communicates with family members	1	2	3	4	5	NA
131503	Communicates with health care team	1	2	3	4	5	NA
131504	Trusts health care providers	1	2	3	4	5	NA
131505	Describes illness or injury	1	2	3	4	5	NA
131506	Recognizes reason for hospitalization	1	2	3	4	5	NA
131507	Participates in decision-making	1	2	3	4	5	NA
131508	Asks questions about illness	1	2	3	4	5	NA
131509	Describes symptoms	1	2	3	4	5	NA
131510	Asks questions about hospital routine	1	2	3	4	5	NA
131511	Asks questions about treatment plan	1	2	3	4	5	NA
131512	Asks questions about surgery	1	2	3	4	5	NA
131513	Asks questions about procedures	1	2	3	4	5	NA
131514	Asks questions about medication	1	2	3	4	5	NA
131515	Describes prescribed treatment	1	2	3	4	5	NA
131516	Reports feeling safe	1	2	3	4	5	NA

Continued

A

Adaptation to Hospitalization: Adolescent—cont'd

		Never Demonstrated	Rarely Demonstrated	Sometimes Demonstrated	Often Demonstrated	Consistently Demonstrated	
131517	Maintains sense of control	1	2	3	4	5	NA
131518	Cooperates with procedures	1	2	3	4	5	NA
131519	Reports pain level	1	2	3	4	5	NA
131520	Takes medication	1	2	3	4	5	NA
131521	Responds to comfort measures	1	2	3	4	5	NA
131522	Responds to diversional activities	1	2	3	4	5	NA
131523	Participates in group therapy	1	2	3	4	5	NA
131524	Participates in teaching activities	1	2	3	4	5	NA
131525	Participates in social interactions	1	2	3	4	5	NA
131526	Interacts with peers	1	2	3	4	5	NA
131527	Maintains pre-admission self-care behaviors	1	2	3	4	5	NA
131528	Participates in discharge planning	1	2	3	4	5	NA

		Consistently Demonstrated	Often Demonstrated	Sometimes Demonstrated	Rarely Demonstrated	Never Demonstrated	
131529	Blames self for admission	1	2	3	4	5	NA
131530	Agitation	1	2	3	4	5	NA
131531	Anxiety	1	2	3	4	5	NA
131532	Fear	1	2	3	4	5	NA
131533	Anger	1	2	3	4	5	NA
131534	Withdrawal	1	2	3	4	5	NA
131535	Aggression	1	2	3	4	5	NA
131536	Sadness	1	2	3	4	5	NA
131537	Apathy	1	2	3	4	5	NA
131538	Loneliness	1	2	3	4	5	NA
131539	Homesickness	1	2	3	4	5	NA

Domain-*Psychosocial Health (III)*   **Class**-*Psychosocial Adaptation (N)*   *7th edition 2024*

OUTCOME CONTENT REFERENCES:

Araújo, Y. B., Santos, S., Neves, N., Cardoso, É., & Nascimento, J. A. (2020). Predictive model of hospitalization for children and adolescents with chronic disease. *Revista Brasileira de Enfermagem, 73*(2), e20180467. https://doi.org/10.1590/0034-7167-2018-0467

Cassemiro, L., Okido, A., Furtado, M., & Lima, R. (2020). The hospital designed by hospitalized children and adolescents. *Revista Brasileira de Enfermagem, 73*(Suppl. 4), e20190399. https://doi.org/10.1590/0034-7167-2019-0399

Esses, S. A., Small, S., Rodemann, A., & Hartman, M. E. (2019). Post-intensive care syndrome: Educational interventions for parents of hospitalized children. *American Journal of Critical Care, 28*(1), 19–27. https://doi.org/10.4037/ajcc2019151

Jamalimoghadam, N., Yektatalab, S., Momennasab, M., Ebadi, A., & Zare, N. (2019). How do hospitalized adolescents feel safe? A qualitative study. *The Journal of Nursing Research, 27*(2), e14. https://doi.org/10.1097/jnr.0000000000000285

Jamalimoghadam, N., Yektatalab, S., Momennasab, M., Ebadi, A., & Zare, N. (2019). Hospitalized adolescents' perception of dignity: A qualitative study. *Nursing Ethics, 26*(3), 728–737. https://doi.org/10.1177/0969733017720828

Lee, S. P., Haycock-Stuart, E., & Tisdall, K. (2019). Participation in communication and decisions with regards to nursing care: The role of children. *Enfermería Clínica, 29*(Suppl. 2), 715–719. https://doi.org/10.1016/j.enfcli.2019.04.109

Mandato, C., Siano, M. A., De Anseris, A., Tripodi, M., Massa, G., De Rosa, R., Buffoli, M., Lamanna, A., Siani, P., & Vajro, P. (2020). Humanization of care in pediatric wards: Differences between perceptions of users and staff according to department type. *Italian Journal of Pediatrics, 46*(1), 65. https://doi.org/10.1186/s13052-020-00824-5

McClowry, S. G., & McLeod, S. M. (1990). The psychosocial responses of school-age children to hospitalization. *Children's Health Care, 19*, 155–161. https://doi.org/10.1207/s15326888chc1903_4

Ridout, B., Kelson, J., Campbell, A., & Steinbeck, K. (2021). Effectiveness of virtual reality interventions for adolescent patients in hospital settings: Systematic review. *Journal of Medical Internet Research, 23*(6), e24967. https://doi.org/10.2196/24967

Smith, W. (2018). Concept analysis of family-centered care of hospitalized pediatric patients. *Journal of Pediatric Nursing, 42*, 57–64. https://doi.org/10.1016/j.pedn.2018.06.014

Thurber, C. A., Patterson, D. R., & Mount, K. K. (2007). Homesickness and children's adjustment to hospitalization: Toward a preliminary model. *Children's Health Care, 36*(1), 1–28. https://doi.org/10.1080/02739610701316753

Vessey, J. A. (2003). Children's psychological responses to hospitalization. *Annual Review of Nursing Research, 21*, 173–203. https://doi.org/10.1891/0739-6686.21.1.173

Adaptation to Hospitalization: Middle Childhood   1314   **A**

Definition: Adaptive response of a child from 6 through 11 years of age to hospitalization

OUTCOME TARGET RATING: Maintain at_____ Increase to_____

		Never Demonstrated	Rarely Demonstrated	Sometimes Demonstrated	Often Demonstrated	Consistently Demonstrated	
OUTCOME OVERALL RATING		1	2	3	4	5	
Indicators:							
131401	Interacts with parents	1	2	3	4	5	NA
131402	Interacts with family members	1	2	3	4	5	NA
131403	Interacts with health care team	1	2	3	4	5	NA
131404	Maintains usual home routine	1	2	3	4	5	NA
131405	Recognizes reason for hospitalization	1	2	3	4	5	NA
131406	Participates in decision-making	1	2	3	4	5	NA
131408	Asks questions about illness	1	2	3	4	5	NA
131409	Asks questions about treatment	1	2	3	4	5	NA
131410	Asks questions about surgery	1	2	3	4	5	NA
131411	Describes illness	1	2	3	4	5	NA
131412	Describes prescribed treatment	1	2	3	4	5	NA
131413	Reports feeling safe	1	2	3	4	5	NA
131414	Maintains sense of control	1	2	3	4	5	NA
131415	Cooperates with procedures	1	2	3	4	5	NA
131416	Reports pain level	1	2	3	4	5	NA
131417	Responds to comfort measures	1	2	3	4	5	NA
131418	Responds to diversional activities	1	2	3	4	5	NA
131419	Participates in social interactions	1	2	3	4	5	NA
131420	Interacts with peers	1	2	3	4	5	NA
131421	Maintains pre-admission self-care behaviors	1	2	3	4	5	NA
131422	Participates in discharge planning	1	2	3	4	5	NA

		Consistently Demonstrated	Often Demonstrated	Sometimes Demonstrated	Rarely Demonstrated	Never Demonstrated	
131423	Agitation	1	2	3	4	5	NA
131424	Anxiety	1	2	3	4	5	NA
131425	Fear	1	2	3	4	5	NA
131426	Anger	1	2	3	4	5	NA
131427	Withdrawal	1	2	3	4	5	NA
131428	Aggression	1	2	3	4	5	NA
131429	Sadness	1	2	3	4	5	NA
131430	Apathy	1	2	3	4	5	NA
131431	Loneliness	1	2	3	4	5	NA
131432	Homesickness	1	2	3	4	5	NA

Domain-*Psychosocial Health (III)*   *Class*-*Psychosocial Adaptation (N)*   *7th edition 2024*

OUTCOME CONTENT REFERENCES:

Azevêdo, A.V. D. S., Lançoni, A. C. Jr., Crepaldi, M. A. (2017). Nursing team, family, and hospitalized child interaction: An integrative review. *Ciência e Saúde Coletiva, 22*(11), 3653–3666. https://doi.org/10.1590/1413-812320172211.26362015

Butler, A. E., Hall, H., & Copnell, B. (2018). Becoming a team: The nature of the parent-healthcare provider relationship when a child is dying in the pediatric intensive care unit. *Journal of Pediatric Nursing, 40,* e26–e32. https://doi.org/10.1016/j.pedn.2018.02.002

Coats, H., Bourget, E., Starks, H., Lindhorst, T., Saiki-Craighill, S., Curtis, J. R., Hays, R., & Doorenbos, A. (2018). Nurses' reflections on benefits and challenges of implementing family-centered care in pediatric intensive care units. *American Journal of Critical Care: An Official Publication, American Association of Critical-Care Nurses, 27*(1), 52–58. https://doi.org/10.4037/ajcc2018353

Esses, S. A., Small, S., Rodemann, A., & Hartman, M. E. (2019). Post-intensive care syndrome: Educational interventions for parents of hospitalized children. *American Journal of Critical Care, 28*(1), 19–27. https://doi.org/10.4037/ajcc2019151

Lee, S. P., Haycock-Stuart, E., & Tisdall, K. (2019). Participation in communication and decisions with regards to nursing care: The role of children. *Enfermería Clínica, 29*(Suppl. 2), 715–719. https://doi.org/10.1016/j.enfcli.2019.04.109

Shields, L. (2001). A review of the literature from developed and developing countries relating to the effects of hospitalization on children and parents. *International Nursing Review, 48*(1), 29–37. https://doi.org/10.1891/0739-6686.21.1.173

Smith, W. (2018). Concept analysis of family-centered care of hospitalized pediatric patients. *Journal of Pediatric Nursing, 42,* 57–64. https://doi.org/10.1016/j.pedn.2018.06.014

Stremler, R., Haddad, S., Pullenayegum, E., & Parshuram, C. (2017). Psychological outcomes in parents of critically ill hospitalized children. *Journal of Pediatric Nursing, 34,* 36–43. https://doi.org/10.1016/j.pedn.2017.01.012

Thurber, C. A., Patterson, D. R., & Mount, K. K. (2007). Homesickness and children's adjustment to hospitalization: Toward a preliminary model. *Children's Health Care, 36*(1), 1–28. https://doi.org/10.1080/02739610701316753

Vessey, J. A. (2003). Children's psychological responses to hospitalization. *Annual Review of Nursing Research, 21*(1), 173–203. https://doi.org/10.1891/0739-6686.21.1.173

Adaptation to Hospitalization: Preschooler   1313

Definition: Adaptive response of a child from 3 through 5 years of age to hospitalization

OUTCOME TARGET RATING: Maintain at_____ Increase to_____

	Never Demonstrated	Rarely Demonstrated	Sometimes Demonstrated	Often Demonstrated	Consistently Demonstrated	
OUTCOME OVERALL RATING	1	2	3	4	5	
Indicators:						
131301 Interacts with parents	1	2	3	4	5	NA
131302 Interacts with health care team	1	2	3	4	5	NA
131303 Maintains usual home routine	1	2	3	4	5	NA
131304 Recognizes reason for hospitalization	1	2	3	4	5	NA
131305 Asks questions about illness	1	2	3	4	5	NA
131306 Asks questions about treatment	1	2	3	4	5	NA
131307 Describes illness	1	2	3	4	5	NA
131308 Describes prescribed treatment	1	2	3	4	5	NA
131309 Reports feeling safe	1	2	3	4	5	NA
131310 Cooperates with procedures	1	2	3	4	5	NA
131311 Reports pain level	1	2	3	4	5	NA
131312 Responds to comfort measures	1	2	3	4	5	NA
131313 Responds to diversional activities	1	2	3	4	5	NA
131314 Participates in social interaction	1	2	3	4	5	NA
131315 Interacts with peers	1	2	3	4	5	NA
131316 Maintains pre-admission self-care behaviors	1	2	3	4	5	NA

Adaptation to Hospitalization: Preschooler—cont'd

	Consistently Demonstrated	Often Demonstrated	Sometimes Demonstrated	Rarely Demonstrated	Never Demonstrated	
131317	Agitation	1	2	3	4	5	NA
131318	Crying	1	2	3	4	5	NA
131319	Separation anxiety	1	2	3	4	5	NA
131320	Regressive behaviors	1	2	3	4	5	NA
131321	Anxiety	1	2	3	4	5	NA
131322	Fear	1	2	3	4	5	NA
131323	Anger	1	2	3	4	5	NA
131324	Withdrawal	1	2	3	4	5	NA
131325	Aggressive behaviors	1	2	3	4	5	NA
131326	Sadness	1	2	3	4	5	NA
131327	Apathy	1	2	3	4	5	NA

Domain-Psychosocial Health (III)   *Class*-Psychosocial Adaptation (N)   7th edition 2024

OUTCOME CONTENT REFERENCES:

Butler, A. E., Hall, H., & Copnell, B. (2018). Becoming a team: The nature of the parent-healthcare provider relationship when a child is dying in the pediatric intensive care unit. *Journal of Pediatric Nursing, 40*, e26–e32. https://doi.org/10.1016/j.pedn.2018.02.002

Esses, S. A, Small, S., Rodemann, A., & Hartman, M. E. (2019). Post-intensive care syndrome: Educational interventions for parents of hospitalized children. *American Journal of Critical Care, 28*(1), 19–27. https://doi.org/10.4037/ajcc2019151

Kasparian, N. A., Kan, J. M., Sood, E., Wray, J., Pincus, H. A., & Newburger, J. W. (2019). Mental health care for parents of babies with congenital heart disease during intensive care unit admission: Systematic review and statement of best practice. *Early Human Development, 139*, 104837. https://doi.org/10.1016/j.earlhumdev.2019.104837

Lee, S. P., Haycock-Stuart, E., & Tisdall, K. (2019). Participation in communication and decisions with regards to nursing care: The role of children. *Enfermería Clínica, 29*(Suppl. 2), 715–719. https://doi.org/10.1016/j.enfcli.2019.04.109

Oh, D. L., Jerman, P., Silvério Marques, S., Koita, K., Purewal Boparai, S. K., Burke Harris, N., & Bucci, M. (2018). Systematic review of pediatric health outcomes associated with childhood adversity. *BMC Pediatrics, 18*(1), 83. https://doi.org/10.1186/s12887-018-1037-7

Smith, W. (2018). Concept analysis of family-centered care of hospitalized pediatric patients. *Journal of Pediatric Nursing, 42*, 57–64. https://doi.org/10.1016/j.pedn.2018.06.014

Vessey, J. A. (2003). Children's psychological responses to hospitalization. *Annual Review of Nursing Research, 21*, 173–203. https://doi.org/10.1891/0739-6686.21.1.173

Adaptation to Physical Disability   **1308**

Definition: Personal actions to adapt to a significant functional and emotional challenges due to a physical disability

OUTCOME TARGET RATING: Maintain at_____ Increase to_____

		Never Demonstrated	Rarely Demonstrated	Sometimes Demonstrated	Often Demonstrated	Consistently Demonstrated	
OUTCOME OVERALL RATING		1	2	3	4	5	
Indicators:							
130801	Verbalizes ability to adjust to disability	1	2	3	4	5	NA
130802	Verbalizes reconciliation to disability	1	2	3	4	5	NA
130803	Adapts to functional limitations	1	2	3	4	5	NA
130804	Modifies lifestyle to accommodate disability	1	2	3	4	5	NA
130825	Selects appropriate assistive devices	1	2	3	4	5	NA
130826	Maintains working condition of assistance devices	1	2	3	4	5	NA
130810	Identifies plan to meet activities of daily living	1	2	3	4	5	NA
130827	Uses strategies to provide self-care	1	2	3	4	5	NA

Continued

A

Adaptation to Physical Disability—cont'd

		Never Demonstrated	Rarely Demonstrated	Sometimes Demonstrated	Often Demonstrated	Consistently Demonstrated	
130811	Identifies plan to meet instrumental activities of daily living	1	2	3	4	5	NA
130828	Uses strategies to complete instrumental activities of daily living (IADL)	1	2	3	4	5	NA
130829	Uses adaptive transportation strategies	1	2	3	4	5	NA
130805	Modifies career goals to accommodate disability	1	2	3	4	5	NA
130830	Modifies home environment to facilitate functioning	1	2	3	4	5	NA
130831	Uses strategies to modify work environment	1	2	3	4	5	NA
130806	Uses strategies to reduce stress related to disability	1	2	3	4	5	NA
130807	Identifies ways to increase sense of control	1	2	3	4	5	NA
130808	Identifies ways to cope with life changes	1	2	3	4	5	NA
130809	Identifies risk of complications associated with disability	1	2	3	4	5	NA
130812	Accepts need for physical assistance	1	2	3	4	5	NA
130821	Obtains information about disability	1	2	3	4	5	NA
130832	Uses strategies to cope with increased symptoms	1	2	3	4	5	NA
130824	Uses personal support system	1	2	3	4	5	NA
130833	Reports stable personal relationships	1	2	3	4	5	NA
130834	Reports positive affect	1	2	3	4	5	NA
130835	Reports increase in resilience	1	2	3	4	5	NA
130817	Reports decrease in stress related to disability	1	2	3	4	5	NA
130836	Reports decrease in fear due to losses	1	2	3	4	5	NA
130837	Reports feeling less of a burden to others	1	2	3	4	5	NA
130838	Reports decrease in negative emotions	1	2	3	4	5	NA
130819	Reports decrease in negative body image	1	2	3	4	5	NA
130820	Reports increase in psychological comfort	1	2	3	4	5	NA
130839	Reports gratitude for remaining abilities	1	2	3	4	5	NA
130840	Reports ability to fulfill needs	1	2	3	4	5	NA
130822	Uses community resources	1	2	3	4	5	NA
130823	Obtains assistance from health professional	1	2	3	4	5	NA

Domain-*Psychosocial Health (III)*   **Class**-*Psychosocial Adaptation (N)*   *3rd edition 2004; revised 2008, 2013, 2024*

OUTCOME CONTENT REFERENCES:

Borade, N., Ingle, A., & Nagarkar, A. (2021). Lived experiences of people with mobility-related disability using assistive devices. *Disability and Rehabilitation: Assistive Technology, 16*(7), 730–734. https://doi.org/10.1080/17483107.2019.1701105

Bužgová, R., & Kozáková, R. (2019). Informing patients with progressive neurological disease of their health status, and their adaptation to the disease. *BMC Neurology, 19*(1), 1–12. https://doi.org/10.1186/s12883-019-1488-y

Freedman, M. E., Healy, B. C., Huffman, J. C., Chitnis, T., Weiner, H. L., & Glanz, B. I. (2021). An at-home positive psychology intervention for individuals with multiple sclerosis. *International Journal of MS Care, 23*(3), 128–134. https://doi.org/10.7224/1537-2073.2020-020

Gómez-Ibáñez, R., Bernabeu-Tamayo, M. D., Aguayo-González, M., Granel, N., Watson, C. E., & Escribano, X. (2021). Early patient experiences of primary above-the-knee amputation for vascular etiologies: A phenomenological study. *Clinical Nursing Research, 30*(5), 539–547. https://doi.org/10.1177/1054773820971873

Hammerlund, C. S., Lexell, J., & Brogårdh, C. (2021). Growing up with a disability following paralytic poliomyelitis: Experiences from persons with late effects of polio. *Disability and Rehabilitation, 43*(7), 960–966. https://doi.org/10.1080/09638288.2019.1647296

Hauschildt, K. E., Seigworth, C., Kamphuis, L. A., Hough, C. L., Moss, M., McPeake, J. M., Harrod, M., & Iwashyna, T. J. (2021). Patients' adaptations after acute respiratory distress syndrome: A qualitative study. *American Journal of Critical Care, 30*(3), 221–229. https://doi.org/10.4037/ajcc2021825

Jörgensen, S., Lennman, E., & Lexell, J. (2021). Sense of coherence and changes over six years among older adults aging with long-term spinal cord injury. *Spinal Cord, 59*, 1278–1284. https://doi.org/10.1038/s41393-021-00713-6

Lewis, M. W., & Wu, L. (2021). Depression and disability among combat veterans' transition to an historically black university. *Journal of Social Work Education, 57*(2), 215–225. https://doi.org/10.1080/10437797.2019.1671258

Adherence Behavior   1600

Definition: Personal actions to promote optimal wellness, recovery, and rehabilitation

OUTCOME TARGET RATING: Maintain at_____ Increase to_____

		Never Demonstrated	Rarely Demonstrated	Sometimes Demonstrated	Often Demonstrated	Consistently Demonstrated	
OUTCOME OVERALL RATING		1	2	3	4	5	
Indicators:							
160001	Asks health-related questions	1	2	3	4	5	NA
160002	Seeks health information from a variety of sources	1	2	3	4	5	NA
160016	Evaluates accuracy of health information obtained	1	2	3	4	5	NA
160003	Uses reputable health information to develop strategies	1	2	3	4	5	NA
160004	Weighs risks/benefits of health behavior	1	2	3	4	5	NA
160007	Provides rationale for adopting a health behavior	1	2	3	4	5	NA
160017	Sets realistic health goals	1	2	3	4	5	NA
160018	Shares health goals with family	1	2	3	4	5	NA
160019	Identifies challenges to meeting personal goals	1	2	3	4	5	NA
160020	Identifies financial restraints on meeting personal goals	1	2	3	4	5	NA
160021	Identifies unhealthy personal behaviors	1	2	3	4	5	NA
160008	Uses strategies to eliminate unhealthy behavior	1	2	3	4	5	NA
160009	Uses strategies to optimize health	1	2	3	4	5	NA
160022	Uses strategies to improve nutrition	1	2	3	4	5	NA
160023	Uses strategies to promote an active lifestyle	1	2	3	4	5	NA
160024	Uses strategies to manage medications	1	2	3	4	5	NA
160010	Uses health care services congruent with need	1	2	3	4	5	NA
160011	Performs activities of daily living consistent with energy and tolerance	1	2	3	4	5	NA
160012	Performs self-screening	1	2	3	4	5	NA
160013	Describes rationale for deviating from a health regimen	1	2	3	4	5	NA
160014	Performs self-monitoring of health status	1	2	3	4	5	NA
160025	Obtains recommended vaccines	1	2	3	4	5	NA
160026	Performs treatment regimen as prescribed	1	2	3	4	5	NA
160027	Follows recommended changes in treatment regimen	1	2	3	4	5	NA
160028	Monitors treatment response	1	2	3	4	5	NA
160029	Keeps appointments with health care professional	1	2	3	4	5	NA

Domain-Health Knowledge & Behavior (IV)   *Class*-Health Behavior (Q)   *1st edition 1997; revised 2004, 2008, 2024*

A

OUTCOME CONTENT REFERENCES:

Burkhart, P. V., Dunbar-Jacob, J. M., & Rohay, J. M. (2001). Accuracy of children's self-reported adherence to treatment. *Journal of Nursing Scholarship, 33*(1), 27–32. https://doi.org/10.1111/j.1547-5069.2001.00027.x

Davoodi, M., Dindamal, B., Dargahi, H., & Faraji-Khiavi, F. (2022). A phenomenological study on barriers of adherence to medical advice among type 2 diabetic patients. *BMC Endocrine Disorders, 22*(1), 1–9. https://doi.org/10.1186/s12902-021-00928-x

Gardner, C. L. (2015). Adherence: A concept analysis. *International Journal of Nursing Knowledge, 26*(2), 96–101. https://doi.org/10.1111/2047-3095.12046

Moreno-Agostino, D., Daskalopoulou, C., Wu, Y.-T., Koukounari, A., Haro, J. M., Tyrovolas, S., Panagiotakos, D. B., Prince, M., & Prina, A. M. (2020). The impact of physical activity on healthy ageing trajectories: Evidence from eight cohort studies. *International Journal of Behavioral Nutrition & Physical Activity, 17*(1), 1–12. https://doi.org/10.1186/s12966-020-00995-8

Pender, N. J. (1990). Expressing health through lifestyle patterns. *Nursing Science Quarterly, 3*(3), 115–122.

Pender, N. J., & Pender, A. R. (1986). Attitudes, subjective norms, and intentions of engagement in health behaviors. *Nursing Research, 35*(1), 15–18.

Potter, P. A., Perry, A. G., Stockert, P., & Hall, A. (2021). *Fundamentals of nursing* (10th ed.). Elsevier.

Shumaker, S. A., Schron, E. B., & Ockene, J. K. (1998). *The handbook of health behavior change* (2nd ed.). Springer.

Sweenie, R., Cushing, C. C., Fleming, K. K., Prabhakaran, S., & Fedele, D. A. (2022). Daily adherence variability and psychosocial differences in adolescents with asthma: A pilot study. *Journal of Behavioral Medicine, 45*(1), 148–158. https://doi.org/10.1007/s10865-021-00247-5

Till, M., Abu-Omar, K., Ferschl, S., Reimers, A. K., & Gelius, P. (2021). Measuring capabilities in health and physical activity promotion: A systematic review. *BMC Public Health, 21*(1), 1–23. https://doi.org/10.1186/s12889-020-10151-3

Adherence Behavior: Clinical Condition   1640

Definition: Personal actions to follow recommendations from a health professional for a specific health problem

OUTCOME TARGET RATING: Maintain at_____ Increase to_____

OUTCOME OVERALL RATING	Never Demonstrated 1	Rarely Demonstrated 2	Sometimes Demonstrated 3	Often Demonstrated 4	Consistently Demonstrated 5	
Indicators:						
164001 Accepts diagnosis	1	2	3	4	5	NA
164002 Shares diagnosis with family	1	2	3	4	5	NA
164003 Seeks reputable information about diagnosis	1	2	3	4	5	NA
164004 Seeks reputable information about treatment options	1	2	3	4	5	NA
164005 Discusses prescribed treatment regimen with health professional	1	2	3	4	5	NA
164006 Develops sense of joint responsibility with health professional	1	2	3	4	5	NA
164007 Discusses prescribed treatment regimen with family	1	2	3	4	5	NA
164008 Performs treatment regimen as prescribed	1	2	3	4	5	NA
164009 Reports positive communication with health professional	1	2	3	4	5	NA
164010 Keeps appointments with health professional	1	2	3	4	5	NA
164011 Reports changes in symptoms to health professional	1	2	3	4	5	NA
164012 Modifies treatment regimen as directed by health professional	1	2	3	4	5	NA
164013 Monitors treatment response	1	2	3	4	5	NA
164014 Monitors medication therapeutic effects	1	2	3	4	5	NA
164015 Obtains needed laboratory tests	1	2	3	4	5	NA
164016 Performs self-screening when directed	1	2	3	4	5	NA
164017 Performs activities of daily living as prescribed	1	2	3	4	5	NA

Adherence Behavior: Clinical Condition—cont'd

	Never Demonstrated	Rarely Demonstrated	Sometimes Demonstrated	Often Demonstrated	Consistently Demonstrated	
164018 Seeks external reinforcement for performance of health behaviors	1	2	3	4	5	NA
1640019 Obtains emotional support from family	1	2	3	4	5	NA

Domain-Health Knowledge & Behavior (IV)   **Class**-Health Behavior (Q)   7th edition 2024

OUTCOME CONTENT REFERENCES:

Davoodi, M., Dindamal, B., Dargahi, H., & Faraji-Khiavi, F. (2022). A phenomenological study on barriers of adherence to medical advice among type 2 diabetic patients. *BMC Endocrine Disorders, 22*(1), 1–9. https://doi.org/10.1186/s12902-021-00928-x

Gardner, C. L. (2015). Adherence: A concept analysis. *International Journal of Nursing Knowledge, 26*(2), 96–101. https://doi.org/10.1111/2047-3095.12046

Menéndez-Colino, R., Martín Maestre, I., González-Montalvo, J. I., & Otero Puime, Á. (2020). Factors affecting exercise program adherence in patients with acute hip fracture and impact on one-year survival. *Brazilian Journal of Physical Therapy, 24*(6), 479–487. https://doi.org/10.1016/j.bjpt.2019.07.008

Murali, K. M., Mullan, J., Roodenrys, S., Hassan, H. C., Lambert, K., & Lonergan, M. (2019). Strategies to improve dietary, fluid, dialysis or medication adherence in patients with end stage kidney disease on dialysis: A systematic review and meta-analysis of randomized intervention trials. *PLOS One, 14*(1), e0211479. https://doi.org/10.1371/journal.pone.0211479

Oliveira, R. S., Primeira, M. R., Santos, W. M., Paula, C. C., & Padoin, S. M. M. (2020). Association between social support and adherence to anti-retroviral treatment in people living with HIV. *Revista Gaúcha de Enfermagem, 41*, e20190290. https://doi.org/10.1590/1983-1447.2020.2019029

Potter, P. A., Perry, A. G., Stockert, P., & Hall, A. (2021). *Fundamentals of nursing* (10th ed.). Elsevier.

Rashidi, A., Kaistha, P., Whitehead, L., & Robinson, S. (2020). Factors that influence adherence to treatment plans amongst people living with cardiovascular disease: A review of published qualitative research studies. *International Journal of Nursing Studies, 110*, 103727. https://doi.org/10.1016/j.ijnurstu.2020.103727

Sousa, H., Ribeiro, O., Paúl, C., Costa, E., Miranda, V., Ribeiro, F., & Figueiredo, D. (2019). Social support and treatment adherence in patients with end-stage renal disease: A systematic review. *Seminars in Dialysis, 32*(6), 562–574. https://doi.org/10.1111/sdi.12831

Adherence Behavior: Healthy Diet   1621

Definition: Personal actions to plan, monitor, and optimize a balanced nutritional dietary pattern

OUTCOME TARGET RATING: Maintain at_____   Increase to_____

	Never Demonstrated	Rarely Demonstrated	Sometimes Demonstrated	Often Demonstrated	Consistently Demonstrated	
OUTCOME OVERALL RATING	1	2	3	4	5	
Indicators:						
162124 Seeks recommendations for a healthy diet pattern	1	2	3	4	5	NA
162101 Sets achievable dietary goals	1	2	3	4	5	NA
162125 Shares dietary goals with family	1	2	3	4	5	NA
162126 Identifies challenges to meeting dietary goals	1	2	3	4	5	NA
162102 Balances caloric intake and caloric requirements	1	2	3	4	5	NA
162103 Seeks information about established nutritional guidelines	1	2	3	4	5	NA
162127 Seeks information about the benefits of organic foods	1	2	3	4	5	NA
162128 Discusses need for nutritional supplements with health professional	1	2	3	4	5	NA
162129 Discusses need for vitamin supplements with health professional	1	2	3	4	5	NA

Continued

A

Adherence Behavior: Healthy Diet—cont'd

		Never Demonstrated	Rarely Demonstrated	Sometimes Demonstrated	Often Demonstrated	Consistently Demonstrated	
162104	Uses recommended nutritional guidelines to plan meals	1	2	3	4	5	NA
162105	Selects foods consistent with recommended nutritional guidelines	1	2	3	4	5	NA
162106	Selects portions consistent with recommended nutritional guidelines	1	2	3	4	5	NA
162107	Selects foods based on nutritional information on food labels	1	2	3	4	5	NA
162108	Washes fresh fruits and vegetables before eating	1	2	3	4	5	NA
162109	Prepares foods following dietary recommendations for fat, sodium, and carbohydrates	1	2	3	4	5	NA
162110	Cooks meat, poultry, fish, and eggs based on safety recommendations	1	2	3	4	5	NA
162111	Eats recommended servings of fruits per day	1	2	3	4	5	NA
162112	Eats recommended servings of vegetables per day	1	2	3	4	5	NA
162113	Eats more whole grain products than refined grain products	1	2	3	4	5	NA
162114	Minimizes foods with high caloric value and little nutritional value	1	2	3	4	5	NA
162130	Minimizes addition of sugar or sweeteners to food and beverages	1	2	3	4	5	NA
162115	Balances fluid intake and fluid loss	1	2	3	4	5	NA
162116	Maintains hydration	1	2	3	4	5	NA
162131	Consumes less than 2300 milligrams of sodium per day	1	2	3	4	5	NA
162117	Selects foods that provide calcium to meet requirements	1	2	3	4	5	NA
162118	Supplements with vitamins/minerals within suggested guidelines	1	2	3	4	5	NA
162119	Chooses foods consistent with cultural religious beliefs	1	2	3	4	5	NA
162120	Discusses use of herbal remedies with health provider	1	2	3	4	5	NA
162121	Avoids foods that interact with medications	1	2	3	4	5	NA
162122	Avoids foods that interact with herbal remedies	1	2	3	4	5	NA
162123	Avoids foods that trigger allergic reactions	1	2	3	4	5	NA
162132	Limits alcohol consumption to 1 (women) to 2 (men) drinks per day	1	2	3	4	5	NA
162133	Practices food safety to prevent bacterial foodborne illness	1	2	3	4	5	NA

Domain-Health Knowledge & Behavior (IV)   *Class*-Health Behavior (Q)   4th edition 2008; revised 2013, 2024

OUTCOME CONTENT REFERENCES:

Cena, H., & Calder, P. C. (2020). Defining a healthy diet: Evidence for the role of contemporary dietary patterns in health and disease. *Nutrients, 12*(2), 334. https://doi.org/10.3390/nu12020334

Downer, S., Berkowitz, S. A., Harlan, T. S., Olstad, D. L., & Mozaffarian, D. (2020). Food is medicine: Actions to integrate food and nutrition into healthcare. *BMJ (Clinical Research ed.), 369*, m2482. https://doi.org/10.1136/bmj.m2482

Dudek, S. G. (2021). *Nutrition essentials for nursing practice* (9th rev. ed.). Wolters Kluwer.

Hockenberry, M. J., Rodgers, C. C., & Wilson, D. (Eds.). (2022). *Wong's essentials of pediatric nursing* (11th ed.). Elsevier.

Marotz, L. R. (2019). *Health, safety, and nutrition for the young child* (10th ed.). Cengage Learning.

Potter, P. A., Perry, A. G., Stockert, P., & Hall, A. (2021). *Fundamentals of nursing* (10th ed.). Elsevier.

U.S. Department of Health and Human Services and U.S. Department of Agriculture. (2020). 2020–2025 *Dietary Guidelines for Americans* (9th ed.). https://www.dietaryguidelines.gov/

Williams, P. (2020). *Basic geriatric nursing*. Elsevier.

Adherence Behavior: Prescribed Activity   1632

Definition: Personal actions to follow daily physical activities recommended by a health professional for a specific health condition

OVERALL TARGET RATING: Maintain at_____ Increase to_____

OVERALL OUTCOME RATING		Never Demonstrated 1	Rarely Demonstrated 2	Sometimes Demonstrated 3	Often Demonstrated 4	Consistently Demonstrated 5	
Indicators:							
163201	Discusses activity recommendations with health professional	1	2	3	4	5	NA
163218	Shares physical activity recommendations with family	1	2	3	4	5	NA
163202	Identifies expected benefits of physical activity	1	2	3	4	5	NA
163203	Identifies barriers to implement prescribed physical activity	1	2	3	4	5	NA
163204	Sets achievable short-term activity goals with health professional	1	2	3	4	5	NA
163205	Sets achievable long-term activity goals with health professional	1	2	3	4	5	NA
163219	Receives instructions on how to perform the activity	1	2	3	4	5	NA
163220	Integrates prescribed activity into daily routine	1	2	3	4	5	NA
163221	Manages pain associated with activity	1	2	3	4	5	NA
163222	Counts steps per day with digital device	1	2	3	4	5	NA
163206	Follows target heart rate set by health professional	1	2	3	4	5	NA
163207	Uses strategies to promote safety	1	2	3	4	5	NA
163223	Uses required assistive devices	1	2	3	4	5	NA
163208	Uses strategies to allocate time for physical activity	1	2	3	4	5	NA
163209	Uses strategies to increase endurance	1	2	3	4	5	NA
163210	Participates in daily prescribed physical activity	1	2	3	4	5	NA
163211	Monitors heart rate	1	2	3	4	5	NA
163212	Monitors respiratory rate	1	2	3	4	5	NA
163224	Monitors fatigue symptoms	1	2	3	4	5	NA
163213	Seeks external reinforcement for performance of health behaviors	1	2	3	4	5	NA

Continued

A

Adherence Behavior: Prescribed Activity—cont'd

		Never Demonstrated	Rarely Demonstrated	Sometimes Demonstrated	Often Demonstrated	Consistently Demonstrated	
163214	Uses diary or app to monitor progress in prescribed physical activity	1	2	3	4	5	NA
163215	Modifies physical activity as directed by health professional	1	2	3	4	5	NA
163216	Identifies symptoms that need to be reported	1	2	3	4	5	NA
163217	Reports symptoms experienced during activity to health professional	1	2	3	4	5	NA

Domain-Health Knowledge & Behavior (IV)   **Class**-Health Behavior (Q)   5th edition 2013; revised 2024

OUTCOME CONTENT REFERENCES:

Gardner, C. L. (2015). Adherence: A concept analysis. *International Journal of Nursing Knowledge, 26*(2), 96–101. https://doi.org/10.1111/2047-3095.12046

Menéndez-Colino, R., Martín Maestre, I., González-Montalvo, J. I., & Otero Puime, Á. (2020). Factors affecting exercise program adherence in patients with acute hip fracture and impact on one-year survival. *Brazilian Journal of Physical Therapy, 24*(6), 479–487. https://doi.org/10.1016/j.bjpt.2019.07.008

Moreno-Agostino, D., Daskalopoulou, C., Wu, Y.-T., Koukounari, A., Haro, J. M., Tyrovolas, S., Panagiotakos, D. B., Prince, M., & Prina, A. M. (2020). The impact of physical activity on healthy ageing trajectories: Evidence from eight cohort studies. *International Journal of Behavioral Nutrition & Physical Activity, 17*(1), 1–12. https://doi.org/10.1186/s12966-020-00995-8

Potter, P. A., Perry, A. G., Stockert, P., & Hall, A. (2021). *Fundamentals of nursing* (10th ed.). Elsevier.

Rai, R., Jongenelis, M. I., Jackson, B., Newton, R. U., & Pettigrew, S. (2020). Factors influencing physical activity participation among older people with low activity levels. *Ageing & Society, 40*(12), 2593–2613. https://doi.org/10.1017/S0144686X1900076X

Riera-Sampol, A., Bennasar-Veny, M., Tauler, P., & Aguilo, A. (2021). Effectiveness of physical activity prescription by primary care nurses using health assets: A randomized controlled trial. *Journal of Advanced Nursing, 77*(3), 1518–1532. https://doi.org/10.1111/jan.14649

Scheerman, K., Schoenmakers, A. H. C., Meskers, C. G. M., & Maier, A. B. (2021). Physical, motivational, and environmental factors influencing physical activity promotion during hospitalization: Older patients' perspective. *Geriatric Nursing, 42*(2), 599–604. https://doi.org/10.1016/j.gerinurse.2021.02.013

Song, Y., Qu, J., Zhang, D., & Zhang, J. (2018). Feasibility and effectiveness of mobile phones in physical activity promotion for adults 50 years and older. *Topics in Geriatric Rehabilitation, 34*(3), 213–222. https://doi.org/10.1097/TGR.0000000000000197

Swann, C., Rosenbaum, S., Lawrence, A., Vella, S. A., McEwan, D., & Ekkekakis, P. (2021). Updating goal-setting theory in physical activity promotion: A critical conceptual review. *Health Psychology Review, 15*(1), 34–50. https://doi.org/10.1080/17437199.2019.1706616

Till, M., Abu-Omar, K., Ferschl, S., Reimers, A. K., & Gelius, P. (2021). Measuring capabilities in health and physical activity promotion: A systematic review. *BMC Public Health, 21*(1), 1–23. https://doi.org/10.1186/s12889-020-10151-3

Williams, P. (2020). *Basic geriatric nursing*. Elsevier.

Adherence Behavior: Prescribed Diet

1622

Definition: Personal actions to follow food and fluid intake recommended by a health professional for a specific health condition

OUTCOME TARGET RATING: Maintain at_____ Increase to_____

		Never Demonstrated	Rarely Demonstrated	Sometimes Demonstrated	Often Demonstrated	Consistently Demonstrated	
OUTCOME OVERALL RATING		1	2	3	4	5	
Indicators:							
162201	Participates in setting achievable dietary goals with health professional	1	2	3	4	5	NA
162221	Discusses need for nutritional supplements with health professional	1	2	3	4	5	NA
162222	Shares dietary goals with family	1	2	3	4	5	NA
162223	Identifies challenges to meeting prescribed dietary goals	1	2	3	4	5	NA
162224	Uses strategies to meet challenges in prescribed dietary goals	1	2	3	4	5	NA
162202	Selects food and fluid consistent with prescribed diet	1	2	3	4	5	NA
162203	Uses nutritional information on labels to guide selections	1	2	3	4	5	NA

Adherence Behavior: Prescribed Diet—cont'd

	Never Demonstrated	Rarely Demonstrated	Sometimes Demonstrated	Often Demonstrated	Consistently Demonstrated	
162204 Selects portions consistent with prescribed diet	1	2	3	4	5	NA
162205 Eats food consistent with prescribed diet	1	2	3	4	5	NA
162206 Drinks fluid consistent with prescribed diet	1	2	3	4	5	NA
162207 Avoids food and fluid not allowed on diet	1	2	3	4	5	NA
162208 Follows recommendations for between-meal food and fluid	1	2	3	4	5	NA
162209 Prepares food and fluid following dietary restrictions	1	2	3	4	5	NA
162210 Follows recommendations for number of meals per day	1	2	3	4	5	NA
162211 Plans meals consistent with prescribed diet	1	2	3	4	5	NA
162212 Plans strategies for situations that affect food and fluid intake	1	2	3	4	5	NA
162213 Alters diet within restrictions when activity level changes	1	2	3	4	5	NA
162214 Follows recommendations for diet staging	1	2	3	4	5	NA
162215 Uses a diary or app to monitor food and fluid intake over time	1	2	3	4	5	NA
162216 Aligns diet with cultural beliefs	1	2	3	4	5	NA
162217 Chooses foods consistent with cultural beliefs	1	2	3	4	5	NA
162218 Avoids food and fluid that interact with medication	1	2	3	4	5	NA
162219 Avoids food and fluid that interact with herbal remedies	1	2	3	4	5	NA
162220 Avoids food and fluid that trigger allergic reactions	1	2	3	4	5	NA

Domain-Health Knowledge & Behavior (IV)   *Class*-Health Behavior (Q)   4th edition 2008; revised 2024

OUTCOME CONTENT REFERENCES:

Dudek, S. G. (2021). *Nutrition essentials for nursing practice* (9th ed.). Wolters Kluwer.

Gardner, C. L. (2015). Adherence: A concept analysis. *International Journal of Nursing Knowledge, 26*(2), 96–101. https://doi.org/10.1111/2047-3095.12046

Murali, K. M., Mullan, J., Roodenrys, S., Hassan, H. C., Lambert, K., & Lonergan, M. (2019). Strategies to improve dietary, fluid, dialysis or medication adherence in patients with end stage kidney disease on dialysis: A systematic review and meta-analysis of randomized intervention trials. *PLOS One, 14*(1), e0211479. https://doi.org/10.1371/journal.pone.0211479

Potter, P. A., Perry, A. G., Stockert, P., & Hall, A. (2021). *Fundamentals of nursing* (10th ed.). Elsevier.

Sousa, H., Ribeiro, O., Paúl, C., Costa, E., Miranda, V., Ribeiro, F., & Figueiredo, D. (2019). Social support and treatment adherence in patients with end-stage renal disease: A systematic review. *Seminars in Dialysis, 32*(6), 562–574. https://doi.org/10.1111/sdi.12831

U.S. Department of Health and Human Services and U.S. Department of Agriculture. (2020). *2020–2025 Dietary Guidelines for Americans* (9th ed.). https://www.dietaryguidelines.gov/

A

Adherence Behavior: Prescribed Medication 1623

Definition: Personal actions to administer medication safely to meet therapeutic effects for a specific or multiple conditions as recommended by a health professional

OUTCOME TARGET RATING: Maintain at_____ Increase to_____

		Never Demonstrated	Rarely Demonstrated	Sometimes Demonstrated	Often Demonstrated	Consistently Demonstrated	
OUTCOME OVERALL RATING		1	2	3	4	5	
Indicators:							
162301	Keeps a list of all prescribed medication with dose and frequency	1	2	3	4	5	NA
162302	Obtains required medication from pharmacy	1	2	3	4	5	NA
162333	Shares beliefs about medication use	1	2	3	4	5	NA
162334	Shares beliefs about the effectiveness of medications	1	2	3	4	5	NA
162335	Shares concerns about risks associated with medications	1	2	3	4	5	NA
162303	Informs health professional of all medication being taken daily	1	2	3	4	5	NA
162336	Takes a list of current medications to each appointment	1	2	3	4	5	NA
162337	Participates in medication reconciliation with health professional	1	2	3	4	5	NA
162338	Shares barriers to medication adherence	1	2	3	4	5	NA
162339	Shares financial concerns about cost of medications	1	2	3	4	5	NA
162340	Shares insurance concerns for medication coverage	1	2	3	4	5	NA
162341	Discusses use of herbal medications with health professional	1	2	3	4	5	NA
162342	Integrates medication into daily routine	1	2	3	4	5	NA
162304	Takes all medication at intervals prescribed	1	2	3	4	5	NA
162305	Takes correct dose	1	2	3	4	5	NA
162306	Modifies dose as instructed	1	2	3	4	5	NA
162307	Takes medication with or without food as prescribed	1	2	3	4	5	NA
162308	Avoids alcohol if contraindicated	1	2	3	4	5	NA
162309	Avoids food and fluids that are contraindicated	1	2	3	4	5	NA
162310	Administers topical medication correctly	1	2	3	4	5	NA
162311	Follows medication precautions	1	2	3	4	5	NA
162312	Monitors medication therapeutic effects	1	2	3	4	5	NA
162313	Monitors medication side effects	1	2	3	4	5	NA
162314	Monitors medication adverse effects	1	2	3	4	5	NA
162315	Uses strategies to minimize side effects	1	2	3	4	5	NA
162316	Reports therapeutic response to health professional	1	2	3	4	5	NA

Adherence Behavior: Prescribed Medication—cont'd

		Never Demonstrated	Rarely Demonstrated	Sometimes Demonstrated	Often Demonstrated	Consistently Demonstrated	
162317	Reports adverse effects to health professional	1	2	3	4	5	NA
162318	Stores medication properly	1	2	3	4	5	NA
162319	Arranges for refills to ensure adequate supply	1	2	3	4	5	NA
162320	Monitors medication expiration date	1	2	3	4	5	NA
162321	Disposes of medication properly	1	2	3	4	5	NA
162322	Disposes of syringes and needles properly	1	2	3	4	5	NA
162323	Administers subcutaneous medication correctly	1	2	3	4	5	NA
162324	Administers intramuscular medication correctly	1	2	3	4	5	NA
162325	Administers intravenous medication correctly	1	2	3	4	5	NA
162326	Maintains asepsis with non-parenteral medication	1	2	3	4	5	NA
162327	Monitors injection insertion sites	1	2	3	4	5	NA
162328	Rotates injection sites	1	2	3	4	5	NA
162329	Maintains needed supplies	1	2	3	4	5	NA
162330	Stores supplies correctly	1	2	3	4	5	NA
162331	Disposes sharps correctly	1	2	3	4	5	NA
162343	Disposes unused medications correctly	1	2	3	4	5	NA
162332	Obtains required laboratory tests	1	2	3	4	5	NA

Domain-Health Knowledge & Behavior (IV)   *Class*-Health Behavior (Q)   4th edition 2008; revised 2013, 2024

OUTCOME CONTENT REFERENCES:
Gardner, C. L. (2015). Adherence: A concept analysis. *International Journal of Nursing Knowledge, 26*(2), 96–101. https://doi.org/10.1111/2047-3095.12046
Huang, Y.-M., Pecanac, K. E., & Shiyanbola, O. O. (2020). "Why am I not taking medications?" Barriers and facilitators of diabetes medication adherence across different health literacy levels. *Qualitative Health Research, 30*(14), 2331–2342. https://doi.org/10.1177/1049732320945296
McQuaid, E. L., & Landier, W. (2018). Cultural issues in medication adherence: Disparities and directions. *Journal of General Internal Medicine, 33*(2), 200–206. https://doi.org/10.1007/s11606-017-4199-3
Mercadante, S., Adile, C., Tirelli, W., Ferrera, P., Penco, I., & Casuccio, A. (2021). Barriers and adherence to pain management in advanced cancer patients. *Pain Practitioner, 2*, 388–393. https://doi.org/10.1111/papr.12965
Murali, K. M., Mullan, J., Roodenrys, S., Hassan, H. C., Lambert, K., & Lonergan, M. (2019). Strategies to improve dietary, fluid, dialysis or medication adherence in patients with end stage kidney disease on dialysis: A systematic review and meta-analysis of randomized intervention trials. *PLOS One, 14*(1), e0211479. https://doi.org/10.1371/journal.pone.0211479
Potter, P. A., Perry, A. G., Stockert, P., & Hall, A. (2021). *Fundamentals of nursing* (10th ed.). Elsevier.
Rathbone, A. P., Jamie, K., Todd, A., & Husband, A. (2021). A qualitative study exploring the lived experience of medication use in different disease states: Linking experiences of disease symptoms to medication adherence. *Journal of Clinical Pharmacy & Therapeutics, 46*(2), 352–362. https://doi.org/10.1111/jcpt.13288
Rosa, W. E., Riegel, B., Ulrich, C. M., & Meghani, S. H. (2020). A concept analysis of analgesic nonadherence for cancer pain in a time of opioid crisis. *Nursing Outlook, 68*(1), 83–93. https://doi.org/10.1016/j.outlook.2019.06.017
Stuart, B. C., Timmons, V., Loh, F. E., Dai, M., & Xu, J. (2021). Can one or two simple questions predict poor medication adherence? *Journal of Evaluation in Clinical Practice, 27*(1), 75–83. https://doi.org/10.1111/jep.13389

Aggression Self-Restraint 1401

Definition: Personal actions to refrain from assaultive, combative, or destructive behaviors toward others

OUTCOME TARGET RATING: Maintain at_____ Increase to_____

		Never Demonstrated	Rarely Demonstrated	Sometimes Demonstrated	Often Demonstrated	Consistently Demonstrated	
OUTCOME OVERALL RATING		1	2	3	4	5	
Indicators:							
140110	Identifies when angry	1	2	3	4	5	NA
140111	Identifies when frustrated	1	2	3	4	5	NA
140112	Identifies situations that precipitate hostility	1	2	3	4	5	NA
140113	Identifies responsibility to maintain control	1	2	3	4	5	NA
140114	Identifies when feeling aggressive	1	2	3	4	5	NA
140115	Identifies alternatives to aggression	1	2	3	4	5	NA
140116	Identifies alternatives to verbal outbursts	1	2	3	4	5	NA
140127	Maintains treatment regimen	1	2	3	4	5	NA
140124	Uses effective conflict resolution skills	1	2	3	4	5	NA
140128	Uses cognitive reappraisal strategies	1	2	3	4	5	NA
140129	Seeks positive peer relationships	1	2	3	4	5	NA
140125	Expresses needs in a non-destructive manner	1	2	3	4	5	NA
140117	Vents negative feelings in a non-destructive manner	1	2	3	4	5	NA
140101	Refrains from verbal outbursts	1	2	3	4	5	NA
140130	Refrains from negative thinking	1	2	3	4	5	NA
140126	Avoids violating others' personal space	1	2	3	4	5	NA
140131	Refrains from cyberbullying	1	2	3	4	5	NA
140103	Refrains from striking others	1	2	3	4	5	NA
140104	Refrains from harming others	1	2	3	4	5	NA
140105	Refrains from harming animals	1	2	3	4	5	NA
140106	Refrains from destroying property	1	2	3	4	5	NA
140132	Refrains from substance abuse	1	2	3	4	5	NA
140109	Controls impulses	1	2	3	4	5	NA
140121	Uses physical activity to reduce pent-up energy	1	2	3	4	5	NA
140122	Uses techniques to control anger	1	2	3	4	5	NA
140123	Uses techniques to control frustration	1	2	3	4	5	NA
140118	Upholds contract to restrain aggressive behaviors	1	2	3	4	5	NA
140119	Maintains self-control without supervision	1	2	3	4	5	NA

Domain-Psychosocial Health (III) *Class*-Self-Control (O) *1st edition 1997; revised 2000, 2004, 2008, 2013, 2024*

OUTCOME CONTENT REFERENCES:

Brochado, S., Fraga, S., Soares, S., Ramos, E., & Barros, H. (2021). Cyberbullying among adolescents: The influence of different modes of inquiry. *Journal of Interpersonal Violence, 36*(3 4), 1933–1950. https://doi.org/10.1177/0886260517744182

Coleman, J. N., & Farrell, A. D. (2021). The influence of exposure to violence on adolescents' physical aggression: The protective influence of peers. *Journal of Adolescence, 90*(C), 53–65. https://doi.org/10.1016/j.adolescence.2021.06.003

Faay, M. D. M., & Sommer, I. E. (2021). Risk and prevention of aggression in patients with psychotic disorders. *American Journal of Psychiatry, 178*(3), 218–220. https://doi.org/10.1176/appi.ajp.2020.21010035

Harrington, A. G., Overall, N. C., & Cross, E. J. (2021). Masculine gender role stress, low relationship power, and aggression toward intimate partners. *Psychology of Men & Masculinities, 22*(1), 48–62. https://doi.org/10.1037/men0000262

Mansueto, G., Cavallo, C., Palmieri, S., Ruggiero, G. M., Sassaroli, S., & Caselli, G. (2021). Adverse childhood experiences and repetitive negative thinking in adulthood: A systematic review. *Clinical Psychology & Psychotherapy, 28*(3), 557–568. https://doi.org/10.1002/cpp.2590

Scheer, J. R., & Mereish, E. H. (2021). Intimate partner violence and illicit substance use among sexual and gender minority youth: The protective role of cognitive reappraisal. *Journal of Interpersonal Violence, 36*(21-22), 9956–9976. https://doi.org/10.1177/0886260519881001

Varcarolis, E. M., & Fosbre, C. D. (2021). *Essential of psychiatric-mental health nursing,* (4th ed.), Elsevier

Agitation Level   1214   **A**

Definition: Severity of disruptive physiological and behavioral manifestations of stress or biochemical triggers

OUTCOME TARGET RATING: Maintain at_____ Increase to_____

		Severe	Substantial	Moderate	Mild	None	
OUTCOME OVERALL RATING		1	2	3	4	5	
Indicators:							
121401	Difficulty processing information	1	2	3	4	5	NA
121402	Restlessness	1	2	3	4	5	NA
121403	Frustration	1	2	3	4	5	NA
121404	Irritability	1	2	3	4	5	NA
121405	Pacing	1	2	3	4	5	NA
121406	Repetitious movements	1	2	3	4	5	NA
121407	Inability to remain seated	1	2	3	4	5	NA
121408	Difficulty staying on tasks	1	2	3	4	5	NA
121409	Resists assistance	1	2	3	4	5	NA
121410	Combativeness	1	2	3	4	5	NA
121411	Thrashing in bed	1	2	3	4	5	NA
121432	Insomnia	1	2	3	4	5	NA
121412	Pulling at tubes or restraints	1	2	3	4	5	NA
121413	Repetitious mannerisms	1	2	3	4	5	NA
121414	Grabbing	1	2	3	4	5	NA
121415	Hoarding	1	2	3	4	5	NA
121416	Hitting	1	2	3	4	5	NA
121417	Kicking	1	2	3	4	5	NA
121418	Throwing	1	2	3	4	5	NA
121419	Spitting	1	2	3	4	5	NA
121420	Biting	1	2	3	4	5	NA
121421	Emotional lability	1	2	3	4	5	NA
121422	Verbal outbursts	1	2	3	4	5	NA
121423	Inappropriate verbalizations	1	2	3	4	5	NA
121424	Inappropriate gestures	1	2	3	4	5	NA
121425	Disinhibition	1	2	3	4	5	NA
121426	Interrupted sleep	1	2	3	4	5	NA
121427	Weight loss	1	2	3	4	5	NA
121428	Dehydration	1	2	3	4	5	NA
121429	Increased blood pressure	1	2	3	4	5	NA
121430	Increased radial pulse rate	1	2	3	4	5	NA
121431	Increased respiratory rate	1	2	3	4	5	NA

Domain-Psychosocial Health (III)   Class-Psychological Well-Being (M)   4th edition 2008; revised 2013

OUTCOME CONTENT REFERENCES:
Cohen-Mansfield, J. (1996). Behavioral and mood evaluations: Assessment of Agitation. *International Psychogeriatrics, 8*(2), 233–245.
Gray, K. F. (2004). Managing agitation and difficult behavior in dementia. *Clinics in Geriatric Medicine, 20*(1), 69–82.
Hamill, R. J. (2006). Managing pain and agitation in the critically ill - Are we there yet? *Critical Care Medicine, 34*(6), 1838–1839. https://doi.org/10.1097/01.ccm.0000220056.92653.3d
Jaber, S., Chanques, G., Altairac, C., Sebbane, M., Vergne, C., Perrigault, P., Eledjam, J. (2005). A prospective study of agitation in a medical-surgical ICU: Incidence, risk factors, and outcomes. *Chest, 128*(4), 2749–2757. https://doi.org/10.1378/chest.128.4.2749
Nott, M. T., Chapparo, C., & Baguley, I. J. (2006). Agitation following traumatic brain injury: An Australian sample. *Brain Injury, 20*(11), 1175–1182. https://doi.org/10.1080/02699050601049114
+Sessler, C. N., Gosnell, M. S., Grap, M. J., Brophy, G. M., O'Neal, P. V., Keane, K. A., Tesoro, E. P., & Elswick, R. K. (2002). The Richmond Agitation-Sedation Scale: Validity and reliability in adult intensive care unit patients. *American Journal of Respiratory Critical Care Medicine, 166*(10), 1338–1344.

A

Alcohol Abuse Cessation Behavior 1629

Definition: Personal actions to eliminate alcohol use that poses a threat to health

OUTCOME TARGET RATING: Maintain at_____ Increase to_____

		Never Demonstrated	Rarely Demonstrated	Sometimes Demonstrated	Often Demonstrated	Consistently Demonstrated	
OUTCOME OVERALL RATING		**1**	**2**	**3**	**4**	**5**	
Indicators:							
162901	Expresses willingness to stop alcohol use	1	2	3	4	5	NA
162902	Expresses belief in the ability to stop alcohol use	1	2	3	4	5	NA
162903	Identifies benefits of eliminating alcohol use	1	2	3	4	5	NA
162931	Identifies co-existence of tobacco and alcohol abuse	1	2	3	4	5	NA
162932	Identifies strategies to control cravings for alcohol	1	2	3	4	5	NA
162904	Identifies negative consequences of alcohol use	1	2	3	4	5	NA
162905	Develops effective strategies to eliminate alcohol use	1	2	3	4	5	NA
162906	Identifies barriers to alcohol elimination	1	2	3	4	5	NA
162907	Identifies emotional states that trigger alcohol use	1	2	3	4	5	NA
162933	Monitors feelings that trigger alcohol use	1	2	3	4	5	NA
162908	Adjusts alcohol elimination strategies as needed	1	2	3	4	5	NA
162909	Commits to alcohol elimination strategies	1	2	3	4	5	NA
162910	Follows selected alcohol elimination strategies	1	2	3	4	5	NA
162911	Participates in screening for associated health problems	1	2	3	4	5	NA
162934	Uses integrative approaches to tobacco-alcohol therapy with medications for nicotine dependence	1	2	3	4	5	NA
162935	Participates in a tailored recovery program	1	2	3	4	5	NA
162912	Uses strategies to cope with withdrawal symptoms	1	2	3	4	5	NA
162936	Uses strategies to control weight	1	2	3	4	5	NA
162937	Uses strategies to control tobacco use	1	2	3	4	5	NA
162913	Uses behavior modification strategies	1	2	3	4	5	NA
162914	Uses effective coping strategies	1	2	3	4	5	NA
162915	Obtains assistance from health professional	1	2	3	4	5	NA

Alcohol Abuse Cessation Behavior—cont'd

		Never Demonstrated	Rarely Demonstrated	Sometimes Demonstrated	Often Demonstrated	Consistently Demonstrated	
162916	Uses personal support system	1	2	3	4	5	NA
162938	Uses reputable health information	1	2	3	4	5	NA
162917	Uses reputable sources of information	1	2	3	4	5	NA
162918	Participates in Alcoholics Anonymous	1	2	3	4	5	NA
162919	Contacts sponsor for cessation support	1	2	3	4	5	NA
162920	Encourages family to participate in Al-Anon	1	2	3	4	5	NA
162922	Adjusts lifestyle to promote alcohol elimination	1	2	3	4	5	NA
162923	Uses prescribed medication as recommended	1	2	3	4	5	NA
162924	Uses non-prescription medication as recommended	1	2	3	4	5	NA
162925	Avoids situations that encourage alcohol use	1	2	3	4	5	NA
162939	Uses available peer recovery support groups	1	2	3	4	5	NA
162927	Uses available community resources	1	2	3	4	5	NA
162928	Participates in counseling	1	2	3	4	5	NA
162929	Monitors for signs of depression	1	2	3	4	5	NA
162940	Abstinence from alcohol use	1	2	3	4	5	NA

Domain-Health Knowledge & Behavior (IV)   *Class*-Health Behavior (Q)   4th edition 2008; revised 2024

OUTCOME CONTENT REFERENCES:

Blackwell, C. W., & Castillo, H. L. (2020). Use of electronic nicotine delivery systems (ENDS) in lesbian, gay, bisexual, transgender and queer persons: Implications for public health nursing. *Public Health Nursing, 37*(4), 569–580. https://doi.org/10.1111/phn.12746

Bold, K. W., Rosen, R. L, Steinberg, M. L., Epstein, E. E., McCrady, B. S., & Williams, J. M. (2020). Smoking characteristics and alcohol use among women in treatment for alcohol use disorder. *Addictive Behaviors, 101*, 1–8. https://doi.org/10.1016/j.addbeh.2019.106137

Case, K. R., Hinds, J. T., Creamer, M. R., Loukas, A., & Perry, C. L. (2020). Who is JUULing and why? An examination of young adult electronic nicotine delivery systems users. *Journal of Adolescent Health, 66*(1), 48–55. https://doi.org/10.1016/j.jadohealth.2019.05.030

DiSilvio, B., Baqdunes, M., Alhajbusain, A., & Cheema, T. (2021). Smoking addiction and strategies for cessation. *Critical Care Nursing Quarterly, 44*(1), 33–48. https://doi.org/10.1097/CNQ.0000000000000338

Haass-Koffler, C. L., Souza, R. D., Wilmott, J. P., Aston, E. R, & Song, J. H. (2021). A combined alcohol and smoking cue-reactivity paradigm in people who drink heavily and smoke cigarettes: Preliminary findings. *Alcohol and Alcoholism, 56*(1), 47–56. https://doi.org/10.1093/alcalc/agaa089

Kelly, J. F., Greene, M. C., Bergman, B. G., White, W. L., & Hoeppner, B. B. (2019). How many recovery attempts does it take to successfully resolve an alcohol or drug problem? *Alcoholism: Clinical and Experimental Research, 43*(7), 1533–1544. https://doi.org/10.1111/acer.14067

Kurti, A. N. (2020). Reducing tobacco use among women of childbearing age: Contributions of tobacco regulatory science and tobacco control. *Experimental and Clinical Psychopharmacology, 28*(5), 501–516. https://doi.org/10.1037/pha0000342

Wootton, R. E., Greenstone, H. S. R., Abdellaoui, A., Denys, D., Verweij, K. J. H., Munafò, M. R., & Treur, J. L. (2020). Bidirectional effects between loneliness, smoking, and alcohol use: Evidence from a mendelian randomization study. *Addiction, 116*, 400–406. https://doi.org/10.1111/add.15142

A

Allergic Response: Localized

0705

Definition: Severity of localized hypersensitive immune response to a specific environmental (exogenous) antigen

OUTCOME TARGET RATING: Maintain at_____ Increase to_____

		Severe	Substantial	Moderate	Mild	None	
OUTCOME OVERALL RATING		1	2	3	4	5	
Indicators:							
070501	Sinus pain	1	2	3	4	5	NA
070502	Headache	1	2	3	4	5	NA
070503	Conjunctivitis	1	2	3	4	5	NA
070504	Lacrimation	1	2	3	4	5	NA
070505	Rhinitis	1	2	3	4	5	NA
070506	Sneezing	1	2	3	4	5	NA
070507	Mucous secretions	1	2	3	4	5	NA
070508	Circumoral edema	1	2	3	4	5	NA
070509	Periorbital edema	1	2	3	4	5	NA
070510	Dark circles under eyes	1	2	3	4	5	NA
070511	Burning sensation of eyes	1	2	3	4	5	NA
070520	Cracked skin	1	2	3	4	5	NA
070512	Localized itching	1	2	3	4	5	NA
070513	Localized rash	1	2	3	4	5	NA
070514	Localized erythema	1	2	3	4	5	NA
070515	Increased localized skin temperature	1	2	3	4	5	NA
070516	Localized edema	1	2	3	4	5	NA
070517	Localized pain	1	2	3	4	5	NA
070518	Localized granuloma	1	2	3	4	5	NA
070519	Localized necrotizing vasculitis	1	2	3	4	5	NA

Domain-Physiologic Health (II)   *Class-Immune Response (H)*   *3rd edition 2004; revised 2018*

OUTCOME CONTENT REFERENCES:

Hinkle, J., & Cheever, K. (Eds.). (2014). *Brunner and Suddarth's textbook of medical-surgical nursing* (13th ed.). Wolters Kluwer Health/Lippincott Williams & Wilkins.

Hohler, S. (2015). Latex allergies: Protecting patients and staff. *OR Nurse, 9*(1), 12–18.

Huether, S. E., & McCance, K. L. (Eds.). (2017). *Understanding pathophysiology* (6th ed.). Elsevier.

Lewis, S. L., Dirksen, S. R., Heitkemper, M. M., & Bucher, L. (2014). *Medical-surgical nursing: Assessment and management of clinical problems* (9th ed.). Elsevier Mosby.

McCance, K. L., & Huether, S. E. (2014). *Pathophysiology: The biological basis for disease in adults and children* (7th ed.). Elsevier.

Prester, L. (2016). Seafood allergy, toxicity, and intolerance: A review. *Journal of the American College of Nutrition, 35*(3), 271–283. https://doi.org/10.1080/07315724.2015.1014120

Proudfoot, C., & Saul, P. (2016). Nut allergy in children: A growing concern. *Practice Nurse, 46*(12), 30–36.

Tomljenovic, D., Baudoin, T., Megla, Z. B., Vagic, D., Hellings, P., & Kalogjera, L. (2016). Nasal and ocular responses after specific and nonspecific nasal challenges in seasonal allergic rhinitis. *Annals of Allergy, Asthma, & Immunology, 116*(3), 199–205. https://doi.org/10.1016/j.anai.2015.12.022

Allergic Response: Systemic   0706

Definition: Severity of systemic hypersensitive immune response to a specific environmental (exogenous) antigen

OUTCOME TARGET RATING: Maintain at_____ Increase to_____

		Severe	Substantial	Moderate	Mild	None	
OUTCOME OVERALL RATING		1	2	3	4	5	
Indicators:							
070601	Laryngeal edema	1	2	3	4	5	NA
070632	Edema of the lips	1	2	3	4	5	NA
070633	Edema of the eyelids	1	2	3	4	5	NA
070634	Edema of the tongue	1	2	3	4	5	NA
070602	Dyspnea at rest	1	2	3	4	5	NA
070603	Wheezing	1	2	3	4	5	NA
070604	Stridor	1	2	3	4	5	NA
070605	Adventitious breath sounds	1	2	3	4	5	NA
070606	Tachycardia	1	2	3	4	5	NA
070607	Decreased blood pressure	1	2	3	4	5	NA
070608	Dysrhythmia(s)	1	2	3	4	5	NA
070609	Pulmonary edema	1	2	3	4	5	NA
070610	Decreased level of consciousness	1	2	3	4	5	NA
070611	Mucous secretions	1	2	3	4	5	NA
070612	Facial edema	1	2	3	4	5	NA
070613	Generalized itching	1	2	3	4	5	NA
070614	Hives	1	2	3	4	5	NA
070615	Body exfoliation	1	2	3	4	5	NA
070616	Petechiae	1	2	3	4	5	NA
070617	Erythema	1	2	3	4	5	NA
070618	Increased skin temperature	1	2	3	4	5	NA
070619	Fever	1	2	3	4	5	NA
070620	Chills	1	2	3	4	5	NA
070621	Nausea	1	2	3	4	5	NA
070622	Vomiting	1	2	3	4	5	NA
070623	Diarrhea	1	2	3	4	5	NA
070624	Abdominal cramping	1	2	3	4	5	NA
070625	Red blood cell hemolysis	1	2	3	4	5	NA
070626	Increased bilirubin	1	2	3	4	5	NA
070627	Enlarged spleen	1	2	3	4	5	NA
070628	Enlarged lymph nodes	1	2	3	4	5	NA
070629	Joint pain	1	2	3	4	5	NA
070630	Muscle pain	1	2	3	4	5	NA
070631	Anaphylactic shock	1	2	3	4	5	NA
070635	Anxiety	1	2	3	4	5	NA

Domain-Physiologic Health (II)   *Class-Immune Response (H)*   *3rd edition 2004; revised 2018*

OUTCOME CONTENT REFERENCES:
Hinkle, J., & Cheever, K. (Eds.). (2014). *Brunner and Suddarth's textbook of medical-surgical nursing* (13th ed.). Wolters Kluwer Health/Lippincott Williams & Wilkins.
Hohler, S. (2015). Latex allergies: Protecting patients and staff. *OR Nurse, 9*(1), 12–18.
Huether, S. E., & McCance, K. L. (Eds.). (2017). *Understanding pathophysiology* (6th ed.). Elsevier.
Lewis, S. L., Dirksen, S. R., Heitkemper, M. M., & Bucher, L. (2014). *Medical-surgical nursing: Assessment and management of clinical problems* (9th ed.). Elsevier Mosby.
McCance, K. L., & Huether, S. E. (2014). *Pathophysiology: The biological basis for disease in adults and children* (7th ed.). Elsevier.
Prester, L. (2016). Seafood allergy, toxicity, and intolerance: A review. *Journal of the American College of Nutrition, 35*(3), 271–283. https://doi.org/10.1080/07315724.2015.1014120
Proudfoot, C., & Saul, P. (2016). Nut allergy in children: A growing concern. *Practice Nurse, 46*(12), 30–36.
Rance, K., & Goldberg, P. (2015). Anaphylaxis overview: Addressing unmet patient needs. *The Journal for Nurse Practitioners, 11*(3), 352–359. https://doi.org/10.1016/j.nurpra.2014.09.006

A

Ambulation

0200

Definition: Personal actions to walk from place to place independently with or without assistive device

OUTCOME TARGET RATING: Maintain at_____ Increase to_____

	Never Demonstrated	Rarely Demonstrated	Sometimes Demonstrated	Often Demonstrated	Consistently Demonstrated	
OUTCOME OVERALL RATING	1	2	3	4	5	
Indicators:						
020018 Bears weight	1	2	3	4	5	NA
020019 Walks with effective gait	1	2	3	4	5	NA
020020 Walks at slow pace	1	2	3	4	5	NA
020021 Walks at moderate pace	1	2	3	4	5	NA
020022 Walks at fast pace	1	2	3	4	5	NA
020023 Walks up steps	1	2	3	4	5	NA
020024 Walks down steps	1	2	3	4	5	NA
020025 Walks up inclines	1	2	3	4	5	NA
020026 Walks down inclines	1	2	3	4	5	NA
020027 Walks short distance (< 1 block)	1	2	3	4	5	NA
020028 Walks moderate distance (> 1 block < 5 blocks)	1	2	3	4	5	NA
020029 Walks long distance (5 blocks or >)	1	2	3	4	5	NA
020030 Walks around room	1	2	3	4	5	NA
020031 Walks around dwelling	1	2	3	4	5	NA
020032 Adjusts to different surface textures	1	2	3	4	5	NA
020033 Walks around obstacles	1	2	3	4	5	NA

Domain-Functional Health (I)   **Class**-Mobility (C)   *1st edition 1997; revised 2004, 2008, 2013, 2024*

OUTCOME CONTENT REFERENCES:

+Akinrolie, O., Webber, S. C., Salbach, N. M., & Barclay, R. (2021). Validation of an adapted questionnaire for outdoor walking among older adults: The CHAMPS-OUTDOORS. *Journal of Aging and Physical Activity, 29*(5), 843–851. https://doi.org/10.1123/japa.2020-0350

Cheng, D. K. Y., Dagenais, M., Alsbury-Nealy, K., Legasto, J. M., Scodras, S., Aravind, G., Takhar, P., & Salbach, N. M. Distance-limited walk tests post-stroke: A systematic review of measurement properties. *Neurorehabilitation, 48*(4), 413–439. https://doi.org/10.3233/NRE-210026

Kim, W., Choi, H. J. J., Yoon, J. S., & Jeoung, J. H. (2021). Asymmetry and variability should be included in the assessment of gait function in poststroke hemiplegia with independent ambulation during early rehabilitation. *Archives of Physical Medicine and Rehabilitation, 102*(4), 611–618. https://doi.org/10.1016/j.apmr.2020.10.115

Mangione, K. K., Posner, M. A., Craik, R. L., Wolff, E. F., Fortinsky, R. H., Beamer, B. A., Binder, E. F., Orwig, D. L., Magaziner, J., & Resnick, B. (2021). Using treatment fidelity measures to understand walking recovery: A secondary analysis from the community ambulation project. *Physical Therapy, 101*(8), 1–9. https://doi.org/10.1093/ptj/pzab109

Master, H., Thoma, L. M., Neogi, T., Dunlop, D. D., LaValley, M., Christiansen, M. B., Voinier, D., & White, D. K. (2021). Daily walking and the risk of knee replacement over 5 years among adults with advance knee osteoarthritis in the United States. *Archives of Physical Medicine and Rehabilitation, 102*(10), 1888–1894. https://doi.org/10.1016/j.apmr.2021.05.014

Rodrigues, I. B., Ponzano, M., Butt, D. A., Bartley, J., Bardai, Z., Ashe, M. C., Chilibeck, P. D., Thabane, L., Wark, J. D., Stapleton, J., & Giangregorio, L. M. (2021). The effects of walking or Nordic walking in adults 50 years and older at elevated risk of fractures: A systematic review and meta-analysis. *Journal of Aging and Physical Activity, 29*(5), 886–899. https://doi.org/10.1123/japa.2020-0262

Rosso, A. L., Harding, A. B., Clarke, P. J., Studenski, S. A., & Rosano, C. (2021). Associations of neighborhood walkability and walking behaviors by cognitive trajectory in older adults. *The Gerontologist, 61*(7), 1053–1061. https://doi.org/10.1093/geront/gnab005

Younesian, H., Legrand, T., Miramand, L., Beausoleil, S., & Turcot, K. (2021). Clinical walking tests and gait pattern characterization during 6-minute walk test using inertial sensors: Follow-up in individuals with lower limb amputation. *Journal of Applied Biomechanics, 37*(5), 440–449. https://doi.org/10.1123/jab.2020-0327

Zajac, J. A., Cavanaugh, J. T., Baker, T., Colón-Semenza, C., DeAngelis, T. R., Duncan, R. P., Fulford, D., Lavalley, M., Nordahl, T., Rawson, K. S., Saint-Hilaire, M., Thomas, C. A., Earhart, G. M., & Ellis, T. D. (2021). Are mobile persons with Parkinson disease necessarily more active? *Journal of Neurologic Therapy, 45*(4), 259–265. https://doi.org/10.1097/NPT.0000000000000362

Ambulation: Wheelchair   0201

Definition: Personal actions to safely move indoors or outdoors in a wheelchair

OUTCOME TARGET RATING: Maintain at_____ Increase to_____

		Never Demonstrated	Rarely Demonstrated	Sometimes Demonstrated	Often Demonstrated	Consistently Demonstrate	
OUTCOME OVERALL RATING		1	2	3	4	5	
Indicators:							
020110	Chooses wheelchair propelling aids	1	2	3	4	5	NA
020111	Chooses chairs for outdoors mobility	1	2	3	4	5	NA
020112	Uses wheelchair propelling aids safely	1	2	3	4	5	NA
020113	Transfers to and from wheelchair	1	2	3	4	5	NA
020114	Propels wheelchair safely	1	2	3	4	5	NA
020115	Propels wheelchair short distance	1	2	3	4	5	NA
020116	Propels wheelchair moderate distance	1	2	3	4	5	NA
020117	Propels wheelchair long distance	1	2	3	4	5	NA
020118	Maneuvers different surface levels	1	2	3	4	5	NA
020119	Maneuvers different surface textures	1	2	3	4	5	NA
020120	Maneuvers curbs	1	2	3	4	5	NA
020121	Maneuvers doorways	1	2	3	4	5	NA
020122	Mancuvers ramps	1	2	3	4	5	NA
020123	Maintains wheelchair function	1	2	3	4	5	NA

**Domain**-Functional Health (I)   _**Class**-Mobility (C)_   _1st edition 1997; revised 2004, 2013, 2024_

OUTCOME CONTENT REFERENCES:

Berthelette, M., Mann, D. D., Ripat, J., & Glazebrook, C. M. (2020). Assessing manual wheelchair caster design for mobility in winter conditions. _Assistive Technology, 32_(1), 31–37. https://doi.org/10.1080/10400435.2018.1464080

Best, K. L., Routhier, F., & Miller, W. C. (2015). A description of manual wheelchair skills training: Current practice in Canadian rehabilitation center. _Disability and Rehabilitation: Assistive Technology,10_(5), 393–400. https://doi.org/10.3109/17483107.2014.907367

Cavallone, P., Bonisoli, E., & Quaglia, G. (2020). Prototyping of manual wheelchair with alternate propulsion system. _Disability and Rehabilitation: Assistive Technology, 15_(8), 945–951. https://doi.org/10.1080/17483107.2019.1629185

Choukou, M. A., Best, K. L., Potvin-Gilbert, M., Routhier, F., Lettre, J., Gamache, S., Borisoff, J. F., & Gagnon, D. (2021). Scoping review of propelling aids for manual wheelchairs. _Assistive Technology, 33_(2), 72–86. https://doi.org/10.1080/10400435.2019.1595789

Croxall, L., Gifford, W., & Jutai, J. (2020). First nations elders who use wheeled mobility: An exploration of culture and health. _Canadian Journal on Aging, 39_(2), 318–327.

D'Souza, C., Paquet, V. L., Lenker, J. A., & Steinfeld, E. (2019). Self-reported difficulty and preferences of wheeled mobility device users for simulated low-floor bus boarding, interior circulation, and disembarking. _Disability and Rehabilitation: Assistive Technology, 14_(2), 109–121. https://doi.org/10.1080/17483107.2017.1401128

De Souza, L. H., & Frank, A. O. (2020). Clinical features of electric powered indoor/outdoor wheelchair users with spinal cord injuries: A cross-sectional study. _Assistive Technology, 32_(3), 117–124. https://doi.org/10.1080/10400435.2018.1503205

Fallot, C., Bascou, J., Pillet, H., & Sauret, C. (2021). Manual wheelchair's turning resistance: Swiveling resistance parameters of front and rear wheels on different surfaces. _Disability and Rehabilitation: Assistive Technology_, _16_(3), 324–331. https://doi.org/10.1080/17483107.2019.1675781

Unsworth, C. A., Rawat, V., Sullivan, J., Tay, R., Naweed, A., & Gudimetla, P. (2019). "I'm very visible but seldom seen": Consumer choice and use of mobility aids on public transport. _Disability and Rehabilitation: Assistive Technology, 14_(2), 122–132. https://doi.org/10.1080/17483107.2017.1407829

A

Anger Self-Restraint

1410

Definition: Personal actions to eliminate or reduce intense hostile thoughts, feelings, and behaviors

OUTCOME TARGET RATING: Maintain at_____ Increase to_____

	Never Demonstrated	Rarely Demonstrated	Sometimes Demonstrated	Often Demonstrated	Consistently Demonstrated	
OUTCOME OVERALL RATING	1	2	3	4	5	
Indicators:						
141001 Identifies when angry	1	2	3	4	5	NA
141002 Identifies when frustrated	1	2	3	4	5	NA
141003 Identifies early signs of anger	1	2	3	4	5	NA
141004 Identifies situations that precipitate anger	1	2	3	4	5	NA
141005 Approaches unpredictable situation with an open mind	1	2	3	4	5	NA
141006 Identifies the basis of angry feelings	1	2	3	4	5	NA
141007 Assumes responsibility for personal behaviors	1	2	3	4	5	NA
141008 Uses effective conflict resolution skills	1	2	3	4	5	NA
141009 Expresses needs in a constructive manner	1	2	3	4	5	NA
141010 Vents negative feelings in a non-threatening manner	1	2	3	4	5	NA
141011 Monitors behavioral manifestations of anger	1	2	3	4	5	NA
141012 Monitors physical manifestations of anger	1	2	3	4	5	NA
141013 Uses physical activity to reduce repressed anger	1	2	3	4	5	NA
141014 Refrains from vacillating between outbursts of anger and passivity	1	2	3	4	5	NA
141015 Avoids imposing one's values on others	1	2	3	4	5	NA
141016 Shares feelings of anger with others	1	2	3	4	5	NA
141017 Uses strategies to control anger	1	2	3	4	5	NA
141018 Uses strategies to control frustration	1	2	3	4	5	NA
141019 Obtains counseling as needed	1	2	3	4	5	NA
141020 Maintains self-control without supervision	1	2	3	4	5	NA

Domain-Psychosocial Health (III)   *Class*-Self-Control (O)   5th edition 2013

OUTCOME CONTENT REFERENCES:

Dunbar, B. (2004). Anger management: A holistic approach. *Journal of the American Psychiatric Nurses Association, 10*(1), 16–23.

Howells, K., & Day, A. (2003). Readiness for anger management: Clinical and theoretical issues. *Clinical Psychology Review, 23*(2), 319–337.

Park, Y.-P., Ryu, H., Han, K. S., Kwon, J. H., Kim, H. K., Kang, H. C., Yoon, J.-W., Cheon, S.-H., & Shin, H. (2010). Anger, anger expression, and suicidal ideation in Korean adolescents. *Archives of Psychiatric Nursing, 24*(3), 168–177. https://doi.org/10.1016/j.apnu.2009.04.004

Puskar, K. R., Stark, K. H., Northcut, T., Williams, R., & Haley, T. (2010). Teaching kids to cope with anger: Peer education. *Journal of Child Health Care, 15*(1), 5–13. https://doi.org/10.1177/1367493510382932

Walker, A. J., Nott, M. T., Doyle, M., Onus, M., McCarthy, K., & Baguley, I. J. (2010). Effectiveness of a group anger management programme after severe traumatic brain injury. *Brain Injury, 24*(3), 517–524. https://doi.org/10.3109/02699051003601721

Anxiety Level   1211   **A**

Definition: Severity of manifested apprehension, tension, or uneasiness arising from an unidentifiable source

OUTCOME TARGET RATING: Maintain at_____ Increase to_____

		Severe	Substantial	Moderate	Mild	None	
OUTCOME OVERALL RATING		1	2	3	4	5	
Indicators:							
121101	Restlessness	1	2	3	4	5	NA
121102	Pacing	1	2	3	4	5	NA
121103	Hand wringing	1	2	3	4	5	NA
121132	Hyperactivity	1	2	3	4	5	NA
121104	Distress	1	2	3	4	5	NA
121105	Uneasiness	1	2	3	4	5	NA
121133	Nervousness	1	2	3	4	5	NA
121134	Excessive worry	1	2	3	4	5	NA
121135	Feeling worthless	1	2	3	4	5	NA
121144	Lack of trust in self	1	2	3	4	5	NA
121136	Guilt	1	2	3	4	5	NA
121106	Muscle tension	1	2	3	4	5	NA
121137	Headache	1	2	3	4	5	NA
121138	Pain	1	2	3	4	5	NA
121107	Facial tension	1	2	3	4	5	NA
121108	Irritability	1	2	3	4	5	NA
121139	Hyperarousal	1	2	3	4	5	NA
121109	Indecisiveness	1	2	3	4	5	NA
121110	Outbursts of anger	1	2	3	4	5	NA
121111	Problem behavior	1	2	3	4	5	NA
121112	Difficulty concentrating	1	2	3	4	5	NA
121113	Difficulty learning	1	2	3	4	5	NA
121114	Difficulty problem-solving	1	2	3	4	5	NA
121140	Difficulty relaxing	1	2	3	4	5	NA
121115	Panic attack	1	2	3	4	5	NA
121116	Verbalized apprehension	1	2	3	4	5	NA
121117	Verbalized anxiety	1	2	3	4	5	NA
121118	Exaggerated concern about life events	1	2	3	4	5	NA
121119	Increased blood pressure	1	2	3	4	5	NA
121120	Increased pulse rate	1	2	3	4	5	NA
121121	Increased respiratory rate	1	2	3	4	5	NA
121122	Dilated pupils	1	2	3	4	5	NA
121123	Sweating	1	2	3	4	5	NA
121124	Dizziness	1	2	3	4	5	NA
121125	Fatigue	1	2	3	4	5	NA
121126	Decreased productivity	1	2	3	4	5	NA
121127	Decreased school achievement	1	2	3	4	5	NA
121141	Interference with social activities	1	2	3	4	5	NA
121142	Interference with family function	1	2	3	4	5	NA
121143	Disinterest in life	1	2	3	4	5	NA
121128	Withdrawal	1	2	3	4	5	NA
121129	Sleep disturbance	1	2	3	4	5	NA
121130	Change in bowel pattern	1	2	3	4	5	NA
121145	Gastric reflux	1	2	3	4	5	NA
121146	Cramping	1	2	3	4	5	NA
121147	Nausea	1	2	3	4	5	NA
121131	Change in eating pattern	1	2	3	4	5	NA

Domain-Psychosocial Health (III)   *Class*-Psychological Well-Being (M)   3rd edition 2004; revised 2018, 2024

OUTCOME CONTENT REFERENCES:

American Psychiatric Association. (2022). *Diagnostic and statistical manual of mental disorders* (5th ed., text rev.). https://doi.org/10.1176/appi.books.9780890425787

Mannes, Z. L., Dunne E. M., Ferguson E. G., Cook, R. L., & Ennis, N. (2021). Symptoms of generalized anxiety disorder as a risk factor for substance use among adults living with HIV. *AIDS Care, 33*(5), 623–632. https://doi.org/10.1080/09540121.2020.1808163

Sampaio, F. M. C., Araújo, O. S. S. L., Sequeira, C. A. da C., Lluch Canut, M. T., & Martins, T. (2018). Evaluation of the psychometric properties of NOC outcomes "Anxiety Level" and "Anxiety Self-Control" in a Portuguese outpatient sample. *International Journal of Nursing Knowledge, 29*(3), 184–191. https://doi.org/10.1111/2047-3095.12169

Santiago, F. J. R., Garduño, M. L. M., Hernández-Aguilera, R. D., & Uscanga, Y. C. (2021). Insecure attachment as a risk factor for the development of anxiety and depression symptoms in a sample of Mexican adults. *Issues in Mental Health Nursing, 42*(8), 768–775. https://doi.org/10.1080/01612840.2020.1836538

Topaz, M., Koleck, T. A., Onorato, N., Smaldone, A., & Bakken, S. (2021). Nursing documentation of symptoms is associated with higher risk of emergency department visits and hospitalizations in homecare patients. *Nursing Outlook, 69*(3), 435–446. https://doi.org/10.1016/j.outlook.2020.12.007

Varcarolis, E. M., & Fosbre, C. D. (2021). *Essentials of psychiatric-mental health nursing* (4th ed.). Elsevier.

Wilson, P. B., Russell, H., & Pugh, J. (2021). Anxiety may be a risk factor for experiencing gastrointestinal symptoms during endurance races: An observational study. *European Journal of Sport Science, 21*(3), 421–427. https://doi.org/10.1080/17461391.2020.1746836

Anxiety Self-Control 1402

Definition: Personal actions to eliminate or reduce feelings of apprehension, tension, or uneasiness from an unidentifiable source

OUTCOME TARGET RATING: Maintain at_____ Increase to_____

		Never Demonstrated	Rarely Demonstrated	Sometimes Demonstrated	Often Demonstrated	Consistently Demonstrated	
OUTCOME OVERALL RATING		1	2	3	4	5	
Indicators:							
140201	Monitors intensity of anxiety	1	2	3	4	5	NA
140202	Eliminates precursors of anxiety	1	2	3	4	5	NA
140219	Identifies triggers of anxiety	1	2	3	4	5	NA
140203	Decreases environmental stimuli when anxious	1	2	3	4	5	NA
140220	Obtains information to reduce anxiety	1	2	3	4	5	NA
140205	Plans coping strategies for stressful situations	1	2	3	4	5	NA
140206	Uses effective coping strategies	1	2	3	4	5	NA
140207	Uses relaxation techniques to reduce anxiety	1	2	3	4	5	NA
140221	Controls breathing when anxious	1	2	3	4	5	NA
140208	Monitors duration of episodes	1	2	3	4	5	NA
140209	Monitors length of time between episodes	1	2	3	4	5	NA
140210	Maintains role performance	1	2	3	4	5	NA
140211	Maintains social relationships	1	2	3	4	5	NA
140222	Shares concerns with others	1	2	3	4	5	NA
140212	Maintains concentration	1	2	3	4	5	NA
140213	Monitors sensory perceptual distortions	1	2	3	4	5	NA
140214	Maintains adequate sleep	1	2	3	4	5	NA
140223	Uses medication as prescribed	1	2	3	4	5	NA
140215	Monitors physical manifestations of anxiety	1	2	3	4	5	NA
140216	Monitors behavioral manifestations of anxiety	1	2	3	4	5	NA
140224	Keeps appointments with health professional	1	2	3	4	5	NA
140217	Controls anxiety response	1	2	3	4	5	NA

Domain-*Psychosocial Health (III)* **Class**-*Self-Control (O)* *1st edition 1997; revised 2000, 2004, 2018*

OUTCOME CONTENT REFERENCES:

American Psychiatric Association. (2013). *Diagnostic and statistical manual of mental disorders* (5th ed.). https://doi.org/10.1176/appi.books.9780890425596

Antai-Otong, D. (2016). Caring for the patient with an anxiety disorder. *Nursing Clinics of North America, 51*(2), 173–183. https://doi.org/10.1016/j.cnur.2016.01.003

+Hudson, W. W. (1992). *The WALMYR assessment scales scoring manual.* WALMYR Publishing.

Sampaio, F. M. C., Araújo, O. S. S. L., Sequeira, C. A. da C., Lluch Canut, M. T., & Martins, T. (2018). Evaluation of the psychometric properties of NOC outcomes "Anxiety Level" and "Anxiety Self-Control" in a Portuguese outpatient sample. *International Journal of Nursing Knowledge, 29*(3), 184–191. https://doi.org/10.1111/2047-3095.12169

Stuart, G. W. (2013). *Principles and practice of psychiatric nursing* (10th ed.). Elsevier Mosby.

Villaggi, B., Provencher, H., Coulombe, S., Meunier, S., Radziszewski, S., Hudon, C., Roberge, P., Provencher, M. D., & Houle, J. (2015). Self-management strategies in recovery from mood and anxiety disorders. *Global Qualitative Nursing Research, 2,* 1–13. https://doi.org/10.1177/2333393615606092

Yearwood, E. L., Pearson, G. S., & Newland, J. A. (Eds.). (2012). *Child and adolescent behavioral health: A resource for advanced practice psychiatric and primary care practitioners in nursing.* Wiley-Blackwell.

Zimmermann, T., Puschmanna, E., van den Busschea, H., Wiesec, B., Ernst, A., Porzelt, S., Daubmann, A., & Scherer, M. (2016). Collaborative nurse-led self-management support for primary care patients with anxiety, depressive or somatic symptoms: Cluster-randomised controlled trial (findings of the SMADS study). *International Journal of Nursing Studies, 63,* 101–111. https://doi.org/10.1016/j.ijnurstu.2016.08.007

Appetite 1014

Definition: Desire to eat

OUTCOME TARGET RATING: Maintain at_____ Increase to_____

	Severely Compromised	Substantially Compromised	Moderately Compromised	Mildly Compromised	Not Compromised	
OUTCOME OVERALL RATING	1	2	3	4	5	
Indicators:						
101401	Desire to eat	1	2	3	4	5	NA
101402	Craving for food	1	2	3	4	5	NA
101403	Enjoyment of food	1	2	3	4	5	NA
101404	Taste of food	1	2	3	4	5	NA
101405	Energy to eat	1	2	3	4	5	NA
101406	Food intake	1	2	3	4	5	NA
101407	Nutrient intake	1	2	3	4	5	NA
101408	Fluid intake	1	2	3	4	5	NA
101409	Stimulus to eat	1	2	3	4	5	NA

Domain-Physiologic Health (II) *Class*-Digestion & Nutrition (K) 3rd edition 2004; revised 2013

OUTCOME CONTENT REFERENCES:

Anderson, K. N. (2002). *Mosby's medical, nursing, & allied health dictionary* (6th ed.). Mosby.

Dudek, S. G. (2001). *Nutrition essentials for nursing practice* (3rd ed.). Lippincott Williams & Wilkins.

Lewis, S. M., Heitkemper, M. M., & Dirksen, S. R. (2011). *Medical-surgical nursing: Assessment and management of clinical problems* (8th ed.). Elsevier Mosby.

McCanse, K. L., Pearson, G. S., & Huether, S. E. (2010). *Pathophysiology: The biological basis for disease in adults and children* (6th ed.). Mosby Elsevier.

Potter, P. A., Perry, A. G., Hall, A., & Stockert, P. A. (2009). *Fundamentals of nursing* (7th ed.). Mosby.

Venes, D. (Ed.). (2013). *Taber's cyclopedic medical dictionary* (22nd ed.). F.A. Davis.

A

Attention Deficit Level

0921

Definition: Severity of persistent patterns of inattention in a child

OUTCOME TARGET RATING: Maintain at_____ Increase to_____

		Severe	Substantial	Moderate	Mild	None	
OUTCOME OVERALL RATING		1	2	3	4	5	
Indicators:							
092101	Inattention	1	2	3	4	5	NA
092102	Difficulty listening	1	2	3	4	5	NA
092103	Inability to pay close attention to details of tasks	1	2	3	4	5	NA
092104	Difficulty organizing tasks	1	2	3	4	5	NA
092105	Inability to stay on task	1	2	3	4	5	NA
092106	Difficulty completing tasks	1	2	3	4	5	NA
092107	Difficulty with tasks that require sustained cognitive effort	1	2	3	4	5	NA
092108	Difficulty resisting temptation	1	2	3	4	5	NA
092109	Careless mistakes completing tasks	1	2	3	4	5	NA
092110	Frequency of losing things	1	2	3	4	5	NA
092111	Excessive internal distractibility	1	2	3	4	5	NA
092112	Excessive external distractibility	1	2	3	4	5	NA
092113	Excessive forgetfulness	1	2	3	4	5	NA
092114	Immaturity relative to chronological age	1	2	3	4	5	NA
092115	Selective inattention to non-preferred tasks	1	2	3	4	5	NA

Domain-Physiologic Health (II)   **Class**-Neurocognitive (J)   *7th edition 2024*

OUTCOME CONTENT REFERENCES:

American Psychiatric Association. (2022). *Diagnostic and statistical manual of mental disorders* (5th ed., text rev.). https://doi.org/10.1176/appi.books.9780890425787

Caldwell, C. L., Wasson, D., Anderson, M. A., Brighton, V., & Dixon, L. (2005). Development of the nursing outcome (NOC) label: Hyperactivity level. *Journal of Child and Adolescent Psychiatric Nursing, 18*(3), 95–102. https://doi.org/10.1111/j.1744-6171.2005.00004.x

Center for Disease Control and Prevention. (2021, September 28). *Attention-Deficit/Hyperactivity Disorder (ADHD).* https://www.cdc.gov/ncbddd/adhd/

Fuller-Thomson, E., Carrique, L., & MacNeil, A. (2022). Generalized anxiety disorder among adults with attention deficit hyperactivity disorder. *Journal of Affective Disorders, 299*, 707–714. https://doi.org/10.1016/j.jad.2021.10.020

He, S., Shuai, L., Wang, Z., Qiu, M., Wilson, A., Xia, W., Cao, X., Lu, L., & Zhang, J. (2021). Online learning performances of children and adolescents with attention deficit hyperactivity disorder during the COVID-19 pandemic. *Inquiry* (00469580), *58*, 1–11. https://doi.org/10.1177/00469580211049065

Hechtman, L. (2000). Assessment and diagnosis of attention deficit/hyperactive disorder. *Child and Adolescent Psychiatric Clinics of North America, 9*(3), 481–498. https://doi.org/10.1016/S1056-4993(18)30102-0

Tandon, M., & Pergjika, A. (2017). Attention deficit hyperactivity disorder in preschool-age children. *Child and Adolescent Psychiatric Clinics of North America, 26*(3), 523–538. https://doi.org/10.1016/j.chc.2017.02.007

Tang, C. H., Chi, M. H., Hsieh, Y. T., Lee, T. I., Tai, Y. C., Lien, Y.-J., Yang, Y. K., & Chen, P. S. (2022). Sex differences in the diagnosis of autism spectrum disorder and effects of comorbid mental retardation and attention-deficit hyperactivity disorder. *Journal of the Formosan Medical Association, 121*(1), 210–217. https://doi.org/10.1016/j.jfma.2021.03.009

Balance   0202

Definition: Ability to maintain body equilibrium

OUTCOME TARGET RATING: Maintain at_____ Increase to_____

		Severely Compromised	Substantially Compromised	Moderately Compromised	Mildly Compromised	Not Compromised	
OUTCOME OVERALL RATING		1	2	3	4	5	
Indicators:							
020202	Maintains balance while sitting without back support	1	2	3	4	5	NA
020214	Maintains balance while bending over	1	2	3	4	5	NA
020212	Maintains balance while rising from sitting position	1	2	3	4	5	NA
020201	Maintains balance while standing	1	2	3	4	5	NA
020203	Maintains balance while walking	1	2	3	4	5	NA
020215	Maintains balance while walking backwards	1	2	3	4	5	NA
020209	Maintains balance while standing on one foot	1	2	3	4	5	NA
020210	Maintains balance while shifting weight from one foot to another	1	2	3	4	5	NA
020213	Maintains balance while turning 360 degrees	1	2	3	4	5	NA
020211	Posture	1	2	3	4	5	NA
		Severe	**Substantial**	**Moderate**	**Mild**	**None**	
020205	Weaving	1	2	3	4	5	NA
020206	Dizziness	1	2	3	4	5	NA
020207	Shakiness	1	2	3	4	5	NA
020208	Stumbling	1	2	3	4	5	NA
020215	Postural sway	1	2	3	4	5	NA

Domain-Functional Health (I)   *Class*-Mobility (C)   *1st edition 1997; revised 2004, 2008, 2013, 2024*

OUTCOME CONTENT REFERENCES:

Haukanes, L., Knapstad, M. K., Kristiansen, L., & Magnussen, L. H. (2021). Association between musculoskeletal function and postural balance in patients with long-lasting dizziness. A cross-sectional study. *Physiotherapy Research International, 26*(3), 1–9. https://doi.org/10.1002/pri.1916

Riis, J., Eika, F., Blomkvist, A. W., Rahbek, M. T., Eikhof, K. D., Hansen, M. D., Søndergaard, M., Ryg, J., Andersen, S., & Jorgensen, M. G. (2020). Lifespan data on postural balance in multiple standing positions. *Gait & Posture, 76*, 68–73. https://doi.org/10.1016/j.gaitpost.2019.11.004

Rodrigues Pereira, N. M., Massé Araya, M. J. P., & Scheicher, M. E. (2021). Improvement of quality of life and postural balance of institutionalized elderly people undergoing to a treadmill walking training. *Journal of Bodywork & Movement Therapies, 28*, 172–179. https://doi.org/10.1016/j.jbmt.2021.07.043

Taulbee, L., Yada, T., Graham, L., O'Halloran, A., Saracino, D., Freund, J., Vallabhajosula, S., & Balasubramanian, C. K. (2021). Use of backward walking speed to screen dynamic balance and mobility deficits in older adults living independently in the community. *Journal of Geriatric Physical Therapy, 44*(4), 189–197. https://doi.org/10.1519/JPT.0000000000000290

Tinetti, M. E. (1986). Performance-oriented assessment of mobility problems in elderly patients. *Journal of the American Geriatric Society, 34*(2), 119–126.

B

Blood Coagulation

Definition: Extent to which blood clots within normal period of time

OUTCOME TARGET RATING: Maintain at_____ Increase to_____

		Severe Deviation from Normal Range	Substantial Deviation from Normal Range	Moderate Deviation from Normal Range	Mild Deviation from Normal Range	No Deviation from Normal Range	
OUTCOME OVERALL RATING		1	2	3	4	5	
Indicators:							
040901	Clot formation	1	2	3	4	5	NA
040912	Prothrombin time (PT)	1	2	3	4	5	NA
040905	Prothrombin time – international normalized ratio (PT-INR)	1	2	3	4	5	NA
040907	Partial thromboplastin time (PTT)	1	2	3	4	5	NA
040913	Hemoglobin (Hgb)	1	2	3	4	5	NA
040908	Platelet count	1	2	3	4	5	NA
040909	Plasma fibrinogen	1	2	3	4	5	NA
040914	Fibrin split products (FSP)	1	2	3	4	5	NA
040910	Hematocrit (Hct)	1	2	3	4	5	NA
040915	Activated clotting time (ACT)	1	2	3	4	5	NA
		Severe	**Substantial**	**Moderate**	**Mild**	**None**	
040902	Bleeding	1	2	3	4	5	NA
040903	Bruising	1	2	3	4	5	NA
040904	Petechiae	1	2	3	4	5	NA
040916	Ecchymosis	1	2	3	4	5	NA
040917	Purpura	1	2	3	4	5	NA
040918	Hematuria	1	2	3	4	5	NA
040919	Blood in stool	1	2	3	4	5	NA
040920	Hemoptysis	1	2	3	4	5	NA
040921	Hematemesis	1	2	3	4	5	NA
040922	Bleeding gums	1	2	3	4	5	NA
040923	Thrombocytopenia	1	2	3	4	5	NA

Domain-Physiologic Health (II)   *Class*-Cardiopulmonary (E)   *2nd edition 2000; revised 2004, 2018*

OUTCOME CONTENT REFERENCES:

Burns, S. M. (Ed.). (2014). *AACN essentials of critical care nursing* (3rd ed.). McGraw-Hill.

Chang, Y., Dabiri, G., Damstetter, E., Ebot, E., Powers, J., & Phillips, T. (2016). Coagulation disorders and their cutaneous presentations: Pathophysiology. *Journal of the American Academy of Dermatology, 74*(5), 783–792. https://doi.org/10.1016/j.jaad.2015.08.072

Christensen, C. R., & Lewis, P. A. (Eds.). (2014). *Core curriculum for vascular nursing.* Wolters Kluwer.

Cremer, M., Sallmon, H., Kling, P., Bührer, C., & Dame, C. (2016). Thrombocytopenia and platelet transfusion in the neonate. *Seminars in Fetal & Neonatal Medicine, 21*(1), 10–18. https://doi.org/10.1016/j.siny.2015.11.001

Dabiri, G., Damstetter, E., Chang, Y., Ebot, E., Powers, J., & Phillips, T. (2016). Coagulation disorders and their cutaneous presentations: Diagnostic work-up and treatment. *Journal of the American Academy of Dermatology, 74*(5), 795–804. https://doi.org/10.1016/j.jaad.2015.08.071

Lewis, S., Dirksen, S., Heitkemper, M., & Bucher, L. (2014). *Medical-surgical nursing: Assessment and management of clinical problems* (9th ed.). Elsevier Mosby.

McCance, K. L., & Huether, S. E. (2014). *Pathophysiology: The biological basis for disease in adults and children* (7th ed.). Elsevier Mosby.

Blood Glucose Control 2300

Definition: Extent to which glucose levels in plasma and urine are maintained in normal range

OUTCOME TARGET RATING: Maintain at_____ Increase to_____

	Severe Deviation from Normal Range	Substantial Deviation from Normal Range	Moderate Deviation from Normal Range	Mild Deviation from Normal Range	No Deviation from Normal Range	
OUTCOME OVERALL RATING	1	2	3	4	5	
Indicators:						
230001	Blood glucose	1	2	3	4	5	NA
230004	Glycosylated hemoglobin	1	2	3	4	5	NA
230005	Fructosamine	1	2	3	4	5	NA
230007	Urine glucose	1	2	3	4	5	NA
230008	Urine ketones	1	2	3	4	5	NA

Domain-Physiologic Health (II)   **Class**-*Therapeutic Response (AA)*   2nd edition 2000; reviewed 2018; revised 2004, 2024

OUTCOME CONTENT REFERENCES:
Martens, T. W., Bergenstal, R. M., Pearson, T., Carlson, A. L., Scheiner, G., Carlos, C., Liao, B., Syring, K., & Pollom, R. D. (2021). Making sense of glucose metrics in diabetes: Linkage between postprandial glucose (PPG), time in range (TIR) & hemoglobin A1c (A1C). *Postgraduate Medicine, 133*(3), 253–264. https://doi.org/10.1080/00325481.2020.1851946

Prentice, J. C., Mohr, D. C., Zhang, L., Li, D., Legler, A., Nelson, R. E., & Conlin, P. R. (2021). Increased hemoglobin A1c time in range reduces adverse health outcomes in older adults with diabetes. *Diabetes Care, 44*(8), 1750–1756. https://doi.org/10.2337/dc21-0292

Sherr, J. L., Schwandt, A., Phelan, H., Clements, M. A., Holl, R. W., Benitez-Aguirre, P. Z., Miller, K. M., Woelfle, J., Dover, T., Maahs, D. M., Fröhlich-Reiterer, E., & Craig, M. E. (2021). Hemoglobin A1c patterns of youth with type 1 diabetes 10 years post diagnosis from 3 continents. *Pediatrics, 148*(2), 1–11. https://doi.org/10.1542/peds.2020-048942

Weiss, T., Edwards, A., Lautsch, D., Rajpathak, S., & Snow, K. (2021). Hemoglobin A1C testing frequency among patients with type 2 diabetes within a U.S. payer system: A retrospective observational study. *Current Medical Research & Opinion, 37*(11), 1859–1866. https://doi.org/10.1080/03007995.2021.1965562

Blood Loss Severity 0413

Definition: Severity of signs and symptoms of internal or external bleeding

OUTCOME TARGET RATING: Maintain at_____ Increase to_____

	Severe	Substantial	Moderate	Mild	None	
OUTCOME OVERALL RATING	1	2	3	4	5	
Indicators:						
041301	Visible blood loss	1	2	3	4	5	NA
041302	Hematuria	1	2	3	4	5	NA
041303	Frank blood from anus	1	2	3	4	5	NA
041304	Hemoptysis	1	2	3	4	5	NA
041305	Hematemesis	1	2	3	4	5	NA
041306	Abdominal distention	1	2	3	4	5	NA
041307	Vaginal bleeding	1	2	3	4	5	NA
041308	Post-surgical bleeding	1	2	3	4	5	NA
041309	Decreased systolic blood pressure	1	2	3	4	5	NA
041310	Decreased diastolic blood pressure	1	2	3	4	5	NA
041311	Increased apical heart rate	1	2	3	4	5	NA
041312	Loss of body heat	1	2	3	4	5	NA
041313	Skin and mucous membrane pallor	1	2	3	4	5	NA
041314	Anxiety	1	2	3	4	5	NA
041315	Decreased cognition	1	2	3	4	5	NA

Continued

Blood Loss Severity—cont'd

		Severe	Substantial	Moderate	Mild	None	
041316	Decreased hemoglobin (Hgb)	1	2	3	4	5	NA
041317	Decreased hematocrit (Hct)	1	2	3	4	5	NA
Estimated blood loss_____(cc)							

Domain-Physiologic Health (II)   *Class*-Cardiopulmonary (E)   *3rd edition 2004; revised 2013*

OUTCOME CONTENT REFERENCES:
American College of Surgeons, Committee on Trauma. (1997). *Advanced trauma life support for doctors.*
Baron, B. J., Sinert, R., Zehtabchi, S., Stavile, K. L., & Scalea, T. M. (2004). Diagnostic utility of sublingual PCO2 for detecting hemorrhage in penetrating trauma patients. *Journal of Trauma, 57*(1), 69–74. https://doi.org/10.1097/01.ta.0000090754.94232.2c
Blankenship, J. C. (1999). Bleeding complications of glycoprotein IIb-IIIa receptor inhibitors. *American Heart Journal, 138*(4 Pt 2), 287–296.
Bose, P., Regan, F., & Paterson-Brown, S. (2006). Improving the accuracy of estimated blood loss at obstetric haemorrhage using clinical reconstructions. *BJOG: An International Journal of Obstetrics & Gynaecology, 113*(8), 919–924. https://doi.org/10.1111/j.1471-0528.2006.01018.x
De Guzman, E., Shankar, M. N., & Mattox, K. L. (1999). Limited volume resuscitation in penetrating thoracoabdominal trauma. *AACN Clinical Issues, 10*(1), 61–68.
Fihn, S. D., Callahan, C. M., Martin, D. C., McDonell, M. B., Henikoff, J. G., & White, R. H. (1996). The risk for and severity of bleeding complications in elderly patients treated with warfarin. *Annals of Internal Medicine, 124*(11), 970–979.
Maxson, J. H. (2000). Management of disseminated intravascular coagulation. *Critical Care Nursing Clinics of North America, 12*(3), 341–352.
Sims, C., Seigne, P., Menconi, M., Monarca, J., Barlow, C., Pettit, J., & Puyana, J. C. (2001). Skeletal muscle acidosis correlates with the severity of blood volume loss during shock and resuscitation. *Journal of Trauma, 51*(6), 1137–1146.
Swearington, P. L., & Keen, J. H. (2001). *Manual of critical care nursing: Nursing interventions and collaborative* management (4th ed.). Mosby.

Blood Product Transfusion Reaction   0700

Definition: Severity of acute complications from blood, plasma, or platelet transfusion

OUTCOME TARGET RATING: Maintain at_____ Increase to_____

		Severe	Substantial	Moderate	Mild	None	
OUTCOME OVERALL RATING		1	2	3	4	5	
Indicators:							
070020	Shortness of breath	1	2	3	4	5	NA
070025	Apprehension	1	2	3	4	5	NA
070012	Anxiety	1	2	3	4	5	NA
070011	Restlessness	1	2	3	4	5	NA
070004	Increased heart rate	1	2	3	4	5	NA
070022	Decreased blood pressure	1	2	3	4	5	NA
070026	Circulatory overload	1	2	3	4	5	NA
070027	Headache	1	2	3	4	5	NA
070028	Wheezing	1	2	3	4	5	NA
070007	Fever	1	2	3	4	5	NA
070008	Chills	1	2	3	4	5	NA
070029	Rigors	1	2	3	4	5	NA
070030	Urticaria	1	2	3	4	5	NA
070009	Itching	1	2	3	4	5	NA
070010	Rash	1	2	3	4	5	NA
070021	Nausea	1	2	3	4	5	NA
070014	Chest pain	1	2	3	4	5	NA
070015	Lumbar pain	1	2	3	4	5	NA
070031	Flank pain	1	2	3	4	5	NA
070032	Abdominal pain	1	2	3	4	5	NA
070003	Decreased urine output	1	2	3	4	5	NA
070017	Hemoglobinuria	1	2	3	4	5	NA
070033	Bronchospasm	1	2	3	4	5	NA
070034	Shock	1	2	3	4	5	NA

Domain-Physiologic Health (II)   *Class*-Immune Response (H)   *1st edition 1997; revised 2004, 2008, 2024*

OUTCOME CONTENT REFERENCES:

Delaney, M., Wendel, S., Bercovitz, R.S., Cid, J., Cohn, C., Dunbar, N. M., Apelseth, T. O., Popovsky, M., Stanworth, S., & Tinmouth, A. (2016). Transfusion reactions: Prevention, diagnosis, and treatment, *The Lancet, 388*, 2825–2836. https://doi.org/10.1016/S0140-6736(15)01313-6

Frazier, S. K., Higgins, J., Bugajski, A., Jones, A. R., & Brown, M. R. (2017). Adverse reactions to transfusion of blood products and best practices for prevention. *Critical Care Nursing Clinics of North America, 29*(3), 271–290. https://doi.org/10.1016/j.cnc.2017.04.002

Hinkle, J. L. (2018). *Brunner & Suddarth's textbook of Medical-surgical nursing* (14th ed.). Wolters Kluwer.

Ignatavicius, D. D., Workman, M. L., Rebar, C. R., & Heimgartner, N. M. (2021). *Medical-surgical nursing: Concepts for interprofessional care* (10th ed.). Elsevier.

McCance, K. L., Huether, S. E., Brashers, V. L., & Rote, N. S. (2019). *Study guide for pathophysiology: The biologic basis for disease in adults and children.* Elsevier.

Raval, J. S., Griggs, J. R., & Fleg, A. (2020). Blood product transfusion in adults: Indications, adverse reactions, and modifications. *American Family Physician, 102*(1), 30–38.

Semple, J. W., Rebetz, J., & Kapur, R. (2019). Transfusion-associated circulatory overload and transfusion-related acute lung injury. *Blood, 133*(17), 1840–1853. https://doi.org/10.1182/blood-2018-10-860809

Sharma, S., Sharma, P., & Tyler, N. L. (2011). Transfusion of blood and blood products: Indications and complications. *American Family Physician, 83*, 719–724.

B

Body Image   1200

Definition: Personal appraisal of own appearance and body functions

OUTCOME TARGET RATING: Maintain at_____ Increase to_____

		Never Positive	Rarely Positive	Sometimes Positive	Often Positive	Consistently Positive	
OUTCOME OVERALL RATING		1	2	3	4	5	
Indicators:							
120001	Internal picture of self	1	2	3	4	5	NA
120002	Congruence between body reality, body ideal, and body presentation	1	2	3	4	5	NA
120019	Attitude towards describing changes in body	1	2	3	4	5	NA
120003	Description of affected body part in positive terms	1	2	3	4	5	NA
120020	Attitude towards looking at affected body part	1	2	3	4	5	NA
120016	Attitude towards touching affected body part	1	2	3	4	5	NA
120017	Attitude towards using strategies to enhance appearance	1	2	3	4	5	NA
120005	Satisfaction with body appearance	1	2	3	4	5	NA
120018	Attitude toward using strategies to enhance function	1	2	3	4	5	NA
120006	Satisfaction with body function	1	2	3	4	5	NA
120007	Adjustment to changes in physical appearance	1	2	3	4	5	NA
120021	Adjustment to changes in body size	1	2	3	4	5	NA
120008	Adjustment to changes in body function	1	2	3	4	5	NA
120009	Adjustment to changes in health status	1	2	3	4	5	NA
120013	Adjustment to body changes due to injury	1	2	3	4	5	NA
120014	Adjustment to body changes due to surgery	1	2	3	4	5	NA
120022	Adjustment to body changes during puberty	1	2	3	4	5	NA
120023	Adjustment to body changes after childbirth	1	2	3	4	5	NA
120015	Adjustment to body changes due to aging	1	2	3	4	5	NA
120024	Focus on abilities rather than disabilities	1	2	3	4	5	NA
120025	Description of personal concerns about body image with others	1	2	3	4	5	NA
120026	Description of personal concerns about body function with others	1	2	3	4	5	NA

Domain-Psychosocial Health (III)   *Class*-Psychological Well-Being (M)   *1st edition 1997; revised 2004, 2008, 2024*

OUTCOME CONTENT REFERENCES:

Bennett, E. V., Hurd, L. C., Pritchard, E. M., Colton, T., & Crocker, P. R. E. (2020). An examination of older men's body image: How men 65 years and older perceive, experience, and cope with their aging bodies. *Body Image, 34*, 27–37. https://doi.org/10.1016/j.bodyim.2020.04.005

Cleary, M., Kornhaber, R., Thapa, D. K., West, S., & Visentin, D. (2020). A quantitative systematic review assessing the impact of burn injuries on body image. *Body Image, 33*, 47–65. https://doi.org/10.1016/j.bodyim.2020.02.008

Fitch, M. (2020). Living with body image changes following completion of cancer treatment. *Canadian Oncology Nursing Journal, 30*(3), 231–234.

Hartman-Munick, S. M., Gordon, A. R., & Guss, C. (2020). Adolescent body image. *Current Opinion in Pediatrics, 32*(4), 455–460. https://doi.org/10.1097/MOP.0000000000000910

Jongenelis, M. I., & Pettigrew, S. (2020). Body image and eating disturbances in children: The role of self-objectification. *Psychology of Women Quarterly, 44*(3), 393–402. https://doi.org/10.1177/0361684320923294

Lee, M., & Damhorst, M. L. (2020). Women's body image throughout the adult life span: A latent growth modeling approach. *International Journal of Aging & Human Development, 91*(3), 317–339. https://doi.org/10.1177/0091415019871206

Markey, C. H., August, K. J., & Dunaev, J. L. (2020). Understanding body image among adults in mid-late life: Considering romantic partners and depressive symptoms in the context of diabetes. *Journal of Health Psychology, 25*(10/11), 1707–1716. https://doi.org/10.1177/1359105318770725

Potter, P. A., Perry, A. G., Stockert, P., & Hall, A. (2021). *Fundamentals of nursing* (10th ed.). Elsevier.

Sklar, E. M. (2015). Body image, weight, and self-concept in men. *American Journal of Lifestyle Medicine, 11*(3), 252–258. https://doi.org/10.1177/1559827615594351

Whitaker, C., Gough, B., Fawkner, H., & Deighton-Smith, N. (2021). Young men's body dissatisfaction: A qualitative analysis of anonymous online accounts. *Journal of Health Psychology, 26*(5), 636–649. https://doi.org/10.1177/1359105319832352

Williams, P. (2020). *Basic geriatric nursing* (7th ed.). Elsevier.

Body Mechanics Performance   1616

Definition: Personal actions to maintain proper body alignment and to prevent muscular skeletal strain or injury

OUTCOME TARGET RATING: Maintain at_____ Increase to_____

		Never Demonstrated	Rarely Demonstrated	Sometimes Demonstrated	Often Demonstrated	Consistently Demonstrated	
OUTCOME OVERALL RATING		1	2	3	4	5	
Indicators:							
161601	Uses correct standing posture	1	2	3	4	5	NA
161602	Uses correct sitting posture	1	2	3	4	5	NA
161603	Uses correct lying posture	1	2	3	4	5	NA
161616	Wears proper shoes	1	2	3	4	5	NA
161617	Maintains center of gravity	1	2	3	4	5	NA
161618	Maintains wide base of support	1	2	3	4	5	NA
161619	Maintains proper alignment	1	2	3	4	5	NA
161604	Uses correct lifting techniques	1	2	3	4	5	NA
161620	Avoids sitting for long periods of time	1	2	3	4	5	NA
161605	Uses correct carrying techniques	1	2	3	4	5	NA
161612	Uses correct pushing techniques	1	2	3	4	5	NA
161607	Uses supportive devices correctly	1	2	3	4	5	NA
161608	Obtains assistance with heavy load	1	2	3	4	5	NA
161613	Maintains muscle strength	1	2	3	4	5	NA
161614	Maintains joint flexibility	1	2	3	4	5	NA
161621	Uses recommended exercises to prevent injury	1	2	3	4	5	NA
161615	Uses proper body mechanics	1	2	3	4	5	NA

Domain-*Health Knowledge & Behavior (IV)*   **Class**-*Health Behavior (Q)*   *3rd edition 2004; revised 2008, 2024*

OUTCOME CONTENT REFERENCES:

Kang, S. W. (2017). The use of body mechanics principle, clinical-practice fatigue, and practice satisfaction of nursing students. *Nursing Plus Open, 3*, 6–10. https://doi.org/10.1016/j.npls.2017.03.001

Potter, P. A., Perry, A. G., Stockert, P. A., & Hall, A. (2021). *Fundamentals of nursing* (10th ed.). Elsevier.

Sorrentino, S. A., & Remmert, L. A. (2021). *Mosby's textbook for nursing assistants.* (10th ed.). Elsevier.

Topcu, S. Y. (2017). Do Turkish patients with lumbar disc herniation know body mechanics? *Journal of Back and Musculoskeletal Rehabilitation, 30*(4), (2017), 835–840. https://doi.org/10.3233/BMR-160542

Body Positioning: Self-Initiated   0203

Definition: Personal actions to change own body position independently with or without assistive device

OUTCOME TARGET RATING: Maintain at_____ Increase to_____

	Severely Compromised	Substantially Compromised	Moderately Compromised	Mildly Compromised	Not Compromised	
OUTCOME OVERALL RATING	1	2	3	4	5	
Indicators:						
020302　Moves from lying to sitting	1	2	3	4	5	NA
020303　Moves from sitting to lying	1	2	3	4	5	NA
020304　Moves from sitting to standing	1	2	3	4	5	NA
020305　Moves from standing to sitting	1	2	3	4	5	NA
020306　Moves from standing to kneeling	1	2	3	4	5	NA
020307　Moves from kneeling to standing	1	2	3	4	5	NA
020308　Moves from standing to squatting	1	2	3	4	5	NA
020309　Moves from squatting to standing	1	2	3	4	5	NA
020314　Moves from floor to standing	1	2	3	4	5	NA
020315　Moves from standing to floor	1	2	3	4	5	NA
020310　Bends at waist while standing	1	2	3	4	5	NA
020311　Moves from side to side while lying	1	2	3	4	5	NA
020301　Moves from front to back while lying	1	2	3	4	5	NA
020313　Moves from back to front while lying	1	2	3	4	5	NA
020316　Upper body strength	1	2	3	4	5	NA
020317　Lower body strength	1	2	3	4	5	NA

Domain-Functional Health (I)   **Class**-Mobility (C)   *1st edition 1997; revised 2000, 2004, 2013, 2024*

OUTCOME CONTENT REFERENCES:

+Berg, K., Wood-Dauphinee, S., Williams, J. I., & Gayton, D. (1989). Measuring balance in the elderly: Preliminary development of an instrument. *Physiotherapy Canada, 41*(6), 304–311.

Chuang, Y.-F., Chen, C.-C., Hsu, M.-J., Huang, N.-J., Huang, Y.-Z., Chan, H.-L., & Chang, Y.-J. (2019). Age related changes of the motor excitabilities and central and peripheral muscle strength. *Journal of Electromyography & Kinesiology, 44*, 132–138. https://doi.org/10.1016/j.jelekin.2018.12.007

Mikulic, M. A., Griffith, E. R., & Jebsen, R. H. (1976). Clinical application of a standardized mobility test. *Archives of Physical Medicine and Rehabilitation, 57*(3), 143–146.

Potter, P. A., Perry, A. G., Stockert, P. A., & Hall, A. M. (2021). *Fundamentals of nursing* (10th ed.). Elsevier.

Rockwood, K., Rockwood, M. R. H., Andrew, M. K., & Mitnitski, A. (2008), Reliability of the hierarchical assessment of balance and mobility in frail older adults. *Journal of the American Geriatrics Society, 56*(7), 1213–1217. https://doi.org/10.1111/j.1532-5415.2008.01773.x

Wu, R., Ditroilo, M., Delahunt, E., & De Vito, G. (2021). Age related changes in motor function (II). Decline in motor performance outcomes. *International Journal of Sports Medicine, 42*(3), 215–226. https://doi.org/10.1055/a-1265-7073

Bone Healing

B

Definition: Extent of regeneration of cells and tissues following bone injury

OUTCOME TARGET RATING: Maintain at_____ Increase to_____

OUTCOME OVERALL RATING		None 1	Limited 2	Moderate 3	Substantial 4	Extensive 5	
Indicators:							
110402	Cellular proliferation	1	2	3	4	5	NA
110403	Callus formation	1	2	3	4	5	NA
110404	Ossification, consolidation, and remodeling	1	2	3	4	5	NA
110405	Intact peripheral circulation	1	2	3	4	5	NA
110406	Return of skeletal function	1	2	3	4	5	NA
		Extensive	Substantial	Moderate	Limited	None	
110401	Hematoma	1	2	3	4	5	NA
110407	Pain	1	2	3	4	5	NA
110408	Edema	1	2	3	4	5	NA
110413	Bone fragments	1	2	3	4	5	NA
110414	Adjacent tissue injury	1	2	3	4	5	NA
110410	Infection in surrounding tissue	1	2	3	4	5	NA
110411	Infection in bone	1	2	3	4	5	NA

Site of fracture (# from skeleton) _____

Domain-Physiologic Health (II) **Class**-Tissue Integrity (L) *1st edition 1997; revised 2004, 2018*

OUTCOME CONTENT REFERENCES:

Bigham-Sadegh, A., & Oryan, A. (2015). Basic concepts regarding fracture healing and the current options and future directions in managing bone fractures. *International Wound Journal, 12*(3), 238–247. https://doi.org/10.1111/iwj.12231

Corrarino, J. E. (2015). Fracture repair: Mechanisms and management. *Journal for Nurse Practitioners, 11*(10), 960–967. https://doi.org/10.1016/j.nurpra.2015.07.009

Grossman, S., & Porth, C. M. (2014). *Porth's pathophysiology: Concepts of altered health states* (9th ed.). Lippincott, Williams & Wilkins.

Potter, P. A., Perry, A. G., Stockert, P. A., & Hall, A. M. (2017). *Fundamentals of nursing* (9th ed.). Elsevier.

B

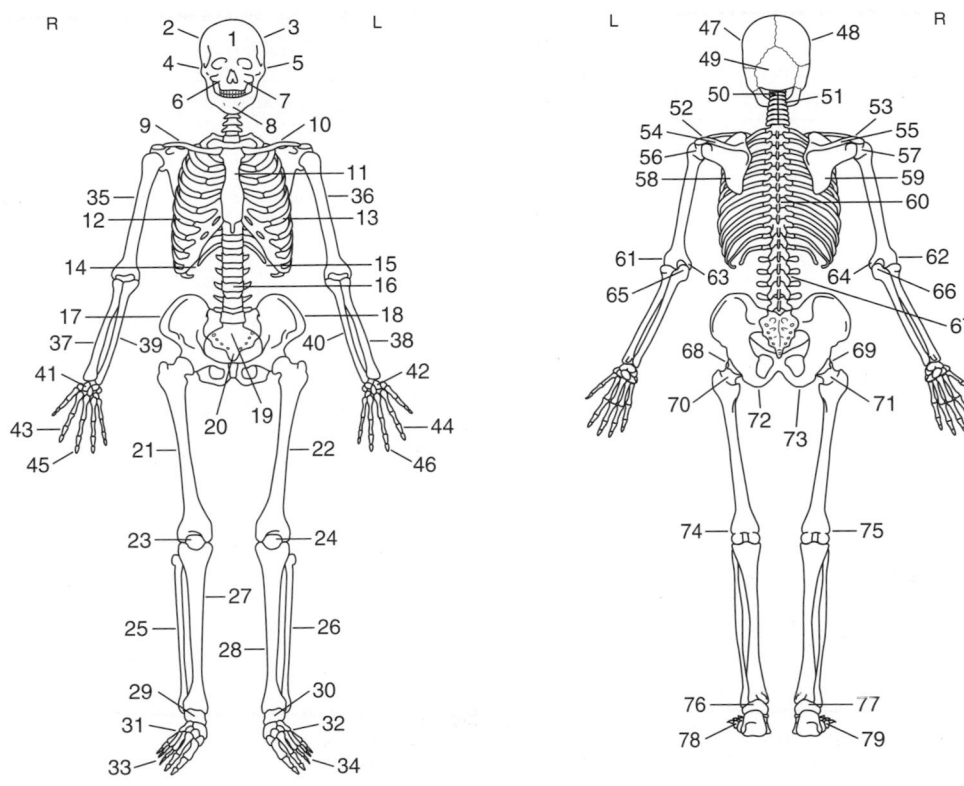

Bones of the head
1. Frontal
2. Right temporal
3. Left temporal
4. Right zygomatic
5. Left zygomatic
6. Right maxilla
7. Left maxilla
8. Mandible
47. Left parietal
48. Right parietal
49. Occipital

Bones of the neck and chest
9. Right clavicle
10. Left clavicle
11. Sternum
12. Right ribs
13. Left ribs
14. Right floating rib
15. Left floating rib
16. Vertebral column
50. Atlas
51. Cervical vertebra(e) specify _____
52. Left acromion
53. Right acromion
54. Left spine of scapula
55. Right spine of scapula
58. Left scapula
59. Right scapula
60. Thoracic vertebra(e) specify _____

Bones of the abdomen
16. Vertebral column
17. Right ilium
18. Left ilium
19. Sacrum
20. Coccyx
72. Left ischium
73. Right ischium
67. Lumbar vertebra(e) specify _____

Bones of the arm
35. Right humerus
36. Left humerus
37. Right radius
38. Left radius
39. Right ulna
40. Left ulna
41. Right carpals
42. Left carpals
43. Right metacarpals
44. Left metacarpals
45. Right phalanges
46. Left phalanges
56. Right head of humerus
57. Left head of humerus
61. Left epicondyle
62. Right epicondyle
63. Left epitrochlea
64. Right epitrochlea
65. Left olecranon
66. Right olecranon

Bones of the leg
21. Right femur
22. Left femur
23. Right patella
24. Left patella
25. Right fibula
26. Left fibula
27. Right tibia
28. Left tibia
29. Right tarsals
30. Left tarsals
31. Right metatarsals
32. Left metatarsals
33. Right phalanges
34. Left phalanges
68. Left head of femur
69. Right head of femur
70. Left neck of femur
71. Right neck of femur
74. Left condyle of femur
75. Right condyle of femur
76. Left talus
77. Right talus
78. Left calcaneus
79. Right calcaneus

B

Bottle Feeding Establishment: Infant

1016

Definition: Establishment of bottle feeding for hydration and nourishment of an infant

OUTCOME TARGET RATING: Maintain at_____ Increase to_____

	Never Demonstrated	Rarely Demonstrated	Sometimes Demonstrated	Often Demonstrated	Consistently Demonstrated	
OUTCOME OVERALL RATING	1	2	3	4	5	
Indicators:						
101613 Proper grasp of nipple	1	2	3	4	5	NA
101614 Effective suck reflex	1	2	3	4	5	NA
101615 Noticeable or audible swallow	1	2	3	4	5	NA
101616 Coordination of suck, swallow, and breath pattern	1	2	3	4	5	NA
101617 Consumes milk or formula from bottle	1	2	3	4	5	NA
101618 Tolerates flow rate of nipple	1	2	3	4	5	NA
101619 Feeding tolerance	1	2	3	4	5	NA
101620 Calm and relaxed during feeding						
101621 Minimum of 6 feedings per day	1	2	3	4	5	NA
101622 Contentment after feeding	1	2	3	4	5	NA
101623 Urine output appropriate for age	1	2	3	4	5	NA
101624 Stools appropriate for age	1	2	3	4	5	NA
101625 Weight gain appropriate for age	1	2	3	4	5	NA

Domain-*Physiologic Health (II)*   **Class**-*Digestion & Nutrition (K)*   5th edition 2013; revised 2024

OUTCOME CONTENT REFERENCES:

Hockenberry, M. J., Wilson, D., & Rodgers, C. C. (Eds.). (2019). *Wong's nursing care of infants and children* (11th ed.). Elsevier.

Kotowski, J., Fowler, C., Hourigan, C., & Orr, F. (2020). Bottle-feeding an infant feeding modality: An integrative literature review. *Maternal Child Nutrition, 16*(2), e12939. https://doi.org/10.1111/mcn.12939

Marshall, J., Clarke, S., Escott, C., & Pados, B. F. (2021). Assessing the flow rate of different bottles and teats for neonates with feeding difficulties: An Australian context. *Journal of Neonatal Nursing, 27*(4), 285–290. https://doi.org/10.1016/j.jnn.2020.11.014

Perry, S. E., Hockenberry, M. J., Lowdermilk, D. J., Wilson, D., Cashion, K., Rodgers, C. C., & Alden, K. R. (2018). *Maternal child nursing care* (6th ed.). Elsevier.

Vollrath, K., Rosenberg, A., Gabrielski, L., Deacon, J., Marshall, S., Rihn, A., & Grover, T. (2019). NICU Discharge feeding bundle improves accuracy of postdischarge feeding preparation and potentially prevents readmission. *Advances in Neonatal Care, 19*(2), 90–96. https://doi.org/10.1097/ANC.0000000000000571

Bottle Feeding Performance

1017

Definition: Caregiver actions to provide fluids to an infant using a bottle

OUTCOME TARGET RATING: Maintain at_____ Increase to_____

	Never Demonstrated	Rarely Demonstrated	Sometimes Demonstrated	Often Demonstrated	Consistently Demonstrated	
OUTCOME OVERALL RATING	1	2	3	4	5	
Indicators:						
101701 Washes hands before preparation of formula	1	2	3	4	5	NA
101702 Prepares formula according to directions	1	2	3	4	5	NA
101703 Uses clean bottles and nipples	1	2	3	4	5	NA
101704 Uses correct size of nipple to regulate fluid flow	1	2	3	4	5	NA
101705 Uses formula before expiration date	1	2	3	4	5	NA
101706 Stores mixed formula correctly	1	2	3	4	5	NA

B

Bottle Feeding Performance—cont'd

		Never Demonstrated	Rarely Demonstrated	Sometimes Demonstrated	Often Demonstrated	Consistently Demonstrated	
101707	Stores breast milk correctly	1	2	3	4	5	NA
101708	Warms bottle in warm water	1	2	3	4	5	NA
101709	Tests temperature of formula prior to feeding	1	2	3	4	5	NA
101710	Responds to infant hunger cues	1	2	3	4	5	NA
101711	Positions infant correctly while feeding	1	2	3	4	5	NA
101712	Positions bottle correctly while feeding	1	2	3	4	5	NA
101714	Responds to infant cues to stop feeding	1	2	3	4	5	NA
101715	Repositions infant in response to choking	1	2	3	4	5	NA

Domain-*Physiologic Health (II)*   **Class**-*Digestion & Nutrition (K)*   *5th edition 2013; revised 2024*

OUTCOME CONTENT REFERENCES:
Hockenberry, M. J., Wilson, D., & Rodgers, C. C. (Eds.). (2019). *Wong's nursing care of infants and children* (11th ed.). Elsevier.
Kotowski, J., Fowler, C., Hourigan, C., & Orr, F. (2020). Bottle-feeding an infant feeding modality: An integrative literature review. *Maternal Child Nutrition, 16*(2), e12939. https://doi.org/10.1111/mcn.12939
+Pados, B. F., Thoyre, S. M., Estrem, H. H., Park, J., & McComish, C. (2018). Factor structure and psychometric properties of the Neonatal Eating Assessment Tool-Bottle-Feeding. *Advances in Neonatal Care, 18*(3), 232–242. https://doi.org/10.1097/ANC.0000000000000494
Perry, S. E., Hockenberry, M. J., Lowdermilk, D. J., Wilson, D., Cashion, K., Rodgers, C. C., & Alden, K. R. (2018). *Maternal child nursing care* (6th ed.). Elsevier.
Vollrath, K., Rosenberg, A., Gabrielski, L., Deacon, J., Marshall, S., Rihn, A., & Grover, T. (2019). NICU Discharge feeding bundle improves accuracy of postdischarge feeding preparation and potentially prevents readmission. *Advances in Neonatal Care, 19*(2), 90–96. https://doi.org/10.1097/ANC.0000000000000571

Bowel Continence   **0500**

Definition: Control of passage of stool from the bowel

OUTCOME TARGET RATING: Maintain at_____ Increase to_____

		Never Demonstrated	Rarely Demonstrated	Sometimes Demonstrated	Often Demonstrated	Consistently Demonstrated	
OUTCOME OVERALL RATING		1	2	3	4	5	
Indicators:							
050008	Recognizes urge to defecate	1	2	3	4	5	NA
050024	Schedules toilet time after morning meal	1	2	3	4	5	NA
050001	Maintains predictable pattern of stool evacuation	1	2	3	4	5	NA
050002	Maintains control of stool passage	1	2	3	4	5	NA
050003	Evacuates stool at least q 3 days	1	2	3	4	5	NA
050006	Sphincter tone adequate to control defecation	1	2	3	4	5	NA
050007	Sphincter innervation functional	1	2	3	4	5	NA
050009	Responds to urge in timely manner	1	2	3	4	5	NA
050012	Gets to toilet between urge and evacuation of stool	1	2	3	4	5	NA
050017	Maintains barrier-free environment for independent toileting	1	2	3	4	5	NA
050013	Ingests adequate amount of fluid	1	2	3	4	5	NA

Continued

Bowel Continence—cont'd

		Never Demonstrated	Rarely Demonstrated	Sometimes Demonstrated	Often Demonstrated	Consistently Demonstrated	
050014	Ingests adequate amount of fiber	1	2	3	4	5	NA
050015	Describes relationship of food intake to stool consistency	1	2	3	4	5	NA
050018	Monitors amount and consistency of stool	1	2	3	4	5	NA
050019	Toilets independently	1	2	3	4	5	NA

		Consistently Demonstrated	Often Demonstrated	Sometimes Demonstrated	Rarely Demonstrated	Never Demonstrated	
050004	Diarrhea	1	2	3	4	5	NA
050005	Constipation	1	2	3	4	5	NA
050025	Impaction	1	2	3	4	5	NA
050020	Overuse of laxatives	1	2	3	4	5	NA
050021	Overuse of enemas	1	2	3	4	5	NA
050022	Soils clothing during day	1	2	3	4	5	NA
050023	Soils clothing or bedding during night	1	2	3	4	5	NA

Domain-Physiologic Health (II)   *Class*-Elimination (F)   1st edition 1997; revised 2004, 2008, 2024

OUTCOME CONTENT REFERENCES:

Collis, D., Kennedy, B. A., & Kearney, L. (2019). The impact of bowel and bladder problems on children's quality of life and their parents: A scoping review. *Child: Care, Health & Development, 45*(1), 1–14. https://doi.org/10.1111/cch.12620

Faleiros, F., Santos, L. M., Bimbatti, K., & Käppler, K. (2021). Bowel emptying methods used by German residents living with Spina Bifida. *Journal of Wound Ostomy & Continence Nursing, 48*(2), 149–152. https://doi.org/10.1097/WON.0000000000000741

Pinto, C. F. C. S., Oliveira, P. da C. M., Fernandes, O. M. F. S. de O., Padilha, J. M. S. C., Machado, P. A. P., Ribeiro, A. L. A., & Ramos, J. L. N. (2020). Nonpharmacological clinical effective interventions in constipation: A systematic review. *Journal of Nursing Scholarship, 52*(3), 261–269. https://doi.org/10.1111/jnu.12555

Richards, D. A., Hilli, A., Pentecost, C., Goodwin, V. A., Frost, J. (2018). Fundamental nursing care: A systematic review of the evidence on the effect of nursing care interventions for nutrition, elimination, mobility and hygiene. *Journal of Clinical Nursing, 27*(11–12), 2179–2188. https://doi.org/10.1111/jocn.14150

Suzuki, M., Okochi, J., Iijima, K., Murata, T., & Kume, H. (2020). Nationwide survey of continence status among older adult residents living in long-term care facilities in Japan: The prevalence and associated risk factors of incontinence and effect of comprehensive care on continence status. *Geriatrics and Gerontology International, 20*(4), 285–290. https://doi.org/10.1111/ggi.13872

Thompson, D. L. (2019). Getting ready for continence certification. *Journal of Wound Ostomy & Continence Nursing, 46*(6), 550–552. https://doi.org/10.1097/WON.0000000000000584

Yates, A. (2019). Basic continence assessment: What community nurses should know. *Journal of Community Nursing, 33*(3), 52–55.

Bowel Elimination

0501

Definition: Formation and evacuation of stool

OUTCOME TARGET RATING: Maintain at_____ Increase to_____

		Severely Compromised	Substantially Compromised	Moderately Compromised	Mildly Compromised	Not Compromised	
OUTCOME OVERALL RATING		1	2	3	4	5	
Indicators:							
050101	Elimination pattern	1	2	3	4	5	NA
050130	Urge to defecate	1	2	3	4	5	NA
050102	Control of bowel movements	1	2	3	4	5	NA
050103	Stool color	1	2	3	4	5	NA
050104	Stool amount for diet	1	2	3	4	5	NA
050105	Stool soft and formed	1	2	3	4	5	NA
050112	Ease of stool passage	1	2	3	4	5	NA
050118	Sphincter tone	1	2	3	4	5	NA
050119	Muscle tone to evacuate stool	1	2	3	4	5	NA
050121	Passage of stool without aids	1	2	3	4	5	NA
050129	Bowel sounds	1	2	3	4	5	NA

Bowel Elimination—cont'd

		Severe	Substantial	Moderate	Mild	None	
050107	Fat in stool	1	2	3	4	5	NA
050108	Blood in stool	1	2	3	4	5	NA
050109	Mucus in stool	1	2	3	4	5	NA
050110	Constipation	1	2	3	4	5	NA
050111	Diarrhea	1	2	3	4	5	NA
050123	Abuse of elimination aids	1	2	3	4	5	NA
050128	Pain with passage of stool	1	2	3	4	5	NA
050131	Burning sensation with passage of stool	1	2	3	4	5	NA

Domain-Physiologic Health (II)   *Class*-Elimination (F)   1st edition 1997; revised 2004, 2008, 2024

OUTCOME CONTENT REFERENCES:

Hogan-Quigley, B., Palm, M. L., & Bickley, L. (2021). *Bates nursing guide to physical examination and history taking* (3rd ed.). Wolters Kluwer.
Nimrouzi, M., & Zarshenas, M. (2019). Holistic approach to functional constipation: Perspective of traditional Persian medicine. *Chinese Journal of Integrative Medicine, 25*(11), 867–872. https://doi.org/10.1007/s11655-015-2302-3
Yates, A. (2019). Basic continence assessment: What community nurses should know. *Journal of Community Nursing, 33*(3), 52–55.

Breastfeeding Establishment: Infant   1000

Definition: Infant's latch and suction on the mother's nipple-areolar complex for nourishment during the first few weeks of breastfeeding

OUTCOME TARGET RATING: Maintain at_____ Increase to_____

		Never Demonstrated	Rarely Demonstrated	Sometimes Demonstrated	Often Demonstrated	Consistently Demonstrated	
OUTCOME OVERALL RATING		1	2	3	4	5	
Indicators:							
100016	Proper latch on	1	2	3	4	5	NA
100017	Proper areolar compression	1	2	3	4	5	NA
100018	Correct tongue placement	1	2	3	4	5	NA
100019	Suck reflex	1	2	3	4	5	NA
100020	Noticeable or audible swallow	1	2	3	4	5	NA
100021	Coordinates suck, swallow, and breathing pattern	1	2	3	4	5	NA
100022	Minimum of 8 feedings per day	1	2	3	4	5	NA
100023	Urinations per day appropriate for age	1	2	3	4	5	NA
100024	Stools per day appropriate for age						
100025	Weight gain appropriate for age	1	2	3	4	5	NA
100026	Infant contentment after feeding	1	2	3	4	5	NA

Domain-Physiologic Health (II)   *Class*-Digestion & Nutrition (K)   1st edition 1997; revised 2004, 2013, 2024

OUTCOME CONTENT REFERENCES:

Barbosa, G. E. F., Silva, V. B., Pereira, J. M., Soares, M. S., Medeiros, R. A., Filho, P. L. B., Pereora, L. B., Pinho, L. & Caldeira, A. P. (2017). Initial breastfeeding difficulties and association with breast disorders among postpartum women. *Revista Paulista de Pediatria, 35*(3), 265–72. https://doi.org/10.1590/1984-0462/;2017;35;3;00004
Dias Emidio, S. C., Barbosa Dias, F. de S., Moorhead, S., Deberg, J., de Souza Oliveira-Kumakura, A. R., & Valentim Carmona, E. (2020). Conceptual and operational definition of nursing outcomes regarding the breastfeeding establishment. *Revista Latino-Americana de Enfermagem (RLAE), 28*, 1–12. https://doi.org/10.1590/1518-8345.3007.3259
Dias Emidio, S. C., Moorhead, S., Oliveira, H. C., Herdman, T. H., Oliveira, K. A. R. de S., & Carmona, E. V. (2020). Validation of nursing outcomes related to breastfeeding establishment. *International Journal of Nursing Knowledge, 31*(2), 134–144. https://doi.org/10.1111/2047-3095.12256
Wambach, K., & Riordan, J. (2015). *Breastfeeding and human lactation* (5th ed.). Jones & Bartlett Learning.
World Health Organization. (2021). Newborn health. https://www.who.int/health-topics/newborn-health#tab=tab_1

B

Breastfeeding Establishment: Maternal   **1001**

Definition: Maternal alignment of infant to mother's nipple-areolar complex for nourishment during the first few weeks of breastfeeding

OUTCOME TARGET RATING: Maintain at_____ Increase to_____

		Never Demonstrated	Rarely Demonstrated	Sometimes Demonstrated	Often Demonstrated	Consistently Demonstrated	
OUTCOME OVERALL RATING		1	2	3	4	5	
Indicators:							
100126	Maintains comfortable position during nursing	1	2	3	4	5	NA
100127	Provides skin to skin contact with infant	1	2	3	4	5	NA
100128	Properly aligns infant to breast	1	2	3	4	5	NA
100129	Supports breast using "C" hold (cupping)	1	2	3	4	5	NA
100130	Experiences breast fullness prior to feeding	1	2	3	4	5	NA
100131	Produces adequate milk	1	2	3	4	5	NA
100132	Senses milk ejection (let-down) reflex	1	2	3	4	5	NA
100133	Recognizes infant swallowing	1	2	3	4	5	NA
100134	Breaks suction before removing infant from breast	1	2	3	4	5	NA
100135	Uses techniques to prevent nipple tenderness	1	2	3	4	5	NA
100136	Avoids artificial nipple use with infant	1	2	3	4	5	NA
100137	Avoids giving water or other liquids to infant	1	2	3	4	5	NA
100138	Provides supplemental feedings if needed	1	2	3	4	5	NA
100139	Bonding between mother and infant	1	2	3	4	5	NA
100140	Recognizes early hunger cues	1	2	3	4	5	NA
100141	Ingests adequate fluid intake	1	2	3	4	5	NA
100142	Pumps breast as needed	1	2	3	4	5	NA
100143	Safely stores breast milk	1	2	3	4	5	NA
100144	Expresses satisfaction with health professional support	1	2	3	4	5	NA
100145	Expresses satisfaction with breastfeeding process	1	2	3	4	5	NA

Domain-Physiologic Health (II)   *Class*-Digestion & Nutrition (K)   *1st edition 1997; revised 2004, 2008, 2024*

OUTCOME CONTENT REFERENCES:
Barbosa, G. E. F., Silva, V. B., Pereira, J. M., Soares, M. S., Medeiros, R. A., Filho, P. L. B., Pereora, L. B., Pinho, L., & Caldeira, A. P. (2017). Initial breastfeeding difficulties and association with breast disorders among postpartum women. *Revista Paulista de Pediatria*, 35(3), 265–72. https://doi.org/10.1590/1984-0462/;2017;35;3;00004
Dias Emidio, S. C., Barbosa Dias, F. de S., Moorhead, S., Deberg, J., de Souza Oliveira-Kumakura, A. R., & Valentim Carmona, E. (2020). Conceptual and operational definition of nursing outcomes regarding the breastfeeding establishment. *Revista Latino-Americana de Enfermagem (RLAE)*, 28, 1–12. https://doi.org/10.1590/1518-8345.3007.3259
Dias Emidio, S. C., Moorhead, S., Oliveira, H. C., Herdman, T. H., Oliveira, K. A. R. de S., & Carmona, E. V. (2020). Validation of nursing outcomes related to breastfeeding establishment. *International Journal of Nursing Knowledge*, 31(2), 134–144. https://doi.org/10.1111/2047-3095.12256
Esterik, V. P. (2012). *Core curriculum for lactation consultant practice* (3rd ed.). Jones & Bartlett Learning.
Wambach, K., & Riordan, J. (2015). *Breastfeeding and human lactation* (5th ed.). Jones & Bartlett Learning.
World Health Organization. (2021). Newborn health. https://www.who.int/health-topics/newborn-health#tab=tab_1

Breastfeeding Maintenance   1002

Definition: Continuation of breastfeeding from establishment to weaning for nourishment of an infant/toddler

B

OUTCOME TARGET RATING: Maintain at_____ Increase to_____

	Never Demonstrated	Rarely Demonstrated	Sometimes Demonstrated	Often Demonstrated	Consistently Demonstrated	
OUTCOME OVERALL RATING	1	2	3	4	5	
Indicators:						
100226 Monitors infant's growth	1	2	3	4	5	NA
100227 Monitors infant's weight	1	2	3	4	5	NA
100228 Monitors infant's development	1	2	3	4	5	NA
100229 Safely collects and stores breast milk	1	2	3	4	5	NA
100230 Safely thaws and warms stored breast milk	1	2	3	4	5	NA
100231 Uses techniques to prevent breast tenderness	1	2	3	4	5	NA
100232 Recognizes signs of decreased milk supply	1	2	3	4	5	NA
100233 Recognizes signs of plugged ducts	1	2	3	4	5	NA
100234 Recognizes signs of mastitis	1	2	3	4	5	NA
100235 Avoids self-medication without checking with health professional	1	2	3	4	5	NA
100236 Perceived family support for breastfeeding	1	2	3	4	5	NA
100237 Perceived support for continuation of lactation on return to work	1	2	3	4	5	NA
100238 Perceived support for continuation of lactation on return to school	1	2	3	4	5	NA
100239 Knowledge of benefits from continued breastfeeding	1	2	3	4	5	NA
100240 Knowledge of resources for support	1	2	3	4	5	NA
100241 Satisfaction with breastfeeding process	1	2	3	4	5	NA

Domain-Physiologic Health (II)   *Class*-Digestion & Nutrition (K)   *1st edition 1997; revised 2004, 2008, 2024*

OUTCOME CONTENT REFERENCES:

Barbosa, G. E. F., Silva, V. B., Pereira, J. M., Soares, M. S., Medeiros, R. A., Filho, P. L. B., Pereora, L. B., Pinho, L., & Caldeira, A. P. (2017). Initial breastfeeding difficulties and association with breast disorders among postpartum women. *Revista Paulista de Pediatria, 35*(3), 265–72. https://doi.org/10.1590/1984-0462/;2017;35;3;00004

Dias Emidio, S. C., Barbosa Dias, F. de S., Moorhead, S., Deberg, J., de Souza Oliveira-Kumakura, A. R., & Valentim Carmona, E. (2020). Conceptual and operational definition of nursing outcomes regarding the breastfeeding establishment. *Revista Latino-Americana de Enfermagem (RLAE), 28*, 1–12. https://doi.org/10.1590/1518-8345.3007.3259

Dias Emidio, S. C., Moorhead, S., Oliveira, H. C., Herdman, T. H., Oliveira, K. A. R. de S., & Carmona, E. V. (2020). Validation of nursing outcomes related to breastfeeding establishment. *International Journal of Nursing Knowledge, 31*(2), 134–144. https://doi.org/10.1111/2047-3095.12256

Esterik, V. P. (2012). *Core curriculum for lactation consultant prac*tice (3rd ed.). Jones & Bartlett Learning.

Henderson, A. M., Pincombe, J., & Stamp, G. E. (2000). Assisting women to establish breastfeeding: Exploring midwives' practices. *Breastfeeding Review, 8*(3), 11–17.

Spatz, D. L. (2021). Proactive planning for breastfeeding assistance and support post birth. *MCN: The American Journal of Maternal Child Nursing, 46*(6), 362. https://doi.org/10.1097/NMC.0000000000000773

Wambach, K., & Riordan, J. (2015). *Breastfeeding and human lactation* (5th ed.). Jones & Bartlett Learning.

World Health Organization. (2021). Newborn health. https://www.who.int/health-topics/newborn-health#tab=tab_1

B

Breastfeeding Weaning

1003

Definition: Progressive discontinuation of breastfeeding of an infant/toddler and substitution of other liquids and foods

OUTCOME TARGET RATING: Maintain at_____ Increase to_____

OUTCOME OVERALL RATING		Never Demonstrated	Rarely Demonstrated	Sometimes Demonstrated	Often Demonstrated	Consistently Demonstrated	
		1	2	3	4	5	
Indicators:							
100324	Recognizes weaning readiness cues	1	2	3	4	5	NA
100325	Recognizes signs of decreased milk supply	1	2	3	4	5	NA
100326	Knowledge of benefits of gradual weaning	1	2	3	4	5	NA
100327	Knowledge of guidelines for rapid "emergency" weaning	1	2	3	4	5	NA
100328	Knowledge of appropriate methods to reduce breast tenderness	1	2	3	4	5	NA
100329	Introduces solids as recommended by health professional	1	2	3	4	5	NA
100330	Replaces one feeding with solids every few days	1	2	3	4	5	NA
100331	Replaces breast milk with other fluids using a bottle or cup	1	2	3	4	5	NA
100332	Introduces new foods one at a time	1	2	3	4	5	NA
100333	Introduces solid foods using a spoon	1	2	3	4	5	NA
100334	Provides additional physical touch during time of weaning	1	2	3	4	5	NA
100335	Knowledge of resources available for support	1	2	3	4	5	NA
100336	Uses reputable resources	1	2	3	4	5	NA
100337	Satisfaction with weaning process	1	2	3	4	5	NA

Domain-*Physiologic Health (II)* **Class**-*Digestion & Nutrition (K)* *1st edition 1997; revised 2004, 2008, 2024*

OUTCOME CONTENT REFERENCES:

Barbosa, G. E. F., Silva, V. B., Pereira, J. M., Soares, M. S., Medeiros, R. A., Filho, P. L. B., Pereora, L. B., Pinho, L., & Caldeira, A. P. (2017). Initial breastfeeding difficulties and association with breast disorders among postpartum women. *Revista Paulista de Pediatria*, 35(3), 265–72. https://doi.org/10.1590/1984-0462/;2017;35;3;00004

Dias Emidio, S. C., Barbosa Dias, F. de S., Moorhead, S., Deberg, J., de Souza Oliveira-Kumakura, A. R., & Valentim Carmona, E. (2020). Conceptual and operational definition of nursing outcomes regarding the breastfeeding establishment. *Revista Latino-Americana de Enfermagem (RLAE), 28*, 1–12. https://doi.org/10.1590/1518-8345.3007.3259

Dias Emidio, S. C., Moorhead, S., Oliveira, H. C., Herdman, T. H., Oliveira, K. A. R. de S., & Carmona, E. V. (2020). Validation of nursing outcomes related to Breastfeeding Establishment. *International Journal of Nursing Knowledge, 31*(2), 134–144. https://doi.org/10.1111/2047-3095.12256

Esterik, V. P. (2012). *Core curriculum for lactation consultant practice* (3rd ed.). Jones & Bartlett Learning.

Wambach, K., & Riordan, J. (2015). *Breastfeeding and human lactation* (5ed.). Jones & Bartlett Learning.

World Health Organization. (2021). Newborn health. https://www.who.int/health-topics/newborn-health#tab=tab_1

Burn Healing   1106

Definition: Extent of healing of a burn injury

OUTCOME TARGET RATING: Maintain at_____ Increase to_____

	None	Limited	Moderate	Substantial	Extensive	
OUTCOME OVERALL RATING	1	2	3	4	5	

Indicators:

		None	Limited	Moderate	Substantial	Extensive	
110601	Percent of graft area healed	1	2	3	4	5	NA
110602	Percent of burn area healed	1	2	3	4	5	NA
110603	Tissue granulation	1	2	3	4	5	NA
110604	Joint movement of affected extremity	1	2	3	4	5	NA
110605	Tissue perfusion of burn area	1	2	3	4	5	NA

		Extensive	Substantial	Moderate	Limited	None	
110606	Pain	1	2	3	4	5	NA
110607	Infection	1	2	3	4	5	NA
110608	Blistered skin	1	2	3	4	5	NA
110609	Purulent drainage	1	2	3	4	5	NA
110610	Foul wound odor	1	2	3	4	5	NA
110611	Burn site edema	1	2	3	4	5	NA
110614	Itching	1	2	3	4	5	NA
110613	Tissue necrosis	1	2	3	4	5	NA
110615	Heat sensitivity in burn area	1	2	3	4	5	NA

Grafted Yes / No

Location of burn _____

001 Head	007 Right upper arm	013 Right thigh
002 Neck	008 Left upper arm	014 Left thigh
003 Anterior trunk	009 Right lower arm	015 Right leg
004 Posterior trunk	010 Left lower arm	016 Left leg
005 Buttock	011 Right hand	017 Right foot
006 Genitalia	012 Left hand	018 Left foot

Domain-*Physiologic Health (II)*   **Class**-*Tissue Integrity (L)*   *4th edition 2008; revised 2024*

OUTCOME CONTENT REFERENCES:

Chong, H. P., Quinn, L., Jeeves, A., Cooksey, R., Lodge, M., Carney, B., & Molony, D. (2020). A comparison study of methods for estimation of a burn surface area: Lund and Browder, e-burn and Mersey Burns. *Burns* (03054179), *46*(2), 483–489. https://doi.org/10.1016/j.burns.2019.08.014

Herndon, D. N. (2018). *Total burn care* (5th ed.). Elsevier.

Jeschke, M. G., van Baar, M. E., Choudhry, M. A., Chung, K. K., Gibran, N. S., & Logsetty, S. (2020). Burn injury. *Nature Reviews. Disease Primers*, *6*(1), 11. https://doi.org/10.1038/s41572-020-0145-5

Partain, K. P., Fabia, R., & Thakkar, R. K. (2020). Pediatric burn care: New techniques and outcomes. *Current Opinion in Pediatrics*, *32*(3), 405–410. https://doi.org/10.1097/MOP.0000000000000902

Burn Recovery

Definition: Extent of overall physical healing and psychological functioning following a major burn injury

OUTCOME TARGET RATING: Maintain at_____ Increase to_____

		None	Limited	Moderate	Substantial	Extensive	
OUTCOME OVERALL RATING		**1**	**2**	**3**	**4**	**5**	
Indicators:							
110701	Tissue granulation	1	2	3	4	5	NA
110702	Tissue perfusion of burn area	1	2	3	4	5	NA
110703	Percent of burn area healed	1	2	3	4	5	NA
110704	Temperature stability	1	2	3	4	5	NA
110705	Electrolyte stability	1	2	3	4	5	NA
110706	Fluid balance	1	2	3	4	5	NA
110707	Self-care ability	1	2	3	4	5	NA
110708	Joint movement of extremities	1	2	3	4	5	NA
110709	Ambulation tolerance	1	2	3	4	5	NA
110729	Fatigue	1	2	3	4	5	NA
110730	Sleep disturbances	1	2	3	4	5	NA
110710	Positive attitude toward touching affected part	1	2	3	4	5	NA
110711	Psychological adjustment to changes in physical appearance	1	2	3	4	5	NA
110712	Psychological adjustment to changes in body function	1	2	3	4	5	NA
110731	Engagement in social activities	1	2	3	4	5	NA
110732	Quality of life	1	2	3	4	5	NA

		Extensive	Substantial	Moderate	Limited	None	
110713	Pain	1	2	3	4	5	NA
110733	Persistent itching	1	2	3	4	5	NA
110714	Decreased cognition	1	2	3	4	5	NA
110715	Pain medication requirements	1	2	3	4	5	NA
110716	Decreased oxygen saturation	1	2	3	4	5	NA
110717	Difficulty breathing	1	2	3	4	5	NA
110718	Weight loss	1	2	3	4	5	NA
110719	Infection	1	2	3	4	5	NA
110720	Blistered skin	1	2	3	4	5	NA
110721	Purulent drainage	1	2	3	4	5	NA
110722	Foul wound odor	1	2	3	4	5	NA
110723	Burn area edema	1	2	3	4	5	NA
110724	Tissue necrosis	1	2	3	4	5	NA
110725	Generalized edema	1	2	3	4	5	NA
110726	Gastrointestinal complications	1	2	3	4	5	NA
110727	Decreased urine output	1	2	3	4	5	NA
110728	Burn site grafting required	1	2	3	4	5	NA
110734	Disfigurement	1	2	3	4	5	NA
110735	Depression	1	2	3	4	5	NA
110736	Anxiety	1	2	3	4	5	NA
110737	Residual physical disability	1	2	3	4	5	NA

Domain-*Physiologic Health (II)* **Class**-*Tissue Integrity (L)* *4th edition 2008; revised 2024*

OUTCOME CONTENT REFERENCES:

Chong, H. P., Quinn, L., Jeeves, A., Cooksey, R., Lodge, M., Carney, B., & Molony, D. (2020). A comparison study of methods for estimation of a burn surface area: Lund and Browder, e-burn and Mersey Burns. *Burns, 46*(2), 483–489. https://doi.org/10.1016/j.burns.2019.08.014

Cimino, S. R., Jorge, N., Rios, J. N., Godleski, M., & Hitzig, S. L. (2020). A scoping review on the long-term outcomes in persons with adult-acquired burn injuries. *Journal of Burn Care & Research, 41*(3), 472–502. https://doi.org/10.1093/jbcr/irz146

Herndon, D. N. (2018). *Total burn care* (5th ed.). Elsevier.

Jeschke, M. G., van Baar, M. E., Choudhry, M. A., Chung, K. K., Gibran, N. S., & Logsetty, S. (2020). Burn injury. *Nature Reviews. Disease Primers, 6*(1), 11. https://doi.org/10.1038/s41572-020-0145-5

Palmieri, T., & ISBI Practice Guidelines Committee. (2018). ISBI Practice Guidelines for burn care, Part 2. *Burns, 44*(7), 1617–1706. https://doi.org/10.1016/j.burns.2018.09.012

Partain, K. P., Fabia, R., & Thakkar, R. K. (2020). Pediatric burn care: New techniques and outcomes. *Current Opinion in Pediatrics, 32*(3), 405–410. https://doi.org/10.1097/MOP.0000000000000902

Romanowski, K. S., Carson, J., Pape, K., Bernal, E., Sharar, S., Wiechman, S., Carter, D., Liu, Y. M., Nitzschke, S., Bhalla, P., Litt, J., Przkora, R., Friedman, B., Popiak, S., Jeng, J., Ryan, C. M., & Joe, V. (2020). American Burn Association Guidelines on the management of acute pain in the adult burn patient: A review of the literature, a compilation of expert opinion, and next steps. *Journal of Burn Care & Research, 41*(6), 1129–1151. https://doi.org/10.1093/jbcr/iraa119

Ryan, C., Schneider, J., Kazis, L., Lee, A., Li, N., Hinson, M., Bauk, H., Peck, M., Meyer, W., Palmieri, T., Pidcock, F., Reilly, D., & Tompkins, R. (2013). Benchmarks for multidimensional recovery after burn injury in young adults. *Journal of Burn Care & Research, 34* (3), e121–e142. https://doi.org/10.1097/BCR.0b013e31827e7ecf

Spronk, I., Legemate, C., Oen, I., van Loey, N., Polinder, S., & van Baar, M. (2018). Health related quality of life in adults after burn injuries: A systematic review. *PLOS One, 13*(5), e0197507. https://doi.org/10.1371/journal.pone.0197507

Spronk, I., Legemate, C. M., Polinder, S., & van Baar, M. E. (2018). Health-related quality of life in children after burn injuries: A systematic review. *Journal of Trauma Acute Care Surgery, 85*(6), 1110–1118. https://doi.org/10.1097/TA.0000000000002072

Tracy, L. M., Edgar, D. W., Schrale, R., Cleland, H., Gabbe, B. J., & BRANZ Adult Long-Term Outcomes Pilot Project participating sites and working party. (2020). Predictors of itch and pain in the 12 months following burn injury: Results from the Burns Registry of Australia and New Zealand (BRANZ) Long-Term Outcomes Project. *Burns & Trauma, 8*, tkz004. https://doi.org/10.1093/burnst/tkz004

Cardiac Pump Effectiveness   0400

Definition: Adequacy of blood volume ejected from the left ventricle of the heart to support systemic perfusion pressure

OUTCOME TARGET RATING: Maintain at_____ Increase to_____

		Severe Deviation from Normal Range	Substantial Deviation from Normal Range	Moderate Deviation from Normal Range	Mild Deviation from Normal Range	No Deviation from Normal Range	
OUTCOME OVERALL RATING		1	2	3	4	5	
Indicators:							
040001	Systolic blood pressure	1	2	3	4	5	NA
040019	Diastolic blood pressure	1	2	3	4	5	NA
040002	Apical heart rate	1	2	3	4	5	NA
040003	Cardiac index	1	2	3	4	5	NA
040004	Ejection fraction	1	2	3	4	5	NA
040006	Peripheral pulses	1	2	3	4	5	NA
040007	Heart size	1	2	3	4	5	NA
040020	Urine output	1	2	3	4	5	NA
040022	24-hour intake and output balance	1	2	3	4	5	NA
040025	Central venous pressure	1	2	3	4	5	NA
		Severe	Substantial	Moderate	Mild	None	
040009	Neck vein distension	1	2	3	4	5	NA
040010	Dysrhythmia	1	2	3	4	5	NA
040011	Abnormal heart sounds	1	2	3	4	5	NA
040012	Angina	1	2	3	4	5	NA
040013	Peripheral edema	1	2	3	4	5	NA
040014	Pulmonary edema	1	2	3	4	5	NA
040015	Diaphoresis	1	2	3	4	5	NA
040016	Nausea	1	2	3	4	5	NA

Continued

C

Cardiac Pump Effectiveness—cont'd

		Severe Deviation from Normal Range	Substantial Deviation from Normal Range	Moderate Deviation from Normal Range	Mild Deviation from Normal Range	No Deviation from Normal Range	
040017	Fatigue	1	2	3	4	5	NA
040023	Dyspnea at rest	1	2	3	4	5	NA
040026	Dyspnea on exertion	1	2	3	4	5	NA
040024	Weight gain	1	2	3	4	5	NA
040027	Ascites	1	2	3	4	5	NA
040028	Hepatomegaly	1	2	3	4	5	NA
040029	Impaired cognition	1	2	3	4	5	NA
040030	Activity intolerance	1	2	3	4	5	NA
040031	Pallor	1	2	3	4	5	NA
040032	Cyanosis	1	2	3	4	5	NA
040033	Flushed	1	2	3	4	5	NA

Domain-*Physiologic Health (II)*   **Class**-*Cardiopulmonary (E)*   *1st edition 1997; revised 2004, 2008, 2024*

OUTCOME CONTENT REFERENCES:

Hinkle, J. L., & Cheever, K. H. (2018). *Brunner & Suddarth's textbook of medical-surgical nursing* (14th ed.). Wolter Kluwer.
Hockenberry, M. J., Rodgers, C. C., & Wilson, D. (Eds.). (2022). *Wong's essentials of pediatric nursing* (11th ed.). Elsevier.
Hravnak, M., Whittle, J., Kelley, M. E., Sereika, S., Good, C. B., Ibrahim, S. A., & Conigliaro, J. (2007). Symptom expression in coronary heart disease and revascularization recommendations for black and white patients. *American Journal of Public Health, 97*(9), 1701–1708. https://doi.org/10.2105/AJPH.2005.084103
Huether, S. E., McCance, K. L., & Brashers, V. L. (2020). *Understanding pathophysiology* (7th ed.). Elsevier.
Ignatavicius, D. D., Workman, M. L., Rebar, C. R., & Heimgartner, N. M. (2021). *Medical-surgical nursing: Concepts for interprofessional care* (10th ed.). Elsevier.
Klabunde, R. E. (2022). *Cardiovascular physiology concepts* (3rd ed.). Wolters Kluwer.
Spinale, F. G. (2015). Assessment of cardiac function--Basic principles and approaches. *Comprehensive Physiology, 5*(4), 1911–46. https://doi.org/10.1002/cphy.c140054

Cardiac Rehabilitation Participation

1636

Definition: Personal actions to perform a prescribed rehabilitation program to recover after a cardiac event and reduce risk factors

OUTCOME TARGET RATING: Maintain at_____ Increase to_____

		Never Demonstrated	Rarely Demonstrated	Sometimes Demonstrated	Often Demonstrated	Consistently Demonstrated	
OUTCOME OVERALL RATING		1	2	3	4	5	
Indicators:							
163601	Collaborates with health provider to create an individualized plan of care	1	2	3	4	5	NA
163602	Attends prescribed exercise sessions	1	2	3	4	5	NA
163603	Performs prescribed exercises	1	2	3	4	5	NA
163604	Increases physical activity through rehabilitation as recommended	1	2	3	4	5	NA
163605	Monitors blood pressure	1	2	3	4	5	NA
163606	Monitors heart rate	1	2	3	4	5	NA
163607	Seeks assistance for transportation to rehabilitation	1	2	3	4	5	NA
163608	Collaborates with health provider to plan an individualized heart healthy diet	1	2	3	4	5	NA
163609	Follows heart healthy diet	1	2	3	4	5	NA

Cardiac Rehabilitation Participation—cont'd

	Never Demonstrated	Rarely Demonstrated	Sometimes Demonstrated	Often Demonstrated	Consistently Demonstrated	
163610 Verbalizes understanding of need for electrocardiogram monitoring during rehabilitation	1	2	3	4	5	NA
163611 Uses medication as prescribed	1	2	3	4	5	NA
163612 Modifies unhealthy behaviors	1	2	3	4	5	NA
163613 Verbalizes commitment to long-term healthy lifestyle	1	2	3	4	5	NA
163614 Maintains optimum weight	1	2	3	4	5	NA
163615 Eliminates tobacco use	1	2	3	4	5	NA
163616 Verbalizes greater ability to manage symptoms related to heart condition	1	2	3	4	5	NA
163617 Uses strategies to manage stress	1	2	3	4	5	NA
163618 Verbalizes benefits of cardiac rehabilitation in conjunction with pharmacologic treatment	1	2	3	4	5	NA
163619 Verbalizes understanding of cholesterol levels	1	2	3	4	5	NA

Domain-Health Knowledge & Behavior (IV)   *Class*-Health Behavior (Q)   6th edition 2018

OUTCOME CONTENT REFERENCES:

Balady, G., Ades, P., Bittner, V., Franklin, B., Gordon, N., Thomas, R., Tomaselli, F., & Yancy, C. (2011). Referral, enrollment, and delivery of cardiac rehabilitation/secondary prevention programs at clinical centers and beyond: A presidential advisory from the American Heart Association. *Circulation, 124*(25), 2951–2960. https://doi.org/10.1161/cir.0b013e31823b21e2

Dalal, H. M., Doherty, P., & Taylor, R. S. (2015). Cardiac rehabilitation. *British Medical Journal, 351*, h5000. https://doi.org/10.1136/bmj.h5000

Gaalema, D., Cutler, A., Higgins, S., & Ades, P. (2015). Smoking and cardiac rehabilitation participation: Associations with referral, attendance, and adherence. *Preventive Medicine, 80*, 67–74. https://doi.org/10.1016/j.ypmed.2015.04.009

Gaalema, D., Savage, P., Rengo, J., Cutler, A., Higgins, S., & Ades, P. (2016). Financial incentives to promote cardiac rehabilitation participation and adherence among Medicaid patients. *Preventive Medicine, 92*, 47–50. https://doi.org/10.1016/j.ypmed.2015.11.032

Sandesara, P., Lambert, C., Gordon, N., Fletcher, G., Franklin, B., Wenger, N., & Sperling, L. (2015). Cardiac rehabilitation and risk reduction: Time to "rebrand and reinvigorate." *Journal of the American College of Cardiology, 65*(4), 389–395. https://doi.org/10.1016/j.jacc.2014.10.059

Cardiopulmonary Function   **0414**

Definition: Ability of the heart to effectively pump blood from the ventricles of the heart and exchange carbon dioxide and oxygen at the alveolar level of the lungs

OUTCOME TARGET RATING: Maintain at_____ Increase to_____

	Severely Compromised	Substantially Compromised	Moderately Compromised	Mildly Compromised	Not Compromised	
OUTCOME OVERALL RATING	1	2	3	4	5	
Indicators:						
041432 Systolic blood pressure	1	2	3	4	5	NA
041433 Diastolic blood pressure	1	2	3	4	5	NA
041434 Ejection fraction	1	2	3	4	5	NA
041435 Pulmonary wedge pressure	1	2	3	4	5	NA
041436 Peripheral pulses	1	2	3	4	5	NA
041437 Apical heart rate	1	2	3	4	5	NA
041438 Cardiac rhythm	1	2	3	4	5	NA
041439 Respiratory rate	1	2	3	4	5	NA
041440 Respiratory rhythm	1	2	3	4	5	NA

Continued

C

Cardiopulmonary Function—cont'd

		Severely Compromised	Substantially Compromised	Moderately Compromised	Mildly Compromised	Not Compromised	
041441	Expulsion of air	1	2	3	4	5	NA
041442	Cardiac index	1	2	3	4	5	NA
041443	Oxygen saturation	1	2	3	4	5	NA
041444	Partial pressure of oxygen in arterial blood (PaO_2)	1	2	3	4	5	NA
041445	Partial pressure of carbon dioxide in arterial blood ($PaCO_2$)	1	2	3	4	5	NA

		Severe	Substantial	Moderate	Mild	None	
041414	Activity intolerance	1	2	3	4	5	NA
041415	Impaired cognition	1	2	3	4	5	NA
041416	Pallor	1	2	3	4	5	NA
041417	Cyanosis	1	2	3	4	5	NA
041418	Flushed	1	2	3	4	5	NA
041419	Neck vein distention	1	2	3	4	5	NA
041420	Chest retraction	1	2	3	4	5	NA
041421	Pursed lip breathing	1	2	3	4	5	NA
041422	Peripheral edema	1	2	3	4	5	NA
041423	Pulmonary edema	1	2	3	4	5	NA
041424	Dyspnea	1	2	3	4	5	NA
041446	Accessory muscle use	1	2	3	4	5	NA
041426	Fatigue	1	2	3	4	5	NA
041427	Restlessness	1	2	3	4	5	NA
041428	Somnolence	1	2	3	4	5	NA
041429	Weight gain	1	2	3	4	5	NA
041430	Weight loss	1	2	3	4	5	NA
041431	Diaphoresis	1	2	3	4	5	NA

Domain-*Physiologic Health (II)*   **Class**-*Cardiopulmonary (E)*   *4th edition 2008; revised 2024*

OUTCOME CONTENT REFERENCES:

Aalders, M., & Kok, W. (2019). Comparison of hemodynamic factors predicting prognosis in heart failure: A systematic review. *Journal of Clinical Medicine,* *8*(10), 1757. https://doi.org/10.3390/jcm8101757

Bauldoff, G., Arno, M. A., Gugrud-Howe, P. M., LeMone, P., & Burke, K. M. (2020). *LeMone and Burke's medical-surgical nursing: Clinical reasoning in patient care* (7th ed.). Pearson.

Hinkle, J. L., & Cheever, K. H. (2018). *Brunner & Suddarth's textbook of medical-surgical nursing* (14th ed.). Wolter Kluwer.

Hockenberry, M. J., Rodgers, C. C., & Wilson, D. (Eds.). (2022). *Wong's essentials of pediatric nursing* (11th ed.). Elsevier.

Hravnak, M., Whittle, J., Kelley, M. E., Sereika, S., Good, C. B., Ibrahim, S. A., & Conigliaro, J. (2007). Symptom expression in coronary heart disease and revascularization recommendations for black and white patients. *American Journal of Public Health, 97*(9), 1701–1708. https://doi.org/10.2105/AJPH.2005.084103

Huether, S. E., McCance, K. L., & Brashers, V. L. (2020). *Understanding pathophysiology* (7th ed.). Elsevier.

Ignatavicius, D. D., Workman, M. L., Rebar, C. R., & Heimgartner, N. M. (2021). *Medical-surgical nursing: Concepts for interprofessional care* (10th ed.). Elsevier.

Klabunde, R. E. (2022). *Cardiovascular physiology concepts* (3rd ed.). Wolters Kluwer.

Theophanous, R., Huang, W., & Ragsdale, L. (2021). Cardiopulmonary emergencies in older adults. *Emergency Medicine Clinics of North America, 39*(2), 323–338. https://doi.org/10.1016/j.emc.2021.01.010

Wiandt, J. V., Winkelman, C., Dolansky, M. A., & Prince-Paul, M. (2020). Patient reported symptom outcomes during medication titration for adult heart failure management. *Applied Nursing Research, 56*, 151342. https://doi.org/10.1016/j.apnr.2020.151342

Caregiver Adaptation to Patient Institutionalization   2200

Definition: Adaptive response of family caregiver when the care recipient is moved to an institution

OUTCOME TARGET RATING: Maintain at_____ Increase to_____

		Never Demonstrated	Rarely Demonstrated	Sometimes Demonstrated	Often Demonstrated	Consistently Demonstrated	
OUTCOME OVERALL RATING		1	2	3	4	5	
Indicators:							
220001	Trusts non-family caregiver	1	2	3	4	5	NA
220018	Cooperates with staff	1	2	3	4	5	NA
220019	Reports positive interactions with staff	1	2	3	4	5	NA
220020	Reports conflict free interaction with staff	1	2	3	4	5	NA
220011	Provides consent for treatment	1	2	3	4	5	NA
220002	Maintains desired control over care	1	2	3	4	5	NA
220003	Participates in care as desired	1	2	3	4	5	NA
220012	Provides information about patient's routine	1	2	3	4	5	NA
220013	Provides patient's comfort items	1	2	3	4	5	NA
220014	Communicates needs of non-verbal patient	1	2	3	4	5	NA
220004	Maintains caregiver-care recipient relationship	1	2	3	4	5	NA
220016	Collaborates with health provider in determining care	1	2	3	4	5	NA
220021	Reports satisfaction with quality of care provided	1	2	3	4	5	NA
220006	Reports decreased need to verbalize feelings about change	1	2	3	4	5	NA
220022	Resolves anxiety about placement	1	2	3	4	5	NA
220007	Resolves feelings of guilt	1	2	3	4	5	NA
220023	Resolves feelings that others overly influenced my decision	1	2	3	4	5	NA
220024	Resolves feelings of ambivalence	1	2	3	4	5	NA
220008	Resolves feelings of anger	1	2	3	4	5	NA
220025	Resolves feelings of betrayal	1	2	3	4	5	NA
220026	Resolves feelings of loss	1	2	3	4	5	NA
220009	Uses conflict resolution strategies	1	2	3	4	5	NA
220017	Reports comfort with role transition	1	2	3	4	5	NA
220027	Reports decrease in caregiver burden	1	2	3	4	5	NA
220028	Reports satisfaction with quality of life	1	2	3	4	5	NA

Domain-Family Health (VI)   *Class*-Family Caregiver Performance (W)   *1st edition 1997; revised 2004, 2008, 2024*

OUTCOME CONTENT REFERENCES:
Alonso, M. S. I., Ursúa, M. P., & Caperos, J. M. (2017). The family caregiver after the institutionalization of the dependent elderly relative. *Educational Gerontology, 43*(12), 650–661. https://doi.org/10.1080/03601277.2017.1386403
Davis, J. D., Hill, B. D., Pillemer, S., Taylor, J., & Tremont, G. (2019). Guilt after placement questionnaire: A new instrument to assess caregiver emotional functioning following nursing home placement. *Aging & Mental Health, 23*(3), 352–356. https://doi.org/10.1080/13607863.2017.1423029
Teng, C., Loy, C. T., Sellars, M., Pond, D., Latt, M. D., Waite, L. M., Sinka, V., Logeman, C., & Tong, A. (2020). Making decisions about long-term institutional care placement among people with dementia and their caregivers: Systematic review of qualitative studies. *The Gerontologist, 60*(4), e329–e346. https://doi.org/10.1093/geront/gnz046

C

Caregiver Emotional Health Status 2506

Definition: Emotional well-being of a care provider while caring for a family member

OUTCOME TARGET RATING: Maintain at_____ Increase to_____

OUTCOME OVERALL RATING		Severely Compromised 1	Substantially Compromised 2	Moderately Compromised 3	Mildly Compromised 4	Not Compromised 5	
Indicators:							
250621	Relationship with care recipient	1	2	3	4	5	NA
250622	Satisfaction with care provided	1	2	3	4	5	NA
250602	Sense of control	1	2	3	4	5	NA
250617	Coping	1	2	3	4	5	NA
250623	Privacy	1	2	3	4	5	NA
250618	Emotional vitality	1	2	3	4	5	NA
250619	Work productivity	1	2	3	4	5	NA
250603	Self-esteem	1	2	3	4	5	NA
250610	Certainty about future	1	2	3	4	5	NA
250624	Family agreement on care provision	1	2	3	4	5	NA
250625	Social connectedness	1	2	3	4	5	NA
250626	Spiritual well-being	1	2	3	4	5	NA
250627	Relationships with health professionals	1	2	3	4	5	NA
250628	Access to respite care	1	2	3	4	5	NA
250629	Adequacy of resources	1	2	3	4	5	NA
250630	Satisfaction with life circumstances	1	2	3	4	5	NA

		Severe	Substantial	Moderate	Mild	None	
250604	Anger	1	2	3	4	5	NA
250605	Resentfulness	1	2	3	4	5	NA
250606	Guilt	1	2	3	4	5	NA
250607	Depression	1	2	3	4	5	NA
250608	Frustration	1	2	3	4	5	NA
250620	Psychological distress	1	2	3	4	5	NA
250631	Daily hassles in care situation	1	2	3	4	5	NA
250609	Ambivalence about situation	1	2	3	4	5	NA
250613	Perceived burden	1	2	3	4	5	NA
250615	Psychotropic medication use	1	2	3	4	5	NA

Domain-Family Health (VI)   *Class*-Family Member Health Status (Z)   *1st edition 1997; revised 2004, 2018, 2024*

OUTCOME CONTENT REFERENCES:

Bangerter, L. R., Liu, Y., & Zarit, S. H. (2019). Longitudinal trajectories of subjective care stressors: The role of personal, dyadic, and family resources. *Aging & Mental Health, 23*(2), 255–262. https://doi.org/10.1080/13607863.2017.1402292

Greenwood, N., Pound, C., Brearly, S., & Smith, R. (2019). A qualitative study of older informal carers' experiences and perceptions of their caring role. *Maturitas, 124*, 1–7. https://doi.org/10.1016/j.maturitas.2019.03.006

Keeton, V. F., Trask, J., Whitney, R., & Bell, J. F. (2020). Overburdened and underprepared: Medical/nursing task performance among informal caregivers in the United States. *Journal of Gerontological Nursing, 46*(90), 25–35. https://doi.org/10.3928/00989134-20200811-05

Leggett, A. N., Polenick, C. A., Maust, D. T., & Kales, H. C. (2018). Falls and hospitalizations among persons with dementia and associated caregiver emotional difficulties. *The Gerontologist, 58*(2), e78–e86. https://doi.org/10.1093/geront/gnx202

Lethin, C., Leino-Kilpi, H., Bleijlevens, M. H. C., Stephan, A., Martin, M. S., Nilsson, K., Nilsson, C., Zabalegui, A., & Karlsson, S. (2020). Predicting caregiver burden in informal caregivers caring for persons with dementia living at home—A follow-up cohort study. *Dementia, 19*(3), 640–660. https://doi.org/10.1177/1471301218782502

Nikzad-Terhune, K., Gaugler, J. E., & Jacobs-Lawson, J. (2019). Dementia caregiving outcomes: The impact of caregiving onset, cognitive impairment and behavioral problems. *Journal of Gerontological Social Work, 62*(5), 543–563. https://doi.org/10.1080/01634372.2019.1625993

Ribeiro, O., Brandão, D., Oliveira, A. F., Teixeira, L., & Paúl, C. (2019). Positive aspects of care in informal caregivers of community-dwelling dementia patients. *Journal of Psychiatry Mental Health Nursing, 27*(4), 330–341. https://doi.org/10.1111/jpm.12582

Shirai, Y., & Koerner, S. S. (2018). Examining the influence of care-recipient resistance on family caregiver emotional and physical well-being: Average frequency versus daily fluctuation. *Journal of Applied Gerontology, 37*(2), 203–227. https://doi.org/10.1177/0733464816631594

Caregiver Home Care Readiness

2202

Definition: Caregiver actions to assume care responsibility for a family member in the home

OUTCOME TARGET RATING: Maintain at_____ Increase to_____

		Never Demonstrated	Rarely Demonstrated	Sometimes Demonstrated	Often Demonstrated	Consistently Demonstrated	
OUTCOME OVERALL RATING		1	2	3	4	5	
Indicators:							
220223	Verbalizes commitment to caregiving role	1	2	3	4	5	NA
220224	Shows positive regard for care recipient	1	2	3	4	5	NA
220225	Learns about the caregiving role	1	2	3	4	5	NA
220226	Obtains reputable information about care recipient's disease	1	2	3	4	5	NA
220227	Obtains reputable information about usual disease trajectory	1	2	3	4	5	NA
220228	Physical stature and strength to provide care	1	2	3	4	5	NA
220229	Participates in individualized discharge plan	1	2	3	4	5	NA
220230	Involves care recipient in planning home care	1	2	3	4	5	NA
220231	Takes responsibility for planning home care	1	2	3	4	5	NA
220232	Takes responsibility for follow-up care	1	2	3	4	5	NA
220233	Obtains training for care activities	1	2	3	4	5	NA
220234	Obtains training for emergency response	1	2	3	4	5	NA
220235	Adapts home environment to abilities of recipient	1	2	3	4	5	NA
220236	Adapts care activities to home setting	1	2	3	4	5	NA
220237	Knowledge of recommended treatment regimen	1	2	3	4	5	NA
220238	Obtains information about medication	1	2	3	4	5	NA
220239	Knowledge of medication management	1	2	3	4	5	NA
220240	Knowledge of recommended procedures	1	2	3	4	5	NA
220241	Knowledge of equipment and supplies required	1	2	3	4	5	NA
220242	Obtains correct supplies for equipment	1	2	3	4	5	NA
220243	Knowledge of equipment operation	1	2	3	4	5	NA
220244	Operates equipment correctly	1	2	3	4	5	NA
220245	Knowledge of prescribed activity	1	2	3	4	5	NA
220246	Knowledge of financial resources	1	2	3	4	5	NA
220247	Obtains financial resources for caregiving	1	2	3	4	5	NA
220248	Partners with health professional	1	2	3	4	5	NA
220249	Plans in place of when to contact health professional	1	2	3	4	5	NA
220250	Perceived social support for caregiving	1	2	3	4	5	NA
220251	Confidence in ability to manage care at home	1	2	3	4	5	NA
220252	Plans for caregiver backup	1	2	3	4	5	NA
220253	Participates in week-end practice leave before discharge	1	2	3	4	5	NA

Domain-Family Health (VI)   *Class*-Family Caregiver Performance (W)   *1st edition 1997; revised 2004, 2008, 2024*

OUTCOME CONTENT REFERENCES:

Milberg, A., Liljeroos, M., Wåhlberg, & Krevers, B. (2020). Sense of support within the family: A cross-sectional study of family members in palliative home care. *BMC Palliative Care, 19*(1), 1–16. https://doi.org/10.1186/s12904-020-00623-z

Vullings, I., Labrie, N., Wammes, J. D., de Bekker-Grob, E. W., & MacNeil-Vroomen, J. (2020). Important components for Dutch in-home care based on qualitative interviews with persons with dementia and informal caregivers. *Health Expectations, 23*(6), 1412–1419. https://doi.org/10.1111/hex.13118

Wu, M.-P., Huang, S.-J., & Tsao, L.-I. (2020). The life experiences among primary family caregivers of home-based palliative care. *American Journal of Hospice & Palliative Medicine, 37*(10), 816–822. https://doi.org/10.1177/1049909 1 20907601

C

Caregiver Lifestyle Disruption 2203

Definition: Severity of disturbances in the lifestyle of a family member due to caregiving

OUTCOME TARGET RATING: Maintain at_____ Increase to_____

OUTCOME OVERALL RATING	Severe 1	Substantial 2	Moderate 3	Mild 4	None 5	
Indicators:						
220315 Disruption of routine activities	1	2	3	4	5	NA
220321 Disruption of activities of daily living (ADL)	1	2	3	4	5	NA
220322 Disruption of instrumental activities of daily living (IADL)	1	2	3	4	5	NA
220323 Sleep deficit	1	2	3	4	5	NA
220324 Nutritional needs deficiency	1	2	3	4	5	NA
220325 Breakdown in family life	1	2	3	4	5	NA
220326 Breakdown in family relationship	1	2	3	4	5	NA
220327 Breakdown in family functioning	1	2	3	4	5	NA
220328 Interference in family time	1	2	3	4	5	NA
220329 Interference with family role responsibilities	1	2	3	4	5	NA
220330 Interference with personal goals	1	2	3	4	5	NA
220331 Interruptions during work hours	1	2	3	4	5	NA
220332 Interference in work productivity	1	2	3	4	5	NA
220333 Interference in work quality	1	2	3	4	5	NA
220343 Interference in pet care	1	2	3	4	5	NA
220334 Hindrance to role flexibility	1	2	3	4	5	NA
220335 Interference in relationships with friends	1	2	3	4	5	NA
220336 Interference in social interactions	1	2	3	4	5	NA
220337 Interruption in social support	1	2	3	4	5	NA
220338 Limitation of diversional activities	1	2	3	4	5	NA
220318 Disruption of living environment	1	2	3	4	5	NA
220319 Financial burden from caregiving	1	2	3	4	5	NA
220339 Delay in career advancement	1	2	3	4	5	NA
220340 Delay in salary increases	1	2	3	4	5	NA
220341 Interference with pet relationship	1	2	3	4	5	NA
220342 Free time constrained	1	2	3	4	5	NA

Domain-Family Health (VI)   **Class**-Family Caregiver Performance (W)   *1st edition 1997; revised 2004, 2008, 2024*

OUTCOME CONTENT REFERENCES:

Alasmee, N., & Hasan, A. A. (2020). Primary caregivers experience of anti-psychotic medication: A qualitative study. *Archives of Psychiatric Nursing, 34*(6), 520–528. https://doi.org/10.1016/j.apnu.2020.09.002

Carlozzi, N. E., Lange, R. T., Boileau, N. R., Kallen, M. A., Sander, A. M., Hanks, R. A., Nakase-Richardson, R., Tulsky, D. S., Massengale, J. P., French, L. A., & Brickell, T. A. (2020). TBI-CareQOL family disruption: Family disruption in caregivers of persons with TBI. *Rehabilitation Psychology, 65*(4), 390–400. https://doi.org/10.1037/rep0000297

Carlozzi, N. E., Sherman, C. W., Angers, K., Belander, M. P., Austin, A. M., & Ryan, K. A. (2018). Caring for an individual with mild cognitive impairment: A qualitative perspective of health-related quality of life from caregivers. *Aging & Mental Health, 22*(9), 1190–1198. https://doi.org/10.1080/13607863.2017.1341468

Coleman, K., Flesch, L., Petiniot, L., Pate, A., Lin, L., Crosby, L., Beebe, D. W., Nelson, A., Alonso, P. B., Davies, S. M., Baker, R. B., & Dondoy, C. E. (2018). Sleep disruption in caregivers of pediatric stem cell recipients. *Pediatric Blood & Cancer, 65*, e26965. https://doi.org/10.1002/pbc.26965

Gray, T. F., Azizoddin, D. R., & Nersesian, P. V. (2020). Loneliness among cancer caregivers: A narrative review. *Palliative and Supportive Care, 18*, 359–367. https://doi.org/10.1017/S1478951519000804

Martsolf, G. R., Kandrack, R., Rodakowski, J., Friedman, E. M., Beach, S., Folb, B., & James, A. E. III. (2020). Work performance among informal caregivers: A review of the literature. *Journal of Aging and Health, 32*(9), 1017–1028. https://doi.org/10.1177/0898264319895374

Schulman-Green, D., & Feder, S. (2018). Integrating family caregivers into palliative oncology care using the self-and family management approach. *Seminars in Oncology Nursing, 34*(3), 252–263. https://doi.org/10.1016/j.soncn.2018.06.006

Schulman-Green, D., Feder, S. L., Dionne-Odom, J. N., Batten, J., En Long, V. J., Harris, Y., Wilpers, A., Wong, T., & Whittemore, R. (2021). Family caregiver support of patient self-management during chronic, life-limiting illness: A qualitative metasynthesis. *Journal of Family Nursing, 27*(1), 1–18. https://doi.org/10.1177/1074840720977180

Caregiver-Patient Relationship   2204

Definition: Positive interactions and connections of the care provider to a family member receiving care

OUTCOME TARGET RATING: Maintain at _____ Increase to _____

	Never Demonstrated	Rarely Demonstrated	Sometimes Demonstrated	Often Demonstrated	Consistently Demonstrated	
OUTCOME OVERALL RATING	**1**	**2**	**3**	**4**	**5**	
Indicators:						
220415 Accepts caregiver role	1	2	3	4	5	NA
220416 Shows respect	1	2	3	4	5	NA
220417 Discusses care needs with family member	1	2	3	4	5	NA
220418 Communicates effectively	1	2	3	4	5	NA
220419 Provides sense of security	1	2	3	4	5	NA
220420 Provides companionship	1	2	3	4	5	NA
220421 Shares emotions	1	2	3	4	5	NA
220422 Uses caring approach	1	2	3	4	5	NA
220423 Responds to care need changes	1	2	3	4	5	NA
220424 Paces care to accommodate needs of family member	1	2	3	4	5	NA
220425 Accepts family member's physical limitations	1	2	3	4	5	NA
220426 Accepts family member's psychological limitations	1	2	3	4	5	NA
220427 Accepts family member's cognitive limitations	1	2	3	4	5	NA
220428 Acknowledges impact of caregiving on relationship with family member	1	2	3	4	5	NA

Domain-Family Health (VI)   *Class*-Family Caregiver Performance (W)   *1st edition 1997; revised 2004, 2008, 2024*

OUTCOME CONTENT REFERENCES:

Bangerter, L. R., Liu, Y., & Zarit, S. H. (2019). Longitudinal trajectories of subjective care stressors: The role of personal, dyadic, and family resources. *Aging & Mental Health, 23*(2), 255–262. https://doi.org/10.1080/13607863.2017.1402292

Greenwood, N., Pound, C., Brearley, S., & Smith, R. (2019). A qualitative study of older informal carers' experiences and perceptions of their caring roles. *Maturitas, 124*, 1–7. https://doi.org/10.1016/j.maturitas.2019.03.006

Junkins, C. C., Kent, E., Litzelman, K., Bevans, M., Cannady, R. S., & Rosenberg, A. R. (2020). Cancer across the ages: A narrative review of caregiver burden for patients of all ages. *Journal of Psychosocial Oncology, 38*(6), 782–798. https://doi.org/10.1080/07347332.2020.1796887

Nikzad-Terhune, K., Gaugler, J. E., & Jacobs-Lawson, J. (2019). Dementia caregiving outcomes: The impact of caregiving onset, cognitive impairment and behavioral problems. *Journal of Gerontological Social Work, 62*(5), 543–563. https://doi.org/10.1080/01634372.2019.1625993

Satherley, R.-M., Coburn, S. S., & Germone, M. (2020). The impact of celiac disease on caregivers' well-being: An integrative review. *Gastroenterology: Celiac Disease, 70*(3), 295–303. https://doi.org/10.1097/MPG.0000000000002572

Shirai, Y., & Koerner, S. S. (2018). Examining the influence of care-recipient resistance on family caregiver emotional and physical well-being: Average frequency versus daily fluctuation. *Journal of Applied Gerontology, 37*(2), 203–227. https://doi.org/10.1177/0733464816631594

C

Caregiver Performance: Direct Care   2205

Definition: Caregiver actions to provide personal and health care services for an individual needing assistance

OUTCOME TARGET RATING: Maintain at_____ Increase to_____

		Never Demonstrated	Rarely Demonstrated	Sometimes Demonstrated	Often Demonstrated	Consistently Demonstrated	
OUTCOME OVERALL RATING		1	2	3	4	5	
Indicators:							
220519	Obtains reputable information about care recipient's disease	1	2	3	4	5	NA
220534	Obtains reputable information about care recipient's disease trajectory	1	2	3	4	5	NA
220520	Obtains reputable information about treatment regimen	1	2	3	4	5	NA
220521	Seeks training for caregiving activities	1	2	3	4	5	NA
220535	Seeks assistance with care tasks as needed	1	2	3	4	5	NA
220513	Performs needed tasks confidently	1	2	3	4	5	NA
220522	Monitors care recipient's adherence to treatment regimen	1	2	3	4	5	NA
220523	Follows protocol for procedures	1	2	3	4	5	NA
220536	Administers medication	1	2	3	4	5	NA
220537	Manages dietary recommendations	1	2	3	4	5	NA
220502	Assists with care recipient's activities of daily living needs	1	2	3	4	5	NA
220506	Assists with care recipient's instrumental activities of daily living needs	1	2	3	4	5	NA
220538	Assists with care recipient's emotional needs	1	2	3	4	5	NA
220524	Monitors health status of care recipient	1	2	3	4	5	NA
220525	Monitors behavior of care recipient	1	2	3	4	5	NA
220510	Anticipates care recipient's needs	1	2	3	4	5	NA
220526	Maintains positive regard for care recipient	1	2	3	4	5	NA
220527	Meets psychosocial needs of care recipient	1	2	3	4	5	NA
220528	Evaluates personal competency to provide care	1	2	3	4	5	NA
220529	Modifies home environment to meet needs	1	2	3	4	5	NA
220530	Uses strategies to promote safety	1	2	3	4	5	NA

Caregiver Performance: Direct Care—cont'd

		Never Demonstrated	Rarely Demonstrated	Sometimes Demonstrated	Often Demonstrated	Consistently Demonstrated	
220531	Contacts health professional when needed	1	2	3	4	5	NA
220532	Uses respite care when needed	1	2	3	4	5	NA
225033	Maintains plan for medical emergencies	1	2	3	4	5	NA
220539	Manages financial resources	1	2	3	4	5	NA

Domain-Family Health (VI)   *Class*-Family Caregiver Performance (W)   *1st edition 1997; revised 2004, 2008, 2018, 2024*

OUTCOME CONTENT REFERENCES:

Adistya, V. K., Nurjannah, I., & Subekti, H. (2018). The interrater reliability of Nursing Outcome Classification (NOC): "Caregiver Performance: Direct Care." *International Journal of Nursing Knowledge, 29*(3), 192–199. https://doi.org/10.1111/2047-3095.12164

Bangerter, L. R., Liu, Y., & Zarit, S. H. (2019). Longitudinal trajectories of subjective care stressors: The role of personal, dyadic, and family resources. *Aging & Mental Health, 23*(2), 255–262. https://doi.org/10.1080/13607863.2017.1402292

Greenwood, N., Pound, C., Brearley, S., & Smith, R. (2019). A qualitative study of older informal carers' experiences and perceptions of their caring role. *Maturitas, 124*, 1–7. https://doi.org/10.1016/j.maturitas.2019.03.006

Head, B. J., Maas, M., & Johnson, M. (2003). Validity and community-health-nursing sensitivity of six outcomes for community health nursing with older clients. *Public Health Nursing, 20*(5), 385–398. https://doi.org/10.1046/j.1525-1446.2003.20507.x

Junkins, C. C., Kent, E., Litzelman, K., Bevans, M., Cannady, R. S., & Rosenberg, A. R. (2020). Cancer across the ages: A narrative review of caregiver burden for patients of all ages. *Journal of Psychosocial Oncology, 38*(6), 782–798. https://doi.org/10.1080/07347332.2020.1796887

Keeton, V. F., Trask, J., Whitney, R., & Bell, J. F. (2020). Overburdened and underprepared: Medical/nursing task performance among informal caregivers in the United States. *Journal of Gerontological Nursing, 46*(9), 25–35. https://doi.org/10.3928/00989134-20200811-05

Kehoe, L. A., Xu, H., Duberstein, P., Loh, K. P., Culakova, E., Canin, B., Hurria, A., Dale, W., Wells, M., Gilmore, N., Kleckner, A. S., Lund, J., Kamen, C., Flannery, M., Hoerger, M., Hopkins, J. O., Liu, J. J., Geer, J., Epstein, R., & Mohile, M. (2019). Quality of life of caregivers of older patients with advanced cancer. *Journal of American Geriatrics Society, 67*(5), 969–977. https://doi.org/10.1111/JGS.15862

Polenick, C. A., Stanz, S., Leggett, A. N., Maust, D. T., Hodgson, N. A., & Kales, H. C. (2020). Stressors and resources related to medication management: Associations with spousal caregivers' role overload. *The Gerontologist, 60*(1), 165–173. https://doi.org/10.1093/geront/gny130

Satherley, R.-M., Coburn, S. S., & Germone, M. (2020). The impact of celiac disease on caregivers' well-being: An integrative review. *Gastroenterology: Celiac Disease, 70*(3), 295–303. https://doi.org/10.1097/MPG.0000000000002572

Caregiver Performance: Indirect Care   2206

Definition: Caregiver actions to arrange and oversee required care for an individual needing assistance

OUTCOME TARGET RATING: Maintain at_____ Increase to_____

		Never Demonstrated	Rarely Demonstrated	Sometimes Demonstrated	Often Demonstrated	Consistently Demonstrated	
OUTCOME OVERALL RATING		**1**	**2**	**3**	**4**	**5**	
Indicators:							
220601	Solves problems confidently	1	2	3	4	5	NA
220616	Monitors changes in health status of care recipient	1	2	3	4	5	NA
220617	Monitors changes in behavior of care recipient	1	2	3	4	5	NA
220614	Anticipates care recipient's needs	1	2	3	4	5	NA
220632	Participates in decision-making	1	2	3	4	5	NA
220633	Provides feedback on impact of care to direct caregiver	1	2	3	4	5	NA
220634	Receives feedback on impact of care from supervisor of direct care	1	2	3	4	5	NA
220618	Obtains needed health care services for care recipient	1	2	3	4	5	NA

Continued

Caregiver Performance: Indirect Care—cont'd

		Never Demonstrated	Rarely Demonstrated	Sometimes Demonstrated	Often Demonstrated	Consistently Demonstrated	
220619	Arranges for needed transportation for care recipient	1	2	3	4	5	NA
220620	Obtains needed equipment for care recipient	1	2	3	4	5	NA
220621	Obtains needed supplies for care recipient	1	2	3	4	5	NA
220622	Obtains required medications for care recipient	1	2	3	4	5	NA
220623	Accepts responsibility for overseeing provision of care	1	2	3	4	5	NA
220624	Provides monetary support	1	2	3	4	5	NA
220635	Monitors school progress	1	2	3	4	5	NA
220625	Monitors provision of care	1	2	3	4	5	NA
220626	Monitors psychosocial needs	1	2	3	4	5	NA
220636	Monitors for emergency care needs	1	2	3	4	5	NA
220627	Maintains positive regard for care recipient	1	2	3	4	5	NA
220628	Coordinates care with other family members	1	2	3	4	5	NA
220629	Promotes communication among family members	1	2	3	4	5	NA
220630	Collaborates in solving problems with health professional	1	2	3	4	5	NA
220637	Collaborates as a resource person	1	2	3	4	5	NA
220609	Performs needed tasks confidently	1	2	3	4	5	NA
220631	Provides for required safety needs	1	2	3	4	5	NA

Domain-Family Health (VI)   **Class**-Family Caregiver Performance (W)   *1st edition 1997; revised 2004, 2008, 2018, 2024*

OUTCOME CONTENT REFERENCES:

Albrecht, E. C., Kaelin, V. C., Rigau, B. L., Dooling-Litfin, J. K., Scully, E. A., Murphy, N. J., McManus, B. M., & Khetani, M. A. (2020). Pilot implementation of an electronic patient-reported outcome measure for planning and monitoring participation-focused care in early intervention. *BMC Medical Informatics and Decision Making, 20*, 189–199. https://doi.org/10.1186/s12911-020-01189-9

Blake, K. V. (2020). Telemedicine and adherence monitoring in children with asthma. *Current Opinion in Pulmonary Medicine, 27*(1), 37–44. https://doi.org/10.1097/MCP.0000000000000739

Davies, S., & Nolan, M. (2006). 'Making it better': Self-perceived roles of family caregivers of older people living in care homes: A qualitative study. *International Journal of Nursing Studies, 43*, 281–291. https://doi.org/10.1016/j.ijnurstu.2005.04.009

deBruin, S. R., Buist, Y., Hassink, J., & Vaandrager, L. (2021). 'I want to make myself useful': The value of nature-based adult day services in urban areas for people with Dementia and their family carers. *Ageing & Society, 41*, 582–604. https://doi.org/10.1017/S0144686X19001168

Soontorn, S., Pongtriang, P., & Songwathana, P. (2020). *Australasian Emergency Care, 23*, 71–76. https://doi.org/10.1016/j.auec.2019.11.002

Vellone, E., Riegel, B., & Alvaro, R. (2018). A situation-specific theory of caregiver contributions to heart failure self-care. *Journal of Cardiovascular Nursing, 34*(2), 166–173. https://doi.org/10.1097/JCN.0000000000000549

Caregiver Physical Health Status   2507

Definition: Physical well-being of a care provider while caring for a family member

OUTCOME TARGET RATING: Maintain at_____ Increase to_____

		Severely Compromised	Substantially Compromised	Moderately Compromised	Mildly Compromised	Not Compromised	
OUTCOME OVERALL RATING		1	2	3	4	5	
Indicators:							
250715	Physical fitness	1	2	3	4	5	NA
250702	Sleep-rest pattern	1	2	3	4	5	NA
250703	Blood pressure	1	2	3	4	5	NA
250704	Energy level	1	2	3	4	5	NA
250705	Physical comfort	1	2	3	4	5	NA
250706	Mobility level	1	2	3	4	5	NA
250707	Resistance to infection	1	2	3	4	5	NA
250708	Physical function	1	2	3	4	5	NA
250709	Weight	1	2	3	4	5	NA
250710	Gastrointestinal function	1	2	3	4	5	NA
250716	Cardiopulmonary function	1	2	3	4	5	NA
250717	Respiratory function	1	2	3	4	5	NA
250718	Nutritional status	1	2	3	4	5	NA
250719	Cognitive status	1	2	3	4	5	NA
250711	Medication use	1	2	3	4	5	NA
250712	Perceived general health	1	2	3	4	5	NA
250720	Perceived access to respite	1	2	3	4	5	NA

Domain-Family Health (VI)   *Class*-Family Member Health Status (Z)   *1st edition 1997; revised 2004, 2008, 2024*

OUTCOME CONTENT REFERENCES:

Abuatiq, A., Brown, R., Wolles, B., & Randall, R. (2020). Perceptions of stress. *Clinical Journal of Oncology Nursing, 24*(10), 51–57. https://doi.org/10.1188/20.cjon.51-57

Greenwood, N., Pound, C., Brearly, S., & Smith, R. (2019). A qualitative study of older informal carers' experiences and perceptions of their caring role. *Maturitas, 124,* 1–7. https://doi.org/10.1016/j.maturitas.2019.03.006

Head, B. J., Maas, M., & Johnson, M. (2003). Validity and community-health-nursing sensitivity of six outcomes for community health nursing with older clients. *Public Health Nursing, 20*(5), 385–398. https://doi.org/10.1046/j.1525-1446.2003.20507.x

Junkins, C. C., Kent, E., Litzelman, K., Bevans, M., Cannady, R. S., & Rosenberg, A. R. (2020). Cancer across the ages: A narrative review of caregiver burden for patients of all ages. *Journal of Psychosocial Oncology, 38*(6), 782–798. https://doi.org/10.1080/07347332.2020.1796887

Kehoe, L. A., Xu, H., Duberstein, P., Loh, K. P., Culakova, E., Canin, B., Hurria, A., Dale, W., Wells, M., Gilmore, N., Kleckner, A. S., Lund, J., Kamen, C., Flannery, M., Hoerger, M., Hopkins, J. O., Liu, J. J., Geer, J., Epstein, R., & Mohile, S. G. (2019). Quality of life of caregivers of older patients with advanced cancer. *Journal of the American Geriatrics Society, 67*(5), 969–977. https://doi.org/10.1111/jgs.15862

Caregiver Role Endurance   **2210**

Definition: Family care provider's capacity to sustain caregiving over an extended period of time

OUTCOME TARGET RATING: Maintain at_____ Increase to_____

		Never Demonstrated	Rarely Demonstrated	Sometimes Demonstrated	Often Demonstrated	Consistently Demonstrated	
OUTCOME OVERALL RATING		1	2	3	4	5	
Indicators:							
221014	Verbally commits to providing care	1	2	3	4	5	NA
221015	Maintains satisfying care recipient-caregiver relationship	1	2	3	4	5	NA
221016	Communicates role expectations clearly to others	1	2	3	4	5	NA
221017	Communicates with family members regularly	1	2	3	4	5	NA
221018	Identifies care recipient's needs	1	2	3	4	5	NA
221019	Gains satisfaction from caregiver role	1	2	3	4	5	NA
221020	Satisfied with care provided	1	2	3	4	5	NA
221021	Receives training to learn care activities	1	2	3	4	5	NA
221022	Masters direct care activities	1	2	3	4	5	NA
221023	Masters indirect care activities	1	2	3	4	5	NA
221024	Masters technical aspects of care	1	2	3	4	5	NA
221025	Identifies services to assist with care	1	2	3	4	5	NA
221026	Shows adaptability to care demands	1	2	3	4	5	NA
221027	Uses supplemental services to assist with care	1	2	3	4	5	NA
221028	Maintains positive communication with health professionals	1	2	3	4	5	NA
221029	Seeks guidance from health professionals about caregiving issues	1	2	3	4	5	NA
221030	Partners with health professionals for support	1	2	3	4	5	NA
221031	Obtains supplies for caregiving	1	2	3	4	5	NA
221032	Secures financial resources for caregiving	1	2	3	4	5	NA
221033	Uses strategies to maintain medication compliance	1	2	3	4	5	NA
220134	Uses social support resources	1	2	3	4	5	NA
221035	Uses respite as needed	1	2	3	4	5	NA
221036	Experiences cooperation from care recipient	1	2	3	4	5	NA
221037	Experiences cooperation from family members	1	2	3	4	5	NA
221038	Maintains caregiver leisure activities	1	2	3	4	5	NA
221039	Maintains own health	1	2	3	4	5	NA
221040	Maintains opportunities to work productively	1	2	3	4	5	NA

Domain-*Family Health (VI)*   **Class**-*Family Caregiver Performance (W)*   *1st edition 1997; revised 2004, 2008, 2024*

OUTCOME CONTENT REFERENCES:

Abuatiq, A., Brown, R., Wolles, B., & Randall, R. (2020). Perceptions of stress. *Clinical Journal of Oncology Nursing, 24*(10), 51–57. https://doi.org/10.1188/20.cjon.51-57

Alasmee, N., & Hasan, A. A. (2020). Primary caregivers experience of anti-psychotic medication: A qualitative study. *Archives of Psychiatric Nursing, 34*, 520–528. https://doi.org/10.1016/j.apnu.2020.09.002

Greenwood, N., Pound, C., Brearly, S., & Smith, R. (2019). A qualitative study of older informal carers' experiences and perceptions of their caring role. *Maturitas, 124*, 1–7. https://doi.org/10.1016/j.maturitas.2019.03.006

Junkins, C. C., Kent, E., Litzelman, K., Bevans, M., Cannady, R. S., & Rosenberg, A. R. (2020). Cancer across the ages: A narrative review of caregiver burden for patients of all ages. *Journal of Psychosocial Oncology, 38*(6), 782–798. https://doi.org/10.1080/07347332.2020.1796887

Nikzad-Terhune, K., Gaugler, J. E., & Jacobs-Lawson, J. (2019). Dementia caregiving outcomes: The impact of caregiving onset, cognitive impairment and behavioral problems. *Journal of Gerontological Social Work, 62*(5), 543–563. https://doi.org/10.1080/01634372.2019.1625993

Ribeiro, O., Brandão, D., Oliverira, A. F., Teixeira, L., & Paúl, C. (2019). Positive aspects of care in informal caregivers of community-dwelling dementia patients. *Journal of Psychiatry Mental Health Nursing, 27*(4), 330–341. https://doi.org/10.1111/jpm.12582

Yu, D. S. F., Cheng, S. T., & Wang, J. (2018). Unravelling positive aspects of caregiving in dementia: An integrative review of research literature. *International Journal of Nursing Studies, 79*, 1–26. https://doi.org/10.1016/j.ijnurstu.2017.10.008

C

Caregiver Stressors 2208

Definition: Severity of biopsychosocial pressure on a family care provider caring for another over an extended period of time

OUTCOME TARGET RATING: Maintain at_____ Increase to_____

		Severe	Substantial	Moderate	Mild	None	
OUTCOME OVERALL RATING		1	2	3	4	5	
Indicators:							
220801	Reported stressors of caregiving	1	2	3	4	5	NA
220802	Physical limitations for caregiving	1	2	3	4	5	NA
220803	Psychological limitations for caregiving	1	2	3	4	5	NA
220804	Cognitive limitations	1	2	3	4	5	NA
220822	Behavioral problems of care recipient	1	2	3	4	5	NA
220823	Care recipient's resistance to care	1	2	3	4	5	NA
220824	Intensive medication management	1	2	3	4	5	NA
220805	Role conflict	1	2	3	4	5	NA
220815	Sense of isolation	1	2	3	4	5	NA
220807	Perceived lack of social support	1	2	3	4	5	NA
220818	Perceived lack of health professional support	1	2	3	4	5	NA
220816	Loss of personal time	1	2	3	4	5	NA
220819	Conflict between work and caregiver responsibilities	1	2	3	4	5	NA
220820	Perceived burden of care recipient's progressive health problems	1	2	3	4	5	NA
220825	Concern over loss of mastery of care activities	1	2	3	4	5	NA
220826	Concern over loss of health insurance	1	2	3	4	5	NA
220827	Financial concerns	1	2	3	4	5	NA
220813	Impairment of caregiver-patient relationship	1	2	3	4	5	NA
220828	Lack of family support	1	2	3	4	5	NA
220821	Impairment of family relationships	1	2	3	4	5	NA

Domain-Family Health (VI)   *Class*-Family Caregiver Performance (W)   *1st edition 1997; revised 2004, 2008, 2024*

OUTCOME CONTENT REFERENCES:

Abuatiq, A., Brown, R., Wolles, B., & Randall, R. (2020). Perceptions of stress. *Clinical Journal of Oncology Nursing, 24*(10), 51–57. https://doi.org/10.1188/20.cjon.51-57

Bangerter, L. R., Liu, Y., & Zarit, S. H. (2019). Longitudinal trajectories of subjective care stressors: The role of personal, dyadic, and family resources. *Aging & Mental Health, 23*(2), 255–262. https://doi.org/10.1080/13607863.2017.1402292

Brown, L. L., Mitchell, U. A., & Ailshire, J. A. (2020). Disentangling the stress process: Race/ethnic differences in the exposure and appraisal of chronic stressors among older adults. *Journal of the American Geriatrics Society, 75*(3), 650–660. https://doi.org/10.1093/geronb/gby072

+Given, C. W., Given, B., Stommel, M., Collins, C., King, S., & Franklin, S. (1992). The caregiver reaction assessment (CRA) for caregivers to persons with chronic physical and mental impairments. *Research in Nursing & Health, 15*(4), 271–283.

Green, A. L., Kutash, K., Ferron, J., Levin, B. L., Debate, R., & Baldwin, J. (2020). Understanding caregiver strain and related constructs in caregivers of youth with emotional and behavioral disorders. *Journal of Child and Family Studies, 29*(3), 761–772. https://doi.org/10.1007/s10826-019-01626-y

Lamborn, P., & Cramer, K. M. (2020). Factors associated with distress in caregivers of people with personality disorders. *Community Mental Health Journal, 56*(7), 1298–1310. https://doi.org/10.1007/s10597-020-00640-5

Polenick, C. A., Stanz, S. D., Leggett, A. N., Maust, D. T., Hodgson, N. A., & Kales, H. C. (2020). Stressors and resources related to medication management: Associations with spousal caregivers' role overload. *The Gerontologist, 60*(1), 165–173. https://doi.org/10.1093/geront/gny130

+Robinson, B. C. (1983). Validation of a caregiver strain index. *Journal of Gerontology, 38*(3), 344–348.

Shirai, Y., & Koerner, S.S. (2018). Examining the influence of care-recipient resistance on family caregiver emotional and physical well-being: Average frequency versus daily fluctuation. *Journal of Applied Gerontology, 37*(2), 203–227. https://doi.org/10.1177/0733464816631594

Caregiver Well-Being

2508

Definition: Extent of positive perception of family care provider's health status

OUTCOME TARGET RATING: Maintain at_____ Increase to_____

OUTCOME OVERALL RATING	Not at All Satisfied	Somewhat Satisfied	Moderately Satisfied	Very Satisfied	Completely Satisfied	
	1	**2**	**3**	**4**	**5**	
Indicators:						
250801 Physical health	1	2	3	4	5	NA
250802 Psychological health	1	2	3	4	5	NA
250803 Lifestyle	1	2	3	4	5	NA
250804 Performance of usual roles	1	2	3	4	5	NA
250805 Social support	1	2	3	4	5	NA
250806 Support for instrumental activities of daily living	1	2	3	4	5	NA
250807 Health professional support	1	2	3	4	5	NA
250815 Availability of training	1	2	3	4	5	NA
250816 Personal meaning received from care	1	2	3	4	5	NA
250808 Social relationships	1	2	3	4	5	NA
250811 Family sharing of responsibilities for caregiving	1	2	3	4	5	NA
250817 Social resource use	1	2	3	4	5	NA
250812 Availability for respite	1	2	3	4	5	NA
250813 Ability to cope	1	2	3	4	5	NA
250818 Personal resilience	1	2	3	4	5	NA
250819 Problem-solving ability	1	2	3	4	5	NA
250809 Caregiver role satisfaction	1	2	3	4	5	NA
250814 Financial resources for caregiving	1	2	3	4	5	NA
250820 Financial stability	1	2	3	4	5	NA

Domain-Family Health (VI)　**Class**-Family Member Health Status (Z)　*1st edition 1997; revised 2004, 2008, 2024*

OUTCOME CONTENT REFERENCES:

Bermejo-Toro, L., Sánchez-Izquierdo, M., Calvete, E., & Roldán, M. A. (2020). Quality of life, psychological well-being, and resilience in caregivers of people with acquired brain injury (ABI). *Brain Injury, 34*(4), 480–488. https://doi.org/10.1080/02699052.2020.1725127

Born, J., Bakx, P., Schut, F., & van Doorslaer, E. (2019). The impact of informal caregiving for older adults on the health of various types of caregivers: A systematic review. *The Gerontologist, 59*(5), e629–e642. https://doi.org/10.1093/geront/gny137

Cavanaugh, D. L., Sutherby, C. G., Sharda, E., Hughes, A. K., & Woodward, A. T. (2020). The relationship between well-being and meaning-making in kinship caregivers. *Children and Youth Services Review, 116*, 105271. https://doi.org/10.1016/j.childyouth.2020.105271

Eaton, J., & Madsen-Wilkerson, N. (2020). Portrait of a caregiver: Ethnodrama development and its influence on caregiver well-being. *The Gerontologist, 60*(6), 1169–1178. https://doi.org/10.1093/geront/gny137

Kissinger, D. B., Grover, K. S., & Turner, R. C. (2020). Pediatric stroke caregiver well-being: A holistic wellness perspective. *Rehabilitation Counseling Bulletin, 63*(4), 245–255. https://doi.org/10.1177/0034355219846653rcb.sagepub.com

Or, R., & Kartal, A. (2019). Influence of caregiver burden on well-being of family member caregivers of older adults. *Psychogeriatrics, 19*, 482–490. https://doi.org/10.1111/psyg.12421

Satherley, R.-M., Coburn, S. S., & Germone, M. (2020). The impact of celiac disease on caregivers' well-being: An integrative review. *Gastroenterology: Celiac Disease, 70*(3), 295–303. https://doi.org/10.1097/MPG.0000000000002572

Chemotherapy: Disruptive Physical Effects   2116

Definition: Severity of physiological adverse effects from chemotherapy

OUTCOME TARGET RATING: Maintain at_____ Increase to_____

OUTCOME OVERALL RATING	Severe 1	Substantial 2	Moderate 3	Mild 4	None 5	
Indicators:						
211601 Nausea	1	2	3	4	5	NA
211602 Vomiting	1	2	3	4	5	NA
211603 Pain	1	2	3	4	5	NA
211604 Loss of appetite	1	2	3	4	5	NA
211605 Food aversion	1	2	3	4	5	NA
211606 Taste changes	1	2	3	4	5	NA
211607 Smell changes	1	2	3	4	5	NA
211608 Diarrhea	1	2	3	4	5	NA
211609 Constipation	1	2	3	4	5	NA
211610 Involuntary weight loss	1	2	3	4	5	NA
211611 Muscle wasting	1	2	3	4	5	NA
211612 Inflamed mucous membranes	1	2	3	4	5	NA
211613 Difficulty swallowing	1	2	3	4	5	NA
211614 Dry mouth	1	2	3	4	5	NA
211615 Abdominal cramping	1	2	3	4	5	NA
211616 Abdominal bloating	1	2	3	4	5	NA
211617 Hair loss	1	2	3	4	5	NA
211618 Fatigue	1	2	3	4	5	NA
211619 Sleep disturbances	1	2	3	4	5	NA
211620 Anemia	1	2	3	4	5	NA
211621 Neutropenia	1	2	3	4	5	NA
211622 Thrombocytopenia	1	2	3	4	5	NA
211623 Altered sensation in the upper extremities	1	2	3	4	5	NA
211624 Altered sensation in the lower extremities	1	2	3	4	5	NA
211625 Abnormal response to cold temperature	1	2	3	4	5	NA
211626 Hypersensitivity reaction to chemotherapy	1	2	3	4	5	NA
211627 Fever	1	2	3	4	5	NA
211628 Compromised immune function	1	2	3	4	5	NA
211629 Cough	1	2	3	4	5	NA
211630 Dyspnea	1	2	3	4	5	NA
211631 Weakness	1	2	3	4	5	NA
211632 Swelling of upper extremities	1	2	3	4	5	NA
211633 Swelling of lower extremities	1	2	3	4	5	NA
211634 Metabolic changes	1	2	3	4	5	NA

Domain-Health & Life Quality (V)   *Class*-Symptom Status (V)   6th edition 2018

OUTCOME CONTENT REFERENCES:
Bonosky, K., & Miller, R. (2005). Hypersensitivity reactions to Oxaliplatin: What nurses need to know. *Clinical Journal of Oncology Nursing, 9*(3), 325–330. https://doi.org/10.1136/bmj.h5000
Given, C., Sikorskii, A., Tamkus, D., Given, B., You, M., McCorkle, R., Champion, V., & Decker, D. (2008). Managing symptoms among patients with breast cancer during chemotherapy: Results of a two-arm behavioral trial. *Journal of Clinical Oncology, 26*(36), 5855–5862. https://doi.org/10.1200/JCO.2008.16.8872
Skolin, I., Hursti, U. K., & Wahlin, Y. B. (2001). Parents' perception of their child's food intake after the start of chemotherapy. *Journal of Pediatric Oncology Nursing, 18*(3), 124–136. https://doi.org/10.1177/104345420101800305
Van Cutsem, E., & Arends, J. (2005). The causes and consequences of cancer-associated malnutrition. *European Journal of Oncology Nursing, 9*(Suppl. 2), S51–S63. https://doi.org/10.1016/j.ejon.2005.09.007

C

Child Development: 1 Month

0120

Definition: Milestones of physical, cognitive, and psychosocial progression by 1 month of age

OUTCOME TARGET RATING: Maintain at_____ Increase to_____

	Never Demonstrated	Rarely Demonstrated	Sometimes Demonstrated	Often Demonstrated	Consistently Demonstrated	
OUTCOME OVERALL RATING	1	2	3	4	5	
Indicators:						
012001 Signals hunger	1	2	3	4	5	NA
012002 Signals discomfort	1	2	3	4	5	NA
012003 Responds to sounds	1	2	3	4	5	NA
012004 Responds to voice	1	2	3	4	5	NA
012005 Responds to face	1	2	3	4	5	NA
012006 Coos	1	2	3	4	5	NA
012007 Smiles spontaneously	1	2	3	4	5	NA
012024 Watches parent intently when speaking	1	2	3	4	5	NA
012008 Eyes follow to mid-line	1	2	3	4	5	NA
012009 Signals overstimulation	1	2	3	4	5	NA
012010 Exhibits five sleep and alert states	1	2	3	4	5	NA
012025 Hands predominately closed	1	2	3	4	5	NA
012011 Flexes extremity	1	2	3	4	5	NA
012012 Holds head erect momentarily	1	2	3	4	5	NA
012013 Turns head side to side when prone	1	2	3	4	5	NA
012014 Holds head in horizontal line with back when prone	1	2	3	4	5	NA
012426 In standing position is limp at knees and hips	1	2	3	4	5	NA
012015 Moro reflex	1	2	3	4	5	NA
012016 Tonic neck reflex	1	2	3	4	5	NA
012017 Dance reflex	1	2	3	4	5	NA
012018 Crawl reflex	1	2	3	4	5	NA
012019 Babinski reflex	1	2	3	4	5	NA
012020 Suck reflex	1	2	3	4	5	NA
012021 Palmer reflex	1	2	3	4	5	NA
012022 Plantar reflex	1	2	3	4	5	NA
012023 Rooting reflex	1	2	3	4	5	NA

Domain-Functional Health (I)   **Class**-Growth & Development (B)   *3rd edition 2004; revised 2024*

OUTCOME CONTENT REFERENCES:

Center for Disease Control and Prevention. (2021, January 22). *CDC's Developmental Milestones.* https://www.cdc.gov/ncbddd/actearly/milestones/index.html

Hagan, J. F., Shaw, J. S., & Duncan, P. M. (Eds.). (2017). *Bright futures: Guidelines for health supervision of infants, children and adolescents* (4th ed.). American Academy of Pediatrics.

Hockenberry, M. J., Rodgers, C. C., & Wilson, D. (Eds.). (2022). *Wong's essentials of pediatric nursing* (11th ed.). Elsevier.

Perry, S. E., Hockenberry, M. J., Lowdermilk, D. J., Wilson, D., Cashion, K., Rodgers, C. C., & Alden, K. R. (2018). *Maternal child nursing care* (6th ed.). Elsevier.

Child Development: 2 Months   0100

Definition: Milestones of physical, cognitive, and psychosocial progression by 2 months of age

OUTCOME TARGET RATING: Maintain at_____ Increase to_____

	Never Demonstrated	Rarely Demonstrated	Sometimes Demonstrated	Often Demonstrated	Consistently Demonstrated	
OUTCOME OVERALL RATING	1	2	3	4	5	
Indicators:						
010002 Crawl reflex disappearance	1	2	3	4	5	NA
010003 Lifts head, neck, and upper chest with support of forearms while in prone position	1	2	3	4	5	NA
010004 Shows some head control in upright position	1	2	3	4	5	NA
010005 Hands frequently open	1	2	3	4	5	NA
010006 Grasp reflex fading	1	2	3	4	5	NA
010007 Coos and vocalizes	1	2	3	4	5	NA
010013 Briefly calms self by sucking on hand or fingers	1	2	3	4	5	NA
010008 Shows interest in auditory stimuli	1	2	3	4	5	NA
010014 Turns head toward sounds	1	2	3	4	5	NA
010009 Shows interest in visual stimuli	1	2	3	4	5	NA
010015 Follows an item with eyes	1	2	3	4	5	NA
010016 Begins to recognize people at a distance	1	2	3	4	5	NA
010010 Smiles	1	2	3	4	5	NA
010011 Shows pleasure in interactions, especially with primary caregivers	1	2	3	4	5	NA

Domain-*Functional Health (I)*   **Class**-*Growth & Development (B)*   1st edition 1997; revised 2004, 2024

OUTCOME CONTENT REFERENCES:

Center for Disease Control and Prevention. (2021, January 22). *CDC's Developmental Milestones.* https://www.cdc.gov/ncbddd/actearly/milestones/index.html
Hagan, J. F., Shaw, J. S., & Duncan, P. M. (Eds.). (2017). *Bright futures: Guidelines for health supervision of infants, children and adolescents* (4th ed.). American Academy of Pediatrics.
Hockenberry, M. J., Rodgers, C. C., & Wilson, D. (Eds.). (2022). *Wong's essentials of pediatric nursing* (11th ed.). Elsevier.
Perry, S. E., Hockenberry, M. J., Lowdermilk, D. J., Wilson, D., Cashion, K., Rodgers, C. C., & Alden, K. R. (2018). *Maternal child nursing care* (6th ed.). Elsevier.

Child Development: 4 Months   0101

Definition: Milestones of physical, cognitive, and psychosocial progression by 4 months of age

OUTCOME TARGET RATING: Maintain at_____ Increase to_____

	Never Demonstrated	Rarely Demonstrated	Sometimes Demonstrated	Often Demonstrated	Consistently Demonstrated	
OUTCOME OVERALL RATING	1	2	3	4	5	
Indicators:						
010101 Holds head erect and raises body on hands while in prone position	1	2	3	4	5	NA
010102 Controls head well	1	2	3	4	5	NA
010103 Rolls over from prone to supine	1	2	3	4	5	NA
010104 Holds own hands	1	2	3	4	5	NA
010105 Grasps rattle	1	2	3	4	5	NA
010106 Reaches for objects	1	2	3	4	5	NA
010117 Uses hands and eyes together	1	2	3	4	5	NA

Continued

C

Child Development: 4 Months—cont'd

		Never Demonstrated	Rarely Demonstrated	Sometimes Demonstrated	Often Demonstrated	Consistently Demonstrated	
010107	Bats at objects	1	2	3	4	5	NA
010108	Babbles and coos	1	2	3	4	5	NA
010118	Different cries to show hunger, pain, or tiredness	1	2	3	4	5	NA
010119	Becomes bored if left alone	1	2	3	4	5	NA
010109	Recognizes parents' voices	1	2	3	4	5	NA
010110	Recognizes parents' touch	1	2	3	4	5	NA
010120	Responds to affection	1	2	3	4	5	NA
010111	Looks at and becomes excited by mobile	1	2	3	4	5	NA
010112	Smiles, laughs, and squeals	1	2	3	4	5	NA
010121	Copies some movements and facial expressions	1	2	3	4	5	NA
010122	Pulls clothing or blanket over face in play	1	2	3	4	5	NA
010116	Exhibits a nocturnal sleep pattern	1	2	3	4	5	NA
010114	Comforts self	1	2	3	4	5	NA

Domain-Functional Health (I)   **Class**-Growth & Development (B)   1st edition 1997; revised 2004, 2008, 2013, 2024

OUTCOME CONTENT REFERENCES:
Center for Disease Control and Prevention. (2021, January 22). *CDC's Developmental Milestones.* https://www.cdc.gov/ncbddd/actearly/milestones/index.html
Hagan, J. F., Shaw, J. S., & Duncan, P. M. (Eds.). (2017). *Bright futures: Guidelines for health supervision of infants, children and adolescents* (4th ed.). American Academy of Pediatrics.
Hockenberry, M. J., Rodgers, C. C., & Wilson, D. (Eds.). (2022). *Wong's essentials of pediatric nursing* (11th ed.). Elsevier.
Perry, S. E., Hockenberry, M. J., Lowdermilk, D. J., Wilson, D., Cashion, K., Rodgers, C. C., & Alden, K. R. (2018). *Maternal child nursing care* (6th ed.). Elsevier.

Child Development: 6 Months

0102

Definition: Milestones of physical, cognitive, and psychosocial progression by 6 months of age

OUTCOME TARGET RATING: Maintain at_____ Increase to_____

		Never Demonstrated	Rarely Demonstrated	Sometimes Demonstrated	Often Demonstrated	Consistently Demonstrated	
OUTCOME OVERALL RATING		1	2	3	4	5	
Indicators:							
010201	Supports head when pulled to sit	1	2	3	4	5	NA
010202	Rolls over both directions	1	2	3	4	5	NA
010203	Sits with support	1	2	3	4	5	NA
010204	Stands when placed and bears weight	1	2	3	4	5	NA
010205	Grasps and mouths objects	1	2	3	4	5	NA
010206	Gestures (e.g., points, shakes head)	1	2	3	4	5	NA
010207	Starts to self-feed	1	2	3	4	5	NA
010217	May begin teething with eruption of lower teeth	1	2	3	4	5	NA
010208	Shows interest in toys	1	2	3	4	5	NA
010218	Holds a bottle	1	2	3	4	5	NA
010209	Transfers small objects from hand to hand	1	2	3	4	5	NA
010219	Tries to get things that are out of reach	1	2	3	4	5	NA

Child Development: 6 Months—cont'd

		Never Demonstrated	Rarely Demonstrated	Sometimes Demonstrated	Often Demonstrated	Consistently Demonstrated	
010220	Likes to play with others, especially parents	1	2	3	4	5	NA
010210	Vocalizes/sings syllables (dada, baba)	1	2	3	4	5	NA
010211	Babbles reciprocally	1	2	3	4	5	NA
010221	Begins to repeat sounds heard	1	2	3	4	5	NA
010212	Smiles, laughs, squeals, imitates noise	1	2	3	4	5	NA
010213	Turns to sounds	1	2	3	4	5	NA
010222	Responds to own name	1	2	3	4	5	NA
010223	Likes to look at self in a mirror	1	2	3	4	5	NA
010224	Holds arms out to be picked up	1	2	3	4	5	NA
010225	Has definite likes and dislikes	1	2	3	4	5	NA
010214	Shows beginning signs of stranger anxiety	1	2	3	4	5	NA
010215	Comforts self	1	2	3	4	5	NA

Domain-*Functional Health (I)*   **Class**-*Growth & Development (B)*   *1st edition 1997; revised 2004, 2024*

OUTCOME CONTENT REFERENCES:

Center for Disease Control and Prevention. (2021, January 22). *CDC's Developmental Milestones.* https://www.cdc.gov/ncbddd/actearly/milestones/index.html
Hagan, J. F., Shaw, J. S., & Duncan, P. M. (Eds.). (2017). *Bright futures: Guidelines for health supervision of infants, children and adolescents* (4th ed.). American Academy of Pediatrics.
Hockenberry, M. J., Rodgers, C. C., & Wilson, D. (Eds.). (2022). *Wong's essentials of pediatric nursing* (11th ed.). Elsevier.
Perry, S. E., Hockenberry, M. J., Lowdermilk, D. J., Wilson, D., Cashion, K., Rodgers, C. C., & Alden, K. R. (2018). *Maternal child nursing care* (6th ed.). Elsevier.

Child Development: 9 Months

0125

Definition: Milestones of physical, cognitive, and psychosocial progression by 9 months of age

OUTCOME TARGET RATING: Maintain at_____ Increase to_____

		Never Demonstrated	Rarely Demonstrated	Sometimes Demonstrated	Often Demonstrated	Consistently Demonstrated	
OUTCOME OVERALL RATING		**1**	**2**	**3**	**4**	**5**	
Indicators:							
012501	Eruption of more teeth	1	2	3	4	5	NA
012502	Creeps or crawls on hands and knees	1	2	3	4	5	NA
012503	Recovers balance when leaning forward	1	2	3	4	5	NA
012504	Pulls self to standing position and holds on to furniture	1	2	3	4	5	NA
012505	Uses thumb and index finger in crude pincer grasp	1	2	3	4	5	NA
012506	Uses fingers to point at things	1	2	3	4	5	NA
012507	Transfers objects from one hand to the other	1	2	3	4	5	NA
012508	Compares 2 cubes by bringing them together	1	2	3	4	5	NA
012509	Watches the path of something as it falls	1	2	3	4	5	NA
012510	Looks for things someone hides	1	2	3	4	5	NA
012511	Plays peek-a-boo	1	2	3	4	5	NA
012512	Puts things in mouth	1	2	3	4	5	NA
012513	Mother is important for own sake	1	2	3	4	5	NA

Continued

Child Development: 9 Months—cont'd

		Never Demonstrated	Rarely Demonstrated	Sometimes Demonstrated	Often Demonstrated	Consistently Demonstrated	
012514	Shows interest in pleasing parent	1	2	3	4	5	NA
012515	Begins to show fear of being alone	1	2	3	4	5	NA
012516	Puts arms in front of face to avoid having it washed	1	2	3	4	5	NA
012517	Turns head directly toward sound	1	2	3	4	5	NA
012518	Sits steadily unsupported	1	2	3	4	5	NA
012519	Has taste preferences	1	2	3	4	5	NA
012520	Increasing fear of strangers	1	2	3	4	5	NA
012521	Frets when parent disappears	1	2	3	4	5	NA
012522	Responds to word "no"	1	2	3	4	5	NA
012523	Copies sounds and gestures of others	1	2	3	4	5	NA
012524	Shows regular pattern in urine elimination	1	2	3	4	5	NA
012525	Shows regular pattern in bowel elimination	1	2	3	4	5	NA

Domain-Functional Health (I)   **Class**-Growth & Development (B)   7th edition 2024

OUTCOME CONTENT REFERENCES:

Center for Disease Control and Prevention. (2021, January 22). *CDC's Developmental Milestones.* https://www.cdc.gov/ncbddd/actearly/milestones/index.html
Hagan, J. F., Shaw, J. S., & Duncan, P. M. (Eds.). (2017). *Bright futures: Guidelines for health supervision of infants, children and adolescents* (4th ed.). American Academy of Pediatrics.
Hockenberry, M. J., Wilson, D., & Rodgers, C. C. (Eds.). (2019). *Wong's nursing care of infants and children* (11th ed.). Elsevier.
Perry, S. E., Hockenberry, M. J., Lowdermilk, D. J., Wilson, D., Cashion, K., Rodgers, C. C., & Alden, K. R. (2018). *Maternal child nursing care* (6th ed.). Elsevier.

Child Development: 12 Months   0103

Definition: Milestones of physical, cognitive, and psychosocial progression by 12 months of age

OUTCOME TARGET RATING: Maintain at_____ Increase to_____

		Never Demonstrated	Rarely Demonstrated	Sometimes Demonstrated	Often Demonstrated	Consistently Demonstrated	
OUTCOME OVERALL RATING		1	2	3	4	5	
Indicators:							
010316	Birth weight tripled	1	2	3	4	5	NA
010317	Equal head and chest circumference	1	2	3	4	5	NA
010301	Pulls to stand	1	2	3	4	5	NA
010302	Cruises around furniture	1	2	3	4	5	NA
010318	Walks with one hand held	1	2	3	4	5	NA
010319	Sits from standing position	1	2	3	4	5	NA
010303	Attempts to take steps alone	1	2	3	4	5	NA
010304	Precise pincer grasp	1	2	3	4	5	NA
010305	Points with index fingers	1	2	3	4	5	NA
010306	Bangs blocks together	1	2	3	4	5	NA
010320	Follow rapidly moving object	1	2	3	4	5	NA
010307	Drinks from cup	1	2	3	4	5	NA
010308	Feeds self finger foods	1	2	3	4	5	NA
010309	Feeds self with spoon	1	2	3	4	5	NA
010321	Turns pages in a book, many at a time	1	2	3	4	5	NA
010310	Uses vocabulary of one to three words in addition to mama, dada	1	2	3	4	5	NA
010322	Recognizes objects by name	1	2	3	4	5	NA

Child Development: 12 Months—cont'd

		Never Demonstrated	Rarely Demonstrated	Sometimes Demonstrated	Often Demonstrated	Consistently Demonstrated	
010311	Imitates vocalizations	1	2	3	4	5	NA
010312	Looks for dropped or hidden object	1	2	3	4	5	NA
010323	Puts out arm or leg to help with dressing	1	2	3	4	5	NA
010324	Responds to simple spoken requests	1	2	3	4	5	NA
010325	Puts things in a container	1	2	3	4	5	NA
010326	Takes things out of a container	1	2	3	4	5	NA
010327	Looks at the right picture or thing when it is named	1	2	3	4	5	NA
010313	Plays social games	1	2	3	4	5	NA
010314	Waves bye-bye	1	2	3	4	5	NA

Domain-*Functional Health (I)*   **Class**-*Growth & Development (B)*   *1st edition 1997; revised 2004, 2024*

OUTCOME CONTENT REFERENCES:
Center for Disease Control and Prevention. (2021, January 22). *CDC's Developmental Milestones.* https://www.cdc.gov/ncbddd/actearly/milestones/index.html
Hagan, J. F., Shaw, J. S., & Duncan, P. M. (Eds.). (2017). *Bright futures: Guidelines for health supervision of infants, children and adolescents* (4th ed.). American Academy of Pediatrics.
Hockenberry, M. J., Rodgers, C. C., & Wilson, D. (Eds.). (2022). *Wong's essentials of pediatric nursing* (11th ed.). Elsevier.
Perry, S. E., Hockenberry, M. J., Lowdermilk, D. J., Wilson, D., Cashion, K., Rodgers, C. C., & Alden, K. R. (2018). *Maternal child nursing care* (6th ed.). Elsevier.

Child Development: 18 Months   0126

Definition: Milestones of physical, cognitive, and psychosocial progression by 18 months of age

OUTCOME TARGET RATING: Maintain at_____ Increase to_____

		Never Demonstrated	Rarely Demonstrated	Sometimes Demonstrated	Often Demonstrated	Consistently Demonstrated	
OUTCOME OVERALL RATING		1	2	3	4	5	
Indicators:							
012601	Runs clumsily with frequent falls	1	2	3	4	5	NA
012602	Walks upstairs with hand held	1	2	3	4	5	NA
012603	Pulls and pushes toys	1	2	3	4	5	NA
012604	Jumps in place with both feet	1	2	3	4	5	NA
012605	Positions self on chair	1	2	3	4	5	NA
012606	Throws ball overhand without falling	1	2	3	4	5	NA
012607	Builds tower of 3 or 4 cubes	1	2	3	4	5	NA
012608	Turns 2 or 3 pages in a book at a time	1	2	3	4	5	NA
012609	Uses spoon without rotation	1	2	3	4	5	NA
012610	Drinks from a cup	1	2	3	4	5	NA
012611	Says 10 or more words	1	2	3	4	5	NA
012612	Points to common objects	1	2	3	4	5	NA
012613	Combines gestures and words	1	2	3	4	5	NA
012614	Scribbles on own	1	2	3	4	5	NA
012615	Imitates others	1	2	3	4	5	NA
012616	Takes off gloves, socks, and shoes	1	2	3	4	5	NA
012617	Unzips zippers	1	2	3	4	5	NA
012618	Exhibits temper tantrums	1	2	3	4	5	NA
012619	Identifies items as "mine"	1	2	3	4	5	NA
012620	Develops dependency on a blanket or toy	1	2	3	4	5	NA
012621	Likes to hand things to others as play	1	2	3	4	5	NA

Continued

Child Development: 18 Months—cont'd

		Never Demonstrated	Rarely Demonstrated	Sometimes Demonstrated	Often Demonstrated	Consistently Demonstrated	
012622	Plays simple pretend games, such as feeding a doll	1	2	3	4	5	NA
012623	Clings to parents in new situations	1	2	3	4	5	NA
012624	Explores alone with parent close by	1	2	3	4	5	NA
012625	Follows 1-step verbal commands	1	2	3	4	5	NA
012626	Shows affection to familiar people	1	2	3	4	5	NA

Domain-Functional Health (I)   **Class**-Growth & Development (B)   7th edition 2024

OUTCOME CONTENT REFERENCES:

Center for Disease Control and Prevention. (2021, January 22). *CDC's Developmental Milestones.* https://www.cdc.gov/ncbddd/actearly/milestones/index.html

Hagan, J. F., Shaw, J. S., & Duncan, P. M. (Eds.). (2017). *Bright futures: Guidelines for health supervision of infants, children and adolescents* (4th ed.). American Academy of Pediatrics.

Hockenberry, M. J., Wilson, D., & Rodgers, C. C. (Eds.). (2019). *Wong's nursing care of infants and children* (11th ed.). Elsevier.

Perry, S. E., Hockenberry, M. J., Lowdermilk, D. J., Wilson, D., Cashion, K., Rodgers, C. C., & Alden, K. R. (2018). *Maternal Child Nursing Care* (6th ed.). Elsevier.

+Provost, B., Crowe, T. K., & McClain, C. (2000). Concurrent validity of the Bayley Scales of Infant Development II Motor Scale and the Peabody Developmental Motor Scales in two-year-old children. *Physical & Occupational Therapy in Pediatrics, 20*(1), 5–18. https://doi.org/10.1080/J006v20n01_02

Child Development: 2 Years   0104

Definition: Milestones of physical, cognitive, and psychosocial progression by 2 years of age

OUTCOME TARGET RATING: Maintain at_____ Increase to_____

		Never Demonstrated	Rarely Demonstrated	Sometimes Demonstrated	Often Demonstrated	Consistently Demonstrated	
OUTCOME OVERALL RATING		**1**	**2**	**3**	**4**	**5**	
Indicators:							
010401	Walks quickly	1	2	3	4	5	NA
010402	Stoops well	1	2	3	4	5	NA
010403	Walks up and down stairs one step at a time	1	2	3	4	5	NA
010404	Walks backward	1	2	3	4	5	NA
010405	Kicks a ball	1	2	3	4	5	NA
010406	Throws a ball	1	2	3	4	5	NA
010419	Runs fairly well using wide stance	1	2	3	4	5	NA
010420	Stands on tiptoe	1	2	3	4	5	NA
010421	Climbs onto and down from furniture without help	1	2	3	4	5	NA
010422	Picks up object without falling	1	2	3	4	5	NA
010407	Makes circular and horizontal strokes with crayon	1	2	3	4	5	NA
010408	Stacks five to six blocks	1	2	3	4	5	NA
010423	Turns door knob	1	2	3	4	5	NA
010424	Unscrews lids	1	2	3	4	5	NA
010425	Feeds self with spoon	1	2	3	4	5	NA
010410	Follows two-step commands	1	2	3	4	5	NA
010411	Indicates wants verbally	1	2	3	4	5	NA
010412	Uses phrases of two to three words	1	2	3	4	5	NA
010413	Listens to story looking at pictures	1	2	3	4	5	NA
010426	Turns pages of book one at a time	1	2	3	4	5	NA
010414	Points to some body parts	1	2	3	4	5	NA

C

Child Development: 2 Years—cont'd

		Never Demonstrated	Rarely Demonstrated	Sometimes Demonstrated	Often Demonstrated	Consistently Demonstrated	
010415	Begins parallel play	1	2	3	4	5	NA
010427	Verbalizes needs for toileting	1	2	3	4	5	NA
010428	Verbalizes needs for food or drink	1	2	3	4	5	NA
010416	Imitates adults	1	2	3	4	5	NA
010417	Interacts with adults in simple games	1	2	3	4	5	NA
010429	Has sustained attention span	1	2	3	4	5	NA
010430	Dresses self in simple clothing	1	2	3	4	5	NA
010431	Increased independence from parent	1	2	3	4	5	NA
010432	Shows defiant behavior	1	2	3	4	5	NA

Domain-*Functional Health (I)*   **Class**-*Growth & Development (B)*   *1st edition 1997; revised 2004, 2024*

OUTCOME CONTENT REFERENCES:
Center for Disease Control and Prevention. (2021, January 22). *CDC's Developmental Milestones.* https://www.cdc.gov/ncbddd/actearly/milestones/index.html
Hagan, J. F., Shaw, J. S., & Duncan, P. M. (Eds.). (2017). *Bright futures: Guidelines for health supervision of infants, children and adolescents* (4th ed.). American Academy of Pediatrics.
Hockenberry, M. J., Rodgers, C. C., & Wilson, D. (Eds.). (2022). *Wong's essentials of pediatric nursing* (11th ed.). Elsevier.
Perry, S. E., Hockenberry, M. J., Lowdermilk, D. J., Wilson, D., Cashion, K., Rodgers, C. C., & Alden, K. R. (2018). *Maternal child nursing care* (6th ed.). Elsevier.

Child Development: 3 Years   0105

Definition: Milestones of physical, cognitive, and psychosocial progression by 3 years of age

OUTCOME TARGET RATING: Maintain at_____ Increase to_____

		Never Demonstrated	Rarely Demonstrated	Sometimes Demonstrated	Often Demonstrated	Consistently Demonstrated	
OUTCOME OVERALL RATING		1	2	3	4	5	
Indicators:							
010501	Balances on one foot	1	2	3	4	5	NA
010502	Pedals a riding toy	1	2	3	4	5	NA
010518	Climbs stairs using alternate feet	1	2	3	4	5	NA
010519	Jumps off bottom step	1	2	3	4	5	NA
010520	Broad jumps	1	2	3	4	5	NA
010521	Tries to dance but loses balance	1	2	3	4	5	NA
010522	Looks to see if anyone is watching	1	2	3	4	5	NA
010503	Dresses self	1	2	3	4	5	NA
010523	Pulls on shoes	1	2	3	4	5	NA
010524	Feeds self	1	2	3	4	5	NA
010525	Prepares simple meal such as cereal and milk	1	2	3	4	5	NA
010526	Helps set the table	1	2	3	4	5	NA
010527	Follows easy commands	1	2	3	4	5	NA
010528	Builds a tower of 9 to 10 cubes	1	2	3	4	5	NA
010504	Manipulates writing/coloring instruments	1	2	3	4	5	NA
010505	Copies a circle	1	2	3	4	5	NA
010506	Copies a cross	1	2	3	4	5	NA
010529	Makes circles with facial features						
010507	Controls bowel in daytime	1	2	3	4	5	NA
010508	Controls bladder in daytime	1	2	3	4	5	NA

Continued

C

Child Development: 3 Years—cont'd

		Never Demonstrated	Rarely Demonstrated	Sometimes Demonstrated	Often Demonstrated	Consistently Demonstrated	
010509	Distinguishes gender differences	1	2	3	4	5	NA
010530	Boys identify with father	1	2	3	4	5	NA
010531	Attempts to please parents	1	2	3	4	5	NA
010532	Aware of family relationships	1	2	3	4	5	NA
010533	Less jealous of siblings	1	2	3	4	5	NA
010534	Separates from parents easily	1	2	3	4	5	NA
010510	Gives own first name	1	2	3	4	5	NA
010511	Gives own age	1	2	3	4	5	NA
010512	Engages in magical thinking/fantasy	1	2	3	4	5	NA
010513	Plays interactive games with peers	1	2	3	4	5	NA
010535	Plays in parallel with others	1	2	3	4	5	NA
010536	Learns simple games	1	2	3	4	5	NA
010514	Begins cooperative group play	1	2	3	4	5	NA
010515	Uses sentences of three or four words	1	2	3	4	5	NA
010537	Asks many questions	1	2	3	4	5	NA
010538	Talks about past and present	1	2	3	4	5	NA
010516	Speech understood by strangers	1	2	3	4	5	NA

Domain-*Functional Health (I)*   **Class**-*Growth & Development (B)*   *1st edition 1997; revised 2004, 2024*

OUTCOME CONTENT REFERENCES:
Center for Disease Control and Prevention. (2021, January 22). *CDC's Developmental Milestones*. https://www.cdc.gov/ncbddd/actearly/milestones/index.html
Hagan, J. F., Shaw, J. S., & Duncan, P. M. (Eds.). (2017). *Bright futures: Guidelines for health supervision of infants, children and adolescents* (4th ed.). American Academy of Pediatrics.
Hockenberry, M. J., Rodgers, C. C., & Wilson, D. (Eds.). (2022). *Wong's essentials of pediatric nursing* (11th ed.). Elsevier.
Perry, S. E., Hockenberry, M. J., Lowdermilk, D. J., Wilson, D., Cashion, K., Rodgers, C. C., & Alden, K. R. (2018). *Maternal child nursing care* (6th ed.). Elsevier.

Child Development: 4 Years   0106

Definition: Milestones of physical, cognitive, and psychosocial progression by 4 years of age

OUTCOME TARGET RATING: Maintain at_____ Increase to_____

		Never Demonstrated	Rarely Demonstrated	Sometimes Demonstrated	Often Demonstrated	Consistently Demonstrated	
OUTCOME OVERALL RATING		1	2	3	4	5	
Indicators:							
010601	Walks, climbs, runs	1	2	3	4	5	NA
010617	Walks up and down stairs using alternative foot	1	2	3	4	5	NA
010603	Hops and jumps on one foot	1	2	3	4	5	NA
010604	Rides tricycle or bicycle with training wheels	1	2	3	4	5	NA
010605	Throws overhand ball	1	2	3	4	5	NA
010606	Builds tower of 10 blocks	1	2	3	4	5	NA
010618	Begins to copy some capital letters	1	2	3	4	5	NA
010607	Draws person with three parts	1	2	3	4	5	NA
010619	Uses scissors to cut out picture	1	2	3	4	5	NA
010620	Laces shoes	1	2	3	4	5	NA
010608	Gives first and last name	1	2	3	4	5	NA
010609	Uses sentences of four to five words, short paragraphs	1	2	3	4	5	NA

Child Development: 4 Years—cont'd

		Never Demonstrated	Rarely Demonstrated	Sometimes Demonstrated	Often Demonstrated	Consistently Demonstrated	
010610	Uses past tense in vocabulary	1	2	3	4	5	NA
010621	Names one or more colors	1	2	3	4	5	NA
010622	Understands the idea of counting	1	2	3	4	5	NA
010611	Describes a recent experience	1	2	3	4	5	NA
010612	Sings a song	1	2	3	4	5	NA
010613	Distinguishes fantasy from reality	1	2	3	4	5	NA
010614	Describes use of common home items	1	2	3	4	5	NA
010616	Engages in creative play	1	2	3	4	5	NA
010623	Plays board or card games	1	2	3	4	5	NA
010624	Protects possessions	1	2	3	4	5	NA
010625	Has an imaginary playmate	1	2	3	4	5	NA
010626	Prefers playing with other children	1	2	3	4	5	NA
010627	Understands sequence of daily events	1	2	3	4	5	NA
010628	Does simple errands	1	2	3	4	5	NA

Domain-Functional Health (I)   *Class*-Growth & Development (B)   *1st edition 1997; revised 2004, 2024*

OUTCOME CONTENT REFERENCES:

Center for Disease Control and Prevention. (2021, January 22). *CDC's Developmental Milestones*. https://www.cdc.gov/ncbddd/actearly/milestones/index.html
Hagan, J. F., Shaw, J. S., & Duncan, P. M. (Eds.). (2017). *Bright futures: Guidelines for health supervision of infants, children and adolescents* (4th ed.). American Academy of Pediatrics.
Hockenberry, M. J., Rodgers, C. C., & Wilson, D. (Eds.). (2022). *Wong's essentials of pediatric nursing* (11th ed.). Elsevier.
Perry, S. E., Hockenberry, M. J., Lowdermilk, D. J., Wilson, D., Cashion, K., Rodgers, C. C., & Alden, K. R. (2018). *Maternal child nursing care* (6th ed.). Elsevier.

Child Development: 5 Years   0107

Definition: Milestones of physical, cognitive, and psychosocial progression by 5 years of age

OUTCOME TARGET RATING: Maintain at_____ Increase to_____

		Never Demonstrated	Rarely Demonstrated	Sometimes Demonstrated	Often Demonstrated	Consistently Demonstrated	
OUTCOME OVERALL RATING		1	2	3	4	5	
Indicators:							
010717	Walks	1	2	3	4	5	NA
010718	Climbs	1	2	3	4	5	NA
010719	Runs	1	2	3	4	5	NA
010702	Skips	1	2	3	4	5	NA
010720	Balances on alternate feet with eyes closed	1	2	3	4		NA
010721	Throws and catches a ball well	1	2	3	4	5	NA
010722	Does a somersault	1	2	3	4	5	NA
010703	Dresses self without assistance	1	2	3	4	5	NA
010723	Ties shoelaces	1	2	3	4	5	NA
010724	Dominant hand is established	1	2	3	4	5	NA
010725	Uses a fork and spoon	1	2	3	4	5	NA
010704	Draws a person with head, body, arms, and legs	1	2	3	4	5	NA
010705	Copies a triangle or square	1	2	3	4	5	NA
010706	Counts using fingers	1	2	3	4	5	NA
010707	Recognizes most letters of alphabet	1	2	3	4	5	NA

Continued

Child Development: 5 Years—cont'd

		Never Demonstrated	Rarely Demonstrated	Sometimes Demonstrated	Often Demonstrated	Consistently Demonstrated	
010726	Names coins						
010708	Prints some letters	1	2	3	4	5	NA
010709	Uses complete sentence of five words	1	2	3	4	5	NA
010710	Uses future tense in vocabulary	1	2	3	4	5	NA
010711	Speaks short paragraphs	1	2	3	4	5	NA
010712	Gives own address	1	2	3	4	5	NA
010727	Knows the days of the week	1	2	3	4	5	NA
010713	Gives own phone number	1	2	3	4	5	NA
010714	Follows simple rules of interactive games with peers	1	2	3	4	5	NA
010716	Engages in creative play	1	2	3	4	5	NA
010728	Eruption of permanent teeth	1	2	3	4	5	NA
010729	Eager to do things right	1	2	3	4	5	NA
010730	Tries to live by the rules	1	2	3	4	5	NA
010731	Questions what parents think by comparing to other adults	1	2	3	4	5	NA
010732	Strongly identifies with parent of same sex	1	2	3	4	5	NA
010733	Shows more independence	1	2	3	4	5	NA
010734	Uses toilet on own	1	2	3	4	5	NA

Domain-Functional Health (I)   **Class**-Growth & Development (B)   1st edition 1997; revised 2004, 2008, 2024

OUTCOME CONTENT REFERENCES:

Center for Disease Control and Prevention. (2021, January 22). *CDC's Developmental Milestones.* https://www.cdc.gov/ncbddd/actearly/milestones/index.html

Hagan, J. F., Shaw, J. S., & Duncan, P. M. (Eds.). (2017). *Bright futures: Guidelines for health supervision of infants, children and adolescents* (4th ed.). American Academy of Pediatrics.

Hockenberry, M. J., Rodgers, C. C., & Wilson, D. (Eds.). (2022). *Wong's essentials of pediatric nursing* (11th ed.). Elsevier.

Perry, S. E., Hockenberry, M. J., Lowdermilk, D. J., Wilson, D., Cashion, K., Rodgers, C. C., & Alden, K. R. (2018). *Maternal child nursing care* (6th ed.). Elsevier.

Child Development: 6–7 Years   0127

Definition: Milestones of physical, cognitive, and psychosocial progression by 6 through 7 years of age

OUTCOME TARGET RATING: Maintain at_____ Increase to_____

		Never Demonstrated	Rarely Demonstrated	Sometimes Demonstrated	Often Demonstrated	Consistently Demonstrated	
OUTCOME OVERALL RATING		1	2	3	4	5	
Indicators:							
012701	Loses first teeth	1	2	3	4	5	NA
012702	Central mandibular incisors erupt	1	2	3	4	5	NA
012703	Gradual increase in dexterity	1	2	3	4	5	NA
012704	Enjoys drawing	1	2	3	4	5	NA
012705	Develops concepts of numbers	1	2	3	4	5	NA
012706	Repeats activities for mastery	1	2	3	4	5	NA
012707	Can count 13 pennies	1	2	3	4	5	NA
012708	Repeats 3 numbers backwards	1	2	3	4	5	NA
012709	Can copy a diamond	1	2	3	4	5	NA
012710	Distinguishes morning from afternoon	1	2	3	4	5	NA
012711	Defines use of common objects	1	2	3	4	5	NA
012712	Notices missing items from a picture	1	2	3	4	5	NA
012713	Obeys triple commands in sequence	1	2	3	4	5	NA
012714	Knows right from left hands	1	2	3	4	5	NA

Child Development: 6–7 Years—cont'd

		Never Demonstrated	Rarely Demonstrated	Sometimes Demonstrated	Often Demonstrated	Consistently Demonstrated	
012715	Takes bath without supervision	1	2	3	4	5	NA
012716	Brushes or combs hair	1	2	3	4	5	NA
012717	Performs nighttime routine alone	1	2	3	4	5	NA
012718	Enjoys board and simple card games	1	2	3	4	5	NA
012719	May cheat to win	1	2	3	4	5	NA
012720	Tries new activities to define abilities	1	2	3	4	5	NA
012721	Enjoys play with children of same age	1	2	3	4	5	NA
012722	Shares with others	1	2	3	4	5	NA
012723	Understands right and wrong	1	2	3	4	5	NA
012724	Has own way of doing things	1	2	3	4	5	NA
012725	Enjoys time alone	1	2	3	4	5	NA
012726	Follows safety rules	1	2	3	4	5	NA
012727	Expresses feelings	1	2	3	4	5	NA
012728	Practices good health habits	1	2	3	4	5	NA
012729	Performs in school to level of ability	1	2	3	4	5	NA

Domain-Functional Health (I)   *Class*-Growth & Development (B)   7th edition 2024

OUTCOME CONTENT REFERENCES:

Hagan, J. F., Shaw, J. S., & Duncan, P. M. (Eds.). (2017). *Bright futures: Guidelines for health supervision of infants, children and adolescents* (4th ed.). American Academy of Pediatrics.
Hockenberry, M. J., Wilson, D., & Rodgers, C. C. (Eds.). (2019). *Wong's nursing care of infants and children* (11th ed.). Elsevier.
Perry, S. E., Hockenberry, M. J., Lowdermilk, D. J., Wilson, D., Cashion, K., Rodgers, C. C., & Alden, K. R. (2018). *Maternal child nursing care* (6th ed.). Elsevier.

Child Development: 8–10 Years   0128

Definition: Milestones of physical, cognitive, and psychosocial progression by 8 through 10 years of age

OUTCOME TARGET RATING: Maintain at_____ Increase to_____

		Never Demonstrated	Rarely Demonstrated	Sometimes Demonstrated	Often Demonstrated	Consistently Demonstrated	
OUTCOME OVERALL RATING		1	2	3	4	5	
Indicators:							
012801	Always on the go	1	2	3	4	5	NA
012802	Bones grow faster than ligaments	1	2	3	4	5	NA
012803	Provides similarities and differences between 2 things from memory	1	2	3	4	5	NA
012804	Understands the concept of reversibility	1	2	3	4	5	NA
012805	Knows the date	1	2	3	4	5	NA
012806	Repeats days of the week in order	1	2	3	4	5	NA
012807	Repeats months of the year in order	1	2	3	4	5	NA
012808	Describes common items in detail	1	2	3	4	5	NA
012809	Makes change for a quarter	1	2	3	4	5	NA
012810	Enjoys reading books and comics	1	2	3	4	5	NA
012811	More aware of time	1	2	3	4	5	NA
012812	Can grasp concept of fractions	1	2	3	4	5	NA
012813	Understands concepts of space	1	2	3	4	5	NA
012814	Understands cause and effect	1	2	3	4	5	NA
012815	Understands conservation	1	2	3	4	5	NA
012816	Classifies objects by more than one characteristic	1	2	3	4	5	NA

Continued

Child Development: 8–10 Years—cont'd

		Never Demonstrated	Rarely Demonstrated	Sometimes Demonstrated	Often Demonstrated	Consistently Demonstrated	
012817	Produces simple paintings or drawings	1	2	3	4	5	NA
012818	Uses common tools	1	2	3	4	5	NA
012819	Uses household utensils	1	2	3	4	5	NA
012820	Responsible for household chores	1	2	3	4	5	NA
012821	Takes music or sport lessons	1	2	3	4	5	NA
012822	Plays computer and video games	1	2	3	4	5	NA
012823	Likes to compete in sports or games	1	2	3	4	5	NA
012824	Gets along with family members	1	2	3	4	5	NA
012825	Is critical of self	1	2	3	4	5	NA
012826	Compares self to others	1	2	3	4	5	NA
012827	Develops close friendships	1	2	3	4	5	NA
012828	Identifies with the same-sex peers	1	2	3	4	5	NA
012829	Displays self confidence	1	2	3	4	5	NA
012830	Likes reward systems	1	2	3	4	5	NA
012831	Understands right from wrong	1	2	3	4	5	NA
012832	Assumes responsibility for homework	1	2	3	4	5	NA
012833	Performs in school to level of ability	1	2	3	4	5	NA

Domain-Functional Health (I)   **Class**-Growth & Development (B)   7th edition 2024

OUTCOME CONTENT REFERENCES:

Hagan, J. F., Shaw, J. S., & Duncan, P. M. (Eds.). (2017). *Bright futures: Guidelines for health supervision of infants, children and adolescents* (4th ed.). American Academy of Pediatrics.

Hockenberry, M. J., Wilson, D., & Rodgers, C. C. (Eds.). (2019). *Wong's nursing care of infants and children* (11th ed.). Elsevier.

Perry, S. E., Hockenberry, M. J., Lowdermilk, D. J., Wilson, D., Cashion, K., Rodgers, C. C., & Alden, K. R. (2018). *Maternal child nursing care* (6th ed.). Elsevier.

Child Development: Early Adolescence   0129

Definition: Milestones of physical, cognitive, and psychosocial progression from 11 years through 14 years of age

OUTCOME TARGET RATING: Maintain at_____ Increase to_____

		Never Demonstrated	Rarely Demonstrated	Sometimes Demonstrated	Often Demonstrated	Consistently Demonstrated	
OUTCOME OVERALL RATING		1	2	3	4	5	
Indicators:							
012901	Experiences accelerating growth spurt	1	2	3	4	5	NA
012902	Preoccupied with rapid body changes	1	2	3	4	5	NA
012903	Displays ability for abstract thinking	1	2	3	4	5	NA
012904	Thinks concretely with little middle ground	1	2	3	4	5	NA
012905	Asks questions	1	2	3	4	5	NA
012906	Expresses interests and curiosity in everyday things	1	2	3	4	5	NA
012907	Develops new values	1	2	3	4	5	NA
012908	Seeks peer relationships with same sex peers	1	2	3	4	5	NA
012909	Compares self with same sex peers	1	2	3	4	5	NA
012910	Measures physical attractiveness by acceptance or rejection by peers	1	2	3	4	5	NA
012911	Struggles for recognition with peers	1	2	3	4	5	NA

C

Child Development: Early Adolescence—cont'd

		Never Demonstrated	Rarely Demonstrated	Sometimes Demonstrated	Often Demonstrated	Consistently Demonstrated	
012912	Conforms to group norms	1	2	3	4	5	NA
012913	Tries out various roles	1	2	3	4	5	NA
012914	Defines independence-dependence boundaries	1	2	3	4	5	NA
012915	Remains dependent on parents while trying to detach	1	2	3	4	5	NA
012916	Displays no major conflicts with parental control	1	2	3	4	5	NA
012917	Accepts reasonable rules	1	2	3	4	5	NA
012918	Uses effective social interaction skills	1	2	3	4	5	NA
012919	Uses effective coping strategies	1	2	3	4	5	NA
012920	Discusses feelings of distress with supportive adult	1	2	3	4	5	NA
012921	Performs in school to level of ability	1	2	3	4	5	NA
012922	Participates in extracurricular school activities	1	2	3	4	5	NA
012923	Expressed anger through moodiness, temper outbursts, and verbal insults	1	2	3	4	5	NA
012924	Observes rules	1	2	3	4	5	NA
012925	Obeys laws	1	2	3	4	5	NA
012926	Exhibits self-esteem	1	2	3	4	5	NA
012927	Experiences intense daydreaming	1	2	3	4	5	NA
012928	Participates in limited dating, usually in groups	1	2	3	4	5	NA

Domain-*Functional Health (I)*   **Class**-*Growth & Development (B)*   7th edition 2024

OUTCOME CONTENT REFERENCES:

Allen, B., & Waterman, H. (2019). Stages of adolescence. https://www.healthychildren.org/English/ages-stages/teen/Pages/Stages-of-Adolescence.aspx
Hagan, J. F., Shaw, J. S., & Duncan, P. M. (Eds.). (2017). *Bright futures: Guidelines for health supervision of infants, children and adolescents* (4th ed.). American Academy of Pediatrics.
Hockenberry, M. J., Wilson, D., & Rodgers, C. C. (Eds.). (2019). *Wong's nursing care of infants and children* (11th ed.). Elsevier.
Ralph, A. (2018). Parenting of adolescents and emerging adults. In Sanders, M. R., & Morawska, A. (Eds.), *Handbook of parenting and child development across the lifespan* (pp. 631–652). Springer International. https://doi.org/10.1007/978-3-319-94598-9_28

Child Development: Late Adolescence   **0130**

Definition: Milestones of physical, cognitive, and psychosocial progression from 18 years through 20 years of age

OUTCOME TARGET RATING: Maintain at_____ Increase to_____

		Never Demonstrated	Rarely Demonstrated	Sometimes Demonstrated	Often Demonstrated	Consistently Demonstrated	
OUTCOME OVERALL RATING		1	2	3	4	5	
Indicators:							
013001	Expresses abstract thoughts	1	2	3	4	5	NA
013002	Acts on long-range choices	1	2	3	4	5	NA
013003	Develops negotiating skills	1	2	3	4	5	NA
013004	Views problems comprehensively	1	2	3	4	5	NA
013005	Displays ability to compromise	1	2	3	4	5	NA
013006	Prepares for chosen career or job	1	2	3	4	5	NA
013007	Expresses a positive body image	1	2	3	4	5	NA

Continued

Child Development: Early Adolescence—cont'd

		Never Demonstrated	Rarely Demonstrated	Sometimes Demonstrated	Often Demonstrated	Consistently Demonstrated	
013008	Expresses positive self-esteem	1	2	3	4	5	NA
013009	Defines social roles	1	2	3	4	5	NA
013010	Establishes independence from family	1	2	3	4	5	NA
013011	Feels emancipated from parents	1	2	3	4	5	NA
013012	Develops individual friendships	1	2	3	4	5	NA
013013	Recognizes feelings of others						
013014	Tests romantic relationships	1	2	3	4	5	NA
013015	Builds personal relationships by giving and sharing with others	1	2	3	4	5	NA
013016	Dates as a romantic couple	1	2	3	4	5	NA
013017	Publicly identifies as heterosexual, gay, lesbian, or bisexual	1	2	3	4	5	NA
013018	Combines intimacy with commitment	1	2	3	4	5	NA
013019	Expresses emotional self-regulation skills	1	2	3	4	5	NA
013020	Describes peer group influence as less important in decision-making	1	2	3	4	5	NA
013021	Judges risk and rewards of actions	1	2	3	4	5	NA
013022	Makes decisions and accepts consequences	1	2	3	4	5	NA
013023	Establishes adult relationship with parents	1	2	3	4	5	NA

Domain-*Functional Health (I)*   **Class**-*Growth & Development (B)*   *7th edition 2024*

OUTCOME CONTENT REFERENCES:

Hagan, J. F., Shaw, J. S., & Duncan, P. M. (Eds.). (2017). *Bright futures: Guidelines for health supervision of infants, children and adolescents* (4th ed.). American Academy of Pediatrics.
Hockenberry, M. J., Wilson, D., & Rodgers, C. C. (Eds.). (2019). *Wong's nursing care of infants and children* (11th ed.). Elsevier.
Ralph, A. (2018). Parenting of adolescents and emerging adults. In Sanders, M. R., & Morawska, A. (Eds.), *Handbook of parenting and child development across the lifespan* (pp. 631–652). Springer International. https://doi.org/10.1007/978-3-319-94598-9_28

Child Development: Middle Adolescence 0131

Definition: Milestones of physical, cognitive, and psychosocial progression from 15 years through 17 years of age

OUTCOME TARGET RATING: Maintain at_____ Increase to_____

		Never Demonstrated	Rarely Demonstrated	Sometimes Demonstrated	Often Demonstrated	Consistently Demonstrated	
OUTCOME OVERALL RATING		1	2	3	4	5	
Indicators:							
013101	Uses effective social interaction skills	1	2	3	4	5	NA
013102	Uses conflict resolution strategies	1	2	3	4	5	NA
013103	Vents negative feelings in a non-destructive manner	1	2	3	4	5	NA
013104	Maintains good peer relationships with same gender	1	2	3	4	5	NA
013105	Maintains good peer relationships with opposite gender	1	2	3	4	5	NA

Child Development: Middle Adolescence—cont'd

		Never Demonstrated	Rarely Demonstrated	Sometimes Demonstrated	Often Demonstrated	Consistently Demonstrated	
013106	Behavioral standards set by peer group	1	2	3	4	5	NA
013107	Respects others	1	2	3	4	5	NA
013108	Uses effective coping strategies	1	2	3	4	5	NA
013109	Discusses feelings of distress with supportive adult	1	2	3	4	5	NA
013110	Displays increasing levels of autonomy	1	2	3	4	5	NA
013111	Major conflicts over independence and control with parents	1	2	3	4	5	NA
013112	Describes personal value system	1	2	3	4	5	NA
013113	Perceives future implications of current behavior	1	2	3	4	5	NA
013114	Uses formal operational thinking	1	2	3	4	5	NA
013115	Uses abstract thinking	1	2	3	4	5	NA
013116	Shows concern for philosophic, political, and social issues	1	2	3	4	5	NA
013117	Idealistic	1	2	3	4	5	NA
013118	Sets academic goals	1	2	3	4	5	NA
013119	Performs in school to level of ability	1	2	3	4	5	NA
013120	Participates in extracurricular school activities	1	2	3	4	5	NA
013121	Performs in work to level of ability	1	2	3	4	5	NA
013122	Spends time on phone or texting friends	1	2	3	4	5	NA
013123	Tries out various roles	1	2	3	4	5	NA
013124	Identifies occupational goals	1	2	3	4	5	NA
013125	Observes rules	1	2	3	4	5	NA
013126	Obeys laws	1	2	3	4	5	NA
013127	Balances self-esteem with feelings of inadequacy	1	2	3	4	5	NA
013128	Shows capacity for intimacy	1	2	3	4	5	NA
013129	Secondary sexual characteristics well advanced	1	2	3	4	5	NA
013130	Internal identification of heterosexual, homosexual or bisexual attractions	1	2	3	4	5	NA
013131	Modified body image	1	2	3	4	5	NA
013132	Expresses comfort with own sexual identity	1	2	3	4	5	NA
013133	Evaluates ability to attract opposite sex	1	2	3	4	5	NA
013134	Expresses feeling of being "in love"	1	2	3	4	5	NA
013135	Multiple plural relationships						
013136	Postpones sexual activity	1	2	3	4	5	NA
013137	Practices good health habits	1	2	3	4	5	NA

Domain-Functional Health (I)   **Class**-Growth & Development (B)   7th edition 2024

OUTCOME CONTENT REFERENCES:

Center for Disease Control and Prevention. (2021, February 22). Teenagers (15–17 years of age).
   https://www.cdc.gov/ncbddd/childdevelopment/positiveparenting/adolescence2.html
Hagan, J. F., Shaw, J. S., & Duncan, P. M. (Eds.). (2017). *Bright futures: Guidelines for health supervision of infants, children and adolescents* (4th ed.). American Academy of Pediatrics.
Hockenberry, M. J., Wilson, D., & Rodgers, C. C. (Eds.). (2019). *Wong's nursing care of infants and children* (11th ed.). Elsevier.

Childhood Bullying Recovery 1312

Definition: Personal actions to promote psychological recovery from adverse effects of childhood bullying

OUTCOME TARGET RATING: Maintain at_____ Increase to_____

		Never Demonstrated	Rarely Demonstrated	Sometimes Demonstrated	Often Demonstrated	Consistently Demonstrated	
OUTCOME OVERALL RATING		1	2	3	4	5	
Indicators:							
131201	Establishes a peer group of friends	1	2	3	4	5	NA
131202	Seeks social support	1	2	3	4	5	NA
131203	Seeks family support	1	2	3	4	5	NA
131204	Develops a safety plan	1	2	3	4	5	NA
131205	Uses effective problem-solving strategies	1	2	3	4	5	NA
131206	Uses effective self-defense strategies	1	2	3	4	5	NA
131207	Participates in activities to build self-esteem	1	2	3	4	5	NA
131208	Participates in activities to build confidence	1	2	3	4	5	NA
131209	Participates in social skill development	1	2	3	4	5	NA
131210	Attends peer group activities	1	2	3	4	5	NA
131211	Participates in structured activities	1	2	3	4	5	NA
131212	Obtains counseling	1	2	3	4	5	NA
131213	Obtains assistance to control anxiety	1	2	3	4	5	NA
131214	Monitors mood	1	2	3	4	5	NA
131215	Eliminates tobacco use	1	2	3	4	5	NA
131216	Refrains from alcohol misuse	1	2	3	4	5	NA
131217	Refrains from substance abuse	1	2	3	4	5	NA
131218	Uses available mental health care services	1	2	3	4	5	NA
131219	Shares suicidal ideas	1	2	3	4	5	NA
131220	Refrains from attempting suicide	1	2	3	4	5	NA
131221	Uses available support groups	1	2	3	4	5	NA
131222	Acknowledges potential to become a bully	1	2	3	4	5	NA
131223	Refrains from abusing others	1	2	3	4	5	NA

Domain-*Psychosocial Health (III)*   **Class**-*Psychosocial Adaptation (N)*   *6th edition 2018*

OUTCOME CONTENT REFERENCES:

Fink-Samnick, E. (2016). The new age of bullying and violence in health care: Part 2. *Professional Case Management, 21*(3), 114–125. https://doi.org/10.1097/NCM.0000000000000146

Hughes, M. R., Gaines, J. S., & Pryor, D. W. (2015). Staying away from school: Adolescents who miss school due to feeling unsafe. *Youth Violence and Juvenile Justice, 13*(3), 270–290. https://doi.org/10.1177/1541204014538067

Niemelä, S., Brunstein-Klomek, A., Sillanmäki, L., Helenius, H., Piha, J., Kumpulainen, K., Moilanen, I., Tamminen, T., Almqvist, F., & Sourander, A. (2011). Childhood bullying behaviors at age eight and substance use at age 18 among males. A nationwide prospective study. *Additive Behaviors, 36*(3), 256–260. https://doi.org/10.1016/j.addbeh.2010.10.012

Circulation Status   **0401**

Definition: Unobstructed, unidirectional blood flow at an appropriate pressure through large vessels of the cardiac systemic and pulmonary circuits

OUTCOME TARGET RATING: Maintain at_____ Increase to_____

		Severe Deviation from Normal Range	Substantial Deviation from Normal Range	Moderate Deviation from Normal Range	Mild Deviation from Normal Range	No Deviation from Normal Range	
OUTCOME OVERALL RATING		1	2	3	4	5	
Indicators:							
040101	Systolic blood pressure	1	2	3	4	5	NA
040102	Diastolic blood pressure	1	2	3	4	5	NA
040103	Pulse pressure	1	2	3	4	5	NA
040104	Mean arterial pressure (MAP)	1	2	3	4	5	NA
040105	Central venous pressure	1	2	3	4	5	NA
040106	Pulmonary wedge pressure	1	2	3	4	5	NA
040141	Right carotid pulse strength	1	2	3	4	5	NA
040142	Left carotid pulse strength	1	2	3	4	5	NA
040143	Right brachial pulse strength	1	2	3	4	5	NA
040144	Left brachial pulse strength	1	2	3	4	5	NA
040145	Right radial pulse strength	1	2	3	4	5	NA
040146	Left radial pulse strength	1	2	3	4	5	NA
040147	Right femoral pulse strength	1	2	3	4	5	NA
040148	Left femoral pulse strength	1	2	3	4	5	NA
040149	Right pedal pulse strength	1	2	3	4	5	NA
040150	Left pedal pulse strength	1	2	3	4	5	NA
040135	Partial pressure of oxygen in arterial blood (PaO$_2$)	1	2	3	4	5	NA
040136	Partial pressure of carbon dioxide in arterial blood (PaCO$_2$)	1	2	3	4	5	NA
040137	Oxygen saturation	1	2	3	4	5	NA
040112	Arterial-venous oxygen difference	1	2	3	4	5	NA
040140	Urine output	1	2	3	4	5	NA
040151	Capillary refill	1	2	3	4	5	NA
		Severe	Substantial	Moderate	Mild	None	
040107	Hypotension	1	2	3	4	5	NA
040163	Tachycardia	1	2	3	4	5	NA
040113	Adventitious breath sounds	1	2	3	4	5	NA
040118	Large vessel bruits	1	2	3	4	5	NA
040119	Neck vein distention	1	2	3	4	5	NA
040120	Peripheral edema	1	2	3	4	5	NA
040121	Ascites	1	2	3	4	5	NA
040123	Fatigue	1	2	3	4	5	NA
040152	Weight gain	1	2	3	4	5	NA
040153	Impaired cognition	1	2	3	4	5	NA
040154	Pallor	1	2	3	4	5	NA
040155	Dependent rubor	1	2	3	4	5	NA
040164	Mottling	1	2	3	4	5	NA
040156	Intermittent claudication	1	2	3	4	5	NA
040157	Decreased skin temperature	1	2	3	4	5	NA
040158	Paresthesia	1	2	3	4	5	NA
040159	Syncope	1	2	3	4	5	NA
040160	Pitting edema	1	2	3	4	5	NA
040161	Lower extremity ulcers	1	2	3	4	5	NA
040162	Numbness	1	2	3	4	5	NA

***Domain**-Physiologic Health (II)*   ***Class**-Cardiopulmonary (E)*   *1st edition 1997; revised 2004, 2008, 2024*

OUTCOME CONTENT REFERENCES:
Hariri, G., Joffre, J., Leblanc, G., Bonsey, M., Lavillegrand, J. R., Urbina, T., Guidet, B., Maury, E., Bakker, J., & Ait-Oufella, H. (2019). Narrative review: Clinical assessment of peripheral tissue perfusion in septic shock. *Annals of Intensive Care, 9*(1), 37. https://doi.org/10.1186/s13613-019-0511-1
Hinkle, J. L., & Cheever, K. H. (2018). *Brunner & Suddarth's textbook of medical-surgical nursing* (14th ed.). Wolter Kluwer.
Hockenberry, M. J., Rodgers, C. C., & Wilson, D. (Eds.). (2022). *Wong's essentials of pediatric nursing* (11th ed.). Elsevier.
Huether, S. E., McCance, K. L., & Brashers, V. L. (2020). *Understanding pathophysiology* (7th ed.). Elsevier.
Ignatavicius, D. D., Workman, M. L., Rebar, C. R., & Heimgartner, N. M. (2021). *Medical-surgical nursing: Concepts for interprofessional care* (10th ed.). Elsevier.
Klabunde, R. E. (2022). *Cardiovascular physiology concepts* (3rd ed.). Wolters Kluwer.

C

Client Satisfaction

3014

Definition: Extent of positive perception of care provided by nursing staff

OUTCOME TARGET RATING: Maintain at_____ Increase to_____

OUTCOME OVERALL RATING	Not at All Satisfied 1	Somewhat Satisfied 2	Moderately Satisfied 3	Very Satisfied 4	Completely Satisfied 5	
Indicators:						
301401 Access to nursing staff	1	2	3	4	5	NA
301402 Access to supplies and equipment needed for care	1	2	3	4	5	NA
301403 Knowledge and expertise of nursing staff	1	2	3	4	5	NA
301404 Competence of nursing staff to perform procedures	1	2	3	4	5	NA
301426 Pleasant relationship with staff	1	2	3	4	5	NA
301405 Protection of legal rights by nursing staff	1	2	3	4	5	NA
301406 Protection of human rights by nursing staff	1	2	3	4	5	NA
301407 Concern for the client by nursing staff	1	2	3	4	5	NA
301408 Concern for the family by nursing staff	1	2	3	4	5	NA
301409 Questions answered completely	1	2	3	4	5	NA
301427 Support in making care choices	1	2	3	4	5	NA
301410 Instruction to improve understanding of illness	1	2	3	4	5	NA
301411 Instruction to improve participation in care	1	2	3	4	5	NA
301428 Provision of needed education	1	2	3	4	5	NA
301429 Clear instructions on procedures	1	2	3	4	5	NA
301412 Integration of cultural beliefs into nursing care	1	2	3	4	5	NA
301413 Integration of values into nursing care	1	2	3	4	5	NA
301414 Assistance to achieve mobility	1	2	3	4	5	NA
301415 Assistance to achieve self-care	1	2	3	4	5	NA
301416 Assistance to cope with emotional concerns	1	2	3	4	5	NA
301417 Assistance to address spiritual needs	1	2	3	4	5	NA
301418 Relief of symptoms of illness	1	2	3	4	5	NA
301419 Care to control pain	1	2	3	4	5	NA
301420 Care to prevent harm or injury	1	2	3	4	5	NA
301421 Care to maintain body functions	1	2	3	4	5	NA
301422 Care to maintain cleanliness	1	2	3	4	5	NA
301423 Cleanliness of care environment	1	2	3	4	5	NA
301424 Coordination of care as the client moves from one care setting to another	1	2	3	4	5	NA
301430 Client included in discharge planning	1	2	3	4	5	NA
301431 Family included in discharge planning	1	2	3	4	5	NA

Domain- *Health & Life Quality (V)*   **Class-***Satisfaction with Care (EE)*   *4th edition 2008; revised 2024*

OUTCOME CONTENT REFERENCES:

DeCola, M. C., Maresca, G., D'Aleo, G., Carnazza, L., Giliberto, S., Maggio, M. G., Bramanti, A., & Calabró, R. S. (2020). Teleassistance for frail elderly people: A usability and customer satisfaction study. *Geriatric Nursing, 41*(4), 463–467. https://doi.org/10.1016/j.gerinurse.2020.01.019

DeSantis, J. P., Cintulova, M., Provencio-Vasquez, E., Rodriguez, A. E., & Cicero, E. C. (2020). Transgender women's satisfaction with healthcare services: A mixed-methods pilot study. *Perspectives in Psychiatric Care, 56*(4), 926–938. https://doi.org/10.1111/ppc.12514

Gimenez-Diez, D., Alía, R. M., Jiménez, S. R., Granel, N., Solá, L. T., & Bernabeu-Tamayo, M. D. (2020). Treating mental health crises at home: Patient satisfaction. *Journal of Psychiatric and Mental Health Nursing, 27*(3), 246–257. https://doi.org/10.1111/jpm.12573

Kortet, S., Melender, H. A., Klemetti, R., Kääriäinen, M., & Kaakinen, P. (2021). Mothers' perceptions of the quality of maternity services at Finnish maternity units: A cross-sectional study. *Nordic Journal of Nursing Research, 41*(1), 14–24. https://doi.org/10.1177/2057158520937541

+Lee, C. F., Wang, X. F., Wong, P. N. F., Koh, Y. L. E., Ngoh, S. H. A., Mohtar, Z. M., Lian, L. G., Ang, K. W., & Tan, N. C. (2020). Psychometric evaluation of a patient satisfaction survey questionnaire to assess advanced practice nurse ambulatory services in primary care. *Journal of Nursing Management, 128*(7), 1481–1488. https://doi.org/10.1111/jonm.13072

Mazurenko, O., Collum, T., Ferdinand, A., & Menachemi, N. (2017). Predictors of hospital patient satisfaction as measured by HCAHPS: A systematic review. *Journal of Healthcare Management, 62*(4), 272–283. https://doi.org/10.1097/JHM-D-15-00050

Meier, A., Erickson, J. I., Snow, N., & Kline, M. (2019). Nurse and patient satisfaction. *The Journal of Nursing Administration, 49*(11), 520–522. https://doi.org/10.1097/NNA.0000000000000814

Räty, V., Haaranen, A., & Rissanen, T. (2019). Patients' satisfaction with child psychiatry. *Scandinavian Journal of Caring Sciences, 34*(1), 62–68. https://doi.org/10.1111/scs.12705

Stamboglis, N., & Jacobs, R. (2020). Factor associated with patient satisfaction of community mental health services: A multilevel approach. *Community Mental Health Journal, 56*(1), 50–64. https://doi.org/10.1007/s10597-019-00449-x

C

Client Satisfaction: Access to Care Resources   3000

Definition: Extent of positive perception of access to nursing staff, supplies, and equipment needed for care

OUTCOME TARGET RATING: Maintain at_____ Increase to_____

		Not at All Satisfied	Somewhat Satisfied	Moderately Satisfied	Very Satisfied	Completely Satisfied	
OUTCOME OVERALL RATING		1	2	3	4	5	
Indicators:							
300001	Availability of registered nurses	1	2	3	4	5	NA
300002	Availability of assistive staff	1	2	3	4	5	NA
300003	Availability of supplies needed for care	1	2	3	4	5	NA
300004	Availability of equipment needed for care	1	2	3	4	5	NA
300005	Informed of registered nurse and assistive staff responsible for care	1	2	3	4	5	NA
300006	Access to registered nurse responsible for care	1	2	3	4	5	NA
300016	Accessibility to services	1	2	3	4	5	NA
300007	Assistance with access to health providers	1	2	3	4	5	NA
300008	Assistance with contacting health provider	1	2	3	4	5	NA
300017	Accommodation of changing needs	1	2	3	4	5	NA
300018	Coordination of care	1	2	3	4	5	NA
300009	Coordination of health care resources	1	2	3	4	5	NA
300010	Coordination of health providers	1	2	3	4	5	NA
300014	Facilitation of appointments with health provider	1	2	3	4	5	NA
300011	Wait times for getting an appointment	1	2	3	4	5	NA
300012	Wait times to be seen at appointment	1	2	3	4	5	NA
300019	Wait times to be seen by specialist	1	2	3	4	5	NA
300015	Access to personal health record	1	2	3	4	5	NA
300013	Access to support group	1	2	3	4	5	NA

Domain- Health & Life Quality(V)   *Class*-Satisfaction with Care (EE)   *3rd edition 2004; revised 2018, 2024*

OUTCOME CONTENT REFERENCES:

Bradshaw, A., & Raphaelson, S. (2021). Improving patient satisfaction with wait times, *Nursing 2021, 51*(4), 67–69. https://doi.org/10.1097/01.NURSE.0000736968.01359.e0

Costa, D. G., Moura, G. M. S. S., Moraes, M. G., Santos, J. L. G., & Magalhães, A. M. M. (2020). Satisfaction attributes related to safety and quality perceived in the experience of hospitalized patients. *Revista Gaúcha de Enfermagem, 41*(esp), e20190152. https://doi.org/10.1590/1983-1447.2020.20190152

De Poli, C., Oyebode, J., Airoldi, M., & Glover, R. (2020). A need-based, multi-level, cross-sectoral framework to explain variations in satisfaction of care needs among people living with dementia. *BMC Health Services Research, 20*(1), 657–670. https://doi.org/10.1186/s12913-020-05416x

Flower, K. B., Wurzelmann, S., Rojas, C., Heredia, K. M., Peereboom, M., Sylvester, F., Agostinelli, K., Ritter, V. S., Fine, J., & Steiner, M. J. (2020). Improving satisfaction and appointment attendance through navigation for Spanish-speaking families. *Journal of Health Care for the Poor and Underserved, 31*(2), 810–826. https://doi.org/10.1353/hpu.2020.0062

Mikocka-Walus, A., Massuger, W., Knowles, S. R., Moore, G. T., Buckton, S., Connell, W., Pavli, P., Raven, L., & Andrews, J. M. (2020). Quality of care in inflammatory bowel disease: Actual health service experiences fall short of the standards. *Internal Medicine Journal, 50*(10), 1216–1225. https://doi.org/10.1111/imj.14683

Räty, V., Haaranen, A., & Rissanen, T. (2019). Patients' satisfaction with child psychiatry. *Scandinavian Journal of Caring Sciences, 34*(1), 62–68. https://doi.org/10.1111/scs.12705

While, C., Winbolt, M., & Nay, R. (2020). Consumer expectations and experiences of quality in Australian home-based community services. *Health & Social Care in the Community, 28*(5), 1459–1467. https://doi.org/10.1111/hsc.12967

Client Satisfaction: Acute Care Transition Process   3017

Definition: Extent of positive perception of staff's preparation for client to transfer to another health care situation

OUTCOME TARGET RATING: Maintain at_____ Increase to_____

		Not at All Satisfied	Somewhat Satisfied	Moderately Satisfied	Very Satisfied	Completely Satisfied	
OUTCOME OVERALL RATING		1	2	3	4	5	
Indicators:							
301701	Discussion of post-acute care options early in hospitalization	1	2	3	4	5	NA
301702	Discussion of post-acute care placement options	1	2	3	4	5	NA
301703	Discussion of insurance coverage for post-acute care placement options	1	2	3	4	5	NA
301704	Personal preferences considered	1	2	3	4	5	NA
301705	Client included in discharge planning	1	2	3	4	5	NA
301706	Family included in discharge planning	1	2	3	4	5	NA
301707	Client assisted to identify facility to support needs	1	2	3	4	5	NA
301708	Discussion of client's functional status	1	2	3	4	5	NA
301709	Discussion of client's rehabilitation potential	1	2	3	4	5	NA
301710	Discussion of client's needs for specialized medications/treatments	1	2	3	4	5	NA
301711	Confirmation of client's care goals	1	2	3	4	5	NA
301712	Discharge plans updated	1	2	3	4	5	NA
301713	Opportunity to express concerns about transition	1	2	3	4	5	NA
301714	Staff suggestions for solutions to concerns	1	2	3	4	5	NA
301715	Questions answered completely	1	2	3	4	5	NA
301716	Discussion of follow-up appointments	1	2	3	4	5	NA
301717	Arrangement for transportation to a new facility	1	2	3	4	5	NA
301718	Staff identify medication required at new facility	1	2	3	4	5	NA
301719	Staff share written and verbal communication with new facility	1	2	3	4	5	NA

Domain-Health & Life Quality (V)   *Class*-Satisfaction with Care (EE)   7th edition 2024

OUTCOME CONTENT REFERENCES:

Achilleos, M., McEwen, J., Hoesly, M., DeAngelo, M., & Jennings, T. (2020). Pharmacist-led program to improve transitions from acute care to skilled facility care. *American Journal of Health-System Pharmacy, 77*(12), 979–984. https://doi.org/10.1093/ajhp/zxaa090

Ayele, R., Manges, K. A., Leonard, C., Lee, M., Galenbeck, E., Molla, M., Levy, C., & Burke, R. E. (2021). How context influences hospital readmissions from skilled nursing facilities: A rapid ethnographic study. *Journal of the American Medical Directors Association, 22*(6), 1248–1254. https://doi.org/10.1016/j.jamda.2020.08.001

Britton, M. C., Petersen-Pickett, J., Hodshon, B., & Chaudhry, S. I. (2019). Mapping the care transition from hospital to skilled nursing facility. *Journal of Evaluation in Clinical Practice, 26*(3), 786–790. https://doi.org/10.1111/jep.13238

Gadbois, E. A., Tyler, D. A., Shield, R., McHugh, J., Winblad, U., Teno, J. M., & Mor, V. (2018). Lost in transition: A qualitative study of patients discharged from hospital to skilled nursing facility. *Journal of General Internal Medicine, 34*(1), 102–109. https://doi.org/10.1007/s11606-018-4695-0

Gupta, S., Perry, J. A., & Kozar, R. (2019). Transitions of care in geriatric medicine. *Clinics in Geriatric Medicine, 35*(1), 45–52. https://doi.org/10.1016/j.cger.2018.08.005

Krol, M. L., Allen, C., Matters, L., Graham, A. J., English, W., & White, H. K. (2018). Health optimization program for elders. *Journal of Nursing Care Quality, 34*(3), 217–222. https://doi.org/10.1097/NCQ.0000000000000375

Oseran, A. S., Lage, D. E., Jernigan, M. C., Metlay, J. P., & Shah, S. J. (2019). A "Hospital-Day-1" model to predict the risk of discharge to a skilled nursing facility. *Journal of the American Medical Directors Association, 20*(6), 689–695. https://doi.org/10.1016/j.jamda.2019.03.035

Richardson, A., Blenkinsopp, A., Downs, M., & Lord, K. (2019). Stakeholder perspectives of care for people living with dementia moving from hospital to care facilities in the community: A systematic review. *BMC Geriatrics, 19*(202), 1–12. https://doi.org/10.1186/s12877-019-1220-1

Thompson, L. R., & Ifejika, N. L. (2019). The transition from the hospital to an inpatient rehabilitation setting for neurological patients. *Nursing Clinics, 54*(3), 357–366. https://doi.org/10.1016/j.cnur.2019.04.004

Client Satisfaction: Caring   3001

Definition: Extent of positive perception of nursing staff's concern for the client

OUTCOME TARGET RATING: Maintain at_____ Increase to_____

		Not at All Satisfied	Somewhat Satisfied	Moderately Satisfied	Very Satisfied	Completely Satisfied	
OUTCOME OVERALL RATING		1	2	3	4	5	
Indicators:							
300101	Courtesy shown by staff	1	2	3	4	5	NA
300102	Compassion shown by staff	1	2	3	4	5	NA
300125	Empathy shown by staff	1	2	3	4	5	NA
300103	Kindness shown by staff	1	2	3	4	5	NA
300104	Respect shown by staff	1	2	3	4	5	NA
300105	Consideration for feelings	1	2	3	4	5	NA
300106	Consideration for opinions	1	2	3	4	5	NA
300126	Consideration of personal preferences	1	2	3	4	5	NA
300107	Concern shown for individual needs	1	2	3	4	5	NA
300108	Relationship with nursing staff	1	2	3	4	5	NA
300109	Frequency checked on by staff	1	2	3	4	5	NA
300110	Promptness answering call light	1	2	3	4	5	NA
300111	Promptness responding to inquires	1	2	3	4	5	NA
300127	Willingness to answer questions	1	2	3	4	5	NA
300123	Follow through with client request	1	2	3	4	5	NA
300112	Emotional support provided	1	2	3	4	5	NA
300124	Assistance to address spiritual needs	1	2	3	4	5	NA
300113	Appropriate use of touch	1	2	3	4	5	NA
300114	Orientation to room, equipment, and routines	1	2	3	4	5	NA
300115	Visiting arrangements	1	2	3	4	5	NA
300116	Family and friends made welcome	1	2	3	4	5	NA
300117	Assistance with letter writing	1	2	3	4	5	NA
300118	Leisure activities provided	1	2	3	4	5	NA
300119	Information provided about options of care	1	2	3	4	5	NA
300128	Information provided about follow-up care	1	2	3	4	5	NA
300120	Consideration for cost of care	1	2	3	4	5	NA
300121	Supplies and equipment not wasted	1	2	3	4	5	NA

***Domain*-Health & Life Quality (V)   *Class*-Satisfaction with Care (EE)   3rd edition 2004; revised 2008, 2024**

OUTCOME CONTENT REFERENCES:

DeCola, M. C., Maresca, G., D'Aleo, G., Carnazza, L., Giliberto, S., Maggio, M. G., Bramanti, A., & Calabró, R. S. (2020). Teleassistance for frail elderly people: A usability and customer satisfaction study. *Geriatric Nursing, 41*(4), 463–467. https://doi.org/10.1016/j.gerinurse.2020.01.019

DeSantis, J. P., Cintulova, M., Provencio-Vasquez, E., Rodriguez, A. E., & Cicero, E. C. (2020). Transgender women's satisfaction with healthcare services: A mixed-methods pilot study. *Perspectives in Psychiatric Care, 56*, 926–938. https://doi.org/10.1111/ppc.12514

Gimenez-Diez, D., Alía, R. M., Jiménez, S. R., Granel, N., Solá, L. T., & Bernabeu-Tamayo, M. D. (2020). Treating mental health crises at home: Patient satisfaction. *Journal of Psychiatric and Mental Health Nursing, 27*, 246–257.

Gustafsson, S., Wälivaara, B. M., & Gabrielsson, S. (2019). Patient satisfaction with telephone nursing. *Journal of Nursing Care Quality, 35*(1), E6–E11. https://doi.or/10.1097/NCQ.0000000000000392

Kortet, S., Melender, H. A., Klemetti, R., Kääriäinen, M., & Kaakinen, P. (2021). Mothers' perceptions of the quality of maternity services at Finnish maternity units: A cross-sectional study. *Nordic Journal of Nursing Research, 41*(1), 14–24. https://doi.org/10.1177/2057158520937541

+Lee, C. F., Wang, X. F., Wong, P. N. F., Koh, Y. L. E., Ngoh, S. H. A., Mohtar, Z. M., Lian, L. G., Ang, K. W., & Tan, N. C. (2020). Psychometric evaluation of a patient satisfaction survey questionnaire to assess advanced practice nurse ambulatory services in primary care. *Journal of Nursing Management, 128*, 1481–1488. https://doi.org/10.1111/jonm.13072

Meier, A., Erickson, J. I., Snow, N., & Kline, M. (2019). Nurse and patient satisfaction. *The Journal of Nursing Administration, 49*(11), 520–522. https://doi.org/10.1097/NNA.0000000000000814

Mensik, J., Leebov, W., & Steinbinder, A. (2019). Caregivers help define a tool to measure cultures of care. *The Journal of Nursing Administration, 49*(3), 138–142. https://doi.org/10.1097/NNA.0000000000000727

Räty, V., Haaranen, A., & Rissanen, T. (2019). Patients' satisfaction with child psychiatry. *Scandinavian Journal of Caring Sciences, 34*(1), 62–68. https://doi.org/10.1111/scs.12705

Simske, N. M., Bendick, A., Rascoe, A. S., Hendrickson, S. B., & Vallier, H. A. (2020). Patient satisfaction is improved with exposure to trauma recovery services. *JAAOS-Journal of the American Academy of Orthopaedic Surgeons, 28*(14), 597–605. https://doi.org/10.5435/JAAOS-D-19-00266

Stamboglis, N., & Jacobs, R. (2020). Factor associated with patient satisfaction of community mental health services: A multilevel approach. *Community Mental Health Journal, 56*(1), 50–64. https://doi.org/10.1007/s10597-019-00449-x

Client Satisfaction: Case Management

3015

Definition: Extent of positive perception of case management services

OUTCOME TARGET RATING: Maintain at_____ Increase to_____

	Not at All Satisfied	Somewhat Satisfied	Moderately Satisfied	Very Satisfied	Completely Satisfied	
OUTCOME OVERALL RATING	1	2	3	4	5	
Indicators:						
301501 Availability of case manager	1	2	3	4	5	NA
301535 Availability of patient navigator	1	2	3	4	5	NA
301536 Accommodation to changing needs	1	2	3	4	5	NA
301502 Availability of supplies needed for care	1	2	3	4	5	NA
301503 Availability of equipment needed for care	1	2	3	4	5	NA
301504 Assistance with contacting physician	1	2	3	4	5	NA
301505 Assistance with gaining access to health providers	1	2	3	4	5	NA
301506 Referrals made to appropriate health providers	1	2	3	4	5	NA
301507 Coordination of health care resources	1	2	3	4	5	NA
301508 Coordination of health providers	1	2	3	4	5	NA
301509 Coordination of care	1	2	3	4	5	NA
301537 Coordination of care at discharge	1	2	3	4	5	NA
301510 Wait times for getting an appointment	1	2	3	4	5	NA
301511 Information provided about support groups	1	2	3	4	5	NA
301538 Appointment scheduling flexibility	1	2	3	4	5	NA
301539 Consideration of transportation needs	1	2	3	4	5	NA
301512 Consideration for feelings	1	2	3	4	5	NA
301513 Consideration of opinions	1	2	3	4	5	NA
301514 Concern shown for individual needs	1	2	3	4	5	NA
301540 Assistance with symptom control	1	2	3	4	5	NA
301515 Information provided about options for care	1	2	3	4	5	NA
301516 Information provided about cost of care	1	2	3	4	5	NA
301517 Consideration of cost of care	1	2	3	4	5	NA
301518 Avoidance of unnecessary treatments and procedures	1	2	3	4	5	NA

Client Satisfaction: Case Management—cont'd

	Not at All Satisfied	Somewhat Satisfied	Moderately Satisfied	Very Satisfied	Completely Satisfied	
301519 Referral regarding costs and finances	1	2	3	4	5	NA
301520 Consistent information provided	1	2	3	4	5	NA
301521 Personal values considered	1	2	3	4	5	NA
301522 Personal preferences considered in care	1	2	3	4	5	NA
301523 Respect for cultural values	1	2	3	4	5	NA
301524 Respect for religious beliefs	1	2	3	4	5	NA
301525 Health providers work as a team	1	2	3	4	5	NA
301526 Safety issues addressed	1	2	3	4	5	NA
301527 Family included in providing care	1	2	3	4	5	NA
301528 Confidentiality of client information maintained	1	2	3	4	5	NA
301529 Explanation provided in understandable terms	1	2	3	4	5	NA
301530 Quality of instructional material provided	1	2	3	4	5	NA
301531 Included in decisions about care	1	2	3	4	5	NA
301532 Support for finding own solutions to problems	1	2	3	4	5	NA
301533 Information provided about legal rights	1	2	3	4	5	NA
301534 Information provided about course of illness	1	2	3	4	5	NA

Domain-Health & Life Health (V)   **Class**-Satisfaction with Care (EE)   4th edition 2008; revised 2024

OUTCOME CONTENT REFERENCES:

Bradshaw, A., & Raphaelson, S. (2021). Improving patient satisfaction with wait times. *Nursing 2021, 51*(4), 67–69. https://doi.org/10.1097/01.NURSE.0000736968. 01359.e0

Costa, D. G., Moura, G. M. S. S., Moraes, M. G., Santos, J. L. G., & Magalhães, A. M. M. (2020). Satisfaction attributes related to safety and quality perceived in the experience of hospitalized patients. *Revista Gaúcha de Enfermagem, 41*(esp), e20190152. https://doi.org/10.1590/1983-1447.2020.20190152

De Poli, C., Oyebode, J., Airoldi, M., & Glover, R. (2020). A need-based, multi-level, cross-sectoral framework to explain variations in satisfaction of care needs among people living with dementia. *BMC Health Services Research, 20*(1), 657–670. https://doi.org/10.1186/s12913-020-05416x

Joo, J. Y, & Huber, D. L. (2014). An integrative review of nurse-led community-based case management effectiveness. *International Nursing Review, 61*(1), 14–24.

Mikocka-Walus, A., Massuger, W., Knowles, S. R., Moore, G. T., Buckton, S., Connell, W., Pavli, P., Raven, L., & Andrews, J. M. (2020). Quality of care in inflammatory bowel disease: Actual health service experiences fall short of the standards. *Internal Medicine Journal, 50*(10), 1216–1225. https://doi.org/10.1111/imj.14683

Schutt, R. K., & Woodford, M. L. (2020). Increasing health service access by expanding disease coverage and adding patient navigation: Challenges for patient satisfaction. *BMC Health Services Research, 20*(1), 175–185. https://doi.org/10.1186/s12913-020-5009-x

Stamboglis, N., & Jacobs, R. (2020). Factors associated with patient satisfaction of community mental health services: A multilevel approach. *Community Mental Health Journal, 56*(1), 50–64. https://doi.org/10.1007/s10597-019-00449-x

Client Satisfaction: Communication   3002

Definition: Extent of positive perception of information exchanged between client and nursing staff

OUTCOME TARGET RATING: Maintain at_____ Increase to_____

	Not at All Satisfied	Somewhat Satisfied	Moderately Satisfied	Very Satisfied	Completely Satisfied	
OUTCOME OVERALL RATING	1	2	3	4	5	
Indicators:						
300201 Staff introduce self and role	1	2	3	4	5	NA
300202 Use of client's preferred name	1	2	3	4	5	NA
300203 Staff speak clearly	1	2	3	4	5	NA
300204 Staff actively listens to client	1	2	3	4	5	NA
300224 Staff maintains eye contact	1	2	3	4	5	NA
300205 Staff encourages questions	1	2	3	4	5	NA
300225 Staff respects privacy	1	2	3	4	5	NA
300206 Staff repeats information as often as needed	1	2	3	4	5	NA

Continued

Client Satisfaction: Communication—cont'd

		Not at All Satisfied	Somewhat Satisfied	Moderately Satisfied	Very Satisfied	Completely Satisfied	
300226	Staff asked thoughtful questions	1	2	3	4	5	NA
300207	Staff takes time when communicating	1	2	3	4	5	NA
300227	Staff gives information about care process	1	2	3	4	5	NA
300208	Staff presents information in understandable way	1	2	3	4	5	NA
300209	Staff makes sure information is understood	1	2	3	4	5	NA
300228	Staff provides material in preferred language	1	2	3	4	5	NA
300210	Staff uses non-judgmental communication	1	2	3	4	5	NA
300219	Staff asks for client's opinion	1	2	3	4	5	NA
300220	Staff uses empathy statements	1	2	3	4	5	NA
300229	Staff acknowledges others' presence	1	2	3	4	5	NA
300221	Staff involves caregiver	1	2	3	4	5	NA
300222	Staff communicates sensitive information in a respectful manner	1	2	3	4	5	NA
300211	Questions answered clearly	1	2	3	4	5	NA
300212	Questions answered completely	1	2	3	4	5	NA
300213	Questions answered in a reasonable length of time	1	2	3	4	5	NA
300214	Consistent information given by staff	1	2	3	4	5	NA
300217	Discrepancies in information are resolved in a timely manner	1	2	3	4	5	NA
300230	Personal concerns considered	1	2	3	4	5	NA
300215	Personal values considered	1	2	3	4	5	NA
300216	Personal preferences considered	1	2	3	4	5	NA
300223	Translator provided	1	2	3	4	5	NA
300218	Alternative communication methods used as needed	1	2	3	4	5	NA
300231	Staff smiles	1	2	3	4	5	NA

Domain-Health & Life Quality (V)   **Class**-Satisfaction with Care (EE)   3rd edition 2004; revised 2018, 2024

OUTCOME CONTENT REFERENCES:

Allen, L. W. (2020). Getting back to basics in communication. *Quality Management in Health Care, 29*(2), 126–127. https://doi.org/10.1097/QMH.0000000000000249

Costa, D. G., Moura, G. M. S. S., Moraes, M. G., Santos, J. L. G., & Magalhães, A. M. M. (2020). Satisfaction attributes related to safety and quality perceived in the experience of hospitalized patients. *Revista Gaúcha de Enfermagem, 41*(esp), e20190152. https://doi.org/10.1590/1983-1447.2020.20190152

De Santis, J. P., Cintulova, M., Provencio-Vasquez, E., Rodriguez, A. E., & Cicero, E. C. (2019). Transgender women's satisfaction with healthcare services: A mixed-methods pilot study. *Perspectives in Psychiatric Care, 56*(4), 926–938. https://doi.org/10.1111/ppc.12514

Flower, K. B., Wurzelmann, S., Rojas, C., Heredia, K. M., Peereboom, M., Sylvester, F., Agostinelli, K., Ritter, V. S., Fine, J., & Steiner, M. J. (2021). Improving satisfaction and appointment attendance through navigation for Spanish-speaking families. *Journal of Health Care for the Poor and Underserved, 31*(2), 810–826. https://doi.org/10.1353/hpu.2020.0062

Gimenez-Diez, D., Alía, R. M., Jiménez, S. R., Granel, N., Solá, L. T., & Bernabeu-Tamayo, M. D. (2020). Treating mental health crises at home: Patient satisfaction with home nursing care. *Journal of Psychiatric Mental Health Nursing, 27*(3), 246–257. https://doi.org/10.1111/jpm.12573

James, S., Desborough, J., McInnes, S., & Halcomb, E. (2020). Nonverbal communication between registered nurses and patients during chronic disease management consultations: Observations from general practice. *Journal of Clinical Nursing, 29*(13/14), 2378–2387. https://doi.org/10.1111/jocn.15249

Jongerius, C., Hessels, R. S., Romijn, J. A., Smets, E. M. A., & Hillen, M. A. (2020). The measurement of eye contact in human interactions: A scoping review. *Journal of Nonverbal Behavior, 44*(3), 363–389. https://doi.org/10.1007/s10919-020-00333-3

Keutchafo, E. L. W., Kerr, J., & Jarvis, M. A. (2020). Evidence of nonverbal communication between nurses and older adults: A scoping review. *BMC Nursing, 19*(1), 53–66. https://doi.org/10.1186/s12912-020-00443-9

Stamboglis, N., & Jacobs, R. (2020). Factors associated with patient satisfaction of community mental health services: A multilevel approach. *Community Mental Health Journal, 56*(1), 50–64. https://doi.org/10.1007/s10597-019-00449-x

Virani, S., Xia, T., Brainch, N., Mitra, S., Ahmed, S., Mutasiigwa, H., Chaudhari, G., & Zaveri, D. (2020). Scaling the great wall: The impact of communication barriers on quality of psychiatric care in Chinese patients. *International Journal of Social Psychiatry, 66*(2), 150–155. https://doi.org/10.1177/0020764019888959

Client Satisfaction: Continuity of Care 3003

Definition: Extent of positive perception of coordination of care as the client moves from one care setting to another

OUTCOME TARGET RATING: Maintain at_____ Increase to_____

C

		Not at All Satisfied	Somewhat Satisfied	Moderately Satisfied	Very Satisfied	Completely Satisfied	
OUTCOME OVERALL RATING		1	2	3	4	5	
Indicators:							
300301	Coordination of care	1	2	3	4	5	NA
300322	Staff, client, and family developed care plan	1	2	3	4	5	NA
300302	Personal preferences included in care plan	1	2	3	4	5	NA
300323	Personal treatment preferences included in care plan	1	2	3	4	5	NA
300305	Safety issues addressed in care plan	1	2	3	4	5	NA
300303	Client and family included in planning care	1	2	3	4	5	NA
300321	Client and family included in discharge planning	1	2	3	4	5	NA
300304	Client resources identified in discharge planning	1	2	3	4	5	NA
300306	Time to prepare for transfer	1	2	3	4	5	NA
300307	Information provided about what to expect when transferred	1	2	3	4	5	NA
300324	Information passed on correctly	1	2	3	4	5	NA
300308	Opportunity provided to express concerns about managing self-care	1	2	3	4	5	NA
300309	Information provided to manage self-care	1	2	3	4	5	NA
300310	Opportunity to demonstrate care activities	1	2	3	4	5	NA
300325	Staff well informed about needs	1	2	3	4	5	NA
300311	Staff offered suggestions for solutions to concerns and questions	1	2	3	4	5	NA
300326	Staff answered questions	1	2	3	4	5	NA
300327	Staff continuity practiced	1	2	3	4	5	NA
300312	Discussion of strategies to meet care needs	1	2	3	4	5	NA
300313	Discussion of strategies to meet household needs	1	2	3	4	5	NA
300314	Personal preparation to deal with potential health problems	1	2	3	4	5	NA
300315	Discussion of guidelines for returning to sexual activities	1	2	3	4	5	NA
300316	Discussion of strategies for returning to work	1	2	3	4	5	NA
300317	Discussion of strategies for returning to homemaking activities	1	2	3	4	5	NA
300318	Discussion of strategies for returning to community activities	1	2	3	4	5	NA
300328	Access to nurse navigator	1	2	3	4	5	NA
300319	Assistance with managing relocation costs and finances	1	2	3	4	5	NA
300329	Assistance accessing services	1	2	3	4	5	NA
300320	Health providers work as a team	1	2	3	4	5	NA

Domain-Health & Life Quality (V)   **Class**-Satisfaction with Care (EE)   3rd edition 2004; revised 2008, 2024

OUTCOME CONTENT REFERENCES:

Kuipers, S. J., Cramm, J. M., & Nieboer, A. P. (2019). The importance of patient-centered care and co-creation of care for satisfaction with care and physical and social well-being of patients with multi-morbidity in the primary care setting. *BMC Health Services Research, 19*(13), 1–9. https://doi.org/10.1186/s12913-018-3818-y

Pfeifer, B. D. (2019). Healthcare consumerism and its impact on rural health. *Frontiers of Health Services Management, 36*(2), 33–36. https://doi.org/10.1097/HAP.0000000000000072

Stamboglis, N., & Jacobs, R. (2020). Factors associated with patient satisfaction of community mental health services: A multilevel approach. *Community Mental Health Journal, 56*(1), 50–64. https://doi.org/10.1007/s10597-019-00449-x

Taylor, K. (2019). Embracing and advancing the consumerist era in healthcare. *Frontiers of Health Services Management, 36*(2), 15–25. https://doi.org/10.1097/HAP.0000000000000069

Tonkikh, O., Zisberg, A., & Shadmi, E. (2020). Association between continuity of nursing care and older adults' hospitalization outcomes: A retrospective observational study. *Journal of Nursing Management. 28*(5), 1062–1069. https://doi.org/10.1111/jonm.13031

C

Client Satisfaction: Cultural Needs Fulfillment   3004

Definition: Extent of positive perception of integration of cultural beliefs, values and social structures into nursing care

OUTCOME TARGET RATING: Maintain at_____ Increase to_____

		Not at All Satisfied	Somewhat Satisfied	Moderately Satisfied	Very Satisfied	Completely Satisfied	
OUTCOME OVERALL RATING		1	2	3	4	5	
Indicators:							
300401	Respect for cultural beliefs	1	2	3	4	5	NA
300402	Respect for cultural health behaviors	1	2	3	4	5	NA
300403	Respect for personal values	1	2	3	4	5	NA
300404	Respect for personal perspectives	1	2	3	4	5	NA
300405	Respect for traditions	1	2	3	4	5	NA
300406	Respect for religious beliefs	1	2	3	4	5	NA
300407	Respect for spiritual beliefs	1	2	3	4	5	NA
300408	Incorporation of cultural beliefs in health teaching	1	2	3	4	5	NA
300409	Care consistent with cultural beliefs	1	2	3	4	5	NA
300410	Use of methods to establish communication for language differences	1	2	3	4	5	NA
300414	Use of preferred language	1	2	3	4	5	NA
300415	Use of preferred language for prescriptions	1	2	3	4	5	NA
300416	Use of language appropriate materials	1	2	3	4	5	NA
300417	Use of bilingual navigators to address language differences	1	2	3	4	5	NA
300411	Consideration for cultural expectations	1	2	3	4	5	NA
300412	Respect for family members' participation in care	1	2	3	4	5	NA
300413	Respect for family members' participation in decisions	1	2	3	4	5	NA

Domain-*Health & Life Quality (V)* · **Class**-*Satisfaction with Care (EE)*   *3rd edition 2004; revised 2024*

OUTCOME CONTENT REFERENCES:

Flower, K. B., Wurzelmann, S., Rojas, C., Heredia, K. M., Peereboom, M., Sylvester, F., Agostinelli, K., Ritter, V. S., Fine, J., & Steiner, M. J. (2021). Improving satisfaction and appointment attendance through navigation for Spanish-speaking families. *Journal of Health Care for the Poor and Underserved, 31*(2), 810–826. https://doi.org/10.1353/hpu.2020.0062

Joo, J. Y., & Liu, M. F. (2020). Nurses' barriers to care of ethnic minorities: A qualitative systematic review. *Western Journal of Nursing Research, 42*(9), 760–771. https://doi.org/10.1177/0193945919883395

Kavukcu, N., & Altintaş, K. H. (2019). The challenges of the health care providers in refugee settings: A systematic review. *Prehospital Disaster Medicine, 34*(2), 188–196. https://doi.org/10.1017/S1049023X19000190

Listerfelt, S., Fridh, I., & Lindahl, B. (2019). Facing the unfamiliar: Nurses' transcultural care in intensive care—A focus group study. *Intensive & Critical Care Nursing, 55*, 1–8. https://doi.org/10.1016/j.iccn.2019.08.002

Phillips, S., Villalobos, A. V. K., Crawbuck, G. S. N., & Pratt-Chapman, M. L. (2019). In their own words: Patient navigator role in culturally sensitive cancer care. *Supportive Care in Cancer, 27*(5), 1655–1662. https://doi.org/10.1007/s00520-018-440-7

Schill, K., & Caxaj, S. (2019). Cultural safety strategies for rural indigenous palliative care: A scoping review. *BMC Palliative Care, 18*(1), 1–13. https://doi.org/10.1186/s12904-019-0404-y

Virani, S., Xia, T., Brainch, N., Mitra, S., Ahmed, S., Mutasiigwa, H., Chaudhari, G., & Zaveri, D. (2020). Scaling the great wall: The impact of communication barriers on quality of psychiatric care in Chinese patients. *International Journal of Social Psychiatry, 66*(2), 150–155. https://doi.org/10.1177/0020764019888959

Client Satisfaction: Discharge Process   3018

Definition: Extent of positive perception of staff's discharge preparation for client and family to independent living

OUTCOME TARGET RATING: Maintain at_____ Increase to_____

		Not at All Satisfied	Somewhat Satisfied	Moderately Satisfied	Very Satisfied	Completely Satisfied	
OUTCOME OVERALL RATING		**1**	**2**	**3**	**4**	**5**	
Indicators:							
301801	Client included in discharge planning	1	2	3	4	5	NA
301802	Family included in discharge planning	1	2	3	4	5	NA
301803	Client assisted to identify support services for care	1	2	3	4	5	NA
301804	Family assisted to identify support services for care	1	2	3	4	5	NA
301805	Personal preferences considered	1	2	3	4	5	NA
301806	Time allowed to prepare for discharge	1	2	3	4	5	NA
301807	Information provided about what to expect when discharged	1	2	3	4	5	NA
301808	Client's resources identified	1	2	3	4	5	NA
301809	Information provided on medications for self-care	1	2	3	4	5	NA
301810	Information provided on treatments for self-care	1	2	3	4	5	NA
301811	Safety issues addressed in providing self-care	1	2	3	4	5	NA
301812	Activity restrictions discussed	1	2	3	4	5	NA
301813	Clear instructions on procedures	1	2	3	4	5	NA
301814	Information on how to obtain supplies	1	2	3	4	5	NA
301815	Staff suggestions for solutions to concerns	1	2	3	4	5	NA
301816	Questions answered completely	1	2	3	4	5	NA
301817	Opportunity to demonstrate procedures	1	2	3	4	5	NA
301818	Opportunity to perform own non-parenteral medication	1	2	3	4	5	NA
301819	Discussion of follow-up treatment	1	2	3	4	5	NA
301820	Assistance with setting appointments	1	2	3	4	5	NA
301821	Discussion of strategies to obtain medication	1	2	3	4	5	NA
301822	Discussion of strategies to address potential complications	1	2	3	4	5	NA
301823	Discussion of home modification for safe functioning	1	2	3	4	5	NA
301824	Discussion of cost of care and insurance coverage	1	2	3	4	5	NA
301825	Discussion of strategies for returning to household duties	1	2	3	4	5	NA
301826	Discussion of strategies for returning to sexual activity	1	2	3	4	5	NA
301827	Discussion of strategies for returning to work	1	2	3	4	5	NA
301828	Discussion of strategies for returning to community activities	1	2	3	4	5	NA
301829	Information for community resources	1	2	3	4	5	NA

Domain-Health & Life Quality (V)   *Class-Satisfaction with Care (EE)*   7th edition 2024

OUTCOME CONTENT REFERENCES:

Bobay, K. L., Conway-Phillips, R., Hughes, R. G., Costa, L., Bahr, S. J., Siclovan, D., Nuccio, S., & Weiss, M. (2020). Clinical nurses' perspectives on discharge practice changes from participating in a translational research study. *Journal of Nursing Management, 29*(3), 553–561. https://doi.org/10.1111/jonm.13171

Casey-Upton, R., Howell, D. M., Kitzman, P. H., Custer, M. G., & Dressler, E. V. (2019). Factors influencing discharge readiness after total knee replacement. *Orthopaedic Nursing, 38*(1), 6–14. https://doi.org/10.1097/NOR.0000000000000513

Fuller, T. E., Pong, D. D., Piniella, N., Pardo, M., Bessa, N., Yoon, C., Boxer, R. B., Schnipper, J. L., & Dalal, A. K. (2020). Interactive digital health tools to engage patients and caregivers in discharge preparation: Implementation study. *Journal of Medical Internet Research, 22*(4), 1–19. https://www.jmir.org/2020/4/e15573/

O'Conner, M., Moriarty, H., Schneider, A., Dowdell, E. B., & Bowles, K. H. (2021). Patients' and caregivers' perspectives in determining discharge readiness from home health. *Geriatric Nursing, 42*(1),151–158. https://doi.org/10.1016/j.gerinurse.2020.12.012

Salmani, N., Marvast, M. Z., Kahdouei, S., & Weiss, M. E. (2020). Adaptation of the parent readiness for hospital discharge scale with mothers of preterm infants discharged from the neonatal intensive care unit. *Journal of Clinical Nursing, 29*(23-24), 4544–4553. https://doi.org/10.1111/jocn.15479

Wallace, A. S., Pierce, N. L., Davisson, E., Manges, K., & Tripp-Reimer, T. (2019). Social resource assessment: Application of a novel communication tool during hospital discharge. *Patient Education and Counseling, 102*(3), 542–549. https://doi.org/10.1016/j.pec.2018.09.022

Weiss, M. E., & Piacentine, L. B. (2006). Psychometric properties of the readiness for hospital discharge scale. *Journal of Nursing Measurement, 14*(3), 163–180. https://doi.org/10.1891/jnm-v14i3a002

Weiss, M. E., Yakusheva, O., Bobay, K. L., Costa, L., Hughes, R. G., Nuccio, S., Hamilton, M., Bahr, S., Siclovan, D., & Bang, J. (2019). Effect of implementing discharge readiness assessment in adult medical-surgical units on 30-day return to hospital: The READI Randomized Clinical Trial. *JAMA Network Open, 2*(1), e187387. https://doi.org/10.1001/jamanetworkopen.2018.7387

Client Satisfaction: Functional Assistance

3005

Definition: Extent of positive perception of nursing assistance to achieve mobility and self-care

OUTCOME TARGET RATING: Maintain at_____ Increase to_____

		Not at All Satisfied	Somewhat Satisfied	Moderately Satisfied	Very Satisfied	Completely Satisfied	
OUTCOME OVERALL RATING		1	2	3	4	5	
Indicators:							
300501	Included in planning for optimal mobility and self-care	1	2	3	4	5	NA
300502	Included in planning time schedule for self-care	1	2	3	4	5	NA
300503	Encouraged to be as active as possible	1	2	3	4	5	NA
300504	Assistance with physical activity	1	2	3	4	5	NA
300505	Exercise routine provided to gain or maintain mobility	1	2	3	4	5	NA
300506	Exercise routine provided to gain or maintain flexibility	1	2	3	4	5	NA
300507	Equipment provided to enhance mobility	1	2	3	4	5	NA
300516	Information provided for correct use of devices	1	2	3	4	5	NA
300509	Room space provided for equipment needed to support functional independence	1	2	3	4	5	NA
300510	Safety taught in all activities	1	2	3	4	5	NA
300511	Opportunity to do self-care unless assistance requested	1	2	3	4	5	NA
300512	Assistance with care	1	2	3	4	5	NA
300517	Encouraged to choose own clothing	1	2	3	4	5	NA
300518	Encouraged to choose food for meals	1	2	3	4	5	NA
300515	Information provided to manage medication	1	2	3	4	5	NA
300519	Information provided to prevent falls	1	2	3	4	5	NA
300520	Handrails provided in bathroom	1	2	3	4	5	NA

Domain-*Health & Life Quality (V)*   **Class**-*Satisfaction with Care (EE)*   *3rd edition 2004; revised 2008, 2024*

OUTCOME CONTENT REFERENCES:

Custer, M. G., & Huebner, R. A. (2019). Identifying homogeneous outcome groups in adult rehabilitation using cluster analysis. *The American Journal of Occupational Therapy, 73*(5), 1–9. https://doi.org/10.5014/ajot.2019.031997

Hsu, S. H., Campbell, C., Weeks, A. K., Herklota, M., Kostelecky, N., Pastores, S. M., Halpern, N. A., & Voigt, L. P. (2020). A pilot survey of ventilated cancer patients' perspectives and recollections of early mobility in the intensive care unit. *Supportive Care in Cancer, 28*(2), 747–753. https://doi.org/10.1007/s00520-019-04867-1

Lake, E. T., Germack, H. D., & Viscardi, M. K. (2016). Missed nursing care is linked to patient satisfaction: A cross-sectional study of U.S. hospitals. *BMJ Quality & Safety, 25*(7), 535–543. https://doi.org/10.1136/bmjqs-2015-003961

Maceri, J., Sekhon, S., Talley, J., Dinnendahl, S., Loseto-Wood, M., & Jasper, D. (2019). Defining patient acuity for nursing assistants and its correlation to patient and staff satisfaction. *Medsurg Nursing, 28*(6), 368–373. https://doi.org/10.1136/bmj.h5000

Ray, G. S., Ekelund, P., Nemes, S., Rolfson, O., & Mohaddes, M. (2020). Changes in health-related quality of life are associated with patient satisfaction following total hip replacement: An analysis of 69,083 patients in the Swedish Hip Arthroplasty Register. *Acta Orthopaedica, 91*(1), 48–52. https://doi.org/10.1080/17453674.2019.1685284

Romero-García, M., Delgado-Hito, P., Cueva-Ariza, L., Martínez-Momblan, M. A., Lluch-Canut, M. T., Trujols-Albet, J., Juvé-Udina, M. E., & Benito, L. (2019). Level of satisfaction of critical care patients regarding the nursing care received: Correlation with sociodemographic and clinical variables. *Australian Critical Care, 32*(6), 486–493. https://doi.org/10.1016/j.aucc.2018.11.002

Spangler, D., Blomqvist, P., Lindberg, Y., & Winblad, U. (2019). Small is beautiful? Explaining resident satisfaction in Swedish nursing home care. *IBMC Health Services Research, 19*(1), 1–12. https://doi.org/10.1186/s12913-019-4694-9

Yildiz, F. T., & Kaşikçi, M. (2020). Impact of training based on Orem's theory on self-care agency and quality of life in patients with coronary artery disease. *The Journal of Nursing Research, 28*(6), e125–137. https://doi.org/10.1097/jnr.0000000000000406

C

Client Satisfaction: Labor & Delivery   3019

Definition: Extent of positive perception of care provided by nursing staff during labor and delivery services

OUTCOME TARGET RATING: Maintain at _____ Increase to _____

		Not at All Satisfied	Somewhat Satisfied	Moderately Satisfied	Very Satisfied	Completely Satisfied	
OUTCOME OVERALL RATING		1	2	3	4	5	
Indicators:							
301901	Staff introductions and explanation of role	1	2	3	4	5	NA
301902	Use of the client's preferred name	1	2	3	4	5	NA
301903	Consideration of personal care preferences	1	2	3	4	5	NA
301904	Orientation to room, equipment, and routines	1	2	3	4	5	NA
301905	Maintenance of privacy	1	2	3	4	5	NA
301906	Courtesy shown by staff	1	2	3	4	5	NA
301907	Protection of client's legal rights	1	2	3	4	5	NA
301908	Respect for family members' participation in care	1	2	3	4	5	NA
301909	Information provided in an understandable way	1	2	3	4	5	NA
301910	Information provided to improve woman's participation in care	1	2	3	4	5	NA
301911	Information provided about status of baby	1	2	3	4	5	NA
301912	Information provided about progress of labor	1	2	3	4	5	NA
301913	Information provided about options for pain relief	1	2	3	4	5	NA
301914	Actions taken to provide comfort	1	2	3	4	5	NA
301915	Non-pharmacological interventions for pain control	1	2	3	4	5	NA
301916	Pharmacological interventions for pain control	1	2	3	4	5	NA
301917	Help with position changes during care	1	2	3	4	5	NA
301918	Coordination of care between care units	1	2	3	4	5	NA
301919	Assistance with selection of food and fluid	1	2	3	4	5	NA
301920	Cleanliness of care environment	1	2	3	4	5	NA
301921	Waiting time to have needs met	1	2	3	4	5	NA
301922	Competence of staff	1	2	3	4	5	NA
301923	Instructions about baby care	1	2	3	4	5	NA
301924	Instructions about breastfeeding	1	2	3	4	5	NA
301925	Instructions about postdelivery care	1	2	3	4	5	NA
301926	Availability of supplies and equipment needed for care	1	2	3	4	5	NA
301927	Care consistent with cultural beliefs	1	2	3	4	5	NA
301928	Client safety measures	1	2	3	4	5	NA
301929	Fall prevention strategies	1	2	3	4	5	NA
301930	Participation in discharge planning	1	2	3	4	5	NA

Domain-Health & Life Quality (V)   *Class*-Satisfaction with Care (EE)   7th edition 2024

OUTCOME CONTENT REFERENCES:

American College of Obstetricians and Gynecologists. (2019). ACOG Committee Opinion No. 766: Approaches to limit intervention during labor and birth. *Obstetrics & Gynecology, 133*(2), e164–e173. https://doi.org/10.1097/AOG.0000000000003074

Baranowska, B., Kajdy, A., Pawlicka, P., Pokropek, E., Rabijewski, M., Sys, D., & Pokropek, A. (2020). What are the critical elements of satisfaction and experience in labor and childbirth—A cross-sectional study. *International Journal of Environmental Research in Public Health, 17*(24), 9295. https://doi.org/10.3390/ijerph17249295

Donate-Manzanares, M., Rodríguez-Cano, T., Gómez-Salgado, J., Rodríguez-Almagro, J., Hernández-Martínez, A., Barrilero-Fernández, E., & Beato-Fernández, L. (2019). Quality of childbirth care in women undergoing labour: Satisfaction with care received and how it changes over time. *Journal of Clinical Medicine, 8*(4),434. https//doi.org/10.3390/jcm8040434

Jolles, M. W., de Vries, M., Hollander, M. H., & van Dillen, J. (2019). Prevalence, characteristics, and satisfaction of women with a birth plan in the Netherlands. *Birth, 46*(4), 686–692. http//doi.org/10.1111/birt.12451

Lopes, F., Nakamura, M. U., & Nomura, R. M. Y. (2021). Women's satisfaction with childbirth in a public hospital in Brazil. *Birth, 48*(2), 251–256. https//doi.org/10.1111/birt.12534

Martins, A. C. M., Giugliani, E. R. J., Nunes, L. N., Bizon, A. M. B. L., de Senna, A, F. K., Paiz, J. C., de Avilla, J. C., & Giugliani, C. (2020). Factors associated with a positive childbirth experience in Brazilian women: A cross-sectional study. *Women and Birth, 34*(4), e337–e345. https://doi.org/10.1016/j.wombi.2020.06.003

Thomson, G., Feeley, C., Moran, V. H., Downe, S., & Oladapo, O. T. (2019). Women's experiences of pharmacological and non-pharmacological pain relief methods for labour and childbirth: A qualitative systematic review. *Reproductive Health, 16*(1), 71. https//doi.org/10.1186/s12978-019-0735-4

World Health Organization. (2018). WHO recommendations intrapartum care for a positive childbirth experience. https://apps.who.int/iris/bitstream/handle/10665/260178/9789241550215-eng.pdf

Client Satisfaction: Pain Management

3016

Definition: Extent of positive perception of nursing care to relieve, minimize, or control pain

OUTCOME TARGET RATING: Maintain at_____ Increase to_____

		Not at All Satisfied	Somewhat Satisfied	Moderately Satisfied	Very Satisfied	Completely Satisfied	
OUTCOME OVERALL RATING		**1**	**2**	**3**	**4**	**5**	
Indicators:							
301601	Pain control	1	2	3	4	5	NA
301602	Pain level regularly monitored	1	2	3	4	5	NA
301618	Actions taken to ask about pain level	1	2	3	4	5	NA
301603	Side effects of medication monitored	1	2	3	4	5	NA
301604	Actions taken to relieve pain	1	2	3	4	5	NA
301605	Actions taken to provide comfort	1	2	3	4	5	NA
301619	Information provided about cause of pain	1	2	3	4	5	NA
301620	Information provided about medication	1	2	3	4	5	NA
301606	Information provided to manage medication use	1	2	3	4	5	NA
301607	Personal preferences considered	1	2	3	4	5	NA
301621	Participation in decision-making on pain management	1	2	3	4	5	NA
301608	Information provided about options for pain management	1	2	3	4	5	NA
301609	Pain management consistent with cultural beliefs	1	2	3	4	5	NA
301610	Preventive approaches used for pain management	1	2	3	4	5	NA
301611	Information provided about activity restrictions	1	2	3	4	5	NA
301612	Information provided about pain relief	1	2	3	4	5	NA
301613	Information provided about options for pain management after discharge	1	2	3	4	5	NA
301614	Referrals made to support groups	1	2	3	4	5	NA
301615	Health providers work as a team to manage pain	1	2	3	4	5	NA
301622	Health providers' knowledge	1	2	3	4	5	NA
301616	Referral to pain management health professionals as needed	1	2	3	4	5	NA
301617	Safety issues addressed with pain medication use	1	2	3	4	5	NA
301623	Addiction issues addressed with pain medication use	1	2	3	4	5	NA

Domain-*Health & Life Quality (V)*   **Class**-*Satisfaction with Care (EE)*   4th edition 2008; revised 2024

OUTCOME CONTENT REFERENCES:

Duncan, R. W., Smith, K. L., Maguire, M., & Stader D. E. III. (2019). Alternative to opioids for pain management in the emergency department decreases opioid usage and maintains patient satisfaction. *American Journal of Emergency Medicine, 37*(1), 38–44. https://doi.org/10.1016/j.ajem.2018.04.043

Elkbuli, A., Stotsenburg, M., Epstein, C., Calvert, K., Boneva, D., McKenney, M., & Deaton, K. (2020). A multidisciplinary approach to improve pain management and satisfaction in a trauma population. *Journal of Trauma Nursing, 27*(2), 96–102. https://doi.org/10.1097/JTN.0000000000000493

Fraser, C., Beasley, M., Macfarlane, G., & Lovell, K. (2019). Telephone cognitive behavioural therapy to prevent the development of chronic widespread pain: A qualitative study of patient perspective and treatment acceptability. *BMC Musculoskeletal Disorder, 20*(1), 1–11. https://doi.org/10.1186/s12891-019-2584-2

Lee, S., Smith, M. L., Dahlke, D. V., Pardo, N., & Ory, M. G. (2020). A cross-sectional examination of patients' perspectives about their pain, pain management, and satisfaction with pain treatment. *Pain Medicine, 21*(2), e164–e171. https://doi.org/10.1093/pm/pnz244

Mazurenko, O., Collum, T., Ferdinand, A., & Menachemi, N. (2017). Predictors of hospital patient satisfaction as measured by HCAHPS: A systematic review. *Journal of Healthcare Management, 62*(4), 272–283. https://doi.org/10.1097/JHM-D-15-00050

Miller, J., MacDermid, J. C., Walton, D. M., & Richardson, J. (2020). Chronic pain self-management support with pain science education and exercise (COMMENCE) for people with chronic pain and multiple comorbidities: A randomized controlled trial. *Archives of Physical Medicine and Rehabilitation, 101*(5), 750–761. https://doi.org/10.1016/j.apmr.2019.12.016

Mohamed, N. S., Castrodad, I. M. D., Gwam, C. U., Etcheson, J. I., Passarello, A. N., George, N. E., Mahajan, A. K., & Delanois, R. E. (2020). Pain intensity in total hip arthroplasty patients: How communication influences satisfaction. *HIP International, 30*(6), 690–694. https://doi.org/10.1177/1120700019851783

Teoh, S. W. K., Payne, C., McDonnell, N., & Petrovski, M. (2021). Postoperative pain management on discharge after day case gynaecologic laparoscopy. *Journal of Pharmacy Practice and Research, 51*(5), 62–66. https://doi.org/10.1002/jppr.1690

Valentine, S., Majer, J., Grant, N., & Taylor, D. (2021). The effect of the consent process on patient satisfaction with pain management: A randomized controlled trial. *Annual of Emergency Medicine, 77*(1), 82–90. https://doi.org/10.1016/j.annemergmed.2020.03.029

Client Satisfaction: Physical Care 3006

Definition: Extent of positive perception of nursing care to maintain body functions and cleanliness

OUTCOME TARGET RATING: Maintain at_____ Increase to_____

		Not at All Satisfied	Somewhat Satisfied	Moderately Satisfied	Very Satisfied	Completely Satisfied	
OUTCOME OVERALL RATING		1	2	3	4	5	
Indicators:							
300601	Assistance with selecting food and fluid	1	2	3	4	5	NA
300602	Assistance with eating	1	2	3	4	5	NA
300603	Designated time for meals	1	2	3	4	5	NA
300604	Fluids available within restriction	1	2	3	4	5	NA
300605	Assistance with mouth care	1	2	3	4	5	NA
300606	Assistance with toileting	1	2	3	4	5	NA
300622	Assistance with maintaining normal bowel habits	1	2	3	4	5	NA
300623	Assistance with maintaining normal bladder habits	1	2	3	4	5	NA
300609	Assistance with bathing	1	2	3	4	5	NA
300624	Assistance with changing clothes	1	2	3	4	5	NA
300610	Assistance with hair care	1	2	3	4	5	NA
300611	Assistance with nail care	1	2	3	4	5	NA
300612	Skin care routine maintained	1	2	3	4	5	NA
300613	Special skin care followed	1	2	3	4	5	NA
300614	Assistance with maintaining comfort	1	2	3	4	5	NA
300615	Time for rest	1	2	3	4	5	NA
300616	Sleep routine maintained	1	2	3	4	5	NA
300617	Assistance with ambulation	1	2	3	4	5	NA
300618	Opportunity for exercise	1	2	3	4	5	NA
300619	Special exercises provided	1	2	3	4	5	NA
300620	Assistance with repositioning	1	2	3	4	5	NA
300621	Assistance with transfer performance	1	2	3	4	5	NA

Domain-Health & Life Quality (V)   **Class**-Satisfaction with Care (EE)   3rd edition 2004; revised 2024

OUTCOME CONTENT REFERENCES:

Bagnasco, A., Dasso, N., Rossi, S., Galanti, C., Varone, G., Catania, G., Zanini, M., Aleo, G., Watson, R., Hayter, M., & Sasso, L. (2019). Unmet nursing care needs on medical and surgical wards: A scoping review of patients' perspectives. *Journal of Clinical Nursing, 29*(3-4), 347–369. https://doi.org/10.1111/jocn.15089

Koskenniemi, J., Leino-Kilpi, H., Puukka, P., Stolt, M., & Suhonen, R. (2018). Being respected by nurses: Measuring older patients' perceptions. *International Journal of Older People Nursing, 13*(3), e12197. https://doi.org/10.1111/opn.12197

Kuipers, S. J., Cramm, J. M., & Nieboer, A. P. (2019). The importance of patient–centered care and co-creation of care for satisfaction with care and physical and social well-being of patients with multi-morbidity in the primary care setting. *BMC Health Services Research, 19*(13), 1–9. https://doi.org/10.1186/s12913-018-3818-y

Mbuzi, V., Fulbrook, P., & Jessup, M. (2017). Indigenous cardiac patients' and relatives' experiences of hospitalisations: A narrative inquiry. *Journal of Clinical Nursing, 26*(23-24), 5052–5064. https://doi.org/10.1111/jocn.14005

New, L., Goodridge, D., Kappel, J., Groot, G., & Dobson, R. (2019). "I just have to take it"- patient safety in acute care: Perspectives and experiences of patients with chronic kidney disease. *BMC Health Services Research, 19*(1), 1–11. https://doi.org/10.1186/s12913-019-4014-4

Radecki, B., Reynolds, S., & Kara, A. (2018). Inpatient fall prevention for the patient's perspective. *Applied Nursing Research, 43*, 114–119. https://doi.org/10.1016/j.apnr.2018.08.001

Client Satisfaction: Physical Environment   3007

Definition: Extent of positive perception of living and treatment environment, equipment, and supplies in acute, rehabilitation, or long-term care settings

OUTCOME TARGET RATING: Maintain at_____ Increase to_____

OUTCOMES OVERALL RATING	Not at All Satisfied	Somewhat Satisfied	Moderately Satisfied	Very Satisfied	Completely Satisfied	
	1	2	3	4	5	
Indicators:						
300701 Cleanliness of room	1	2	3	4	5	NA
300702 Cleanliness of bathroom	1	2	3	4	5	NA
300703 Cleanliness of equipment	1	2	3	4	5	NA
300704 Control of room lighting	1	2	3	4	5	NA
300705 Control of room temperature	1	2	3	4	5	NA
300721 Control of odors	1	2	3	4	5	NA
300706 Control of bathroom temperature	1	2	3	4	5	NA
300707 Comfort of treatment room temperature	1	2	3	4	5	NA
300708 Comfort of room humidity	1	2	3	4	5	NA
300709 Control of noise	1	2	3	4	5	NA
300710 Control of number of people in room	1	2	3	4	5	NA
300711 Supplies and equipment within reach	1	2	3	4	5	NA
300722 Food quality	1	2	3	4	5	NA
300723 Food service	1	2	3	4	5	NA
300724 Nurse call system within reach	1	2	3	4	5	NA
300725 Homelike surroundings	1	2	3	4	5	NA
300726 Sense of safety in personal space	1	2	3	4	5	NA
300713 Access to telephone	1	2	3	4	5	NA
300714 Access to television	1	2	3	4	5	NA
300715 Access to radio	1	2	3	4	5	NA
300716 Attractiveness of room	1	2	3	4	5	NA
300727 Availability of areas for privacy	1	2	3	4	5	NA
300728 Availability of area to visit with patients	1	2	3	4	5	NA
300729 Availability of adjustable furniture	1	2	3	4	5	NA
300717 Availability of chairs for family and visitors	1	2	3	4	5	NA
300730 Availability of rest area for parents and family	1	2	3	4	5	NA
300718 Availability of space nearby for family and visitors	1	2	3	4	5	NA
300719 Orientation of family and visitors to facilities	1	2	3	4	5	NA
300720 Space in room for personal items	1	2	3	4	5	NA

Domain-*Health & Life Quality (V)*   **Class**-*Satisfaction with Care (EE)*   *3rd edition 2004; revised 2008, 2024*

OUTCOME CONTENT REFERENCES:

Kortet, S., Melender, H. L., Klemetti, R., Kääriäinen, M., & Kaakinen, P. (2021). Mothers' perceptions of the quality of maternity services at Finnish maternity units: A cross-sectional study. *Nordic Journal of Nursing Research, 41*(1), 14–24. https://doi.org/10.1177/2057158520937541

McLaughlan, R., Sadek, A., & Willis, J. (2019). Attractions to fuel the imagination: Reframing understandings of the role of distraction relative to well-being in the pediatric hospital. *Health Environments Research & Design Journal, 12*(2), 130–146. https://doi.org/10.1177/1937586718810878

Mazurenko, O., Collum, T., Ferdinand, A., & Menachemi, N. (2017). Predictors of hospital patient satisfaction as measured by HCAHPS: A systematic review. *Journal of Healthcare Management, 62*(4). https://doi.org/10.1097/JHM-D-15-00050

Sadek, A. H., & Willis, J. (2020). Ways to harness the built environment of ambulatory cancer facilities for comprehensive patient support: A review of the literature. *International Journal of Nursing Studies, 101*, 1–13. https://doi.org/10.1016/j.ijnurstu.2019.05.004

Simske, N. M., Benedick, A., Bascoe, A. S., Hendrickson, S. B., & Vallier, H. A. (2020). Patient satisfaction is improved with exposure to trauma recovery services. *JAAOS-Journal of the American Academy of Orthopaedic Surgeons, 28*(14), 597–605. https://doi.org/10.5435/JAAOS-D-19-00266

Client Satisfaction: Protection of Rights   3008

Definition: Extent of positive perception of protection of a client's legal and moral rights provided by nursing staff

OUTCOME TARGET RATING: Maintain at_____ Increase to_____

C

		Not at All Satisfied	Somewhat Satisfied	Moderately Satisfied	Very Satisfied	Completely Satisfied	
OUTCOME OVERALL RATING		1	2	3	4	5	
Indicators:							
300801	Maintenance of privacy	1	2	3	4	5	NA
300802	Care consistent with religious and spiritual needs	1	2	3	4	5	NA
300803	Confidentiality of information maintained	1	2	3	4	5	NA
300804	Requests respected	1	2	3	4	5	NA
300805	Personal preferences for care considered	1	2	3	4	5	NA
300816	Treatment approaches aligned with personal preferences	1	2	3	4	5	NA
300806	Use of client's preferred name	1	2	3	4	5	NA
300807	Introduced to staff	1	2	3	4	5	NA
300808	Introduced to roommate(s)	1	2	3	4	5	NA
300809	Information provided about available services of other disciplines	1	2	3	4	5	NA
300810	Information provided about support groups	1	2	3	4	5	NA
300811	Allowed to choose between care options	1	2	3	4	5	NA
300812	Included in decisions about care	1	2	3	4	5	NA
300817	Information on designating surrogate decision maker	1	2	3	4	5	NA
300818	Information provided about informed consent	1	2	3	4	5	NA
300813	Information provided about legal rights	1	2	3	4	5	NA
300814	Information provided about advance directives	1	2	3	4	5	NA
300819	Information provided about parental rights	1	2	3	4	5	NA
300820	Information provided about palliative care	1	2	3	4	5	NA
300821	Information provided to family about advance directives	1	2	3	4	5	NA
300815	Avoidance of repetitive questions by more than one provider	1	2	3	4	5	NA

Domain-Health & Life Quality (V)   **Class**-Satisfaction with Care (EE)   *3rd edition 2004; revised 2024*

OUTCOME CONTENT REFERENCES:

Allen, L. W. (2020). Getting back to basics in communication. *Quality Management in Health Care, 29*(2), 126–127. https://doi.org/10.1097/QMH.0000000000000249

Arstein-Kerslake, A., & Black, J. (2020). Right to legal capacity in therapeutic jurisprudence: Insights form critical disability theory and the convention on the rights of persons with disabilities. *International Journal of Law and Psychiatry, 68*, 1–10. https://doi.org/10.1016/j.ijlp.2019.101535

Chang, K. H., Chi, W. C., Liao, H. F., Chen, S. C., Chiou, H. Y., Escorpizo, R., & Liou, T. H. (2020). Development of indicators to assure disability evaluation based on the International Classification of Functioning, Disability, and Health in Taiwan: A Delphi consensus. *Disability and Rehabilitation, 42*(7), 975–982. https://doi.org/10.1080/09638288.2018.1514536

Costa, D. G., Moura, G. M. S. S., Moraes, M. G., Santos, J. L. G., & Magalhães, A. M. M. (2020). Satisfaction attributes related to safety and quality perceived in the experience of hospitalized patients. *Revista Gaúcha de Enfermagem, 41*(esp), e20190152. https://doi.org/10.1590/1983-1447.2020.20190152

Luo, H., Liu, G., Lu, J., & Xue, J. (2021). Association of shared decision-making with inpatient satisfaction: A cross-sectional study. *BMC Medical Informatics and Decision Making, 21*, 1–11. https://doi.org/10.1186/s12911-021-01385-1

Martinez Tapia, C., Canoui-Poitrine, F., Caillet, P., Bastuji-Garin, S., Tournigand, C., Assaf, E., Varnier, G., Pamoukdjian, F., Brain, E., Rollot-Trad, F., & Laurent, M., Paillaud, E. (2019). Preferences for surrogate designation and decision-making process in older versus younger adults with cancer: A comparative cross-sectional study. *Patient Education and Counseling, 102*(3), 429–435. https://doi.org/10.1016/j.pec.2018.09.024

Sona, C., Pollard, K. A., Schallom, M., Schrupp, A., & Wessman, B. T. (2020). Implementation of a standardized patient/family communication bundle. *Critical Care Nursing Clinics, 32*(2), 243–251. https://doi.org/10.1016/j.cnc.2020.02.006

Zahrai, A., Bhanot, K., Mei, X. Y., Crawford, E., Tan, Z., Yee, A., & Palda, V. (2020). Surgeon clinical practice variation and patient preferences during the informed consent discussion: A mixed methods analysis in lumbar spine surgery. *Canadian Journal of Surgery, 63*(3), E284–E297. https://doi.org/10.1503/cjs.005619

Client Satisfaction: Psychological Care 3009

Definition: Extent of positive perception of nursing assistance to cope with emotional issues and perform mental activities

OUTCOME TARGET RATING: Maintain at_____ Increase to_____

		Not at All Satisfied	Somewhat Satisfied	Moderately Satisfied	Very Satisfied	Completely Satisfied	
OUTCOME OVERALL RATING		1	2	3	4	5	
Indicators:							
300921	Respected as a person	1	2	3	4	5	NA
300901	Information provided about course of illness	1	2	3	4	5	NA
300902	Information provided about expected improvement	1	2	3	4	5	NA
300917	Information provided about usual emotional responses to disease	1	2	3	4	5	NA
300918	Information provided about usual emotional responses to treatment regimen	1	2	3	4	5	NA
300922	Discussion of impact of illness on private life	1	2	3	4	5	NA
300904	Assistance with identifying community support groups for client	1	2	3	4	5	NA
300905	Assistance with identifying community support groups for family	1	2	3	4	5	NA
300906	Discussion of strategies to cope with mental impairments	1	2	3	4	5	NA
300923	Discussion of strategies to cope with emotional issues	1	2	3	4	5	NA
300924	Assistance with decision-making about care	1	2	3	4	5	NA
300925	Attention to safety concerns	1	2	3	4	5	NA
300907	Emotional support provided	1	2	3	4	5	NA
300908	Counseling provided to improve mental functioning	1	2	3	4	5	NA
300909	Counseling provided to improve emotional stability	1	2	3	4	5	NA
300910	Counseling provided to improve social interactions	1	2	3	4	5	NA
300919	Assistance with finding counseling services	1	2	3	4	5	NA
300912	Support for finding own solutions to problems	1	2	3	4	5	NA
300926	Attention paid to emotions	1	2	3	4	5	NA
300913	Support for expressing feelings	1	2	3	4	5	NA
300914	Support for working through feelings of loss	1	2	3	4	5	NA
300915	Support for identifying ways to cope with stress	1	2	3	4	5	NA
300916	Support for adjusting to functional changes	1	2	3	4	5	NA
300920	Assistance to address spiritual needs	1	2	3	4	5	NA

Domain-Health & Life Quality (V) **Class**-Satisfaction with Care (EE) *3rd edition 2004; revised 2008, 2024*

OUTCOME CONTENT REFERENCES:

Bagnasco, A., Dasso, N., Rossi, S., Galanti, C., Varone, G., Catania, G., Zanini, M., Aleo, G., Watson, R., Hayter, M., & Sasso, L. (2019). Unmet nursing care needs on medical and surgical wards: A scoping review of patients' perspectives. *Journal of Clinical Nursing, 29*(3-4), 347–369. https://doi.org/10.1111/jocn.15089

Koskenniemi, J., Leino-Kilpi, H., Puukka, P., Stolt, M., & Suhonen, R. (2018). Being respected by nurses: Measuring older patients' perceptions. *International Journal of Older People Nursing, 13*(3), e12197. https://doi.org/10.1111/opn.12197

Kuipers, S. J., Cramm, J. M., & Nieboer, A. P. (2019). The importance of patient–centered care and co-creation of care for satisfaction with care and physical and social well-being of patients with multi-morbidity in the primary care setting. *BMC Health Services Research, 19*(13), 1–9. https://doi.org/10.1186/s12913-018-3818-y

Mbuzi, V., Fulbrook, P., & Jessup, M. (2017). Indigenous cardiac patients' and relatives' experiences of hospitalisations: A narrative inquiry. *Journal of Clinical Nursing, 26*(23-24), 5052–5064. https://doi.org/10.1111/jocn.14005

New, L., Goodridge, D., Kappel, J., Groot, G., & Dobson, R. (2019). "I just have to take it"- patient safety in acute care: Perspectives and experiences of patients with chronic kidney disease. *BMC Health Services Research, 19*(1), 1–11. https://doi.org/10.1186/s12913-019-4014-4

Pitrou, I., Berbiche, D., & Vasiliadis, H. M. (2020). Mental health and satisfaction with primary care services in older adults: A study from the patient perspective on four dimensions of care. *Family Practice, 37*(4), 459–464. https://doi.org/10.1093/fampra/cmaa019

Radecki, B., Reynolds, S., & Kara, A. (2018). Inpatient fall prevention for the patient's perspective. *Applied Nursing Research, 43*, 114–119. https://doi.org/10.1016/j.apnr.2018.08.001

Romero-García, M., Delgado-Hito, P., Cueva-Ariza, L., Martínez-Momblan, M. A., Lluch-Canut, M. T., Trujols-Albet, J., Juvé-Udina, M. E., & Benito, L. (2019). Level of satisfaction of critical care patients regarding the nursing care received: Correlation with sociodemographic and clinical variables. *Australian Critical Care, 32*(6), 486–493. https://doi.org/10.1016/j.aucc.2018.11.002

Client Satisfaction: Safety   3010

Definition: Extent of positive perception of procedures, information, and nursing care to prevent harm or injury

OUTCOME TARGET RATING: Maintain at_____ Increase to_____

	Not at All Satisfied	Somewhat Satisfied	Moderately Satisfied	Very Satisfied	Completely Satisfied	
OUTCOME OVERALL RATING	1	2	3	4	5	
Indicators:						
301001 Explanation of safety rules and procedures	1	2	3	4	5	NA
301016 Explanation of emergency evacuation plan and procedures	1	2	3	4	5	NA
301017 Information shared about reporting errors in care	1	2	3	4	5	NA
301002 Prompt response to injury by staff	1	2	3	4	5	NA
301003 Client identified before receiving medication	1	2	3	4	5	NA
301018 Client encouraged to ask questions	1	2	3	4	5	NA
301014 Protective devices used to prevent harm	1	2	3	4	5	NA
301019 Use of personal protection strategies	1	2	3	4	5	NA
301020 Equitable treatment and care	1	2	3	4	5	NA
301005 Assistance with transfer performance	1	2	3	4	5	NA
301006 Assistance with ambulation	1	2	3	4	5	NA
301007 Assistance with toileting	1	2	3	4	5	NA
301008 Assistance with bathing	1	2	3	4	5	NA
301009 Warning signs of high-risk environment clearly displayed	1	2	3	4	5	NA
301015 Fall prevention strategies	1	2	3	4	5	NA
301011 Information provided about treatment risks and complications	1	2	3	4	5	NA
301012 Maintenance of safe environment when cognitive function is impaired	1	2	3	4	5	NA
301021 Maintenance of crowd-free environment	1	2	3	4	5	NA
301013 Maintenance of protective environment when at risk for self-injury	1	2	3	4	5	NA
301022 Maintenance of a protective environment when at risk from others	1	2	3	4	5	NA

Domain-Health & Life Quality (V)   *Class*-Satisfaction with Care (EE)   *3rd edition 2004; revised 2008, 2024*

OUTCOME CONTENT REFERENCES:

Bagnasco, A., Dasso, N., Rossi, S., Galanti, C., Varone, G., Catania, G., Zanini, M., Aleo, G., Watson, R., Hayter, M., & Sasso, L. (2019). Unmet nursing care needs on medical and surgical wards: A scoping review of patients' perspectives. *Journal of Clinical Nursing, 29*(3-4), 347–369. https://doi.org/10.1111/jocn.15089

Koskenniemi, J., Leino-Kilpi, H., Puukka, P., Stolt, M., & Suhonen, R. (2018). Being respected by nurses: Measuring older patients' perceptions. *International Journal of Older People Nursing, 13*(3), e12197. https://doi.org/10.1111/opn.12197

Kuipers, S. J., Cramm, J. M., & Nieboer, A. P. (2019). The importance of patient–centered care and co-creation of care for satisfaction with care and physical and social well-being of patients with multi-morbidity in the primary care setting. *BMC Health Services Research, 19*(13), 1–9. https://doi.org/10.1186/s12913-018-3818-y

Mbuzi, V., Fulbrook, P., & Jessup, M. (2017). Indigenous cardiac patients' and relatives' experiences of hospitalisations: A narrative inquiry. *Journal of Clinical Nursing, 26*(23-24), 5052–5064. https://doi.org/10.1111/jocn.14005

New, L., Goodridge, D., Kappel, J., Groot, G., & Dobson, R. (2019). "I just have to take it"- patient safety in acute care: Perspectives and experiences of patients with chronic kidney disease. *BMC Health Services Research, 19*(1), 1–11. https://doi.org/10.1186/s12913-019-4014-4

Radecki, B., Reynolds, S., & Kara, A. (2018). Inpatient fall prevention for the patient's perspective. *Applied Nursing Research, 43*, 114–119. https://doi.org/10.1016/j.apnr.2018.08.001

Client Satisfaction: Symptom Control 3011

Definition: Extent of positive perception of nursing care to relieve symptoms of illness

OUTCOME TARGET RATING: Maintain at_____ Increase to_____

OUTCOME OVERALL RATING	Not at All Satisfied 1	Somewhat Satisfied 2	Moderately Satisfied 3	Very Satisfied 4	Completely Satisfied 5	
Indicators:						
301101 Patterns of symptoms identified	1	2	3	4	5	NA
301117 Symptom cluster identified	1	2	3	4	5	NA
301102 Severity of symptoms identified	1	2	3	4	5	NA
301103 Duration of symptoms identified	1	2	3	4	5	NA
301104 Investigation of cause of symptoms	1	2	3	4	5	NA
301105 Actions taken to prevent symptoms	1	2	3	4	5	NA
301118 Recognized need for goal for symptom management	1	2	3	4	5	NA
301106 Symptoms responded to promptly	1	2	3	4	5	NA
301115 Care to control symptoms	1	2	3	4	5	NA
301119 Medication offered to control symptoms	1	2	3	4	5	NA
301112 Monitored for control of symptoms	1	2	3	4	5	NA
301109 Actions taken to provide comfort	1	2	3	4	5	NA
301113 Monitored for comfort	1	2	3	4	5	NA
301110 Symptoms regularly monitored	1	2	3	4	5	NA
301120 Monitored for new symptoms	1	2	3	4	5	NA
301111 Monitored for unusual symptoms	1	2	3	4	5	NA
301121 Recognized worsening symptoms	1	2	3	4	5	NA
301122 Monitored for need of additional treatment	1	2	3	4	5	NA
301123 Recognized when relief present	1	2	3	4	5	NA
301124 Actions to deal with symptom unpredictability	1	2	3	4	5	NA
301114 Referrals made to other health providers	1	2	3	4	5	NA

Domain-Health & Life Quality (V)   **Class**-Satisfaction with Care (EE)   *3rd edition 2004; revised 2008, 2024*

OUTCOME CONTENT REFERENCES:

Corwin, E. J., Berg, J. A., Armstrong, T. S., DeVito Dabbs, A., Lee, K. A., Meek, P., & Redeker, N. (2014). Envisioning the future in symptom science. *Nursing Outlook, 62*, 346–351. https://doi.org/10.1016/j.outlook.2014.06.006

Cowman, S. (2018). Bedside to bench: Re-thinking nursing research. *Journal of Advance Nursing, 74*, 235–236. https://doi.org/10.1111/jan.13254

Hogan-Quigley, B., Palm, M. L., & Bickley, L. (2020). *Nursing guide to physical examination and history taking.* Wolters Kluwer.

Mansutti, I., Saiani, L., Morandini, M., & Palese, A. (2020). Post-stroke delirium risk factors, signs and symptoms of onset and outcomes as perceived by expert nurses: A focus group study. *Journal of Stroke and Cerebrovascular diseases, 29*(9), 1–11. https://doi.org/10.1016/j.jstrokecerebrovasdis.2020.105013

Salvetti, M. G., Donato, S. C. T., Machado, C. S. P., Almeida, N. G., Dos Santos, D. V., & Kurita, G. P. (2021). Psychoeducational nursing interventions for symptom management in cancer patients: A randomized clinical trial. *Asia-Pacific Journal of Oncology Nursing, 8*(2), 156–63. https://doi.org/10.4103/apjon.apjon_56_20

Schmid-Mohler, G., Caress, A. L., Spirig, R., & Yorke, J. (2018). Introducing a model for emotional distress in respiratory disease: A systematic review and synthesis of symptom management models. *Journal of Advanced Nursing, 75*(9), 1854–1867. https://doi.org/10.1111/jan.13968

Tripp-Reimer, T., Williams, J. K., Gardner, S. E., Rakel, B., Herr, K., McCarthy, A. M., Hand, L. L., Gilbertson-White, S., & Cherwin, C. (2020). An integrated model of multimorbidity and symptom science. *Nursing Outlook, 68*(4), 430–439. https://doi.org/10.1016/j.outlook.2020.03.003

Client Satisfaction: Teaching   3012

Definition: Extent of positive perception of instruction provided by nursing staff to improve knowledge, understanding, and participation in care

OUTCOME TARGET RATING: Maintain at_____ Increase to_____

		Not at All Satisfied	Somewhat Satisfied	Moderately Satisfied	Very Satisfied	Completely Satisfied	
OUTCOME OVERALL RATING		1	2	3	4	5	
Indicators:							
301210	Personal knowledge considered before teaching	1	2	3	4	5	NA
301224	Material presented in preferred language	1	2	3	4	5	NA
301219	Explanations provided in understandable terms	1	2	3	4	5	NA
301225	Information presented in small amounts	1	2	3	4	5	NA
301218	Time for client learning	1	2	3	4	5	NA
301226	Uses teach-back method	1	2	3	4	5	NA
301227	Session involves others as desired	1	2	3	4	5	NA
301220	Quality of instruction material	1	2	3	4	5	NA
301222	Explanation of medical diagnosis	1	2	3	4	5	NA
301223	Explanation of nursing care	1	2	3	4	5	NA
301203	Explanation of diagnostic tests and preparation	1	2	3	4	5	NA
301204	Explanation of results of diagnostic tests	1	2	3	4	5	NA
301205	Explanation of medication therapeutic effects	1	2	3	4	5	NA
301206	Explanation of medication side effects	1	2	3	4	5	NA
301207	Explanation of reasons for treatment	1	2	3	4	5	NA
301208	Explanation of self-care responsibilities for treatment	1	2	3	4	5	NA
301209	Explanation of self-care responsibilities for medication management	1	2	3	4	5	NA
301212	Explanation of activity restrictions	1	2	3	4	5	NA
301215	Discussion of strategies to improve health	1	2	3	4	5	NA
301211	Information provided about signs of complications	1	2	3	4	5	NA
301216	Explanation of available health resources	1	2	3	4	5	NA
301228	Explanation of treatment costs	1	2	3	4	5	NA
301221	Staff supportive of learning process	1	2	3	4	5	NA
301229	Staff provided consistent information	1	2	3	4	5	NA
301230	Opportunity for evaluation of teaching methods	1	2	3	4	5	NA

Domain-Health & Life Quality (V)   *Class*-Satisfaction with Care (EE)   *3rd edition 2004; revised 2008, 2024*

OUTCOME CONTENT REFERENCES:

Nickels, D., Dolansky, M., Marek, J., & Burke, K. (2020). Nursing students use of teach-back to improve patients' knowledge and satisfaction: A quality improvement project. *Journal of Professional Nursing, 36*(2), 70–76. https://doi.org/10.1016/j.profnurs.2019.08.005

Peters, C., Bowen, B., Jusino-Leon, G., Kooran, S., Smith, D., Higgins, M., & Spinks, K. R. (2019). Structured DVD education. *Clinical Journal of Oncology Nursing, 23*(2), 181–190. https://doi.org/10.1188/19.CJON.181-190

Scott, C., Andrews, D., Bulla, S., & Loerzel, V. (2019). Teach-back method: Using a nursing education intervention to improve discharge instructions on an adult oncology unit. *Clinical Journal of Oncology Nursing, 23*(3), 288–294. https://doi.org/10.1188/19.CJON.288-294

Solberg, B. S., Haavik, J., & Halmay, A. (2019). Health care services for adults with ADHD: Patient satisfaction and the role of psycho-education. *Journal of Attention Disorders, 23*(1), 99–108. https://doi.org/10.1177/1087054715587941

St. John, I. J., & Englund, H. (2020). Improving patient discharge education through daily educational bursts. *Journal of Professional Development, 36*(5), 283–287. https://doi.org/10.1097/NND.0000000000000627

Client Satisfaction: Technical Aspects of Care   3013

Definition: Extent of positive perception of nursing staff's knowledge and expertise in providing care

OUTCOME TARGET RATING: Maintain at_____ Increase to_____

		Not at All Satisfied	Somewhat Satisfied	Moderately Satisfied	Very Satisfied	Completely Satisfied	
OUTCOME OVERALL RATING		1	2	3	4	5	
Indicators:							
301301	Correct care provided	1	2	3	4	5	NA
301302	Organization of care	1	2	3	4	5	NA
301303	Thoroughness of care	1	2	3	4	5	NA
301318	Explanation of medical terms	1	2	3	4	5	NA
301304	Capability of staff	1	2	3	4	5	NA
301305	Registered nurse knowledge of disease process	1	2	3	4	5	NA
301316	Registered nurse knowledge of procedures	1	2	3	4	5	NA
301307	Registered nurse knowledge of medication	1	2	3	4	5	NA
301308	Registered nurse knowledge of health history	1	2	3	4	5	NA
301319	Competent in performing physical exams	1	2	3	4	5	NA
301320	Competence in providing treatments	1	2	3	4	5	NA
301321	Competence in administrating medications	1	2	3	4	5	NA
301322	Competent in operating equipment	1	2	3	4	5	NA
301309	Consistency in performance of care	1	2	3	4	5	NA
301310	Consistency of staff providing care	1	2	3	4	5	NA
301311	Comfort attended to during treatments	1	2	3	4	5	NA
301312	Gentleness of staff	1	2	3	4	5	NA
301323	Competence of supportive staff	1	2	3	4	5	NA
301314	Responsiveness of staff to emergencies	1	2	3	4	5	NA
301324	Access to needed equipment	1	2	3	4	5	NA
301325	Knowledgeable about equipment	1	2	3	4	5	NA
301315	Supplies and equipment not wasted	1	2	3	4	5	NA

Domain-Health & Life Quality (V)   **Class**-Satisfaction with Care (EE)   *3rd edition 2004; revised 2008, 2024*

OUTCOME CONTENT REFERENCES:

Costa, D. G., Moura, G. M. S. S., Moraes, M. G., Santos, J. L. G., & Magalhães, A. M. M. (2020). Satisfaction attributes related to safety and quality perceived in the experience of hospitalized patients. *Revista Gaúcha de Enfermagem, 41*(esp), e20190152. https://doi.org/10.1590/1983-1447.2020.20190152

Jakobsson, S., Ringström, G., Andersson, E., Eliasson, B., Johannsson, G., Simrén, M., & Ung, E. J. (2019). Patient safety before and after implementing person-centred inpatient care—A quasi-experimental study. *Journal of Clinical Nursing, 28*(3-4), 602–612. https://doi.org/10.1111/jocn.15120

Reyes, P., Puelle, F., & Barria, R. M. (2020). Perception of the quality of physiotherapy care provided to outpatients from primary health care in Chile. *Evaluation & the Health Professions, 43*(1), 16–22. https://doi.org/10.1177/0163278718770711

Roulin, M.-J., Jonniaux, S., Guisado, H., & Séchaud, L. (2020). Perceptions of inpatients and nurses towards the importance of nurses' caring behaviours in rehabilitation: A comparative study. *International Journal of Nursing Practice, 26*(4), e12835. https://doi.org/10.1111/ijn.12835

Usmani, O. S. (2019). Choosing the right inhaler for your asthma or COPD patient. *Therapeutics and Clinical Risk Management, 15*, 461–472. https://doi.org/10.2147/TCRM.S160365

Client Satisfaction: Telehealth Services

3020

Definition: Extent of positive perception of information and care received through telehealth

OUTCOME TARGET RATING: Maintain at_____ Increase to_____

	Not at All Satisfied	Somewhat Satisfied	Moderately Satisfied	Very Satisfied	Completely Satisfied	
OUTCOME OVERALL RATING	1	2	3	4	5	
Indicators:						
302001 Staff introduce self and role	1	2	3	4	5	NA
302002 Courtesy shown by staff	1	2	3	4	5	NA
302003 Compassion shown by staff	1	2	3	4	5	NA
302004 Concern shown for individual needs	1	2	3	4	5	NA
302005 Staff readily available	1	2	3	4	5	NA
302006 Staff respectful of privacy	1	2	3	4	5	NA
302007 Staff knowledge of medical history	1	2	3	4	5	NA
302008 Confidentiality of information maintained	1	2	3	4	5	NA
302009 Staff actively listening to what was said	1	2	3	4	5	NA
302010 Staff comfortable to communicate with	1	2	3	4	5	NA
302011 Staff took time to communicate	1	2	3	4	5	NA
302012 Staff spoke clearly to be heard	1	2	3	4	5	NA
302013 Staff understood feelings	1	2	3	4	5	NA
302014 Personal values were considered	1	2	3	4	5	NA
302015 Personal preferences were considered	1	2	3	4	5	NA
302016 Opportunity provided to express concerns	1	2	3	4	5	NA
302017 Staff offered suggestions to address concerns	1	2	3	4	5	NA
302018 Opportunity provided to ask questions	1	2	3	4	5	NA
302019 Staff offered suggestions to address questions	1	2	3	4	5	NA
302020 Information provided about options for care	1	2	3	4	5	NA
302021 Information provided about cost of care	1	2	3	4	5	NA
302022 Information provided to manage self-care	1	2	3	4	5	NA
302023 Information provided to manage follow-up visits	1	2	3	4	5	NA
302024 Safety issues addressed	1	2	3	4	5	NA
302025 Promptness in responding to inquires	1	2	3	4	5	NA
302026 Staff help to get appointment time to fit schedule	1	2	3	4	5	NA
302027 Staff help to get appointment that accommodates family	1	2	3	4	5	NA
302028 Staff involved family members	1	2	3	4	5	NA
302029 Wait time for getting an appointment	1	2	3	4	5	NA
302030 Wait time for health professional interaction at appointment time	1	2	3	4	5	NA

Domain-Health & Life Quality (V)   *Class*-Satisfaction with Care (EE)   7th edition 2024

OUTCOME CONTENT REFERENCES:
Bushey, M. A., Kroenke, K., Weiner, J., Porter, B., Evans, E., Baye, F., Lourens, S., & Weitlauf, S. (2020). Telecare management of pain and mood symptoms: Adherence, utility, and patient satisfaction. *Journal of Telemedicine and Telecare, 26*(10), 619–626. https://doi.org/10.1177/1357633X19856156

Gentry, M. T., Lapid, M. I., Clark, M. M., & Rummans, T. A. (2019). Evidence for telehealth group-based treatment: A systematic review. *Journal of Telemedicine and Telecare, 25*(6), 327–342. https://doi.org/10.1177/1357633X18775855

Hajesmaeel-Gohari, S., & Bahaadinbeigy, K. (2021). The most used questionnaires for evaluating telemedicine services. *BMC Medical Informatics and Decision Making, 21*(36), 3–11. https://doi.org/10.1186/s12911-021-01407-y

Le, L. B., Rahal, H. K., Viramontes, M. R., Meneses, K. G., Dong, T .S., & Saab, S. (2019). Patient satisfaction and healthcare utilization using telemedicine in liver transplant recipients. *Digestive Diseases and* Sciences, 64(5), 1150–1157. https://doi.org/10.1007/s10620-018-5397-5

Manz, W. J., Goel, R., Fakunle, O. P., Labib, S. A., & Bariteau, J. T. (2021). Feasibility of rapid development and deployment of a telemedicine program in a foot and ankle orthopedic practice. *Foot & Ankle Internationals, 42*(3), 320–328. https://doi.org/10.1177/1071100720963059

+Parmanto, B., Lewis, A. N. Jr., Graham, K. M., & Bertolet, M. H. (2016). Development of the telehealth usability questionnaire (TUQ). *International Journal of Telerehabilitation, 8*(1), 3–10. https://doi.org/10.5195/ijt.2016.6196

Serhal, E., Kirvan, A., Sanches, M., & Crawford, A. (2020). Client satisfaction and experience with telepsychiatry: Development and validation of a survey using clinical quality domains. *Journal of Medical Internet Research, 22*(9), e19198. https://doi.org/10.2196/19198

Slightam, C., Gregory, A. J., Hu, J., Jacobs, J., Gurmessa, T., Kimerling, R., Blonigen, D., & Zulman, D. (2020). Patient perceptions of video visits using Veterans Affairs telehealth tablets: Survey study. *Journal of Medical Internet Research, 22*(4), e15682. https://doi.org/10.2196/15682

Tenforde, A. S., Borgstrom, H., Polich, G., Steere, H., Davis, I. S., Cotton, K., O'Donnell, M., & Silver, J. K. (2020). Outpatient physical, occupational, and speech therapy synchronous telemedicine. *American Journal of Physical Medicine & Rehabilitation, 99*(11), 977–981. https://doi.org/10.1097/PHM.0000000000001571

Wynn, S. T. (2021). Achieving patient satisfaction: Utilizing telehealth via an academic-practice partnership. *Journal of the American Psychiatric Nurses Association, 27*(2), 143–147. https://doi.org/10.1177/1078390320902828

C

Cognition   0900

Definition: Ability to execute complex mental processes

OUTCOME TARGET RATING: Maintain at_____ Increase to_____

OUTCOME OVERALL RATING		Never Demonstrated	Rarely Demonstrated	Sometimes Demonstrated	Often Demonstrated	Consistently Demonstrated	
		1	2	3	4	5	
Indicators:							
090017	Communicates clearly for age	1	2	3	4	5	NA
090018	Communicates appropriately for age	1	2	3	4	5	NA
090019	Comprehends meaning of situations	1	2	3	4	5	NA
090020	Exhibits attentiveness	1	2	3	4	5	NA
090021	Concentrates	1	2	3	4	5	NA
090022	Cognitive orientation	1	2	3	4	5	NA
090023	Exhibits immediate memory	1	2	3	4	5	NA
090024	Exhibits recent memory	1	2	3	4	5	NA
090025	Exhibits remote memory	1	2	3	4	5	NA
090026	Processes information	1	2	3	4	5	NA
090027	Explains similarity between two items	1	2	3	4	5	NA
090028	Alternatives weighed when making decisions	1	2	3	4	5	NA
090029	Makes appropriate decisions	1	2	3	4	5	NA
090030	Exhibits complex calculations skills	1	2	3	4	5	NA
090031	Draws a complex figure	1	2	3	4	5	NA

Domain-*Physiologic Health (II)*   **Class**-*Neurocognitive (J)*   *1st edition 1997; revised 2004, 2008, 2024*

OUTCOME CONTENT REFERENCES:

Ashrafi, F., Taheri, M. S., Farzaneh, A., Behnam, B., & Ahmadi, M. A. (2019). Cognitive functions and white matter lesion on magnetic resonance images in a sample of normal Iranian population with cardiovascular risk factors. *The Neuroradiology Journal, 32*(2), 108–116. https://doi.org/10.1177/1971400919825862

Coelho, J. C. F., Ribeiro, A. R. M., Sampaio, F. M. C., Sequeira, C. A., da C., Fortuño, M., del M. L., & Merino, J. R. (2019). Cultural adaptation and psychometric properties assessment of the NOC outcome "Cognition" in a sample of Portuguese adults with mental illness. *International Journal of Nursing Knowledge, 31*(3), 180–187. https://doi.org/10.1111/2047-3095.12268

Cordell, C. B., Borson, S., Boustani, M., Chodosh, J., Reuben, D., Verghese, J., Thies, W., & Fried, L. B. (2013). Alzheimer's Association recommendations for operationalizing the detection of cognitive impairment during the Medicare annual wellness visit in a primary care setting. *Alzheimer's & Dementia, 9*(5), 141–150. https://doi.org/10.1016/j.jalz.2012.09.011

Fletcher, K. A., Hicks, V. L., Johnson, R. H., Laverentz, D. M., Phillips, C. J., Pierce, L., N. B., Wilhoite, D. L., & Gay, J. E. (2019). A concept analysis of conceptual learning: A guide for educators. *Journal of Nursing Education, 58*(1), 7–15. https://doi.org/10.3928/01484834-201900103-03

Hogan-Quigley, B., Palm, M. L., & Bickley, L. (2021). *Bates nursing guide to physical examination and history taking* (3rd ed.). Wolters Kluwer.

Norris, D. (2017). Short-term memory and long-term memory are still different. *Psychological Bulletin, 143*(9), 992–1009. https://doi.org/10.1037/bul0000108

Őnal, G., & Huri, M. (2021). Cognitive functions of children with brain tumor in the treatment process. *British Journal of Occupational Therapy, 84*(3), 164–172. https://doi.org/10.1177/0308022620941396

Shin, J. (2020). A meta-analysis of the relationship between working memory and second language reading comprehension: Does task type matter? *Applied Psycholinguistics, 41*(4), 873–900. https://doi.org/10.1017/S0142716420000272

Cognitive Orientation 0901

Definition: Ability to identify person, place, and time accurately

OUTCOME TARGET RATING: Maintain at_____ Increase to_____

	Never Demonstrated	Rarely Demonstrated	Sometimes Demonstrated	Often Demonstrated	Consistently Demonstrated	
OUTCOME OVERALL RATING	1	2	3	4	5	
Indicators:						
090110 Identifies self	1	2	3	4	5	NA
090111 Identifies significant other	1	2	3	4	5	NA
090112 Identifies current place	1	2	3	4	5	NA
090113 Identifies correct day	1	2	3	4	5	NA
090114 Identifies correct month	1	2	3	4	5	NA
090115 Identifies correct year	1	2	3	4	5	NA
090116 Identifies correct season	1	2	3	4	5	NA
090117 Identifies current leader of the country	1	2	3	4	5	NA
090118 Identifies significant current events	1	2	3	4	5	NA

Domain-*Physiologic Health (II)*   **Class**-*Neurocognitive (J)*   *1st edition 1997; reviewed 2018; revised 2004, 2024*

OUTCOME CONTENT REFERENCES:

+Folstein, M., Folstein S., & McHugh, P. (1975). "Mini-mental state": A practical method for grading the cognitive state of patients for the clinician. *Journal of Psychiatric Research, 12*(3), 189–198. https://doi.org/10.1016/0022-3956(75)90026-6

Ichii, S., Nakamura, T., Kawarabayashi, T., Takatama, M., Ohgami, T., Ihara, K., & Shoji, M. (2019). CogEvo, a cognitive function balancer, is a sensitive and easy psychiatric test battery for age-related cognitive decline. *Geriatrics & Gerontology International, 20*(3), 248–255. https://doi.org/10.1111/ggi.13847

+Jórgensen, K., Nielsen, T. R., Nielsen, A., Walldorf, F. B., & Waldemar, G. (2019). Brief assessment of impaired cognition questionnaire (BASIC-Q)—Development and validation of a new tool for identification of cognitive impairment in community settings. *International Journal of Geriatric Psychiatry, 35*(7), 693–701. https://doi.org/10.1002/gps.5286

McKay, A., Love, J., Trevena-Peters, J., Gracey, J., & Ponsford, J. (2020). The relationship between agitation and impairments of orientation and memory during the PTA period after traumatic brain injury. *Neuropsychological Rehabilitation, 30*(4), 579–590. https://doi.org/10.1080/09602011.2018.1479276

Mitchell, A. J. (2017). The mini-mental state examination (MMSE): Update on its diagnostic accuracy and clinical utility for cognitive disorders. In A. J. Larner (Ed.), *Cognitive screening instruments: A practical approach* (2nd ed., pp. 37–48). Springer International.

Muniz-Terrera, G., Robitaille, A., Goerdten, J., Massa, F., & Johansson, B. (2021). Do I lose cognitive function as fast as my twin partner? Analyses based on classes of MMSE trajectories of twins aged 80 and older. *Age and Aging, 50*(3), 847–853. https://doi.org/10.1093/ageing/afaa239

Oh, E. S., Rosenberg, P. B., Rattinger, G. B., Stuart, E. A., Lyketson, C. G., & Leoutsakos, J. M. S. (2021). Psychotropic medication and cognitive, functional, and neuropsychiatric outcomes in Alzheimer's disease (AD). *Journal of the American Geriatrics Society, 69*(4), 955–963. https://doi.org/10.1111/jgs.16970

Van Steenwinkel, I., Van Audenhove. C., & Heylighen. A. (2019). Offering architects insights into experiences of living with dementia: A case study on orientation in space, time, and identity. *Dementia, 18*(2), 742–756. https://doi.org/10.1177/1471301217692905

Comfort Status 2008

Definition: Overall physical, psychospiritual, sociocultural, and environmental ease and safety of an individual

OUTCOME TARGET RATING: Maintain at_____ Increase to_____

	Severely Compromised	Substantially Compromised	Moderately Compromised	Mildly Compromised	Not Compromised	
OUTCOME OVERALL RATING	1	2	3	4	5	
Indicators:						
200801 Physical well-being	1	2	3	4	5	NA
200802 Symptom control	1	2	3	4	5	NA
200803 Psychological well-being	1	2	3	4	5	NA
200804 Physical surroundings	1	2	3	4	5	NA
200805 Room temperature	1	2	3	4	5	NA
200813 Noise level	1	2	3	4	5	NA
200814 Privacy	1	2	3	4	5	NA

Continued

C

Comfort Status—cont'd

		Severely Compromised	Substantially Compromised	Moderately Compromised	Mildly Compromised	Not Compromised	
200806	Social support from family	1	2	3	4	5	NA
200807	Social support from friends	1	2	3	4	5	NA
200808	Social relationships	1	2	3	4	5	NA
200809	Spiritual life	1	2	3	4	5	NA
200810	Care consistent with cultural beliefs	1	2	3	4	5	NA
200811	Care consistent with needs	1	2	3	4	5	NA
200812	Ability to communicate needs	1	2	3	4	5	NA

Domain-Health & Life Quality (V)   **Class**-Perceived Health & Life Situation (U)   4th edition 2008; revised 2024

OUTCOME CONTENT REFERENCES:

Aksoy Derya, Y., & Pasinlioğlu, T. (2017). The effect of nursing care based on comfort theory on women's postpartum comfort levels after caesarean sections. *International Journal of Nursing Knowledge, 28*(3), 138–144. https://doi.org/10.1111/2047-3095.12122

Bice, A. A., Hall, J., & Devereaux, M. J. (2018). Exploring holistic comfort in children who experience a clinical venipuncture procedure. *Journal of Holistic Nursing, 36*(2), 108–122. https://doi.org/10.1177/0898010117692719

Ignatavicius, D. D., Workman, M. L., Rebar, C. R., & Heimgartner, N. M. (2021). *Medical-surgical nursing: Concepts for interprofessional care* (10th ed.). Elsevier.

Kolcaba, K. (2003). *Comfort theory and practice: A vision for holistic health care and research.* Springer.

Kolcaba, K., & Crawford, C. L. (2020). Comfort. In S. J. Peterson & T. S. Bredow, *Middle range theories: Application to nursing research and practice.* (pp. 196–207). Wolters Kluwer.

Krinsky, R., Murillo, I., & Johnson, J. (2014). A practical application of Katharine Kolcaba's Comfort Theory to cardiac patients. *Applied Nursing Research, 27*(2), 147–150. https://doi.org/10.1016/j.apnr.2014.02.004

Lafond, D. A., Bowling, S., Fortkiewicz, J. M., Reggio, C., & Hinds, P. S. (2019). Integrating the Comfort Theory™ into pediatric primary palliative care to improve access to care. *Journal of Hospice & Palliative Nursing, 21*(5), 382–389. https://doi.org/10.1097/NJH.0000000000000538

Sharma, M. C., & Kalia, R. (2021). Testing Katharine Kolcaba Theory of Comfort: Effectiveness of integrative comfort care interventions on discomfort experienced by children (aged 5–10 years) during postoperative period. *Journal of Pediatric Surgical Nursing, 10*(4), 168–175. https://doi.org/10.1097/JPS.0000000000000320

Vicdan, A. K. (2020). The effect of training given to hemodialysis patients according to the Comfort Theory. *Clinical Nurse Specialist: The Journal for Advanced Nursing Practice, 34*(1), 30–37. https://doi.org/10.1097/NUR.0000000000000495

Wensley, C., Botti, M., McKillop, A., & Merry, A. F. (2017). A framework of comfort for practice: An integrative review identifying the multiple influences on patients' experience of comfort in healthcare settings. *International Journal of Quality Health Care, 29*(2), 151–162. https://doi.org/10.1093/intqhc/mzw158

Comfort Status: Environment

2009

Definition: Environmental ease, comfort, and safety of surroundings

OUTCOME TARGET RATING: Maintain at_____ Increase to_____

		Severely Compromised	Substantially Compromised	Moderately Compromised	Mildly Compromised	Not Compromised	
OUTCOME OVERALL RATING		1	2	3	4	5	
Indicators:							
200901	Needed supplies and equipment within reach	1	2	3	4	5	NA
200902	Room temperature	1	2	3	4	5	NA
200918	Room humidity	1	2	3	4	5	NA
200903	Environment conducive to sleep	1	2	3	4	5	NA
200904	Contentment with physical surroundings	1	2	3	4	5	NA
200905	Orderliness of environment	1	2	3	4	5	NA
200906	Cleanliness of environment	1	2	3	4	5	NA
200907	Floor free of clutter	1	2	3	4	5	NA
200908	Safety devices used appropriately	1	2	3	4	5	NA

C

Comfort Status: Environment—cont'd

		Severely Compromised	Substantially Compromised	Moderately Compromised	Mildly Compromised	Not Compromised	
200909	Room lighting	1	2	3	4	5	NA
200910	Privacy	1	2	3	4	5	NA
200911	Availability of space for visitors	1	2	3	4	5	NA
200912	Comfortable bed	1	2	3	4	5	NA
200913	Comfortable furniture	1	2	3	4	5	NA
200914	Needed environmental adaptations	1	2	3	4	5	NA
200915	Peaceful environment	1	2	3	4	5	NA
200916	Control of noise	1	2	3	4	5	NA
200917	Control of odors	1	2	3	4	5	NA
200919	Control of electronic alarms	1	2	3	4	5	NA

Domain-Health & Life Quality (V)   *Class*-Perceived Health & Life Situation (U)   4th edition 2008; revised 2024

OUTCOME CONTENT REFERENCES:

Aksoy Derya, Y., & Pasinlioğlu, T. (2017). The effect of nursing care based on comfort theory on women's postpartum comfort levels after caesarean sections. *International Journal of Nursing Knowledge, 28*(3), 138–144. https://doi.org/10.1111/2047-3095.12122

Ignatavicius, D. D., Workman, M. L., Rebar, C. R., & Heimgartner, N. M. (2021). *Medical-surgical nursing: Concepts for interprofessional care* (10th ed.). Elsevier.

Kolcaba, K. (2003). *Comfort theory and practice: A vision for holistic health care and research*. Springer.

Kolcaba, K., & Crawford, C. L. (2020). Comfort. In S. J. Peterson & T. S. Bredow. *Middle range theories: Application to nursing research and practice*. (pp. 189–207). Wolkers Kluwer.

Lafond, D. A., Bowling, S., Fortkiewicz, J. M., Reggio, C., & Hinds, P. S. (2019). Integrating the Comfort Theory™ into pediatric primary palliative care to improve access to care. *Journal of Hospice & Palliative Nursing, 21*(5), 382–389. https://doi.org/10.1097/NJH.0000000000000538

Sharma, M. C., & Kalia, R. (2021). Testing Katharine Kolcaba Theory of Comfort: Effectiveness of integrative comfort care interventions on discomfort experienced by children (aged 5–10 years) during postoperative period. *Journal of Pediatric Surgical Nursing, 10*(4), 168–175. https://doi.org/10.1097/JPS.0000000000000320

Wensley, C., Botti, M., McKillop, A., & Merry, A. F. (2017). A framework of comfort for practice: An integrative review identifying the multiple influences on patients' experience of comfort in healthcare settings. *International Journal of Quality Health Care, 29*(2), 151–162. https://doi.org/10.1093/intqhc/mzw158

Comfort Status: Physical   2010

Definition: Physical ease related to bodily sensations and homeostatic mechanisms

OUTCOME TARGET RATING: Maintain at_____ Increase to_____

		Severely Compromised	Substantially Compromised	Moderately Compromised	Mildly Compromised	Not Compromised	
OUTCOME OVERALL RATING		1	2	3	4	5	
Indicators:							
201001	Symptom control	1	2	3	4	5	NA
201002	Physical well-being	1	2	3	4	5	NA
201003	Muscular relaxation	1	2	3	4	5	NA
201004	Comfortable position	1	2	3	4	5	NA
201005	Comfortable clothing	1	2	3	4	5	NA
201006	Personal grooming and hygiene	1	2	3	4	5	NA
201007	Food intake	1	2	3	4	5	NA
201008	Fluid intake	1	2	3	4	5	NA
201009	Energy level	1	2	3	4	5	NA
201010	Body temperature	1	2	3	4	5	NA
201011	Airway patency	1	2	3	4	5	NA
201012	Oxygen saturation	1	2	3	4	5	NA

Continued

Comfort Status: Physical—cont'd

		Severe	Substantial	Moderate	Mild	None	
201013	Itching	1	2	3	4	5	NA
201014	Labored breathing	1	2	3	4	5	NA
201016	Restless legs syndrome	1	2	3	4	5	NA
201017	Muscle aches	1	2	3	4	5	NA
201018	Headache	1	2	3	4	5	NA
201025	Pain	1	2	3	4	5	NA
201019	Nausea	1	2	3	4	5	NA
201020	Vomiting	1	2	3	4	5	NA
201021	Urinary incontinence	1	2	3	4	5	NA
201022	Bowel incontinence	1	2	3	4	5	NA
201023	Diarrhea	1	2	3	4	5	NA
201024	Constipation	1	2	3	4	5	NA

Domain-Health & Life Quality (V) **Class**-Perceived Health & Life Situation (U) 4th edition 2008; revised 2024

OUTCOME CONTENT REFERENCES:

Aksoy Derya, Y., & Pasinlioğlu, T. (2017). The effect of nursing care based on comfort theory on women's postpartum comfort levels after caesarean sections. *International Journal of Nursing Knowledge, 28*(3), 138–144. https://doi.org/10.1111/2047-3095.12122

Bice, A. A., Hall, J., & Devereaux, M. J. (2018). Exploring holistic comfort in children who experience a clinical venipuncture procedure. *Journal of Holistic Nursing, 36*(2), 108–122. https://doi.org/10.1177/0898010117692719

Bice, A. A., & Wyatt, T. H. (2016). Holistic comfort interventions for pediatric nursing procedures: A systematic review. *Journal of Holistic Nursing, 35*(3), 280–295. https://doi.org/10.1177/0898010116660397

Ignatavicius, D. D., Workman, M. L., Rebar, C. R., & Heimgartner, N. M. (2021). *Medical-surgical nursing: Concepts for interprofessional care* (10th ed.). Elsevier.

Kolcaba, K. (2003). *Comfort theory and practice: A vision for holistic health care and research.* Springer.

Kolcaba, K., & Crawford, C. L. (2020). Comfort. In S. J. Peterson & T. S. Bredow, *Middle range theories: Application to nursing research and practice.* (pp. 189–207). Wolters Kluwer.

Kolcaba, K., Dowd, T., Steiner, R., & Mitzel, A. (2004). Efficacy of hand massage for enhancing the comfort of hospice patients, *Journal of Hospice and Palliative Nursing, 6*(2), 91–102. https://doi.org/10.1097/00129191-200404000-00012

Krinsky, R., Murillo, I., & Johnson, J. (2014). A practical application of Katharine Kolcaba's Comfort Theory to cardiac patients. *Applied Nursing Research, 27*(2), 147–150. https://doi.org/10.1016/j.apnr.2014.02.004

Lafond, D. A., Bowling, S., Fortkiewicz, J. M., Reggio, C., & Hinds, P. S. (2019). Integrating the Comfort Theory™ into pediatric primary palliative care to improve access to care. *Journal of Hospice & Palliative Nursing, 21*(5), 382–389. https://doi.org/10.1097/NJH.0000000000000538

Sharma, M. C., & Kalia, R. (2021). Testing Katharine Kolcaba Theory of Comfort: Effectiveness of integrative comfort care interventions on discomfort experienced by children (aged 5–10 years) during postoperative period. *Journal of Pediatric Surgical Nursing, 10*(4), 168–175. https://doi.org/10.1097/JPS.0000000000000320

Wensley, C., Botti, M., McKillop, A., & Merry, A. F. (2017). A framework of comfort for practice: An integrative review identifying the multiple influences on patients' experience of comfort in healthcare settings. *International Journal of Quality Health Care, 29*(2), 151–162. https://do.org/:10.1093/intqhc/mzw158

Comfort Status: Psychospiritual

2011

Definition: Psychospiritual ease related to self-concept, emotional well-being, source of inspiration, and meaning and purpose in one's life

OUTCOME TARGET RATING: Maintain at_____ Increase to_____

		Severely Compromised	Substantially Compromised	Moderately Compromised	Mildly Compromised	Not Compromised	
OUTCOME OVERALL RATING		1	2	3	4	5	
Indicators:							
201101	Psychological well-being	1	2	3	4	5	NA
201102	Faith	1	2	3	4	5	NA
201103	Hope	1	2	3	4	5	NA
201104	Self-concept	1	2	3	4	5	NA
201119	Self-esteem	1	2	3	4	5	NA
201105	Internal picture of self	1	2	3	4	5	NA
201106	Calm and tranquil affect	1	2	3	4	5	NA
201107	Expressions of optimism	1	2	3	4	5	NA

Comfort Status: Psychospiritual—cont'd

		Severely Compromised	Substantially Compromised	Moderately Compromised	Mildly Compromised	Not Compromised	
201108	Goal setting	1	2	3	4	5	NA
201109	Meaning and purpose in life	1	2	3	4	5	NA
201110	Spiritual contentment	1	2	3	4	5	NA
201111	Connectedness with inner self	1	2	3	4	5	NA
		Severe	**Substantial**	**Moderate**	**Mild**	**None**	
201112	Depression	1	2	3	4	5	NA
201113	Anxiety	1	2	3	4	5	NA
201114	Stress	1	2	3	4	5	NA
201115	Fear	1	2	3	4	5	NA
201116	Loss of faith	1	2	3	4	5	NA
201117	Sense of spiritual abandonment	1	2	3	4	5	NA
201118	Suicidal thoughts	1	2	3	4	5	NA

Domain-*Health & Life Quality (V)*   **Class**-*Perceived Health & Life Situation (U)*   *4th edition 2008; revised 2024*

OUTCOME CONTENT REFERENCES:

Aksoy Derya, Y., & Pasinlioğlu, T. (2017). The effect of nursing care based on comfort theory on women's postpartum comfort levels after caesarean sections. *International Journal of Nursing Knowledge, 28*(3), 138–144. https://doi.org/10.1111/2047-3095.12122

Ignatavicius, D. D., Workman, M. L., Rebar, C. R., & Heimgartner, N. M. (2021). *Medical-surgical nursing: Concepts for interprofessional care* (10th ed.). Elsevier.

Kolcaba, K. (2003). *Comfort theory and practice: A vision for holistic health care and research*. Springer.

Kolcaba, K., & Crawford, C. L. (2020). Comfort. In S. J. Peterson & T. S. Bredow (Eds.), *Middle range theories: Application to nursing research and practice*. (pp.189–207). Wolters Kluwer.

Lafond, D. A., Bowling, S., Fortkiewicz, J. M., Reggio, C., & Hinds, P. S. (2019). Integrating the Comfort Theory™ into pediatric primary palliative care to improve access to care. *Journal of Hospice & Palliative Nursing, 21*(5), 382–389. https://doi.org/10.1097/NJH.0000000000000538

Sharma, M. C., & Kalia, R. (2021). Testing Katharine Kolcaba Theory of Comfort: Effectiveness of integrative comfort care interventions on discomfort experienced by children (aged 5–10 years) during postoperative period. *Journal of Pediatric Surgical Nursing, 10*(4), 168–175. https://doi.org/10.1097/JPS.0000000000000320

Wensley, C., Botti, M., McKillop, A., & Merry, A. F. (2017). A framework of comfort for practice: An integrative review identifying the multiple influences on patients' experience of comfort in healthcare settings. *International Journal of Quality Health Care, 29*(2), 151–162. https://doi.org/10.1093/intqhc/mzw158

Comfort Status: Sociocultural   2012

Definition: Social ease related to interpersonal, family, and societal relationships within a cultural context

OUTCOME TARGET RATING: Maintain at_____ Increase to_____

		Severely Compromised	Substantially Compromised	Moderately Compromised	Mildly Compromised	Not Compromised	
OUTCOME OVERALL RATING		1	2	3	4	5	
Indicators:							
201201	Social support from family	1	2	3	4	5	NA
201202	Social support from friends	1	2	3	4	5	NA
201203	Relationships with family	1	2	3	4	5	NA
201204	Relationships with friends	1	2	3	4	5	NA
201205	Trust in relationships with family	1	2	3	4	5	NA
201206	Trust in relationships with friends	1	2	3	4	5	NA
201207	Social interactions with others	1	2	3	4	5	NA
201216	Participation of family in decision-making	1	2	3	4	5	NA
201208	Care consistent with cultural beliefs	1	2	3	4	5	NA
201209	Availability of culture-specific foods	1	2	3	4	5	NA
201210	Incorporation of cultural beliefs into daily activities	1	2	3	4	5	NA
201211	Use of spoken language	1	2	3	4	5	NA
201212	Ability to communicate needs	1	2	3	4	5	NA

Continued

Comfort Status: Sociocultural—cont'd

		Severely Compromised	Substantially Compromised	Moderately Compromised	Mildly Compromised	Not Compromised	
201213	Use of strategies to enhance communication	1	2	3	4	5	NA
201214	Willingness to call on others for help	1	2	3	4	5	NA
201215	Use of disclosure	1	2	3	4	5	NA

Domain-Health & Life Quality (V) **Class**-Perceived Health & Life Situation (U) 4th edition 2008; revised 2024

OUTCOME CONTENT REFERENCES:

Aksoy Derya, Y., & Pasinlioğlu, T. (2017). The effect of nursing care based on comfort theory on women's postpartum comfort levels after caesarean sections. *International Journal of Nursing Knowledge, 28*(3), 138–144. https://doi.org/10.1111/2047-3095.12122

Kolcaba, K. (2003). *Comfort theory and practice: A vision for holistic health care and research.* Springer.

Kolcaba, K., & Crawford, C. L. (2020). Comfort. In S. J. Peterson & T. S. Bredow, *Middle range theories: Application to nursing research and practice.* (pp. 189–207). Wolters Kluwer.

Lafond, D. A., Bowling, S., Fortkiewicz, J. M., Reggio, C., & Hinds, P. S. (2019). Integrating the Comfort Theory™ into pediatric primary palliative care to improve access to care. *Journal of Hospice & Palliative Nursing, 21*(5), 382–389. https://doi.org/10.1097/NJH.0000000000000538

Sharma, M. C., & Kalia, R. (2021). Testing Katharine Kolcaba Theory of Comfort: Effectiveness of integrative comfort care interventions on discomfort experienced by children (aged 5–10 years) during postoperative period. *Journal of Pediatric Surgical Nursing, 10*(4), 168–175. https://doi.org/10.1097/JPS.0000000000000320

Wensley, C., Botti, M., McKillop, A., & Merry, A. F. (2017). A framework of comfort for practice: An integrative review identifying the multiple influences on patients' experience of comfort in healthcare settings. *International Journal of Quality Health Care, 29*(2), 151–162. https://doi.org/10.1093/intqhc/mzw158

Communication

0902

Definition: Ability to receive, interpret, and express spoken, written, and non-verbal messages

OUTCOME TARGET RATING: Maintain at_____ Increase to_____

		Severely Compromised	Substantially Compromised	Sometimes Compromised	Often Compromised	Consistently Compromised	
OUTCOME OVERALL RATING		1	2	3	4	5	
Indicators:							
090201	Use of written language	1	2	3	4	5	NA
090217	Use of text-messaging	1	2	3	4	5	NA
090202	Use of spoken language	1	2	3	4	5	NA
090203	Use of pictures and drawings	1	2	3	4	5	NA
090204	Use of sign language	1	2	3	4	5	NA
090215	Use of mouth and sign language synchronization	1	2	3	4	5	NA
090205	Use of non-verbal language	1	2	3	4	5	NA
090216	Use of enhanced gestures	1	2	3	4	5	NA
090214	Use of empathic online communication	1	2	3	4	5	NA
090211	Use of alternative communication device	1	2	3	4	5	NA
090212	Use of augmentative communication device	1	2	3	4	5	NA
090206	Acknowledgement of messages received	1	2	3	4	5	NA
090210	Accurate interpretation of messages	1	2	3	4	5	NA
090207	Directs message to correct recipient	1	2	3	4	5	NA
090208	Exchanges messages accurately with others	1	2	3	4	5	NA
090213	Environment receptive to communication	1	2	3	4	5	NA

Domain-Physiologic Health (II) **Class**-Neurocognitive (J) 1st edition 1997; revised 2004, 2018, 2024

C

OUTCOME CONTENT REFERENCES:
Chazin, K. T., Ledford, J. R., & Pak, N. S. (2021). A systematic review of augmented input interventions and exploratory analysis of moderators. *American Journal of Speech-Language Pathology, 30*(3), 1210–1223. https://doi.org/10.1044/2020_AJSLP-20-00102

Han, J. Y., Kim, E., Lee, Y., Shah, D. V., & Gustafson, D. (2019). A longitudinal investigation of empathic exchanges in online cancer support groups: Message reception and expression effects on patients' psychosocial health outcomes. *Journal of Health Communications, 24*(6), 615–623. https://doi.org/10.1080/10810730.2019.1644401

Krause, J. C., & Hague, A. K. (2020). Signing exact English transliteration: Effects of accuracy and lag time on message intelligibility. *The Journal of Deaf Studies and Deaf Education, 25*(2), 199–211. https://doi.org/10.1093/deafed/enz042

Quick, N., Erickson, K., & Mccright, J. (2019). The most frequently used words: Comparing child-directed speech and young children's speech to inform vocabulary selection for aided input. *Augmentative and Alternative Communication, 35*(2), 120–131. https://doi.org/10.1080/07434618.2019.1576225

Roberts, M. Y., Curtis, P. R., Sone, B. J., & Hampton, L. H. (2019). Association of parent training with child language development: A systematic review and meta-analysis. *JAMA Pediatrics, 173*(7), 671–680. https://doi.org/10.1001/jamapediatrics.2019.1197

Shuter, J., Rosander, C., Kim, R. S., & Brownstein, J. S. (2019). Passenger or patient? The automobile: A new frontier in health promotion. *Health Promotion Practice, 20*(3), 328–332. https://doi.org/10.1177/1524839919830653

Sparrow, K., Lind, C., & van Steenbrugge, W. (2020). Gesture, communication, and adult acquired hearing loss. *Journal of Communication Disorders, 87*, 1–14. https://doi.org/10.1016/j.jcomdis.2020.106030

Thiessen, A., Brown, J., Freeland, T., & Brewer, C. H. (2019). Identification and expression of themes depicted in visual scene and grid displays by adults with traumatic brain injury. *American Journal of Speech-Language Pathology, 28*(2), 664–675. https://doi.org/10.1044/2018_AJSLP-18-0086

Tsinivits, D., & Unsworth, S. (2021). The impact of older siblings on the language environment and language development of bilingual toddlers. *Applied Psycholinguistics, 42*(2), 325–344. https://doi.org/10.1017/S0142716420000570

Communication: Expressive   **0903**

Definition: Ability to express meaningful verbal and/or non-verbal messages

OUTCOME TARGET RATING: Maintain at_____ Increase to_____

	Severely Compromised	Substantially Compromised	Moderately Compromised	Mildly Compromised	Not Compromised	
OUTCOME OVERALL RATING	**1**	**2**	**3**	**4**	**5**	
Indicators:						
090301 Use of written language	1	2	3	4	5	NA
090302 Use of spoken language: vocal	1	2	3	4	5	NA
090303 Use of spoken language: esophageal	1	2	3	4	5	NA
090305 Use of pictures and drawings	1	2	3	4	5	NA
090311 Use of online communication	1	2	3	4	5	NA
090306 Use of sign language	1	2	3	4	5	NA
090312 Use of mouth and sign language synchronization	1	2	3	4	5	NA
090307 Use of non-verbal language	1	2	3	4	5	NA
090313 Use of enhanced gestures	1	2	3	4	5	NA
090314 Use of text-messaging	1	2	3	4	5	NA
090310 Use of alternative communication device	1	2	3	4	5	NA
090304 Clarity of message	1	2	3	4	5	NA
090308 Directs messages to correct recipient	1	2	3	4	5	NA
090315 Respect in expression	1	2	3	4	5	NA
090316 Empathy in expression	1	2	3	4	5	NA

Domain-Physiologic Health (II)   *Class*-Neurocognitive (J)   *1st edition 1997; revised 2004, 2018, 2024*

OUTCOME CONTENT REFERENCES:

Braillon, A., & Taiebi, F. (2020). Practicing "reflective listening" is a mandatory prerequisite for empathy. *Patient Education and Counseling, 103*(9), 1866–1867. https://doi.org/10.1016/j.pec.2020.03.024

Burkitt, E., Watling, D., & Message, H. (2019). Expressivity in children's drawings of themselves for adult audiences with varied authority and familiarity. *British Journal of Developmental Psychology, 37*(3), 354–368. https:doi.org/10.1111/bjdp.12278

Han, J. Y., Kim, E., Lee, Y., Shah, D. V., & Gustafson, D. (2019). A longitudinal investigation of empathic exchanges in online cancer support groups: Message reception and expression effects on patients' psychosocial health outcomes. *Journal of Health Communications, 24*(6), 615–623. https://doi.org/10.1080/10810730.2019.1644401

Krause, J. C., & Hague, A. K. (2020). Signing exact English transliteration: Effects of accuracy and lag time on message intelligibility. *The Journal of Deaf Studies and Deaf Education, 25*(2), 199–211. https://doi.org/10.1093/deafed/enz042

Pearson, E., Wilde, L., Heald, M., Royston, R., & Oliver, C. (2019). Communication in angelman syndrome: A scoping review. *Developmental Medicine & Child Neurology, 61*(11), 1266–1274. https://doi.org/10.1111/dmcn.14257

Richardson, L., McCoy, A., & McNaughton, D. (2019). "He's worth the extra work": The employment experiences of adults with ASD who use augmentative and alternative communication (AAC) as reported by adults with ASD, family members, and employers. *Work, 62*(2), 205–219. https://doi.org/10.3233/WOR-192856

Shuter, J., Rosander, C., Kim, R. S., & Brownstein, J. S. (2019). Passenger or patient? The automobile: A new frontier in health promotion. *Health Promotion Practice, 20*(3), 328–332. https://doi.org/10.1177/1524839919830653

Sparrow, K., Lind, C., & van Steenbrugge, W. (2020). Gesture, communication, and adult acquired hearing loss. *Journal of Communication Disorders, 87*, 1–14. https://doi.org/10.1016/j.jcomdis.2020.106030

Sutton, A., Trudeau, N., Morford, J. P., & Smith, M. M. (2021). Expressive and receptive use of speech and graphic symbols by typically developing children: What skills contribute to performance on structured sentence-level tasks? *International Journal of Speech-Language Pathology, 23*(2), 155–167. https://doi.org/10.1080/17549507.2020.1756406

Thiessen, A., Brown, J., Freeland, T., & Brewer, C. H. (2019). Identification and expression of themes depicted in visual scene and grid displays by adults with traumatic brain injury. *American Journal of Speech-Language Pathology, 28*(2), 664–675. https://doi.org/10.1044/2018_AJSLP-18-0086

Communication: Receptive 0904

Definition: Ability to receive and interpret verbal and/or non-verbal messages

OUTCOME TARGET RATING: Maintain at_____ Increase to_____

		Severely Compromised	Substantially Compromised	Moderately Compromised	Mildly Compromised	Not Compromised	
OUTCOME OVERALL RATING		1	2	3	4	5	
Indicators:							
090401	Interpretation of written language	1	2	3	4	5	NA
090402	Interpretation of spoken language	1	2	3	4	5	NA
090403	Interpretation of pictures and drawings	1	2	3	4	5	NA
090404	Interpretation of sign language	1	2	3	4	5	NA
090410	Interpretation of text messages	1	2	3	4	5	NA
090411	Interpretation of online exchanges	1	2	3	4	5	NA
090405	Interpretation of non-verbal language	1	2	3	4	5	NA
090408	Use of augmentative communication device	1	2	3	4	5	NA
090409	Environment conducive to reception of communication	1	2	3	4	5	NA
090406	Acknowledgement of messages received	1	2	3	4	5	NA

Domain-*Physiologic Health (II)*   **Class**-*Neurocognitive (J)*   *1st edition 1997; revised 2000, 2004, 2018, 2024*

OUTCOME CONTENT REFERENCES:

Chazin, K. T., Ledford, J. R., & Pak, N. S. (2021). A systematic review of augmented input interventions and exploratory analysis of moderators. *American Journal of Speech-Language Pathology, 30*(3), 1210–1223. https://doi.org/10.1044/2020_AJSLP-20-00102

Han, J. Y., Kim, E., Lee, Y., Shah, D. V., & Gustafson, D. (2019). A longitudinal investigation of empathic exchanges in online cancer support groups: Message reception and expression effects on patients' psychosocial health outcomes. *Journal of Health Communications, 24*(6), 615–623. https://doi.org/10.1080/10810730.2019.1644401

Krause, J. C., & Hague, A. K. (2020). Signing exact English transliteration: Effects of accuracy and lag time on message intelligibility. *The Journal of Deaf Studies and Deaf Education, 25*(2), 199–211. https://doi.org/10.1093/deafed/enz042

Quick, N., Erickson, K., & Mccright, J. (2019). The most frequently used words: Comparing child-directed speech and young children's speech to inform vocabulary selection for aided input. *Augmentative and Alternative Communication, 35*(2), 120–131. https://doi.org/10.1080/07434618.2019.1576225

C

Roberts, M. Y., Curtis, P. R., Sone, B. J., & Hampton, L. H. (2019). Association of parent training with child language development A systematic review and meta-analysis. *JAMA Pediatrics, 173*(7), 671–680. https://doi.org/10.1001/jamapediatrics.2019.1197

Shuter, J., Rosander, C., Kim, R. S., Brownstein, J. S. (2019). Passenger or patient? The automobile: A new frontier in health promotion. *Health Promotion Practice, 20*(3), 328–332. https://doi.org/10.1177/1524839919830653

Thiessen, A., Brown, J., Freeland, T., & Brewer, C. H. (2019). Identification and expression of themes depicted in visual scene and grid displays by adults with traumatic brain injury. *American Journal of Speech-Language Pathology, 28*(2), 664–675. https://doi.org/10.1044/2018_AJSLP-18-0086

Tsinivits, D., & Unsworth, S. (2021). The impact of older siblings on the language environment and language development of bilingual toddlers. *Applied Psycholinguistics, 42*(2), 325–344. https://doi.org/10.1017/S0142716420000570

C

Community Competence 2700

Definition: Capacity of a community to use social capital to collectively problem-solve to achieve community goals

OUTCOME TARGET RATING: Maintain at_____ Increase to_____

		Poor	Fair	Good	Very Good	Excellent	
OUTCOME OVERALL RATING		1	2	3	4	5	
Indicators:							
270001	Participation rates in community activities	1	2	3	4	5	NA
270003	Consideration of common and competing interests among groups when solving problems	1	2	3	4	5	NA
270004	Representation of all segments of the community in problem-solving	1	2	3	4	5	NA
270005	Community issues articulated in media	1	2	3	4	5	NA
270006	Community issues articulated in community forums	1	2	3	4	5	NA
270007	Focus on community versus individual agendas	1	2	3	4	5	NA
270021	Collaboration among community groups to resolve problems	1	2	3	4	5	NA
270009	Consensus on goals and priorities	1	2	3	4	5	NA
270010	Consensus on actions to implement goals	1	2	3	4	5	NA
270011	Communication among members and groups	1	2	3	4	5	NA
270022	Level of social capital among members	1	2	3	4	5	NA
270023	Level of social capital among groups in the community	1	2	3	4	5	NA
270012	Effective use of conflict management strategies	1	2	3	4	5	NA
270013	Procurement of resources	1	2	3	4	5	NA
270014	Use of external resources to meet goals	1	2	3	4	5	NA
270015	Flexibility of structures and processes that guide community decision-making	1	2	3	4	5	NA
270016	Participation rate in local government elections	1	2	3	4	5	NA
270017	Participation rate in school elections	1	2	3	4	5	NA
270018	Members attendance at community forums	1	2	3	4	5	NA
270019	Attainment of community goals	1	2	3	4	5	NA

Domain-Community Health (VII)   **Class**-Community Well-Being (BB)   2nd edition 2000; revised 2004, 2008, 2024

OUTCOME CONTENT REFERENCES:

Carroll, L. D., Wetherill, M. S., Teasdale, T. A., & Salvatore, A. L. (2021). Community health improvement plans. *Journal of Public Health Management and Practice, 28*(1), e291–298. https://doi.org/10.1097/PHH.0000000000001279

Castle, B., Wendel, M., Kelly Pryor, B. N., & Ingram, M. (2017). Assessing community leadership: Understanding community capacity for health improvement. *Journal of Public Health Management and Practice, 23*(Suppl 4), S47–S52. https://doi.org/10.1097/PHH.0000000000000587

García, A. A., West Ohueri, C., & Garay, R., Guzmán, M., Hanson, K., Vasquez, M., Zunñiga, J., & Tierney, W. (2021). Community engagement as a foundation for improving neighborhood health. *Public Health Nursing, 38*(2), 223–231. https://doi.org/10.1111/phn.12870

Lee, S., & Jung, M. (2018). Social capital, community capacity, and health. *The Health Care Manager, 37*(4), 290–298. https://doi.org/10.1097/HCM.0000000000000233

Reyes, D., & Meyer, K. (2020). Identifying community priorities for neighborhood livability: Engaging neighborhood residents to facilitate community assessment. *Public Health Nursing, 37*(1), 87–95. https://doi.org/10.1111/phn.1267

Stanhope, M., & Lancaster, J. (2020). *Public health nursing: Population-centered health care in the community* (10th ed.). Elsevier.

Westphaln, K. K., Fry-Bowers, E. K., & Georges, J. M. (2020). Social capital. *Advances in Nursing Science, 43*(2), E80–E111. https://doi.org/10.1097/ANS.0000000000000296

Community Disaster Readiness

2804

Definition: Community preparedness to respond to a natural or man-made calamitous event

OUTCOME TARGET RATING: Maintain at_____ Increase to_____ .

		Poor	Fair	Good	Very Good	Excellent	
OUTCOME OVERALL RATING		1	2	3	4	5	
Indicators:							
280401	Identification of potential types of community disasters	1	2	3	4	5	NA
280445	Identification of local experts in health and environmental arenas	1	2	3	4	5	NA
280432	Plan to protect water sources	1	2	3	4	5	NA
280433	Plan to protect food supplies	1	2	3	4	5	NA
280404	Policy designating temporary administrative authority	1	2	3	4	5	NA
280405	Public health laboratory facilities	1	2	3	4	5	NA
280406	Public health disease surveillance system	1	2	3	4	5	NA
280446	Environmental surveillance system	1	2	3	4	5	NA
280447	Weather surveillance system	1	2	3	4	5	NA
280434	Plan to access electronic health records	1	2	3	4	5	NA
280408	Mass immunization plan	1	2	3	4	5	NA
280409	Surge capacity of hospital resources	1	2	3	4	5	NA
280435	Written plan for mobilization of personnel	1	2	3	4	5	NA
280436	Written plan for evacuation	1	2	3	4	5	NA
280437	Written plan for triage	1	2	3	4	5	NA
280448	Written plan to engage all health care professionals	1	2	3	4	5	NA
280449	Written agreements with community health workers for disaster response	1	2	3	4	5	NA
280438	Current written plan for communication	1	2	3	4	5	NA
280439	Current written plan for resource appropriation	1	2	3	4	5	NA
280411	Essential agency involvement in planning	1	2	3	4	5	NA
280412	Assignment of agency responsibilities in the event of disaster	1	2	3	4	5	NA
280413	Ongoing training for disaster response personnel	1	2	3	4	5	NA
280414	Plan to protect health and safety of response personnel	1	2	3	4	5	NA
280415	Notification network to alert response personnel	1	2	3	4	5	NA
280416	Notification network to alert government and support agencies	1	2	3	4	5	NA
280417	Operational communication equipment	1	2	3	4	5	NA
280440	Plan for alternative communication among disaster personnel	1	2	3	4	5	NA
280441	Plan for alternative communication among agency networks	1	2	3	4	5	NA
280419	Functional community warning mechanisms	1	2	3	4	5	NA
280420	Operational alternative utility resources	1	2	3	4	5	NA
280421	Emergency power backup	1	2	3	4	5	NA
280422	Equipment and supply availability	1	2	3	4	5	NA
280423	Equipment and supply maintenance	1	2	3	4	5	NA
280424	Designated, equipped shelters	1	2	3	4	5	NA
280425	Emergency shelter capacity	1	2	3	4	5	NA
280450	Plan to shelter farm animals	1	2	3	4	5	NA
280451	Plan to shelter pets	1	2	3	4	5	NA
280426	Regular mass casualty drills with evaluation	1	2	3	4	5	NA
280427	Public education on disaster warning and response	1	2	3	4	5	NA
280428	Media plan for public information updates	1	2	3	4	5	NA
280452	Plan for evacuation of community members	1	2	3	4	5	NA
280453	Designation of helicopter landing areas in the community	1	2	3	4	5	NA
280454	Plan for decontamination of victims	1	2	3	4	5	NA
280443	Plan for coordination of victim health care	1	2	3	4	5	NA
280444	Plan for documentation of victim health care	1	2	3	4	5	NA
280455	Plan for morgue facilities	1	2	3	4	5	NA
280430	Plan for mental health care services	1	2	3	4	5	NA
280456	Plans for post-disaster physical and mental follow-up of volunteers	1	2	3	4	5	NA
280431	Written post-disaster plan	1	2	3	4	5	NA

Domain-*Community Health (VII)*   **Class**-*Community Health Protection (CC)*   *3rd edition 2004; revised 2008, 2024*

OUTCOME CONTENT REFERENCES:

Charnley, G., Kelman, I., Gaythorpe, K., & Murray, K. A. (2021). Traits and risk factors of post-disaster infectious disease outbreaks: A systematic review. *Scientific Reports, 11*(1), 5616. https://doi.org/10.1038/s41598-021-85146-0

Khan, Y., Brown, A. D., Gagliardi, A. R., O'Sullivan, T., Lacarte, S., Henry, B., & Schwartz, B. (2019). Are we prepared? The development of performance indicators for public health emergency preparedness using a modified Delphi approach. *PLOS One, 14*(12), e0226489. https://doi.org/10.1371/journal.pone.0226489

Lichtveld, M., & Birnbaum, L. (2020). Advances in environmental health and disaster research 15 years after Hurricane Katrina. *American Journal of Public Health 110*(10), 1478–1479. https://doi.org/10.2105/AJPH.2020.305739

Ryan, B., Johnston, K. A., Taylor, M., & McAndrew, R. (2020). Community engagement for disaster preparedness: A systematic literature review. *International Journal of Disaster Risk Reduction, 49*, 101655. https://doi.org/10.1016/j.ijdrr.2020.101655

Salmani, I., Seyedin, H., Ardalan, A., & Farajkhoda, T. (2019). Conceptual model of managing health care volunteers in disasters: A mixed method study. *BMC Health Services Research, 19*(1), 241. https://doi.org/10.1186/s12913-019-4073-6

Stanhope, M., & Lancaster, J. (2020). *Public health nursing: Population-centered health care in the community* (10th ed.). Elsevier.

Sutton, J., Fischer, L., James, L. E., & Sheff, S. E. (2020). Earthquake early warning message testing: Visual attention, behavioral responses, and message perceptions. *International Journal of Disaster Risk Reduction, 49*, 101664. https://doi.org/10.1016/j.ijdrr.2020.101664

Veenema, T. G., Lavin, R. P., Bender, A., Thornton, C. P., & Schneider-Firestone, S. (2019). National nurse readiness for radiation emergencies and nuclear events: A systematic review of the literature. *Nursing Outlook, 67*(1), 54–88. https://doi.org/10.1016/j.outlook.2018.10.005

Community Disaster Recovery   2705

Definition: Community actions to help members cope, recover, and return to a new normal after a disaster

OUTCOME TARGET RATING: Maintain at_____ Increase to_____

		Poor	Fair	Good	Very Good	Excellent	
OUTCOME OVERALL RATING		**1**	**2**	**3**	**4**	**5**	
Indicators:							
270501	Support provided by community leaders to help members recover	1	2	3	4	5	NA
270502	Estimates of extent of damage caused by disaster	1	2	3	4	5	NA
270503	Gradual transition from response to recovery efforts	1	2	3	4	5	NA
270504	Shift from short-term goals to long-term recovery	1	2	3	4	5	NA
270505	Assistance from government agencies for disaster relief	1	2	3	4	5	NA
270506	Establishment of priorities for available disaster recovery resources	1	2	3	4	5	NA
270507	Rebuilding of destroyed infrastructure	1	2	3	4	5	NA
270508	Rebuilding of destroyed homes and businesses	1	2	3	4	5	NA
270509	Restoration of public services	1	2	3	4	5	NA
270510	Level of perceived social support experienced by members impacted by disaster	1	2	3	4	5	NA
270511	Plan to strengthen community resilience	1	2	3	4	5	NA
270512	Availability of faith leaders to provide spiritual comfort	1	2	3	4	5	NA
270513	Availability of bereavement support groups after the disaster	1	2	3	4	5	NA
270514	Focus on mental health issues created by the disaster event	1	2	3	4	5	NA
270515	Plan for remembrances for those who died	1	2	3	4	5	NA
270516	Analysis of injury patterns	1	2	3	4	5	NA
270517	Evaluation of emergency response by key groups	1	2	3	4	5	NA
270518	Evaluation of support organizations to disaster recovery efforts	1	2	3	4	5	NA
270519	Analysis of the economic impact of the disaster by government leaders	1	2	3	4	5	NA
270520	Analysis of the health care challenges for the future disaster preparation	1	2	3	4	5	NA
270521	Post-disaster evaluation process	1	2	3	4	5	NA

***Domain**-Community Health (VII)*   ***Class**-Community Well-Being (BB)*   *7th edition 2024*

OUTCOME CONTENT REFERENCES:

Aoun, S. M., Breen, L. J., White, I., Rumbold, B., & Kellehear, A. (2018). What sources of bereavement support are perceived helpful by bereaved people and why? Empirical evidence for the compassionate communities approach. *Palliative Medicine, 32*(8), 1378–1388. https://doi.org/10.1177/0269216318774995

Bhattarai, S., Maycock, B., Alfonso, H., & Reid, A. (2020). Development of an integrated pathways model of factors influencing the progress of recovery after a disaster. *Asia-Pacific Journal of Public Health, 32*(5), 226–234. https://doi.org/10.1177/1010539520935386

Koebele, E. A., Crow, D. A., & Albright, E. A. (2020). Building resilience during recovery: Lessons from Colorado's watershed resilience pilot program. *Environmental Management, 66*(1), 1–15. https://doi.org/10.1007/s00267-020-01296-3

Ntontis, E., Drury, J., Amlôt, R., Rubin, G. J., Williams, R., & Saavedra, P. (2021). Collective resilience in the disaster recovery period: Emergent social identity and observed social support are associated with collective efficacy, well-being, and the provision of social support. *British Journal of Social Psychology, 60*(3), 1075–1095. https://doi.org/10.1111/bjso.12434

Stanhope, M., & Lancaster, J. (2020). *Public health nursing: Population-centered health care in the community* (10th ed.). Elsevier.

Yabe, T., Tsubouchi, K., Fujiwara, N., Sekimoto, Y., & Ukkusuri, S. V. (2020). Understanding post-disaster population recovery patterns. *Journal of the Royal Society Interface, 17*(163), 20190532. https://doi.org/10.1098/rsif.2019.0532

Community Disaster Response 2806

Definition: Community response following a natural or man-made calamitous event

OUTCOME TARGET RATING: Maintain at_____ Increase to_____

		Poor	Fair	Good	Very Good	Excellent	
OUTCOME OVERALL RATING		1	2	3	4	5	
Indicators:							
280609	Command authority identified	1	2	3	4	5	NA
280613	Operation of communication system	1	2	3	4	5	NA
280608	Mobilization of personnel	1	2	3	4	5	NA
280617	Information provided to public	1	2	3	4	5	NA
280611	Triage of injured individuals	1	2	3	4	5	NA
280612	Evacuation of injured individuals	1	2	3	4	5	NA
280610	Evacuation of population	1	2	3	4	5	NA
280601	Availability of safe water	1	2	3	4	5	NA
280602	Availability of safe food	1	2	3	4	5	NA
280603	Availability of medication	1	2	3	4	5	NA
280604	Availability of supplies	1	2	3	4	5	NA
280605	Availability of shelters	1	2	3	4	5	NA
280606	Availability of hospital resources	1	2	3	4	5	NA
280607	Availability of personnel	1	2	3	4	5	NA
280637	Availability of sanitation activities	1	2	3	4	5	NA
280623	Availability of functional equipment	1	2	3	4	5	NA
280614	Government agencies notified of needs	1	2	3	4	5	NA
280615	Support agencies notified of needs	1	2	3	4	5	NA
280618	Response of government agencies in carrying out responsibilities	1	2	3	4	5	NA
280619	Response of support agencies in carrying out responsibilities	1	2	3	4	5	NA
280620	Coordination efforts of local, state, federal, international and non-governmental agencies	1	2	3	4	5	NA
280621	Performance of response personnel	1	2	3	4	5	NA
280622	Operation of emergency power	1	2	3	4	5	NA
280624	Availability of decontamination equipment	1	2	3	4	5	NA
280625	Access to electronic health records	1	2	3	4	5	NA
280626	Mental health care available for population	1	2	3	4	5	NA
280627	Mental health care available for response personnel	1	2	3	4	5	NA
280628	Response of public health laboratory facilities	1	2	3	4	5	NA
280629	Accurate disposition logs of patients and evacuees	1	2	3	4	5	NA
280630	Data collected on injury patterns	1	2	3	4	5	NA
280631	Data collected on disease incidence	1	2	3	4	5	NA
280632	Mass immunization plan	1	2	3	4	5	NA
280633	Availability of morgue facilities	1	2	3	4	5	NA

Community Disaster Response—cont'd

		Poor	Fair	Good	Very Good	Excellent	
280638	Provision shelter for farm animals	1	2	3	4	5	NA
280639	Provision of shelter for pets	1	2	3	4	5	NA
280635	Replacement of prescribed medication for individuals	1	2	3	4	5	NA
280636	Post-disaster follow-up	1	2	3	4	5	NA
280640	Post-disaster evaluation	1	2	3	4	5	NA

Domain-*Community Health (VII)*   **Class**-*Community Health Protection (CC)*   *4th edition 2008; revised 2013, 2024*

OUTCOME CONTENT REFERENCES:

Charnley, G., Kelman, I., Gaythorpe, K., & Murray, K. A. (2021). Traits and risk factors of post-disaster infectious disease outbreaks: A systematic review. *Scientific Reports, 11*(1), 5616. https://doi.org/10.1038/s41598-021-85146-0

Khan, Y., Brown, A. D., Gagliardi, A. R., O'Sullivan, T., Lacarte, S., Henry, B., & Schwartz, B. (2019). Are we prepared? The development of performance indicators for public health emergency preparedness using a modified Delphi approach. *PLOS One, 14*(12), e0226489. https://doi.org/10.1371/journal.pone.0226489

Lichtveld, M., & Birnbaum, L. (2020). Advances in environmental health and disaster research 15 years after Hurricane Katrina. *American Journal of Public Health 110*(10), 1478–1479. https://doi.org/10.2105/AJPH.2020.305739

Ryan, B., Johnston, K. A., Taylor, M., & McAndrew, R. (2020). Community engagement for disaster preparedness: A systematic literature review. *International Journal of Disaster Risk Reduction, 49*, 101655, https://doi.org/10.1016/j.ijdrr.2020.101655

Salmani, I., Seyedin, H., Ardalan, A., & Farajkhoda, T. (2019). Conceptual model of managing health care volunteers in disasters: A mixed method study. *BMC Health Services Research, 19*(1), 241. https://doi.org/10.1186/s12913-019-4073-6

Stanhope, M., & Lancaster, J. (2020). *Public health nursing: Population centered health care in the community* (10th ed.). Elsevier.

Sutton, J., Fischer, L., James, L. E., & Sheff, S. E. (2020). Earthquake early warning message testing: Visual attention, behavioral responses, and message perceptions. *International Journal of Disaster Risk Reduction, 49*, 101664. https://doi.org/10.1016/j.ijdrr.2020.101664

Veenema, T. G., Lavin, R. P., Bender, A., Thornton, C. P., & Schneider-Firestone, S. (2019). National nurse readiness for radiation emergencies and nuclear events: A systematic review of the literature. *Nursing Outlook, 67*(1), 54–88. https://doi.org/10.1016/j.outlook.2018.10.005

Community Grief Recovery   2706

Definition: Community actions to help members cope and return to a new normal after a significant loss of life or property

OUTCOME TARGET RATING: Maintain at_____ Increase to_____

		Poor	Fair	Good	Very Good	Excellent	
OUTCOME OVERALL RATING		1	2	3	4	5	
Indicators:							
270601	Support provided by community leaders to help members grieve	1	2	3	4	5	NA
270602	Gradual transition from response to grief recovery efforts	1	2	3	4	5	NA
270603	Shift from short-term goals to long-term grief recovery	1	2	3	4	5	NA
270604	Assistance from government agencies	1	2	3	4	5	NA
270605	Establishment of priorities for available recovery resources	1	2	3	4	5	NA
270606	Opportunities for community recovery activities	1	2	3	4	5	NA
270607	Members' participation in recovery activities	1	2	3	4	5	NA
270608	Identification of long-term challenges faced by community	1	2	3	4	5	NA
270609	Activation of available vertical and horizontal communication networks	1	2	3	4	5	NA
270610	Availability of grief counselors	1	2	3	4	5	NA
270611	Plan to strengthen community resilience	1	2	3	4	5	NA
270612	Availability of faith leaders to provide spiritual comfort	1	2	3	4	5	NA
270613	Availability of bereavement support groups	1	2	3	4	5	NA
270614	Creation of new jobs	1	2	3	4	5	NA
270615	Plan for rebuilding infrastructure	1	2	3	4	5	NA
270616	Revitalization of neighborhoods	1	2	3	4	5	NA
270617	Plan for community recognition of the event such as a grief ritual	1	2	3	4	5	NA
270618	Plan for remembrances for those who lost their lives	1	2	3	4	5	NA
270619	Plan for reunion of survivors	1	2	3	4	5	NA

Domain-*Community Health (VII)*   **Class**-*Community Well-Being (BB)*   *7th edition 2024*

OUTCOME CONTENT REFERENCES:
Aoun, S. M., Breen, L. J., Rumbold, B., Christian, K. M., Same, A., & Abel, J. (2019). Matching response to need: What makes social networks fit for providing bereavement support? *PLOS One, 14*(3), e0213367. https://doi.org/10.1371/journal.pone.0213367
Aoun, S. M., Breen, L. J., White, I., Rumbold, B., & Kellehear, A. (2018). What sources of bereavement support are perceived helpful by bereaved people and why? Empirical evidence for the compassionate communities approach. *Palliative Medicine, 32*(8), 1378-1388. https://doi.org/10.1177/0269216318774995
Cherry, K. E., & Gibson, A. (2021). *The intersection of trauma and disaster behavioral health.* Springer.
Mueller, D., Bacalso, E., Ortega-Williams, A., Pate, D. J., & Topitzes, J. (2021). A mutual process of healing self and healing the community: A qualitative study of coping with and healing from stress, adversity, and trauma among diverse residents of a midwestern city. *Journal of Community Psychology, 49*(5), 1169–1194. https://doi.org/10.1002/jcop.22530
Schultz, K., Cattaneo, L. B., Sabina, C., Brunner, L., Jackson, S., & Serrata, J. V. (2016). Key roles of community connectedness in healing from trauma. *Psychology of Violence, 6*(1), 42–48. https://doi.org/10.1037/vio0000025
Stanhope, M., & Lancaster, J. (2020). *Public health nursing: Population-centered health care in the community* (10th ed.). Elsevier.
Zuniga-Villanueva, G., Ramirez-Garcia Luna, J. L., & Villafranca-Andino, R. I. (2021). A compassionate communities approach in a grief and bereavement support program: Bridging the gap in palliative care. *Journal of Social Work in End-of-Life & Palliative Care, 17*(1), 9–18. https://doi.org/10.1080/15524256.2021.1894309

Community Grief Response

2703

Definition: Community immediate response to members' grief that involves loss of life or property

OUTCOME TARGET RATING: Maintain at_____ Increase to_____

		Poor	Fair	Good	Very Good	Excellent	
OUTCOME OVERALL RATING		1	2	3	4	5	
Indicators:							
270301	Assessment of members' needs by leaders	1	2	3	4	5	NA
270302	Coordination of grief response efforts	1	2	3	4	5	NA
270303	Cooperation among members	1	2	3	4	5	NA
270304	Identification of mental health needs of members	1	2	3	4	5	NA
270305	Availability of mental health services	1	2	3	4	5	NA
270308	Community post-trauma response program	1	2	3	4	5	NA
270309	Availability of humanitarian aid	1	2	3	4	5	NA
270310	Community information articulated in media	1	2	3	4	5	NA
270311	Community needs articulated in community forums	1	2	3	4	5	NA
270312	Recognition of members' problems	1	2	3	4	5	NA
270313	Resettlement options	1	2	3	4	5	NA
270314	Community psychosocial integration	1	2	3	4	5	NA
270315	Members' engagement in response to event	1	2	3	4	5	NA
270316	Use of psychosocial support systems	1	2	3	4	5	NA
270317	Availability of group interventions	1	2	3	4	5	NA
270318	Availability of stabilizing processes	1	2	3	4	5	NA
270319	Availability of coping support groups	1	2	3	4	5	NA
270320	Ability of community to adapt to traumatic losses	1	2	3	4	5	NA
270322	Preservation of jobs	1	2	3	4	5	NA
270324	Distribution of economic resources	1	2	3	4	5	NA

Domain-*Community Health (VII)* **Class**-*Community Well-Being (BB)* 5th edition 2013; revised 2024

OUTCOME CONTENT REFERENCES:
Cherry, K. E., & Gibson, A. (2021). *The intersection of trauma and disaster behavioral health.* Springer.
Hilliker, L. (2008). The reporting of grief by one newspaper of record for the U.S.: The New York Times. Omega: *Journal of Death & Dying, 57*(3), 261–278.
Kropf, N. P., & Jones, B. L. (2014). When public tragedies happen: Community practice approaches in grief, loss, and recovery. *Journal of Community Practice, 22*(3), 281–298. https://doi.org/10.1080/10705422.2014.929539
Lebowitz A. J. (2015). Community collaboration as a disaster mental health competency: A systematic literature review. *Community Mental Health Journal, 51*(2), 125–131. https://doi.org/10.1007/s10597-014-9751-6
Lee, J. Y., Kim, S. W., & Kim, J. M. (2020). The impact of community disaster trauma: A focus on emerging research of PTSD and other mental health outcomes. *Chonnam Medical Journal, 56*(2), 99–107. https://doi.org/10.4068/cmj.2020.56.2.99

Macy, R. D., Behar, L., Paulson, R., Delman, J., Schmid, L., & Smith, S. F. (2004). Community-based, acute posttraumatic stress management: A description and evaluation of a psychosocial-intervention continuum. *Harvard Review of Psychiatry, 12*(4), 217–228.

Stanhope, M., & Lancaster, J. (2020). *Public health nursing: Population-centered health care in the community* (10th ed.). Elsevier.

van den Berg, B., Grievink, L., Gutschmidt, K., Lang, T., Palmer, S., Ruijten, M., Stumpel, R., & Yzermans, J. (2008). The public health dimension of disasters-health outcome assessment of disasters. *Prehospital & Disaster Medicine, 23*(4), s55–s59.

Wayment, H. A., & Silver, R. C. (2021). Grief and solidarity reactions 1 week after an on-campus shooting. *Journal of Interpersonal Violence, 36*(5/6), NP2423–NP2442. https://doi.org/10.1177/0886260518766431

C

Community Health Screening Effectiveness   2807

Definition: Quality of community actions to screen members for potential health risks or presymptomatic conditions

OUTCOME TARGET RATING: Maintain at_____ Increase to_____

		Poor	Fair	Good	Very good	Excellent	
OUTCOME OVERALL RATING		1	2	3	4	5	
Indicators:							
280701	Identification of high-risk conditions prevalent in the population	1	2	3	4	5	NA
280702	Identification of conditions that can benefit from early detection and treatment	1	2	3	4	5	NA
280703	Selection of screening focused on early detection	1	2	3	4	5	NA
280704	Identification of screening needs for infants	1	2	3	4	5	NA
280705	Identification of screening needs for toddlers and preschoolers	1	2	3	4	5	NA
280706	Identification of screening needs for school age children	1	2	3	4	5	NA
280707	Identification of screening needs for adults	1	2	3	4	5	NA
280708	Education of members of importance of screening	1	2	3	4	5	NA
280709	Identification of screening frequency requirements	1	2	3	4	5	NA
280710	Advertisement of screening opportunities	1	2	3	4	5	NA
280711	Identification of resources needed for screening	1	2	3	4	5	NA
280712	Coordination with health care organizations that provide screening	1	2	3	4	5	NA
280713	Outreach to target populations	1	2	3	4	5	NA
280714	Identification of cultural implications of screening	1	2	3	4	5	NA
280715	Evaluation of cost-to-benefit ratio for specific screening	1	2	3	4	5	NA
280716	Provision of screening for prevalent conditions in the community	1	2	3	4	5	NA
280717	Provision of screening for infants	1	2	3	4	5	NA
280718	Provision of screening for toddlers and preschoolers	1	2	3	4	5	NA
280719	Provision of screening for school age children	1	2	3	4	5	NA
280720	Provision of screening for adults	1	2	3	4	5	NA
280721	Provision of screening for elders	1	2	3	4	5	NA
280722	Mechanism for follow-up	1	2	3	4	5	NA
280723	Mechanism for referral	1	2	3	4	5	NA
280724	Support from influential community members	1	2	3	4	5	NA
280725	Target population participation rates in screening	1	2	3	4	5	NA

Domain-*Community Health (VII)*   **Class**-*Community Health Protection (CC)*   *5th edition 2013*

OUTCOME CONTENT REFERENCES:

Macha, K., & McDonough, J. P. (2012). *Epidemiology for advanced nursing practice*. Jones & Bartlett.

Nguyen, T., Tanjasiri, S., Kagawa-Singer, M., Tran, J., & Foo, M. (2008). Community health navigators for breast- and cervical-cancer screening among Cambodian and Laotian women: Intervention strategies and relationship-building processes. *Health Promotion Practice, 9*(4), 356–357.

Nies, M. A., & McEwen, M. (2007). *Community/public health nursing: Promoting the health of populations* (4th ed.). Saunders Elsevier.

Raz, A. E. (2009). Can population-based carrier screening be left to the community? *Journal of Genetic Counseling, 18*(2), 114–118.

Shannon, P., & Anderson, P. R. (2008). Developmental screening in community health care centers and pediatric practices: An evaluation of the baby steps program. *Intellectual and Developmental Disabilities, 46*(4), 281–289.

Community Health Status   **2701**

Definition: General state of well-being of a community or population

OUTCOME TARGET RATING: Maintain at_____ Increase to_____

		Poor	Fair	Good	Very Good	Excellent	
OUTCOME OVERALL RATING		**1**	**2**	**3**	**4**	**5**	
Indicators:							
270111	Health status of infants	1	2	3	4	5	NA
270112	Health status of children	1	2	3	4	5	NA
270113	Health status of adolescents	1	2	3	4	5	NA
270140	Health status of pregnant women	1	2	3	4	5	NA
270114	Health status of adults	1	2	3	4	5	NA
270115	Health status of elders	1	2	3	4	5	NA
270132	Health status of minority populations	1	2	3	4	5	NA
270141	Health status of disadvantaged populations	1	2	3	4	5	NA
270142	Health status of low-income families	1	2	3	4	5	NA
270101	Participation rates in preventive health care services	1	2	3	4	5	NA
270102	Prevalence of health promotion programs	1	2	3	4	5	NA
270103	Prevalence of health protection programs	1	2	3	4	5	NA
270104	School enrollment rate	1	2	3	4	5	NA
270105	School attendance rate	1	2	3	4	5	NA
270106	Participation rates in worksite health programs	1	2	3	4	5	NA
270107	Participation rates in community health programs	1	2	3	4	5	NA
270108	Participation rates in school health programs	1	2	3	4	5	NA
270109	Evidence of health protection measures	1	2	3	4	5	NA
270110	Members with adequate health insurance coverage	1	2	3	4	5	NA
270116	Attendance at programs for healthy pregnancy	1	2	3	4	5	NA
270117	Compliance with environmental health standards	1	2	3	4	5	NA
270124	Mortality rates	1	2	3	4	5	NA
270133	Maternal mortality rates	1	2	3	4	5	NA
270143	Infant mortality rates	1	2	3	4	5	NA
270119	Morbidity rates	1	2	3	4	5	NA
270144	Immunization rates	1	2	3	4	5	NA
270120	Mental health illness rates	1	2	3	4	5	NA
270125	Chronic disease rates	1	2	3	4	5	NA
270145	Air pollution levels	1	2	3	4	5	NA
270134	Substance abuse rates for adults	1	2	3	4	5	NA
270135	Substance abuse rates for adolescents	1	2	3	4	5	NA
270136	Smoking rates	1	2	3	4	5	NA
270126	Sexually transmitted disease rates	1	2	3	4	5	NA
270137	Preterm birth rates	1	2	3	4	5	NA
270138	Low birth weight rates	1	2	3	4	5	NA
270121	Injury rates	1	2	3	4	5	NA
270122	Crime statistics	1	2	3	4	5	NA
270146	Suicide rates	1	2	3	4	5	NA
270139	Homicide rates	1	2	3	4	5	NA
270127	Health surveillance data systems in place	1	2	3	4	5	NA
270128	Community health standards for health measurement and evaluation are defined	1	2	3	4	5	NA
270129	Monitoring of community health standards for health measurement and evaluation	1	2	3	4	5	NA
270130	Community demographics represented in health care planning and evaluation	1	2	3	4	5	NA

Domain-Community Health (VII)   *Class*-Community Well-Being (BB)   *2nd edition 2000; revised 2004, 2008, 2024*

OUTCOME CONTENT REFERENCES:

Comer, K. F., Gibson, P. J., Zou, J., Rosenman, M., & Dixon, B. E. (2018). Electronic health record (EHR)-based community health measures: An exploratory assessment of perceived usefulness by local health departments. *BMC Public Health, 18,* Article 647. https://doi.org/10.1186/s12889-018-5550-2

Savage, C. (2019). *Community health and nursing practice: Caring for populations.* F.A. Davis.

Stanhope, M., & Lancaster, J. (2020). *Public health nursing: Population-centered health care in the community* (10th ed.). Elsevier.

U.S. Department of Health and Human Services, Office of Disease Prevention and Health Promotion. (n.d.). *Healthy people 2030.* https://health.gov/healthypeople?_ga=2.211075605.126410647.1643675115-1263545106.1641401162

C

Community Immune Status   2800

Definition: Resistance of community members to the invasion and spread of an infectious agent that could threaten public health

OUTCOME TARGET RATING: Maintain at_____ Increase to_____

	Poor	Fair	Good	Very Good	Excellent	
OUTCOME OVERALL RATING	1	2	3	4	5	
Indicators:						
280001 Immunization rates equal to or greater than current national standards	1	2	3	4	5	NA
280002 Incidence of vaccine preventable disease at or below recommended national rate	1	2	3	4	5	NA
280003 Prevalence of vaccine preventable disease at or below recommended national rate	1	2	3	4	5	NA

Domain *Community Health (VII)*   **Class**-*Community Well-Being (BB)*   *2nd edition 2000; revised 2004, 2013, 2024*

OUTCOME CONTENT REFERENCES:

Bauer, K. E., Agruss, J. C., & Mayefsky, J. H. (2021). Partnering with parents to remove barriers and improve influenza immunization rates for young children. *Journal of the American Association of Nurse Practitioners, 33*(6), 470–475. https://doi.org/10.1097/JXX.0000000000000381

Dong, M., He, F., & Deng, Y. (2021). How to understand herd immunity in the context of COVID-19. *Viral Immunology, 34*(3), 174–181. https://doi.org/10.1089/vim.2020.0195

Frederiksen, L., Zhang, Y., Foged, C., & Thakur, A. (2020). The long road toward COVID-19 herd immunity: Vaccine platform technologies and mass immunization strategies. *Frontiers in Immunology, 11,* 1817. https://doi.org/10.3389/fimmu.2020.01817

Recommendations for prevention and control of influenza in children, 2020–2021. (2020). *Pediatrics, 146*(4), 1–29. https://doi.org/10.1542/peds.2020-024588

Saad-Roy, C. M., Levin, S. A., Metcalf, C. J. E., & Grenfell, B. T. (2021). Trajectory of individual immunity and vaccination required for SARS-CoV-2 community immunity: A conceptual investigation. *Journal of the Royal Society Interface, 18,* (175), 20200683. https://doi.org/10.1098/rsif.2020.0683

Strengthening the effectiveness of national, state, and local efforts to improve HPV vaccination coverage in the United States: Recommendations from the National Vaccine Advisory Committee. (2018). *Public Health Reports, 133*(5), 543–550. https://doi.org/10.1177/0033354918793629

Willis, E., Gundacker, C., Harris, M., & Mameledzija, M. (2020). Improving immunization and health literacy through a community-based approach. *Studies in Health Technology and Informatics, 269,* 142–152. https://doi.org/10.3233/SHTI200028

Community Immune Status: Adult   2796

Definition: Immunization rates of community members through vaccination

OUTCOME TARGET RATING: Maintain at_____ Increase to_____

	Poor	Fair	Good	Very Good	Excellent	
OUTCOME OVERALL RATING	1	2	3	4	5	
Indicators:						
279601 Immunization rates for Tetanus, Diphtheria, and Pertussis (Tdap or Td) equal to or greater than current national standards	1	2	3	4	5	NA
279602 Immunization rates for Measles, Mumps & Rubella (MMR) equal to or greater than current national standards	1	2	3	4	5	NA
279603 Immunization rates for Varicella (VAR) equal to or greater than current national standards	1	2	3	4	5	NA

Continued

C

Community Immune Status: Adult—cont'd

		Poor	Fair	Good	Very Good	Excellent	
279604	Immunization rates for Zoster recombinant (RZV) equal to or greater than current national standards (individuals over 50 years old)	1	2	3	4	5	NA
279605	Immunization rates for Pneumococcal conjugate (PCV 13) equal to or greater than current national standards (individuals 19–26 years old)	1	2	3	4	5	NA
279606	Immunization rates for Pneumococcal polysaccharide (PPSV23) equal to or greater than current national standards (individuals over 65 years old)	1	2	3	4	5	NA
279607	Immunization rates for Influenza inactivated (IIV) or Influenza recombinant (RIV4) equal to or greater than current national standards	1	2	3	4	5	NA
279608	Immunization rates for COVID-19 equal to or greater than current national standards	1	2	3	4	5	NA

Domain-Community Health (VII)   **Class**-Community Well-Being (BB)   7th edition 2024

OUTCOME CONTENT REFERENCES:

Center for Disease Control and Prevention. (2021, February 12). *Recommended adult immunization schedule for ages 19 years or older—United States 2020*. U.S. Department of Health and Human Services. https://www.cdc.gov/vaccines/schedules/downloads/adult/adult-combined-schedule.pdf

Dong, M., He, F., & Deng, Y. (2021). How to understand herd immunity in the context of COVID-19. *Viral Immunology, 34*(3), 174–181. https://doi.org/10.1089/vim.2020.0195

Frederiksen, L., Zhang, Y., Foged, C., & Thakur, A. (2020). The long road toward COVID-19 herd immunity: Vaccine platform technologies and mass immunization strategies. *Frontiers in Immunology, 11*, 1817. https://doi.org/10.3389/fimmu.2020.01817

Saad-Roy, C. M., Levin, S. A., Metcalf, C. J. E., & Grenfell, B. T. (2021). Trajectory of individual immunity and vaccination required for SARS-CoV-2 community immunity: A conceptual investigation. *Journal of the Royal Society Interface, 18*, 20200683. https://doi.org/10.1098/rsif.2020.0683

Willis, E., Gundacker, C., Harris, M., & Mameledzija, M. (2020). Improving immunization and health literacy through a community-based approach. *Studies in Health Technology and Informatics, 269*, 142–152. https://doi.org/10.3233/SHTI200028

Community Immune Status: School Age Child   2797

Definition: Immunization rates of children 7 to 18 years old for protection from the invasion and spread of an infectious agent through vaccination

OUTCOME TARGET RATING: Maintain at_____ Increase to_____

		Poor	Fair	Good	Very Good	Excellent	
OUTCOME OVERALL RATING		**1**	**2**	**3**	**4**	**5**	
Indicators:							
279701	Immunization rates for Tetanus, Diphtheria, and Pertussis (Tdap or Td) equal to or greater than current national standards for ages 11–12 years old	1	2	3	4	5	NA
279702	Immunization rates for Human Papillomavirus (HPV) equal to greater than current national standards for ages 11–12 years old	1	2	3	4	5	NA
279703	Immunization rates for Meningococcal conjugate (MenACWY) equal to or greater than current national standards for ages 11–12 years old	1	2	3	4	5	NA
279704	Immunization rates for Meningococcal conjugate booster (MenACWY) equal to or greater than current national standards for age 16 years (booster)	1	2	3	4	5	NA
279705	Immunization rates for Influenza inactivated (IIV) or Influenza recombinant (RIV4) equal to or greater than current national standards	1	2	3	4	5	NA
279706	Immunization rates for COVID-19 equal to or greater than current national standards	1	2	3	4	5	NA

Domain-Community Health (VII)   **Class**-Community Well-Being (BB)   7th edition 2024

OUTCOME CONTENT REFERENCES:

Centers for Disease Control and Prevention. (2021). *2021 Recommended vaccinations for children (7–18 Years Old) parent-friendly version.* U.S. Department of Health and Human Services. https://www.cdc.gov/vaccines/schedules/easy-to-read/adolescent-easyread.html

Dong, M., He, F., & Deng, Y. (2021). How to understand herd immunity in the context of COVID-19. *Viral Immunology, 34*(3), 174–181. https://doi.org/10.1089/vim.2020.0195

Frederiksen, L., Zhang, Y., Foged, C., & Thakur, A. (2020). The long road toward COVID-19 herd immunity: Vaccine platform technologies and mass immunization strategies. *Frontiers in Immunology, 11,* 1817. https://doi.org/10.3389/fimmu.2020.01817

Hockenberry, M. J., Wilson, D., & Rodgers, C. C. (Eds.). (2019). *Wong's nursing care of infants and children* (11th ed.). Elsevier.

Saad-Roy, C. M., Levin, S. A., Metcalf, C. J. E., & Grenfell, B. T. (2021). Trajectory of individual immunity and vaccination required for SARS-CoV-2 community immunity: A conceptual investigation. *Journal of the Royal Society Interface, 18,* 20200683. https://doi.org/10.1098/rsif.2020.0683

Willis, E., Gundacker, C., Harris, M., & Mameledzija, M. (2020). Improving immunization and health literacy through a community-based approach. *Studies in Health Technology and Informatics, 269,* 142–152. https://doi.org/10.3233/SHTI200028

C

Community Immune Status: Young Child   2798

Definition: Immunization rates of infants and children from birth to 6 years old for protection from the invasion and spread of an infectious agent through vaccination

OUTCOME TARGET RATING: Maintain at_____ Increase to_____

		Poor	Fair	Good	Very Good	Excellent	
OUTCOME OVERALL RATING		1	2	3	4	5	
Indicators:							
279801	Immunization rates for Hepatitis B equal to or greater than current standards (1–2 months)	1	2	3	4	5	NA
279802	Immunization rates for Rotavirus equal to or greater than current standards (2, 4, & 6 months)	1	2	3	4	5	NA
279803	Immunization rates for Tetanus, Diphtheria, and Pertussis (Tdap or Td) equal to or greater than current standards (2, 4, & 6 months)	1	2	3	4	5	NA
279804	Immunization rates for Pneumococcal disease (PC13) equal to or greater than current standards (2, 4, & 6 months)	1	2	3	4	5	NA
279805	Immunization rates for Polio (IPV) equal to or greater than current standards (2, 4, & 6–18 months)	1	2	3	4	5	NA
279806	Immunization rates for Varicella (VAR) equal to or greater than current national standards (12–15 months)	1	2	3	4	5	NA
279807	Immunization rates for Hepatitis A equal to or greater than current standards (12–24 months)	1	2	3	4	5	NA
279808	Immunization rates for second dose Hepatitis A equal to or greater than current standards (6 months after initial dose)	1	2	3	4	5	NA
279809	Immunization rates for Pneumococcal disease (PC13) equal to or greater than current standards (12–15 months)	1	2	3	4	5	NA
279810	Immunization rates for Tetanus, Diphtheria, and Pertussis (Tdap or Td) equal to or greater than current standards (12–15 months)	1	2	3	4	5	NA
279811	Immunization rates for Measles, Mumps, & Rubella (MMR) equal to or greater than current standards (12–15 months)	1	2	3	4	5	NA
279812	Immunization rates for Measles, Mumps, & Rubella (MMR) equal to or greater than current standards (4–6 years)	1	2	3	4	5	NA
279813	Immunization rates for second dose Polio (IPV) equal to or greater than current standards (4–6 years)	1	2	3	4	5	NA
279814	Immunization rates for second dose Varicella (VAR) equal to or greater than current standards (4–6 years)	1	2	3	4	5	NA
279815	Immunization rates for Influenza inactivated (IIV) or Influenza recombinant (RIV4) equal to or greater than current standards (6 months and annually)	1	2	3	4	5	NA
279816	Immunization rates for COVID-19 equal to or greater than current national standards (5–6 years)	1	2	3	4	5	NA

Domain-Community Health (VII)   *Class-Community Well-Being (BB)*   *7th edition 2024*

OUTCOME CONTENT REFERENCES:
Centers for Disease Control and Prevention. (2021). 2021 Recommended vaccinations for infants and children (birth through 6 years) parent-friendly version. U.S. Department of Health and Human Services. https://www.cdc.gov/vaccines/schedules/easy-to-read/child-easyread.html
Dong, M., He, F., & Deng, Y. (2021). How to understand herd immunity in the context of COVID-19. *Viral Immunology, 34*(3), 174–181. https://doi.org/10.1089/vim.2020.0195
Frederiksen, L., Zhang, Y., Foged, C., & Thakur, A. (2020). The long road toward COVID-19 herd immunity: Vaccine platform technologies and mass immunization strategies. *Frontiers in Immunology, 11*, 1817. https://doi.org/10.3389/fimmu.2020.01817
Hockenberry, M. J., Wilson, D., & Rodgers, C. C. (Eds.). (2019). *Wong's nursing care of infants and children* (11th ed.). Elsevier.
Saad-Roy, C. M., Levin, S. A., Metcalf, C. J. E., & Grenfell, B. T. (2021). Trajectory of individual immunity and vaccination required for SARS-CoV-2 community immunity: A conceptual investigation. *Journal of the Royal Society Interface, 18*, 20200683. https://doi.org/10.1098/rsif.2020.0683
Willis, E., Gundacker, C., Harris, M., & Mameledzija, M. (2020). Improving immunization and health literacy through a community-based approach. *Studies in Health Technology and Informatics, 269*, 142–152. https://doi.org/10.3233/SHTI200028

Community Immunity Effectiveness   2799

Definition: Community actions to increase resistance of community members to the invasion and spread of an infectious agent that could threaten public health

OUTCOME TARGET RATING: Maintain at_____ Increase to_____

OUTCOME OVERALL RATING		Poor	Fair	Good	Very Good	Excellent	
		1	2	3	4	5	
Indicators:							
279901	Education on the role of vaccines in preventing illness or death	1	2	3	4	5	NA
279902	Education through public service announcements	1	2	3	4	5	NA
279903	Education on the risks and benefits of specific vaccines	1	2	3	4	5	NA
279904	Education addressing misperception of vaccination	1	2	3	4	5	NA
279905	Education on herd immunity to protect those who cannot be vaccinated	1	2	3	4	5	NA
279906	Education on available immunizations for specific age groups	1	2	3	4	5	NA
279907	Availability of low-cost immunizations	1	2	3	4	5	NA
279908	Availability of immunizations in neighborhood	1	2	3	4	5	NA
279909	Surveillance of communicable disease incidence in community	1	2	3	4	5	NA
279910	Screening of at-risk populations for infections	1	2	3	4	5	NA
279911	Surveillance of required immunization status in school systems	1	2	3	4	5	NA
279912	Surveillance of immunization status in group living facilities (e.g., jails, group homes, long-term care)	1	2	3	4	5	NA
279913	Surveillance of immunization status among health professionals	1	2	3	4	5	NA
279914	Adherence with annual flu immunization recommendations	1	2	3	4	5	NA
279915	Adherence to travel immunization requirements	1	2	3	4	5	NA
279916	Maintenance of accurate immunizations records by individuals or parents	1	2	3	4	5	NA
279917	Reminder programs for required vaccines from health professionals	1	2	3	4	5	NA

Domain-*Community Health (VII)*   **Class**-*Community Health Protection (CC)*   *7th edition 2024*

OUTCOME CONTENT REFERENCES:
Abdullahi, L. H., Kagina, B. M., Ndze, V. N., Hussey, G. D., & Wiysonge, C. S. (2020). Improving vaccination uptake among adolescents. *The Cochrane Database of Systematic Reviews, 1*(1), CD011895. https://doi.org/10.1002/14651858.CD011895.pub2
Anderson, E. J., Daugherty, M. A., Pickering, L. K., Orenstein, W. A., & Yogev, R. (2018). Protecting the community through child vaccination. *Clinical Infectious Diseases: An official publication of the Infectious Diseases Society of America, 67*(3), 464–471. https://doi.org/10.1093/cid/ciy142
Bauer, K. E., Agruss, J. C., & Mayefsky, J. H. (2021). Partnering with parents to remove barriers and improve influenza immunization rates for young children. *Journal of the American Association of Nurse Practitioners, 33*(6), 470–475. https://doi.org/10.1097/JXX.0000000000000381
Dong, M., He, F., & Deng, Y. (2021). How to understand herd immunity in the context of COVID-19. *Viral Immunology, 34*(3), 174–181. https://doi.org/10.1089/vim.2020.0195
Frederiksen, L., Zhang, Y., Foged, C., & Thakur, A. (2020). The long road toward COVID-19 herd immunity: Vaccine platform technologies and mass immunization strategies. *Frontiers in Immunology, 11*, 1817. https://doi.org/10.3389/fimmu.2020.01817
Hakim, H., Provencher, T., Chambers, C. T., Driedger, S. M., Dube, E., Gavaruzzi, T., Giguere, A., Ivers, N. M., MacDonald, S., Paquette, J. S., Wilson, K., Reinharz, D., & Witteman, H. O. (2019). Interventions to help people understand community immunity: A systematic review. *Vaccine, 37*(2), 235–247. https://doi.org/10.1016/j.vaccine.2018.11.016
Recommendations for prevention and control of influenza in children, 2020–2021. (2020). *Pediatrics, 146*(4), 1–29. https://doi.org/10.1542/peds.2020-024588
Saad-Roy, C. M., Levin, S. A., Metcalf, C. J. E., & Grenfell, B. T. (2021). Trajectory of individual immunity and vaccination required for SARS-CoV-2 community immunity: A conceptual investigation. *Journal of the Royal Society Interface, 18*, 20200683. https://doi.org/10.1098/rsif.2020.0683
Strengthening the effectiveness of national, state, and local efforts to improve HPV vaccination coverage in the United States: Recommendations from the National Vaccine Advisory Committee. (2018). *Public Health Reports, 133*(5), 543–550. https://doi.org/10.1177/0033354918793629
Willis, E., Gundacker, C., Harris, M., & Mameledzija, M. (2020). Improving immunization and health literacy through a community-based approach. *Studies in Health Technology and Informatics, 269*, 142–152. https://doi.org/10.3233/SHTI200028

Community Pandemic Readiness 2707

Definition: Community preparedness to respond to an epidemic or pandemic event

OUTCOME TARGET RATING: Maintain at_____ Increase to_____

		Poor	Fair	Good	Very Good	Excellent	
OUTCOME OVERALL RATING		1	2	3	4	5	
Indicators:							
270701	Identification of potential types of infectious agents	1	2	3	4	5	NA
270702	Identification of local experts	1	2	3	4	5	NA
270703	Identification of high-risk groups	1	2	3	4	5	NA
270704	Plan for social distancing guidelines	1	2	3	4	5	NA
270705	Plan for quarantine guidelines	1	2	3	4	5	NA
270706	Plan for travel restrictions within geographic areas	1	2	3	4	5	NA
270707	Plan for required personal protective equipment distribution	1	2	3	4	5	NA
270708	Availability of public health laboratory facilities	1	2	3	4	5	NA
270709	Availability of public health disease surveillance system	1	2	3	4	5	NA
270710	Plan to access electronic health records of community members	1	2	3	4	5	NA
270711	Written plan for mass immunization	1	2	3	4	5	NA
270712	Surge capacity of hospital resources	1	2	3	4	5	NA
270713	Written plan for mobilization of health care personnel	1	2	3	4	5	NA
270714	Written plan for creation of expanded testing centers	1	2	3	4	5	NA
270715	Written plan for communication with community members	1	2	3	4	5	NA
270716	Written plan for resource appropriation	1	2	3	4	5	NA
270717	Essential agencies involvement in planning	1	2	3	4	5	NA
270718	Assignment of agency responsibilities	1	2	3	4	5	NA
270719	Plan for contacting available service organizations for support	1	2	3	4	5	NA
270720	Plan for contact tracing	1	2	3	4	5	NA
270721	Plan to protect health and safety of response personnel	1	2	3	4	5	NA
270722	Functional community warning mechanisms	1	2	3	4	5	NA
270723	Guidelines for hospital equipment and supply availability	1	2	3	4	5	NA
270724	Guidelines for long-term care facilities	1	2	3	4	5	NA
270725	Plan for public education on pandemic warning and response	1	2	3	4	5	NA
270726	Plan for public education on prevention of infection transmission	1	2	3	4	5	NA
270727	Media plan for public information updates	1	2	3	4	5	NA
270728	Plan for coordination of health care	1	2	3	4	5	NA
270729	Plan for documentation of health care	1	2	3	4	5	NA
270730	Plan for expanded morgue facilities	1	2	3	4	5	NA
270731	Plan for expanded mental health care services	1	2	3	4	5	NA
270732	Written post-pandemic plan for community recovery	1	2	3	4	5	NA

Domain-*Community Health (VII)*   **Class**-*Community Health Protection (CC)*   *7th edition 2024*

OUTCOME CONTENT REFERENCES:

Bennett, J. (2020). *Mandell, Douglas, and Bennett's principals and practice of infectious diseases* (9th ed.). Elsevier.

Chaabna, K., Doraiswamy, S., Mamtani, R., & Cheema, S. (2021). Facemask use in community settings to prevent respiratory infection transmission: A rapid review and meta-analysis. *International Journal of Infectious Diseases, 104*, 198–206. https://doi.org/10.1016/j.ijid.2020.09.1434

Charnley, G., Kelman, I., Gaythorpe, K., & Murray, K. A. (2021). Traits and risk factors of post-disaster infectious disease outbreaks: A systematic review. *Scientific Reports, 11*(1), 5616. https://doi.org/10.1038/s41598-021-85146-0

Chu, D. K., Akl, E. A., Duda, S., Solo, K., Yaacoub, S., & Schünemann, H. J. (2020). Physical distancing, face masks, and eye protection to prevent person-to-person transmission of SARS-CoV-2 and COVID-19: A systematic review and meta-analysis. *Lancet, 395*, 1973–1987.

Forman, R., Atun, R., McKee, M., & Mossialos, E. (2020). 12 Lessons learned from the management of the coronavirus pandemic. *Health Policy (Amsterdam, Netherlands), 124*(6), 577–580. https://doi.org/10.1016/j.healthpol.2020.05.008

Khan, Y., Brown, A. D., Gagliardi, A. R., O'Sullivan, T., Lacarte, S., Henry, B., & Schwartz, B. (2019). Are we prepared? The development of performance indicators for public health emergency preparedness using a modified Delphi approach. *PLOS One, 14*(12), e0226489. https://doi.org/10.1371/journal.pone.0226489

Lichtveld, M., & Birnbaum, L. (2020). Advances in environmental health and disaster research 15 years after Hurricane Katrina. *American Journal of Public Health, 110*(10), 1478–1479. https://doi.org/10.2105/AJPH.2020.305739

Stanhope, M., & Lancaster, J. (2020). *Public health nursing: Population-centered health care in the community* (10th ed.). Elsevier.

U.S. Department of Health and Human Services, Office of Disease Prevention and Health Promotion. (n.d.). *Healthy people 2030.* https://health.gov/healthypeople?_ga=2.211075605.126410647.1643675115-1263545106.1641401162

Community Pandemic Recovery   **2708**

Definition: Community actions to help members cope, recover, and return to a new normal after a pandemic

OUTCOME TARGET RATING: Maintain at_____ Increase to_____

		Poor	Fair	Good	Very Good	Excellent	
OUTCOME OVERALL RATING		1	2	3	4	5	
Indicators:							
270801	Support provided by community leaders to help members regain health	1	2	3	4	5	NA
270802	Support from community leaders to ensure equitable treatment of aged, minorities, lower class citizens	1	2	3	4	5	NA
270803	Gradual transition from response to recovery efforts as infection rates decrease	1	2	3	4	5	NA
270804	Shift from short-term goals to long-term recovery	1	2	3	4	5	NA
270805	Assistance from government agencies for unemployment issues	1	2	3	4	5	NA
270806	Stabilization of available housing	1	2	3	4	5	NA
270807	Establishment of priorities for available pandemic recovery resources	1	2	3	4	5	NA
270808	Opportunities for community socialization activities after quarantine	1	2	3	4	5	NA
270809	Members' participation in economic recovery activities	1	2	3	4	5	NA
270810	Identification of long-term health challenges faced by community	1	2	3	4	5	NA
270811	Availability of grief counselors to assist those who lost family members	1	2	3	4	5	NA
270812	Plan to strengthen community resilience	1	2	3	4	5	NA
270813	Availability of faith leaders to provide spiritual comfort	1	2	3	4	5	NA
270814	Availability of bereavement support groups after the pandemic	1	2	3	4	5	NA
270815	Focus on mental health issues created by the pandemic response	1	2	3	4	5	NA
270816	Creation of new jobs to strengthen the economy	1	2	3	4	5	NA
270817	Plan for rebuilding infrastructure	1	2	3	4	5	NA
270818	Plan for community recognition of the pandemic such as a grief ritual	1	2	3	4	5	NA
270819	Plan for remembrances for those who lost their lives	1	2	3	4	5	NA
270820	Analysis of the social impact of the pandemic by government leaders	1	2	3	4	5	NA
270821	Analysis of the economic impact of the pandemic by government leaders	1	2	3	4	5	NA
270822	Analysis of the health care changes needed for the future pandemic preparation	1	2	3	4	5	NA

Domain-Community Health (VII)   *Class*-Community Well-Being (BB)   7th edition 2024

OUTCOME CONTENT REFERENCES:

Aoun, S. M., Breen, L. J., White, I., Rumbold, B., & Kellehear, A. (2018). What sources of bereavement support are perceived helpful by bereaved people and why? Empirical evidence for the compassionate communities approach. *Palliative Medicine, 32*(8), 1378–1388. https://doi.org/10.1177/0269216318774995

Corbie-Smith, G., Wolfe, M. K., Hoover, S. M., & Dave, G. (2021). Centering equity and community in the recovery of the COVID-19 pandemic. *North Carolina Medical Journal, 82*(1), 62–67. https://doi.org/10.18043/ncm.82.1.62

McCartan, C., Adell, T., Cameron, J., Davidson, G., Knifton, L., McDaid, S., & Mulholland, C. (2021). A scoping review of international policy responses to mental health recovery during the COVID-19 pandemic. *Health Research Policy and Systems, 19*(1), 58. https://doi.org/10.1186/s12961-020-00652-3

Morrow-Howell, N., Galucia, N., & Swinford, E. (2020). Recovering from the COVID-19 pandemic: A focus on older adults. *Journal of Aging & Social Policy, 32*(4-5), 526–535. https://doi.org/10.1080/08959420.2020.1759758

Murphy, L., Markey, K., O' Donnell, C., Moloney, M., & Doody, O. (2021). The impact of the COVID-19 pandemic and its related restrictions on people with pre-existent mental health conditions: A scoping review. *Archives of Psychiatric Nursing, 35*(4), 375–394. https://doi.org/10.1016/j.apnu.2021.05.002

Nicola, M., Alsafi, Z., Sohrabi, C., Kerwan, A., Al-Jabir, A., Iosifidis, C., Agha, M., & Agha, R. (2020). The socio-economic implications of the coronavirus pandemic (COVID-19): A review. *International Journal of Surgery (London, England), 78*, 185–193. https://doi.org/10.1016/j.ijsu.2020.04.018

Stanhope, M., & Lancaster, J. (2020). *Public health nursing: Population-centered health care in the community* (10th ed.). Elsevier.

Trump, B. D., Bridges, T. S., Cegan, J. C., Cibulsky, S. M., Greer, S. L., Jarman, H., Lafferty, B. J., Surette, M. A., & Linkov, I. (2020). An analytical perspective on pandemic recovery. *Health Security, 18*(3), 250–256. https://doi.org/10.1089/hs.2020.0057

Community Pandemic Response   2709

Definition: Community actions to eliminate or reduce the spread of infectious diseases during an epidemic or pandemic that threatens public health

OUTCOME TARGET RATING: Maintain at_____ Increase to_____

		Poor	Fair	Good	Very Good	Excellent	
OUTCOME OVERALL RATING		1	2	3	4	5	
Indicators:							
270901	Priority care for high-risk groups	1	2	3	4	5	NA
270902	Easy access to testing by individuals	1	2	3	4	5	NA
270903	Adherence to mandated social distancing	1	2	3	4	5	NA
270904	Adherence to mandated quarantine periods	1	2	3	4	5	NA
270905	Adherence to mandated travel restrictions	1	2	3	4	5	NA
270906	Availability of personal protective equipment	1	2	3	4	5	NA
270907	Use of personal protective equipment to decrease disease spread	1	2	3	4	5	NA
270908	Education about the importance of hand hygiene and disinfecting of common surfaces	1	2	3	4	5	NA
270909	Adherence to visitor restrictions in health care facilities	1	2	3	4	5	NA
270910	Adherence to visitor restrictions in elderly housing complexes	1	2	3	4	5	NA
270911	Adherence to mandated business operation restrictions	1	2	3	4	5	NA
270912	Notification of known contacts concerning risk for infection	1	2	3	4	5	NA
270913	Disease occurrences reported as mandated	1	2	3	4	5	NA
270914	Availability of health care services for infected individuals	1	2	3	4	5	NA
270915	Availability of needed hospital equipment	1	2	3	4	5	NA
270916	Use of masks and eye protection by health professionals	1	2	3	4	5	NA
270917	Promotion of community wide immunization	1	2	3	4	5	NA
270918	Plan for mass immunization	1	2	3	4	5	NA
270919	Enforcement of infection surveillance programs	1	2	3	4	5	NA
270920	Enforcement of infection control programs	1	2	3	4	5	NA
270921	Identification of mental health needs	1	2	3	4	5	NA
270922	Access to mental health care services	1	2	3	4	5	NA
270923	Culturally appropriate public education about infection transmission	1	2	3	4	5	NA
270924	Public education focused on strategies to prevent infection	1	2	3	4	5	NA
270925	Monitoring of communicable disease morbidity	1	2	3	4	5	NA
270926	Monitoring of communicable disease mortality	1	2	3	4	5	NA
270927	Monitoring of hospitalizations related to infectious agent	1	2	3	4	5	NA
270928	Monitoring of communicable disease complications	1	2	3	4	5	NA

Domain-*Community Health (VII)*   **Class**-*Community Health Protection (CC)*   *7th edition 2024*

OUTCOME CONTENT REFERENCES:

Bennett, J. (2020). *Mandell, Douglas, and Bennett's principals and practice of infectious diseases* (9th ed.). Elsevier.

Chaabna, K., Doraiswamy, S., Mamtani, R., & Cheema, S. (2021). Facemask use in community settings to prevent respiratory infection transmission: A rapid review and meta-analysis. *International Journal of Infectious Diseases, 104*, 198–206. https://doi.org/10.1016/j.ijid.2020.09.1434

Chu, D. K., Akl, E. A., Duda, S., Solo, K., Yaacoub, S., & Schünemann, H. J. (2020). Physical distancing, face masks, and eye protection to prevent person-to-person transmission of SARS-CoV-2 and COVID-19: A systematic review and meta-analysis. *Lancet, 395*, 1973–1987.

Forman, R., Atun, R., McKee, M., & Mossialos, E. (2020). 12 Lessons learned from the management of the coronavirus pandemic. *Health Policy, 124*(6), 577–580. https://doi.org/10.1016/j.healthpol.2020.05.008

Stanhope, M., & Lancaster, J. (2020). *Public health nursing: Population-centered health care in the community* (10th ed.). Elsevier.

U.S. Department of Health and Human Services, Office of Disease Prevention and Health Promotion. (n.d.). *Healthy people 2030.* https://health.gov/healthypeople?_ga=2.211075605.126410647.1643675115-1263545106.1641401162

Veenema, T. G., & Toke, J. (2006). Early detection and surveillance for biopreparedness and emerging infectious diseases. *Online Journal of Issues in Nursing, 11*(1), 47–59.

Weber, D. J., Babcock, H., Hayden, M. K., Wright, S. B., Murthy, A. R., Guzman-Cottrill, J., Haessler, S., Rock, C., Van Schooneveld, T., Forde, C. A., Logan, L. K., Malani, A., Henderson, D. K. (2020). Universal pandemic precautions—An idea ripe for the times. *Infection Control & Hospital Epidemiology, 41*(11), 1321–1322. https://doi.org/10.1017/ice.2020.327

Community Program Effectiveness 2808

Definition: Quality of coordinated program activities that promote health and prevent, reduce, or eliminate health problems for an aggregate or population

OUTCOME TARGET RATING: Maintain at_____ Increase to_____

		Poor	Fair	Good	Very Good	Excellent	
OUTCOME OVERALL RATING		1	2	3	4	5	
Indicators:							
280820	Assessment of need for the program	1	2	3	4	5	NA
280801	Program goals consistent with community assessment	1	2	3	4	5	NA
280821	Programs tailored to current infection threat	1	2	3	4	5	NA
280822	Program adaptable to changing situation	1	2	3	4	5	NA
280802	Achievable program goals	1	2	3	4	5	NA
280803	Consistency of content with program goals	1	2	3	4	5	NA
280804	Consistency of methods with program goals	1	2	3	4	5	NA
280805	Quality of program methods	1	2	3	4	5	NA
280806	Timetable for program activities	1	2	3	4	5	NA
280807	Marketing plans for the program	1	2	3	4	5	NA
280808	Participation rate in program	1	2	3	4	5	NA
280809	Reduction in targeted health risks for participants	1	2	3	4	5	NA
280810	Improvement of health status of participants	1	2	3	4	5	NA
280811	Financial resources for program	1	2	3	4	5	NA
280812	Qualified program personnel	1	2	3	4	5	NA
280813	Program goals supported by data	1	2	3	4	5	NA
280823	Monitoring of program goals	1	2	3	4	5	NA
280815	Measurement of program goals	1	2	3	4	5	NA
280824	Modification of goals based on program outcomes	1	2	3	4	5	NA
280814	Cost-benefit analyses support program	1	2	3	4	5	NA
280816	Participants' satisfaction with program	1	2	3	4	5	NA
280817	Community members' satisfaction with program	1	2	3	4	5	NA
280818	Support from influential community representatives	1	2	3	4	5	NA
280825	Modification of program goals based on demographic changes	1	2	3	4	5	NA
280826	Modification of program approaches based on demographics	1	2	3	4	5	NA
280819	Plans for sustaining successful program	1	2	3	4	5	NA

Domain-*Community Health (VII)* **Class**-*Community Health Protection (CC)* 5th edition 2013; revised 2024

OUTCOME CONTENT REFERENCES:

Chugg, B., Lu, L., Ouyand, D., Anderson, B., Ha, R., D'Agostino, A., Sujeer, A., Rudman, S., Garcia, A., & Ho, D. E. (2021). Evaluation of allocation schemes of COVID-19 testing resources in a community-based door-to-door testing program. *JAMA Health Forum, 2*(8), 1–11. https://doi.org/10.1001/jamahealthforum.2021.2260

Del Rios, M., Giachello, A., Khosla, S., Luna, G., Pobee, R., Vergara-Rodriguez, P., & Sugrue, N. (2021). Illinois unidos: A community demands equity, justice, and inclusion. *American Journal of Public Health, 111*(S3), S204–S207. https://doi.org/10.2105/AJPH.2021.306407

Mertens, D. M., & Wilson, A. T. (2019). *Program evaluation theory and practice* (2nd ed.). Guilford Press.

Michener, L., Aguilar-Gaxiola. S., Alberti. P. M., Castaneda, M. J., Castrucci, B. C., Harrison, L. M., Hughes, L. S., Richmond. A., & Wallerstein. N. (2020). Engaging with communities—Lessons (re) learned from COVID-19, *Prevention Chronic Disease, 17*, 1–8. https://doi.org/10.5888/pcd17.200250

Newcomer, K. E., Hatry, H. P., & Wholey, J. S. (2015). *Handbook of practical program evaluation* (4th ed.). Jossey-Bass.

Rossi, P. H., Lipsey, M. W., & Henry, G. T. (2019). *Evaluation: A systematic approach* (8th ed.). Sage.

Stanhope, M., & Lancaster, J. (2020). *Public health nursing: Population-centered health care in the community* (10th ed.). Elsevier.

Community Resilience 2704

Definition: Community actions to collectively adapt and function in response to adverse health, socio-economic, geopolitical, and physical environmental challenges

OUTCOME TARGET RATING: Maintain at_____ Increase to_____

	Poor	Fair	Good	Very Good	Excellent	
OUTCOME OVERALL RATING	1	2	3	4	5	
Indicators:						
270401 Community assessment plan	1	2	3	4	5	NA
270402 Community resources prepared to respond	1	2	3	4	5	NA
270403 Ongoing training for communication requirements	1	2	3	4	5	NA
270431 Community response plan	1	2	3	4	5	NA
270405 Community mobilization following adversity	1	2	3	4	5	NA
270406 Key leaders monitoring of socio-economic environment	1	2	3	4	5	NA
270432 Key leaders building trust with community members	1	2	3	4	5	NA
270433 Key leaders provision of frequent information updates	1	2	3	4	5	NA
270407 Key leaders monitoring of geopolitical environment	1	2	3	4	5	NA
270408 Key leaders monitoring of physical environment	1	2	3	4	5	NA
270434 Key leaders monitoring of business environment	1	2	3	4	5	NA
270435 Key leaders monitoring of housing environment	1	2	3	4	5	NA
270409 Key leaders coordination response	1	2	3	4	5	NA
270410 Key leaders conflict resolution strategies	1	2	3	4	5	NA
270411 Key leaders encouragement of hope for the future	1	2	3	4	5	NA
270412 Continuation of routine community services	1	2	3	4	5	NA
270413 Availability of health care services	1	2	3	4	5	NA
270414 Availability of mental health care services	1	2	3	4	5	NA
270415 Availability of resources to maintain basic needs	1	2	3	4	5	NA
270436 Accurate information provided by media and social media platforms	1	2	3	4	5	NA
270417 Use of communication networks	1	2	3	4	5	NA
270418 Inter-organizational collaboration within the community	1	2	3	4	5	NA
270419 Collaboration with state agencies	1	2	3	4	5	NA
270420 Collaboration with federal agencies	1	2	3	4	5	NA
270421 Support agencies notified of needs	1	2	3	4	5	NA
270422 Access to external resources	1	2	3	4	5	NA
270423 Policies that enable participation of grass root organizations	1	2	3	4	5	NA
270424 Support of members affected by change in environment	1	2	3	4	5	NA
270437 Support of disadvantaged members of the community	1	2	3	4	5	NA
270438 Community level of social cohesion	1	2	3	4	5	NA
270439 Community discussion of impact of changes in health	1	2	3	4	5	NA
270425 Community discussion of impact of changes in environment	1	2	3	4	5	NA
270426 Community expression of confidence in overcoming adversity	1	2	3	4	5	NA
270427 Community cooperation to meet challenges	1	2	3	4	5	NA
270428 Community support groups	1	2	3	4	5	NA
270429 Community adaptation to changes	1	2	3	4	5	NA
270440 Community identification of future needs	1	2	3	4	5	NA
270430 Community preparation for future challenges	1	2	3	4	5	NA

Domain-Community Health (VII) *Class-Community Well-Being (BB)* *5th edition 2013; revised 2024*

OUTCOME CONTENT REFERENCES:

Fan, C., Jiang, Y., & Mostafavi, A. (2020). Emergent social cohesion for coping with community disruptions in disasters. *Journal of the Royal Society Interface, 17*(164), 20190778. https://doi.org/10.1098/rsif.2019.0778

García, A. A., West Ohueri, C., Garay, R., Guzmán, M., Hanson, K., Vasquez, M., Zunñiga, J., & Tierney, W. (2021). Community engagement as a foundation for improving neighborhood health. *Public Health Nursing, 38*(2), 223–231. https://doi.org/10.1111/phn.12870

Jewett, R. L., Mah, S. M., Nicholas Howell, N., & Larsen, M. M. (2021). Social cohesion and community resilience during COVID-19 and pandemics: A rapid scoping review to inform the United Nations Research Roadmap for COVID-19 Recovery. *International Journal of Health Services, 51*(3), 325–336. https://doi.org/10.1111/phn.12870

Ludin, S. M., Rohaizat, M., & Arbon, P. (2019). The association between social cohesion and community disaster resilience: A cross-sectional study. *Health and Social Care in the Community, 27*(3), 621–631. https://doi.org/10.1111/hsc.12674

Patel, S. S., Rogers, M. B., Amlôt, R., & Rubin, G. J. (2017). What do we mean by 'community resilience'? A systematic literature review of how it is defined in the literature. *PLOS Currents, 9,* 1–48. https://doi.org/10.1371/currents.dis.db775af25efc5a c4f0660ad9c9f7db2

Sobeck, J., Smith-Darden, J., Hicks, M., Kernsmith, P., Kilgore, P. E., Treemore-Spears, L., & McElmurry, S. (2020). Stress, coping, resilience and trust during the Flint water crisis. *Behavioral Medicine, 46*(3/4), 202–216. https://doi.org/10.1080/08964289.2020.1729085

Stanhope, M., & Lancaster, J. (2020). *Public health nursing: Population-centered health care in the community* (10th ed.). Elsevier.

Vaughan, E., & Tinker, T. (2009). Effective health risk communication about pandemic influenza for vulnerable populations. *American Journal of Public Health, 99*(Suppl. 2), S324–S332. https://doi.org/10.2105/AJPH.2009.162537

Wyche, K., Pfefferbaum, R., Pfefferbaum, B., Norris, F., Wisnieski, D., & Younger, H. (2011). Exploring community resilience in workforce communities of first responders serving Katrina survivors. *American Journal of Orthopsychiatry, 81*(1), 18–30. https://doi.org/10.1111/j.1939-0025.2010.01068.x

Community Risk Control: Bullying　　　　2811

Definition: Community actions to prevent or eliminate repeated verbal, social, physical, or cyber intimidation of vulnerable persons

OUTCOME TARGET RATING: Maintain at_____ Increase to_____

		Poor	Fair	Good	Very Good	Excellent	
OUTCOME OVERALL RATING		1	2	3	4	5	
Indicators:							
281101	Problem assessment by community stakeholders and policy makers	1	2	3	4	5	NA
281102	Representation of all segments of the community	1	2	3	4	5	NA
281103	Mobilization of community members to eliminate bullying	1	2	3	4	5	NA
281104	Provision of bullying prevention programs	1	2	3	4	5	NA
281105	Identification of high-risk groups	1	2	3	4	5	NA
281106	Identification of prevalent types of bullying	1	2	3	4	5	NA
281107	Educational opportunities focused on bullying prevention	1	2	3	4	5	NA
281108	Competence in managing bullying by community leaders	1	2	3	4	5	NA
281109	Identification of groups who are being bullied	1	2	3	4	5	NA
281110	Identification of groups who are bullying others	1	2	3	4	5	NA
281111	Funds dedicated to bullying prevention programs	1	2	3	4	5	NA
281112	Adoption of a zero tolerance for bullying policy in the community	1	2	3	4	5	NA
281113	Enforcement of a zero tolerance for bullying policy in the community	1	2	3	4	5	NA
281114	Availability of referral systems for counseling	1	2	3	4	5	NA
281115	Educational programs presented in schools	1	2	3	4	5	NA
281116	Participation of school leaders in anti-bullying campaign	1	2	3	4	5	NA
281117	Available media coverage to highlight bullying prevention	1	2	3	4	5	NA
281118	Systematic monitoring of bullying levels	1	2	3	4	5	NA

Domain-Community Health (VII)　**Class**-Community Health Protection (CC)　6th edition 2018

OUTCOME CONTENT REFERENCES:

Brandau, M. S. (2016). *Adolescent victims' experiences with cyberbullying: A grounded theory study* (Publication No. 10125546) [Doctoral dissertation, The University of North Dakota] ProQuest Dissertations & Theses Global.

Gibson, J., Flaspohler, P., & Watts, V. (2015). Engaging youth in bullying prevention through community-based participatory research. *Community Health, 38*(1), 120–130.

Gradinger, P., Yanagida, T., & Strohmeir, D. (2015). Prevention of cyberbullying and cyber victimization: Evaluation of the ViSC social competence program. *Journal of School Violence, 14*(1), 87–110.

Olweus, D., & Limber, S. (2010). Bullying in school: Evaluation and dissemination of the Olweus bullying prevention program. *American Journal of Orthopsychiatry, 80*(1), 124–134.

Wong-Lo, M., Bullock, L., & Gable, R. (2011). Cyber bullying practices to face digital aggression. *Emotional and Behavioral Difficulties, 16*(3), 317–325.

C

Community Risk Control: Chronic Disease   2801

Definition: Community actions to eliminate or reduce the incidence of chronic diseases and related complications

OUTCOME TARGET RATING: Maintain at_____ Increase to_____

		Poor	Fair	Good	Very Good	Excellent	
OUTCOME OVERALL RATING		**1**	**2**	**3**	**4**	**5**	
Indicators:							
280101	Provision of public education programs on chronic disease	1	2	3	4	5	NA
280102	Target population participation rates in risk reduction programs	1	2	3	4	5	NA
280103	Availability of preventive screening programs	1	2	3	4	5	NA
280104	Target population participation rates in preventive screening programs	1	2	3	4	5	NA
280105	Availability of chronic disease self-management education programs	1	2	3	4	5	NA
280106	Proportion of target population participation rates in chronic disease self-management education programs	1	2	3	4	5	NA
280107	Availability of health care services to treat chronic disease	1	2	3	4	5	NA
280118	Provision of health care services to fit target population	1	2	3	4	5	NA
280119	Monitoring of incidence of chronic disease	1	2	3	4	5	NA
280120	Monitoring of prevalence of chronic disease	1	2	3	4	5	NA
280121	Monitoring of chronic disease morbidity	1	2	3	4	5	NA
280122	Monitoring of chronic disease mortality	1	2	3	4	5	NA
280123	Monitoring of chronic disease complications	1	2	3	4	5	NA
280128	Monitoring of costs of chronic diseases	1	2	3	4	5	NA
280129	Monitoring of access to health care services	1	2	3	4	5	NA
280111	Compliance with national standards for chronic disease prevention and management	1	2	3	4	5	NA
280112	Incidence of chronic disease at or below state or national rates	1	2	3	4	5	NA
280114	Prevalence of chronic disease at or below state or national rates	1	2	3	4	5	NA
280124	Public policies that promote health	1	2	3	4	5	NA
280125	Public policies that prevent disease	1	2	3	4	5	NA
280116	Procurement and allocation of funding for chronic disease prevention programs	1	2	3	4	5	NA
280126	Evidence of advocacy efforts for prevention of chronic illness	1	2	3	4	5	NA
280127	Evidence of advocacy efforts for management of chronic illness	1	2	3	4	5	NA

Domain-*Community Health (VII)*   **Class**-*Community Health Protection (CC)*   *2nd edition 2000; revised 2004, 2008, 2013, 2024*

OUTCOME CONTENT REFERENCES:

Calo, W. A., Murray, A., Francis, E., Bermudez, M., & Kraschnewski, J. (2020). Reaching the Hispanic community about COVID-19 through existing chronic disease prevention programs. *Preventing Chronic Disease, 17*, 1–7. https://doi.org/10.5888/pcd17.200165

Centers for Disease Control and Prevention, National Center for Chronic Disease Prevention and Health Promotion. *About chronic diseases.* https://www.cdc.gov/chronicdisease/about/index.htm

Frejuk, K. L., Harasemiw, O., Komenda, P., Lavallee, B., McLeod, L., Chartrand, C., Di Nella, M., Ferguson, T. W., Martin, H., Wicklow, B., & Dart, A. B. (2021). Impact of a screen, triage and treat program for identifying chronic disease risk in Indigenous children. *CMAJ: Canadian Medical Association Journal, 193*(36), E1415–E1422. https://doi.org/10.1503/cmaj.210507

Greer, A. E., Faber, M., Smith, G., Pendley, S., & Kamdar, N. (2021). Objectively measured chronic disease risk among food pantry patrons. *Public Health Nursing, 38*(5), 920–925. https://doi.org/10.1111/phn.12915

Leser, K. A., Liu, S. T., Smathers, C. A., Graffagnino, C. L., & Pirie, P. L. (2021). Adoption, sustainability, and dissemination of chronic disease prevention policies in community-based organizations. *Health Promotion Practice, 22*(1), 72–81. https://doi.org/10.1177/1524839919850757

Matheson, A., Walton, M., Gray, R., Wehipeihana, N., & Wistow, J. (2020). Strengthening prevention in communities through systems change: Lessons from the evaluation of Healthy Families NZ. *Health Promotion International, 35*(5), 947–957. https://doi.org/10.1093/heapro/daz092

O'Rourke, T. W. (2020). Applying the concepts of "community spread" and "flatten the curve" to chronic conditions and their prevention. *American Journal of Health Education, 51*(4), 199–202. https://doi.org/10.1080/19325037.2020.1766605

Robinson, K. L., Driedger, M. S., Elliot, S. J., & Eyles, J. (2006). Understanding facilitators of and barriers to health promotion practice. *Health Promotion Practice, 7*(4), 467–476.

Stanhope, M., & Lancaster, J. (2020). *Public health nursing: Population-centered health care in the community* (10th ed.). Elsevier.

U.S. Department of Health and Human Services, Office of Disease Prevention and Health Promotion. (n.d.). *Healthy people 2030.* https://health.gov/healthypeople?_ga=2.211075605.126410647.1643675115-1263545106.1641401162

Community Risk Control: Communicable Disease   2802

Definition: Community actions to eliminate or reduce the spread of infectious agents that threaten public health

OUTCOME TARGET RATING: Maintain at_____ Increase to_____

OUTCOME OVERALL RATING	Poor	Fair	Good	Very Good	Excellent	
	1	2	3	4	5	
Indicators:						
280225 Easy access to testing by individuals	1	2	3	4	5	NA
280201 Screening of all targeted high-risk groups	1	2	3	4	5	NA
280202 Surveillance for infectious disease outbreaks including a system of data collection, reporting, and follow-up	1	2	3	4	5	NA
280203 Investigation and notification of contacts concerning risk for infectious disease	1	2	3	4	5	NA
280204 Disease occurrences reported as mandated	1	2	3	4	5	NA
280205 Availability of treatment services for infected individuals	1	2	3	4	5	NA
280206 Provision of products to decrease disease spread	1	2	3	4	5	NA
280207 Established polices and surveillance for assuring safe food storage, handling, and preparation	1	2	3	4	5	NA
280208 Water testing consistent with local, state, and federal regulations	1	2	3	4	5	NA
280226 Enforcement of mandated quarantine	1	2	3	4	5	NA
280209 Promotion of community wide immunization	1	2	3	4	5	NA
280220 Plan for mass immunization	1	2	3	4	5	NA
280210 Enforcement of infection surveillance programs	1	2	3	4	5	NA
280221 Enforcement of infection control programs	1	2	3	4	5	NA
280211 Availability of chemoprophylaxis for travelers	1	2	3	4	5	NA
280212 Evidence of environmental controls	1	2	3	4	5	NA
280213 Enforcement of environmental monitoring policies	1	2	3	4	5	NA
280214 Enforcement of domestic animal vaccination	1	2	3	4	5	NA
280215 Availability of health care services to treat communicable diseases	1	2	3	4	5	NA
280216 Access to health care services	1	2	3	4	5	NA
280217 Culturally appropriate public education about transmission of infectious disease	1	2	3	4	5	NA
280127 Public education focused on strategies to prevent infection	1	2	3	4	5	NA
280218 Policies supporting control of infectious disease	1	2	3	4	5	NA
280222 Monitoring of communicable disease morbidity	1	2	3	4	5	NA

C

C

Community Risk Control: Communicable Disease—cont'd

	Poor	Fair	Good	Very Good	Excellent	
280223 Monitoring of communicable disease mortality	1	2	3	4	5	NA
280228 Monitoring of hospitalizations related to infectious agent	1	2	3	4	5	NA
280224 Monitoring of communicable disease complications	1	2	3	4	5	NA

Domain-Community Health (VII)   **Class**-Community Health Protection (CC)   2nd edition 2000; revised 2004, 2008, 2024

OUTCOME CONTENT REFERENCES:

Bennett, J. (2020). *Mandell, Douglas, and Bennett's principals and practice of infectious diseases* (9th ed.). Elsevier.
McArthur, D. B. (2019). Emerging infectious diseases. *The Nursing Clinics of North America, 54*(2), 297–311. https://doi.org/10.1016/j.cnur.2019.02.006
Stanhope, M., & Lancaster, J. (2020). *Public health nursing: Population-centered health care in the community* (10th ed.). Elsevier.
U.S. Department of Health and Human Services, Office of Disease Prevention and Health Promotion. (n.d.). *Healthy people 2030*.
   https://health.gov/healthypeople?_ga=2.211075605.126410647.1643675115-1263545106.1641401162
Veenema, T. G., & Toke, J. (2006). Early detection and surveillance for biopreparedness and emerging infectious diseases. *Online Journal of Issues in Nursing,* *11*(1), 47–59.
6 Infection Protection Strategies. (2020). *Consumer Reports on Health, 32*(6), 6–8.

Community Risk Control: Environmental Hazards   2812

Definition: Community actions to monitor, eliminate, or reduce environmental hazards

OUTCOME TARGET RATING: Maintain at_____ Increase to_____

	Poor	Fair	Good	Very Good	Excellent	
OUTCOME OVERALL RATING	1	2	3	4	5	
Indicators:						
281201 Problem assessment by community stakeholders and policy makers	1	2	3	4	5	NA
281202 Surveillance for sources of environmental hazards	1	2	3	4	5	NA
281203 Ground level ozone concentration	1	2	3	4	5	NA
281204 Air particulate matter level	1	2	3	4	5	NA
281205 Enforcement of industry emissions standards	1	2	3	4	5	NA
281206 Agricultural pesticide levels in ground waters	1	2	3	4	5	NA
281207 Traffic-related air pollution level	1	2	3	4	5	NA
281208 Diesel particulate matter level	1	2	3	4	5	NA
281209 Enforcement of vehicle emissions standards	1	2	3	4	5	NA
281210 Strategies to reduce traffic noise	1	2	3	4	5	NA
281211 Provision of culturally-appropriate public education	1	2	3	4	5	NA
281212 Abatement of environmental hazards	1	2	3	4	5	NA
281213 Compliance with regulatory standards	1	2	3	4	5	NA
281214 Water quality	1	2	3	4	5	NA
281215 Availability of green space	1	2	3	4	5	NA
281216 Radon elimination program	1	2	3	4	5	NA
281217 Community recycling program	1	2	3	4	5	NA
281218 Community electronic waste recycling program	1	2	3	4	5	NA
281219 Funds dedicated to elimination of environmental hazards	1	2	3	4	5	NA

Domain-Community Health (VII)   **Class**-Community Health Protection (CC)   6th edition 2018

OUTCOME CONTENT REFERENCES:

Apollonio, D., Wolfe, N., & Bero, L. (2016). Realist review of policy intervention studies aimed at reducing exposures to environmental hazards in the United States. *BMC Public Health, 16*(1). https://doi.org/10.1186/s12889-016-3461-7
Borthakur, A. (2016). Health and environmental hazards of electronic waste in India. *Journal of Environmental Health, 78*(8), 18–23.
Heacock, M., Kelly, C., Asante, K., Birnbaum, L., Bergman, Å., Bruné, M.-N., Buka, I., Carpenter, D. O., Chen, A., Huo, X., Kamel, M., Landrigan, P. J., Magalini, F., Diaz-Barriga, F., Neira, M., Omar, M., Pascale, A., Ruchirawat, M., Sly, L., & Sly, P. D. (2016). E-waste and harm to vulnerable populations: A growing global problem. *Environmental Health Perspectives, 124*(5), 550–555. https://doi.org/10.1289/ehp.1509699
Woods, M., Crabbe, H., Close, R., Studden, M., Milojevic, A., Leonardi, G., & Chalabi, Z. (2016). Decision support for risk prioritisation of environmental health hazards in a UK city. *Environmental Health: A Global Access Science Source, 15*(Suppl. 1), 35–47. https://doi.org/10.1186/s12940-016-0099-y

Community Risk Control: Lead Exposure 2803

Definition: Community actions to eliminate or reduce lead exposure and poisoning

OUTCOME TARGET RATING: Maintain at_____ Increase to_____

OUTCOME OVERALL RATING	Poor	Fair	Good	Very Good	Excellent	
	1	2	3	4	5	
Indicators:						
280314 Problem assessment by community stakeholders and policy makers	1	2	3	4	5	NA
280315 Organization of lead screening programs that includes focus on preschools	1	2	3	4	5	NA
280316 Culturally appropriate marketing of screening programs to high-risk groups	1	2	3	4	5	NA
280301 Use of lead screening programs by targeted high-risk groups	1	2	3	4	5	NA
280317 Organization of referral and treatment services for exposed individuals	1	2	3	4	5	NA
280302 Referral of exposed individuals to treatment	1	2	3	4	5	NA
280318 Treatment of individuals with exposure to lead	1	2	3	4	5	NA
280303 Surveillance for sources of lead	1	2	3	4	5	NA
280304 Abatement of known lead sources in the community	1	2	3	4	5	NA
280305 Programs to identify nutritional deficiencies in targeted high-risk groups	1	2	3	4	5	NA
280306 Programs to correct nutritional deficiencies in targeted high-risk groups	1	2	3	4	5	NA
280307 Provision of culturally appropriate public education about lead poisoning prevention	1	2	3	4	5	NA
280319 Participation rates of high-risk groups in education programs	1	2	3	4	5	NA
280308 Policies that require the removal of lead-based paint from all buildings	1	2	3	4	5	NA
280321 Funds dedicated to screening of lead hazards	1	2	3	4	5	NA
280322 Funds dedicated to elimination of lead hazards	1	2	3	4	5	NA
280310 Incidence of elevated lead levels at or below recommended national standards	1	2	3	4	5	NA
280311 Enforcement of home-buyer notification	1	2	3	4	5	NA
280320 Advocacy on behalf of renters of pre-1950 homes	1	2	3	4	5	NA
280312 Enforcement of emission standards	1	2	3	4	5	NA

Domain-Community Health (VII)   **Class**-Community Health Protection (CC)   *2nd edition 2000; revised 2004, 2008, 2013*

OUTCOME CONTENT REFERENCES:

Kincl, L. D., Dietrich, K. N., & Bhattacharya, A. (2006). Injury trends for adolescents with early childhood lead exposure. *Journal of Adolescent Health, 39*(4), 604–606. https://doi.org/10.1016/j.jadohealth.2006.02.008

Morgan, L. (1996). Children and lead: A model of care for community health providers. *Family and Community Health, 19*(1), 42–48.

Needleman, H. (1998). Childhood lead poisoning: The promise and abandonment of primary prevention. *American Journal of Public Health, 88*(12), 1871–1876.

Needleman, H., Schell, A., Bellinger, D., Leviton, A., & Allred, E. (1990). The long-term effects of exposure to low doses of lead in childhood. *The New England Journal of Medicine, 22*(2), 83–90.

Rischitelli, G., Nygren, P., Biougatsos, C., Feeman, M., & Helfand, M. (2006). Screening for elevated lead levels in childhood and pregnancy: An update summary of evidence for the U.S. Preventive Services Task Force. *Pediatrics, 118*(6), 1867–1895. https://doi.org/10.1542/peds.2006-2284

Schwartz, J. (1994). Societal benefits of reducing lead exposure. *Environmental Research, 66*(1), 105–124.

Shih, R. A., Glass, T. A., Bandeen-Roche, K., Carlson, M. C., Bolla, K. I., Todd, A. C., & Schwartz, B. S. (2006). Environmental lead exposure and cognitive function in community-dwelling older adults. *Neurology, 67*(9), 1556–1562. https://doi.org/10.1212/01.wnl.0000239836.26142.c5

Community Risk Control: Obesity   2809

Definition: Community actions to reduce obesity and related chronic diseases

OUTCOME TARGET RATING: Maintain at_____ Increase to_____

		Poor	Fair	Good	Very Good	Excellent	
OUTCOME OVERALL RATING		1	2	3	4	5	
Indicators:							
280901	Identification of cultural components of the obesity epidemic	1	2	3	4	5	NA
280902	Screening of high-risk members across the lifespan	1	2	3	4	5	NA
280903	Provision of community education programs on prevention of obesity	1	2	3	4	5	NA
280904	Participation rates of high-risk members in educational programs	1	2	3	4	5	NA
280905	Provision of children's programs to encourage physical activity	1	2	3	4	5	NA
280906	Participation rates in children's programs that encourage physical activity	1	2	3	4	5	NA
280907	Education of parents on importance of physical activity	1	2	3	4	5	NA
280908	Provision of healthy meals in lunch programs	1	2	3	4	5	NA
280909	Provision of family events that encourage active lifestyles	1	2	3	4	5	NA
280910	Provision of school-based obesity prevention programs	1	2	3	4	5	NA
280911	Provision of community programs to encourage activity	1	2	3	4	5	NA
280912	Provision of educational programs focused on healthy diet	1	2	3	4	5	NA
280913	Availability of community resources to support weight loss	1	2	3	4	5	NA
280914	Availability of affordable healthy food and beverages in public service venues	1	2	3	4	5	NA
280915	Limitation of unhealthy food and beverage advertisement	1	2	3	4	5	NA
280916	Incentives for food retailers to offer healthy food and beverage choices	1	2	3	4	5	NA
280917	Availability of fresh produce for purchase	1	2	3	4	5	NA
280918	Access to recreational facilities	1	2	3	4	5	NA
280919	Community facilities for physical activities	1	2	3	4	5	NA
280920	Availability of bicycle paths	1	2	3	4	5	NA
280921	Availability of walking paths	1	2	3	4	5	NA
280922	Availability of parks	1	2	3	4	5	NA
280923	Community coalitions to address obesity epidemic	1	2	3	4	5	NA
280924	Monitoring the incidence of obesity	1	2	3	4	5	NA
280925	Monitoring the incidence of diabetes	1	2	3	4	5	NA
280926	Monitoring the incidence of cardiovascular disease	1	2	3	4	5	NA
280927	Monitoring obesity complications	1	2	3	4	5	NA
280928	Public policies that promote healthy living	1	2	3	4	5	NA
280929	Procurement and allocation of funding for obesity prevention programs	1	2	3	4	5	NA

Domain-Community Health (VII)   *Class*-Community Health Protection (CC)   5th edition 2013

OUTCOME CONTENT REFERENCES:
Anderson, S., & Whitaker, R. (2010). Household routines and obesity in U.S. preschool-aged children. *Pediatrics, 125*(3), 420–428. https://doi.org/10.1542/peds.2009-0417
Bauer, K., Neumark-Sztainer, D., Hannan, P., Fulkerson, J., & Story, M. (2011). Relationships between the family environment and school-based obesity prevention efforts: Can school programs help adolescents who are most in need? *Health Education Research, 26*(4), 675–688. https://doi.org/10.1093/her/cyr027
Cappellano, K. (2011). Let's move-tools to fuel a healthier population. *Nutrition Today, 46*(3), 149–154. https://doi.org/10.1097/NT.0b013e3181ec6a6d
Khan, L., Sobush, K., Keener, D., Goodman, K., Lowry, A., Kakierek, J., & Zaro, S. (2009). Recommended community strategies and measurements to prevent obesity in the United States. *Morbidity and Mortality Weekly Report, 58*(RR-7), 1–26.
Kwapiszewski, R., & Wallace, A. (2011). A pilot program to identify and reverse childhood obesity in a primary care clinic. *Clinical Pediatrics, 50*(7), 630–635. https://doi.org/10.1177/0009922811398389
Tucker, S., Foster, L., Murphy, J., Olsen, G., Orth, K., Voss, J., Aleman, M., & Lohse, C. (2011). A school based community partnership for promoting healthy habits for life. *Journal of Community Health, 36*(3), 414–422. https://doi.org/10.1007/s10900-010-9323-9
Uusitupa, M., Tuomilehto, J., & Puska, P. (2011). Are we really active in the prevention of obesity and type 2 diabetes at the community level? *Nutrition, Metabolism, & Cardiovascular Diseases, 21*(5), 380–389. https://doi.org/10.1016/j.numecd.2010.12.007

Community Risk Control: Suicide

C

Definition: Community actions to prevent suicides

OUTCOME TARGET RATING: Maintain at_____ Increase to_____

		Poor	Fair	Good	Very Good	Excellent	
OUTCOME OVERALL RATING		1	2	3	4	5	
Indicators:							
281301	Sustained commitment to community suicide prevention strategies	1	2	3	4	5	NA
281302	Systematic assessment of at-risk groups	1	2	3	4	5	NA
281303	Maintenance of social support for at-risk groups	1	2	3	4	5	NA
281304	Availability of mental health care services	1	2	3	4	5	NA
281305	Provision of community suicide crisis line	1	2	3	4	5	NA
281306	Enforcement of weapon control policies	1	2	3	4	5	NA
281307	Provision of psychosocial suicide prevention programs	1	2	3	4	5	NA
281308	Enforcement of lethal drug control program	1	2	3	4	5	NA
281309	Use of consciousness raising strategies	1	2	3	4	5	NA
281310	Provision of universal school-based interventions	1	2	3	4	5	NA
281311	Referral of individuals with suicide ideation to mental health services	1	2	3	4	5	NA
281312	Provision of public information during seasonal high-risk periods	1	2	3	4	5	NA
281313	Social support programs for veterans after deployment	1	2	3	4	5	NA
281314	Use of social media for educational programs to increase awareness of suicide risk	1	2	3	4	5	NA
281315	Support for suicide prevention programs from influential community representatives	1	2	3	4	5	NA
281316	Identification of cultural components of suicide risk	1	2	3	4	5	NA
281317	Systematic monitoring of community suicide rate	1	2	3	4	5	NA
281318	Systematic monitoring of community suicide prevention strategies	1	2	3	4	5	NA

Domain-Community Health (VII)   *Class*-Community Health Protection (CC)   6th edition 2018

OUTCOME CONTENT REFERENCES:

Calear, A., Christensen, H., Freeman, A., Fenton, K., Grant, J., van Spijker, B., & Donker, T. (2016). A systematic review of psychosocial suicide prevention interventions for youth. *European Child & Adolescent Psychiatry, 25*(5), 467–482. https://doi.org/10.1007/s00787-015-0783-4

Flannery, D., Singer, M. I., & Wester, K. (2001). Violence exposure, psychological trauma, and suicide risk in a community sample of dangerously violent adolescents. *Journal of the American Academy of Child and Adolescent Psychiatry, 40*(4), 435–442. https://doi.org/10.1097/00004583-200104000-00012

Fountoulaskis, K. N., Gonda, X., & Rihmer, Z. (2011). Suicide prevention programs through community intervention. *Journal of Affective Disorders, 30*(1-2), 10–16. https://doi.org/10.1016/j.jad.2010.06.009

Marutani, M., Yamamoto-Mitani, N., & Kodama, S. (2016). Public health nurses' activities for suicide prevention in Japan. *Public Health Nursing, 33*(4), 325–334. https://doi.org/10.1111/phn.12247

Oyama, H., Watanabe, N., Ono, Y., Sakashita, T., Takenoshita, Y., Taguchi, M., Takizawa, T., Mura, R., & Kumagai, M. (2005). Community-based suicide prevention through group activity for the elderly successfully reduced the high suicide rate for females. *Psychiatry and Clinical Neurosciences, 59*(3), 337–344. https://doi.org/10.1111/j.1440-1819.2005.01379.x

C

Community Risk Control: Unhealthy Cultural Traditions   2810

Definition: Community actions to promote customs, beliefs, values, and laws that support members' health and lifestyle modifications within the culture

OUTCOME TARGET RATING: Maintain at_____ Increase to_____

	Poor	Fair	Good	Very Good	Excellent	
OUTCOME OVERALL RATING	1	2	3	4	5	
Indicators:						
281001 Systematic assessment of cultural practices within the community	1	2	3	4	5	NA
281002 Representation of all segments of the community	1	2	3	4	5	NA
281003 Mobilization of community members to identify healthy cultural practices	1	2	3	4	5	NA
281004 Mobilization of community members to identify harmful cultural practices	1	2	3	4	5	NA
281005 Mobilization of community members to eliminate harmful cultural practices	1	2	3	4	5	NA
281006 Use of influential community representatives to foster recommended changes	1	2	3	4	5	NA
281007 Availability of financial resources	1	2	3	4	5	NA
281008 Educational programs for reinforcement of healthy cultural practices	1	2	3	4	5	NA
281009 Educational opportunities to discuss harmful cultural practices	1	2	3	4	5	NA
281010 Promotion of laws against harmful practices	1	2	3	4	5	NA
281011 Enforcement of existing legislation	1	2	3	4	5	NA
281012 Incentives for healthy behavior	1	2	3	4	5	NA
281013 Treatment of members with conditions related to harmful practice	1	2	3	4	5	NA
281014 Availability of referral systems for counseling	1	2	3	4	5	NA
281015 Availability of culturally relevant resources	1	2	3	4	5	NA
281016 Capacity of the community to monitor harmful practices	1	2	3	4	5	NA
281017 Modifications of harmful cultural practices to make them safe	1	2	3	4	5	NA
281018 Elimination of harmful cultural practices	1	2	3	4	5	NA
281019 Reinforcement of healthy cultural practices	1	2	3	4	5	NA

Domain-Community Health (VII)   **Class**-Community Health Protection (CC)   5th edition 2013

OUTCOME CONTENT REFERENCES:

Al-Qattan, M., & Al-Zahrani, K. (2009). A review of burns related to traditions, social habits, religious activities, festivals and traditional medical practices. *Burns, 35*(4), 476–481. https://doi.org/10.1016/j.burns.2008.03.001

Bell, R., Hillers, V., & Thomas, T. (1999). Hispanic grandmothers preserve cultural traditions and reduce foodborne illness by conducting safe cheese workshops. *Journal of the American Dietetic Association, 99*(9), 1114–1116. https://doi.org/10.1016/S0002-8223(99)00269-2

Natoli, L., Renzaho, A., & Rinaudo, T. (2008). Reducing harmful traditional practices in Adjibar, Ethiopia: Lessons learned from the Adjibar safe motherhood project. *Contemporary Nurse, 29*(1), 110–119. https://doi.org/10.5172/conu.673.29.1.110

Smeltzer, S., Bare, B., Hinkle, J., & Cheever, K. (2008). *Brunner and Sudarth's textbook of medical-surgical nursing* (11th ed., pp. 127–138). Lippincott Williams & Wilkins.

The United Nations Children's Fund. (2005). *Female genital mutilation/cutting: A statistical exploration 2005.*

World Health Organization. (2001). *Female genital mutilation: Integrating the prevention and the management of the health complications into the curricula of nursing and midwifery; A teacher's guide.*

Community Risk Control: Violence 2805

Definition: Community actions to eliminate or reduce intentional violent acts resulting in serious physical or psychological harm

OUTCOME TARGET RATING: Maintain at_____ Increase to_____

		Poor	Fair	Good	Very Good	Excellent	
OUTCOME OVERALL RATING		1	2	3	4	5	
Indicators:							
280501	Systematic assessment of at-risk groups	1	2	3	4	5	NA
280502	Support programs for high-risk groups	1	2	3	4	5	NA
280503	Intervention programs for high-risk groups	1	2	3	4	5	NA
280504	Existence of weapon control policies	1	2	3	4	5	NA
280505	Enforcement of weapon control policies	1	2	3	4	5	NA
280506	Strategies to reduce violent content in the media	1	2	3	4	5	NA
280507	Control of violent content in the media	1	2	3	4	5	NA
280508	Educational programs on violence prevention	1	2	3	4	5	NA
280509	Competence in recognizing violence by community leaders	1	2	3	4	5	NA
280510	Competence in managing violence by community leaders	1	2	3	4	5	NA
280514	Strategies to maintain a culture of respect	1	2	3	4	5	NA
280511	Acceptance of population diversity	1	2	3	4	5	NA
280512	Enforcement of laws against hate crimes by community leaders	1	2	3	4	5	NA
280513	Systematic monitoring of community violence levels	1	2	3	4	5	NA
280515	Enforcement of a non-violence policy	1	2	3	4	5	NA

Domain-*Community Health (VII)* **Class**-*Community Health Protection (CC)* *3rd edition 2004; revised 2018*

OUTCOME CONTENT REFERENCES:

Black, S., Weinles, D., & Washington, E. (2010). Victim strategies to stop bullying. *Youth Violence and Juvenile Justice, 8*(2), 138–147.

Mann, M., Kristjansson, A., Sigfusdottir, I., & Smith, M. (2015). The role of community, family, peer, and school factors in group bullying: Implications for school-based intervention. *Journal of School Health, 85*(7), 477–486. https://doi.org/10.1111/josh.12270

McCartan, K., Kemshall, H., & Tabachnick, J. (2015). The construction of community understandings of sexual violence: Rethinking public, practitioner and policy discourses. *Journal of Sexual Aggression, 21*(1), 100–116.

Milam, A., Buggs, S., Furr-Holden, D., Leaf, P., Bradshaw, C., & Webster, D. (2016). Changes in attitudes toward guns and shootings following implementation of the Baltimore safe streets intervention. *Journal of Urban Health, 93*(4), 609–626. https://doi.org/10.1007/s11524-016-0060-y

Morrel-Samuels, S., Bacallao, M., Brown, S., Bower, M., & Zimmerman, M. (2015). Community engagement in youth violence prevention: Crafting methods to context. *Journal of Primary Prevention, 37*(2), 189–207. https://doi.org/10.1007/s10935-016-0428-5

Reidy, D., Kearns, M., DeGue, S., Lilienfeld, S., Massetti, G., & Kiehl, K. (2015). Why psychopathy matters: Implications for public health and violence prevention. *Aggression and Violent Behavior, 24*, 214–225. https://doi.org/10.1016/j.avb.2015.05.018

Smokowski, P., & Kopasz, K. (2005). Bullying in school: An overview of types, effects, family characteristics, and intervention strategies. *Children & Schools, 27*(2), 101–109.

Zeoli, A., Grady, S., Pizarro, J., & Melde, C. (2015). Modeling the movement of homicide by type to inform public health prevention efforts. *American Journal of Public Health, 105*(10), 2035–2041. https://doi.org/10.2105/AJPH.2015.302732

Community Violence Level 2702

Definition: Incidence of violent acts compared with local, state, or national values

OUTCOME TARGET RATING: Maintain at_____ Increase to_____

		Poor	Fair	Good	Very Good	Excellent	
OUTCOME OVERALL RATING		1	2	3	4	5	
Indicators:							
270201	Homicide rate	1	2	3	4	5	NA
270202	Suicide rate	1	2	3	4	5	NA
270203	Sexual assault rate	1	2	3	4	5	NA

Community Violence Level—cont'd

		Poor	Fair	Good	Very Good	Excellent	
270204	Physical assault rate	1	2	3	4	5	NA
270205	Child abuse rate	1	2	3	4	5	NA
270206	Elder abuse rate	1	2	3	4	5	NA
270207	Partner abuse rate	1	2	3	4	5	NA
270208	Hate crime rate	1	2	3	4	5	NA
270209	Gun violence rate	1	2	3	4	5	NA
270210	High-school violence rate	1	2	3	4	5	NA
270211	Murder-suicide rate	1	2	3	4	5	NA

Domain-Community Health (VII)   *Class*-Community Well-Being (BB)   *3rd edition 2004; revised 2018*

OUTCOME CONTENT REFERENCES:

Bushman, B. J., Newman, K., Calvert, S. L., Downey, G., Dredze, M., Gottfredson, M., Jablonski, N. G., Masten, A. S., Morrill, C., Neill, D. B., Romer, D., & Webster, D. W. (2016). Youth violence: What we know and what we need to know. *American Psychologist, 71*(1), 17–39. https://doi.org/10.1037/a0039687

Marvicsin, D., Boucher, N., & Eagle, M. (2013). Youth bullying: Implications for primary care providers. *Journal for Nurse Practitioners, 9*(8), 523–527.

Sumner, S., Mercy, J., Dahlberg, L., Hillis, S., Klevens, J., & Houry, D. (2015). Violence in the United States: Status, challenges, and opportunities. *JAMA: Journal of the American Medical Association, 314*(5), 478–488. https://doi.org/10.1001/jama.2015.8371

U.S. Department of Health and Human Services, Office of Disease Prevention and Health Promotion. (2016). *Healthy people 2020.* https://www.healthypeople.gov

Waasdorp, T., Pas, E., O'Brennan, L., & Bradshaw, C. (2011). A multilevel perspective on the climate of bullying: Discrepancies among students, school staff, and parents. *Journal of School Violence, 10*(2), 115–132. https://doi.org/10.1080/15388220.2010.539164

Concentration   **0905**

Definition: Ability to focus on a specific stimulus

OUTCOME TARGET RATING: Maintain at_____ Increase to_____

		Never Demonstrated	Rarely Demonstrated	Sometimes Demonstrated	Often Demonstrated	Consistently Demonstrated	
OUTCOME OVERALL RATING		1	2	3	4	5	
Indicators:							
090501	Maintains attention	1	2	3	4	5	NA
090502	Maintains focus	1	2	3	4	5	NA
090517	Follows three-step commands	1	2	3	4	5	NA
090503	Responds to visual cues	1	2	3	4	5	NA
090504	Responds to auditory cues	1	2	3	4	5	NA
090505	Responds to tactile cues	1	2	3	4	5	NA
090506	Responds to olfactory cues	1	2	3	4	5	NA
090507	Responds to language cues	1	2	3	4	5	NA
090508	Spells "world" backwards	1	2	3	4	5	NA
090518	Adds totals of three coins	1	2	3	4	5	NA
090515	Counts backward from 20 by 3s	1	2	3	4	5	NA
090516	Counts backward from 100 by 7s	1	2	3	4	5	NA
090510	Names the months of the year backward, starting with January	1	2	3	4	5	NA
090511	Draws a circle	1	2	3	4	5	NA
090514	Draws a triangle	1	2	3	4	5	NA
090512	Draws a pentagon	1	2	3	4	5	NA

Domain-Physiologic Health (II)   *Class*-Neurocognitive (J)   *1st edition 1997; revised 2004, 2008, 2024*

OUTCOME CONTENT REFERENCES:

+Cercy, S. P., Simakhodskaya, Z., & Elliott, A. (2010). Diagnostic accuracy of a new instrument for detecting cognitive dysfunction in an emergent psychiatric population: The Brief Cognitive Screen. *Academic Emergency Medicine, 17*, 307–315. https://doi.org/10.1111/j.1553-2712.2010. 00682.x

Cordell, C. B., Borson, S., Boustani, M., Chodosh, J., Reuben, D., Verghese, J., Thies, W., & Fried, L. B. (2013). Alzheimer's Association recommendations for operationalizing the detection of cognitive impairment during the Medicare annual wellness visit in a primary care setting. *Alzheimer's & Dementia, 9*(5), 141–150. https//doi.org/10.1016/j.jalz.2012.09.011

Fletcher, K. A., Hicks, V. L., Johnson, R. H., Laverentz, D. M., Phillips, C. J., Pierce, L. N. B., Wilhoite, D. L., & Gay, J. E. (2019). A concept analysis of conceptual learning: A guide for educators. *Journal of Nursing Education, 58*(1), 7–15. https://doi.org/10.3928/01484834-201900103-03

Folstein, M. F., Folstein, S. E., & McHugh, P. R. (1975). "Mini-Mental State": A practical method for grading the cognitive state of patients for the clinician. *Journal of Psychiatric Research, 12*(3), 189–198. https://doi.org/10.1016/0022-3956(75)90026-6

Hogan-Quigley, B., Palm, M. L., & Bickley, L. (2021). *Bates nursing guide to physical examination and history taking* (3rd ed.). Wolters Kluwer.

Norris, D. (2017). Short-term memory and long-term memory are still different. *Psychological Bulletin, 143*(9), 992–1009. https://doi.org/10.1037/bul0000108

Parkhurst, D., Wyatt, R., Andary, M., & Sylvain, J. (2020). Validation of a Brief Cognitive Screening Examination in an adult acute inpatient rehabilitation population. *Topics in Geriatric Rehabilitation, 36*(2), 122–126. https://doi.org/10.1097/TGR.0000000000000267

Shin, J. (2020). A meta-analysis of the relationship between working memory and second language reading comprehension: Does task type matter? *Applied Psycholinguistics, 41*(4), 873–900. https://doi.org/10.1017/S0142716420000272

Coordinated Movement — 0212

Definition: Ability of muscles to work together voluntarily for purposeful movement

OUTCOME TARGET RATING: Maintain at_____ Increase to_____

OUTCOME OVERALL RATING		Severely Compromised	Substantially Compromised	Moderately Compromised	Mildly Compromised	Not Compromised	
		1	2	3	4	5	
Indicators:							
021201	Strength of muscle contraction	1	2	3	4	5	NA
021202	Muscle tone	1	2	3	4	5	NA
021203	Speed of movement	1	2	3	4	5	NA
021204	Smooth movement	1	2	3	4	5	NA
021205	Control of movement	1	2	3	4	5	NA
021206	Steadiness of movement	1	2	3	4	5	NA
021207	Balanced movement	1	2	3	4	5	NA
021208	Muscle tension	1	2	3	4	5	NA
021209	Movement in desired direction	1	2	3	4	5	NA
021210	Movement with desired timing	1	2	3	4	5	NA
021211	Movement at desired speed	1	2	3	4	5	NA
021212	Movement with desired precision	1	2	3	4	5	NA

Domain-Functional Health (I)   **Class**-Mobility (C)   *3rd edition 2004; reviewed 2018*

OUTCOME CONTENT REFERENCES:

Andani, M., & Bahrami, F. (2012). COMAP: A new computational interpretation of human movement planning level based on coordinated minimum angle jerk policies and six universal movement elements. *Human Movement Science, 31*(5), 1037–1055. https://doi.org/10.1016/j.humov.2012.01.001

Crawford, S. G., Wilson, B. N., & Dewey, D. (2001). Identifying developmental coordination disorder: Consistency between tests. *Physical & Occupational Therapy in Pediatrics, 20*(2/3), 29–50.

+Junaid, K., Harris, S. R., Fulmer, K. A., & Carswell, A. (2000). Teachers' use of the MABC checklist to identify children with motor coordination difficulties. *Pediatric Physical Therapy, 12*(4), 158–163.

Mokhtarinia, H., Sanjari, M., Chehrehrazi, M., Kahrizi, S., & Parnianpour, M. (2016). Trunk coordination in healthy and chronic nonspecific low back pain subjects during repetitive flexion-extension tasks: Effects of movement asymmetry, velocity and load. *Human Movement Science, 45*, 182–192. https://doi.org/10.1016/j.humov.2015.11.007

Preece, S., Mason, D., & Bramah, C. (2016). The coordinated movement of the spine and pelvis during running. *Human Movement Science, 45*, 110–118. https://doi.org/10.1016/j.humov.2015.11.014

Schmitz, T. J., & O'Sullivan, S. B. (2014). Examination of coordination and balance. In S. O'Sullivan, T. Schmitz, & G. Fulk (Eds.), *Physical rehabilitation* (6th ed., pp. 206–250). F.A. Davis.

Coping   1302

Definition: Personal actions to manage stressors that tax an individual's resources

OUTCOME TARGET RATING: Maintain at_____ Increase to_____

		Never Demonstrated	Rarely Demonstrated	Sometimes Demonstrated	Often Demonstrated	Consistently Demonstrated	
OUTCOME OVERALL RATING		1	2	3	4	5	
Indicators:							
130224	Verbalizes self-confidence	1	2	3	4	5	NA
130203	Verbalizes sense of control	1	2	3	4	5	NA
130225	Identifies problem-focused coping strategies	1	2	3	4	5	NA
130226	Identifies emotional-focused coping strategies	1	2	3	4	5	NA
130227	Identifies avoidant coping strategies	1	2	3	4	5	NA
130205	Verbalizes acceptance of situation	1	2	3	4	5	NA
130220	Seeks reputable information about diagnosis	1	2	3	4	5	NA
130221	Seeks reputable information about treatment	1	2	3	4	5	NA
130207	Modifies lifestyle to reduce stress	1	2	3	4	5	NA
130208	Adapts to life changes	1	2	3	4	5	NA
130228	Relies of family for support	1	2	3	4	5	NA
130229	Relies on friends for support	1	2	3	4	5	NA
130230	Relies on coworkers for support						
130231	Relies on health care professionals for support	1	2	3	4	5	NA
130232	Expresses emotions triggered by stressful situations	1	2	3	4	5	NA
130210	Uses effective behaviors to reduce stress	1	2	3	4	5	NA
130233	Uses distraction to cope with stress	1	2	3	4	5	NA
130234	Uses animal-assisted therapy	1	2	3	4	5	NA
130235	Relies on spiritual beliefs and prayer	1	2	3	4	5	NA
130212	Uses effective coping strategies	1	2	3	4	5	NA
130213	Avoids unduly stressful situations	1	2	3	4	5	NA
130214	Verbalizes need for assistance	1	2	3	4	5	NA
130223	Obtains assistance from health professional	1	2	3	4	5	NA
130216	Reports decrease in physical symptoms of stress	1	2	3	4	5	NA
130217	Reports decrease in negative feelings	1	2	3	4	5	NA
130204	Reports decrease in stressful situations	1	2	3	4	5	NA
130218	Reports increase in psychological comfort	1	2	3	4	5	NA

Domain-Psychosocial Health (III)   *Class*-Psychosocial Adaptation (N)   *1st edition 1997; revised 2004, 2008, 2024*

OUTCOME CONTENT REFERENCES:

Bakan, G., & Inci, F. H. (2021). Predictor of self-efficacy in individuals with chronic disease: Stress-coping strategies. *Journal of Clinical Nursing, 30*(5/6), 874–881. https://doi.org/10.1111/jocn.15633

Bassi, M., Cilia, S., Falautano, M., Grobberio, M., Niccolai, C., Pattini, M., Pietrolongo, E., Quartuccio, M. E., Viterbo, R. G., Allegri, B., Amato, M. P., Benin, M., De Luca, G., Gasperini, C., Minacapelli, E., Patti, F., Trojano, M., & Delle Fave, A. (2020). Illness perceptions and psychological adjustment among persons with multiple sclerosis: The mediating role of coping strategies and social support. *Disability & Rehabilitation, 42*(26), 3780–3792. https://doi.org/10.1080/09638288.2019.1610511

Konaszewski, K., Niesiobędzka, M., & Surzykiewicz, J. (2021). Resilience and mental health among juveniles: Role of strategies for coping with stress. *Health & Quality of Life Outcomes, 19*(1), 1–12. https://doi.org/10.1186/s12955-021-01701-3

Kozusznik, M. W., Puig-Perez, S., Kożusznik, B., & Pulopulos, M. M. (2021). The relationship between coping strategies and sleep problems: The role of depressive symptoms. *Annals of Behavioral Medicine, 55*(3), 253–265. https://doi.org/10.1093/abm/kaaa048

Ling, T. W. (2021). Coping strategies of patients with end stage kidney disease on hemodialysis: A systematic review. *Nephrology Nursing Journal, 48*(1), 31–48. https://doi.org/10.37526/1526-744X.2021.48.1.31

Shin, H., Bartlett, R., & De Gagne, J. C. (2020). Integrative literature review on psychological distress and coping strategies among survivors of adolescent cancer. *Oncology Nursing Forum, 47*(5), E131–E148. https://doi.org/10.1188/20.ONF.E131-E148

Skinner, E. A., Edge, K., Altman, J., & Sherwood, H. (2003). Searching for the structure of coping: A review and critique of category systems for classifying ways of coping. *Psychological Bulletin, 129*(2), 216–269. https://doi.org/10.1037/0033-2909.129.2.216

Tan, R., Koh, S., Wong, M. E., Rui, M., & Shorey, S. (2020). Caregiver stress, coping strategies, and support needs of mothers caring for their children who are undergoing active cancer treatments. *Clinical Nursing Research, 29*(7), 460–468. https://doi.org/10.1177/1054773819888099

Cup Feeding Establishment: Infant 1018

Definition: Establishment of cup feeding for hydration and nourishment of an infant

OUTCOME TARGET RATING: Maintain at_____ Increase to_____

		Never Demonstrated	Rarely Demonstrated	Sometimes Demonstrated	Often Demonstrated	Consistently Demonstrated	
OUTCOME OVERALL RATING		1	2	3	4	5	
Indicators:							
101801	Placement of tongue in cup	1	2	3	4	5	NA
101802	Laps or sips milk or formula	1	2	3	4	5	NA
101803	Produces noisy splashing sounds	1	2	3	4	5	NA
101812	Noticeable or audible swallow	1	2	3	4	5	NA
101806	Feeding tolerance	1	2	3	4	5	NA
101813	Eight or more feedings per day	1	2	3	4	5	NA
101808	Contentment after feeding	1	2	3	4	5	NA
101809	Urine output appropriate for age	1	2	3	4	5	NA
101810	Stools appropriate for age	1	2	3	4	5	NA
101811	Weight gain appropriate for age	1	2	3	4	5	NA

Domain-Physiologic Health (II)   *Class-Digestion & Nutrition (K)*   *5th edition 2013; revised 2024*

OUTCOME CONTENT REFERENCES:

Flint, A., New, K., & Davies, M. W. (2016). Cup feeding versus other forms of supplemental enteral feeding for newborn infants unable to fully breastfeed. *The Cochrane Database of Systematic Reviews.* https://doi.org/10.1002/14651858.CD005092.pub3

Lang, S., Lawrence, C., & Orme, R. (1994). Cup feeding: An alternative method of infant feeding. *Archives of Disease in Childhood, 71*(4), 365–369. https://doi.org/10.1136/adc.71.4.365

McKinney, C. M., Robin, P., Glass, R. P., Coffey, P., Rue, T., Vaughn, M. G., & Cunningham, M. (2016). Feeding neonates by cup: A systematic review of the literature. *Maternal Child Health Journal, 20*(8), 1620–1633. https://doi.org/10.1007/s10995-016-1961-9

Penny, F., Judge, M., Brownell, E., & McGrath, J. M. (2018). Cup feeding as a supplemental, alternative feeding method for preterm breastfed infants: An integrative review. *Maternal and Child Health Journal, 22*(8), 1568–1579. https://doi.org/10.1007/s10995-018-2632-9

Cup Feeding Performance   1019

Definition: Caregiver actions to provide fluids to an infant using a cup

OUTCOME TARGET RATING: Maintain at_____ Increase to_____

		Never Demonstrated	Rarely Demonstrated	Sometimes Demonstrated	Often Demonstrated	Consistently Demonstrated	
OUTCOME OVERALL RATING		1	2	3	4	5	
Indicators:							
101901	Washes hands before feeding	1	2	3	4	5	NA
101902	Prepares formula according to directions	1	2	3	4	5	NA
101903	Uses a small clean cup without a spout	1	2	3	4	5	NA
101904	Uses formula before expiration date	1	2	3	4	5	NA
101905	Stores mixed formula correctly	1	2	3	4	5	NA
101906	Stores breast milk correctly	1	2	3	4	5	NA
101907	Tests temperature of fluid prior to feeding	1	2	3	4	5	NA
101908	Responds to infant hunger cues	1	2	3	4	5	NA
101909	Positions infant correctly while feeding	1	2	3	4	5	NA
101910	Positions cup correctly while feeding	1	2	3	4	5	NA
101912	Allows infant to pace feeding	1	2	3	4	5	NA
101913	Responds to infant cues to stop feeding	1	2	3	4	5	NA
101914	Repositions infant in response to choking	1	2	3	4	5	NA

Domain-*Physiologic Health (II)*   **Class**-*Digestion & Nutrition (K)*   *5th edition 2013; revised 2024*

OUTCOME CONTENT REFERENCES:

Flint, A., New, K., & Davies, M. W. (2016). Cup feeding versus other forms of supplemental enteral feeding for newborn infants unable to fully breastfeed. *The Cochrane Database of Systematic Reviews.* https://doi.org/10.1002/14651858.CD005092

Lang, S., Lawrence, C., & Orme, R. (1994). Cup feeding: An alternative method of infant feeding. *Archives of Disease in Childhood, 71*(4), 365–369.

McKinney, C. M., Robin, P., Glass, R. P., Coffey, P., Rue, T., Vaughn, M. G., & Cunningham, M. (2016). Feeding neonates by cup: A systematic review of the literature. *Maternal Child Health Journal 20,* 1620–1633. https://doi.org/10.1007/s10995-016-1961-9

Penny, F., Judge, M., Brownell, E., & McGrath, J. M. (2018). Cup feeding as a supplemental, alternative feeding method for preterm breastfed infants: An integrative review. *Maternal and Child Health Journal, 22,* 1568–1579. https://doi.org/10.1007/s10995-018-2632-9

Vollrath, K., Rosenberg, A., Gabrielski, L., Deacon, J., Marshall, S., Rihn, A., & Grover, T. (2019). NICU discharge feeding bundle improves accuracy of post-discharge feeding preparation and potentially prevents readmission. *Advances in Neonatal Care, 19*(2), 90–96. https://doi.org/10.1097/ANC.0000000000000571

Yilmaz, G., Caylan, N., Karacan, C. D., Bodur, I., & Gokcay, G. (2014). Effect of cup feeding and bottle feeding on breastfeeding in late preterm infants: A randomized controlled study. *Journal of Human Lactation, 30*(2), 174–179. https://doi.org/10.1177/0890334413 517940

Decision-Making   0906

Definition: Ability to make judgments and choose between two or more alternatives

OUTCOME TARGET RATING: Maintain at_____ Increase to_____

		Never Demonstrated	Rarely Demonstrated	Sometimes Demonstrated	Often Demonstrated	Consistently Demonstrated	
OUTCOME OVERALL RATING		1	2	3	4	5	
Indicators:							
090613	Identifies the problem	1	2	3	4	5	NA
090614	Identifies preferences for selecting option	1	2	3	4	5	NA
090601	Identifies relevant information	1	2	3	4	5	NA
090602	Identifies alternatives	1	2	3	4	5	NA
090603	Identifies potential consequences of each alternative	1	2	3	4	5	NA
090615	Identifies potential benefits of each alternative	1	2	3	4	5	NA

Continued

Decision-Making—cont'd

		Never Demonstrated	Rarely Demonstrated	Sometimes Demonstrated	Often Demonstrated	Consistently Demonstrated	
090604	Identifies resources necessary to support each alternative	1	2	3	4	5	NA
090611	Identifies time frame necessary to support each alternative	1	2	3	4	5	NA
090612	Identifies sequence necessary to support each alternative	1	2	3	4	5	NA
090605	Recognizes contradiction with others' desires	1	2	3	4	5	NA
090616	Recognizes what others are doing	1	2	3	4	5	NA
090617	Acknowledges emotional factors in selecting alternatives	1	2	3	4	5	NA
090606	Acknowledges social context of the situation	1	2	3	4	5	NA
090607	Acknowledges relevant legal implications	1	2	3	4	5	NA
090608	Weighs alternatives	1	2	3	4	5	NA
090609	Selects final decision among alternatives	1	2	3	4	5	NA

Domain-*Physiologic Health (II)*   **Class**-*Neurocognitive (J)*   *1st edition 1997; revised 2004, 2008, 2024*

OUTCOME CONTENT REFERENCES:

Bruch, E., & Feinberg, F. (2017). Decision-making processes in social context. *Annal Review of Sociology, 43*(1), 207–227. https://doi.org/10.1146/annurev-soc-060116-053622

Del Missier, F., Hansson, P., Parker, A. M., & de Bruin, W. B. (2020). *Psychology and Aging, 35*(4), 553–564. https://doi.org/10.1037/pag0000443.supp

Guo, K. L. (2020). DECIDE. A decision-making model for more effective decision making by health care managers. *The Health Care Manager, 39*(3), 133–141. https://doi.org/10.1097/HCM.0000000000000299

Manetti, W. (2019). Sound clinical judgment in nursing: A concept analysis. *Nursing Forum, 54*(1), 102–110. https://doi.org/10.1111/nuf.12303

Dehydration Severity   0621

Definition: Severity of fluid loss from the body

OUTCOME TARGET RATING: Maintain at_____ Increase to_____

		Severe	Substantial	Moderate	Mild	None	
OUTCOME OVERALL RATING		1	2	3	4	5	
Indicators:							
062101	Thirst	1	2	3	4	5	NA
062102	Dry mouth and tongue	1	2	3	4	5	NA
062103	Halitosis	1	2	3	4	5	NA
062104	Infrequent urination	1	2	3	4	5	NA
062105	Dark colored urine	1	2	3	4	5	NA
062106	Reduced urine output	1	2	3	4	5	NA
062107	Reduced axillary sweating	1	2	3	4	5	NA
062108	Sunken eyes	1	2	3	4	5	NA
062109	Sunken fontanel (infants)	1	2	3	4	5	NA
062110	Sunken cheeks	1	2	3	4	5	NA
062111	Dry skin	1	2	3	4	5	NA
062112	Loss of skin turgor	1	2	3	4	5	NA
062113	Decreased blood pressure	1	2	3	4	5	NA
062114	Rapid thready pulse	1	2	3	4	5	NA

D

Dehydration Severity—cont'd

	Severe	Substantial	Moderate	Mild	None	
062115 Dizziness	1	2	3	4	5	NA
062116 Headache	1	2	3	4	5	NA
062117 Irritability	1	2	3	4	5	NA
062118 Cries without tears	1	2	3	4	5	NA
062119 Decreased capillary refill	1	2	3	4	5	NA
062120 Increased hematocrit	1	2	3	4	5	NA
062121 Increased blood urea nitrogen	1	2	3	4	5	NA
062122 Increased blood glucose	1	2	3	4	5	NA
062123 Increased serum creatinine	1	2	3	4	5	NA
062124 Weight loss	1	2	3	4	5	NA
062125 Fatigue	1	2	3	4	5	NA
062126 Muscle cramps	1	2	3	4	5	NA
062127 Muscle twitching	1	2	3	4	5	NA
062128 Constipation	1	2	3	4	5	NA
062129 Body temperature elevation	1	2	3	4	5	NA
062130 Confusion	1	2	3	4	5	NA

Domain-Physiologic Health (II)   **Class**-Fluid & Electrolytes (G)   7th edition 2024

OUTCOME CONTENT REFERENCES:

Ashraf, M. M., & Rea, R. (2017). Effect of dehydration on blood tests. *Practical Diabetes, 34*(5), 169–171. https://doi.org/10.1002/pdi.2111

Bahouth, M. N., Gottesman, R. F., & Szanton, S. L. (2018). Primary 'dehydration' and acute stroke: A systematic research review. *Journal of Neurology, 265*(10), 2167–2181. https://doi.org/10.1007/s00415-018-8799-6

Barrado, M. Y., Hatter, L., Moore, K. J., Sampson, E. L., Rait, G., Manthorpe, J., Smith, C. H., Nair, P., & Davies, N. (2021). Nutrition and hydration for people living with dementia near the end of life: A qualitative systematic review. *Journal of Advanced Nursing, 77*(2), 664–680. https://doi.org/10.1111/jan.14654

Huether, S. E., McCance, K. L., & Brashers, V. L. (2020). *Understanding pathophysiology* (7th ed.). Elsevier.

Ignatavicius, D. D., Workman, M. L., Rebar, C. R., & Heimgartner, N. M. (2021). *Medical-surgical nursing: Concepts for interprofessional care* (10th ed.). Elsevier.

Kear, T. M. (2017). Fluid and electrolyte management across the age continuum. *Nephrology Nursing Journal, 44*(6), 491–497.

Potter, P. A., & Perry, A. G. (2021). *Fundamentals of nursing* (10th ed.). Elsevier.

Perrier, E. T., Armstrong, L. E., Bottin, J. H., Clark, W. F., Dolci, A., Guelinckx, I., Iroz, A., Kavouras, S. A., Lang, F., Lieberman, H. R., Melander, O., Morin, C., Seksek, I., Stookey, J. D., Tack, I., Vanhaecke, T., Vecchio, M., & Péronnet, F. (2021). Hydration for health hypothesis: A narrative review of supporting evidence. *European Journal of Nutrition, 60*(3), 1167–1180. https://doi.org/10.1007/s00394-020-02296-z

Reddi, A. S. (2018). *Fluid, electrolyte, and acid-base disorders: Clinical evaluation and management* (2nd ed.). Springer.

Delirium Level   0916

Definition: Severity of disturbance in consciousness and cognition that develops over a short period of time and is reversible

OUTCOME TARGET RATING: Maintain at_____ Increase to_____

	Severe	Substantial	Moderate	Mild	None	
OUTCOME OVERALL RATING	**1**	**2**	**3**	**4**	**5**	
Indicators:						
091601 Disorientation of time	1	2	3	4	5	NA
091602 Disorientation of place	1	2	3	4	5	NA
091603 Disorientation of person	1	2	3	4	5	NA
091604 Psychomotor activity	1	2	3	4	5	NA
091605 Impaired cognition	1	2	3	4	5	NA
091606 Impaired memory	1	2	3	4	5	NA
091607 Difficulty following complex commands	1	2	3	4	5	NA
091608 Difficulty interpreting environmental stimuli	1	2	3	4	5	NA
091609 Difficulty maintaining focus	1	2	3	4	5	NA

Continued

Delirium Level—cont'd

		Severe	Substantial	Moderate	Mild	None	
091610	Difficulty maintaining conversation	1	2	3	4	5	NA
091611	Misinterpretation of cues	1	2	3	4	5	NA
091612	Meaningless verbalizations	1	2	3	4	5	NA
091613	Altered level of consciousness	1	2	3	4	5	NA
091614	Reduction in abstract reasoning	1	2	3	4	5	NA
091615	Restlessness	1	2	3	4	5	NA
091616	Agitation	1	2	3	4	5	NA
091617	Disruption of sleep-wake pattern	1	2	3	4	5	NA
091618	Labile mood	1	2	3	4	5	NA
091619	Sundowning	1	2	3	4	5	NA
091620	Hallucinations	1	2	3	4	5	NA
091621	Delusions	1	2	3	4	5	NA

Domain-*Physiologic Health (II)*   **Class**-*Neurocognitive (J)*   *4th edition 2008; revised 2013*

OUTCOME CONTENT REFERENCES:
Foreman, M. D., Mion, L. C., Tryostad, L., & Fletcher, K. (1999). Standard of practice protocol: Acute confusion/delirium. *Geriatric Nursing, 20*(3), 147–152.
Johnson, M. (2001). Assessing confused patients. *Journal of Neurology Neurosurgery and Psychiatry, 71*(Suppl. 1), i7–i12.
Miller, J., Neelon, V., Champagne, M., Bailey, D., Ng'andu, N., Belyea, M., Jarrell, E., Montoya, L., & Williams, A. (1997). The assessment of acute confusion as part of nursing care. *Applied Nursing Research, 10*(3), 143–151.
Rapp, C. G., Wakefield, B., Kundrat, M., Mentes, J., Tripp-Reimer, T., Culp, K., Mobiliy, P. Akins, J., & Onega, L. L. (2000). Acute confusion assessment instruments: Clinical versus research usability. *Applied Nursing Research, 13*(1), 37–45.
Trzepacz, P. T. (1999). The delirium rating scale: Its use in consultation-liaison research. *Psychosomatics, 40*(3), 193–204.
Wakefield, B., Mentes, J., Mobily, P., Tripp-Reimer, T., Culp, K. R., Rapp, C. G., Gaspar, P., Kundrat, M., Wadle, K. R., & Akins, J. (2001). Acute confusion. In M. L. Maas, K. C. Buckwalter, M. D, Hardy, T. Tripp-Reimer, M. G, Titler, & J. P. Specht (Eds.), *Nursing care of older adults: Diagnoses, outcomes & interventions* (pp. 442–454). Mosby.

Dementia Level

0920

Definition: Severity of irreversible disturbances in consciousness and cognition that leads to mental, physical, and social functional losses over an extended period of time

OUTCOME TARGET RATING: Maintain at_____ Increase to_____

		Severe	Substantial	Moderate	Mild	None	
OUTCOME OVERALL RATING		1	2	3	4	5	
Indicators:							
092001	Difficulty remembering recent events	1	2	3	4	5	NA
092002	Difficulty remembering names	1	2	3	4	5	NA
092003	Difficulty recognizing family members	1	2	3	4	5	NA
092004	Difficulty remembering names of familiar objects	1	2	3	4	5	NA
092005	Difficulty finding way to familiar places	1	2	3	4	5	NA
092006	Difficulty maintaining conversation	1	2	3	4	5	NA
092007	Difficulty interpreting physiological cues	1	2	3	4	5	NA
092008	Difficulty processing information	1	2	3	4	5	NA
092009	Difficulty following complex commands	1	2	3	4	5	NA
092010	Difficulty problem-solving	1	2	3	4	5	NA
092011	Difficulty expressing needs	1	2	3	4	5	NA
092012	Difficulty performing basic activities of daily living	1	2	3	4	5	NA
092013	Difficulty performing instrumental activities of daily living	1	2	3	4	5	NA
092014	Difficulty interpreting environmental stimuli	1	2	3	4	5	NA
092032	Difficulty receiving basic care	1	2	3	4	5	NA

Dementia Level—cont'd

		Severe	Substantial	Moderate	Mild	None	
092033	Difficulty controlling own behavior	1	2	3	4	5	NA
092015	Unsafe wandering	1	2	3	4	5	NA
092016	Immobility	1	2	3	4	5	NA
092017	Disorientation of time	1	2	3	4	5	NA
092018	Disorientation of place	1	2	3	4	5	NA
092019	Disorientation of person	1	2	3	4	5	NA
092020	Bowel incontinence	1	2	3	4	5	NA
092021	Urinary incontinence	1	2	3	4	5	NA
092022	Disruption of sleep/wake pattern	1	2	3	4	5	NA
092023	Disruption of social activities	1	2	3	4	5	NA
092024	Depression	1	2	3	4	5	NA
092025	Agitation	1	2	3	4	5	NA
092026	Restlessness	1	2	3	4	5	NA
092027	Aggression	1	2	3	4	5	NA
092028	Suspiciousness	1	2	3	4	5	NA
092029	Social withdrawal	1	2	3	4	5	NA
092030	Change in personality	1	2	3	4	5	NA
092031	Altered level of consciousness	1	2	3	4	5	NA

Domain-*Physiologic Health (II)*   **Class**-*Neurocognitive (J)*   *5th edition 2013; revised 2024*

OUTCOME CONTENT REFERENCES:

Al Ghassani, A., Rababa, M., & Abu Khait, A. (2021). Agitation in people with dementia: A concept analysis. *Nursing Forum, 56*(4), 1015–1023. https://doi.org/10.1111/nuf.12629

Corté-Beringola, A., Vicent, L., Martin-Asenjo, R., Puerto, E., Domínguez-Pérez, L., Maruri, R., Moreno, G., Vidán, M. T., Arribas, F., & Bueno, H. (2021). Diagnosis, prevention, and management of delirium in the intensive cardiac care unit. *American Heart Journal, 232*, 164-176. https://doi.org/10.1016/j.ahj.2020.11.011

Dunphy, L., Akin-Komolafe, T., & Etheridge, Z. (2021). Mixed dementia and hyperactive delirium: A diagnostic challenge. *BMJ Case Report, 14*(5), 1–6. https://doi.org/10.1136/bcr-2020-238542

Galik, E. M., Resnick, B., Holmes, S. D., Vigne, E., Lynch, K., Ellis, J., Zhu, S., & Barr, E. (2021). A cluster randomized controlled trial testing the impact of function and behavior focused care for nursing home residents with dementia. *Journal of the American Medical Directors Association, 22*(7), 1421–1428. https://doi.org/10.1016/j.jamda.2020.12.020

Ignatavicius, D. D., Workman, M. L., Rebar, C. R., & Heimgartner, N. M. (2021). *Medical-surgical nursing: Concepts for interprofessional collaborative care* (10th ed.), Elsevier.

Lee, S. J., Park, M. S., Choi, Y. R., & Chang, S. O. (2021). Concept development of identification of discomfort for nursing home patients with advanced dementia. *International Journal of Nursing Knowledge, 32*(4), 274–285. https://doi.org/10.1111/2047-3095.12277

Watson, K., & Hatcher, D. (2020). Factors influencing management of agitation in aged care facilities: A qualitative study of staff perceptions. *Journal of Clinical Nursing, 30*(1-2), 136–144. https://doi.org/10.1111/jocn.15530

Williams, P. (2020). *Basic geriatrics nursing.* (7th ed.). Elsevier.

Depression Level   1208

Definition: Severity of melancholic mood and loss of interest in life events

OUTCOME TARGET RATING: Maintain at_____ Increase to_____

		Severe	Substantial	Moderate	Mild	None	
OUTCOME OVERALL RATING		1	2	3	4	5	
Indicators:							
120837	Anxiety	1	2	3	4	5	NA
120801	Depressed mood	1	2	3	4	5	NA
120802	Loss of interest in activities	1	2	3	4	5	NA
120827	Negative life events	1	2	3	4	5	NA
120803	Lack of pleasure in activities	1	2	3	4	5	NA

Continued

Depression Level—cont'd

		Severe	Substantial	Moderate	Mild	None	
120838	Social withdrawal	1	2	3	4	5	NA
120804	Impaired concentration	1	2	3	4	5	NA
120805	Inappropriate guilt	1	2	3	4	5	NA
120828	Excessive guilt	1	2	3	4	5	NA
120806	Fatigue	1	2	3	4	5	NA
120807	Feelings of worthlessness	1	2	3	4	5	NA
120808	Psychomotor retardation	1	2	3	4	5	NA
120829	Psychomotor agitation	1	2	3	4	5	NA
120839	Obsessed over events	1	2	3	4	5	NA
120840	Worry	1	2	3	4	5	NA
120841	Increased physical complaints	1	2	3	4	5	NA
120842	Helplessness	1	2	3	4	5	NA
120809	Insomnia	1	2	3	4	5	NA
120830	Hypersomnia	1	2	3	4	5	NA
120843	Decreased productivity	1	2	3	4	5	NA
120810	Weight gain	1	2	3	4	5	NA
120831	Weight loss	1	2	3	4	5	NA
120811	Increased appetite	1	2	3	4	5	NA
120832	Decreased appetite	1	2	3	4	5	NA
120835	Recurrent thoughts of death	1	2	3	4	5	NA
120836	Recurrent thoughts of suicide	1	2	3	4	5	NA
120813	Indecisiveness	1	2	3	4	5	NA
120844	Impulsiveness	1	2	3	4	5	NA
120814	Sadness	1	2	3	4	5	NA
120815	Crying spells	1	2	3	4	5	NA
120816	Anger	1	2	3	4	5	NA
120817	Hopelessness	1	2	3	4	5	NA
120818	Loneliness	1	2	3	4	5	NA
120819	Low self-esteem	1	2	3	4	5	NA
120845	Rejection sensitivity	1	2	3	4	5	NA
120820	Decreased libido	1	2	3	4	5	NA
120821	Decreased activity level	1	2	3	4	5	NA
120822	Lack of spontaneity	1	2	3	4	5	NA
120823	Irritability	1	2	3	4	5	NA
120846	Disruptive behavior	1	2	3	4	5	NA
120833	Recreational drug use	1	2	3	4	5	NA
120834	Increased alcohol use	1	2	3	4	5	NA
120825	Poor personal hygiene	1	2	3	4	5	NA

Domain-Psychosocial Health (III)   **Class**-Psychological Well-Being (M)   2nd edition 2000; revised 2004, 2008, 2024

OUTCOME CONTENT REFERENCES:

American Psychiatric Association. (2022). *Diagnostic and statistical manual of mental disorders* (5th ed., text rev.). https://doi.org/10.1176/appi.books.9780890425787

Beck, A. T., Steer, R. A., & Carbin, M. G. 1988). Psychometric properties of the Beck Depression Inventory: Twenty-five years of evaluation. *Clinical Psychology Review, 8*(1), 77–100. https://doi.org/10.1016/0272-7358(88)90050-5

Gillitzer, M. (2019). Implementing a depression screening algorithm in a memory clinic. *Archives of Psychiatric Nursing, 33*(6), 123–129. https://doi.org/10.1016/j.apnu.2019.10.003

Hazell, C. M., Smith, H. E., & Jones, C. J. (2019). The blurred line between physical ageing and mental health in older adults: Implications for the measurement of depression. *Clinical Medicine Insights: Psychiatry, 10*, 1–5. https://doi.org/10.1177/1179557319885634

Hockberry, M. J., Rodgers, C. C., & Wilson, D. (2022). *Wong's essential of pediatric nursing* (11th ed.). Elsevier.

Potter, P. A., Perry, A. G., Stockert, P. A., & Hall, A. M. (2021). *Fundamentals of nursing* (10th ed.). Elsevier.

Thordardottir, E. B., Gudmundsdottir, H., Gudmundsdottir, B., Hrólfsdóttir, A. M., Aspelund, T., & Hauksdottir, A. (2019). Development and predictors of psychological outcomes following the 2008 earthquake in Iceland: A longitudinal cohort study. *Scandinavian Journal of Public Health, 47*(2), 269–279. https://doi.org/10.1177/1403494818771444

Varcarolis, E. M., & Fosbre, C. D. (2021). *Essentials of psychiatric-mental health nursing* (4th ed.). Elsevier.

Williams, P. (2020). *Basic geriatric nursing* (7th ed.). Elsevier.

Yu, Y., Yu, Y., & Lin, Y. (2020). Anxiety and depression aggravate impulsiveness: the mediating and moderating role of cognitive flexibility. *Psychology, Health & Medicine, 25*(1), 25–36. https://doi.org/10.1080/13548506.2019.1601748

Depression Self-Control   1409

Definition: Personal actions to minimize melancholy and maintain interest in life events

OUTCOME TARGET RATING: Maintain at_____ Increase to_____

		Never Demonstrated	Rarely Demonstrated	Sometimes Demonstrated	Often Demonstrated	Consistently Demonstrated	
OUTCOME OVERALL RATING		1	2	3	4	5	
Indicators:							
140901	Monitors ability to concentrate	1	2	3	4	5	NA
140902	Monitors intensity of depression	1	2	3	4	5	NA
140903	Identifies precursors of depression	1	2	3	4	5	NA
140904	Plans strategies to reduce effects of precursors	1	2	3	4	5	NA
140905	Monitors behavioral manifestations of depression	1	2	3	4	5	NA
140927	Uses a behavioral log	1	2	3	4	5	NA
140928	Monitors mood	1	2	3	4	5	NA
140909	Reports improved mood	1	2	3	4	5	NA
140929	Engages in self-evaluation	1	2	3	4	5	NA
140930	Engages in self-rewards	1	2	3	4	5	NA
140931	Practices problem-solving approaches	1	2	3	4	5	NA
140925	Delays big decision until feeling better	1	2	3	4	5	NA
140906	Reports adequate sleep	1	2	3	4	5	NA
140932	Engages in relaxation techniques	1	2	3	4	5	NA
140933	Follows sleep promoting behavior pattern	1	2	3	4	5	NA
140934	Uses light therapy	1	2	3	4	5	NA
140907	Reports improved libido	1	2	3	4	5	NA
140908	Monitors physical manifestations of depression	1	2	3	4	5	NA
140910	Maintains stable weight	1	2	3	4	5	NA
140924	Sets realistic goals	1	2	3	4	5	NA
140911	Follows treatment regimen	1	2	3	4	5	NA
140923	Uses medication as prescribed	1	2	3	4	5	NA
140935	Participates in Cognitive Behavioral Therapy (CBT)	1	2	3	4	5	NA
140914	Adheres to psychotherapy schedule	1	2	3	4	5	NA
140936	Participates in mindfulness training	1	2	3	4	5	NA
140937	Considers complementary therapies	1	2	3	4	5	NA
140926	Participates in enjoyable activities	1	2	3	4	5	NA
140938	Participates in purposeful activities	1	2	3	4	5	NA
140913	Follows exercise plan	1	2	3	4	5	NA
140915	Reports symptom changes to a health provider	1	2	3	4	5	NA
140920	Avoids alcohol misuse	1	2	3	4	5	NA
140921	Avoids non-prescription drug misuse	1	2	3	4	5	NA
140922	Avoids recreational drug use	1	2	3	4	5	NA
140918	Maintains personal hygiene	1	2	3	4	5	NA

Domain-Psychosocial Health (III)   *Class*-Self-Control (O)   *2nd edition 2000; revised 2004, 2008, 2024*

OUTCOME CONTENT REFERENCES:

American Psychiatric Association. (2022). *Diagnostic and statistical manual of mental disorders* (5th ed., text rev.). https://doi.org/10.1176/appi.books.9780890425787

Duncan, M. J., Rayward, A. T., Holliday, E. G., Brown, W. J., Vanelanotte, C., Murawski, B., & Plotnikoff, R. C. (2021). Effect of a physical activity and sleep m-health intervention on a composite activity-sleep behavior score and mental health: A mediation analysis of two randomised controlled trials. *International Journal of Behavioral Nutrition and Physical Activity, 18*(45), 1–12. https://doi.org/10.1186/s12966-021-01112-z

Hockberry, M. J., Rodgers, C. C., & Wilson, D. (2022). *Wong's essential of pediatric nursing* (11th ed.). Elsevier.

Lewis, C. C., Marti, C. N., Marriott, B. R., Scott, K., & Ayer, D. (2019). Patterns of practice in community mental health treatment of adult depression. *Psychotherapy Research, 29*(1), 70–77. https://doi.org/10.1080/10503307.2017.1303210

Ogata, K., Ataka, K., Suzuki, H., Yagi, T., Okawa, A., Fukumoto, T., Zhang, B., Nakata, M., Yada, T., & Asakawa, A. (2020). Lavender oil reduces depressive mood in healthy individuals and enhances the activity of single oxytocin neurons of the hypothalamus isolated from mice: A preliminary study. *Evidence-Based Complementary and Alternative Medicine, 4,* 1–9. https://doi.org/10.1155/2020/5418586

Thummathai, K., Sethabouppha, H., Chanprasit, C., & Lasuka, D. (2020). Depression prevention in adolescents based on Buddhism and sufficiency economy philosophy. *Archives of Psychiatric Nursing, 34*(1), 70–74. https://doi.org/10.1016/j.apnu.2019.10.005

Varcarolis, E. M., & Fosbre, C. D. (2021). *Essentials of psychiatric-mental health nursing* (4th ed.). Elsevier.

Williams, P. (2020). *Basic geriatric nursing* (7th ed.). Elsevier.

Wood, M., Griffiths, J., & Paltoglou, A. E. (2021). Exploring difficulties in men's experience of self and agency during antidepressant use. *Psychology of Men & Masculinities, 22*(2), 2298–2305. https://doi.org/10.1037/men0000330

D

Development: Established Adulthood   0124

Definition: Cognitive, physical, psychosocial, and moral progression from 30 through 44 years of age

OUTCOME TARGET RATING: Maintain at_____ Increase to_____

OUTCOME OVERALL RATING		Never Demonstrated	Rarely Demonstrated	Sometimes Demonstrated	Often Demonstrated	Consistently Demonstrated	
		1	2	3	4	5	
Indicators:							
012001	Maintains lifelong learning	1	2	3	4	5	NA
012002	Exhibits high level cognitive function	1	2	3	4	5	NA
012003	Uses expanded language skills	1	2	3	4	5	NA
012004	Uses accumulated knowledge in decision-making	1	2	3	4	5	NA
012005	Maintains gainful employment	1	2	3	4	5	NA
012006	Seeks advancement in work status	1	2	3	4	5	NA
012007	Acquires professional skills and credentials in a career	1	2	3	4	5	NA
012008	Selects a career mentor	1	2	3	4	5	NA
012009	Seeks career-building opportunities	1	2	3	4	5	NA
012010	Assumes increasing responsibility in work role	1	2	3	4	5	NA
012011	Develops mutually gratifying adult friendships	1	2	3	4	5	NA
012012	Develops positive relationships with co-workers	1	2	3	4	5	NA
012013	Develops more compassionate relationships with siblings	1	2	3	4	5	NA
012014	Maintains positive relationships with immediate family	1	2	3	4	5	NA
012015	Maintains positive relationships with extended family	1	2	3	4	5	NA
012016	Establishes personal residence	1	2	3	4	5	NA
012017	Embraces sexual identity	1	2	3	4	5	NA
012018	Establishes intimate relationships	1	2	3	4	5	NA
012019	Practices safe sex	1	2	3	4	5	NA
012020	Makes decisions about marriage vs. single life	1	2	3	4	5	NA
012021	Makes decisions about parenthood	1	2	3	4	5	NA
012022	Negotiates tasks and roles with partner	1	2	3	4	5	NA

Development: Established Adulthood—cont'd

		Never Demonstrated	Rarely Demonstrated	Sometimes Demonstrated	Often Demonstrated	Consistently Demonstrated	
012023	Discusses personal needs with partner	1	2	3	4	5	NA
012024	Copes with extended family care needs	1	2	3	4	5	NA
012025	Starts a family	1	2	3	4	5	NA
012026	Adapts to parental role	1	2	3	4	5	NA
012027	Copes with competing demands of family vs. career	1	2	3	4	5	NA
012028	Maintains positive partner relationship during parenting challenges	1	2	3	4	5	NA
012029	Exhibits positive self-esteem	1	2	3	4	5	NA
012030	Exhibits personal responsibility	1	2	3	4	5	NA
012031	Avoids substance misuse	1	2	3	4	5	NA
012032	Adheres to laws that protect welfare of others	1	2	3	4	5	NA
012033	Acknowledges personal values	1	2	3	4	5	NA
012034	Acknowledges values of others	1	2	3	4	5	NA
012035	Acknowledges personal opinions	1	2	3	4	5	NA
012036	Acknowledges opinions of others	1	2	3	4	5	NA
012037	Creates a niche in society through family, occupational, and community commitments	1	2	3	4	5	NA

Domain-Functional Health (I)   **Class**-Growth & Development (B)   7th edition 2024

OUTCOME CONTENT REFERENCES:

Arnett, J. J., Robinson, O., & Lachman, M. E. (2020). Rethinking adult development: Introduction to the special issue. *American Psychologist*, *75*(4), 425–430. https://doi.org/10.1037/amp0000633

Athan, A. M. (2020). Reproductive identity: An emerging concept. *American Psychologist*, *75*(4), 445–456. https://doi.org/10.1037/amp0000623

Berk, L. (2018). *Development across the lifespan* (7th ed.). Pearson Education.

Bühler, J. L., & Nikitin, J. (2020). Sociohistorical context and adult social development: New directions for 21st century research. *American Psychologist*, *75*(4), 457–469. https://doi.org/10.1037/amp0000611

Mehta, C. M., Arnett, J. J., Palmer, C. G., & Nelson, L. J. (2020). Established adulthood: A new conception of ages 30 to 45. *American Psychologist*, *75*(4), 431–444. https://doi.org/10.1037/amp0000600

Development: Late Adulthood   0121

Definition: Cognitive, physical, psychosocial, and moral progression from 65 years of age and older

OUTCOME TARGET RATING: Maintain at_____ Increase to_____

		Never Demonstrated	Rarely Demonstrated	Sometimes Demonstrated	Often Demonstrated	Consistently Demonstrated	
OUTCOME OVERALL RATING		1	2	3	4	5	
Indicators:							
012101	Maintains cognitive function	1	2	3	4	5	NA
012102	Maintains language skills	1	2	3	4	5	NA
012103	Maintains problem-solving skills	1	2	3	4	5	NA
012104	Maintains lifelong learning	1	2	3	4	5	NA
012106	Compensates if deterioration in memory occurs	1	2	3	4	5	NA
012149	Exhibits stable personality traits	1	2	3	4	5	NA
012105	Exhibits realistic outlook about abilities	1	2	3	4	5	NA
012107	Copes with personal loss	1	2	3	4	5	NA
012108	Copes with own mortality	1	2	3	4	5	NA

Continued

Development: Late Adulthood—cont'd

		Never Demonstrated	Rarely Demonstrated	Sometimes Demonstrated	Often Demonstrated	Consistently Demonstrated	
012109	Maintains life interests	1	2	3	4	5	NA
012110	Exhibits sense of pride	1	2	3	4	5	NA
012111	Exhibits sense of accomplishment	1	2	3	4	5	NA
012150	Maintains positive relationships with immediate family	1	2	3	4	5	NA
012151	Maintains positive relationships with extended family	1	2	3	4	5	NA
012114	Maintains close relationships with friends	1	2	3	4	5	NA
012115	Copes with adult children in the home	1	2	3	4	5	NA
012116	Performs positive role in lives of grandchildren	1	2	3	4	5	NA
012117	Adjusts to parenting role of grandchildren	1	2	3	4	5	NA
012152	Chooses to continue working beyond retirement age	1	2	3	4	5	NA
012119	Develops new interests	1	2	3	4	5	NA
012128	Adapts to functional impairment	1	2	3	4	5	NA
012120	Adapts to changing needs for assistance	1	2	3	4	5	NA
012121	Accepts assistance from others	1	2	3	4	5	NA
012153	Evaluates personal fall risk	1	2	3	4	5	NA
012154	Plans for retirement based on finances	1	2	3	4	5	NA
012122	Adjusts to change in financial income	1	2	3	4	5	NA
012118	Adjusts to retirement	1	2	3	4	5	NA
012155	Finalizes a will and estate planning	1	2	3	4	5	NA
012156	Evaluates safety of current home environment	1	2	3	4	5	NA
012123	Adjusts to change in living arrangements	1	2	3	4	5	NA
012124	Adjusts to change in marital status	1	2	3	4	5	NA
012125	Adjusts to change in marital relationship	1	2	3	4	5	NA
012126	Adjusts to sexual function changes	1	2	3	4	5	NA
012127	Practices safe sex	1	2	3	4	5	NA
012129	Avoids substance misuse	1	2	3	4	5	NA
012130	Challenges ageism stereotypes	1	2	3	4	5	NA
012131	Derives support from religious or spiritual beliefs	1	2	3	4	5	NA
012132	Seeks understanding to meaning of own life	1	2	3	4	5	NA
012133	Adheres to laws that protect welfare of others	1	2	3	4	5	NA
012134	Acknowledges personal values	1	2	3	4	5	NA
012135	Acknowledges values of others	1	2	3	4	5	NA
012136	Acknowledges personal opinions	1	2	3	4	5	NA
012137	Acknowledges opinions of others	1	2	3	4	5	NA
012138	Refrains from violating the rights of others	1	2	3	4	5	NA
012139	Respects others	1	2	3	4	5	NA
012140	Respects the environment	1	2	3	4	5	NA
012141	Supports equality in treatment of others	1	2	3	4	5	NA
012142	Recognizes that mutual trust is necessary in healthy relationships	1	2	3	4	5	NA
012157	Continues involvement in community activities	1	2	3	4	5	NA

Domain-Functional Health (I)   **Class**-Growth & Development (B)   4th edition 2008; revised 2024

OUTCOME CONTENT REFERENCES:

Arnett, J. J., Robinson, O., & Lachman, M. E. (2020). Rethinking adult development: Introduction to the special issue. *American Psychologist, 75*(4), 425–430. https://doi.org/10.1037/amp0000633

Berk, L. (2018). *Development across the lifespan* (7th ed.). Pearson Education.

Bühler, J. L., & Nikitin, J. (2020). Sociohistorical context and adult social development: New directions for 21st century research. *American Psychologist, 75*(4), 457–469. https://doi.org/10.1037/amp0000611

Williams, P. (2020). *Basic geriatric nursing* (7th ed.). Elsevier.

D

Development: Middle Adulthood   0122

Definition: Cognitive, physical, psychosocial, and moral progression from 45 through 64 years of age

OUTCOME TARGET RATING: Maintain at_____ Increase to_____

		Never Demonstrated	Rarely Demonstrated	Sometimes Demonstrated	Often Demonstrated	Consistently Demonstrated	
OUTCOME OVERALL RATING		1	2	3	4	5	
Indicators:							
012201	Exhibits high level cognitive function	1	2	3	4	5	NA
012203	Uses accumulated knowledge in decision-making	1	2	3	4	5	NA
012242	Adapts to vision changes	1	2	3	4	5	NA
012243	Adapts to hearing loss	1	2	3	4	5	NA
012244	Adapts to mobility changes	1	2	3	4	5	NA
012204	Exhibits high level problem-solving skills	1	2	3	4	5	NA
012205	Exhibits creativity	1	2	3	4	5	NA
012206	Maintains lifelong learning	1	2	3	4	5	NA
012207	Exhibits success in chosen occupation	1	2	3	4	5	NA
012208	Exhibits occupational flexibility	1	2	3	4	5	NA
012209	Copes with personal loss	1	2	3	4	5	NA
012210	Copes with career burnout	1	2	3	4	5	NA
012211	Expresses optimism about the present	1	2	3	4	5	NA
012212	Expresses optimism about the future	1	2	3	4	5	NA
012213	Adjusts to children leaving home	1	2	3	4	5	NA
012245	Pursues new interests or educational opportunities	1	2	3	4	5	NA
012214	Copes with adult children in the home	1	2	3	4	5	NA
012215	Performs positive role in lives of grandchildren	1	2	3	4	5	NA
012216	Adjusts to parenting role of grandchildren	1	2	3	4	5	NA
012217	Exhibits strong sense of self	1	2	3	4	5	NA
012218	Maintains a healthy intimate relationship with partner	1	2	3	4	5	NA
012246	Develops closer relationships with parents	1	2	3	4	5	NA
012247	Maintains positive relationships with immediate family	1	2	3	4	5	NA
012248	Maintains positive relationships with extended family	1	2	3	4	5	NA
012249	Provides social support for aging parents	1	2	3	4	5	NA
012250	Provides caregiving for elder family member	1	2	3	4	5	NA
012251	Maintains close relationships with friends	1	2	3	4	5	NA

Continued

Development: Middle Adulthood—cont'd

		Never Demonstrated	Rarely Demonstrated	Sometimes Demonstrated	Often Demonstrated	Consistently Demonstrated	
012222	Adjusts to sexual function changes	1	2	3	4	5	NA
012223	Practices safe sex	1	2	3	4	5	NA
012224	Adjusts to midlife physical changes	1	2	3	4	5	NA
012252	Plans for retirement activities	1	2	3	4	5	NA
012253	Evaluates retirement living needs	1	2	3	4	5	NA
012254	Considers early retirement	1	2	3	4	5	NA
012255	Develops a financial plan for retirement	1	2	3	4	5	NA
012256	Finalizes a will and estate planning	1	2	3	4	5	NA
012257	Recognizes increased risk for cancer and heart disease	1	2	3	4	5	NA
012225	Avoids substance misuse	1	2	3	4	5	NA
012226	Adheres to laws that protect welfare of others	1	2	3	4	5	NA
012227	Acknowledges personal values	1	2	3	4	5	NA
012228	Acknowledges values of others	1	2	3	4	5	NA
012229	Acknowledges personal opinions	1	2	3	4	5	NA
012230	Acknowledges opinions of others	1	2	3	4	5	NA
012231	Refrains from violating rights of others	1	2	3	4	5	NA
012232	Respects others	1	2	3	4	5	NA
012233	Respects the environment	1	2	3	4	5	NA
012234	Supports equality in treatment of others	1	2	3	4	5	NA
012235	Recognizes that mutual trust is necessary in healthy relationships	1	2	3	4	5	NA
012258	Volunteers in the community	1	2	3	4	5	NA

Domain-Functional Health (I)   **Class**-Growth & Development (B)   4th edition 2008; revised 2024

OUTCOME CONTENT REFERENCES:

Arnett, J. J., Robinson, O., & Lachman, M. E. (2020). Rethinking adult development: Introduction to the special issue. *American Psychologist*, 75(4), 425–430. https://doi.org/10.1037/amp0000633

Berk, L. (2018). *Development across the lifespan* (7th ed.). Pearson Education.

Bühler, J. L., & Nikitin, J. (2020). Sociohistorical context and adult social development: New directions for 21st century research. *American Psychologist*, 75(4), 457–469. https://doi.org/10.1037/amp0000611

Development: Young Adulthood

0123

Definition: Cognitive, physical, psychosocial, and moral progression from 21 through 29 years of age as an emerging adult

OUTCOME TARGET RATING: Maintain at_____ Increase to_____

		Never Demonstrated	Rarely Demonstrated	Sometimes Demonstrated	Often Demonstrated	Consistently Demonstrated	
OUTCOME OVERALL RATING		1	2	3	4	5	
Indicators:							
012301	Expresses complex thoughts	1	2	3	4	5	NA
012337	Seeks new knowledge for problem-solving	1	2	3	4	5	NA
012338	Considers context of the situation	1	2	3	4	5	NA

Development: Young Adulthood—cont'd

		Never Demonstrated	Rarely Demonstrated	Sometimes Demonstrated	Often Demonstrated	Consistently Demonstrated	
012302	Expands language skills	1	2	3	4	5	NA
012339	Examines occupational options and required skills	1	2	3	4	5	NA
012303	Makes educational choices	1	2	3	4	5	NA
012304	Makes occupational choices	1	2	3	4	5	NA
012340	Chooses a career	1	2	3	4	5	NA
012305	Establishes gainful employment	1	2	3	4	5	NA
012306	Establishes pattern of lifelong learning	1	2	3	4	5	NA
012341	Acknowledges importance of close friends	1	2	3	4	5	NA
012342	Relies on friends for support	1	2	3	4	5	NA
012343	Expands friendship network	1	2	3	4	5	NA
012307	Exhibits stable personality traits	1	2	3	4	5	NA
012308	Adjusts lifestyle according to life events	1	2	3	4	5	NA
012309	Embraces sexual identity	1	2	3	4	5	NA
012344	Establishes intimate relationships	1	2	3	4	5	NA
012310	Practices safe sex	1	2	3	4	5	NA
012345	Maintains positive relationships with immediate family	1	2	3	4	5	NA
012346	Maintains positive relationships with extended family	1	2	3	4	5	NA
012347	Exhibits conflict-resolutions skills	1	2	3	4	5	NA
012348	Exhibits positive self-esteem	1	2	3	4	5	NA
012317	Exhibits autonomy	1	2	3	4	5	NA
012318	Exhibits self-control	1	2	3	4	5	NA
012319	Exhibits personal responsibility	1	2	3	4	5	NA
012320	Avoids substance misuse	1	2	3	4	5	NA
012321	Adheres to laws that protect the welfare of others	1	2	3	4	5	NA
012322	Acknowledges personal values	1	2	3	4	5	NA
012323	Acknowledges values of others	1	2	3	4	5	NA
012324	Acknowledges personal opinions	1	2	3	4	5	NA
012325	Acknowledges opinions of others	1	2	3	4	5	NA
012326	Refrains from violating the rights of others	1	2	3	4	5	NA
012327	Respects others	1	2	3	4	5	NA
012349	Contributes to the community	1	2	3	4	5	NA
012328	Respects the environment	1	2	3	4	5	NA

Domain-Functional Health (I)   **Class**-Growth & Development (B)   4th edition 2008; revised 2013, 2024

OUTCOME CONTENT REFERENCES:

Arnett, J. J., Robinson, O., & Lachman, M. E. (2020). Rethinking adult development: Introduction to the special issue. *American Psychologist, 75*(4), 425–430. https://doi.org/10.1037/amp0000633

Athan, A. M. (2020). Reproductive identity: An emerging concept. *American Psychologist, 75*(4), 445–456. https://doi.org/10.1037/amp0000623

Barry, C. M., Madsen, S. D., & DeGrace, A. (2015). Growing up with a little help from their friends in emerging adulthood. In J.J. Arnett, *The Oxford handbook of emerging adulthood* (pp.215–229). Oxford University Press. https://doi.org/10.1093/oxfordhb/9780199795574.013.008

Berk, L. (2018). *Development across the lifespan* (7th ed.). Pearson Education.

Bühler, J. L., & Nikitin, J. (2020). Sociohistorical context and adult social development: New directions for 21st century research. *American Psychologist, 75*(4), 457–469. https://doi.org/10.1037/amp0000611

King, P., M., & Kitchener, K. S. (2015). Cognitive development in the emerging adult: The emergence of complex cognitive skills. In J. J. Arnett (Ed.), *The Oxford handbook of emerging adulthood* (pp. 105–125). Oxford University Press. https://doi.org/10.1093/oxfordhb/9780199795574.013.14

Digital Literacy Behavior

2040

Definition: Personal actions to use information and communication technologies to find, evaluate, create, store, and communicate information using cognitive and technical skills

OUTCOME TARGET RATING: Maintain at_____ Increase to_____

		Never Demonstrated	Rarely Demonstrated	Sometimes Demonstrated	Often Demonstrated	Consistently Demonstrated	
OUTCOME OVERALL RATING		1	2	3	4	5	
Indicators:							
204001	Identifies types of electronic devices	1	2	3	4	5	NA
204002	Identifies types of output devices	1	2	3	4	5	NA
204003	Identifies types of electronic storage devices	1	2	3	4	5	NA
204004	Identifies types of input devices	1	2	3	4	5	NA
204005	Develops effective mouse and keyboarding skills	1	2	3	4	5	NA
204006	Uses a variety of software products	1	2	3	4	5	NA
204007	Navigates the worldwide web	1	2	3	4	5	NA
204008	Uses a global browser	1	2	3	4	5	NA
204009	Uses an electronic device to gather health information	1	2	3	4	5	NA
204010	Shares content using the internet	1	2	3	4	5	NA
204011	Uses attachments to share information	1	2	3	4	5	NA
204012	Uses critical thinking skills to evaluate information from internet sites	1	2	3	4	5	NA
204013	Compares collected information from multiple sites for accuracy	1	2	3	4	5	NA
204014	Identifies advertising approaches used online	1	2	3	4	5	NA
204015	Communicates effectively using electronic applications	1	2	3	4	5	NA
204016	Uses virtual networking tools	1	2	3	4	5	NA
204017	Develops strong passwords for devices and applications	1	2	3	4	5	NA
204018	Stores passwords for all applications	1	2	3	4	5	NA
204019	Protects personal identity using multiple strategies	1	2	3	4	5	NA
204020	Uses applications to scan documents for viruses	1	2	3	4	5	NA
204021	Uses safe practices for social media applications	1	2	3	4	5	NA
204022	Identifies bullying on social media	1	2	3	4	5	NA
204023	Identifies scam messages received	1	2	3	4	5	NA
204024	Purchases items using safe internet sites	1	2	3	4	5	NA
204025	Uses appropriate digital etiquette	1	2	3	4	5	NA
204026	Understands copyright issues	1	2	3	4	5	NA
204027	Increases creativity using the internet	1	2	3	4	5	NA

Domain-Health Knowledge & Behavior (IV)   Class-Health Supporting Life Skills (II)   7th edition 2024

OUTCOME CONTENT REFERENCES:

Dadaczynski, K., Okan, O., Messer, M., Leung, A., Rosário, R., Darlington, E., & Rathmann, K. (2021). Digital health literacy and web-based information-seeking behaviors of university students in Germany during the COVID-19 pandemic: Cross-sectional survey study. *Journal of Medical Internet Research, 23*(1), e24097. https://doi.org/10.2196/24097

Feuchtwang, A. (2018). Good quality digital literacy: Making online life safer for pupils. *British Journal of School Nursing, 13*(6), 276–277. https://doi.org/10.12968/bjsn.2018.13.6.276

Hobbs, R. (2017). *Create to learn: Introduction to digital literacy.* J. Wiley & Sons.

Khanlou, N., Khan, A., Vazquez, L. M., & Zangeneh, M. (2021). Digital literacy, access to technology and inclusion for young adults with developmental disabilities. *Journal of Developmental & Physical Disabilities, 33*(1), 1–25. https://doi.org/10.1007/s10882-020-09738-w

Nouri, S. S., Adler-Milstein, J., Thao, C., Acharya, P., Barr-Walker, J., Sarkar, U., & Lyles, C. (2020). Patient characteristics associated with objective measures of digital health tool use in the United States: A literature review. *Journal of the American Medical Informatics Association, 27*(5), 834–841. https://doi.org/10.1093/jamia/ocaa02

Oh, S. S., Kim, K.-A., Kim, M., Oh, J., Chu, S. H., & Choi, J. (2021). Measurement of digital literacy among older adults: Systematic review. *Journal of Medical Internet Research, 23*(2). https://doi.org/10.2196/26145

Suslo, R., Paplicki, M., Dopierala, K., & Drobnik, J. (2018). Fostering digital literacy in the elderly as a means to secure their health needs and human rights in the reality of the twenty-first century. *Family Medicine & Primary Care Review, 20*(3), 271–275. https://doi.org/10.5114/fmpcr.2018.78273

Vincent, L. (2021). Preventing identity theft: Don't let thieves damage your credit or disrupt your life. *AJN, American Journal of Nursing, 16*(7), 24–25, 43.

Dignified Life Closure

1307

Definition: Personal actions to maintain control of end-of-life decisions and desired care

OUTCOME TARGET RATING: Maintain at_____ Increase to_____

OUTCOME OVERALL RATING	Never Demonstrated	Rarely Demonstrated	Sometimes Demonstrated	Often Demonstrated	Consistently Demonstrated	
	1	**2**	**3**	**4**	**5**	
Indicators:						
130702 Expresses hopefulness	1	2	3	4	5	NA
130726 Shares cultural beliefs important to care	1	2	3	4	5	NA
130703 Participates in decisions related to care	1	2	3	4	5	NA
130704 Participates in decisions about hospitalization	1	2	3	4	5	NA
130705 Participates in decisions about resuscitation status	1	2	3	4	5	NA
130727 Considers palliative care or hospice services	1	2	3	4	5	NA
130706 Controls decisions about organ donation	1	2	3	4	5	NA
130728 Communicates care needs with health professional	1	2	3	4	5	NA
130707 Participates in planning funeral	1	2	3	4	5	NA
130708 Maintains current will	1	2	3	4	5	NA
130709 Maintains advance directives	1	2	3	4	5	NA
130729 Puts financial affairs in order	1	2	3	4	5	NA
130710 Resolves important life issues	1	2	3	4	5	NA
130711 Shares feelings about dying with others	1	2	3	4	5	NA
130730 Makes decisions to reduce burden on family	1	2	3	4	5	NA
130712 Reconciles relationships	1	2	3	4	5	NA
130713 Completes meaningful goals	1	2	3	4	5	NA
130714 Maintains sense of control of remaining time	1	2	3	4	5	NA
130715 Exchanges affection with others	1	2	3	4	5	NA
130716 Disengages gradually from significant others	1	2	3	4	5	NA
130717 Recalls lifetime memories	1	2	3	4	5	NA
130718 Reviews life's accomplishments	1	2	3	4	5	NA
130719 Discusses spiritual experiences	1	2	3	4	5	NA

Continued

D

Dignified Life Closure—cont'd

	Never Demonstrated	Rarely Demonstrated	Sometimes Demonstrated	Often Demonstrated	Consistently Demonstrated	
130720 Discusses spiritual concerns	1	2	3	4	5	NA
130721 Maintains physical independence as much as possible	1	2	3	4	5	NA
130722 Controls treatment choices	1	2	3	4	5	NA
130731 Chooses pain control strategies	1	2	3	4	5	NA
130723 Controls food/drink intake	1	2	3	4	5	NA
130724 Controls personal possessions	1	2	3	4	5	NA
130725 Expresses readiness for death	1	2	3	4	5	NA

Domain-Psychosocial Health (III) **Class**-Psychosocial Adaptation (N) 3rd edition 2004; revised 2013, 2024

OUTCOME CONTENT REFERENCES:

Bloomer, M. J., Botti, M., Runacres, F., Poon, P., Barnfield, J., & Hutchinson, A. M. (2019). Cultural considerations at end of life in a geriatric inpatient rehabilitation setting. *Collegian, 26*(1), 165–170. https://doi.org/10.1016/j.colegn.2018.07.004

Bovero, A., Gottardo, F., Botto, R., Tosi, C., Selvatico, M., & Torta, R. (2020). Definition of a good death, attitudes toward death, and feelings of interconnectedness among people taking care of terminally ill patients with cancer: An exploratory study. *American Journal of Hospice & Palliative Medicine, 37*(5), 343–349. https://doi.org/10.1177/1049909119883835

Broden, E. G., Deatrick, J., Ulrich, C., & Curley, M. A. Q. (2020). Defining a "good death" in the pediatric intensive care unit. *American Journal of Critical Care, 29*(2), 111–121. https://doi.org/10.4037/ajcc2020466

Cha, E., Kim, J., Sohn, M. K., Lee, B. S., Jung, S. S., Lee, S., & Lee, I. (2021). Perceptions on good-life, good-death, and advance care planning in Koreans with non-cancerous chronic diseases. *Journal of Advanced Nursing, 77*(2), 889–898. https://doi.org/10.1111/jan.14633

Fleming, J., Calloway, R., Perrels, A., Farquhar, M., Barclay, S., & Brayne, C. (2017). Dying comfortably in very old age with or without dementia in different care settings—A representative "older old" population study. *BMC Geriatrics, 17*(1), 222. https://doi.org/10.1186/s12877-017-0605-2

Krikorian, A., Maldonado, C., & Pastrana, T. (2020). Patient's perspectives on the notion of a good death: A systematic review of the literature. *Journal of Pain & Symptom Management, 59*(1), 152–164. https://doi.org/10.1016/j.jpainsymman.2019.07.033

Li, T., Pei, X., Chen, X., & Zhang, S. (2021). Identifying end-of-life preferences among Chinese patients with cancer using the Heart to Heart Card Game. *American Journal of Hospice & Palliative Medicine, 38*(1), 62–67. https://doi.org/10.1177/1049909120917361

Puente, F. D., Palma, A. E., Sánchez, G. M. R., Hueso, M. C., Esteban, B. A. A., & Montoya, J. R. (2020). Development of a scale based on Nursing Outcome Classification "Dignified Life Closure" (1307) to assess end-of-life dignity of patients in care homes for the elderly. *International Journal of Nursing Knowledge, 31*(1), 44–49. https://doi.org/10.1111/2047-3095.12264

Takahashi, Z., Yamakawa, M., Nakanishi, M., Fukahori, H., Igarashi, N., Aoyama, M., Sato, K., Sakai, S., Nagae, H., & Miyashita, M. (2021). Defining a good death for people with dementia: A scoping review. *Japanese Journal of Nursing Science, 18*(2), e12402. https://doi.org/10.1111/jjns.12402

Discharge Readiness: Independent Living   0311

Definition: Preparedness of a patient to relocate from a health care institution to living independently

OUTCOME TARGET RATING: Maintain at_____ Increase to_____

	Never Demonstrated	Rarely Demonstrated	Sometimes Demonstrated	Often Demonstrated	Consistently Demonstrated	
OUTCOME OVERALL RATING	1	2	3	4	5	
Indicators:						
031118 Reports confidence in ability to participate in discharge teaching	1	2	3	4	5	NA
031119 Reports physically ready to go home	1	2	3	4	5	NA
031120 Reports pain controlled	1	2	3	4	5	NA
031121 Reports emotionally ready to go home	1	2	3	4	5	NA
031122 Reports confidence in ability to live independently	1	2	3	4	5	NA
031117 Participates in discharge planning with caregiver	1	2	3	4	5	NA
031123 Describes how to get community resources	1	2	3	4	5	NA
031124 Reports access to trained caregivers	1	2	3	4	5	NA

Discharge Readiness: Independent Living—cont'd

		Never Demonstrated	Rarely Demonstrated	Sometimes Demonstrated	Often Demonstrated	Consistently Demonstrated	
031113	Reports able to obtain needed assistance when experiencing problems	1	2	3	4	5	NA
031114	Describes personal support system	1	2	3	4	5	NA
031106	Describes signs and symptoms to health professional of potential complications	1	2	3	4	5	NA
031125	Describes physical ability to care for self	1	2	3	4	5	NA
031126	Describes emotional ability to care for self	1	2	3	4	5	NA
031127	Describes how home modified for safe functioning	1	2	3	4	5	NA
031116	Describes how to manage own parenteral medication	1	2	3	4	5	NA
031115	Describes how to manage own non-parenteral medication	1	2	3	4	5	NA
031128	Describes plan for medication adherence	1	2	3	4	5	NA
031107	Describes prescribed treatments	1	2	3	4	5	NA
031129	Describes how to do treatments	1	2	3	4	5	NA
031130	Describes activity restrictions	1	2	3	4	5	NA
031108	Describes risks for complications	1	2	3	4	5	NA
031131	Describes follow-up therapy	1	2	3	4	5	NA
031132	Describes plan for emergencies	1	2	3	4	5	NA
031133	Performs activities of daily living (ADLs) independently	1	2	3	4	5	NA
031134	Plans support for instrumental activities of daily living (IADLs) independently	1	2	3	4	5	NA
031112	Makes appropriate judgments	1	2	3	4	5	NA

Domain-Functional Health (I)   **Class**-Self-Care (D)   3rd edition 2004; revised 2008, 2024

OUTCOME CONTENT REFERENCES:

Bobay, K. L., Conway-Phillips, R., Hughes, R. G., Costa, L., Bahr, S. J., Siclovan, D., Nuccio, S., & Weiss, M. (2020). Clinical nurses' perspectives on discharge practice changes from participating in a translational research study. *Journal of Nursing Management, 29*(3), 553–561. https://doi.org/10.1111/jonm.13171

Casey-Upton, R., Howell, D. M., Kitzman, P. H., Custer, M. G., & Dressler, E. V. (2019). Factors influencing discharge readiness after total knee replacement. *Orthopaedic Nursing, 38*(1), 6–14. https://doi.org/10.1097/NOR.0000000000000513

Dharmarajan, K., Han, L., Gahbauer, E. A., Leo-Summers, L. S., & Gill, T. M. (2020). Disability and recovery after hospitalization for medical illness among community-living older persons: A prospective cohort study. *Journal of the American Geriatrics Society, 68*(3), 486–495. https://doi.org/10.1111/jgs.16350

Fuller, T. E., Pong, D. D., Piniella, N., Pardo, M., Bessa, N., Yoon, C., Boxer, R. B., Schnipper, J. L., & Dalal, A. K. (2020). Interactive digital health tools to engage patients and caregivers in discharge preparation: Implementation study. *Journal of Medical Internet Research, 22*(4), 1–19. https://www.jmir.org/2020/4/e15573

Hua, W., Wang, L., Li, C., Simoni, J. M., Yuwen, W., & Jiang, L. (2021). Understanding preparation for preterm infant discharge from parents' and healthcare providers' perspectives: Challenges and opportunities. *Journal of Advanced Nursing, 77*(3), 1379–1390. https://doi.org/10.1111/jan.14676

O'Conner, M., Moriarty, H., Schneider, A., Dowdell, E. B., & Bowles, K. H. (2021). Patients' and caregivers' perspectives in determining discharge readiness from home health. *Geriatric Nursing, 42*(1), 151–158. https://doi.org/10.1016/j.gerinurse.2020.12.012

Pellet, J., Weiss, M., Rapin, J., Jaques, C., & Mabire, C. (2020). Nursing discharge teaching for hospitalized older people: A rapid realist review. *Journal of Advanced Nursing, 76*(4), 2885–2896. https://doi.org/10.1111/jan.14511

Salmani, N., Marvast, M. Z., Kahdouei, S., & Weiss, M. E. (2020). Adaptation of the parent readiness for hospital discharge scale with mothers of preterm infants discharged from the neonatal intensive care unit. *Journal of Clinical Nursing, 29*(23-24), 4544–4553. https://doi.org/10.1111/jocn.15479

Smith, V. C., Mao, W., & McCormick, M. C. (2021). Changes in assessment of and satisfaction with discharge preparation from the neonatal intensive care unit. *Advances in Neonatal Care, 21*(5), E144–E151. https://doi.org/10.1097/ANC.0000000000000862

Wallace, A. S., Pierce, N. L., Davisson, E., Manges, K., & Tripp-Reimer, T. (2019). Social resource assessment: Application of a novel communication tool during hospital discharge. *Patient Education and Counseling, 102*(3), 542–549. https://doi.org/10.1016/j.pec.2018.09.022

Wang, M., Wang, Y., Meng, N., & Li, X. (2021). The factors of patient-reported readiness for hospital discharge in patients with depression: A cross-sectional study. *Journal of Psychiatric Mental Health Nursing, 28*(3), 409–421. https://doi.org/10.1111/jpm.12693

Weiss, M. E., Lerret, S. M., Sawin, K. J., & Schiffman, R. F. (2020). Parent readiness for hospital discharge scale: Psychometrics and association with post discharge outcomes. *Journal of Pediatric Health Care,34*(1), 30–37. https://doi.org/10.1016/j.pedhc.2019.06.011

Weiss, M. E., & Piacentine, L. B. (2006). Psychometric properties of the readiness for hospital discharge scale. *Journal of Nursing Measurement, 14*(3), 163–180. https://doi.org/10.1891/jnm-v14i3a002

Weiss, M. E., Yakusheva, O., Bobay, K. L., Costa, L., Hughes, R. G., Nuccio, S., Hamilton, M., Bahr, S., Siclovan, D., & Bang, J. (2019). Effect of implementing discharge readiness assessment in adult medical-surgical units on 30-day return to hospital The READI Randomized Clinical Trial. *JAMA Network Open, 2*(1), e187387. https://doi.org/10.1001/jamanetworkopen.2018.7387

Discharge Readiness: Supported Living 0312

Definition: Preparedness of the patient for relocation from a health care institution to a lower level of supported living

OUTCOME TARGET RATING: Maintain at_____ Increase to_____

OUTCOME OVERALL RATING	Never Demonstrated	Rarely Demonstrated	Sometimes Demonstrated	Often Demonstrated	Consistently Demonstrated	
	1	2	3	4	5	
Indicators:						
031209 Participates in discharge planning	1	2	3	4	5	NA
031210 Family involved in discharge planning	1	2	3	4	5	NA
031204 Accepts transfer to new facility	1	2	3	4	5	NA
031201 Patient needs consistent with available staff support	1	2	3	4	5	NA
031211 Describes a transition plan for the new facility	1	2	3	4	5	NA
031212 Describes rehabilitation potential	1	2	3	4	5	NA
031213 Describes level of family support	1	2	3	4	5	NA
031214 Describes medication needs	1	2	3	4	5	NA
031215 Describes mobility needs	1	2	3	4	5	NA
031216 Describes functional status needs	1	2	3	4	5	NA
031217 Describes dietary needs	1	2	3	4	5	NA
031218 Describes treatment goals	1	2	3	4	5	NA
031219 Describes self-care goals	1	2	3	4	5	NA
031208 Describes plan for continuity of care	1	2	3	4	5	NA
031220 Describes advanced care planning	1	2	3	4	5	NA
031203 Oriented to care at new facility	1	2	3	4	5	NA

Domain-Functional Health (I)   *Class*-Self-Care (D)   *3rd edition 2004; revised 2008, 2024*

OUTCOME CONTENT REFERENCES:

Britton, M. C., Petersen-Pickett, J., Hodshon, B., & Chaudhry, S. I. (2020). Mapping the care transition from hospital to skilled nursing facility. *Journal of Evaluation in Clinical Practice, 26*(3), 786–790. https://doi.org/10.1111/jep.13238

Dalal, A. K., Piniella, N., Fuller, T. E., Pong, D., Pardo, M., Bessa, N., Yoon, C., Lipsitz, S., & Schnipper, J. L. (2021). Evaluation of electronic health record-integrated digital health tools to engage hospitalized patients in discharge preparation. *Journal of the American Medical Informatics Association, 28*(4), 704–712. https://doi.org/10.1093/jamia/ocaa321

Mabire, C., Bachnick, S., Ausserhofer, D., & Simon, M. (2019). Patient readiness for hospital discharge and its relationship to discharge preparation and structural factors: A cross-sectional study. *International Journal of Nursing Studies, 90*, 13–20. https://doi.org/10.1016/j.ijnurstu.2018.09.016

Popejoy, L. L., Wakefield, B. J., Vogelsmeier, A. A., Galambos, C. M., Lewis, A. M., Huneke, D., Petroski, G., & Mehr, D. R. (2019). Reengineering skilled nursing facility discharge. *Journal of Nursing Care Quality, 35*(2), 158–164. https://doi.org/10.1097/NCQ.0000000000000413

Smith, V. C., Mao, W., & McCormick, M. C. (2021). Changes in assessment of and satisfaction with discharge preparation from the neonatal intensive care unit. *Advances in Neonatal Care, 21*(5), E144–E151. https://doi.org/10.1097/ANC.0000000000000862

Toles, M., Leeman, J., Colón-Emeric, C., & Hanson, L. C. (2020). Implementing a standardized transition care plan in skilled nursing facilities. *Journal of Applied Gerontology, 39*(8), 855–862. https://doi.org/10.1177/0733464818783689

Wales, L., Dunford, C., & Davis, K. (2020). Following severe childhood stroke, specialised residential rehabilitation improvise self-care independence but there are ongoing needs at discharge. *British Journal of Occupational Therapy, 83*(8), 530–537. https://doi.org/10.1177/0308022619894870

Discomfort Level **2109**

Definition: Severity of observed or reported mental or physical discomfort

OUTCOME TARGET RATING: Maintain at_____ Increase to_____

OUTCOME OVERALL RATING		Severe	Substantial	Moderate	Mild	None	
		1	2	3	4	5	
Indicators:							
210901	Pain	1	2	3	4	5	NA
210938	Headache	1	2	3	4	5	NA
210939	Tachycardia	1	2	3	4	5	NA
210902	Anxiety	1	2	3	4	5	NA
210903	Moaning	1	2	3	4	5	NA
210904	Suffering	1	2	3	4	5	NA
210905	Thrashing	1	2	3	4	5	NA
210940	Agitation	1	2	3	4	5	NA
210906	Stress	1	2	3	4	5	NA
210907	Fear	1	2	3	4	5	NA
210908	Depression	1	2	3	4	5	NA
210941	Fatigue	1	2	3	4	5	NA
210909	Hallucinations	1	2	3	4	5	NA
210910	Delusions	1	2	3	4	5	NA
210911	Paranoid thoughts	1	2	3	4	5	NA
210942	Confusion	1	2	3	4	5	NA
210912	Obsessive compulsive behaviors	1	2	3	4	5	NA
210913	Hyperactivity	1	2	3	4	5	NA
210914	Restlessness	1	2	3	4	5	NA
210915	Restless legs syndrome	1	2	3	4	5	NA
210916	Itching	1	2	3	4	5	NA
210943	Hives	1	2	3	4	5	NA
210944	Rash	1	2	3	4	5	NA
210917	Muscle aches	1	2	3	4	5	NA
210945	Muscle cramps	1	2	3	4	5	NA
210918	Grimacing	1	2	3	4	5	NA
210919	Facial tension	1	2	3	4	5	NA
210921	Jerking	1	2	3	4	5	NA
210946	Inability to move	1	2	3	4	5	NA
210922	Poor body positioning	1	2	3	4	5	NA
210923	Labored breathing	1	2	3	4	5	NA
210924	Air hunger	1	2	3	4	5	NA
210947	Choking	1	2	3	4	5	NA
210948	Coughing	1	2	3	4	5	NA
210949	Wheezing	1	2	3	4	5	NA
210950	Mucous secretions	1	2	3	4	5	NA
210926	Chilling	1	2	3	4	5	NA
210927	Hypothermia	1	2	3	4	5	NA
210951	Fever	1	2	3	4	5	NA
210952	Edema	1	2	3	4	5	NA
210953	Abdominal distention	1	2	3	4	5	NA
210920	Rebound tenderness	1	2	3	4	5	NA
210954	Ascites	1	2	3	4	5	NA
210955	Dry mouth and mucous membranes	1	2	3	4	5	NA
210956	Dehydration	1	2	3	4	5	NA
210925	Loss of appetite	1	2	3	4	5	NA
210957	Heartburn	1	2	3	4	5	NA

Continued

Discomfort Level—cont'd

		Severe	Substantial	Moderate	Mild	None	
210928	Nausea	1	2	3	4	5	NA
210929	Vomiting	1	2	3	4	5	NA
210930	Diarrhea	1	2	3	4	5	NA
210931	Bowel incontinence	1	2	3	4	5	NA
210932	Constipation	1	2	3	4	5	NA
210933	Urinary incontinence	1	2	3	4	5	NA
210934	Inability to communicate	1	2	3	4	5	NA
210935	Suicidal thoughts	1	2	3	4	5	NA
210958	Loneliness	1	2	3	4	5	NA
210959	Sadness	1	2	3	4	5	NA
210936	Loss of faith	1	2	3	4	5	NA
210937	Sense of spiritual abandonment	1	2	3	4	5	NA

Domain-Perceived Health (V)   **Class**-Symptom Status (V)   4th edition 2008; revised 2024

OUTCOME CONTENT REFERENCES:

Berntzen, H., Bjørk, I. T., Storsveen, A., & Wøien, H. (2020). "Please mind the gap": A secondary analysis of discomfort and comfort in intensive care. *Journal of Clinical Nursing, 29*(13/14), 2441–2454. https://doi.org/10.1111/jocn.15260

Ignatavicius, D. D., Workman, M. L., Rebar, C. R., & Heimgartner, N. M. (2021). *Medical-surgical nursing: Concepts for interprofessional care* (10th ed.). Elsevier.

Kalfon, P., Baumstarck, K., Estagnasie, P., Geantot, M.-A., Berric, A., Simon, G., Floccard, B., Signouret, T., Boucekine, M., Fromentin, M., Nyunga, M., Sossou, A., Venot, M., Robert, R., Follin, A., Audibert, J., Renault, A., Garrouste-Orgeas, M., Collange, O., Levat, Q., Villard, I., Thevenin, D., Pottecher. J., Patrigeon. R.-G., Revel, N., Vigne, C., Azoulay, E., Mimoz, O., Auquier, P., & IPREA Study Group. (2017). A tailored multicomponent program to reduce discomfort in critically ill patients: A cluster-randomized controlled trial. *Intensive Care Medicine, 43*(12), 1829–1840. https://doi.org/10.1007/s00134-017-4991-x

Kolcaba, K. (2003). *Comfort theory and practice: A vision for holistic health care and research.* Springer.

Kolcaba, K., & Crawford, C. L. (2020). Comfort. In S. J. Peterson & T. S. Bredow, *Middle range theories: Application to nursing research and practice.* (pp. 189–207). Wolters Kluwer.

Distorted Thought Self-Control

1403

Definition: Self-restraint of disruptions in perception, thought processes, and thought content

OUTCOME TARGET RATING: Maintain at_____ Increase to_____

		Never Demonstrated	Rarely Demonstrated	Sometimes Demonstrated	Often Demonstrated	Consistently Demonstrated	
OUTCOME OVERALL RATING		1	2	3	4	5	
Indicators:							
140301	Recognizes hallucinations or delusions are occurring	1	2	3	4	5	NA
140302	Refrains from attending to hallucinations or delusions	1	2	3	4	5	NA
140303	Refrains from responding to hallucinations or delusions	1	2	3	4	5	NA
140304	Monitors frequency of hallucinations or delusions	1	2	3	4	5	NA
140305	Describes content of hallucinations or delusions	1	2	3	4	5	NA
140306	Reports decrease in hallucinations or delusions	1	2	3	4	5	NA
140316	Shares emotional response to hallucinations or delusions	1	2	3	4	5	NA
140307	Asks for validation of reality	1	2	3	4	5	NA
140308	Maintains affect consistent with mood	1	2	3	4	5	NA
140309	Interacts with others appropriately	1	2	3	4	5	NA
140317	Communicates willingly with others	1	2	3	4	5	NA

D

Distorted Thought Self-Control—cont'd

	Never Demonstrated	Rarely Demonstrated	Sometimes Demonstrated	Often Demonstrated	Consistently Demonstrated	
140310 Perceives environment accurately	1	2	3	4	5	NA
140311 Exhibits logical thought flow patterns	1	2	3	4	5	NA
140312 Exhibits reality-based thinking	1	2	3	4	5	NA
140313 Exhibits appropriate thought content	1	2	3	4	5	NA
140318 Uses organized speech	1	2	3	4	5	NA
140319 Uses customary sentence construction	1	2	3	4	5	NA
140314 Exhibits ability to grasp ideas of others	1	2	3	4	5	NA

Domain-Psychosocial Health (III)   **Class**-Self-Control (O)   1st edition 1997; revised 2000, 2004, 2018

OUTCOME CONTENT REFERENCES:
Ayer, A., Yahnçentin, B., Aydinli, E., Sevilmis, S., Ulas, H., Binbay, T., Akdede, B. B., & Alptekin, K. (2016). Formal thought disorder in first-episode psychosis. Comprehensive Psychiatry, 70, 209–215. https://doi.org/10.1016/j.comppsych.2016.08.005
Black, D., & Adreasen, N. C. (2014). Introductory textbook of psychiatry (6th ed.). American Psychiatric.
+Cummings, J. L. (1997). The Neuropsychiatric Inventory: Assessing psychopathology in dementia patients. Neurology, 48 (Suppl. 6), S10–S16.
Frederick, J., & Cotanch, P. (1995). Self-help techniques for auditory hallucinations in schizophrenia. Issues in Mental Health Nursing, 16(3), 213–224.
Ólafsson, R., Snorrason, Í., Bjarnason, R., Emmelkamp, P., Ólason, D., & Kristjánsson, Á. (2014). Replacing intrusive thoughts: Investigating thought control in relation of OCD symptoms. Journal of Behavior Therapy and Experimental Psychiatry, 45(4), 506–515. https://doi.org/10.1016/j.jbtep.2014.07.007
Price, B. (2016). Hallucinations: Insights and supportive first care. Nursing Standard, 30(21), 49–58. https://doi.org/10.7748/ns.30.21.49.s45
Sousa, P., Sellwood, W., Spray, A., Fernyhough, C., & Bentall, R. (2016). Inner speech and clarity of self-concept in thought disorder and auditory-verbal hallucinations. Journal of Nervous and Mental Disease, 204(12), 885–893. https://doi.org/10.1097/NMD.0000000000000584
Stuart, G. W. (2013). Principles and practice of psychiatric nursing (10th ed.). Elsevier Mosby.

Drug Abuse Cessation Behavior   1630

Definition: Personal actions to eliminate drug use that poses a threat to health

OUTCOME TARGET RATING: Maintain at_____ Increase to_____

	Never Demonstrated	Rarely Demonstrated	Sometimes Demonstrated	Often Demonstrated	Consistently Demonstrated	
OUTCOME OVERALL RATING	1	2	3	4	5	
Indicators:						
163001 Expresses willingness to stop drug use	1	2	3	4	5	NA
163002 Expresses belief in the ability to stop drug use	1	2	3	4	5	NA
163003 Identifies benefits of eliminating harmful drug use	1	2	3	4	5	NA
163004 Identifies negative consequences of drug use	1	2	3	4	5	NA
163005 Develops effective strategies to eliminate drug use	1	2	3	4	5	NA
163006 Identifies barriers to harmful drug use elimination	1	2	3	4	5	NA
163007 Adjusts drug use elimination strategies as needed	1	2	3	4	5	NA
163029 Confirms the need for treatment	1	2	3	4	5	NA
163008 Commits to drug elimination strategies	1	2	3	4	5	NA
163009 Follows selected drug elimination strategies	1	2	3	4	5	NA
163010 Participates in screening for associated health problems	1	2	3	4	5	NA
163030 Participates in screening for use of other substances	1	2	3	4	5	NA

Continued

Drug Abuse Cessation Behavior—cont'd

		Never Demonstrated	Rarely Demonstrated	Sometimes Demonstrated	Often Demonstrated	Consistently Demonstrated	
163011	Uses strategies to cope with withdrawal symptoms	1	2	3	4	5	NA
163031	Uses strategies to distance self from other users	1	2	3	4	5	NA
163012	Uses behavior modification strategies	1	2	3	4	5	NA
163013	Uses effective coping strategies	1	2	3	4	5	NA
163032	Uses effective strategies to control pain	1	2	3	4	5	NA
163033	Uses strategies to increase social interaction	1	2	3	4	5	NA
163014	Obtains assistance from health professional	1	2	3	4	5	NA
163015	Uses personal support system	1	2	3	4	5	NA
163016	Uses reputable sources of information	1	2	3	4	5	NA
163034	Uses reputable eHealth resources	1	2	3	4	5	NA
163017	Uses drug replacement therapy	1	2	3	4	5	NA
163035	Uses cognitive behavioral therapy	1	2	3	4	5	NA
163036	Uses family therapy	1	2	3	4	5	NA
163037	Uses Mindfulness-Oriented Recovery Enhancement therapy	1	2	3	4	5	NA
163019	Identifies emotional states that affect drug use	1	2	3	4	5	NA
163020	Adjusts lifestyle to promote drug elimination	1	2	3	4	5	NA
163038	Adjusts to change in career	1	2	3	4	5	NA
163039	Uses strategies to adjust to career change	1	2	3	4	5	NA
163040	Uses strategies to adjust to changes in living situation	1	2	3	4	5	NA
163021	Participates in drug withdrawal program	1	2	3	4	5	NA
163022	Participates in counseling	1	2	3	4	5	NA
163023	Monitors for signs of depression	1	2	3	4	5	NA
163024	Uses prescribed medication as recommended	1	2	3	4	5	NA
163025	Uses non-prescription medication as recommended	1	2	3	4	5	NA
163026	Uses available support groups	1	2	3	4	5	NA
163027	Uses available community resources	1	2	3	4	5	NA
163041	Abstinence from drug use	1	2	3	4	5	NA

Domain-Health Knowledge & Behavior (IV)   **Class**-Health Behavior (Q)   4th edition 2008; revised 2024

OUTCOME CONTENT REFERENCES:

Anyimukwu, C., & Omondi, A. (2020). Assessment of psychosocial interventions in opioid cessation: A systematic review. *Journal of Alcohol & Drug Education, 64*(2), 62–86.

Gueta, K., & Chen, G. (2021). "You have to start normalizing": Identity construction among self-changers and treatment changers in the context of drug use normalization. *Social Science & Medicine, 275*(1), 1–9. https://doi.org/10.1016/j.socscimed.2021.113828

Lefebvre-Durel, C., Bailly, I., Hunault, J., Jovic, L., Novic, M., Vorspan, F., Bellivier, F., Drunat, O., & Kerever, S. (2021). Benzodiazepine and Z drug cessation in elderly patients: A qualitative study on the perception of healthcare providers and the place of advanced practice nurses. *International Journal of Mental Health Nursing, 30*(3), 646–660. https://doi.org/10.1111/inm.12831

Pergolizzi, J. V. Jr., Raffa, R. B., & Rosenblatt, M. H. (2020). Opioid withdrawal symptoms, a consequence of chronic opioid use and opioid use disorder: Current understanding and approaches to management. *Journal of Clinical Pharmacy and Therapeutics. 45*(5), 892–903. https://doi.org/10.1111/jcpt.13114

Pericot-Valverde, I., Heo, M., Akiyama, M. J., Norton, B. L., Agyemang, L., Niu, J., & Litwin, A. H. (2020). Factors and HCV treatment outcomes associated with smoking among people who inject drugs on opioid agonist treatment: Secondary analysis of the PREV AIL randomized clinical trial. *BMC Infectious Diseases, 20*(1), 928–939. https://doi.org/10.1186/s12879-020-05667-3

Rudolph, A. E., Upton, E., Young, A. M., & Havens, J. R. (2020). Social network predictors of recent and sustained injection drug use cessation: Findings from a longitudinal cohort study. *Addiction, 116*(40, 856–864. https://doi.org/10.1111/add.15218

Vandenbussche, N., Paemeleire, K., & Katsarava, Z. (2020). The many faces of medication-overuse headache in clinical practice. *Headache: The Journal of Head and Face Pain, 60*(5), 1021–1036. https://doi.org/10.1111/head.13785

Dry Eye Severity   2110

Definition: Severity of signs and symptoms of insufficient tears

OUTCOME TARGET RATING: Maintain at_____ Increase to_____

		Severe	Substantial	Moderate	Mild	None	
OUTCOME OVERALL RATING		1	2	3	4	5	
Indicators:							
211001	Decreased tear production	1	2	3	4	5	NA
211002	Incomplete eyelid closure	1	2	3	4	5	NA
211003	Redness of conjunctiva	1	2	3	4	5	NA
211004	Burning eye sensation	1	2	3	4	5	NA
211005	Itchy eye sensation	1	2	3	4	5	NA
211006	Gritty sensation	1	2	3	4	5	NA
211007	Foreign body sensation	1	2	3	4	5	NA
211008	Eye pain	1	2	3	4	5	NA
211009	Excessive watering	1	2	3	4	5	NA
211010	Blurred vision	1	2	3	4	5	NA
211011	Excessive mucous secretions	1	2	3	4	5	NA
211012	Sensitivity to light	1	2	3	4	5	NA

Domain-*Health & Life Quality (V)*   **Class**-*Symptom Status (V)*   *5th edition 2013*

OUTCOME CONTENT REFERENCES:

Dawson, D. (2005). Development of a new eye care guideline for critically ill patients. *Intensive Critical Care Nursing, 21*(2), 119–122. https://doi.org/10.1016/j.iccn.2005.01.004

Tavares, F., Fernandes, R. S., Bernardes, T. F., Bonfioli, A. A., & Soares, E. J. (2010). Dry eye disease. *Seminars in Ophthalmology, 25*(3), 84–93.

Versura, P., Nanni, P., Bavelloni, A., Blalock, W. L., Piazzi, M., Roda, A., & Campos, E. C. (2010). Tear proteomics in evaporative dry eye disease. *Eye, 24*(8), 1396–1402. https://doi.org/10.1038/eye.2010.7

Eating Disorder Self-Control
1411

Definition: Personal actions to eliminate maladaptive behaviors and to adopt and maintain healthy eating patterns and optimum body weight

OUTCOME TARGET RATING: Maintain at_____ Increase to_____

	Never Demonstrated	Rarely Demonstrated	Sometimes Demonstrated	Often Demonstrated	Consistently Demonstrated	
OUTCOME OVERALL RATING	1	2	3	4	5	
Indicators:						
141101 Selects a healthy target weight	1	2	3	4	5	NA
141102 Participates in setting achievable dietary goals with health professional	1	2	3	4	5	NA
141103 Sets achievable weight gain goals	1	2	3	4	5	NA
141104 Sets achievable weight loss goals	1	2	3	4	5	
141105 Monitors body weight	1	2	3	4	5	NA
141106 Maintains progress toward target weight	1	2	3	4	5	NA
141107 Follows a healthy eating plan	1	2	3	4	5	NA
141108 Identifies emotional states that affect food and fluid intake	1	2	3	4	5	NA
141109 Identifies social situations that affect food and fluid intake	1	2	3	4	5	NA
141110 Plans strategies for situations that affect food and fluid intake	1	2	3	4	5	NA
141111 Identifies maladaptive eating behaviors	1	2	3	4	5	NA
141112 Verbalizes a desire to decrease maladaptive eating behaviors	1	2	3	4	5	NA
141113 Eliminates maladaptive eating behaviors	1	2	3	4	5	NA
141114 Follows treatment plan	1	2	3	4	5	NA
141115 Identifies daily food and fluid intake that meets nutritional needs	1	2	3	4	5	NA
141116 Consumes daily caloric intake appropriate for metabolic needs	1	2	3	4	5	NA
141117 Consumes daily nutrient intake appropriate for metabolic needs	1	2	3	4	5	NA
141118 Maintains body weight appropriate for height	1	2	3	4	5	NA
141119 Uses strategies to manage stress	1	2	3	4	5	NA
141120 Engages in recommended exercise routine	1	2	3	4	5	NA
141121 Identifies an accurate perception of body image	1	2	3	4	5	NA
141122 Expresses satisfaction with body image	1	2	3	4	5	NA
141123 Expresses positive esteem	1	2	3	4	5	NA
141124 Expresses satisfaction with personal self-control	1	2	3	4	5	NA
141125 Identifies supportive family relationships	1	2	3	4	5	NA
141126 Uses medication as prescribed	1	2	3	4	5	NA
141127 Expresses determination to recover from eating disorder	1	2	3	4	5	NA

Eating Disorder Self-Control—cont'd

		Consistently Demonstrated	Often Demonstrated	Sometimes Demonstrated	Rarely Demonstrated	Never Demonstrated	
141128	Nutritional deficits	1	2	3	4	5	NA
141129	Preoccupation with food	1	2	3	4	5	NA
141130	Preoccupation with weight	1	2	3	4	5	NA
141131	Purging	1	2	3	4	5	NA
141132	Bingeing	1	2	3	4	5	NA
141133	Overuse of diuretics	1	2	3	4	5	NA
141134	Overuse of laxatives	1	2	3	4	5	NA
141135	Depression	1	2	3	4	5	NA
141136	Substance abuse	1	2	3	4	5	NA
141137	Suicidal thoughts	1	2	3	4	5	NA
141138	Irregular menstrual cycles	1	2	3	4	5	NA
141139	Excessive exercise	1	2	3	4	5	NA

Domain-*Psychosocial Health (III)*　　**Class**-*Self-Control (O)*　　*5th edition 2013*

OUTCOME CONTENT REFERENCES:

Berkman, N. D., Bulik, C. M., Brownley, K. A., Lohr, K. N., Sedway, J. A., Rooks, A., & Gartlehner, G. (2006). Management of eating disorders. Evidence report/technology assessment No. 135. (Prepared by the RTI International-University of North Carolina Evidence-Based Practice Center under Contract No. 290-02-0016.) Publication No. 06-E010. *Agency for Healthcare Research and Quality.*

Berkman, N., Lohr, K., & Bulik, C. (2007). Outcomes of eating disorder: A systematic review of the literature. *International Journal of Eating Disorders, 40*(4), 293–309. https://doi.org/10.1002/eat.20369

Fichter, M., Quadflieg, N., & Hedlund, S. (2006). Twelve-year course and outcome predictors of anorexia nervosa. *International Journal of Eating Disorders, 39*(2), 87–100. https://doi.org/10.1002/eat.20215

Kong, S. (2005). Day treatment programme for patients with eating disorders: Randomized controlled trial. *Journal of Advanced Nursing, 51*(1), 5–14. https://doi.org/10.1111/j.1365-2648.2005.03454.x

Patching, J., & Lawler, J. (2009). Understanding women's experiences of developing an eating disorder and recovering: A life-history approach. *Nursing Inquiry, 16*(1), 10–21. https://doi.org/10.1111/j.1440-1800.2009.00436.x

Sadock, B. J., & Sadock V. A. (2007). *Kaplan & Sadock's synopsis of psychiatry: Behavioral sciences/clinical psychiatry* (10th ed.). Lippincott, Williams, & Wilkins.

Stuart, G. W. (2009). *Principles and practice of psychiatric nursing* (9th ed.). Mosby Elsevier.

Electrolyte & Acid/Base Balance　　　　　**0600**

Definition: Balance of electrolytes and non-electrolytes in the intracellular and extracellular compartments of the body

OUTCOME TARGET RATING: Maintain at_____ Increase to_____

		Severe Deviation from Normal Range	Substantial Deviation from Normal Range	Moderate Deviation from Normal Range	Mild Deviation from Normal Range	No Deviation from Normal Range	
OUTCOME OVERALL RATING		1	2	3	4	5	
Indicators:							
060001	Apical heart rate	1	2	3	4	5	NA
060002	Apical heart rhythm	1	2	3	4	5	NA
060003	Respiratory rate	1	2	3	4	5	NA
060004	Respiratory rhythm	1	2	3	4	5	NA
060005	Serum sodium	1	2	3	4	5	NA
060006	Serum potassium	1	2	3	4	5	NA
060007	Serum chloride	1	2	3	4	5	NA
060008	Serum calcium	1	2	3	4	5	NA
060009	Serum magnesium	1	2	3	4	5	NA
060010	Serum pH	1	2	3	4	5	NA
060011	Serum albumin	1	2	3	4	5	NA

Continued

Electrolyte & Acid/Base Balance—cont'd

		Severe Deviation from Normal Range	Substantial Deviation from Normal Range	Moderate Deviation from Normal Range	Mild Deviation from Normal Range	No Deviation from Normal Range	
060012	Serum creatinine	1	2	3	4	5	NA
060013	Serum bicarbonate	1	2	3	4	5	NA
060024	Serum carbon dioxide	1	2	3	4	5	NA
060025	Serum phosphorus	1	2	3	4	5	NA
060026	Serum glucose	1	2	3	4	5	NA
060027	Serum hematocrit	1	2	3	4	5	NA
060014	Blood urea nitrogen	1	2	3	4	5	NA
060028	Blood urea nitrogen to creatinine ratio	1	2	3	4	5	NA
060015	Urine pH	1	2	3	4	5	NA
060029	Urine sodium	1	2	3	4	5	NA
060030	Urine chloride	1	2	3	4	5	NA
060031	Urine creatinine	1	2	3	4	5	NA
060032	Urine osmolarity	1	2	3	4	5	NA
060022	Urine specific gravity	1	2	3	4	5	NA

		Severe	Substantial	Moderate	Mild	None	
060033	Impaired cognition	1	2	3	4	5	NA
060034	Fatigue	1	2	3	4	5	NA
060035	Muscle weakness	1	2	3	4	5	NA
060036	Muscle cramps	1	2	3	4	5	NA
060037	Abdominal cramps	1	2	3	4	5	NA
060038	Nausea	1	2	3	4	5	NA
060039	Dysrhythmia	1	2	3	4	5	NA
060040	Restlessness	1	2	3	4	5	NA
060041	Paresthesia	1	2	3	4	5	NA

Domain-Physiologic Health (II) **Class**-Fluid & Electrolytes (G) 1st edition 1997; revised 2004, 2008, 2024

OUTCOME CONTENT REFERENCES:
Huether, S. E., McCance, K. L., & Brashers, V. L. (2020). *Understanding pathophysiology* (7th ed.). Elsevier.
Reddi, A. S. (2018). *Fluid, electrolyte and acid-base disorders clinical evaluation and management* (2nd ed.). Springer. https://doi.org/10.1007/978-3-319-60167-0
Seifter, J. L. (2019). Body fluid compartments, cell membrane ion transport, electrolyte concentrations, and acid-base balance. *Seminars in Nephrology, 39*(4), 368–379. https://doi.org/10.1016/j.semnephrol.2019.04.006

Electrolyte Balance

0606

Definition: Concentration of serum ions necessary to maintain equilibrium among electrolytes

OUTCOME TARGET RATING: Maintain at_____ Increase to_____

		Severe Deviation from Normal Range	Substantial Deviation from Normal Range	Moderate Deviation from Normal Range	Mild Deviation from Normal Range	No Deviation from Normal Range	
OUTCOME OVERALL RATING		1	2	3	4	5	
Indicators:							
060601	Decreased serum sodium	1	2	3	4	5	NA
060602	Increased serum sodium	1	2	3	4	5	NA
060603	Decreased serum potassium	1	2	3	4	5	NA

Electrolyte Balance—cont'd

		Severe Deviation from Normal Range	Substantial Deviation from Normal Range	Moderate Deviation from Normal Range	Mild Deviation from Normal Range	No Deviation from Normal Range	
060604	Increased serum potassium	1	2	3	4	5	NA
060605	Decreased serum chloride	1	2	3	4	5	NA
060606	Increased serum chloride	1	2	3	4	5	NA
060607	Decreased serum calcium	1	2	3	4	5	NA
060608	Increased serum calcium	1	2	3	4	5	NA
060609	Decreased serum magnesium	1	2	3	4	5	NA
060610	Increased serum magnesium	1	2	3	4	5	NA
060611	Decreased serum phosphorus	1	2	3	4	5	NA
060612	Increased serum phosphorus	1	2	3	4	5	NA

Domain-*Physiologic Health (II)*   **Class**-*Fluid & Electrolytes (G)*   *5th edition 2013; reviewed 2024*

OUTCOME CONTENT REFERENCES:

Bauldoff, G., Gubrud, P., & Carno, M. (2019). *Medical-surgical nursing: Critical thinking in patient care* (7th ed.). Pearson.
Hinkle, J. L., & Cheever, K. H. (2018). *Brunner & Suddarth's textbook of medical-surgical nursing* (14th ed.). Wolter Kluwer.
Hockenberry, M. J., Wilson, D., & Rodgers, C. C. (Eds.). (2019). *Wong's nursing care of infants and children* (11th ed.). Elsevier.
Huether, S. E., McCance, K. L., & Brashers, V. L. (2020). *Understanding pathophysiology* (7th ed.). Elsevier.
Ignatavicius, D. D., Workman, M. L., Rebar, C. R., & Heimgartner, N. M. (2021). *Medical-surgical nursing: Concepts for interprofessional care* (10th ed.). Elsevier.
Kear, T. M. (2017). Fluid and electrolyte management across the age continuum. *Nephrology Nursing Journal, 44*(6), 491–497.
Potter, P. A., & Perry, A. G. (2021). *Fundamentals of nursing* (10th ed.). Elsevier.
Reddi, A. S. (2018). *Fluid, electrolyte, and acid-base disorders: Clinical evaluation and management* (2nd ed.). Springer.

Elopement Occurrence   1919

Definition: Number of times an individual with a cognitive impairment leaves a secure area

OUTCOME TARGET RATING: Maintain at_____ Increase to_____

		10 and over	7–9	4–6	1–3	None	
OUTCOME OVERALL RATING		1	2	3	4	5	

Indicators:

191901	Leaves place of residence unattended	1	2	3	4	5	NA
191902	Leaves secure area unattended	1	2	3	4	5	NA
191903	Opens exterior door	1	2	3	4	5	NA
191904	Slips away from group activities	1	2	3	4	5	NA
191905	Leaves with visitors	1	2	3	4	5	NA
191906	Leaves with others	1	2	3	4	5	NA
191907	Climbs out window	1	2	3	4	5	NA
191908	Infringes on others' space	1	2	3	4	5	NA

Specify period of time 24 hours /1 week /1 month

Domain-*Health Knowledge & Behavior (IV)*   **Class**-*Safety (HH)*   *4th edition 2008; revised 2024*

OUTCOME CONTENT REFERENCES:

Aud, M. A. (2004). Dangerous wandering: Elopements of older adults with dementia from long-term care facilities. *American Journal of Alzheimer's Disorders and Other Dementias, 19*(6), 361–368. https://doi.org/10.1177/153331750401900602
MacAndrew, M., Beattie, E., O'Reilly, M., Kolanowski, A., & Windsor, C. (2017). The trajectory of tolerance for wandering-related boundary transgression: An exploration of care staff and family perceptions. *The Gerontologist, 57*(3), 451–460. https://doi.org/10.1093/geront/gnv136
MacAndrew, M., Brooks, D., & Beattie, E. (2017). Nonpharmacological interventions for managing wandering in the community: A narrative review of the evidence base. *Health and Social Care, 27*(2), 306–319. https://doi.org/10.1111/hsc.12590

Elopement Propensity Risk — 1920

Definition: The propensity of an individual with cognitive impairment to escape a secure area

OUTCOME TARGET RATING: Maintain at_____ Increase to_____

OUTCOME OVERALL RATING	Consistently Demonstrated 1	Often Demonstrated 2	Sometimes Demonstrated 3	Rarely Demonstrated 4	Never Demonstrated 5	
Indicators:						
192016 History of elopement	1	2	3	4	5	NA
192001 Wanders	1	2	3	4	5	NA
192017 Pacing	1	2	3	4	5	NA
192018 Lapping	1	2	3	4	5	NA
192019 Infringes on others' space	1	2	3	4	5	NA
192002 Appears agitated	1	2	3	4	5	NA
192020 Asks for directions	1	2	3	4	5	NA
192003 Refuses to remove coat	1	2	3	4	5	NA
192004 Packs bag to leave	1	2	3	4	5	NA
192005 Attempts to leave secure area	1	2	3	4	5	NA
192021 Tests doors and windows	1	2	3	4	5	NA
192006 Leaves secure area unobserved	1	2	3	4	5	NA
192007 Leaves yard when outside	1	2	3	4	5	NA
192008 Appears sad	1	2	3	4	5	NA
192010 Appears frightened	1	2	3	4	5	NA
192011 Asks others for assistance to leave	1	2	3	4	5	NA
192012 Attempts to leave with visitors	1	2	3	4	5	NA
192013 States wants to go home	1	2	3	4	5	NA
192022 States wants to go to work	1	2	3	4	5	NA
192014 Announces intent to leave	1	2	3	4	5	NA
192015 Tampers with alarm	1	2	3	4	5	NA

Domain-Health Knowledge & Behavior (IV) **Class-**Safety (HH) 4th edition 2008; revised 2024

OUTCOME CONTENT REFERENCES:

Aud, M. A. (2004). Dangerous wandering: Elopements of older adults with dementia from long-term care facilities. *American Journal of Alzheimer's Disorders and Other Dementias, 19*(6), 361–368. https://doi.org/10.1177/153331750401900602

Barrett, B., Bulat, T., Schultz, S. K., & Luther, S. (2018). Factors associated with wandering behaviors in veterans with mild dementia: A prospective longitudinal community-based study. *American Journal of Alzheimer's Disease & Other Dementias, 33*(2), 100–111. https://doi.org/10.1177/1533317517735168

MacAndrew, M., Beattie, E., O'Reilly, M., Kolanowski, A., & Windsor, C. (2017). The trajectory of tolerance for wandering-related boundary transgression: An exploration of care staff and family perceptions. *The Gerontologist, 57*(3), 451–460. https://doi.org/10.1093/geront/gnv136

MacAndrew, M., Brooks, D., & Beattie, E. (2017). Nonpharmacological interventions for managing wandering in the community: A narrative review of the evidence base. *Health and Social Care, 27*, 306–319. https://doi.org/10.1111/hsc.12590

Endurance — 0001

Definition: Capacity of muscles and cardiovascular system to sustain activity

OUTCOME TARGET RATING: Maintain at_____ Increase to_____

OUTCOME OVERALL RATING	Severely Compromised 1	Substantially Compromised 2	Moderately Compromised 3	Mildly Compromised 4	Not Compromised 5	
Indicators:						
000101 Performance of usual routine	1	2	3	4	5	NA
000102 Physical activity	1	2	3	4	5	NA
000106 Muscle endurance	1	2	3	4	5	NA

Endurance—cont'd

	Severely Compromised	Substantially Compromised	Moderately Compromised	Mildly Compromised	Not Compromised	
000619	Muscle strength	1	2	3	4	5	NA
000620	Muscle flexibility	1	2	3	4	5	NA
000108	Libido	1	2	3	4	5	NA
000109	Energy restored after rest	1	2	3	4	5	NA
000112	Blood oxygen level with activity	1	2	3	4	5	NA
000113	Hemoglobin	1	2	3	4	5	NA
000114	Hematocrit	1	2	3	4	5	NA
000115	Blood glucose	1	2	3	4	5	NA
000116	Serum electrolytes	1	2	3	4	5	NA

		Severe	Substantial	Moderate	Mild	None	
000621	Breathlessness	1	2	3	4	5	NA
0111	Lethargy	1	2	3	4	5	NA
000118	Physical fatigue	1	2	3	4	5	NA
000110	Exhaustion	1	2	3	4	5	NA
000622	Physical deconditioning	1	2	3	4	5	NA

Domain-Functional Health (I)   **Class**-Energy Maintenance (A)   1st edition 1997; revised 2004, 2008, 2013, 2024

OUTCOME CONTENT REFERENCES:

Dallaway, N., Lucas, S. J. E., & Ring, C. (2021). Concurrent brain endurance training improves endurance exercise performance. *Journal of Science and Medicine in Sport, 24*(4), 405–411. https://doi.org/10.1016/j.jsama.2020.10.008

Feter, N., Caputo, E. L., Koth, F. M., Delpino, F. M., Tomaz, G. D. S., Doring, I. R., Leite, J. S., Cassuriaga, J., Treptow, J. G., Weymar, M. K., Alt, R., Reichert, F. F., da Silva, M. C., & Rombaldi, A. J. (2021). Association between specific types of physical activity during the COVID-19 pandemic and the risk of subjective memory decline: Findings from the PAMPA Cohort. *Public Health, 200*, 49–55. https://doi.org/10.1016/j.puhw.2021.09.014

Loureiro, L. M. R., dos Santos Neto, E., Molina, G. E., Amato, A. A., Arruda, S. F., Reis, C. E. G., & da Costa, T. H. M. (2021). Coffee increases post-exercise muscle glycogen recovery in endurance athletes: A randomized clinical trial. *Nutrients, 13*(10), 1–13. https://doi.org/10.3390/nu13103335

McCarthy, D., Desbrow, B., & Irwin, C. (2021). Cognitive effects of acute aerobic exercise: Exploring the influence of exercise duration, exhaustion, task complexity and expectancies in endurance-trained individuals. *Journal of Sport Sciences, 39*(2), 183–191. https://doi.org/10.1080/02640414.2020.1809976

Maltais, F., de la Hoz, A., Casaburi, R., & O'Donnell, D. (2021). Effects of Tiotropium/Olodaterol on activity-related breathlessness, exercise endurance and physical activity in patients with COPD: Narrative review with meta-pooled analyses. *Advanced Therapy, 38*(2), 835–853. https://doi.org/10.1007/s12325-020-01557-x

Souabni, M., Hammouda, O., Romdhani, M., Trabelsi, K., Ammar, A., & Driss, T. (2021). Benefits of daytime napping opportunity on physical and cognitive performances in physically active participants: A systematic review. *Sports Medicine, 51*(10), 2215–2146. https://doi.org/10.1007/s40279-021-01482-1

Energy Conservation   0002

Definition: Personal actions to manage energy for initiating and sustaining activity

OUTCOME TARGET RATING: Maintain at_____ Increase to_____

		Never Demonstrated	Rarely Demonstrated	Sometimes Demonstrated	Often Demonstrated	Consistently Demonstrated	
OUTCOME OVERALL RATING		1	2	3	4	5	
Indicators:							
000210	Prioritizes activities for the day	1	2	3	4	5	NA
000209	Organizes activities to conserve energy	1	2	3	4	5	NA
000211	Delegates tasks	1	2	3	4	5	NA
000201	Balances activity and rest	1	2	3	4	5	NA
000202	Uses naps to restore energy	1	2	3	4	5	NA
000203	Recognizes energy limitations	1	2	3	4	5	NA
000204	Uses energy conservation techniques	1	2	3	4	5	NA

Continued

Energy Conservation—cont'd

		Never Demonstrated	Rarely Demonstrated	Sometimes Demonstrated	Often Demonstrated	Consistently Demonstrated	
000212	Uses proper body mechanics	1	2	3	4	5	NA
000205	Adapts lifestyle to energy level	1	2	3	4	5	NA
000206	Maintains adequate nutrition	1	2	3	4	5	NA
000207	Reports adequate endurance for activity	1	2	3	4	5	NA

Domain-*Functional Health (I)*   **Class**-*Energy Maintenance (A)*   *1st edition 1997; revised 2004, 2018*

OUTCOME CONTENT REFERENCES:

Blikman, L., Huisstede, B., Kooijmans, H., Stam, H., Bussmann, J., & van Meeteren, J. (2013). Effectiveness of energy conservation treatment in reducing fatigue in multiple sclerosis: A systematic review and meta-analysis. *Archives of Physical Medicine and Rehabilitation, 94*(7), 1360–1376. https://doi.org/10.1016/j.apmr.2013.01.025
Dreiling, D. (2009). Energy conservation. *Home Health Care Management & Practice, 22*(1), 26–33.
Larsen, P. D. (Ed.). (2016). *Lubkin's chronic illness: Impact and intervention* (9th ed.). Jones & Bartlett Learning.
+Lee, K. A., Hicks, G., & Nino-Murcia, G. (1991). Validity and reliability of a scale to assess fatigue. *Psychiatry Research, 36*(3), 291–298.
McCance, K. L., & Huether, S. E. (2014). *Pathophysiology: The biological basis for disease in adults and children* (7th ed.). Elsevier Mosby.
Potter, P. A., Perry, A. G., Stockert, P. A., & Hall, A. M. (2017). *Fundamentals of nursing* (9th ed.). Elsevier.

Exercise Participation

1633

Definition: Personal actions to perform a self-planned, structured, and repetitive regimen to maintain or advance the level of fitness and health

OUTCOME TARGET RATING: Maintain at_____ Increase to_____

		Never Demonstrated	Rarely Demonstrated	Sometimes Demonstrated	Often Demonstrated	Consistently Demonstrated	
OUTCOME OVERALL RATING		**1**	**2**	**3**	**4**	**5**	
Indicators:							
163301	Plans appropriate exercise with health provider before starting exercise	1	2	3	4	5	NA
163302	Identifies barriers to exercise program	1	2	3	4	5	NA
163303	Sets realistic short-term goals	1	2	3	4	5	NA
163304	Sets realistic long-term goals	1	2	3	4	5	NA
163305	Sets target heart rate based on health status	1	2	3	4	5	NA
163306	Achieves target heart rate during exercise	1	2	3	4	5	NA
163307	Balances life routine to include exercise	1	2	3	4	5	NA
163308	Participates in regular exercise	1	2	3	4	5	NA
163309	Performs exercise correctly	1	2	3	4	5	NA
163310	Wears appropriate clothing for exercise	1	2	3	4	5	NA
163311	Uses strategies to overcome exercise barriers	1	2	3	4	5	NA
163312	Performs exercise in safe environment	1	2	3	4	5	NA
163313	Uses strategies to prevent physical injury	1	2	3	4	5	NA
163314	Uses equipment correctly	1	2	3	4	5	NA
163315	Uses protective devices	1	2	3	4	5	NA
163316	Uses proper warm-up techniques	1	2	3	4	5	NA
163317	Uses proper cool-down techniques	1	2	3	4	5	NA
163318	Monitors heart rate	1	2	3	4	5	NA
163319	Monitors respiratory rate	1	2	3	4	5	NA
163320	Monitors progress	1	2	3	4	5	NA
163321	Engages in moderate-intensity aerobic exercise to increase endurance	1	2	3	4	5	NA

E

Exercise Participation—cont'd

		Never Demonstrated	Rarely Demonstrated	Sometimes Demonstrated	Often Demonstrated	Consistently Demonstrated	
163322	Engages in exercises to increase strength	1	2	3	4	5	NA
163323	Engages in exercises to maintain flexibility	1	2	3	4	5	NA
163324	Engages in exercises to maintain balance	1	2	3	4	5	NA
163325	Plans for disruption in exercise program	1	2	3	4	5	NA
163326	Varies exercise	1	2	3	4	5	NA
163327	Adheres to exercise program	1	2	3	4	5	NA
163328	Optimizes opportunities to exercise	1	2	3	4	5	NA
163329	Uses strategies to make exercise interesting	1	2	3	4	5	NA
163330	Maintains fluid balance	1	2	3	4	5	NA
163331	Maintains caloric requirements based on exercise	1	2	3	4	5	NA
163332	Uses personal support system	1	2	3	4	5	NA
163333	Uses community resources	1	2	3	4	5	NA
163334	Contacts a health provider as needed	1	2	3	4	5	NA

Domain-Health Knowledge & Behavior (IV)   *Class*-Health Behavior (Q)   5th edition 2013

OUTCOME CONTENT REFERENCES:

Haskell, W., Lee, I-M., Pate, R., Powell, K., Blair, S., Franklin, B., Macera, C., Heath, G., Thompson, P., & Bauman, A. (2007). Physical activity and public health: Updated recommendation for adults from the American College of Sports Medicine and the American Heart Association. *Circulation, 116*(9), 1081–1093.

Jung, M. E., & Brawley, L. R. (2010). Concurrent management of exercise with other valued life goals: Comparison of frequent and less frequent exercisers. *Psychology of Sport and Exercise, 11*(5), 372–377.

National Institute on Aging. (2009). *Exercise & physical activity: Your everyday guide from the National Institute on Aging.*

Resnick, B., & D'Adamo, C. (2011). Factors associated with exercise among older adults in a continuing care retirement community. *Rehabilitation Nursing, 36*(2), 47–53, 82.

Shields, C. A., & Brawley, L. R. (2006). Preferring proxy-agency: Impact on self-efficacy for exercise. *Journal of Health Psychology, 11*(6), 904–914. https://doi.org/10.1177/1359105306069092

Fall Prevention Behavior 1909

Definition: Personal or family caregiver actions to minimize risk factors that might precipitate falls in the personal environment

OUTCOME TARGET RATING: Maintain at_____ Increase to_____

		Never Demonstrated	Rarely Demonstrated	Sometimes Demonstrated	Often Demonstrated	Consistently Demonstrated	
OUTCOME OVERALL RATING		1	2	3	4	5	
Indicators:							
190923	Asks for assistance	1	2	3	4	5	NA
190924	Conducts home assessment for risk	1	2	3	4	5	NA
190925	Modifies home hazards	1	2	3	4	5	NA
190903	Places barriers to prevent falls	1	2	3	4	5	NA
190905	Uses handrails as needed	1	2	3	4	5	NA
190915	Uses grab bars as needed	1	2	3	4	5	NA
190914	Uses non-skid mats in tub/shower	1	2	3	4	5	NA
190926	Wears loose clothing of correct size and length	1	2	3	4	5	NA
190910	Uses well-fitting shoes	1	2	3	4	5	NA
190901	Uses assistive devices correctly	1	2	3	4	5	NA
190918	Uses vision correcting devices	1	2	3	4	5	NA

Continued

Fall Prevention Behavior—cont'd

		Never Demonstrated	Rarely Demonstrated	Sometimes Demonstrated	Often Demonstrated	Consistently Demonstrated	
190927	Uses hearing aid correctly	1	2	3	4	5	NA
190928	Pays attention to surroundings	1	2	3	4	5	NA
190929	Pays attention to pavement evenness	1	2	3	4	5	NA
190930	Provides assistance with activities of daily living	1	2	3	4	5	NA
190902	Provides assistance with mobility	1	2	3	4	5	NA
190931	Assesses mobility level	1	2	3	4	5	NA
190932	Participates in exercise sessions	1	2	3	4	5	NA
190933	Participates in supervised therapy	1	2	3	4	5	NA
190919	Uses safe transfer procedure	1	2	3	4	5	NA
190935	Uses caution on stairs	1	2	3	4	5	NA
190922	Uses adequate lighting	1	2	3	4	5	NA
190936	Avoid using step stools and ladders	1	2	3	4	5	NA
190937	Eliminates clutter from floors	1	2	3	4	5	NA
190938	Clears spills from floors	1	2	3	4	5	NA
190907	Removes rugs	1	2	3	4	5	NA
190908	Arranges for removal of snow and ice from walking surfaces	1	2	3	4	5	NA
190911	Adjusts toilet seat height as needed	1	2	3	4	5	NA
190912	Adjusts chair height as needed	1	2	3	4	5	NA
190913	Adjusts bed height as needed	1	2	3	4	5	NA
190916	Controls restlessness	1	2	3	4	5	NA
190939	Reviews medication for side effects	1	2	3	4	5	NA
190917	Uses precautions when taking medication that increase risk for falls	1	2	3	4	5	NA
190940	Reviews disease condition with health professional on fall risk	1	2	3	4	5	NA

Domain-Health Knowledge & Behavior (IV)   **Class**-Safety (HH)   1st edition 1997; revised 2004, 2013, 2024

OUTCOME CONTENT REFERENCES:

Araújo, J. N. M., Fernandes, A. P. N. L., Silva, A. B., Moura, L. A., Ferreira, M. A. Jr., & Vitor, A. F. (2018). Clinical validation of Fall Prevention Behavior in a hospital environment. *Revista Brasileira de Enfermagem, 71*(4), 1841–1849. https://doi.org/10.1590/0034-7167-2017-0212

Araújo, J. N. M., Nunes de Lima Fernandes, A. P., Moura, L. A., Palhano dos Santos, M. M., Ferreira, M, A. Jr., & Fortes Vitor, A. (2017). Validation of nursing outcome content Fall Prevention Behavior in a hospital environment. *Revista da Rede de Enfermagem do Nordeste , 18*(3), 337–344. https://doi.org/10.15253/2175-6783.2017000300008

Bolding, D. J., & Corman, E. (2019). Falls in the geriatric patient. *Clinics Geriatric Medicine, 35*(1), 115–126 https://doi.org/10.1016/j.cger.2018.08.010

Chippendale, T. (2019). Predicting use of outdoor fall prevention strategies: Considerations for prevention practices. *Journal of Applied Gerontology, 38*(6), 775–790. https://doi.org/10.1177/0733464817751199

de Freitas Luzia, M., Duarte Vidor, I., Eilert da Silva, A. C. F., & de Fátima Lucena, A. (2020). Fall prevention in hospitalized patients: Evaluation through the nursing classification/ NOC. *Applied Nursing Research, 54*, 1–5. https://doi.org/10.1016/j.apnr.2020.151273

Flint, J., Morris, M., Nguyen, A. T., Keglovits, M., Somerville, E. K., Hu, Y.-L., & Stark, S. L. (2020). Fall prevention bingo: effects of a novel community-based education tool on older adults' knowledge and readiness to reduce risks for falls. *American Journal of Health Education, 51*(6), 406–412. https://doi.org/10.1080/19325037.2020.1822236

Hunter, S. W., Higa, J., Frengopoulos, C., Viana, R., & Payne, M. P. C. (2020). Evaluating knowledge of falls risk factors and falls prevention strategies among lower extremity amputees after inpatient prosthetic rehabilitation: A prospective study. *Disability and Rehabilitation, 42*(16), 2252–2261. https://doi.org/10.1080/09638288.2018.1555721

Iaboni, A., & Mulsant, B. H. (2020). Why do older adults taking antidepressants fall? *The American Journal of Geriatric Psychiatry, 28*(3), 285–287. https://doi.org/10.1016/j.jagp.2019.11.001

Naseri, C., McPhail, S. M., Haines, T. P., Morris, M. E., Shorr, R., Etherton-Beer, C., Netto, J., Flicker, L., Bulsara, M., Lee, D.-C. A., Francis-Coad, J., Waldron, N., Boudville, A., & Hill, A.-M. (2020). Perspectives of older adults regarding barriers and enables to engaging in fall prevention activities after hospital discharge. *Health and Social Care in the Community, 28*(5), 1710–1722. https://doi.org/10.1111/hsc.12996

Sherrington, C., Fairhall, N., Kwok, W., Wallbank, G., Tiedemann, A., Michaleff, Z. A., Ng, C. A. C. M., & Bauman, A. (2020). Evidence on physical activity and fall prevention for people aged 65+ years: Systematic review to inform the WHO guidelines on physical activity and sedentary behavior. *International Journal of Behavioral Nutrition and Physical Activity, 17*(1),144. https://doi.org/10.1186/s12966-020-01041-3

Yunchuan, Z., Alderden, J., Lind, B., & Stibrany, J. (2019). Risk factors for falls in homebound community-dwelling older adults. *Public Health Nursing, 36*(6), 772–778. https://doi.org/10.1111/phn.12651

Falls Occurrence   1912

Definition: Number of times an individual falls

OUTCOME TARGET RATING: Maintain at_____ Increase to_____

		10 and over	7–9	4–6	1–3	None	
OUTCOME OVERALL RATING		1	2	3	4	5	
Indicators:							
191201	Falls while standing still	1	2	3	4	5	NA
191202	Falls while walking	1	2	3	4	5	NA
191211	Falls while using assistive devices	1	2	3	4	5	NA
191212	Falls while on hard surfaces	1	2	3	4	5	NA
191213	Falls while on uneven surfaces	1	2	3	4	5	NA
191203	Falls while sitting	1	2	3	4	5	NA
191204	Falls from bed	1	2	3	4	5	NA
191214	Falls from heights	1	2	3	4	5	NA
191205	Falls while transferring	1	2	3	4	5	NA
191206	Falls climbing steps	1	2	3	4	5	NA
191207	Falls descending steps	1	2	3	4	5	NA
191215	Falls going to toilet	1	2	3	4	5	NA
191210	Falls while bending over	1	2	3	4	5	NA

Specify period of time 24 hours/1 week/1 month

Domain-*Health Knowledge & Behavior (IV)*   **Class**-*Safety (HH)*   1st edition 1997; revised 2004, 2008, 2024

OUTCOME CONTENT REFERENCES:
Cruz, A. O., Santana, S. M. M., Costa, C. M., Gomes da Costa, L. A., & Ferraz, D. D. (2020). Prevalence of falls in frail elderly users of ambulatory assistive devices: A comparative study. *Disability and Rehabilitation: Assistive Technology, 15*(5), 510–514. https://doi.org/10.1080/17483107.2019.1587016
Kim, M., Chang, M., Nam, E., Kim, S. G., Cho, S., Ryu, D. H., Kam, S., Choi, Y. B., Kim, M. J., & Kun, X. (2020). Fall characteristics among elderly populations in urban and rural areas in Korea. *Medicine, 99*(46), pe 23106. https://doi.org/10.1097/MD.0000000000023106
Soto-Varela, A., Gayoso-Diz, P., Faraldo-García, A., Rossi-Izquierdo, M., Vaamonde-Sánchez-Andrade, I., del-Río-Valeiras, M., Lirola-Delgado, A., & Santos-Pérez, S. (2019). Optimizing costs in reducing rate of falls in older people with the improvement of balance by means of vestibular rehabilitation (ReFOVeRe study): A randomized controlled trial comparing computerized dynamic posturography vs mobile vibrotactile posturography system. *BMC Geriatrics, 19*(1), 1–8. https://doi.org/10.1186/s12877-018-1019-5S
Yokota, M., Fujita, T., Nakahara, S., & Sakamoto, T. (2020). Clarifying differences in injury patterns between ground-level falls and falls from heights among elderly in Japan. *Public Health, 181*, 114–118. https://doi.org/10.1016/j.puhe.2019.11.020
Yoo, J. S., Kim, C. G., Yim, J. E., & Jeon, M. Y. (2016). Factors influencing falls in the frail elderly individuals in urban and rural areas. *Aging Clinical and Experimental Research, 28*(4), 687–697. https://doi.org/10.1007/s40520-015-0469-2

Family Coping   2600

Definition: Capacity of the family to manage stressors that tax family resources

OUTCOME TARGET RATING: Maintain at_____ Increase to_____

		Never Demonstrated	Rarely Demonstrated	Sometimes Demonstrated	Often Demonstrated	Consistently Demonstrated	
OUTCOME OVERALL RATING		1	2	3	4	5	
Indicators:							
260020	Establishes role flexibility	1	2	3	4	5	NA
260002	Enables member role flexibility	1	2	3	4	5	NA
260003	Confronts family problems	1	2	3	4	5	NA
260005	Manages family problems	1	2	3	4	5	NA

Continued

Family Coping—cont'd

		Never Demonstrated	Rarely Demonstrated	Sometimes Demonstrated	Often Demonstrated	Consistently Demonstrated	
260006	Involves family members in decision-making	1	2	3	4	5	NA
260007	Expresses feelings and emotions openly among members	1	2	3	4	5	NA
260021	Uses strategies to manage family conflict	1	2	3	4	5	NA
260009	Uses family-centered stress reduction strategies	1	2	3	4	5	NA
260010	Cares for needs of all family members	1	2	3	4	5	NA
260011	Establishes family priorities	1	2	3	4	5	NA
260012	Establishes schedule for family routines and activities	1	2	3	4	5	NA
260019	Shares responsibility for family tasks	1	2	3	4	5	NA
260013	Arranges for respite care	1	2	3	4	5	NA
260014	Plans for emergencies	1	2	3	4	5	NA
260015	Maintains financial stability	1	2	3	4	5	NA
260022	Reports need for family assistance	1	2	3	4	5	NA
260023	Obtains family assistance	1	2	3	4	5	NA
260024	Uses available family support system	1	2	3	4	5	NA
260026	Uses available support from friends	1	2	3	4	5	NA
260025	Uses available community resources	1	2	3	4	5	NA
260027	Uses available spiritual support	1	2	3	4	5	NA

Domain-Family Health (VI)   **Class**-Family Well-Being (X)   *2nd edition 2000; revised 2004, 2008, 2013, 2024*

OUTCOME CONTENT REFERENCES:

Anderson, L. M., Smith, K. E., Nuñez, M. C., & Farrell, N. R. (2021). Family accommodation in eating disorders: A preliminary examination of correlates with familial burden and cognitive-behavioral treatment outcome. *Eating Disorders, 29*(4), 327–343. https://doi.org/10.1080/10640266.2019.1652473

Laghi, F., Bianchi, D., Pompili, S., Lonigro, A., & Baiocco, B. (2021). Binge eating and binge drinking behaviors: the role of family functioning. *Psychology, Health & Medicine, 26*(4), 408–420. https://doi.org/10.1080/13548506.2020.1742926

Li, Y., Ying, J., Zhang, X., Li, H., Ma, D., Zhao, Y., & Sun, J. (2021). Coping strategies mediate the association between family functioning and posttraumatic growth in family caregivers of people with dementia. *Aging & Mental Health, 25*(9), 1684–1691. https://doi.org/10.1080/13607863.2020.1786800

Liu, Y., & Merritt, D. H. (2021). Family routines and child problem behaviors in fragile families: The role of social demographic and contextual factors. *Children and Youth Services Review, 129*, 1–12. https://doi.org/10.1016/j.childyouth.2021.106187

Mussatto, K. A., Van Rompay, M. I., Trachtenberg, F. L., Pemberton, V., Young-Borkowski, L., Uzark, K., Hollenbeck-Pringle, D., Dunbar-Masterson, C., Infinger, P., Walter, P., & Sawin, K. (2021). Family function, quality of life, and well-being in parents of infants with hypoplastic left heart syndrome. *Journal of Family Nursing, 27*(3), 222–234. https://doi.org/10.1177/1074840720987309

Nadrowska, N., Blazek, M., & Lewandowska-Walter, A. (2021). Polish adaptation of the family resilience assessment scale (FRAS). *Community Mental Health Journal, 57*(1), 153–160. https://doi.org/10.1007/s10597-020-00626-3

Neugebauer, C., & Mastergeorge, A. M. (2021). The family stress model in the context of pediatric cancer: A systematic review. *Journal of Child and Family Studies, 30*(5), 1099–1122. https://doi.org/10.1007/s10826-021-01928-0

Smith, S. L., & McQuade, H. B. (2021). Exploring the health of families with a child with autism. *Autism, 25*(5), 1203–1215. https://doi.org/10.1177/1362361320986354

Tulagan, N., & Eccles, J. S. (2021). African American mothers' socialization strategies to address adolescent-related academic expectations and risk concerns. *Journal of Child and Family Studies, 30*, 855–869. https://doi.org/10.1007/s10826-021-01922-6

Van Riper, M., Knafl, G. J., Barbieri-Figueiredo, M. D. C., Caples, M., Choi, H., de Graaf, G., Duarte, E. D., Honda, J., Marta, E., Phetrasuwan, S., Alfieri, S., Amdelo, M., Deoisres, W., Fleming, L., dos Santos, A. S., Rocha da Silva, M. J., Skelton, B., van der Veek, S., & Knafl, K. A. Measurement of family management in families of individuals with down syndrome: A cross-cultural investigation. *Journal of Family Nursing, 27*(1), 8–22. https://doi.org/10.1177/107484072975167

Family Functioning 2602

Definition: Capacity of a family to evolve and meet the needs of its members

OUTCOME TARGET RATING: Maintain at_____ Increase to_____

		Never Demonstrated	Rarely Demonstrated	Sometimes Demonstrated	Often Demonstrated	Consistently Demonstrated	
OUTCOME OVERALL RATING		1	2	3	4	5	
Indicators:							
260224	Accepts new members through marriage	1	2	3	4	5	NA
260225	Accepts new members through birth or adoption	1	2	3	4	5	NA
260201	Socializes new family members	1	2	3	4	5	NA
260226	Members communicate effectively with other members	1	2	3	4	5	NA
260227	Members promote self-management disease strategies	1	2	3	4	5	NA
260228	Provides care for dependent adult members	1	2	3	4	5	NA
260229	Provides care for children	1	2	3	4	5	NA
260203	Regulates behavior of members	1	2	3	4	5	NA
260204	Allocates responsibilities among members	1	2	3	4	5	NA
260206	Maintains stable core of traditions	1	2	3	4	5	NA
260208	Adapts to developmental transitions	1	2	3	4	5	NA
260209	Adapts to unexpected crises	1	2	3	4	5	NA
260230	Adapts to changes in health status of members	1	2	3	4	5	NA
260210	Obtains adequate resources to meet needs of members	1	2	3	4	5	NA
260211	Creates environment where members can openly express feelings	1	2	3	4	5	NA
260231	Creates environment for learning	1	2	3	4	5	NA
260212	Accepts diversity among members	1	2	3	4	5	NA
260232	Teaches respect for others	1	2	3	4	5	NA
260233	Develops sense of trust among members	1	2	3	4	5	NA
260234	Develops sense of shared responsibility	1	2	3	4	5	NA
260213	Involves members in problem-solving	1	2	3	4	5	NA
260214	Involves members in conflict resolution	1	2	3	4	5	NA
260235	Teaches sense of right and wrong	1	2	3	4	5	NA
260236	Balances interactions between members	1	2	3	4	5	NA
260221	Members receptive to new ideas	1	2	3	4	5	NA
260205	Members perform expected roles	1	2	3	4	5	NA
260237	Members accept new roles	1	2	3	4	5	NA
260222	Members support one another	1	2	3	4	5	NA
260223	Members assist one another	1	2	3	4	5	NA
260216	Members spend time with one another	1	2	3	4	5	NA
260217	Members express commitment to family	1	2	3	4	5	NA
260238	Members express positivity	1	2	3	4	5	NA
260239	Members share common religious core values	1	2	3	4	5	NA
260218	Members express loyalty to family	1	2	3	4	5	NA
260240	Members express appreciation to other members	1	2	3	4	5	NA
260241	Members value service to others	1	2	3	4	5	NA
260219	Members participate in community activities	1	2	3	4	5	NA

Domain-Family Health (VI)   *Class*-Family Well-Being (X)   *2nd edition 2000; revised 2004, 2008, 2013, 2024*

OUTCOME CONTENT REFERENCES:

Friedmann, M. L. (1991). An instrument to evaluate effectiveness in family functioning. *Western Journal of Nursing Research, 13*(2), 220–241.

Kaakinen, J. R., Coehlo, D. P., Robinson, M., & Daves, F. A. (2018). *Family health care nursing: Theory, practice, and research* (6th ed.). F. A. Davis.

Knafl, K. A., Deatrick, J. A., Gallo, A. M., & Skelton, B. (2021). Tracing the use of the Family Management Framework and Measure: A scoping review. *Journal of Family Nursing, 27*(2), 87–106. https://doi.org/10.1177/1074840721994331

Leeman, J., Crandell, J. L., Lee, A., Bai, J., Sandelowski, M., & Knafl, K. (2016). Family functioning and the well-being of children with chronic conditions: A meta-analysis. *Research in Nursing & Health, 39*(4), 229–243. https://doi.org/10.1002/nur.21725

Oltean, I. I., Perlman, C., Meyer, S., & Ferro, M. A. (2020). Child mental illness and mental health service use: Role of family functioning. *Journal of Child & Family Studies, 29*(9), 2602–2613. https://doi.org/10.1007/s10826-020-01784-4

Shamali, M., Konradsen, H., Svavarsdottir, E. K., Shahriari, M., Ketilsdottir, A., & Østergaard, B. (2021). Factors associated with family functioning in patients with heart failure and their family members: An international cross-sectional study. *Journal of Advanced Nursing, 77*(7), 3034–3045. https://doi.org/10.1111/jan.14810

Tulagan, N., & Eccles, J. S. (2021). African American mothers' socialization strategies to address adolescent-related academic expectations and risk concerns. *Journal of Child and Family Studies, 30*(2135), 855–869. https://doi.org/10.1007/s10826-021-01922-6

Van Schoors, M., Caes, L., Knoble, N. B., Goubert, L., Verhofstadt, L. L., & Alderfer, M. A. (2017). Systematic review: Associations between family functioning and child adjustment after pediatric cancer diagnosis: A meta-analysis. *Journal of Pediatric Psychology, 42*(1), 6–18. https://doi.org/10.1093/jpepsy/jsw070

Zhang, Y. (2018). Family functioning in the context of an adult family member with illness: A concept analysis. *Journal of Clinical Nursing, 27*(15-16), 3205–3224. https://doi.org/10.1111/jocn.14500

Family Health Status

2606

Definition: Overall health and social competence of a family

OUTCOME TARGET RATING: Maintain at_____ Increase to_____

		Severely Compromised	Substantially Compromised	Moderately Compromised	Mildly Compromised	Not Compromised	
OUTCOME OVERALL RATING		1	2	3	4	5	
Indicators:							
260605	Physical health of members	1	2	3	4	5	NA
260606	Physical activity of members	1	2	3	4	5	NA
260618	Mental health of members	1	2	3	4	5	NA
260601	Immunization of members	1	2	3	4	5	NA
260628	Screening for infections of members	1	2	3	4	5	NA
260612	Physical development of members	1	2	3	4	5	NA
260613	Psychosocial development of members	1	2	3	4	5	NA
260617	Adjustment to disabilities	1	2	3	4	5	NA
260602	Appropriate childcare provisions	1	2	3	4	5	NA
260603	Appropriate dependent adult care provisions	1	2	3	4	5	NA
260604	Access to health care	1	2	3	4	5	NA
260632	Access to dental care	1	2	3	4	5	NA
260633	Access to mental health services	1	2	3	4	5	NA
260629	Age-appropriate health screening of members	1	2	3	4	5	NA
260607	School attendance of members	1	2	3	4	5	NA
260608	School achievement of members	1	2	3	4	5	NA
260609	Parental employment	1	2	3	4	5	NA
260610	Appropriate housing	1	2	3	4	5	NA
260634	Residential stability	1	2	3	4	5	NA
260611	Nutritious food supply	1	2	3	4	5	NA
260630	Financial resources	1	2	3	4	5	NA
260615	Appropriate health care resources	1	2	3	4	5	NA
260616	Appropriate social services resources	1	2	3	4	5	NA
		Severe	**Substantial**	**Moderate**	**Mild**	**None**	
260620	Domestic violence	1	2	3	4	5	NA
260635	Sibling conflict	1	2	3	4	5	NA
260621	Physical abuse of members	1	2	3	4	5	NA
260624	Psychological abuse of members	1	2	3	4	5	NA

Family Health Status—cont'd

		Severe	Substantial	Moderate	Mild	None	
260636	Patterns of overeating	1	2	3	4	5	NA
260625	Alcohol abuse	1	2	3	4	5	NA
260626	Tobacco use	1	2	3	4	5	NA
260627	Recreational drug use	1	2	3	4	5	NA
260631	Gambling addiction	1	2	3	4	5	NA
260637	Stress	1	2	3	4	5	NA

Domain-Family Health (VI)   *Class*-Family Well-Being (X)   2nd edition 2000; revised 2004, 2008, 2013, 2024

OUTCOME CONTENT REFERENCES:

Geerts-Perry, A. T., Riggs, S. A., Kaminski, P. L., & Murrell, A. (2021). Psychological well-being and family functioning in middle childhood: The unique role of sibling relational dynamics. *Journal of Family Issues, 42*(12), 2965–2985. https://doi.org/10.1177/0192513X21993191

Kava, C. M., Thompson, L. E., Vo, T., Shockley, D., Sabourin, J., & Afifi, R. A. (2021). "I like to try my hardest to keep my small family together": Housing as a key resource for academic success of pregnant and parenting college-aged students. *Health Promotion Practice, 22*(4), 469–474. https://doi.org/10.1177/1524839920981957

Laghi, F., Bianchi, D., Pompili, S., Lonigro, A., & Baiocco, B. (2021). Binge eating and binge drinking behaviors: the role of family functioning. *Psychology, Health & Medicine, 26*(4), 408–420. https://doi.org/10.1080/13548506.2020.1742926

Li, Y., Ying, J., Zhang, X., Li, H., Ma, D., Zhao, Y., & Sun, J. (2021). Coping strategies mediate the association between family functioning and posttraumatic growth in family caregivers of people with dementia. *Aging & Mental Health, 25*(9), 1684–1691. https://doi.org/10.1080/13607863.2020.1786800

Liu, Y., & Merritt, D. H. (2021). Family routines and child problem behaviors in fragile families: The role of social demographic and contextual factors. *Children and Youth Services Review, 129*, 1–12. https://doi.org/10.1016/j.childyouth.2021.106187

Meland, E., Breidablik, H. J., & Thuen, F. (2021). Family factors predicting self-rated health during early adolescence. *Scandinavian Journal of Public Health, 49*(5), 546–554. https://doi.org/10.1177/1403494820972282

Sievert, E. D. C., Schweizer, K., Barkmann, C., Fahrenkrug, S., & Becker-Hebly, I. (2021). Not social transition status, but peer relations and family functioning predict psychological functioning in a German clinical sample of children with gender dysphoria. *Clinical Child Psychology and Psychiatry, 26*(1), 79–95. https://doi.org/10.1177/1359104520964530

Smith, S. L., & McQuade, H. B. (2021). Exploring the health of families with a child with autism. *Autism, 25*(5), 1203–1215. https://doi.org/10.1177/1362361320986354

Tulagan, N., & Eccles, J. S. (2021). African American mothers' socialization strategies to address adolescent-related academic expectations and risk concerns. *Journal of Child and Family Studies, 30*(2135), 855–869. https://doi.org/10.1007/s10826-021-01922-6

F

Family Integrity   **2603**

Definition: Capacity of family members to maintain cohesion and emotional bonding

OUTCOME TARGET RATING: Maintain at_____ Increase to_____

		Never Demonstrated	Rarely Demonstrated	Sometimes Demonstrated	Often Demonstrated	Consistently Demonstrated	
OUTCOME OVERALL RATING		1	2	3	4	5	
Indicators:							
260317	Uses strategies to maintain communication	1	2	3	4	5	NA
260308	Involves members in conflict resolution	1	2	3	4	5	NA
260309	Involves members in problem-solving	1	2	3	4	5	NA
260310	Encourages individual autonomy and independence	1	2	3	4	5	NA
260318	Eats meals together	1	2	3	4	5	NA
260312	Participates in leisure-time activities together	1	2	3	4	5	NA
260313	Participates in family rituals	1	2	3	4	5	NA
260314	Participates in family traditions	1	2	3	4	5	NA
260315	Members provide support during times of crisis	1	2	3	4	5	NA

Continued

Family Integrity—cont'd

		Never Demonstrated	Rarely Demonstrated	Sometimes Demonstrated	Often Demonstrated	Consistently Demonstrated	
260301	Members express loyalty	1	2	3	4	5	NA
260302	Members express strong ties to family	1	2	3	4	5	NA
260319	Members express support of stepchildren	1	2	3	4	5	NA
260320	Siblings express warmth to one another	1	2	3	4	5	NA
260303	Members express affection to one another	1	2	3	4	5	NA
260306	Members share thoughts, feelings, interests, concerns	1	2	3	4	5	NA
260321	Members express positive emotions	1	2	3	4	5	NA
260307	Members communicate openly and honestly with one another	1	2	3	4	5	NA
260305	Interacts frequently with extended family	1	2	3	4	5	NA
260304	Members assist one another in performing roles and daily tasks	1	2	3	4	5	NA
260322	Members plan for future	1	2	3	4	5	NA

Domain-Family Health (VI)   **Class**-Family Well-Being (X)   2nd edition 2000; revised 2004, 2013, 2024

OUTCOME CONTENT REFERENCES:

Chua, R. Y., Kadirvelu, A., Yasin, S., & Park, M. S. A. (2021). An exploratory model of family resilience processes and functioning: A cultural perspective of the Semai indigenous communities in Perak, Malaysia. *Journal of Cross-Cultural Psychology, 52*(6), 567–582. https://doi.org/10.1177/00220221211028297

Dang, Q., Bai, R., Zhang, B., & Lin, Y. (2021). Family functioning and negative emotions in older adults: the mediating role of self-integrity and the moderating role of self-stereotyping. *Aging & Mental Health, 25*(11), 2124–2131. https://doi.org/10.1080/1307863.2020.1799940

Geerts-Perry, A. T., Riggs, S. A., Kaminski, P. L., & Murrell, A. (2021). Psychological well-being and family functioning in middle childhood: The unique role of sibling relational dynamics. *Journal of Family Issues, 42*(12), 2965–2985. https://doi.org/10.1177/0192513X21993191

Jarana-Díaz, T., Romero-Martín, M., Ponce-Blandón, J. A., & Jiménez-Picón, N. (2021). Integrative review of related factors and defining characteristics of lack of family integrity. *International Journal of Nursing Knowledge, 32*(1), 44–52. https://doi.org/10.1111/2047-3095.12289

Laghi, F., Bianchi, D., Pompili, S., Lonigro, A., & Baiocco, B. (2021). Binge eating and binge drinking behaviors: The role of family functioning. *Psychology, Health & Medicine, 26*(4), 408–420. https://doi.org/10.1080/13548506.2020.1742926

Meland, E., Breidablik, H. J., & Thuen, F. (2021). Family factors predicting self-rated health during early adolescence. *Scandinavian Journal of Public Health, 49*(5), 546–554. https://doi.org/10.1177/1403494820972282

Family Normalization

2604

Definition: Capacity of a family to develop strategies for optimal functioning when a member has a chronic illness or disability

OUTCOME TARGET RATING: Maintain at_____ Increase to_____

		Never Demonstrated	Rarely Demonstrated	Sometimes Demonstrated	Often Demonstrated	Consistently Demonstrated	
OUTCOME OVERALL RATING		**1**	**2**	**3**	**4**	**5**	
Indicators:							
260417	Acknowledges potential of impairment to alter family routines	1	2	3	4	5	NA
260403	Maintains usual family routines	1	2	3	4	5	NA
260405	Adapts family routines to accommodate needs of affected member	1	2	3	4	5	NA
260406	Meets physical needs of family members	1	2	3	4	5	NA
260421	Maintains parental alliance	1	2	3	4	5	NA

Family Normalization—cont'd

		Never Demonstrated	Rarely Demonstrated	Sometimes Demonstrated	Often Demonstrated	Consistently Demonstrated	
260407	Meets psychosocial needs of family members	1	2	3	4	5	NA
260408	Meets developmental needs of family members	1	2	3	4	5	NA
260418	Reports family life returned to precrisis state	1	2	3	4	5	NA
260419	Maintains activities and routines as appropriate	1	2	3	4	5	NA
260420	Maintains usual expectations for member	1	2	3	4	5	NA
260412	Provides activities appropriate to age and ability for affected member	1	2	3	4	5	NA
260413	Structures activities to avoid embarrassment of affected member	1	2	3	4	5	NA
260414	Structures environment to avoid embarrassment of affected member	1	2	3	4	5	NA
260422	Uses available respite care	1	2	3	4	5	NA
260415	Uses community support groups	1	2	3	4	5	NA

Domain-*Family Health (VI)*   **Class**-*Family Well-Being (X)*   *2nd edition 2000; revised 2004, 2008, 2013, 2024*

OUTCOME CONTENT REFERENCES:

Anderson, L. M., Smith, K. E., Nuñez, M. C., & Farrell, N. R. (2021). Family accommodation in eating disorders: A preliminary examination of correlates with familial burden and cognitive-behavioral treatment outcome. *Eating Disorders, 29*(4), 327–343. https://doi.org/10.1080/10640266.2019.1652473

Baena, S., Jiménez, L., Lorence, B., & Hidalgo, M. V. (2021). Family functioning in families of adolescents with mental health disorders: The role of parenting alliance. *Children, 8*(3), 222–231. https://doi.org/10.3390/children8030222

Im, Y., & Kim, D. H. (2021). Family management style and psychosocial health of children with chronic conditions. *Journal of Child and Family Studies, 30*(1), 483–492. https://doi.org/10.1007/s10826-020-01870-7

Kelm, M. C., Fladeboe, K., Galtieri, L., Kawamura, J., King, K., Friedman, D., Compas, B., Breiger, D., Lengua, L., & Katz, L. F. (2021). Primary and secondary caregiver depressive symptoms and family functioning following a pediatric cancer diagnosis: An exploration of the buffering hypothesis. *Psycho-Oncology, 30*(6), 928–935. https://doi.org/10.1002/pon.5676

Stough, C. O., & Origlio, J. (2021). Family functioning in pediatric functional gastrointestinal disorders: A systematic review. *Journal of Pediatric Psychology, 46*(5), 485–500. https://doi.org/10.1093/jpepsy/jsab007

Family Normalization: Autism Spectrum Disorder   **2613**

Definition: Capacity of a family to develop strategies for optimal functioning when a member has autism spectrum disorder

OUTCOME TARGET RATING: Maintain at_____ Increase to_____

		Never Demonstrated	Rarely Demonstrated	Sometimes Demonstrated	Often Demonstrated	Consistently Demonstrated	
OUTCOME OVERALL RATING		1	2	3	4	5	
Indicators:							
261301	Accepts diagnosis of affected member	1	2	3	4	5	NA
261302	Consults with health professional regarding care of affected member	1	2	3	4	5	NA
261303	Communicates diagnosis with family members	1	2	3	4	5	NA
261304	Provides basic information about autism spectrum disorder to family members	1	2	3	4	5	NA

Continued

Family Normalization: Autism Spectrum Disorder—cont'd

		Never Demonstrated	Rarely Demonstrated	Sometimes Demonstrated	Often Demonstrated	Consistently Demonstrated	
261305	Communicates behavioral strategies with relevant individuals	1	2	3	4	5	NA
261306	Communicates importance of routine schedule with relevant individuals	1	2	3	4	5	NA
261307	Acknowledges abilities of affected member	1	2	3	4	5	NA
261308	Recognizes relationship between stress and disruptive behaviors	1	2	3	4	5	NA
261309	Adapts family routines to accommodate needs of affected member	1	2	3	4	5	NA
261310	Identifies psychosocial needs of family members	1	2	3	4	5	NA
261311	Identifies developmental needs of family members	1	2	3	4	5	NA
261312	Uses strategies to meet physical needs of affected member	1	2	3	4	5	NA
261313	Uses strategies to meet psychosocial needs of each member	1	2	3	4	5	NA
261314	Uses strategies to foster positive self-esteem of affected member	1	2	3	4	5	NA
261315	Maintains routine	1	2	3	4	5	NA
261316	Provides appropriate activities for ability of affected member	1	2	3	4	5	NA
261317	Structures activities to avoid embarrassment of members	1	2	3	4	5	NA
261318	Structures environment to avoid embarrassment of affected member	1	2	3	4	5	NA
261319	Alters family roles to meet treatment requirements	1	2	3	4	5	NA
261320	Provides peer activities for siblings	1	2	3	4	5	NA
261321	Uses respite to relieve care burden of family members	1	2	3	4	5	NA
261322	Plans for guardianship of affected member	1	2	3	4	5	NA
261323	Plans for financial support of affected member's care needs	1	2	3	4	5	NA
261324	Uses community support groups	1	2	3	4	5	NA

Domain-Family Health (VI)   **Class**-Family Well-Being (X)   6th edition 2018

OUTCOME CONTENT REFERENCES:

Althoff, C. E., Dammann, C. P., Hope, S. J., & Ausderau, K. K. (2019). Parent-mediated interventions for children with autism spectrum disorder: A systematic review. *The American Journal of Occupational Therapy: Official Publication of the American Occupational Therapy Association, 73*(3), 7303205010p1–7303205010p13. https://doi.org/10.5014/ajot.2019.030015

Baghdadli, A., Pry, R., Michelon, C., & Rattaz, C. (2014). Impact of autism in adolescents on parental quality of life. *Quality Life Research 23*(6), 1859–1868. https://doi.org/10.1007/s11136-014-0635-6

Cridland, E. K., Jones, S. C., Stoyles, G., Caputi, P., & Magee, C. A. (2016). Families living with autism spectrum disorder: Roles and responsibilities of adolescent sisters. *Focus on Autism and Other Developmental Disabilities, 31*(3), 196–207. https://doi.org/10.1177/1088357615583466

Gorlin, J. B., McAlpine, C. P., Garwick, A., & Wieling, E. (2016). Severe childhood autism: The family lived experience. *Journal of Pediatric Nursing, 31*(6), 580–597. https://doi.org/10.1016/j.pedn.2016.09.002

O'Brien, S. (2016). Families of adolescents with autism: Facing the future. *Journal of Pediatric Nursing, 31*(2), 204–213. https://doi.org/10.1016/j.pedn.2015.10.019

Schlebusch, L., Samuels, A. E., & Dada, S. (2016). South African families raising children with autism spectrum disorders: Relationship between family routines, cognitive appraisal and family quality of life. *Journal of Intellectual Disability Research, 60*(5), 412–423. https://doi.org/10.1111/jir.12292

Turcotte, P., Mathew, M., Shea, L. L., Brusilovskiy, E., & Nonnemacher, S. L. (2016). Services needs across the lifespan for individuals with autism. *Journal of Autism and Developmental Disabilities, 46*(7), 2480–2489. https://doi.org/10.1007/s10803-016-2787-4

Family Normalization: Dementia   2611

Definition: Capacity of a family to develop strategies for optimal functioning when a member has dementia

OUTCOME TARGET RATING: Maintain at_____ Increase to_____

		Never Demonstrated	Rarely Demonstrated	Sometimes Demonstrated	Often Demonstrated	Consistently Demonstrated	
OUTCOME OVERALL RATING		1	2	3	4	5	
Indicators:							
261101	Accepts diagnosis based on comprehensive neurological exam	1	2	3	4	5	NA
261102	Obtains consultation with health professional experts regarding care of affected member	1	2	3	4	5	NA
261103	Develops consensus regarding needs of affected member	1	2	3	4	5	NA
261104	Recognizes importance of supporting affected member's abilities	1	2	3	4	5	NA
261105	Recognizes relationship between stress and disruptive behaviors	1	2	3	4	5	NA
261106	Acknowledges needed change in family roles	1	2	3	4	5	NA
261107	Adapts family routine to accommodate needs of affected member	1	2	3	4	5	NA
261108	Divides care responsibilities among members	1	2	3	4	5	NA
261109	Meets physical needs of affected member	1	2	3	4	5	NA
261110	Meets psychosocial needs of affected member	1	2	3	4	5	NA
261111	Adjusts expectations based on current abilities of affected member	1	2	3	4	5	NA
261112	Provides activities appropriate for affected member	1	2	3	4	5	NA
261113	Structures activities to avoid stress overload of affected member	1	2	3	4	5	NA
261114	Structures environment to engage affected member	1	2	3	4	5	NA
261115	Uses respite to relieve care burden of family members	1	2	3	4	5	NA
261116	Maintains family involvement in care decisions	1	2	3	4	5	NA
261117	Maintains family involvement in care activities	1	2	3	4	5	NA
261118	Evaluates the capacity of the family to provide care of affected member as disease progresses	1	2	3	4	5	NA
261119	Uses community support groups	1	2	3	4	5	NA

Domain-Family Health (VI)   *Class*-Family Well-Being (X)   6th edition 2018

OUTCOME CONTENT REFERENCES:

Deist, M., & Greeff, A. P. (2017). Living with a parent with dementia: A family resilience study. *Dementia, 16*(1), 126–141. https://doi.org/10.1177/1471301215621853

Epps, F., Skemp, L., & Specht, J. (2016). How do we promote health? From the words of African American older adults with dementia and their family members. *Research in Gerontological Nursing, 9*(6), 278–287. https://doi.org/10.3928/19404921-20160928-01

Kiriake, A., & Moriyama, M. (2016). Development and testing of the partnership scale for primary family caregivers caring for patients with dementia. *Journal of Family Nursing, 22*(3), 339–367. https://doi.org/10.1177/1074840716656450

Steiner, V., Pierce, L. L., & Salvador, D. (2016). Information needs of family caregivers of people with dementia. *Rehabilitation Nursing, 41*(3), 162–169. https://doi.org/10.1002/rnj.214

F

Family Participation in Professional Care

Definition: Capacity of a family to be involved in decision-making, care delivery, and evaluation of care provided by health care personnel

OUTCOME TARGET RATING: Maintain at_____ Increase to_____

	Never Demonstrated	Rarely Demonstrated	Sometimes Demonstrated	Often Demonstrated	Consistently Demonstrated	
OUTCOME OVERALL RATING	1	2	3	4	5	
Indicators:						
260514 Participates in selecting health care professional	1	2	3	4	5	NA
260501 Participates in planning care	1	2	3	4	5	NA
260502 Participates in providing care	1	2	3	4	5	NA
260503 Provides relevant information	1	2	3	4	5	NA
260504 Obtains required information	1	2	3	4	5	NA
260505 Identifies factors that affect care	1	2	3	4	5	NA
260506 Collaborates in determining treatment	1	2	3	4	5	NA
260515 Collaborates in determining need for second opinion	1	2	3	4	5	NA
260507 Defines needs and problems relevant to care	1	2	3	4	5	NA
260508 Makes decisions when patient is unable to do so	1	2	3	4	5	NA
260509 Participates in decisions with patient	1	2	3	4	5	NA
260510 Participates in mutual goal setting for care	1	2	3	4	5	NA
260511 Evaluates effectiveness of care	1	2	3	4	5	NA
260513 Participates in discharge planning	1	2	3	4	5	NA

***Domain**-Family Health (VI)*   ***Class**-Family Well-Being (X)*   *2nd edition 2000; revised 2008, 2013, 2024*

OUTCOME CONTENT REFERENCES:

Chasson, G. S., Eskow, K. G., Summers, J. A., & Dreher, T. M. (2021). Characterization of family-directed care coordination and involvement in behavioral treatments in an autism-specific Medicaid waiver. *Journal of Autism and Developmental Disorders, 51*(40), 715–724. https://doi.org/10.1007/s10803-020-04583-4

Klostermann, S., Iskander, J., Enlow, P., Delamater, A. M., Dolan, L., & Pendley, J. S. (2021). Predicting healthcare utilization in youth with type 1 diabetes: The importance of family level variables. *Pediatric Diabetes, 22*(1), 294–302. https://doi.org/10.1111/pedi.13146

Østergaard, B., Mahrer-Imhof, R., Shamali, M., Nørgaard, B., Jeune, B., Pedersen, K. S., & Lauridsen, J. (2020). Effect of family nursing therapeutic conversations on patients with heart failure and their family members: Secondary outcomes of a randomized multicenter trial. *Journal of Clinical Nursing, 30*(5-6), 742–756. https://doi.org/10.1111/jocn.15603

Shamali, M., Konradsen, H., Svavarsdottir, E. K., Shahriari, M., Ketilsdottir, A., & Østergaard, B. (2021). Factors associated with family functioning in patients with heart failure and their family members: An international cross-sectional study. *Journal of Advanced Nursing, 77*(7), 3034–3045. https://doi.org/10.1111/jan.14810

Family Performance: Dementia Care   2212

Definition: Capacity of a family to provide a member with dementia a safe, nurturing, and positive physical, emotional, spiritual, and social environment

OUTCOME TARGET RATING: Maintain at_____ Increase to_____

		Never Demonstrated	Rarely Demonstrated	Sometimes Demonstrated	Often Demonstrated	Consistently Demonstrated	
OUTCOME OVERALL RATING		1	2	3	4	5	
Indicators:							
221201	Seeks reputable sources of dementia information	1	2	3	4	5	NA
221202	Makes decision when affected member is unable to do so	1	2	3	4	5	NA
221203	Provides for affected member's needs	1	2	3	4	5	NA
221204	Evaluates level of supervision needed for affected member	1	2	3	4	5	NA
221205	Monitors progression of disease	1	2	3	4	5	NA
221206	Monitors signs and symptoms	1	2	3	4	5	NA
221207	Monitors for pain	1	2	3	4	5	NA
221208	Monitors medication	1	2	3	4	5	NA
221209	Uses strategies to deal with confusion	1	2	3	4	5	NA
221210	Uses strategies to deal with forgetfulness	1	2	3	4	5	NA
221211	Uses strategies to manage behavioral responses	1	2	3	4	5	NA
221212	Uses strategies to manage cognitive changes	1	2	3	4	5	NA
221213	Uses strategies to manage functional changes	1	2	3	4	5	NA
221214	Uses strategies to promote communication	1	2	3	4	5	NA
221215	Uses strategies to control pain	1	2	3	4	5	NA
221216	Uses strategies to promote adequate food intake	1	2	3	4	5	NA
221217	Uses strategies to promote adequate fluid intake	1	2	3	4	5	NA
221218	Uses strategies to promote safety	1	2	3	4	5	NA
221219	Uses strategies to accomplish activities of daily living	1	2	3	4	5	NA
221220	Uses strategies to manage procedures	1	2	3	4	5	NA
221221	Uses strategies for medication administration	1	2	3	4	5	NA
221222	Promotes communication among family members	1	2	3	4	5	NA
221223	Adapts family routines to accommodate needs of affected member	1	2	3	4	5	NA
221224	Uses strategies to manage family conflict	1	2	3	4	5	NA
221225	Uses strategies to involve all family members in decision-making	1	2	3	4	5	NA
221226	Uses strategies to involve all family members in care	1	2	3	4	5	NA
221227	Uses respite care for family members	1	2	3	4	5	NA
221228	Uses strategies to make home modifications	1	2	3	4	5	NA
221229	Manages personal property	1	2	3	4	5	NA
221230	Monitors legal issues	1	2	3	4	5	NA

Continued

F

Family Performance: Dementia Care—cont'd

		Never Demonstrated	Rarely Demonstrated	Sometimes Demonstrated	Often Demonstrated	Consistently Demonstrated	
221231	Monitors insurance issues	1	2	3	4	5	NA
221232	Monitors financial issues	1	2	3	4	5	NA
221233	Collaborates in determining treatment plan	1	2	3	4	5	NA
221234	Coordinates care provided by health professionals	1	2	3	4	5	NA
221235	Uses strategies to deal with unpredictable behavior	1	2	3	4	5	NA
221236	Uses available community resources	1	2	3	4	5	NA
221237	Keeps appointments with health professional	1	2	3	4	5	NA
221238	Maintains plan for medical emergencies	1	2	3	4	5	NA
221239	Maintains plan for end-of-life care	1	2	3	4	5	NA
221240	Evaluates the capacity of the family to provide care of affected member as disease progresses	1	2	3	4	5	NA

Domain-Family Health (VI)   **Class**-Family Caregiver Performance (W)   6th edition 2018

OUTCOME CONTENT REFERENCES:

Beeber, A., & Zimmerman, S. (2012). Adapting the family management style framework for families caring for older adults with dementia. *Journal of Family Nursing, 18*(1), 123–145. https://doi.org/10.1177/1074840711427144

Gilhooly, K. J., Gilhooly, M. L., Sullivan, M. P., McIntyre, A., Wilson, L., Harding, E., Woodbridge, R., & Crutch, S. (2016). A meta-review of stress, coping and interventions in dementia and dementia caregiving. *BMC Geriatrics, 16*, 106. https://doi.org/10.1186/s12877-016-0280-8

Ma, K., & Saw, A. (2020). An international systematic review of dementia caregiving interventions for Chinese families. *International Journal of Geriatric Psychiatry, 35*(11), 1263–1284. https://doi.org/10.1002/gps.5400

Matthews, J., Campbell, G., Husaker, A., Klinger, J., Mecca, L., Hu, L. Hostein, S., & Lingler, J. (2016). Wearable technology to garner the perspective of dementia family caregivers. *Journal of Gerontological Nursing, 42*(4), 16–22. https://doi.org/10.3928/00989134-20151008-65

McCabe, M., You, E., & Tatangelo, G. (2016). Hearing their voice: A systematic review of dementia family caregivers' needs. *Gerontological Society of America, 56*(5), e70–e88. https://doi.org/10.1093/geront/gnw078

Messina, A., Lattanzi, M., Albanese, E., & Fiordelli, M. (2022). Caregivers of people with dementia and mental health during COVID-19: Findings from a cross-sectional study. *BMC Geriatrics, 22*(1), 56. https://doi.org/10.1186/s12877-022-02752-x

Steiner, V., Pierce, L., & Salvador, D. (2016). Information needs of family caregivers of people with dementia. *Rehabilitation Nursing, 41*(3), 162–169. https://doi.org/10.1002/rnj.214

Family Resilience 2608

Definition: Capacity of a family to positively adapt and function following a significant adversity or crisis

OUTCOME TARGET RATING: Maintain at_____ Increase to_____

		Never Demonstrated	Rarely Demonstrated	Sometimes Demonstrated	Often Demonstrated	Consistently Demonstrated	
OUTCOME OVERALL RATING		1	2	3	4	5	
Indicators:							
260801	Mobilizes quickly following adversity	1	2	3	4	5	NA
260833	Maintains optimism	1	2	3	4	5	NA
260802	Proposes practical, constructive solutions for disputes	1	2	3	4	5	NA
260803	Adapts to adversities as challenges	1	2	3	4	5	NA
260804	Tolerates separations when required	1	2	3	4	5	NA
260805	Discusses meaning of crisis	1	2	3	4	5	NA
260806	Expresses confidence in overcoming adversities	1	2	3	4	5	NA
260807	Maintains values, goals, and dreams	1	2	3	4	5	NA

Family Resilience—cont'd

		Never Demonstrated	Rarely Demonstrated	Sometimes Demonstrated	Often Demonstrated	Consistently Demonstrated	
260809	Supports members	1	2	3	4	5	NA
260810	Cooperates to meet challenges	1	2	3	4	5	NA
260811	Nurtures members	1	2	3	4	5	NA
260812	Protects members	1	2	3	4	5	NA
260813	Communicates clearly among members	1	2	3	4	5	NA
260814	Clarifies ambiguous communication	1	2	3	4	5	NA
260815	Uses conflict resolution strategies	1	2	3	4	5	NA
260816	Shares humor	1	2	3	4	5	NA
260817	Reports learning and growth	1	2	3	4	5	NA
260818	Maintains usual family routines	1	2	3	4	5	NA
260819	Prepares for future challenges	1	2	3	4	5	NA
260820	Supports individuality and independence among members	1	2	3	4	5	NA
260821	Accepts respite from extended family	1	2	3	4	5	NA
260822	Accepts respite from friends	1	2	3	4	5	NA
260834	Accepts financial support from others	1	2	3	4	5	NA
260823	Accepts assistance with direct care from extended family	1	2	3	4	5	NA
260824	Accepts assistance with direct care from friends	1	2	3	4	5	NA
260825	Accepts assistance with instrumental activities of daily living from extended family	1	2	3	4	5	NA
260826	Accepts assistance with instrumental activities of daily living from friends	1	2	3	4	5	NA
260835	Seeks emotional support from partner	1	2	3	4	5	NA
260827	Seeks emotional support from extended family	1	2	3	4	5	NA
260828	Seeks emotional support from friends	1	2	3	4	5	NA
260836	Participates in religious traditions	1	2	3	4	5	NA
260829	Uses community resources for assistance	1	2	3	4	5	NA
260830	Uses community groups for emotional support	1	2	3	4	5	NA
260831	Adjusts schedules to support and assist members	1	2	3	4	5	NA
260832	Uses health care team for information and assistance	1	2	3	4	5	NA

Domain-Family Health (VI)   **Class**-Family Well-Being (X)   3rd edition 2004; revised 2008, 2013, 2024

OUTCOME CONTENT REFERENCES:

Al-Jadiri, A., Tybor, D. J., Mulé, C., & Sakai, C. (2021). Factors associated with resilience in families of children with autism spectrum disorder. *Journal of Developmental & Behavioral Pediatrics, 42*(1), 16–22. https://doi.org/10.1097/DBP.0000000000000867

Coffield, C., Michael, S., & Srinivasavaradan, D. (2021). Building resilience: Resources to help families grow from challenging times. *Exceptional Parent, 51*(1), 33–38.

Fong, V., Gardiner, E., & Iarocci, G. (2021). Satisfaction with informal supports predicts resilience in families of children with autism spectrum disorder. *Autism: The International Journal of Research & Practice, 25*(2), 452–463. https://doi.org/10.1177/1362361320962677

Herbell, K., Breitenstein, S. M., Melnyk, B. M., & Guo, J. (2020). Family resilience and flourishment: Well-being among children with mental, emotional, and behavioral disorders. *Research in Nursing & Health, 43*(5), 465–477. https://doi.org/10.1002/nur.22066

Kim, G. M., Lim, J. Y., Kim, E. J., & Kim, S. S. (2018). A model of adaptation for families of elderly patients with dementia: Focusing on family resilience. *Aging & Mental Health, 22*(10), 1295–1303. https://doi.org/10.1080/13607863.2017.1354972

Maurović, I., Liebenberg, L., & Ferić, M. (2020). A review of family resilience: Understanding the concept and operationalization challenges to inform research and practice. *Child Care in Practice, 26*(4), 337–357. https://doi.org/10.1080/13575279.2020.1792838

Patterson, J. M. (2002). Integrating family resilience and family stress theory. *Journal of Marriage and Family. 64*(2), 349–360. https://doi.org/10.1111/j.1741-3737.2002.00349.x

Zhou, J., He, B., He, Y., Huang, W., Zhu, H., Zhang, M., & Wang, Y. (2020). Measurement properties of family resilience assessment questionnaires: A systematic review. *Family Practice, 37*(5), 581–591. https://doi.org/10.1093/fampra/cmaa027

F

Family Risk Control: Bullying   2612

Definition: Capacity of a family to understand, prevent, or eliminate repeated verbal, social, physical, or cyber intimidation of members

OUTCOME TARGET RATING: Maintain at_____ Increase to_____

		Never Demonstrated	Rarely Demonstrated	Sometimes Demonstrated	Often Demonstrated	Consistently Demonstrated	
OUTCOME OVERALL RATING		1	2	3	4	5	
Indicators:							
261201	Obtains information about bullying	1	2	3	4	5	NA
261202	Discusses information about bullying among members	1	2	3	4	5	NA
261203	Provides examples of bullying among members	1	2	3	4	5	NA
261204	Defines bullying with children	1	2	3	4	5	NA
261205	Discusses risk factors of bullying with children	1	2	3	4	5	NA
261206	Communicates family values	1	2	3	4	5	NA
261207	Communicates socially responsible behavior among members	1	2	3	4	5	NA
261208	Models socially responsible behavior	1	2	3	4	5	NA
261209	Communicates with members in a positive manner	1	2	3	4	5	NA
261210	Provides safe family environment	1	2	3	4	5	NA
261211	Uses resilience strategies	1	2	3	4	5	NA
261212	Participates in family activities	1	2	3	4	5	NA
261213	Participates in family meals	1	2	3	4	5	NA
261214	Engages in school activities	1	2	3	4	5	NA
261215	Observes children in social group	1	2	3	4	5	NA
261216	Adopts zero tolerance for bullying	1	2	3	4	5	NA
261217	Monitors children for bullying behavior	1	2	3	4	5	NA
261218	Monitors changes in participation in social activities	1	2	3	4	5	NA
261219	Monitors behavior of siblings	1	2	3	4	5	NA
261220	Monitors online social behavior	1	2	3	4	5	NA
261221	Facilitates positive social experiences	1	2	3	4	5	NA
261222	Confronts member with bullying behavior	1	2	3	4	5	NA
261223	Obtains psychological evaluation of member with bullying behavior	1	2	3	4	5	NA
261224	Enrolls member in professional counseling	1	2	3	4	5	NA
261225	Participates in intervention strategies	1	2	3	4	5	NA

Domain-Family Health (VI)   **Class**-Family Well-Being (X)   6th edition 2018

OUTCOME CONTENT REFERENCES:

Brandau, M. S. (2016). *Adolescent victims' experiences with cyberbullying: A grounded theory study* (Publication No. 10125546) [Doctoral dissertation, The University of North Dakota] ProQuest Dissertations & Theses Global.

Elfmam, J. (Ed.). (2009). *NAMI Iowa children's mental health resources* (pp. 70–72). National Alliance on Mental Illness Iowa.

Lösel, F., & Bender, D. (2014). Aggressive, delinquent, and violent outcomes of school bullying: Do family and individual factors have a protective function? *Journal of School Violence, 13*(1), 59–79. https://doi.org/10.1080/15388220.2013.840644

Mann, M. J., Kristjansson, A. L., Sigfusdottir, I. D., & Smith, M. L. (2015). The role of community, family, peer, and school factors in group bullying: Implications for school-based intervention. *Journal of School Health, 85*(7), 477–486. https://doi.org/10.1111/josh.12270

Smokowski, P. R., & Kopasz, K. H. (2005). Bullying in school: An overview of types, effects, family characteristics, and intervention strategies. *Children & Schools, 27*(2), 101–110. https://doi.org/10.1093/cs/27.2.101

Wolke, D., & Skew, A. J. (2012). Bullying among siblings. *International Journal of Adolescent Medicine & Health, 24*(1), 17–25. https://doi.org/10.1515/ijamh.2012.004

Wong-Lo, M., Bullock, L. M., & Gable, R. A. (2011). Cyber bullying: Practices to face digital aggression. *Emotional and Behavioural Difficulties, 16*(3), 317–325. https://doi.org/10.1080/13632752.2011.595098

Family Risk Control: Elopement   2614

Definition: Capacity of the family to understand, prevent, or limit repeated wandering from a secure area of an individual with cognitive impairment

OUTCOME TARGET RATING: Maintain at_____ Increase to_____

		Never Demonstrated	Rarely Demonstrated	Sometimes Demonstrated	Often Demonstrated	Consistently Demonstrated	
OUTCOME OVERALL RATING		1	2	3	4	5	
Indicators:							
261401	Defines elopement for family members	1	2	3	4	5	NA
261402	Identifies history of elopement	1	2	3	4	5	NA
261403	Obtains information about elopement	1	2	3	4	5	NA
261404	Discusses risk factors of elopement	1	2	3	4	5	NA
261405	Identifies individual's pattern of activity	1	2	3	4	5	NA
261406	Identifies strategies to limit individual's agitation	1	2	3	4	5	NA
261407	Identifies situations fearful for the individual	1	2	3	4	5	NA
261408	Identifies strategies to manage threatening situations for all members	1	2	3	4	5	NA
261409	Identifies behaviors to be tolerated	1	2	3	4	5	NA
261410	Promotes safe physical activity	1	2	3	4	5	NA
261411	Observes individual's behaviors occurring prior to wandering episodes	1	2	3	4	5	NA
261412	Provides protected space for wandering, if needed	1	2	3	4	5	NA
261413	Provides safe home environment	1	2	3	4	5	NA
261414	Uses alarm system for exit door	1	2	3	4	5	NA
261415	Participates in intervention strategies	1	2	3	4	5	NA
261416	Communicates with individual in a positive manner	1	2	3	4	5	NA
261417	Teaches family members constructive ways to interact with individual	1	2	3	4	5	NA
261418	Facilitates positive social experiences for individual	1	2	3	4	5	NA
261419	Monitors changes in behavior	1	2	3	4	5	NA

Domain-Family Health (VI)   *Class*-Family Well-Being (X)   7th edition 2024

OUTCOME CONTENT REFERENCES:

Aud, M. A. (2004). Dangerous wandering: Elopements of older adults with dementia from long-term care facilities. *American Journal of Alzheimer's Disorders and Other Dementias, 19*(6), 361–368. https://doi.org/10.1177/153331750401900602

Barrett, B., Bulat, T., Schultz, S. K., & Luther, S. (2018). Factors associated with wandering behaviors in veterans with mild dementia: A prospective longitudinal community-based study. *American Journal of Alzheimer's Disease & Other Dementias, 33*(2), 100–111. https://doi.org/10.1177/1533317517735168

MacAndrew, M., Beattie, E., O'Reilly, M., Kolanowski, A., & Windsor, C. (2017). The trajectory of tolerance for wandering-related boundary transgression: An exploration of care staff and family perceptions. *The Gerontologist, 57*(3), 451–460. https://doi.org/10.1093/geront/gnv136

MacAndrew, M., Brooks, D., & Beattie, E. (2017). Nonpharmacological interventions for managing wandering in the community: A narrative review of the evidence base. *Health and Social Care, 27*, 306–319. https://doi.org/10.1111/hsc.12590

Family Risk Control: Household Food Insecurity 2620

Definition: Capacity of a family to understand, prevent, eliminate, or reduce the threat of inadequate access to quality, affordable, nutritious food due to financial restrictions

OUTCOME TARGET RATING: Maintain at_____ Increase to_____

		Never Demonstrated	Rarely Demonstrated	Sometimes Demonstrated	Often Demonstrated	Consistently Demonstrated	
OUTCOME OVERALL RATING		1	2	3	4	5	
Indicators:							
262001	Acknowledges family risk of food insecurity	1	2	3	4	5	NA
262002	Acknowledges potential consequences of food insecurity	1	2	3	4	5	NA
262003	Acknowledges impact of food insecurity on family members	1	2	3	4	5	NA
262004	Seeks current information on healthy food choices	1	2	3	4	5	NA
262005	Seeks current information on how to reduce food costs	1	2	3	4	5	NA
262006	Identifies neighborhood food stores	1	2	3	4	5	NA
262007	Attends nutrition education classes	1	2	3	4	5	NA
262008	Takes advantage of school lunch programs for children	1	2	3	4	5	NA
262009	Uses supplemental nutrition assistance programs (SNAP)	1	2	3	4	5	NA
262010	Attends congregate meal sites	1	2	3	4	5	NA
262011	Uses local food pantries	1	2	3	4	5	NA
262012	Shares food needs with support network	1	2	3	4	5	NA
262013	Participates in senior meal programs	1	2	3	4	5	NA
262014	Monitors body weight of family members	1	2	3	4	5	NA
262015	Monitors changes in general health status of family members	1	2	3	4	5	NA
262016	Uses available community resources	1	2	3	4	5	NA
262017	Acquires food for current short-term needs	1	2	3	4	5	NA
262018	Stabilizes access to food over time	1	2	3	4	5	NA

Domain-Family Health (IV) **Class-** *Family Well-being (X)* *7th edition 2024*

OUTCOME CONTENT REFERENCES:

Ashby, S., Kleve, S., McKechnie, R., & Palermo, C. (2016). Measurement of the dimensions of food insecurity in developed countries: A systematic literature review. *Public Health Nutrition,19*(16), 2887–2896. https://doi.org/10.1017/S1368980016001166

Banerjee, S., Radak, T., Khubchandani, J., & Dunn, P. (2021). Food insecurity and mortality in American adults: Results From the NHANES-linked mortality study. *Health Promotion Practice, 22*(2), 204–214. https://doi.org/10.1177/1524839920945927

Cockerham, M., Camel, S., James, L., & Neill, D. (2021). Food insecurity in baccalaureate nursing students: A cross-sectional survey. *Journal of Professional Nursing, 37*(2), 249–254. https://doi.org/10.1016/j.profnurs.2020.12.015

Coleman-Jensen, A., Rabbitt, C. A., & Singh, G. A. (2019). Household food security in the United States in 2018. *U.S. Department of Agriculture Economic Research Service.* https://www.ers.usda.gov/webdocs/publications/94849/err-270.pdf?v=963.1

Diallo, A. F., Falls, K., Hicks, K., Gibson, E. M., Obaid, R., Slattum, P., Zanjani, F., Price, E., & Parsons, P. (2020). The Healthy Meal Program: A food insecurity screening and referral program for urban dwelling older adults. *Public Health Nursing, 37*(5), 671–676. https://doi.org/10.1111/phn.12778

Dush, J. L. (2020). Adolescent food insecurity: A review of contextual and behavioral factors. *Public Health Nursing, 37*(3), 327–338. https://doi.org/10.1111/phn.12708

Hawkins, M., & Panzera, A. (2021). Food insecurity: A key determinant of health. *Archives of Psychiatric Nursing, 35*(1), 113–117. https://doi.org/10.1016/j.apnu.2020.10.01

+Johnson, C. M., Ammerman, A., Adair, L. S., Aiello, A. E., Flax, V. L., Elliott, S., Hardison-Moody, A., & Bowen, S. K. (2020). The Four Domain Food Insecurity Scale (4D-FIS): Development and evaluation of a complementary food insecurity measure. *Translational Behavioral Medicine, 10*(6), 1255–1265. https://doi.org/10.1093/tbm/ibaa125

Kamdar, N., Lester, H. F., Daundasekara, S. S., Greer, A. E., Hundt, N. E., Utech, A., & Hernandez, D. C. (2021). Food insecurity: Comparing odds between working-age veterans and nonveterans with children. *Nursing Outlook, 69*(2), 212–220. https//doi.org/10.1016/j.oulook.2020.08.011

Leung, C. W., Stewart, A. L., Portela-Parra, E. T., Adler, N. E., Laraia, B. A., & Epel, E. S. (2020). Understanding the psychological distress of food insecurity: A qualitative study of children's experiences and related coping strategies. *Journal of the Academy of Nutrition & Dietetics, 120*(3), 395–403. https://doi.org/10.1016/j.jand.2019.10.012

+Pinstrup-Andersen, P. (2009). Food security: Definition and measurement. *Food Security,1,* 5–7. https://doi.org/10.1007/s12571-008-0002-y

Potter, P. A., Perry, A. G., Stockert, P. A., & Hall, A. (2021). *Fundamentals of nursing* (10th ed.). Elsevier.

U.S. Department of Agriculture. (2019). *Definitions of food security.* https://www.ers.usda.gov/topics/food-nutrition-assistance/food-security-in-the-us/definitions-of-food-security.aspx

Family Risk Control: Obesity   2610

Definition: Capacity of a family to understand, prevent, or eliminate obesity among members

OUTCOME TARGET RATING: Maintain at_____ Increase to_____

		Never Demonstrated	Rarely Demonstrated	Sometimes Demonstrated	Often Demonstrated	Consistently Demonstrated	
OUTCOME OVERALL RATING		1	2	3	4	5	
Indicators:							
261001	Acknowledges risk factors	1	2	3	4	5	NA
261002	Acknowledges consequences of obesity	1	2	3	4	5	NA
261003	Seeks reputable information about obesity prevention	1	2	3	4	5	NA
261004	Obtains reputable information about weight loss strategies	1	2	3	4	5	NA
261005	Identifies target weight for members	1	2	3	4	5	NA
261006	Members commit to healthy eating plan	1	2	3	4	5	NA
261007	Monitors environmental factors that encourage overeating	1	2	3	4	5	NA
261008	Monitors family eating patterns	1	2	3	4	5	NA
261009	Monitors food portion sizes to maintain healthy weight	1	2	3	4	5	NA
261010	Prepares healthy meals together	1	2	3	4	5	NA
261011	Eats meals together	1	2	3	4	5	NA
261012	Understands importance of eating breakfast	1	2	3	4	5	NA
261013	Provides healthy breakfast choices	1	2	3	4	5	NA
261014	Provides healthy snacks	1	2	3	4	5	NA
261015	Drinks water for adequate hydration	1	2	3	4	5	NA
261016	Adjusts recipes to decrease calories	1	2	3	4	5	NA
261017	Reads food labels for nutritional content	1	2	3	4	5	NA
261018	Introduces healthy new items into family's diet	1	2	3	4	5	NA
261019	Makes healthy choices when eating out	1	2	3	4	5	NA
261020	Limits availability of high caloric food	1	2	3	4	5	NA
261021	Limits availability of high caloric fluid	1	2	3	4	5	NA
261022	Limits saturated fat intake	1	2	3	4	5	NA
261023	Limits consumption of sweetened beverages	1	2	3	4	5	NA
261024	Eliminates using food as reward	1	2	3	4	5	NA
261025	Limits electronic screen time	1	2	3	4	5	NA
261026	Encourages involvement in regular exercise	1	2	3	4	5	NA
261027	Promotes active family activities	1	2	3	4	5	NA
261028	Encourages involvement in sports	1	2	3	4	5	NA
261029	Modifies family routine to increase activity level of members	1	2	3	4	5	NA
261030	Maintains healthy sleep routines of members	1	2	3	4	5	NA
261031	Uses available community resources to increase activity level	1	2	3	4	5	NA

Domain-Family Health (VI)   *Class*-Family Well-Being (X)   5th edition 2013

OUTCOME CONTENT REFERENCES:
Anderson, S. E., & Whitaker, R. C. (2010). Household routines and obesity in U.S. preschool-aged children. *Pediatrics, 125*(3), 420–428. https://doi.org/10.1542/peds.2009-0417
Blanson Henkemans, O. A., van der Boog, P. J., Lindenberg, J., van der Mast, C. A., Neerinex, M. A., & Zwetsloot-Schonk, B. J. (2009). An online lifestyle diary with a persuasive computer assistant providing feedback on self-management. *Technology and Health Care, 17*(3), 253-267. https://doi.org/10.3233/THC-2009-0545
Cappellano, K. L. (2011). Let's move-tools to fuel a healthier population. *Nutrition Today, 46*(3), 149–154. https://doi.org/10.1097/NT.0b013e3181ec6a6d
Cowart, L. W., Biro, D. J., Wasserman, T., Stein, R. F., Reider, L. R., & Brown, B. (2010). Designing and pilot-testing a church based community program to reduce obesity among African Americans. *The ABNF Journal, 21*(1), 4–10.
Jordan-Welch, M. (2008). End the epidemic of childhood obesity one family at a time. *American Nurse Today, 3*(6), 26–31.
Kitzman-Ulrich, H., Wilson, D. K., St. George, S. M., Lawman, H., Segal, M., & Fairchild, A. (2010). The integration of a family systems approach for understanding youth obesity, physical activity, and dietary programs. *Clinical Child & Family Psychology Review, 13*(3), 231–253. https://doi.org/10.1007/s10567-010-0073-0
Wen, L. M., Simpson, J. M., Baur, L. A., Rissel, C., & Flood, V. M. (2011). Family functioning and obesity risk behaviors: Implications for early obesity intervention. *Obesity, 19*(6), 1252–1258. https://doi.org/10.1038/oby.2010.285

F

Family Risk Control: Violence   2615

Definition: Capacity of family to understand, prevent, eliminate, or reduce the threat of exposure to violence within the family unit

OUTCOME TARGET RATING: Maintain at_____ Increase to_____

		Never Demonstrated	Rarely Demonstrated	Sometimes Demonstrated	Often Demonstrated	Consistently Demonstrated	
OUTCOME OVERALL RATING		1	2	3	4	5	
Indicators:							
261501	Obtains information about positive parenting	1	2	3	4	5	NA
261502	Obtains information about positive caregiving	1	2	3	4	5	NA
261503	Identifies personal risk factors	1	2	3	4	5	NA
261504	Identifies children with propensity toward violence	1	2	3	4	5	NA
261505	Identifies children at risk of violence	1	2	3	4	5	NA
261506	Identifies sibling risk factors	1	2	3	4	5	NA
261507	Identifies parental relationship risk factors	1	2	3	4	5	NA
261508	Identifies caregiver relationship risk factors	1	2	3	4	5	NA
261509	Identifies supportive family relationships	1	2	3	4	5	NA
261510	Identifies supportive community relationships	1	2	3	4	5	NA
261511	Maintains psychological stability	1	2	3	4	5	NA
261512	Identifies the power balance between persons	1	2	3	4	5	NA
261513	Develops non-tolerance violence stance	1	2	3	4	5	NA
261514	Develops positive peer relationships	1	2	3	4	5	NA
261515	Develops social competence	1	2	3	4	5	NA
261516	Maintains financial stability	1	2	3	4	5	NA
261517	Uses effective problem-solving strategies	1	2	3	4	5	NA
261518	Uses non-violent disciplinary strategies	1	2	3	4	5	NA
261519	Uses strategies to avoid violent behavior	1	2	3	4	5	NA
261520	Uses strategies to avoid isolation	1	2	3	4	5	NA
261521	Uses strategies to abstain from substance use	1	2	3	4	5	NA
261522	Uses personal support system to control violence	1	2	3	4	5	NA
261523	Encourages members to report violence in family	1	2	3	4	5	NA

Family Risk Control: Violence—cont'd

		Never Demonstrated	Rarely Demonstrated	Sometimes Demonstrated	Often Demonstrated	Consistently Demonstrated	
261524	Uses community resources to control violence	1	2	3	4	5	NA
261525	Monitors mental health of members	1	2	3	4	5	NA
261526	Respects the laws of country	1	2	3	4	5	NA

Domain-*Family Health (VI)*   **Class**-*Family Well-Being (X)*   *7th edition 2024*

OUTCOME CONTENT REFERENCES:

Chan, K. L., Lo, R., & Ip, P. (2021). From exposure to family violence during childhood to depression in adulthood: A path analysis on the mediating effects of intimate partner violence. *Journal of Interpersonal Violence, 36*(9-10), 4431–4450. https://doi.org/10.1177/0886260518790596

Choi, S., Lee, M., Lee, E., Park, S., & Kim, H. (2021). A gambling addiction process in adults who experienced domestic violence in childhood. *Journal of Korean Academy of Psychiatric and Mental Health Nursing, 30*(2), 168–179. https://doi.org/10.12934/jkpmhn.2021.30.2,168

Ebert, C., & Steinert, J. I. (2021). Prevalence and risk factors of violence against women and children during COVID-19, Germany. *Bulletin of the World Health Organization, 99*, 429–438. https://doi.org/10.2471/BLT20.270983

Haj-Yahia, M. M., Sousa, C. A., & Lugassi, R. (2021). The relationship between exposure to violence in the family of origin during childhood, psychological distress, and perpetrating violence in intimate relationships among male university students. *Journal of Interpersonal Violence, 36*(15-16), NP8347–NP8372. https://doi.org/10.1177/088626051943280

Hautala, D., & Sittner, K. (2021). Moderators of the association between exposure to violence in community, family, dating contexts and substance use disorder risk among North American Indigenous adolescents. *Journal of Interpersonal Violence, 36*(9-10), 4615–4640. https://doi.org/10.1177/0886260518792255

Jungari, S. (2021). Violent motherhood: Prevalence and factors affecting violence against pregnant women in India. *Journal of Interpersonal Violence, 3*(11-12), NP6322–NP6342. https://doi.org/10.1177/0886260518815134

Memiah, P., Mu, T. A., Prevot, K., Cook, C. K., Mwangi, M. M., Mwangi, E. W., Owuor, K., & Biadgilign, S. (2021). The prevalence of intimate partner violence, associated risk factors, and other moderating effects: Findings from the Kenya national health demographic survey. *Journal of Interpersonal Violence, 36*(11-12), 5297–5317. https://doi.org/10.1177/0886260518804177

Ramsay, D., Steeves, M., Feng, C., & Farag, M. (2021). Protective and risk factors associated with youth attitudes toward violence in Canada. *Journal of Interpersonal Violence, 36*(1-2), NP871–NP895. https://doi.org/10.1177/0886260517736275

Reif, K., & Jaffe, P. (2020). Risk factors and agency involvement associated with children present in domestic homicides. *Journal of Child and Family Studies, 30*, 591–602. https://doi.org/10.1007/s10826-020-01857-4

Ridings, L. E., Beasley, L. O., Bohora. S., Espeleta, H. C., & Silovsky, J. F. (2021). The role of social support on depression among vulnerable caregivers reporting bidirectional physical violence. *Journal of Interpersonal Violence, 36*(5-6), NP2800–NP2822. https://doi.org/10.1177/0886260518767913

Schaefer, L. M., Howell, K. H., Thurston, I. B., Kaufman, C. C., & Hasselle, A. J. (2021). Protective factors associated with fewer generalized anxiety disorder symptoms among women exposed to intimate partner violence. *Journal of Interpersonal Violence, 36*(13-14), 5923–5947. https://doi.org/10.1177/0886260518817027

Skinner, G. C. M., Bywaters, P. W. B., Bilson, A., Duschinsky, R., Clements, K., & Hutchinson, D. (2021). The 'toxic trio' (domestic violence, substance misuse and mental ill-health): How good is the evidence base? *Children and Youth Services Review, 120*, 1–11. https://doi.org/10.1016/j.childyouth.2020.105678

Sutton, T. E., & Simons, L. G. (2021). Examining adolescent family experiences as risks for young adulthood intimate partner violence in two longitudinal samples. *Journal of Youth and Adolescence, 50*(9), 1797–1810. https://doi.org/10.1007/s10964-021-01473-3

Wildman, E. K., MacManus, D., Kuipers, E., & Onwumere, J. (2021). COVID-19, severe mental illness, and family violence. *Psychological Medicine, 51*(5), 705–706. https://doi.org/10.1017/S0033291721000490

Family Social Climate   2601

Definition: Capacity of a family to provide a supportive milieu as characterized by family member relationships and goals

OUTCOME TARGET RATING: Maintain at_____ Increase to_____

		Never Demonstrated	Rarely Demonstrated	Sometimes Demonstrated	Often Demonstrated	Consistently Demonstrated	
OUTCOME OVERALL RATING		1	2	3	4	5	
Indicators:							
260127	Communicates warmth and support to members	1	2	3	4	5	NA
260128	Uses positive communication strategies	1	2	3	4	5	NA
260101	Participates in activities together	1	2	3	4	5	NA
260102	Participates in family traditions	1	2	3	4	5	NA

Continued

Family Social Climate—cont'd

		Never Demonstrated	Rarely Demonstrated	Sometimes Demonstrated	Often Demonstrated	Consistently Demonstrated	
260129	Participates in family meals	1	2	3	4	5	NA
260103	Attends religious services together	1	2	3	4	5	NA
260121	Maintains relationships with extended family members	1	2	3	4	5	NA
260122	Maintains relationships with friends	1	2	3	4	5	NA
260105	Participates in leisure activities	1	2	3	4	5	NA
260119	Participates in community events	1	2	3	4	5	NA
260106	Establishes family rules	1	2	3	4	5	NA
260123	Establishes family routine	1	2	3	4	5	NA
260124	Maintains family routine	1	2	3	4	5	NA
260108	Maintains clean home	1	2	3	4	5	NA
260109	Supports one another	1	2	3	4	5	NA
260110	Provides privacy for members	1	2	3	4	5	NA
260111	Supports individuality and independence among members	1	2	3	4	5	NA
260125	Encourages maturity enhancing activities	1	2	3	4	5	NA
260126	Encourages life-long learning	1	2	3	4	5	NA
260112	Shares the decision-making process	1	2	3	4	5	NA
260113	Works cooperatively to meet family goals	1	2	3	4	5	NA
260114	Shares feelings with one another	1	2	3	4	5	NA
260120	Shares problems with one another	1	2	3	4	5	NA
260130	Shares behavioral expectations for family members	1	2	3	4	5	NA
260115	Discusses issues relevant to family	1	2	3	4	5	NA
260116	Solves problems together	1	2	3	4	5	NA
260117	Promotes cohesion	1	2	3	4	5	NA

Domain-*Family Health (VI)*   **Class**-*Family Well-Being (X)*   *2nd edition 2000; revised 2004, 2008, 2013, 2018*

OUTCOME CONTENT REFERENCES:

Alderfer, M. A. (2017). Commentary: Family processes and outcomes research advances and future directions. *Journal of Pediatric Psychology, 42*(1), 125–129. https://doi.org/10.1093/jpepsy/jsw100

Burston, A., Puckering, C., & Kearney, E. (2005). At HOME in Scotland: Validation of the home observation for measurement of the environment inventory. *Child: Care, Health & Development, 31*(5), 533–538. https://doi.org/10.1111/j.1365-2214.2005.00546.x

Gerhardt, C. A., Berg, C. A., Wiebe, D. J., & Holmbeck, G. N. (2017). Introduction to special issues on family processes and outcomes in pediatric psychology. *Journal of Pediatric Psychology, 42*(1), 1–5. https://doi.org/10.1093/jpepsy/jsw104

Moos, R. H. (1974). *Family environment scale-form R.* Consulting Psychologists Press.

Murphy, L. K., Murray, C. B., & Compas, B. E. (2017). Topical review: Integrating findings on direct observation of family communication in studies comparing pediatric chronic illness and typically developing samples. *Journal of Pediatric Psychology, 42*(1), 85–94. https://doi.org/10.1093/jpepsy/jsw051

Sawin, K. J., & Harrigan, M. P. (1995). *Measures of family functioning for research and practice.* Springer.

Family Social Network Support 2630

Definition: Capacity of a family to obtain reliable assistance and encouragement from others outside the immediate family

OUTCOME TARGET RATING: Maintain at _____ Increase to _____

		Never Demonstrated	Rarely Demonstrated	Sometimes Demonstrated	Often Demonstrated	Consistently Demonstrated	
OUTCOME OVERALL RATING		1	2	3	4	5	
Indicators:							
263001	Positive social interaction skills of members with others	1	2	3	4	5	NA
263002	Individuals who care about family members	1	2	3	4	5	NA
263003	Members willingness to ask others for assistance	1	2	3	4	5	NA
263004	Members willingness to share needs with others	1	2	3	4	5	NA
263005	Members willingness to share experiences with others	1	2	3	4	5	NA
263006	Tangible assistance by extended family members	1	2	3	4	5	NA
263007	Tangible assistance by neighbors	1	2	3	4	5	NA
263008	Tangible assistance by friends	1	2	3	4	5	NA
263009	Tangible assistance by co-workers	1	2	3	4	5	NA
263010	Tangible assistance from members of faith group	1	2	3	4	5	NA
263011	Information provided by others	1	2	3	4	5	NA
263012	Members acceptance of advice provided by others	1	2	3	4	5	NA
263013	Members acceptance of assistance provided by others	1	2	3	4	5	NA
263014	Emotional support from extended family	1	2	3	4	5	NA
263015	Emotional support from friends	1	2	3	4	5	NA
263016	Emotional support from neighbors	1	2	3	4	5	NA
263017	Emotional support from co-workers	1	2	3	4	5	NA
263018	Spiritual support from members of faith group	1	2	3	4	5	NA
263019	Supportive social media contacts of members	1	2	3	4	5	NA

Domain-Family Health (VI)   **Class**-Family Well-Being (X)   7th edition 2024

OUTCOME CONTENT REFERENCES:

Biegel, D. E., Pernice-Duca, F., Chang, C.-W., Chung, C.-L., Min, M. O., & D'Angelo, L. (2013). Family social networks and recovery from severe mental illness of clubhouse members. *Journal of Family Social Work, 16*(4), 274–296. https://doi.org/10.1080/10522158.2013.794379

Kumar, N., Oles, W., Howell, B. A., Janmohamed, K., Lee, S. T., Funaro, M. C., O'Connor, P. G., & Alexander, M. (2021). The role of social network support in treatment outcomes for medication for opioid use disorder: A systematic review. *Journal of Substance Abuse Treatment, 127*, 108367. https://doi.org/10.1016/j.jsat.2021.108367

Murillo, R., Pirzada, A., Wu, D., Gallo, L. C., Davis, S., Ostrovsky, N. W., Penedo, F. J., Perreira, K., Reina, S. A., Van Horn, L., Stamler, J., & Daviglus, M. L. (2020). The association between family social network size and healthy lifestyle factors: Results from the Hispanic Community Health Study/Study of Latinos (HCHS/SOL). *Journal of Behavioral Medicine, 43*(2), 198–208. https://doi.org/10.1007/s10865-019-00082-9

Nevard, I., Green, C., Bell, V., Gellatly, J., Brooks, H., & Bee, P. (2021). Conceptualizing the social networks of vulnerable children and young people: A systematic review and narrative synthesis. *Social Psychiatry & Psychiatric Epidemiology, 56*(2), 169–182. https://doi.org/10.1007/s00127-020-01968-9

Park, N. S., Jang, Y., Chiriboga, D. A., & Chung, S. (2021). The role of social networks on depressive symptoms: A comparison of older Koreans in three geographic areas. *International Journal of Aging & Human Development, 92*(3), 364–382. https://doi.org/10.1177/0091415020905553

Sharifian, N., Kraal, A. Z., Zaheed, A. B., Sol, K., & Zahodne, L. B. (2020). The longitudinal association between social network composition and episodic memory in older adulthood: The importance of contact frequency with friends. *Aging & Mental Health, 24*(11), 1789–1795. https://doi.org/10.1080/13607863.2019.1660850

Sharifian, N., Manly, J. J., Brickman, A. M., & Zahodne, L. B. (2019). Social network characteristics and cognitive functioning in ethnically diverse older adults: The role of network size and composition. *Neuropsychology, 33*(7), 956–963. https://doi.org/10.1037/neu0000564

Slesnick, N., Zhang, J., & Walsh, L. (2021). Youth experiencing homelessness with suicidal ideation: Understanding risk associated with peer and family social networks. *Community Mental Health Journal, 57*(1), 128–135. https://doi.org/10.1007/s10597-020-00622-7

Family Support During Treatment   2609

Definition: Capacity of a family to be present and to provide emotional support for an individual undergoing treatment

OUTCOME TARGET RATING: Maintain at_____ Increase to_____

		Never Demonstrated	Rarely Demonstrated	Sometimes Demonstrated	Often Demonstrated	Consistently Demonstrated	
OUTCOME OVERALL RATING		1	2	3	4	5	
Indicators:							
260901	Members express desire to support ill member	1	2	3	4	5	NA
260902	Members express feelings and emotions of concern for ill member	1	2	3	4	5	NA
260903	Members ask how they may assist	1	2	3	4	5	NA
260904	Requests information about procedure	1	2	3	4	5	NA
260905	Requests information about patient condition	1	2	3	4	5	NA
260906	Members maintain communication with ill member	1	2	3	4	5	NA
260907	Members encourage ill member	1	2	3	4	5	NA
260908	Members provide comforting touch to ill member	1	2	3	4	5	NA
260915	Seeks social support for ill member	1	2	3	4	5	NA
260916	Seeks spiritual support for ill member	1	2	3	4	5	NA
260910	Collaborates with ill member in determining care	1	2	3	4	5	NA
260911	Collaborates with health providers in determining care	1	2	3	4	5	NA
260912	Members verbalize meaning of health crisis	1	2	3	4	5	NA
260913	Contacts other members as desired by ill member	1	2	3	4	5	NA
260914	Provides accurate information to other members	1	2	3	4	5	NA
260917	Participates in discharge planning	1	2	3	4	5	NA

Domain-Family Health (VI)   **Class**-Family Well-Being (X)   *3rd edition 2004; revised 2008, 2013*

OUTCOME CONTENT REFERENCES:

American Heart Association. (2000). Part 2: Ethical aspects of CPR and ECC. *Circulation, 102*(Suppl. 8), I12–I21.

Breen, M., Coombes, L., & Bradbourne, C. (2009). Supportive care for children and young people during cancer treatment. *Community Practitioner, 82*(9), 28–31.

Bull, M. J., Hansen, H. E., & Gross, C. R. (2000). Differences in family caregiver outcomes by their level of involvement in discharge planning. *Applied Nursing Research, 13*(2), 76–82.

Eichhorn, D. J., Meyers, T. A., Guzzetta, C. E., Clark, A. P., Klein, J. D., & Calvin, A. O. (2001). During invasive procedures and resuscitation: Hearing the voice of the patient. *AJN, American Journal of Nursing, 101*(5), 48–55. https://doi.org/10.1097/00000446-200105000-00020

Emergency Nurses Association. (2000). *Presenting the option for family presence* (2nd ed.).

Meyers, T. A., Eichhorn, D. J., & Guzzetta, C. E. (1998). Do families want to be present during CPR? A retrospective survey. *Journal of Emergency Nursing, 24*(5), 400–405.

Meyers, T. A., Eichhorn, D. J., Guzzetta, C. E., Clark, A. P., Klein, J. D., Taliaferro, E., & Calvin, A. (2000). Family presence during invasive procedures and resuscitation. *AJN, American Journal of Nursing, 100*(2), 32–42.

Rhee, H., Belyea, M., & Brasch, J. (2010). Family support and asthma outcomes in adolescents: Barriers to adherence as a mediator. *Journal of Adolescent Health, 47*(5), 472–478. https://doi.org/10.1016/j.jadohealth.2010.03.009

Fatigue: Disruptive Effects   **0008**

Definition: Severity of observed or reported disruptive effects of chronic fatigue on daily functioning

OUTCOME TARGET RATING: Maintain at_____ Increase to_____

		Severe	Substantial	Moderate	Mild	None	
OUTCOME OVERALL RATING		**1**	**2**	**3**	**4**	**5**	
Indicators:							
000801	Chronic malaise	1	2	3	4	5	NA
000802	Chronic lethargy	1	2	3	4	5	NA
000824	Chronic sleep disturbance	1	2	3	4	5	NA
000803	Decreased energy level	1	2	3	4	5	NA
000825	Decreased physical conditioning	1	2	3	4	5	NA
000826	Exercise intolerance	1	2	3	4	5	NA
000804	Interference with activities of daily living	1	2	3	4	5	NA
000827	Interference with instrumental activities of daily living	1	2	3	4	5	NA
000805	Impaired home maintenance	1	2	3	4	5	NA
000806	Disruption of routine	1	2	3	4	5	NA
000807	Interference with treatment regimen	1	2	3	4	5	NA
000808	Decreased appetite	1	2	3	4	5	NA
000809	Altered nutritional status	1	2	3	4	5	NA
000810	Impaired physical activity	1	2	3	4	5	NA
000811	Impaired role performance	1	2	3	4	5	NA
000812	Impaired work performance	1	2	3	4	5	NA
000813	Impaired school performance	1	2	3	4	5	NA
000814	Absenteeism from work	1	2	3	4	5	NA
000815	Absenteeism from school	1	2	3	4	5	NA
000816	Disruption of interpersonal relationships	1	2	3	4	5	NA
000817	Interference with leisure activities	1	2	3	4	5	NA
000818	Pessimistic about current health status	1	2	3	4	5	NA
000819	Pessimistic about future health status	1	2	3	4	5	NA
000820	Impaired recall	1	2	3	4	5	NA
000821	Impaired mood	1	2	3	4	5	NA
000822	Impaired life enjoyment	1	2	3	4	5	NA
000823	Psychological comorbidity	1	2	3	4	5	NA

Domain-Health & Life Quality (V)   *Class*-Symptom Status (V)   5th edition 2013; revised 2024

OUTCOME CONTENT REFERENCES:
Ba, J., Chen, Y., & Liu, D. (2021). Fatigue in adults with type 2 diabetes: A systematic review and meta-analysis. *Western Journal of Nursing Research, 43*(2), 172–181. https://doi.org/10.1177/0193945920938636
Brunton, L. K., McPhee, P. G., & Gorter, J. W. (2021). Self-reported factors contributing to fatigue and its management in adolescents and adults with cerebral palsy. *Disability & Rehabilitation, 43*(7), 929–935. https://doi.org/10.1080/09638288.2019.1647294
Gaber, T. (2021). Assessment and management of post-COVID fatigue. *Progress in Neurology & Psychiatry, 25*(1), 36–39. https://doi.org/10.1002/pnp.698
Kuo, H.-J., Huang, Y.-C., & García, A. A. (2020). Fatigue, pain, sleep difficulties, and depressive symptoms in Mexican Americans and Chinese Americans with type 2 diabetes. *Journal of Immigrant & Minority Health, 22*(5), 895–902. https://doi.org/10.1007/s10903-020-01001-w
Muthanna, F. M. S., Karuppannan, M., Hassan, B. A. R., & Mohammed, A. H. (2021). Impact of fatigue on quality of life among breast cancer patients receiving chemotherapy. *Osong Public Health & Research Perspectives, 12*(2), 115–125. https://doi.org/10.24171/j.phrp.2021.12.2.09
Rodríguez-Muguruza, S., Combe, B., Guillemin, F., Fautrel, B., Olive, A., Marsal, S., Valero, O., Rincheval, N., & Lukas, C. (2020). Predictors of fatigue and persistent fatigue in early rheumatoid arthritis: A longitudinal observational study, data from the ESPOIR cohort. *Scandinavian Journal of Rheumatology, 49*(4), 259–266. https://doi.org/10.1080/03009742.2020.1726449

Fatigue Level

0007

Definition: Severity of observed or reported overwhelming feeling of tiredness, lack of energy, and exhaustion associated with impaired physical and cognitive functioning

OUTCOME TARGET RATING: Maintain at_____ Increase to_____

		Severe	Substantial	Moderate	Mild	None	
OUTCOME OVERALL RATING		1	2	3	4	5	
Indicators:							
000701	Exhaustion	1	2	3	4	5	NA
000702	Lassitude	1	2	3	4	5	NA
000729	Insufficient energy	1	2	3	4	5	NA
000703	Depressed mood	1	2	3	4	5	NA
000730	Apathy	1	2	3	4	5	NA
000731	Daytime drowsiness	1	2	3	4	5	NA
000732	Disturbed sleep-wake cycle	1	2	3	4	5	NA
000733	Tiredness	1	2	3	4	5	NA
000734	Weakness	1	2	3	4	5	NA
000704	Loss of appetite	1	2	3	4	5	NA
000705	Decreased libido	1	2	3	4	5	NA
000706	Impaired concentration	1	2	3	4	5	NA
000735	Impaired memory	1	2	3	4	5	NA
000707	Decreased motivation	1	2	3	4	5	NA
000708	Headaches	1	2	3	4	5	NA
000709	Sore throat	1	2	3	4	5	NA
000710	Tender lymph nodes	1	2	3	4	5	NA
000711	Muscle pain	1	2	3	4	5	NA
000712	Joint pain	1	2	3	4	5	NA
000713	Postexertional malaise	1	2	3	4	5	NA
000714	Stress level	1	2	3	4	5	NA
000736	Anxiety level	1	2	3	4	5	NA

Domain-*Functional Health (I)*   **Class**-*Energy Maintenance (A)*   *4th edition 2008; revised 2024*

OUTCOME CONTENT REFERENCES:

+Aaronson, L. S., Teel, C., Cassmeyer, V., Neuberger, G. B., Pallikkathayil, L., Pierce, J., Press, A. N., Williams, P. D., & Wingate, A. (1999). Defining and measuring fatigue. *Image—Journal of Nursing Scholarship, 31*(1), 45–51.

Dukes, J. C., Chakan, M., Mills, A., & Marcaurd, M. (2021). Approach to fatigue: Best practice. *Medical Clinics of North America, 105*(1), 137–148. https://doi.org/10.1016/j.mcna.2020.09.007

Gaber, T. (2021). Assessment and management of post-COVID fatigue. *Progress in Neurology & Psychiatry, 25*(1), 36–39. https://doi.org/10.1002/pnp.698

+Krupp, L. B., LaRocca, N. G., Muir Nash, J., & Steinberg, A. D. (1989). The Fatigue Severity Scale: Application to patients with multiple sclerosis and systemic lupus erythematosus. *Archives of Neurology, 46*(10), 1121–1123.

Ma, Y., He, B., Jiang, M., Yang, Y., Wang, C., Huang, C., & Han, L. (2020). Prevalence and risk factors of cancer-related fatigue: A systematic review and meta-analysis. *International Journal of Nursing Studies, 111*, 103707. https://doi.org/10.1016/j.ijnurstu.2020.103707

Menzies, V., Kelly, D. L., Yang, G. S., Starkweather, A., & Lyon, D. E. (2021). A systematic review of the association between fatigue and cognition in chronic noncommunicable diseases. *Chronic Illness, 17*(2), 129–150. https://doi.org/10.1177/1742395319836472

+Michielsen, H. J., De Vries, J., Van Heck, G., Van de Vijven, F. J., Sijtsma, K. (2004). Examination of the dimensionality of fatigue: The construction of the Fatigue Assessment Scale (FAS). *European Journal of Psychological Assessment, 20*(1), 39–48.

+Okuyama, T., Akechi, T., Kugaya, A., Okamura, H., Shima, Y., Maruguchi, M., Hosaka, T., & Uchitomi, Y. (2000). Development and validation of the Cancer Fatigue Scale: A brief, three-dimensional, self-rating scale for assessment of fatigue in cancer patients. *Journal of Pain and Symptom Management, 19*(1), 5–14.

+Piper, B. F., Dibble, S. L., Dodd, M. J., Weiss, M. C., Slaughter, R. E., & Paul, S. M. (1998). The revised Piper Fatigue Scale: Psychometric evaluation in women with breast cancer. *Oncology Nursing Forum, 25*(4), 67–84.

Shen, J., Barbera, J., & Shapiro, C. M. (2006). Distinguishing sleepiness and fatigue: Focus on definition and measurement. *Sleep Medicine Reviews, 10*(1), 63–76. https://doi.org/10.1016/j.smrv.2005.05.004

+Smets, E. M., Garssen, B., Bonke, B., & De Haes, J. C. (1995). The Multidimensional Fatigue Inventory (MFI) psychometric qualities of an instrument to assess fatigue. *Journal of Psychosomatic Research, 39*(3), 315–325.

+Tiesinga, L., Dassen, T., Halfens, R., & van Den Heuvel, W. (2001). Sensitivity, specificity, and usefulness of the Dutch Fatigue Scale. *Nursing Diagnosis, 12*(3), 93–106.

Torossian, M., & Jacelon, C. S. (2021). Chronic illness and fatigue in older individuals: A systematic review. *Rehabilitation Nursing, 46*(3), 125–136. https://doi.org/10.1097/RNJ.0000000000000278

Fear Level 1210

Definition: Severity of manifested apprehension, tension, or uneasiness arising from an identifiable source

OUTCOME TARGET RATING: Maintain at_____ Increase to_____

		Severe	Substantial	Moderate	Mild	None	
OUTCOME OVERALL RATING		1	2	3	4	5	
Indicators:							
121001	Distress	1	2	3	4	5	NA
121002	Tendency to blame others	1	2	3	4	5	NA
121003	Self-absorption	1	2	3	4	5	NA
121004	Lack of self-confidence	1	2	3	4	5	NA
121005	Restlessness	1	2	3	4	5	NA
121036	Nervousness	1	2	3	4	5	NA
121006	Irritability	1	2	3	4	5	NA
121007	Outbursts of anger	1	2	3	4	5	NA
121008	Difficulty concentrating	1	2	3	4	5	NA
121009	Difficulty learning	1	2	3	4	5	NA
121010	Difficulty problem-solving	1	2	3	4	5	NA
121011	Decreased perceptual field	1	2	3	4	5	NA
121012	Perceived inadequacy in interpersonal relationships	1	2	3	4	5	NA
121013	Exaggerated concern about life events	1	2	3	4	5	NA
121014	Preoccupation with life events	1	2	3	4	5	NA
121015	Preoccupation with source of fear	1	2	3	4	5	NA
121016	Increased blood pressure	1	2	3	4	5	NA
121037	Chest pain	1	2	3	4	5	NA
121017	Increased radial pulse rate	1	2	3	4	5	NA
121018	Increased respiratory rate	1	2	3	4	5	NA
121038	Dyspnea	1	2	3	4	5	NA
121019	Dilated pupils	1	2	3	4	5	NA
121020	Sweating	1	2	3	4	5	NA
121039	Dry mouth	1	2	3	4	5	NA
121021	Feeling faint	1	2	3	4	5	NA
121022	Muscle tension	1	2	3	4	5	NA
121023	Facial tension	1	2	3	4	5	NA
121024	Frequent urination	1	2	3	4	5	NA
121025	Diarrhea	1	2	3	4	5	NA
121040	Nausea	1	2	3	4	5	NA
121041	Upset stomach	1	2	3	4	5	NA
121026	Inability to sleep	1	2	3	4	5	NA
121027	Skin pallor	1	2	3	4	5	NA
121028	Fatigue	1	2	3	4	5	NA
121029	Withdrawal	1	2	3	4	5	NA
121030	Avoidance behavior	1	2	3	4	5	NA
121031	Verbalized fear	1	2	3	4	5	NA
121032	Crying	1	2	3	4	5	NA
121033	Dread	1	2	3	4	5	NA
121034	Panic	1	2	3	4	5	NA
121042	Inability to act	1	2	3	4	5	NA
121035	Terror	1	2	3	4	5	NA
121043	Sense of impending doom	1	2	3	4	5	NA

F

Domain-Psychosocial Health (III)   *Class*-Psychological Well-Being (M)   *3rd edition 2004; revised 2008, 2024*

OUTCOME CONTENT REFERENCES:

Botkin, T. N., Makol, B. A., Racz, S. J., & De Los Reyes, A. (2021). Multi-informant assessments of adolescents' fears of negative and positive evaluation: Criterion and incremental validity in relation to observed behavior. *Journal of Psychopathology and Behavioral Assessment, 43*(1), 58–69. https://doi.org/10.1007/s10862-020-09855

Cardinale, E. M., Ryan, R. M., & Marsh, A. A. (2021). Maladaptive fearlessness: An examination of the association between subjective fear experience and antisocial behaviors linked with callous unemotional traits. *Journal of Personality Disorders, 35*(Suppl. A), 39–56. https://doi.org/10.1521/pedi_2020_34_486

Herdman, T. H., Kamitsuru, S., & Lopes, C. T. (2021). *Nursing diagnoses: Definitions and classification, 2021-2023* (12th ed.). Thieme

Molgora, S., Fenaroli, V., & Saita, E. (2020). Psychological distress profiles in expectant mothers: What is the association with pregnancy-related and relational variable? *Journal of Affective Disorders, 262*, 83–89. https://doi.org/10.1016/j.jad.2019.10.045

F

Fear Level: Adolescent   1218

Definition: Severity of manifested apprehension, tension, or uneasiness arising from an identifiable source in a child from 12 through 17 years of age

OUTCOME TARGET RATING: Maintain at_____   Increase to_____

		Severe	Substantial	Moderate	Mild	None	
OUTCOME OVERALL RATING		1	2	3	4	5	
Indicators:							
121801	Increased heart rate	1	2	3	4	5	NA
121802	Headaches	1	2	3	4	5	NA
121803	Stomachaches	1	2	3	4	5	NA
121804	Nervousness	1	2	3	4	5	NA
121805	Frequent urination	1	2	3	4	5	NA
121806	Frequent diarrhea	1	2	3	4	5	NA
121807	Fatigue	1	2	3	4	5	NA
121808	Weight loss	1	2	3	4	5	NA
121809	Sweating	1	2	3	4	5	NA
121810	Crying	1	2	3	4	5	NA
121811	Emotional lability	1	2	3	4	5	NA
121812	Stammering	1	2	3	4	5	NA
121813	Irritability	1	2	3	4	5	NA
121814	Excessive giggling	1	2	3	4	5	NA
121815	Avoidance behavior	1	2	3	4	5	NA
121816	Withdrawal	1	2	3	4	5	NA
121817	Increased school absence	1	2	3	4	5	NA
121818	Cheating	1	2	3	4	5	NA
121819	Difficulty staying on task	1	2	3	4	5	NA
121820	Difficulty concentrating	1	2	3	4	5	NA
121821	Tics	1	2	3	4	5	NA
121822	Fidgeting	1	2	3	4	5	NA
121827	Rocking motion	1	2	3	4	5	NA
121828	Shaking	1	2	3	4	5	NA
121829	Social avoidance behavior	1	2	3	4	5	NA
121830	Violent behavior	1	2	3	4	5	NA
121831	Violence displayed in drawings	1	2	3	4	5	NA
121832	Destructive behavior	1	2	3	4	5	NA
121833	Stealing	1	2	3	4	5	NA
121834	Regressive behavior	1	2	3	4	5	NA
121835	Excessive approval seeking behavior	1	2	3	4	5	NA
121836	Demanding behavior	1	2	3	4	5	NA

Fear Level: Adolescent—cont'd

		Severe	Substantial	Moderate	Mild	None	
121837	Fabrication of stories	1	2	3	4	5	NA
121838	Continuous questioning	1	2	3	4	5	NA
121839	Uncertainty intolerance	1	2	3	4	5	NA
121840	Injury faking behavior	1	2	3	4	5	NA
121841	Self-destructive behavior	1	2	3	4	5	NA
121842	Recreational drug use	1	2	3	4	5	NA
121843	Alcohol use	1	2	3	4	5	NA
121844	Excessive self-denigration	1	2	3	4	5	NA
121845	Dread	1	2	3	4	5	NA
121846	Panic	1	2	3	4	5	NA
121847	Terror	1	2	3	4	5	NA

Domain-Psychosocial Health (III) **Class**-Psychological Well-Being (M) 7th edition 2024

OUTCOME CONTENT REFERENCES:
Birnie, K. A., Heathcote, L. C., Bhandari, R. P., Feinstein, A., Yoon, I. A., & Simons, L. E. (2020). Parent physical and mental health contributions to interpersonal fear avoidance processes in pediatric pain. *PAIN, 161,* 1202–1211. https://doi.org/10.1097/j.pain.0000000000001820
Herdman, T. H., Kamitsuru, S., & Lopes, C. T. (2021). *Nursing diagnoses: Definitions and classification, 2021-2023* (12th ed.). Thieme.
Hockenberry, M., Rodgers, C., & Wilson, D. (2022). *Wong's essential of pediatric nursing* (11th ed.). Elsevier.
Hunt, C., Cooper, S. E., Hartnell, M. P., & Lissek, S. (2019). Anxiety sensitivity and intolerance of uncertainty facilitate associations between generalized Pavlovian fear and maladaptive avoidance decisions. *Journal of Abnormal Psychology, 128*(4), 315–326. https://doi.org/10.1037/abn0000422
Lei, J., & Russell, A. (2021). I have a fear of negative evaluation, get me out of here! Examining latent constructs of social anxiety and autistic traits in neurotypical and autistic young people. *Journal of Autism and Developmental Disorders, 51*(5), 1729–1747. https://doi.org/10.1007/s10803-020-04657-3
Rafihi-Ferreira, R. E., Lewis, K. M., McFayden, T., & Ollendick, T. H. (2019). Predictors of nighttime fears and sleep problems in young children. *Journal of Child and Family Studies, 28*(4), 941–949. https://doi.org/10.1007/s10826-019-01332-9
Varcarolis, E. M., & Fosbre, C. D. (2021). *Essentials of psychiatric-mental health nursing,* (4th ed.). Elsevier.

Fear Level: Middle Childhood — 1219

Definition: Severity of manifested apprehension, tension, or uneasiness arising from an identifiable source in a child from 6 through 11 years of age

OUTCOME TARGET RATING: Maintain at_____ Increase to_____

		Severe	Substantial	Moderate	Mild	None	
OUTCOME OVERALL RATING		1	2	3	4	5	
Indicators:							
121901	Increased heart rate	1	2	3	4	5	NA
121902	Headaches	1	2	3	4	5	NA
121903	Stomachaches	1	2	3	4	5	NA
121904	Frequent urination	1	2	3	4	5	NA
121905	Frequent diarrhea	1	2	3	4	5	NA
121906	Fatigue	1	2	3	4	5	NA
121907	Change in eating habits	1	2	3	4	5	NA
121908	Sweating	1	2	3	4	5	NA
121909	Crying	1	2	3	4	5	NA
121910	Nightmares	1	2	3	4	5	NA
121911	Emotional lability	1	2	3	4	5	NA
121912	Stammering	1	2	3	4	5	NA
121913	Irritability	1	2	3	4	5	NA

Continued

Fear Level: Middle Childhood—cont'd

		Severe	Substantial	Moderate	Mild	None	
121914	Excessive giggling	1	2	3	4	5	NA
121915	Avoidance behavior	1	2	3	4	5	NA
121916	Withdrawal	1	2	3	4	5	NA
121917	School absence	1	2	3	4	5	NA
121918	Cheating	1	2	3	4	5	NA
121919	Difficulty staying on task	1	2	3	4	5	NA
121920	Difficulty concentrating	1	2	3	4	5	NA
121921	Tics	1	2	3	4	5	NA
121922	Nail biting	1	2	3	4	5	NA
121923	Hair chewing	1	2	3	4	5	NA
121924	Chewing clothing	1	2	3	4	5	NA
121925	Fidgeting	1	2	3	4	5	NA
121926	Rocking motion	1	2	3	4	5	NA
121927	Shaking	1	2	3	4	5	NA
121928	Violent behavior	1	2	3	4	5	NA
121929	Violence displayed in drawings	1	2	3	4	5	NA
121930	Destructive behavior	1	2	3	4	5	NA
121931	Stealing	1	2	3	4	5	NA
121932	Regressive behavior	1	2	3	4	5	NA
121933	Excessive approval seeking behavior	1	2	3	4	5	NA
121934	Demanding behavior	1	2	3	4	5	NA
121935	Fabrication of stories	1	2	3	4	5	NA
121936	Continuous questioning	1	2	3	4	5	NA
121937	Injury faking behavior	1	2	3	4	5	NA
121938	Self-destructive behavior	1	2	3	4	5	NA
121939	Recreational drug use	1	2	3	4	5	NA
121940	Alcohol use	1	2	3	4	5	NA
121941	Excessive self-denigration	1	2	3	4	5	NA
121942	Dread	1	2	3	4	5	NA
121943	Panic	1	2	3	4	5	NA
121944	Terror	1	2	3	4	5	NA

***Domain**-Psychosocial Health (III)*   ***Class**-Psychological Well-Being (M)*   *7th edition 2024*

OUTCOME CONTENT REFERENCES:
Herdman, T. H., Kamitsuru, S., & Lopes, C. T. (2021). *Nursing diagnoses: Definitions and classification, 2021-2023* (12th ed.). Thieme.
Hockenberry, M., Rodgers, C., & Wilson, D. (2022). *Wong's essential of pediatric nursing* (11th ed.). Elsevier.
Rafihi-Ferreira, R. E., Lewis, K. M., McFayden, T., & Ollendick, T. H. (2019). Predictors of nighttime fears and sleep problems in young children. *Journal of Child and Family Studies, 28*(4), 941–949. https//doi.org/10.1007/s10826-019-01332-9
Varcarolis, E. M., & Fosbre, C. D. (2021). *Essentials of psychiatric-mental health nursing* (4th ed.). Elsevier.

Fear Level: Preschooler   1220

Definition: Severity of manifested apprehension, tension, or uneasiness arising from an identifiable source in a child from 3 through 5 years of age

OUTCOME TARGET RATING: Maintain at_____ Increase to_____

		Severe	Substantial	Moderate	Mild	None	
OUTCOME OVERALL RATING		1	2	3	4	5	
Indicators:							
122001	Increased heart rate	1	2	3	4	5	NA
122002	Headaches	1	2	3	4	5	NA
122003	Stomachaches	1	2	3	4	5	NA
122004	Nightmares	1	2	3	4	5	NA
122005	Bedwetting	1	2	3	4	5	NA
122006	Change in eating habits	1	2	3	4	5	NA
122007	Crying	1	2	3	4	5	NA
122008	Freezing	1	2	3	4	5	NA
122009	Stammering	1	2	3	4	5	NA
122010	Excessive giggling	1	2	3	4	5	NA
122011	Avoidance behavior	1	2	3	4	5	NA
122012	Withdrawal	1	2	3	4	5	NA
122013	Difficulty concentrating	1	2	3	4	5	NA
122014	Nail biting	1	2	3	4	5	NA
122015	Finger sucking	1	2	3	4	5	NA
122016	Hair chewing	1	2	3	4	5	NA
122017	Chewing clothing	1	2	3	4	5	NA
122018	Fidgeting	1	2	3	4	5	NA
122019	Rocking motion	1	2	3	4	5	NA
122020	Shaking	1	2	3	4	5	NA
122021	Violence displayed in drawings	1	2	3	4	5	NA
122022	Excessive approval seeking behavior	1	2	3	4	5	NA
122023	Demanding behavior	1	2	3	4	5	NA
122024	Continuous questioning	1	2	3	4	5	NA
122025	Clinging behavior	1	2	3	4	5	NA
122026	Separation anxiety	1	2	3	4	5	NA

Domain-*Psychosocial Health (III)*   **Class**-*Psychological Well-Being (M)(F)*   *7th edition 2024*

OUTCOME CONTENT REFERENCES:
Herdman, T. H., Kamitsuru, S., & Lopes, C. T. (2021). *Nursing diagnoses: Definitions and classification, 2021-2023* (12th ed.). Thieme.
Hockenberry, M., Rodgers, C., & Wilson, D. (2022). *Wong's essential of pediatric nursing* (11th ed.). Elsevier.
Rafihi-Ferreira, R. E., Lewis, K. M., McFayden, T., & Ollendick, T. H. (2019). Predictors of nighttime fears and sleep problems in young children. *Journal of Child and Family Studies, 28*(4), 941–949. https//doi.org/10.1007/s10826-019-01332-9
Shewark, E. A., Brick, T. R., & Buss, K. A. (2020). Capturing temporal dynamics of fear behaviors on a moment-to-moment basis. *Infancy, 25*(3), 264–285. https://doi.org/10.1111/infa.12328

Fear Self-Control 1404

Definition: Personal actions to eliminate or reduce disabling feelings of apprehension, tension, or uneasiness from an identifiable source

OUTCOME TARGET RATING: Maintain at_____ Increase to_____

OUTCOME OVERALL RATING		Never Demonstrated 1	Rarely Demonstrated 2	Sometimes Demonstrated 3	Often Demonstrated 4	Consistently Demonstrated 5	
Indicators:							
140401	Monitors intensity of fear	1	2	3	4	5	NA
140402	Eliminates precursors of fear	1	2	3	4	5	NA
140419	Recognizes source of fear	1	2	3	4	5	NA
140420	Obtains information to reduce fear	1	2	3	4	5	NA
140404	Avoids source of fear when possible	1	2	3	4	5	NA
140405	Plans coping strategies for fearful situations	1	2	3	4	5	NA
140406	Uses effective coping strategies	1	2	3	4	5	NA
140407	Uses relaxation techniques to reduce fear	1	2	3	4	5	NA
140421	Controls breathing when fearful	1	2	3	4	5	NA
140408	Monitors duration of episodes	1	2	3	4	5	NA
140409	Monitors length of time between episodes	1	2	3	4	5	NA
140422	Monitors physical manifestations of fear	1	2	3	4	5	NA
140423	Monitors behavioral manifestations of fear	1	2	3	4	5	NA
140410	Maintains role performance	1	2	3	4	5	NA
140411	Maintains social relationships	1	2	3	4	5	NA
140412	Maintains concentration	1	2	3	4	5	NA
140413	Maintains control over life	1	2	3	4	5	NA
140414	Maintains physical functioning	1	2	3	4	5	NA
140415	Maintains a sense of purpose despite fear	1	2	3	4	5	NA
140416	Remains productive	1	2	3	4	5	NA
140417	Controls fear response	1	2	3	4	5	NA
140424	Uses medication as prescribed	1	2	3	4	5	NA
140425	Keeps appointments with health professional	1	2	3	4	5	NA
140426	Maintains social support	1	2	3	4	5	NA

Domain-*Psychosocial Health (III)* **Class**-*Self Control (O)* *1st edition 1997; revised 2000, 2004, 2018*

OUTCOME CONTENT REFERENCES:
American Psychiatric Association. (2013). *Diagnostic and statistical manual of mental disorders* (5th ed.). https://doi.org/10.1176/appi.books.9780890425596
Kim, B. H., Choi, J. E., Cho, J. A., Cho, J. H., & Kim, M. S. (2015). Death, fear, and readiness as factors associated with successful aging. *Journal of Hospice & Palliative Nursing, 17*(2), 149–156.
+Marks, I. M., & Mathews, A. M. (1979). Brief standard self-rating for phobic patients. *Behavior Research and Therapy, 17*(3), 263–267.
Posner, M. I., & Rothbart, M. K. (2019). Controlling fear over the lifespan. *American Journal of Psychiatry, 176*(12), 974–975. https://doi.org/10.1176/appi.ajp.2019.19101037
Salmela, M., Salanterä, S., & Aronen, T. (2010). Coping with hospital-related fears: Experiences of pre-school-aged children. *Journal of Advanced Nursing, 66*(6), 1222–1231.
Stuart, G. W. (2013). *Principles and practice of psychiatric nursing* (10th ed.). Elsevier Mosby.

Fetal Status: Antepartum   **0111**

Definition: Extent to which fetal signs are within normal limits from conception to the onset of labor

OUTCOME TARGET RATING: Maintain at_____ Increase to_____

		Severe Deviation from Normal Range	Substantial Deviation from Normal Range	Moderate Deviation from Normal Range	Mild Deviation from Normal Range	No Deviation from Normal Range	
OUTCOME OVERALL RATING		1	2	3	4	5	
Indicators:							
011101	Fetal heart rate (120–160 bpm)	1	2	3	4	5	NA
011102	Deceleration patterns in electronic fetal monitor findings	1	2	3	4	5	NA
011122	Fetal heart rate variability between 5 and 25 bpm above and below baseline	1	2	3	4	5	NA
011104	Fetal ultrasound findings	1	2	3	4	5	NA
011105	Fetal movement frequency	1	2	3	4	5	NA
011106	Fetal movement pattern	1	2	3	4	5	NA
011107	Nonstress test	1	2	3	4	5	NA
011108	Contraction stress test	1	2	3	4	5	NA
011109	Auscultated acceleration test	1	2	3	4	5	NA
011110	Biophysical profile score	1	2	3	4	5	NA
011111	Amniotic fluid sample findings	1	2	3	4	5	NA
011112	Umbilical artery blood flow velocity	1	2	3	4	5	NA
011114	Doppler umbilical flow study	1	2	3	4	5	NA
011115	Surfactant levels/ratio	1	2	3	4	5	NA
011116	Chorionic villi sampling	1	2	3	4	5	NA
011117	Quadruple screen	1	2	3	4	5	NA
011118	Echocardiography	1	2	3	4	5	NA
011119	Nuchal translucency testing (NTT)	1	2	3	4	5	NA
011120	Acoustic stimulation test	1	2	3	4	5	NA
011121	First-trimester combined screening	1	2	3	4	5	NA
011123	Cardiotocography (CTG) results	1	2	3	4	5	NA

Domain-*Functional Health (I)*   **Class**-*Growth & Development (B)*   *2nd edition 2000; revised 2004, 2013, 2024*

OUTCOME CONTENT REFERENCES:
Casanova, R., Chuang, A., Goepfert, A. R., Hueppchen, N. A., & Weiss, P. M. (2019). *Beckmann and Ling's obstetrics and gynecology* (8th ed.). Wolters Kluwer.
Mengistu, T. S., Schreiber, V., Flatley, C., Fox, J., & Kumar, S. (2021). Factors associated with increased risk of early severe neonatal morbidity in late preterm and early term infants. *Journal of Clinical Medicine. 10*(6), 1319. https://doi.org/10.3390/jcm10061319
Simpson, K. R., Lyndon, A., & Davidson, L. A. (2018). Patient safety implications of electronic alerts and alarms of maternal-fetal status during labor. *Nursing for Women's Health, 20*(4), 358–66. https://doi.org/10.1016/j.nwh.2016.07.004
Sung, S., & Abramovitz, A. (2021). Variable decelerations. In *StatPearls*. StatPearls Publishing. https://www.ncbi.nlm.nih.gov/books/NBK546627/
Tamber, K. K., Hayes, D. J. L., Carey, S. J., Wijekoon, J. H. B., & Heazell, A. E. P. (2020). A systematic scoping review to identify the design and assess the performance of devices for antenatal continuous fetal monitoring. *PLOS One. 15*(12), e0242983. https://doi.org/10.1371/journal.pone.0242983

Fetal Status: Intrapartum 0112

Definition: Extent to which fetal signs are within normal limits from onset of labor to delivery

OUTCOME TARGET RATING: Maintain at_____ Increase to_____

		Severe Deviation from Normal Range	Substantial Deviation from Normal Range	Moderate Deviation from Normal Range	Mild Deviation from Normal Range	No Deviation from Normal Range	
OUTCOME OVERALL RATING		1	2	3	4	5	
Indicators:							
011201	Baseline fetal heart rate (120–160 bpm)	1	2	3	4	5	NA
011213	Periodic fetal heart rate deceleration	1	2	3	4	5	NA
011218	Fetal heart rate variability between 5 and 25 bpm above and below baseline	1	2	3	4	5	NA
011204	Amniotic fluid color	1	2	3	4	5	NA
011205	Amniotic fluid amount	1	2	3	4	5	NA
011206	Fetal position	1	2	3	4	5	NA
011207	Fetal presenting part	1	2	3	4	5	NA
011209	Fetal scalp blood pH	1	2	3	4	5	NA
011210	Fetal scalp stimulation response	1	2	3	4	5	NA
011212	Fetal pulse oximetry	1	2	3	4	5	NA
011215	Episodic fetal heart rate patterns	1	2	3	4	5	NA
011216	Fetal heart rate accelerations with movement	1	2	3	4	5	NA
011217	Fetal heart rate accelerations with stimulation	1	2	3	4	5	NA
011219	Intermittent fetal auscultation	1	2	3	4	5	NA
011220	Cardiotocography (CTG) results	1	2	3	4	5	NA

Domain-Functional Health (I)   *Class*-Growth & Development (B)   2nd edition 2000; revised 2004, 2008, 2013, 2024

OUTCOME CONTENT REFERENCES:

Furuya, N., Hasegawa, J., Imai, H., Homma, C., Kurasaki, A., Kondo, H., & Suzuki, N. (2021). Accuracy of predicting neonatal distress using a five-level classification of fetal heart rate monitoring. *Journal of Obstetrics and Gynaecology Research*, 47(1), 254–261. https://doi.org/10.1111/jog.14490

Kaplan, R., & Adams, S. (2018), Incidental fetal ultrasound findings: Interpretation and management. *Journal of Midwifery & Women's Health*, 63(3), 323–329. https://doi.org/10.1111/jmwh.12754

Murray, M., & Huelsmann, G. (2020). *Labor and delivery nursing: A guide to evidence-based practice* (2nd ed.). Springer.

Puertas, A., Góngora, J., Valverde, M., Revelles, L., Manzanares, S., & Carrillo, M. P. (2019). Cardiotocography alone vs. cardiotocography with ST segment analysis for intrapartum fetal monitoring in women with late-term pregnancy. A randomized controlled trial. *European Journal of Obstetrics & Gynecology and Reproductive Biology*, 234, 213–217. https://doi.org/10.1016/j.ejogrb.2019.01.023

Triebwasser, J. E., Colvin, R., Macones, G. A., & Cahill, A. G. (2016). Nonreassuring fetal status in the second stage of labor: Fetal monitoring features and association with neonatal outcomes. *American Journal of Perinatology*, 33(7), 665–670. https://doi.org/10.1055/s-0036-1571316

Uchida, T., Kanayama, N., Kawai, K., Mukai, M., Suzuki, K., Itoh, H., & Niwayama, M. (2018). Reevaluation of intrapartum fetal monitoring using fetal oximetry: A review. *Journal of Obstetrics and Gynaecology*, 44(12), 2127–2134. https://doi.org/10.1111/jog.13761

Wang, I. T., Tsai, M. T., Erickson, S. R., & Wu, C. H. (2019). Tocolysis and the risk of nonreassuring fetal status among pregnant women in labor: Findings from a population-based retrospective cohort study. *Medicine*, 98(50), e18190. https://doi.org/10.1097/MD.0000000000018190

Financial Literacy Behavior   2014

Definition: Personal actions to understand key financial concepts, evaluate information, manage assets, and make strategic decisions

OUTCOME TARGET RATING: Maintain at_____ Increase to_____

		Never Demonstrated	Rarely Demonstrated	Sometimes Demonstrated	Often Demonstrated	Consistently Demonstrated	
OUTCOME OVERALL RATING		1	2	3	4	5	
Indicators:							
201401	Identifies short-term financial goals	1	2	3	4	5	NA
201402	Identifies long-term financial goals	1	2	3	4	5	NA
201403	Keeps financial records	1	2	3	4	5	NA
201404	Identifies current expenses	1	2	3	4	5	NA
201405	Identifies sources of income	1	2	3	4	5	NA
201406	Develops personal budget	1	2	3	4	5	NA
201407	Calculates total value of financial assets from all sources	1	2	3	4	5	NA
201408	Uses financial planning resources	1	2	3	4	5	NA
201409	Saves for unexpected expenses	1	2	3	4	5	NA
201410	Handles financial transactions	1	2	3	4	5	NA
201411	Pays bills on time	1	2	3	4	5	NA
201412	Balances personal records with financial statement	1	2	3	4	5	NA
201413	Interprets personal credit score	1	2	3	4	5	NA
201414	Identifies types of loans	1	2	3	4	5	NA
201415	Identifies types of credit cards	1	2	3	4	5	NA
201416	Identifies types of bankruptcies	1	2	3	4	5	NA
201417	Identifies payroll deduction categories	1	2	3	4	5	NA
201418	Identifies types of health care coverage	1	2	3	4	5	NA
201419	Selects health care coverage	1	2	3	4	5	NA
201420	Identifies types of insurance	1	2	3	4	5	NA
201421	Reviews benefits of insurance plans	1	2	3	4	5	NA
201422	Plans for retirement	1	2	3	4	5	NA
201423	Saves for retirement	1	2	3	4	5	NA
201424	Plans for estate assets	1	2	3	4	5	NA
201425	Identifies future financial needs	1	2	3	4	5	NA

Domain-Health Knowledge & Behavior (IV)   *Class-Health Supporting Life Skills (II)*   6th edition 2018

OUTCOME CONTENT REFERENCES:

Han, S. D., Boyle, P. A., James, B. D., Yu, L., & Bennett, D. A. (2015). Poorer financial and health literacy among community-dwelling older adults with mild cognitive impairment. *Journal of Aging and Health, 27*(6), 1105–1117. https://doi.org/10.1177/0898264315577780

Meyer, M. (2016). Is financial literacy a determinant of health? *The Patient: Patient-centered Outcome Research, 10,* 381–387. https://doi.org/10.1007/s40271-016-0205-9

Meyer, M., & Hudak, R. (2016). Assessing the effects of financial literacy on patient engagement. *American Journal of Health Behavior, 40*(4), 523–533. https://doi.org/10.5993/AJHB.40.4.14

Patel, M., Kruger, D., Cupal, S., & Zimmerman, M. (2016). Effect of financial stress and positive financial behaviors on cost-related nonadherence to health regimens among adults in a community-based setting. *Preventing Chronic Disease, 13,* E46. https://doi.org/10.5888/pcd13.160005

Yates, D., & Ward, C. (2011). Financial literacy: Examining the knowledge transfer of personal finance from high school to college to adulthood. *American Journal of Business Education, 4*(1), 65–78. https://doi.org/10.19030/ajbe.v4i1.1274

F

Fluid Balance 0601

Definition: Balance of the input and output of fluids in the body

OUTCOME TARGET RATING: Maintain at_____ Increase to_____

		Severely Compromised	Substantially Compromised	Moderately Compromised	Mildly Compromised	Not Compromised	
OUTCOME OVERALL RATING		1	2	3	4	5	
Indicators:							
060107	24-hour intake and output balance	1	2	3	4	5	NA
060109	Stable body weight	1	2	3	4	5	NA
060131	Capillary refill time	1	2	3	4	5	NA
060101	Blood pressure	1	2	3	4	5	NA
060122	Radial pulse rate	1	2	3	4	5	NA
060125	Respiratory rate	1	2	3	4	5	NA
060102	Mean arterial pressure (MAP)	1	2	3	4	5	NA
060103	Central venous pressure	1	2	3	4	5	NA
060104	Pulmonary wedge pressure	1	2	3	4	5	NA
060105	Peripheral pulses	1	2	3	4	5	NA
060132	Skin moisture	1	2	3	4	5	NA
060116	Skin turgor	1	2	3	4	5	NA
060117	Mucous membrane moisture	1	2	3	4	5	NA
060118	Serum electrolytes	1	2	3	4	5	NA
060126	Kidney function	1	2	3	4	5	NA
060133	Gastrointestinal function	1	2	3	4	5	NA
060119	Hematocrit	1	2	3	4	5	NA
060134	Urine color	1	2	3	4	5	NA
060120	Urine specific gravity	1	2	3	4	5	NA
060135	Fluid intake	1	2	3	4	5	NA
060127	Urine output	1	2	3	4	5	NA

Domain-*Physiologic Health (II)* **Class**-*Fluid & Electrolytes (G)* *1st edition 1997; revised 2004, 2018, 2024*

OUTCOME CONTENT REFERENCES:

Davies, H., Leslie, G., Jacob, E., & Morgan, D. (2019). Estimation of body fluid status by fluid balance and body weight in critically ill adult patients: A systematic review. *Worldviews on Evidence-Based Nursing, 16*(6), 470–477. https://doi.org/10.1111/wvn.12394

Hockenberry, M. J., Wilson, D., & Rodgers, C. C. (Eds.). (2019). *Wong's nursing care of infants and children* (11th ed.). Elsevier.

Holroyd, S. (2020). Frequency volume charts and fluid balance monitoring: Getting it right. *Journal of Community Nursing, 34*(1), 55–58. https://doi.org/10.5888/cd13.160005

Huether, S. E., McCance, K. L., & Brashers, V. L. (2020). *Understanding pathophysiology* (7th ed.). Elsevier.

Ignatavicius, D. D., Workman, M. L., Rebar, C. R., & Heimgartner, N. M. (2021). *Medical-surgical nursing: Concepts for interprofessional care* (10th ed.). Elsevier.

Kavouras, S. A. (2002). Assessing hydration status. *Current Opinion in Clinical Nutrition and Metabolic Care, 5*(5), 519–524.

Kear, T. M. (2017). Fluid and electrolyte management across the age continuum. *Nephrology Nursing Journal, 44*(6), 491–497.

Potter, P. A., & Perry, A. G. (2021). *Fundamentals of nursing* (10th ed.). Elsevier.

Reddi, A. S. (2018). *Fluid, electrolyte, and acid-base disorders: Clinical evaluation and management* (2nd ed.). Springer.

F

Fluid Overload Severity   **0603**

Definition: Severity of signs and symptoms of excess intracellular and extracellular fluids

OUTCOME TARGET RATING: Maintain at_____ Increase to_____

		Severe	Substantially	Moderately	Mild	None	
OUTCOME OVERALL RATING		1	2	3	4	5	
Indicators:							
060301	Periorbital edema	1	2	3	4	5	NA
060302	Hand edema	1	2	3	4	5	NA
060303	Sacral edema	1	2	3	4	5	NA
060304	Ankle edema	1	2	3	4	5	NA
060305	Leg edema	1	2	3	4	5	NA
060306	Ascites	1	2	3	4	5	NA
060307	Increased abdominal girth	1	2	3	4	5	NA
060308	Generalized edema	1	2	3	4	5	NA
060309	Venous congestion	1	2	3	4	5	NA
060324	Neck vein distention	1	2	3	4	5	NA
060325	Pleural effusion	1	2	3	4	5	NA
060326	Tachypnea	1	2	3	4	5	NA
060327	Orthopnea	1	2	3	4	5	NA
060310	Rales	1	2	3	4	5	NA
060311	Malaise	1	2	3	4	5	NA
060312	Lethargy	1	2	3	4	5	NA
060313	Headache	1	2	3	4	5	NA
060328	Irritability	1	2	3	4	5	NA
060314	Confusion	1	2	3	4	5	NA
060315	Seizures	1	2	3	4	5	NA
060316	Coma	1	2	3	4	5	NA
060317	Increased blood pressure	1	2	3	4	5	NA
060318	Weight gain	1	2	3	4	5	NA
060319	Decreased urine output	1	2	3	4	5	NA
060320	Decreased urine specific gravity	1	2	3	4	5	NA
060321	Decreased urine color	1	2	3	4	5	NA
060322	Decreased serum sodium	1	2	3	4	5	NA
060323	Increased serum sodium	1	2	3	4	5	NA
060329	Increased blood urea nitrogen (BUN)	1	2	3	4	5	NA
060330	Increased creatinine (CRT)	1	2	3	4	5	NA
060331	Increased brain natriuretic peptide (NT pro-BNP)	1	2	3	4	5	NA

Domain-*Physiologic Health (II)*   **Class**-*Fluid & Electrolytes (G)*   *3rd edition 2004; revised 2013, 2024*

OUTCOME CONTENT REFERENCES:
Alobaidi, R., Morgan, C., Basu, R. K., Stenson, E., Featherstone, R., Majumdar, S. R., & Bagshaw, S. M. (2018). Association between fluid balance and outcomes in critically ill children: A systematic review and meta-analysis. *Journal of American Medical Association of Pediatrics*, 172(3), 257–268. https://doi.org/10.1001/jamapediatrics.2017.4540
Gomes, J., Pesavento, M. L., de Freitas, F. F. M., & Coelho, F. U. de A. (2019). Fluid overload and risk of mortality in critically ill patients. *Dimensions of Critical Care Nursing*, 38(6), 293–299. https://doi.org/10.1097/DCC.0000000000000383
Hockenberry, M. J., Wilson, D., & Rodgers, C. C. (Eds.). (2019). *Wong's nursing care of infants and children* (11th ed.). Elsevier.
Huether, S. E., McCance, K. L., & Brashers, V. L. (2020). *Understanding pathophysiology* (7th ed.). Elsevier.
Ignatavicius, D. D., Workman, M. L., Rebar, C. R., & Heimgartner, N. M. (2021). *Medical-surgical nursing: Concepts for interprofessional* care (10th ed.). Elsevier.
Miller, W. L. (2016). Fluid volume overload and congestion in heart failure: Time to reconsider pathophysiology and how volume is assessed. *Circulation: Heart Failure*, 9(8), e002922. https://doi.org/10.1161/circheartfailure.115.002922
Potter, P. A., & Perry, A. G. (2021). *Fundamentals of nursing* (10th ed.). Elsevier.
Reddi, A. S. (2018). *Fluid, electrolyte, and acid-base disorders: Clinical evaluation and management* (2nd ed.). Springer.

F

Foot Health 1108

Definition: Condition of the feet

OUTCOME TARGET RATING: Maintain at_____ Increase to_____

OUTCOME OVERALL RATING	Severely Compromised	Substantially Compromised	Moderately Compromised	Mildly Compromised	Not Compromised	
	1	2	3	4	5	
Indicators:						
110801 Cleanliness of feet	1	2	3	4	5	NA
110802 Grooming of nails	1	2	3	4	5	NA
110803 Skin moisture right foot	1	2	3	4	5	NA
110804 Skin moisture left foot	1	2	3	4	5	NA
110805 Skin temperature right foot	1	2	3	4	5	NA
110806 Skin temperature left foot	1	2	3	4	5	NA
110807 Palpable pedal pulse right foot	1	2	3	4	5	NA
110808 Palpable pedal pulse left foot	1	2	3	4	5	NA
110809 Color of toes of right foot	1	2	3	4	5	NA
110810 Color of toes of left foot	1	2	3	4	5	NA
110811 Sensation right foot	1	2	3	4	5	NA
110812 Sensation left foot	1	2	3	4	5	NA
110813 Condition of nails right foot	1	2	3	4	5	NA
110814 Condition of nails left foot	1	2	3	4	5	NA

	Severe	Substantial	Moderate	Mild	None	
110815 Edema right foot	1	2	3	4	5	NA
110816 Edema left foot	1	2	3	4	5	NA
110817 Pain right foot	1	2	3	4	5	NA
110818 Pain left foot	1	2	3	4	5	NA
110819 Foot ulcer right foot	1	2	3	4	5	NA
110820 Foot ulcer left foot	1	2	3	4	5	NA
110821 Neuropathy right foot	1	2	3	4	5	NA
110822 Neuropathy left foot	1	2	3	4	5	NA
110823 Calluses or corns on right foot	1	2	3	4	5	NA
110824 Calluses or corns on left foot	1	2	3	4	5	NA
110825 Dry cracks in right heel	1	2	3	4	5	NA
110826 Dry cracks in left heel	1	2	3	4	5	NA

Domain-Physiologic Health (II)   **Class-** Tissue Integrity (L)   7th edition 2024

OUTCOME CONTENT REFERENCES:

Aronson, R., Chu, L., Joseph, N., & Brown, R. (2021). Prevalence and risk evaluation of diabetic complications of the foot among adults with type 1 and type 2 diabetes in a large Canadian population (PEDAL Study). *Canadian Journal of Diabetes, 45*(7), 588–593. https://doi.org/10.1016/j.jcjd.2020.11.011

Fernández-Torres, R., Ruiz-Muñoz, M., Pérez-Panero, A. J., García-Romero, J. C., & Gónzalez-Sánchez, M. (2020). Clinician assessment tools for patients with diabetic foot disease: A systematic review. *Journal of Clinical Medicine, 9*(5), 1487. https://doi.org/10.3390/jcm9051487

O'Connor, J. J., Deroche, C. B., & Wipke-Tevis, D. D. (2021). Foot care self-management in non-diabetic older adults: A pilot controlled trial. *Western Journal of Nursing Research, 43*(8), 751–761. https://doi.org/10.1177/0193945920962712

+Persaud, R., Coutts, P. M., Brandon, A., Verma, L., Elliott, J. A., & Sibbald, R. G. (2018). Validation of the Healthy Foot Screen: A novel assessment tool for common clinical abnormalities. *Advances in Skin & Wound Care, 31*(4),154–162. https://doi.org/10.1097/01.ASW.0000530686.16243.d5

Shazadeh Safavi, P., Janney, C., Jupiter, D., Kunzler, D., Bui, R., Panchbhavi, V. K. (2018). A systematic review of the outcome evaluation tools for the foot and ankle. *Foot & Ankle Specialist, 12*(5), 461–470. https://doi.org/10.1177/1938640018803747

Gait 0222

Definition: Ability to walk with correct body alignment, with smooth gait cycle, and at a steady pace

OUTCOME TARGET RATING: Maintain at_____ Increase to_____

		Severely Compromised	Substantially Compromised	Moderately Compromised	Mildly Compromised	Not Compromised	
OUTCOME OVERALL RATING		1	2	3	4	5	
Indicators:							
022201	Steadiness of gait	1	2	3	4	5	NA
022202	Balance while walking	1	2	3	4	5	NA
022208	Base of support	1	2	3	4	5	NA
022203	Walking posture	1	2	3	4	5	NA
022204	Walks in straight line	1	2	3	4	5	NA
022205	Length of stride	1	2	3	4	5	NA
022206	Step symmetry	1	2	3	4	5	NA
022225	Head turning	1	2	3	4	5	NA
022226	Stride time variability	1	2	3	4	5	NA
022227	Cadence	1	2	3	4	5	NA
022209	Arm swing	1	2	3	4	5	NA
022228	Bone integrity	1	2	3	4	5	NA
022210	Range of right knee flexion	1	2	3	4	5	NA
022229	Range of right knee extension	1	2	3	4	5	NA
022211	Range of left knee flexion	1	2	3	4	5	NA
022230	Range of left knee extension	1	2	3	4	5	NA
022212	Range of right hip flexion	1	2	3	4	5	NA
022213	Range of left hip flexion	1	2	3	4	5	NA
022231	Dorsiflexion of right ankle	1	2	3	4	5	NA
022232	Dorsiflexion of left ankle	1	2	3	4	5	NA
		Severe	**Substantial**	**Moderate**	**Mild**	**None**	
		1	2	3	4	5	NA
022214	Hesitancy	1	2	3	4	5	NA
022215	Limping	1	2	3	4	5	NA
022216	Shuffling gait	1	2	3	4	5	NA
022217	Weaving	1	2	3	4	5	NA
022218	Stumbling	1	2	3	4	5	NA
022219	Hopping	1	2	3	4	5	NA
022220	Leaning from side to side	1	2	3	4	5	NA
022221	Twisting hips	1	2	3	4	5	NA
022222	Lifting of knees as in marching	1	2	3	4	5	NA
022223	Stiff-legged walk	1	2	3	4	5	NA
022224	Forward stooped posture	1	2	3	4	5	NA

Domain-Functional Health (I)   **Class**-Mobility (C)   5th edition 2013; revised 2018

OUTCOME CONTENT REFERENCES:

Arcolin, I., Godi, M., & Corna, S. (2022). Which model best assesses gait in healthy elderly? A confirmatory factor analysis of existing conceptual gait models. *Gait & Posture, 91*, 94–98. https://doi.org/10.1016/j.gaitpost.2021.10.007

Borowicz, A., Zasadzka, E., Gaczkowska, A., Gawkiwsjam O., & Pawlaczyk, N. (2016). Assessing gait and balance impairment in elderly residents of nursing homes. *Journal of Physical Therapy Science, 28*(9), 2486–2490. https://doi.org/10.1589/jpts.28.2486

Harris, M. H., Holden, M. K., Cahalin, L. P., Fitzpatrick, D., Lowe, S., & Canavan, P. K. (2008). Gait in older adults: A review of the literature with an emphasis toward achieving favorable clinical outcomes, part I. *Clinical Geriatrics, 16*(7), 32–44.

Kozinc, Ž., Löfler, S., Hofer, C., Carraro, U., & Šarabon, N. (2020). Diagnostic balance tests for assessing risk of falls and distinguishing older adult fallers and non-fallers: A systematic review with meta-analysis. *Diagnostics* (Basel, Switzerland), *10*(9), 667. https://doi.org/10.3390/diagnostics10090667

Lyons, R. (2015). Acute limping in a young child: Evaluation and management review. *Journal of Nurse Practitioners, 11*(10), 1004–1010. https://doi.org/10.1016/j.nurpra.2015.08.023

Moon, Y., Sung, J., An, R., Hernandez, M. E., & Sosnoff, J. J. (2016). Gait variability in people with neurological disorders: A systematic review and meta-analysis. *Human Movement Science, 11*(10), 197–208. https://doi.org/10.1016/j.humov.2016.03.010

Romei, M., Galli, M., Motta, F., Schwartz, M., & Crivellni, M. (2004). Use of the normalcy index for the evaluation of gait pathology. *Gait & Posture, 19*(1), 85–90.

Salzman, B. (2010). Gait and balance disorders in older adults. *American Family Physician, 82*(1), 61–68.

Gastrointestinal Function

1015

Definition: Ability of the gastrointestinal tract to ingest and digest food products, absorb nutrients, and eliminate waste

OUTCOME TARGET RATING: Maintain at_____ Increase to_____

		Severely Compromised	Substantially Compromised	Moderately Compromised	Mildly Compromised	Not Compromised	
OUTCOME OVERALL RATING		**1**	**2**	**3**	**4**	**5**	
Indicators:							
101501	Food tolerance	1	2	3	4	5	NA
101524	Appetite	1	2	3	4	5	NA
101525	Gastric emptying time	1	2	3	4	5	NA
101503	Frequency of stools	1	2	3	4	5	NA
101504	Color of stool	1	2	3	4	5	NA
101505	Consistency of stool	1	2	3	4	5	NA
101506	Amount of stool	1	2	3	4	5	NA
101508	Bowel sounds	1	2	3	4	5	NA
101509	Color of gastric aspirates	1	2	3	4	5	NA
101510	Amount of residual gastric aspirates	1	2	3	4	5	NA
101526	pH of gastric aspirates	1	2	3	4	5	NA
101527	Serum albumin	1	2	3	4	5	NA
101528	Hematocrit	1	2	3	4	5	NA
101529	Blood glucose	1	2	3	4	5	NA
		Severe	**Substantial**	**Moderate**	**Mild**	**None**	
101513	Abdominal pain	1	2	3	4	5	NA
101514	Abdominal distention	1	2	3	4	5	NA
101515	Abdominal tenderness	1	2	3	4	5	NA
101516	Regurgitation	1	2	3	4	5	NA
101530	Gastric reflux	1	2	3	4	5	NA
101517	Increase in visible peristalsis	1	2	3	4	5	NA
101520	Blood in stool	1	2	3	4	5	NA
101521	White blood count elevation	1	2	3	4	5	NA
101522	White blood count depression	1	2	3	4	5	NA
101523	White blood count differential	1	2	3	4	5	NA
101531	Indigestion	1	2	3	4	5	NA
101532	Nausea	1	2	3	4	5	NA
101533	Vomiting	1	2	3	4	5	NA
101534	Hematemesis	1	2	3	4	5	NA
101535	Diarrhea	1	2	3	4	5	NA
101536	Constipation	1	2	3	4	5	NA
101537	Weight loss	1	2	3	4	5	NA
101538	Gastrointestinal bleeding	1	2	3	4	5	NA

Domain-Physiologic Health (II)   *Class*-Digestion & Nutrition (K)   4th edition 2008; revised 2013

OUTCOME CONTENT REFERENCES:

Chowdhury, A., & Lobo, D. (2011). Fluids and gastrointestinal function. *Current Opinion in Clinical Nutrition & Metabolic Care, 14*(5), 469–476.

Hockenberry, M., & Wilson, D. (2011). *Wong's nursing care of infants and children* (9th ed.). Mosby.

LeMone, P., Burke, K., & Bauldoff, G. (2011). *Medical-surgical nursing: Critical thinking in patient care* (5th ed., pp. 560–587). Pearson Education.

Smeltzer, S., Bare, B., Hinkle, J., & Cheever, K. (2010). Assessment of digestive and gastrointestinal function. In *Brunner & Suddarrth's textbook of medical-surgical nursing* (12th ed., pp. 978–996). Lippincott Williams & Wilkins.

Viteri, F. (2010). INCAP studies of hematologic and gastrointestinal function in healthy individuals and those with protein-energy malnutrition and infection. *Food and Nutrition Bulletin, 31*(1), 130–140. https://doi.org/10.1177/156482651003100113

Gender Identity   1221

Definition: Acceptance, acknowledgment, and expression of a deeply felt sense of one's own gender identity as male, female, a blend of both, or neither

OUTCOME TARGET RATING: Maintain at _____ Increase to _____

	Never Demonstrated	Rarely Demonstrated	Sometimes Demonstrated	Often Demonstrated	Consistently Demonstrated	
OUTCOME OVERALL RATING	1	2	3	4	5	
Indicators:						
122101 Reconciles differences between biological sex at birth and gender identity	1	2	3	4	5	NA
122102 Exhibits clear sense of gender identity	1	2	3	4	5	NA
122103 Chooses preferred term to express gender identity	1	2	3	4	5	NA
122104 Exhibits comfort with gender identity	1	2	3	4	5	NA
122105 Shares gender identity with others	1	2	3	4	5	NA
122106 Shares preferred pronouns with others	1	2	3	4	5	NA
122107 Uses healthy coping behaviors to resolve gender identity issues	1	2	3	4	5	NA
122108 Exhibits external behaviors consistent with gender identity	1	2	3	4	5	NA
122109 Chooses clothing and hairstyle to express gender identity	1	2	3	4	5	NA
122110 Seeks social support	1	2	3	4	5	NA
122111 Reports healthy relationships with significant others	1	2	3	4	5	NA

Domain-*Psychosocial Health (III)*   **Class**-*Psychological Well-Being (M)*   *7th edition 2024*

OUTCOME CONTENT REFERENCES:
Bjarnadottir, R. I., Bockting, W., Trifilio, M., & Dowding, D. W. (2019). Assessing sexual orientation and gender identity in home health care: Perceptions and attitudes of nurses. *LGBT Health*, 6(8), 409–416. https://doi.org/10.1089/lgbt.2019.0030

Luctkar-Flude, M., Tyerman, J., Ziegler, E., Carroll, B., Shortall, C., Chumbley, L., & Tregunno, D. (2020). Developing a sexual orientation and gender identity nursing education toolkit. *Journal of Continuing Education in Nursing*, 51(9), 412–419. https://doi.org/10.3928/00220124-20200812-06

Porta, C. M., Gower, A. L., Brown, C., Wood, B., & Eisenberg, M. E. (2020). Perceptions of sexual orientation and gender identity minority adolescents about labels. *Western Journal of Nursing Research*, 42(2), 81–89. https://doi.org/10.1177/0193945919838618

Suen, L. W., Lunn, M. R., Katuzny, K., Finn, S., Duncan, L., Sevelius, J., Flentje, A., Capriotti, M. R., Lubensky, M. E., Hunt, C., Weber, S., Bibbins-Domingo, K., & Obedin-Maliver, J. (2020). What sexual and gender minority people want researchers to know about sexual orientation and gender identity questions: A qualitative study. *Archives of Sexual Behavior*, 49(7), 2301–2318. https://doi.org/10.1007/s10508-020-01810-y

G

Grief Resolution 1304

Definition: Personal actions to adjust thoughts, feelings, and behaviors to actual or impending loss

OUTCOME TARGET RATING: Maintain at_____ Increase to_____

	Never Demonstrated	Rarely Demonstrated	Sometimes Demonstrated	Often Demonstrated	Consistently Demonstrated	
OUTCOME OVERALL RATING	**1**	**2**	**3**	**4**	**5**	
Indicators:						
130401 Resolves feelings about loss	1	2	3	4	5	NA
130402 Expresses spiritual beliefs about death	1	2	3	4	5	NA
130403 Verbalizes reality of loss	1	2	3	4	5	NA
130404 Verbalizes acceptance of loss	1	2	3	4	5	NA
130423 Verbalizes acceptance of unexpected loss	1	2	3	4	5	NA
130405 Describes meaning of the loss	1	2	3	4	5	NA
130406 Participates in planning service	1	2	3	4	5	NA
130409 Discusses unresolved conflict(s)	1	2	3	4	5	NA
130410 Reports absence of somatic distress	1	2	3	4	5	NA
130424 Reports decreased anger	1	2	3	4	5	NA
130411 Reports decreased preoccupation with loss	1	2	3	4	5	NA
130412 Maintains living environment	1	2	3	4	5	NA
130413 Maintains personal grooming and hygiene	1	2	3	4	5	NA
130414 Reports adequate sleep	1	2	3	4	5	NA
130415 Reports adequate nutrition intake	1	2	3	4	5	NA
130416 Reports normal sexual desire	1	2	3	4	5	NA
130417 Seeks social support	1	2	3	4	5	NA
130425 Shares loss through social media	1	2	3	4	5	NA
130418 Shares loss with significant others	1	2	3	4	5	NA
130419 Reports increased involvement in social activities	1	2	3	4	5	NA
130426 Reports feeling satisfied with life	1	2	3	4	5	NA
130421 Expresses positive expectations about the future	1	2	3	4	5	NA

Domain-Psychosocial Health (III)   **Class**-Psychosocial Adaptation (N)   *1st edition 1997; revised 2004, 2013, 2024*

OUTCOME CONTENT REFERENCES:

Lundorff, M., Johannsen, M., & O'Connor, M. (2021). Time elapsed since loss of grief persistency? Prevalence and predictors of ICD-11 prolonged grief disorder using difference applications of the duration criterion. *Journal of Affective Disorders, 279*, 89–97. https://doi.org/10.1016/j.jad.2020.09.116

Paloma-Castro, O., Pastor-Montero, S. M., Fuentes, C. C., Albar-Marín, M. J., Bas-Sarmiento, P., Moreno-Corral, L. J., & Romero-Sánchez, J. M. (2021). Nursing diagnosis of grieving in cases of perinatal loss: A preliminary clinical validation. *International Journal of Nursing Knowledge, 32*(3), 157–165. https://doi.org/10.1111/2047-3095.12305

Romero, M. M. (2021). Meaning reconstruction in bereaved family caregivers of person's with Alzheimer's disease: A mixed-methods study. *OMEGA—Journal of Death and Dying, 82*(4), 548–569. https://doi.org/10.1177/0030222818821024

Scheinfeld, E., Barney, K., Gangi, K., Nelson, E. C., & Sinardi, C. C. (2021). Filling the void: Grieving and healing during a socially isolating global pandemic. *Journal of Social and Personal Relationships, 38*(10), 2817–2837. https//doi.org/10.1177/02654075211034914

Tang, S., Chen Q., Fan, M., & Eisma, M. C. (2021). Correlates of mental health after COVID-19 bereavement in mainland China. *Journal of Pain and Symptom Management, 61*(6), e1–e4. https://doi.org/10.1016/j.jpainsymman.2021.02.016

Varga, M. A., & Varga, M. (2021). Grieving college students use of social media. *Illness, Crisis & Loss, 29*(4), 290–300. https://doi.org/10.1177/1054137319827426

Yap, J. F. C., Garcia, L. L., & Alfaro, R. A. (2021). Anticipatory grieving and loss during the COVID-19 pandemic. *Journal of Public Health, 43*(2), e279–e280. https://doi.org/10.1093/pubmed/fdaa211

Group Therapy Participation   1641

Definition: Personal involvement in the reciprocal interactions guided by a group facilitator

OUTCOME TARGET RATING: Maintain at_____ Increase to_____

OUTCOME OVERALL RATING	Never Demonstrated 1	Rarely Demonstrated 2	Sometimes Demonstrated 3	Often Demonstrated 4	Consistently Demonstrated 5	
Indicators:						
164101 Attentive during session	1	2	3	4	5	NA
164102 Exhibits a relaxed presence	1	2	3	4	5	NA
164103 Uses respectful language	1	2	3	4	5	NA
164104 Shows unconditional regard	1	2	3	4	5	NA
164105 Shows empathy	1	2	3	4	5	NA
164106 Stays on topic	1	2	3	4	5	NA
164107 Focuses on group tasks	1	2	3	4	5	NA
164108 Exhibits listening skills	1	2	3	4	5	NA
164109 Exhibits non-verbal behavior congruent with verbal communication	1	2	3	4	5	NA
164110 Encourages members to participate	1	2	3	4	5	NA
164111 Encourages members to ask questions	1	2	3	4	5	NA
164112 Shares information about self	1	2	3	4	5	NA
164113 Shares personal issues with members	1	2	3	4	5	NA
164114 Shares personal feelings with members	1	2	3	4	5	NA
164115 Identifies with members	1	2	3	4	5	NA
164116 Provides feedback to members	1	2	3	4	5	NA
164117 Receives support from members	1	2	3	4	5	NA
164118 Receives encouragement from members	1	2	3	4	5	NA
164119 Acknowledges suggestions from others	1	2	3	4	5	NA
164120 Suggests a possible solution	1	2	3	4	5	NA
164121 Shares strategies on how to cope	1	2	3	4	5	NA
164122 Helps members gain insight	1	2	3	4	5	NA
164123 Complies with established group expectations	1	2	3	4	5	NA
164124 Complies with facilitator requests	1	2	3	4	5	NA

Domain-Health Knowledge & Behavior (IV)   *Class*-Health Behavior (Q)   7th edition 2024

OUTCOME CONTENT REFERENCES:

Chouliara, Z., Karatzias, T., Gullone, A., Ferguson, S., Cosgrove, K., & Draucker, C. B. (2020). Therapeutic change in group therapy for interpersonal trauma: A relational framework for research and clinical practice. *Journal of Interpersonal Violence, 35*(15/16), 2897–2916. https://doi.org/10.1177/0886260517696860

Fawcett, E., Neary, M., Ginsburg, R., & Cornish, P. (2020). Comparing the effectiveness of individual and group therapy for students with symptoms of anxiety and depression: A randomized pilot study. *Journal of American College Health, 68*(4), 430–437. https://doi.org/10.1080/07448481.2019.1577862

Hartley-Bangs, L. (2017). Treating women with substance use disorders: The woman's recovery group manual, by Shelly. F. Greenfield. *Social Work with Groups, 40*(4), 391–392. https://doi.org/10.1080/01609513.2016.1232120

Ripley, D., & Welfare, L. E. (2021). Reflections on person-centered group therapy from clients in opioid treatment. *Journal for Specialists in Group Work, 46*(4), 322–338. https://doi.org/10.1080/01933922.2021.1950879

Sugarman, D. E., Wigderson, S. B., Iles, B., Kaufman, J. S., Fitzmaurice, G. M., Hilario, E. Y., Robbins, M. S., & Greenfield, S. F. (2016). Measuring affiliation in group therapy for substance use disorders in the women's recovery group study: Does it matter whether the group is all-women or Mixed-Gender? *The American Journal on Addiction, 25*(7), 573–580. https://doi.org/10.1111/ajad.12443

Valeri, L., Sugarman, D. E., Reilly, M. E., McHugh, R. K., Fitzmaurice, G. M., & Greenfield, S. R. (2018). Group therapy for women with substance use disorders: In-session affiliation predicts women's substance use treatment outcomes. *Journal of Substance Abuse Treatment, 94*, 60–68. https://doi.org/10.1016/j.jsat.2018.08.008

Growth   0110

Definition: Normal increase in height and body weight from infancy through adolescence

OUTCOME TARGET RATING: Maintain at_____ Increase to_____

OUTCOME OVERALL RATING	Severe Deviation from Normal Range 1	Substantial Deviation from Normal Range 2	Moderate Deviation from Normal Range 3	Mild Deviation from Normal Range 4	No Deviation from Normal Range 5	
Indicators:						
011001 Weight percentile for sex	1	2	3	4	5	NA
011002 Weight percentile for age	1	2	3	4	5	NA
011003 Weight percentile for height	1	2	3	4	5	NA
011004 Rate of weight gain	1	2	3	4	5	NA
011005 Rate of height gain	1	2	3	4	5	NA
011006 Length/height percentile for age	1	2	3	4	5	NA
011007 Length/height percentile for sex	1	2	3	4	5	NA
011008 Head circumference percentile for age	1	2	3	4	5	NA
011009 Bone mass index	1	2	3	4	5	NA
011010 Mean body mass	1	2	3	4	5	NA
011012 Change in growth pattern over time	1	2	3	4	5	NA
011013 Triceps skinfold thickness	1	2	3	4	5	NA
011014 Subscapular skinfold thickness	1	2	3	4	5	NA

Domain-*Functional Health (I)*   **Class**-*Growth & Development (B)*   *1st edition 1997; revised 2004, 2018*

OUTCOME CONTENT REFERENCES:

Carter, R., Jacobson, J., Molteno, C., Dodge, N., Meintjes, E., & Jacobson, S. (2016). Fetal alcohol growth restriction and cognitive impairment. *Pediatrics, 138*(2). https://doi.org/10.1542/peds.2016-0775

Foote, J. (2014). Optimizing linear growth measurement in children. *Journal of Pediatric Healthcare, 28*(5), 413–419. https://doi.org/10.1016/j.pedhc.2014.01.001

Foote, J., Brady, L., Burke, A., Cook, J., Dutcher, M., Gradoville, K., Groos, J. A., Kinkade, K. M., Meeks, R. A., Mohr, P. J., Schultheis, D. S., Walker, B. S., & Phillips, K. T. (2011). Development of an evidence-based clinical practice guideline on linear growth measurement of children. *Journal of Pediatric Nursing, 26*(4), 312–324. https://doi.org/10.1016/j.pedn.2010.09.002

Hernandez, R., Marcell, A., Garcia, J., Amankwah, E., & Cheng, T. (2015). Predictors of favorable growth patterns during the obesity epidemic among U.S. school children. *Clinical Pediatrics, 54*(5), 458–468. https://doi.org/10.1177/0009922815570579

Hutcheon, J., Jacobsen, G., Kramer, M., Martinussen, M., & Platt, R. (2016). Small size at birth or abnormal intrauterine growth trajectory: Which matters more for child growth? *American Journal of Epidemiology, 183*(12), 1107–1113.

Schrieken, M., Visser, J., Oosterling, I., van Steijn, D., Bons, D., Draaisma, J., van der Gaag, R.-J., Buitelaar, J., Donders, R., & Rommelse, N. (2013). Small size at birth or abnormal intrauterine growth trajectory: Which matters more for child growth. *European Child & Adolescent Psychiatry, 22*(1), 35–43. https://doi.org/10.1093/aje/kwv310

Guilt Resolution   1310

Definition: Personal actions to adjust intense and frequent thoughts, feelings, and behaviors due to actual or perceived self-blame

OUTCOME TARGET RATING: Maintain at_____ Increase to_____

OUTCOME OVERALL RATING	Never Demonstrated 1	Rarely Demonstrated 2	Sometimes Demonstrated 3	Often Demonstrated 4	Consistently Demonstrated 5	
Indicators:						
131001 Expresses the causes of guilt	1	2	3	4	5	NA
131002 Identifies feelings of guilt	1	2	3	4	5	NA
131003 Monitors intensity of feelings	1	2	3	4	5	NA
131004 Monitors frequency of feelings	1	2	3	4	5	NA

Guilt Resolution—cont'd

		Never Demonstrated	Rarely Demonstrated	Sometimes Demonstrated	Often Demonstrated	Consistently Demonstrated	
131005	Expresses the personal meaning of guilt	1	2	3	4	5	NA
131006	Identifies a realistic perception of the cause of guilt	1	2	3	4	5	NA
131007	Identifies guilt as a common reaction	1	2	3	4	5	NA
131008	Identifies exaggerated negative feelings	1	2	3	4	5	NA
131009	Identifies irrational thoughts	1	2	3	4	5	NA
131010	Shares feelings of guilt with significant others	1	2	3	4	5	NA
131011	Shares feelings of guilt with health providers	1	2	3	4	5	NA
131012	Uses strategies to decrease guilt	1	2	3	4	5	NA
131013	Reports absence of somatic distress	1	2	3	4	5	NA
131014	Follows recommended treatment	1	2	3	4	5	NA
131015	Uses effective coping strategies	1	2	3	4	5	NA
131016	Uses support services	1	2	3	4	5	NA
131017	Reports improved mood	1	2	3	4	5	NA
131018	Reports increased involvement in social activities	1	2	3	4	5	NA
131019	Expresses positive expectations about the future	1	2	3	4	5	NA
131020	Reports decreased preoccupation with guilt	1	2	3	4	5	NA
131021	Resolves feelings of guilt	1	2	3	4	5	NA
131022	Verbalizes acceptance of guilt	1	2	3	4	5	NA
131023	Adapts to life changes	1	2	3	4	5	NA

Domain-Psychosocial Health (III)   **Class**-Psychosocial Adaption (N)   5th edition 2013

OUTCOME CONTENT REFERENCES:

Abrams, R. D., & Finesinger, J. E. (1953). Guilt reactions in patients with cancer. *Cancer, 6*(3), 474–482.

Antai-Otong, D. (2008). Crisis intervention and management: The role of adaptation. In *Psychiatric nursing: Biological & behavioral concepts* (2nd ed., pp. 961–983). Thomson Delmar Learning.

Arnold, E. C., & Boggs, K. U. (2011). Communicating with clients in crisis. In *Interpersonal relationships: Professional communication skills for nurses* (6th ed., pp. 415–435). Elsevier/Saunders.

Fortinash, K. M. (2008). Grief and loss. In K. M. Fortinash, & P. A. Holoday Worret (Eds.), *Psychiatric mental health nursing* (4th ed., pp. 591–606). Mosby Elsevier.

Nishith, P., Nixon, R. D. V., & Resick, P. A. (2005). Resolution of trauma-related guilt following treatment of PTSD in female rape victims: A result of cognitive processing therapy targeting comorbid depression? *Journal of Affective Disorders, 86*(2-3), 259–265.

Health Beliefs

1700

Definition: Personal convictions that influence health behaviors

OUTCOME TARGET RATING: Maintain at_____ Increase to_____

		Very Weak	Weak	Moderate	Strong	Very Strong	
OUTCOME OVERALL RATING		1	2	3	4	5	
Indicators:							
170001	Perceived importance of taking action	1	2	3	4	5	NA
170002	Perceived threat from inaction	1	2	3	4	5	NA
170012	Perceived threat of hospitalization	1	2	3	4	5	NA
170003	Perceived benefits of action	1	2	3	4	5	NA
170004	Perceived internal control of action	1	2	3	4	5	NA

Continued

H

Health Beliefs—cont'd

		Very Weak	Weak	Moderate	Strong	Very Strong	
170005	Perceived control of health outcome	1	2	3	4	5	NA
170006	Perceived reduction of threat from action	1	2	3	4	5	NA
170007	Perceived improvement in lifestyle from action	1	2	3	4	5	NA
170008	Perceived ability to perform action	1	2	3	4	5	NA
170009	Perceived resources to perform action	1	2	3	4	5	NA
170010	Perceived absence of barriers to action	1	2	3	4	5	NA
170013	Perceived trust in information sources	1	2	3	4	5	NA

Domain-*Health Knowledge & Behavior (IV)*   **Class**-*Health Beliefs (R)*   *1st edition 1997; revised 2024*

OUTCOME CONTENT REFERENCES:

Carpenter, C. J. (2010). A meta-analysis of the effectiveness of Health Belief Model variables in predicting behavior. *Health Communication, 25*(8), 661–669. https://doi.org/10.1080/10410236.2010.521906

+Champion, V. L. (1993). Instrument refinement for breast cancer screening behaviors. *Nursing Research, 42*(3), 139–143. https://doi.org/10.1097/00006199-199305000-00003

Chen, Y., Zhou, R., Chen, B., Chen, H., Li, Y., Chen, Z., Zhu, H., & Wang, H. (2020). Knowledge, perceived beliefs, and preventive behaviors related to COVID-19 among Chinese older adults: Cross-sectional web-based survey. *Journal of Medical Internet Research, 22*(12), e23729. https://doi.org/10.2196/23729

Costa, M. F. (2020). Health Belief Model for coronavirus infection risk determinants. *Revista de Saude Publica, 54*, 47. https://doi.org/10.11606/s1518-8787.2020054002494

Fridman, I., Lucas, N., Henke, D., & Zigler, C. K. (2020). Association between public knowledge about COVID-19, trust in information sources, and adherence to social distancing: Cross-sectional survey. *JMIR Public Health and Surveillance, 6*(3), e22060. https://doi.org/10.2196/22060

Maykrantz, S. A., Gong, T., Petrolino, A. V., Nobiling, B. D., & Houghton, J. D. (2021). How trust in information sources influences preventative measures compliance during the COVID-19 pandemic. *International Journal of Environmental Research and Public Health, 18*(11), 5867. https://doi.org/10.3390/ijerph18115867

Nobiling, B. D., & Maykrantz, S. A. (2017). Exploring perceptions about and behaviors related to mental illness and mental health service utilization among college students using the Health Belief Model (HBM). *American Journal of Health Education, 48*(5), 306–319. https://doi.org/10.1080/19325037.2017.1335628

O'Connor, P. J., Martin, B., Weeks, C. S., & Ong, L. (2014). Factors that influence young people's mental health help-seeking behaviors: A study based on the Health Belief Model. *Journal of Advanced Nursing, 70*(11), 2577–2587. https://doi.org/10.1111/jan.12423

Rosenstock, I. M. (1974). Historical origins of the Health Belief Model. *Health Education & Behavior, 2*(4), 328–335. https://doi.org/10.1177/109019817400200403

Rosenstock, I. M., Strecher, V. J., & Becker, M. H. (1988). Social learning theory and the Health Belief Model. *Health Education Quarterly, 15*(2), 175–183. https://doi.org/10.1177/109019818801500203

Shmueli, L. (2021). Predicting intention to receive COVID-19 vaccine among the general population using the Health Belief Model and the Theory of Planned Behavior Model. *BMC Public Health, 21*(1), 804. https://doi.org/10.1186/s12889-021-10816-7

Zampetakis, L. A., & Melas, C. (2021). The Health Belief Model predicts vaccination intentions against COVID-19: A survey experiment approach. *Applied Psychology, Health and Well-Being, 13*(2), 469–484. https://doi.org/10.1111/aphw.12262

Zhang, K. C., Fang, Y., Cao, H., Chen, H., Hu, T., Chen, Y. Q., Zhou, X., & Wang, Z. (2020). Parental acceptability of COVID-19 vaccination for children under the age of 18 years: Cross-sectional online survey. *JMIR Pediatrics and Parenting, 3*(2), e24827. https://doi.org/10.2196/24827

Health Beliefs: Perceived Ability to Perform   **1701**

Definition: Personal conviction that one can carry out a given health behavior

OUTCOME TARGET RATING: Maintain at_____ Increase to_____

		Very Weak	Weak	Moderate	Strong	Very Strong	
OUTCOME OVERALL RATING		1	2	3	4	5	
Indicators:							
170101	Perception that health behavior is not too complex	1	2	3	4	5	NA
170102	Perception that health behavior requires reasonable effort	1	2	3	4	5	NA
170110	Perception of positive impact of health behavior on lifestyle	1	2	3	4	5	NA
170103	Perception that the frequency of health behavior is not excessive	1	2	3	4	5	NA
170104	Perception of likelihood of performing health behavior over time	1	2	3	4	5	NA
170105	Confidence related to past experience with health behavior	1	2	3	4	5	NA

Health Beliefs: Perceived Ability to Perform—cont'd

	Very Weak	Weak	Moderate	Strong	Very Strong	
170106 Confidence related to past experience with similar health behaviors	1	2	3	4	5	NA
170107 Confidence related to observation of successful experiences of others	1	2	3	4	5	NA
170108 Confidence in ability to perform health behavior	1	2	3	4	5	NA

Domain*-Health Knowledge & Behavior (IV)*   ***Class****-Health Beliefs (R)*   *1st edition 1997; revised 2004, 2024*

OUTCOME CONTENT REFERENCES:

Al-Sabbagh, M. Q., Al-Ani, A., Mafrachi, B., Siyam, A., Isleem, U., Massad, F. I., Alsabbagh, Q., & Abufaraj, M. (2022). Predictors of adherence with home quarantine during COVID-19 crisis: The case of Health Belief Model. *Psychology, Health & Medicine, 27*(1), 215–227. https://doi.org/10.1080/13548506.2021.1871770

Aschwanden, D., Strickhouser, J. E., Sesker, A. A., Lee, J. H., Luchetti, M., Terracciano, A., & Sutin, A. R. (2021). Preventive behaviors during the COVID-19 pandemic: Associations with perceived behavioral control, attitudes, and subjective norm. *Frontiers in Public Health, 9*, 662835. https://doi.org/10.3389/fpubh.2021.662835

Bauer, M. S., Williford, W. O., McBride, L., McBride, K., & Shea, N. M. (2005). Perceived barriers to health care access in a treated population. *International Journal of Psychiatry in Medicine, 35*(1), 13–26. https://doi.org/10.2190/U1D5-8B1D-UW69-U1Y4

Calfee, C. S., Katz, P. P., Yelin, E. H., Iribarren, C., & Eisner, M. D. (2007). The influence of perceived control of asthma on health outcomes. *Chest, 130*(5), 1312–1318.

Carpenter, C. J. (2010). A meta-analysis of the effectiveness of Health Belief Model variables in predicting behavior. *Health Communication, 25*(8), 661–669.

Chen, Y., Zhou, R., Chen, B., Chen, H., Li, Y., Chen, Z., Zhu, H., & Wang, H. (2020). Knowledge, perceived beliefs, and preventive behaviors related to COVID-19 among Chinese older adults: Cross-sectional web-based survey. *Journal of Medical Internet Research, 22*(12), e23729. https://doi.org/10.2196/23729

Kim, K. K., Horan, M. L., Gendler, P., & Patel, M. K. (1991). Development and evaluation of the Osteoporosis Health Belief Scale. *Research in Nursing & Health, 14*(2), 155–163.

O'Connor, P. J., Martin, B., Weeks, C. S., & Ong, L. (2014). Factors that influence young people's mental health help-seeking behaviors: A study based on the Health Belief Model. *Journal of Advanced Nursing, 70*(11), 2577–2587. https://doi.org/10.1111/jan.12423

Ramos, A. K., Carvajal-Suarez, M., Trinidad, N., Quintero, S. A., Molina, D., Johnson-Beller, R., & Rowland, S. A. (2021). Health and well-being of Hispanic/Latino meatpacking workers in Nebraska: An application of the Health Belief Model. *Workplace Health & Safety, 69*(12), 564–572. https://doi.org/10.1177/21650799211016907

Ritchie, D., Van den Broucke, S., & Van Hal, G. (2021). The Health Belief Model and Theory of Planned Behavior applied to mammography screening: A systematic review and meta-analysis. *Public Health Nursing, 38*, 482–492. https://doi.org/10.1111/phn.12842

Robertson, D., & Keller, C. (1992). Relationships among health beliefs, self-efficacy, and exercise adherence in patients with coronary artery disease. *Heart & Lung, 21*(1), 56–63.

Rosenstock, I. M. (1974). Historical origins of the Health Belief Model. *Health Education & Behavior, 2*(4), 328–335. https://doi.org/10.1177/109019817400200403

Rosenstock, I. M., Strecher, V. J., & Becker, M. H. (1988). Social learning theory and the Health Belief Model. *Health Education Quarterly, 15*(2), 175–183. https://doi.org/10.1177/109019818801500203

+Smith, M. S., Wallston, K. A., & Smith, C. A. (1995). The development and validation of the Perceived Health Competence Scale. *Health Education Research, 10*(1), 51–64.

Zhang, K. C., Fang, Y., Cao, H., Chen, H., Hu, T., Chen, Y., Zhou, X., & Wang, Z. (2021). Behavioral intention to receive a COVID-19 vaccination among Chinese factory workers: Cross-sectional online survey. *Journal of Medical Internet Research, 23*(3), e24673. https://doi.org/10.2196/24673

Health Beliefs: Perceived Control   1702

Definition: Personal conviction that one can influence a health outcome

OUTCOME TARGET RATING: Maintain at_____ Increase to_____

	Very Weak	Weak	Moderate	Strong	Very Strong	
OUTCOME OVERALL RATING	1	2	3	4	5	
Indicators:						
170201 Perceived responsibility for health decisions	1	2	3	4	5	NA
170202 Requested involvement in health decisions	1	2	3	4	5	NA
170203 Efforts at gathering information	1	2	3	4	5	NA
170204 Belief that own decisions control health outcomes	1	2	3	4	5	NA
170205 Belief that own actions control health outcomes	1	2	3	4	5	NA
170206 Willingness to designate surrogate decision-maker	1	2	3	4	5	NA
170207 Willingness to have current living will	1	2	3	4	5	NA

Domain*-Health Knowledge & Behavior (IV)*   ***Class****-Health Beliefs (R)*   *1st edition 1997; reviewed 2024*

OUTCOME CONTENT REFERENCES:

Aschwanden, D., Strickhouser, J. E., Sesker, A. A., Lee, J. H., Luchetti, M., Terracciano, A., & Sutin, A. R. (2021). Preventive behaviors during the COVID-19 pandemic: Associations with perceived behavioral control, attitudes, and subjective norm. *Frontiers in Public Health, 9*, 662835. https://doi.org/10.3389/fpubh.2021.662835

Carpenter, C. J. (2010). A meta-analysis of the effectiveness of Health Belief Model variables in predicting behavior. *Health Communication, 25*, 661–669. https://doi.org/10.1080/10410236.2010.521906

+Champion, V. L. (1993). Instrument refinement for breast cancer screening behaviors. *Nursing Research, 42*(3), 139–143. https://doi.org/10.1097/00006199-199305000-00003

Gillis, A. J. (1993). Determinants of health promoting lifestyle: An integrative review. *Journal of Advanced Nursing, 18*(3), 345–353. https://doi.org/10.1046/j.1365-2648.1993.18030345.x

Rosenstock, I. M. (1974). Historical origins of the Health Belief Model. *Health Education & Behavior, 2*(4), 328–335. https://doi.org/10.1177/109019817400200403.

Rosenstock, I. M., Strecher, V. J., & Becker, M. H. (1988). Social learning theory and the Health Belief Model. *Health Education Quarterly, 15*(2), 175–183. https://doi.org/10.1177/109019818801500203

+Wallston, K. A., & Wallston, B. S. (1981). Health locus of control scales. In H. Lefcourt (Ed.), *Research with the locus of control construct* (Vol. 1, pp. 189–243). Academic Press.

+Wallston, K. A., Wallston, B. S., & DeVellis, R. (1978). Development of the Multidimensional Health Locus of Control (MHLC) Scales. *Health Education Monographs, 6*(2), 160–170. https://doi.org/10.1177/109019817800600107

Zhang, K. C., Fang, Y., Cao, H., Chen, H., Hu, T., Chen, Y. Q., Zhou, X., & Wang, Z. (2020). Parental acceptability of COVID-19 vaccination for children under the age of 18 years: Cross-sectional online survey. *JMIR Pediatrics and Parenting, 3*(2), e24827. https://doi.org/10.2196/24827

H

Health Beliefs: Perceived Resources 1703

Definition: Personal conviction that one has adequate means to carry out a health behavior

OUTCOME TARGET RATING: Maintain at_____ Increase to_____

OUTCOME OVERALL RATING		Very Weak	Weak	Moderate	Strong	Very Strong	
		1	2	3	4	5	
Indicators:							
170301	Perceived support of significant others	1	2	3	4	5	NA
170302	Perceived support of friends	1	2	3	4	5	NA
170303	Perceived support of neighbors	1	2	3	4	5	NA
170304	Perceived support of health provider	1	2	3	4	5	NA
170305	Perceived support of self-help groups	1	2	3	4	5	NA
170306	Perceived functional ability	1	2	3	4	5	NA
170307	Perceived energy to act	1	2	3	4	5	NA
170309	Perceived adequacy of time	1	2	3	4	5	NA
170310	Perceived adequacy of personal finances	1	2	3	4	5	NA
170311	Perceived adequacy of health insurance	1	2	3	4	5	NA
170319	Perceived access to laboratory testing	1	2	3	4	5	NA
170320	Perceived access to vaccine	1	2	3	4	5	NA
170318	Perceived access to medication	1	2	3	4	5	NA
170312	Perceived access to equipment	1	2	3	4	5	NA
170313	Perceived access to supplies	1	2	3	4	5	NA
170314	Perceived access to health care services	1	2	3	4	5	NA
170315	Perceived access to transportation	1	2	3	4	5	NA
170316	Perceived access to physical assistance	1	2	3	4	5	NA

Domain-Health Knowledge & Behavior (IV)   *Class*-Health Beliefs (R)   *1st edition 1997; revised 2004, 2024*

OUTCOME CONTENT REFERENCES:

+Becker, H., Stuifbergen, A. K., & Sands, D. (1991). Development of a scale to measure barriers to health promotion activities among persons with disabilities. *American Journal of Health Promotion, 5*(6), 449–454.

Gillis, A. J. (1993). Determinants of health promoting lifestyle: An integrative review. *Journal of Advanced Nursing, 18*(3), 345–353.

Kim, K. K., Horan, M. L., Gendler, P., & Patel, M. K. (1991). Development and evaluation of the Osteoporosis Health Belief Scale. *Research in Nursing & Health, 14*(2), 155–163.

O'Connor, P. J., Martin, B., Weeks, C. S., & Ong, L. (2014). Factors that influence young people's mental health help-seeking behaviors: A study based on the Health Belief Model. *Journal of Advanced Nursing, 70*, 2577–2587. https://doi.org/10.1111/jan.12423

Robertson, D., & Keller, C. (1992). Relationships among health beliefs, self-efficacy, and exercise adherence in patients with coronary artery disease. *Heart & Lung, 21*(1), 56–63.

Rosenstock, I. M. (1974). Historical origins of the Health Belief Model. *Health Education & Behavior, 2*(4), 328–335. https://doi.org/10.1177/109019817400200403

Rosenstock, I. M., Strecher, V. J., & Becker, M. H. (1988). Social learning theory and the Health Belief Model. *Health Education Quarterly, 15*(2), 175–183. https://doi.org/10.1177/109019818801500203

Zampetakis, L. A., & Melas, C. (2021). The Health Belief Model predicts vaccination intentions against COVID-19: A survey experiment approach. *Applied Psychology. Health and Well-Being, 13*(2), 469–484. https://doi.org/10.1111/aphw.12262

Health Beliefs: Perceived Threat   1704

Definition: Personal conviction that a threatening health problem is serious and has potential negative consequences for lifestyle

OUTCOME TARGET RATING: Maintain at_____ Increase to_____

	Very Weak	Weak	Moderate	Strong	Very Strong	
OUTCOME OVERALL RATING	1	2	3	4	5	
Indicators:						
170401 Perceived threat to health	1	2	3	4	5	NA
170415 Perceived threat of hospitalization	1	2	3	4	5	NA
170403 Perceived vulnerability to progressive health problems	1	2	3	4	5	NA
170404 Concern regarding illness or injury	1	2	3	4	5	NA
170405 Concern regarding potential complications	1	2	3	4	5	NA
170406 Perceived severity of illness or injury	1	2	3	4	5	NA
170407 Perceived severity of complications	1	2	3	4	5	NA
170408 Perceived threat of discomfort from illness or injury	1	2	3	4	5	NA
170409 Perception that condition may be of long duration	1	2	3	4	5	NA
170410 Perceived impact on current lifestyle	1	2	3	4	5	NA
170411 Perceived impact on future lifestyle	1	2	3	4	5	NA
170412 Perceived impact on functional status	1	2	3	4	5	NA
170414 Perceived threat of death	1	2	3	4	5	NA

Domain-Health Knowledge & Behavior (IV)   *Class*-Health Beliefs (R)   *1st edition 1997; revised 2004, 2024*

OUTCOME CONTENT REFERENCES:

Carpenter, C. J. (2010). A meta-analysis of the effectiveness of Health Belief Model variables in predicting behavior. *Health Communication, 25*, 661–669. https://doi.org/10.1080/10410236.2010.521906

+Champion, V. L. (1993). Instrument refinement for breast cancer screening behaviors. *Nursing Research, 42*(3), 139–143. https://doi.org/10.1097/00006199-199305000-00003

Chen, Y., Zhou, R., Chen, B., Chen, H., Li, Y., Chen, Z., Zhu, H., & Wang, H. (2020). Knowledge, perceived beliefs, and preventive behaviors related to COVID-19 among Chinese older adults: Cross-sectional web-based survey. *Journal of Medical Internet Research, 22*(12), e23729. https://doi.org/10.2196/23729

Costa M. F. (2020). Health Belief Model for coronavirus infection risk determinants. *Revista de Saude Publica, 54*, 47. https://doi.org/10.11606/s1518-8787.2020054002494

Fridman, I., Lucas, N., Henke, D., & Zigler, C. K. (2020). Association between public knowledge about COVID-19, trust in information sources, and adherence to social distancing: Cross-sectional survey. *JMIR Public Health and Surveillance, 6*(3), e22060. https://doi.org/10.2196/22060

Maykrantz, S. A., Gong, T., Petrolino, A. V., Nobiling, B. D., & Houghton, J. D. (2021). How trust in information sources influences preventative measures compliance during the COVID-19 pandemic. *International Journal of Environmental Research and Public Health, 18*(11), 5867. https://doi.org/10.3390/ijerph18115867

O'Connor, P. J., Martin, B., Weeks, C. S., & Ong, L. (2014). Factors that influence young people's mental health help-seeking behaviors: A study based on the Health Belief Model. *Journal of Advanced Nursing, 70*, 2577–2587.

Ritchie, D., Van den Broucke, S., & Van Hal, G. (2021). The Health Belief Model and Theory of Planned Behavior applied to mammography screening: A systematic review and meta-analysis. *Public Health Nursing, 38*, 482–492. https://doi.org/10.1111/phn.12842

Rosenstock, I. M. (1974). Historical origins of the Health Belief Model. *Health Education & Behavior, 2*(4), 328–335. https://doi.org/10.1177/109019817400200403.

Rosenstock, I. M., Strecher, V. J., & Becker, M. H. (1988). Social Learning Theory and the Health Belief Model. *Health Education Quarterly, 15*(2), 175–183. https://doi.org/10.1177/109019818801500203

Shmueli, L. (2021). Predicting intention to receive COVID-19 vaccine among the general population using the Health Belief Model and the Theory of Planned Behavior Model. *BMC Public Health, 21*(1), 804. https://doi.org/10.1186/s12889-021-10816-7

Zampetakis, L. A., & Melas, C. (2021). The Health Belief Model predicts vaccination intentions against COVID-19: A survey experiment approach. *Applied Psychology. Health and Well-Being, 13*(2), 469–484. https://doi.org/10.1111/aphw.12262

Zhang, K. C., Fang, Y., Cao, H., Chen, H., Hu, T., Chen, Y. Q., Zhou, X., & Wang, Z. (2020). Parental acceptability of COVID-19 vaccination for children under the age of 18 years: Cross-sectional online survey. *JMIR Pediatrics and Parenting, 3*(2), e24827. https://doi.org/10.2196/24827

Health Insurance Literacy Behavior

2041

Definition: Personal actions to obtain, understand, and evaluate information about health insurance plans, eligibility, coverage, costs, and utilization

OUTCOME TARGET RATING: Maintain at_____ Increase to_____

		Never Demonstrated	Rarely Demonstrated	Sometimes Demonstrated	Often Demonstrated	Consistently Demonstrated	
OUTCOME OVERALL RATING		1	2	3	4	5	
Indicators:							
204101	Verbalizes understanding of benefits of health insurance coverage	1	2	3	4	5	NA
204102	Identifies type of insurance needed based on health needs	1	2	3	4	5	NA
204103	Verbalizes understanding of basic insurance terms	1	2	3	4	5	NA
204104	Explores employer supported plans	1	2	3	4	5	NA
204105	Explores government supported plans	1	2	3	4	5	NA
204106	Determines eligibility for specific insurance plans	1	2	3	4	5	NA
204107	Identifies benefits provided	1	2	3	4	5	NA
204108	Identifies coverage provided	1	2	3	4	5	NA
204109	Identifies premium monthly costs	1	2	3	4	5	NA
204110	Identifies copays required	1	2	3	4	5	NA
204111	Identifies annual benefit limit	1	2	3	4	5	NA
204112	Identifies deductible requirements	1	2	3	4	5	NA
204113	Identifies in-network health providers	1	2	3	4	5	NA
204114	Makes insurance coverage choices based on values	1	2	3	4	5	NA
204115	Makes insurance coverage choices based on medical history	1	2	3	4	5	NA
204116	Makes insurance coverage needs based on family needs	1	2	3	4	5	NA
204117	Asks questions about coverage of specific treatments	1	2	3	4	5	NA
204118	Asks about coverage before obtaining services	1	2	3	4	5	NA
204119	Accesses health care services using insurance coverage	1	2	3	4	5	NA
204120	Competes required insurance forms	1	2	3	4	5	NA

Domain- *Health Knowledge & Behavior (IV)*   **Class-***Health Supporting Life Skills (II)*   *7th edition 2024*

OUTCOME CONTENT REFERENCES:

Adepoju, O., Mask, A., & McLeod, A. (2019). Factors associated with health insurance literacy: Proficiency in finding, selecting, and making appropriate decisions. *Journal of Healthcare Management, 64*(2), 79–89. https://doi.org/10.1097/JHM-D-18-00021

Call, K. T., Conmy, A., Alarcón, G., Hagge, S. L., & Simon, A. H. (2020). Health insurance literacy: How best to measure and does it matter to health care access and affordability? *Research in Social and Administrative Pharmacy, 17*(6), 1166–1173. https://doi.org/10.1016/j.sapharm.2020.09.002

Feinberg, I., Greenberg, D., Tighe, E. L., & Ogrodnick, M. M. (2019). Health insurance literacy and low wage earners: Why reading matters. *Adult Literacy Education, 1*(2), 4–18.

James, T. G., Sullivan, M. K., Dumeny, L., Lindsey, K., Cheong J., & Nicolette, G. (2020). Health insurance literacy and health service utilization among college students. *Journal of American College Health, 68*(2), 200–206. https://doi.org/10.1080/07448481.2018.1538151

McCormack, L., Bann, C., Uhrig, J., Berkman, N., & Rudd, R. (2009). Health insurance literacy of older adults. *The Journal of Consumer Affairs, 43*, 223–248.

Nobles, A. L., Curtis, B. A., Ngo, D. A., Vardell, E., & Holstege, C. P. (2019). Health insurance literacy: A mixed methods study of college students. *Journal of American College Health, 67*(5), 469–478. https://doi.org/10.1080/07448481.2018.1486844

+Paez, K. A., Mallery, C. J., Noel, H., Pugliese, C., McSorley, V. E., Lucado, J. L., & Ganachari, D. (2014). Development of the Health Insurance Literacy Measure (HILM): Conceptualizing and measuring consumer ability to choose and use private health insurance. *Journal of Health Communication, 19* (Suppl 2), 225–239. https://doi.org/10.1080/10810730.2014.936568

Villagra, V. G., Bhuva, B., Coman, E., Smith, D. O., & Fifield, J. (2019). Health insurance literacy: Disparities by race, ethnicity, and language preference. *American Journal of Managed Care, 25*(3), e71–e75.

Yagi, B. F., Luster, J. E., Scherer, A. M., Farron, M. R., Smith, J. E., & Tipirneni, R. (2021). Association of health insurance literacy with health care utilization: A systematic review. *Journal of General Internal Medicine, 37*(2), 375–389. https://doi.org/10.1007/s11606-021-06819-0

Health Literacy Behavior   2015

Definition: Personal actions to obtain, understand, and evaluate information related to health, illness, and available services to make care decisions

OUTCOME TARGET RATING: Maintain at_____ Increase to_____

		Never Demonstrated	Rarely Demonstrated	Sometimes Demonstrated	Often Demonstrated	Consistently Demonstrated	
OUTCOME OVERALL RATING		1	2	3	4	5	
Indicators:							
201501	Identifies personal health needs	1	2	3	4	5	NA
201502	Obtains reputable information relevant to health	1	2	3	4	5	NA
201503	Verbalizes understanding of written information relevant to health	1	2	3	4	5	NA
201504	Verbalizes understanding of verbal information relevant to health	1	2	3	4	5	NA
201505	Verbalizes understanding of visual information relevant to health	1	2	3	4	5	NA
201506	Verbalizes understanding of recommended medication	1	2	3	4	5	NA
201507	Verbalizes understanding of recommended treatment	1	2	3	4	5	NA
201508	Evaluates information relevant to personal health	1	2	3	4	5	NA
201509	Acknowledges patient rights	1	2	3	4	5	NA
201510	Acknowledges patient responsibilities	1	2	3	4	5	NA
201511	Completes health-related documents	1	2	3	4	5	NA
201512	Identifies personal health care preferences	1	2	3	4	5	NA
201513	Identifies health providers	1	2	3	4	5	NA
201514	Identifies preventive services	1	2	3	4	5	NA
201515	Shares questions	1	2	3	4	5	NA
201516	Shares concerns	1	2	3	4	5	NA
201517	Accesses health care services congruent with needs	1	2	3	4	5	NA
201518	Uses personal support system	1	2	3	4	5	NA
201519	Applies health information to personal situation	1	2	3	4	5	NA
201520	Makes informed decisions about health care	1	2	3	4	5	NA
201521	Shares decisions regarding health care	1	2	3	4	5	NA

Domain-Health Knowledge & Behavior (IV)   *Class*-Health Supporting Life Skills (II)   6th edition 2018

OUTCOME CONTENT REFERENCES:

+Chinn, D., & McCarthy, C. (2013). All aspects of Health Literacy Scale (AAHLS): Developing a tool to measure functional, communicative and critical health literacy in primary healthcare settings. *Patient Education and Counseling, 90*(2), 247–253. https://doi.org/10.1016/j.pec.2012.10.019

Macabasco-O'Connell, A., & Fry-Bowers, E. K. (2011). Knowledge and perceptions of health literacy among nursing professionals. *Journal of Health Communication, 16*(9), 295–307. https://doi.org/10.1080/10810730.2011.604389

Nielsen-Bohlman, L., Panzer, A. M., & Kindig, D. A. (Eds.). (2004). *Health literacy: As prescription to end confusion.* National Academies Press.

Nutbeam, D. (2000). Health literacy as a public health goal: A challenge for contemporary health education and communication strategies into the 21st century. *Health Promotion International, 15*(3), 259–267. https://doi.org/10.1093/heapro/15.3.259

Osborne, R., Batterham, R., Elsworth, G., Hawkins, M., & Buchbinder, R. (2013). The grounded psychometric development and initial validation of the Health Literacy Questionnaire (HLQ). *BMC Public Health, 13*(1), 658. https://doi.org/10.1186/1471-2458-13-658

Rosenkilde, L. K., Rowlands, G., Protheroe, J., & Wolf, M. S. (2014, April). Developing a method to derive indicative health literacy from routine socio-economic data. Paper presented at the 2nd European Health Literacy Conference, Aarhus, Denmark.

Rudd, R. E., Groene, O. R., & Navarro-Rubio, M. D. (2013). On health literacy and health outcomes: Background, impact, and future directions. *Revista de Calidad Asistecial, 28*(3), 188–192. https://doi.org/10.1186/s12939-019-1057-4

Schwartzberg, J. G., Cowett, A., VanGeest, J., & Wolf, M. (2007). Communication techniques for patients with low health literacy: A survey of physicians, nurses, and pharmacists. *American Journal of Health Behavior, 31*(Suppl. 1), S96–S104.

H

Sørensen, K., Van den Broucke, S., Fullam, J., Doyle, G., Pelikan, J., Slonska, Z., & Brand, H. (2012). Health literacy and public health: A systematic review and integration of definitions and models. *BMC Public Health, 12*, 80. https://doi.org/10.1186/1471-2458-12-80

Sørensen, K., Van den Broucke, S., Pelikan, J., Fullam, J., Doyle, G., Slonska, Z., Kondilils, B., Stoffels, V., Osborne, R., & Brand, H. (2013). Measuring health literacy in populations: Illuminating the design and development process of the European Health Literacy Survey Questionnaire (HLS-EU-Q), *BMC Public Health, 13*. https://doi.org/10.1186/1471-2458-13-948

Health Orientation 1705

Definition: Personal attitudes and commitment to health behaviors as lifestyle priorities

OUTCOME TARGET RATING: Maintain at_____ Increase to_____

OUTCOME OVERALL RATING	Very Weak	Weak	Moderate	Strong	Very Strong	
	1	2	3	4	5	
Indicators:						
170501 Focus on wellness	1	2	3	4	5	NA
170514 Focus on maintaining health behaviors	1	2	3	4	5	NA
170502 Focus on disease prevention	1	2	3	4	5	NA
170503 Focus on maintaining role performance	1	2	3	4	5	NA
170504 Focus on maintaining functional abilities	1	2	3	4	5	NA
170505 Focus on adjustment to life situations	1	2	3	4	5	NA
170506 Focus on overall well-being	1	2	3	4	5	NA
170516 Focus on paying attention to one's health	1	2	3	4	5	NA
170517 Focus on obtaining reputable health information	1	2	3	4	5	NA
170518 Focus on positive attitude towards health	1	2	3	4	5	NA
170507 Expectation that individual is responsible for health-related choices	1	2	3	4	5	NA
170508 Perception that health behavior is relevant to one's health	1	2	3	4	5	NA
170515 Perception of the importance of incorporating health behaviors with cultural beliefs	1	2	3	4	5	NA
170512 Perception that health is a high priority in making lifestyle choices	1	2	3	4	5	NA

Domain-Health Knowledge & Behavior (IV)   *Class*-Health Beliefs (R)   *1st edition 1997; revised 2004; reviewed 2018*

OUTCOME CONTENT REFERENCES:

Chae, J., & Quick, B. L. (2015). An examination of the relationship between health information use and health orientation in Korean mothers: Focusing on the type of health information. *Journal of Health Communication, 20*(3), 275–284. https://doi.org/10.1080/10810730.2014.925016

Dutta, M. J. (2007). Health information processing from television: The role of health orientation. *Health Communication, 21*(1), 1–9. https://doi.org/10.1080/10410230701283256

Gillis, A. J. (1993). Determinants of health promoting lifestyle: An integrative review. *Journal of Advanced Nursing, 18*(3), 345–353.

Kulbok, P., & Baldwin, J. (1992). From preventive health behavior to health promotion: Advancing a positive construct of health. *Advances in Nursing Science, 14*(4), 50–64.

Pender, N. J., Murdaugh, C. L., & Parsons, M. A. (2014). *Health promotion in nursing practice* (7th ed.). Prentice Hall.

+Walker, S. N., Sechrist, K. R., & Pender, N. J. (1987). The Health-Promoting Lifestyle Profile: Development and psychometric characteristics. *Nursing Research, 36*(2), 76–81.

+Walker, S. N., Sechrist, K. R., & Pender, N. J. (1995). *The Health-Promoting Lifestyle Profile II*. University of Nebraska at Omaha.

Health Promoting Behavior   **1602**

Definition: Personal actions to sustain or increase wellness

OUTCOME TARGET RATING: Maintain at_____ Increase to_____

		Never Demonstrated	Rarely Demonstrated	Sometimes Demonstrated	Often Demonstrated	Consistently Demonstrated	
OUTCOME OVERALL RATING		1	2	3	4	5	
Indicators:							
160201	Uses risk avoidance behaviors	1	2	3	4	5	NA
160202	Monitors environment for risks	1	2	3	4	5	NA
160203	Monitors personal behavior for risks	1	2	3	4	5	NA
160221	Balances activity and rest	1	2	3	4	5	NA
160222	Maintains adequate sleep	1	2	3	4	5	NA
160205	Uses effective stress reduction techniques	1	2	3	4	5	NA
160206	Maintains social relationships	1	2	3	4	5	NA
160207	Performs healthy behaviors routinely	1	2	3	4	5	NA
160208	Supports healthful public policy	1	2	3	4	5	NA
160209	Uses financial resources to promote health	1	2	3	4	5	NA
160210	Uses social support to promote health	1	2	3	4	5	NA
160212	Obtains recommended immunizations	1	2	3	4	5	NA
160213	Obtains recommended health screenings	1	2	3	4	5	NA
160214	Follows healthy diet	1	2	3	4	5	NA
160223	Drinks eight glasses of water daily	1	2	3	4	5	NA
160224	Obtains regular check-ups	1	2	3	4	5	NA
160215	Uses effective weight control strategies	1	2	3	4	5	NA
160216	Uses effective exercise routine	1	2	3	4	5	NA
160226	Practices safe sex	1	2	3	4	5	NA
160227	Maintains oral health	1	2	3	4	5	NA
160217	Avoids exposure to infectious disease	1	2	3	4	5	NA
160225	Avoids exposure to second-hand smoke	1	2	3	4	5	NA
160228	Practices safe driving	1	2	3	4	5	NA
160218	Avoids alcohol misuse	1	2	3	4	5	NA
160219	Avoids tobacco use	1	2	3	4	5	NA
160220	Avoids recreational drug use	1	2	3	4	5	NA

Domain-*Health Knowledge & Behavior (IV)*   **Class**-*Health Behavior (Q)*   *1st edition 1997; revised 2004, 2008, 2024*

OUTCOME CONTENT REFERENCES:

Arif, N., & Qayyum, S. (2019). Health orientation and health-promoting behaviors in women. *Journal of Postgraduate Medical Institute, 33*(1), 34–40.

Daley, E. M., Marhefka, S. L., Wang, W., Noble, C. A., Mahony, H., Arzola, S., Singleton, A., Malmi, M., Ziemba, R., Turner, D., Marwah, E., & Walsh-Buhi, E. R. (2019). Longitudinal evaluation of the Teen Outreach Programme: Impacts of a health promotion programme on risky sexual behaviours. *Health Education Journal, 78*(8), 916–930. https://doi.org/10.1177/0017896919857777

Karataş, T., & Polat, Ü. (2021). Effect of nurse-led program on the exercise behavior of coronary artery patients: Pender's Health Promotion Model. *Patient Education & Counseling, 104*(5), 1183–1192. https://doi.org/10.1016/j.pec.2020.10.003

Maglione, J. L. (2021). Health-promoting behaviors of low-income adults in a community health center. *Journal of Community Health Nursing, 38*(2), 61–72. https://doi.org/10.1080/07370016.2021.1887563

Murdaugh, C. L., Parsons, M. A., & Pender, N. J. (2019). *Health promotion in nursing practice* (8th ed.). Pearson Education.

Park, E., & Chang, Y. (2020). Using digital media to empower adolescents in smoking prevention: Mixed methods study. *JMIR Pediatrics and Parenting, 3*(1), e13031. https://doi.org/10.2196/13031

Ruiz-Palomino, E., Giménez-García, C., Ballester-Arnal, R., & Gil-Llario, M. D. (2020). Health promotion in young people: Identifying the predisposing factors of self-care health habits. *Journal of Health Psychology, 25*(10/11), 1410–1424. https://doi.org/10.1177/1359105318758858

Trisnowati, H., Ismail, D., & Padmawati, R. S. (2021). Health promotion through youth empowerment to prevent and control smoking behavior: A conceptual paper. *Health Education, 121*(3), 275–294. https://doi.org/10.1108/HE-09-2020-0092

+Walker, S. N., Sechrist, K. R., & Pender, N. J. (1987). The Health Promoting Lifestyle Profile: Development and psychometric characteristics. *Nursing Research, 36*(2), 76–81.

+Walker, S. N., Sechrist, K. R., & Pender, N. J. (1995). *The Health Promoting Lifestyle Profile II*. University of Nebraska at Omaha.

Health Seeking Behavior

1603

Definition: Personal actions to promote optimal wellness, recovery, and rehabilitation

OUTCOME TARGET RATING: Maintain at_____ Increase to_____

	Never Demonstrated	Rarely Demonstrated	Sometimes Demonstrated	Often Demonstrated	Consistently Demonstrated	
OUTCOME OVERALL RATING	**1**	**2**	**3**	**4**	**5**	
Indicators:						
160301 Asks health-related questions	1	2	3	4	5	NA
160302 Completes health-related tasks	1	2	3	4	5	NA
160303 Performs self-screening	1	2	3	4	5	NA
160313 Obtains assistance from health professional	1	2	3	4	5	NA
160305 Performs activities of daily living consistent with tolerance	1	2	3	4	5	NA
160306 Describes strategies to eliminate unhealthy behavior	1	2	3	4	5	NA
160314 Performs self-initiated health behavior	1	2	3	4	5	NA
160308 Performs prescribed health behavior	1	2	3	4	5	NA
160315 Uses reputable health information	1	2	3	4	5	NA
160310 Describes strategies to optimize health	1	2	3	4	5	NA
160316 Seeks assistance when needed	1	2	3	4	5	NA

Domain-*Health Knowledge & Behavior (IV)*   **Class**-*Health Behavior (Q)*   *1st edition 1997; revised 2004, 2008, 2013*

OUTCOME CONTENT REFERENCES:

Folden, S. L. (1993). Definitions of health and health goals of participants in a community-based pulmonary rehabilitation program. *Public Health Nursing, 10*(1), 31–35.

Frich, J. C., Ose, L., Malterud, K., & Fugelli, P. (2006). Perceived vulnerability to heart disease in patients with familial hypercholesterolemia: A qualitative interview study. *Annals of Family Medicine, 4*(3), 198–204. https://doi.org/10.1370/afm.529

Jensen, L., & Allen, M. (1993). Wellness: The dialect of illness. *Image—The Journal of Nursing Scholarship, 25*(3), 220–224.

Kaplan, M., Kiernan, N. E., & James, L. (2006). Intergenerational family conversations and decision making about eating healthfully. *Journal of Nutrition Education & Behavior, 38*(5), 298–306. https://doi.org/10.1016/j.jneb.2006.02.010

Macnee, C. L., Edwards, J., Kaplan, A., Reed, S., Bradford, S., Walls, J., & Schaller-Ayers, J. M. (2006). Evaluation of NOC standardized outcome of "Health Seeking Behavior" in nurse-managed clinics. *Journal of Nursing Care Quality, 21*(3), 242–247. https://doi.org/10.1097/00001786-200607000-00009

Mansfield, A. K., Addis, M. E., & Mahalik, J. R. (2003). "Why won't he go to the doctor?" The psychology of men's help seeking. *International Journal of Men's Health, 2*(2), 93–109.

Nicoteri, J. A., & Arnold, E. C. (2005). The development of health care-seeking behaviors in traditional-age undergraduate college students. *Journal of the American Academy of Nurse Practitioners, 17*(10), 411–415. https://doi.org/10.1111/j.1745-7599.2005.00071.x

Pender, N. J. (1990). Expressing health through lifestyle patterns. *Nursing Science Quarterly, 3*(3), 115–122.

Pender, N. J., & Pender, A. R. (1986). Attitudes, subjective norms, and intentions of engage in health behaviors. *Nursing Research, 35*(1), 15–18.

Stevenson, J. S. (2001). Health seeking behaviors. In M. L. Maas, K. C. Buckwalter, M. D. Hardy, T. Tripp-Reimer, M. G. Titler, & J. P. Specht (Eds.), *Nursing care of older adults: Diagnoses, outcomes & interventions* (pp. 75–85). Mosby.

+Walker, S. N., Sechrist, K. R., & Pender, N. J. (1987). The Health Promoting Lifestyle Profile: Development and psychometric characteristics. *Nursing Research, 36*(2), 76–81.

+Walker, S. N., Sechrist, K. R., & Pender, N. J. (1995). *The Health Promoting Lifestyle Profile II*. University of Nebraska at Omaha.

Woods, N. (1989). Conceptualizations of self-care: Toward health-oriented models. *Advances in Nursing Science, 12*(1), 1–13.

Hearing Compensation Behavior   **1610**

Definition: Personal actions to identify, monitor, and compensate for hearing loss

OUTCOME TARGET RATING: Maintain at_____ Increase to_____

		Never Demonstrated	Rarely Demonstrated	Sometimes Demonstrated	Often Demonstrated	Consistently Demonstrated	
OUTCOME OVERALL RATING		1	2	3	4	5	
Indicators:							
161016	Accepts diagnosis of hearing loss	1	2	3	4	5	NA
161017	Obtains reputable information about hearing loss	1	2	3	4	5	NA
161018	Identifies cause of hearing loss with health professional	1	2	3	4	5	NA
161001	Monitors symptoms of hearing deterioration	1	2	3	4	5	NA
161002	Positions self to advantage hearing	1	2	3	4	5	NA
161003	Reminds others to use techniques that advantage hearing	1	2	3	4	5	NA
161004	Eliminates background noise	1	2	3	4	5	NA
161019	Evaluates impact of tinnitus	1	2	3	4	5	NA
161020	Identifies strategies to enhance hearing in public locations	1	2	3	4	5	NA
161005	Uses sign language	1	2	3	4	5	NA
161006	Uses lip reading	1	2	3	4	5	NA
161007	Uses closed captioning for television viewing	1	2	3	4	5	NA
161009	Uses hearing supportive devices	1	2	3	4	5	NA
161012	Uses hearing aids correctly	1	2	3	4	5	NA
161010	Cares for internal hearing assistive devices correctly	1	2	3	4	5	NA
161011	Cares for external hearing assistive devices correctly	1	2	3	4	5	NA
161021	Protects hearing assistive devices from heat and moisture	1	2	3	4	5	NA
161022	Avoids loud noise exposure	1	2	3	4	5	NA
161013	Uses support services for hearing impaired	1	2	3	4	5	NA
161023	Uses smoke alarm with strobe light or vibrating features	1	2	3	4	5	NA
161024	Obtains annual hearing evaluation	1	2	3	4	5	NA

Domain-Health Knowledge & Behavior (IV)   ***Class***-Health Behavior (Q)   2nd edition 2000; revised 2004, 2008, 2024

OUTCOME CONTENT REFERENCES:

Cunningham, L. L., & Tucci, D. L. (2017). Hearing loss in adults. *New England Journal of Medicine, 377*(25), 2465–2473. https://doi.org/10.1056/NEJMra1616601

Hinkle, J. L., & Cheever, K. H. (Eds.). (2018). *Brunner and Suddarth's textbook of medical-surgical nursing* (14th ed.). Wolters Kluwer.

+Houmøller, S. S., Wolff, A., Möller, S., Narne, V. K., Narayanan, S. K., Godballe, C., Hougaard, D. D., Loquet, G., Gaihede, M., Hammershøi, D., & Schmidt, J. H. (2022). Prediction of successful hearing aid treatment in first-time and experienced hearing aid users: Using the International Outcome Inventory for Hearing Aids. *International Journal of Audiology, 61*(2), 119–129. https://doi.org/10.1080/14992027.2021.1916632

Lieu, J. E. C., Kenna, M., Anne, S., & Davidson, L. (2020). Hearing loss in children: A review. *Journal of American Medical Association, 324*(21), 2195–2205. https://doi.org/10.1001/jama.2020.17647

Weycker, J. M., Dillard, L. K., Pinto, A., Fischer, M. E., Cruickshanks, K. J., & Tweed, T. S. (2021). Factors affecting hearing aid adoption by adults with high-frequency hearing loss: The Beaver Dam Offspring Study. *American Journal of Audiology, 30,* 1067–1075. https://doi.org/10.1044/2021_AJA-21-00050

Yuan, Y., Wang, H., Chen, Q., Xie, C., Li, H., Lin, L., & Tian, L. (2021). Illness experience and coping styles of young and middle-aged patients with sudden sensorineural hearing loss: A qualitative study. *BMC Health Services Research, 21*(1), 1–10. https://doi.org/10.1186/s12913-021-06763-z

Heedfulness of Affected Side

0918

Definition: Personal actions to acknowledge, protect, and cognitively integrate affected body part(s) into self

OUTCOME TARGET RATING: Maintain at_____ Increase to_____

		Never Demonstrated	Rarely Demonstrated	Sometimes Demonstrated	Often Demonstrated	Consistently Demonstrated	
OUTCOME OVERALL RATING		1	2	3	4	5	
Indicators:							
091801	Acknowledges affected side as being integral to self	1	2	3	4	5	NA
091802	Protects affected side when ambulating	1	2	3	4	5	NA
091803	Protects affected side when positioning	1	2	3	4	5	NA
091804	Protects affected side when transferring	1	2	3	4	5	NA
091805	Protects affected side during rest or sleep	1	2	3	4	5	NA
091806	Performs daily care to affected side	1	2	3	4	5	NA
091807	Arranges environment to compensate for physical or sensory deficits	1	2	3	4	5	NA
091808	Changes body orientation to enable unaffected side to compensate for physical or sensory deficits	1	2	3	4	5	NA
091809	Uses visual scanning as a compensatory strategy	1	2	3	4	5	NA
091810	Promotes strength and dexterity of affected limb	1	2	3	4	5	NA
091811	Prevents under use of affected limb	1	2	3	4	5	NA
091812	Maintains postural control	1	2	3	4	5	NA

Domain-Physiologic Health (II)   *Class*-Neurocognitive (J)   *4th edition 2008; revised 2013*

OUTCOME CONTENT REFERENCES:

Duncan, P. W., Zorowitz, R., Bates, B., Choi, J. Y., Glasberg, J. J., Graham, G. D., Kats, R. C., Lamberty, K., & Reker, D. (2005). Management of adult stroke rehabilitation care: A clinical practice guideline. *Stroke, 36*(9), e100–143.

Intercollegiate Stroke Working Party. (2004). *National clinical guidelines for stroke* (2nd ed.). Clinical Effectiveness and Evaluation Unit of the Royal College of Physicians.

Punt, T. D., & Riddoch, M. J. (2006). Motor neglect: Implications for movement and rehabilitation following stroke. *Disability and Rehabilitation, 28*(13-14), 857–864. https://doi.org/10.1080/09638280500535025

Slater, D. I., Curtin, S., Johns, J. S., Schmidt, C., Tipton, J. L., & Newbury, R. E. (2006). *Middle cerebral artery stroke.* https://www.emedicine.com/pmr/topic77.htm

Perennou, D. A., Leblond, C., Amblard, B., Micallef, J. P., Herisson, C., & Pelissier, Y. (2001). Transcutaneous electric nerve stimulation reduces neglect-related postural instability after stroke. *Archives of Physical Medicine and Rehabilitation, 82*(4), 440–448.

Ringman, J. M., Saver, J. L., Woolson, R. F., Clarke, W. R., & Adams, H. P. (2004). Frequency, risk factors, anatomy, and course of unilateral neglect in an acute stroke cohort. *Neurology, 63*(3), 468–474. https://doi.org/10.1212/01.wnl.0000133011.10689.ce

Weitzel, E. A. (2001). Unilateral neglect. In M. L. Maas, K. C. Buckwalter, M. D. Hardy, T. Tripp-Reimer, M. G. Titler, & J. P. Specht (Eds.), *Nursing care of older adults: Diagnosis, outcomes, and interventions* (pp. 492–502). Mosby.

Hemodialysis Access   1105

Definition: Functionality of a dialysis access site and health of surrounding tissues

OUTCOME TARGET RATING: Maintain at_____ Increase to_____

		Severely Compromised	Substantially Compromised	Moderately Compromised	Mildly Compromised	Not Compromised	
OUTCOME OVERALL RATING		**1**	**2**	**3**	**4**	**5**	
Indicators:							
110501	Blood volume flow through fistula/shunt	1	2	3	4	5	NA
110502	Site skin color	1	2	3	4	5	NA
110517	Access site skin temperature	1	2	3	4	5	NA
110505	Bruit	1	2	3	4	5	NA
110506	Thrill	1	2	3	4	5	NA
110509	Distal peripheral pulses	1	2	3	4	5	NA
110510	Distal peripheral skin temperature	1	2	3	4	5	NA
110511	Distal peripheral skin color	1	2	3	4	5	NA
110514	Clotting time	1	2	3	4	5	NA
		Severe	**Substantial**	**Moderate**	**Mild**	**None**	
110503	Drainage at site	1	2	3	4	5	NA
110507	Hematoma at site	1	2	3	4	5	NA
110508	Bleeding at site	1	2	3	4	5	NA
110512	Distal peripheral edema	1	2	3	4	5	NA
110515	Tenderness at site	1	2	3	4	5	NA
110513	Cannula displacement	1	2	3	4	5	NA

Domain-Physiologic Health (II)   **Class-***Tissue Integrity (L)*   *2nd edition 2000; revised 2004, 2013*

OUTCOME CONTENT REFERENCES:

Broscious, S. K., & Castagnola, J. (2006). Chronic kidney disease: Acute manifestations and role of critical care nurses. *Critical Care Nurse, 26*(4), 17-28. https://doi.org/10.4037/ccn2006.26.4.17

Eisenbud, M. D. (1996). *The handbook of dialysis access.* Columbus, OH: Anadem.

Gutch, C. F., Stoner, M. H., & Corea, A. L. (1999). *Review of hemodialysis for nurses and dialysis personnel* (6th ed.). Mosby.

Lancaster, L. E. (Ed.). (1995). *ANNA's core curriculum for nephrology nurses* (3rd ed.) (Section X).

Levine, D. Z. (1997). *Caring for the renal patient* (3rd ed.). W.B. Saunders.

Rabani, A., & Jafarian, A. (2005). Function and complications of arteriovenous fistula in chronic hemodialysis patients (a report from two referral centers). *Journal of Medical Council of Islamic Republic of Iran, 22*(4), 369.

Hemodialysis: Disruptive Effects   2306

Definition: Severity of observed or reported disruptive effects of hemodialysis treatments

OUTCOME TARGET RATING: Maintain at _____ Increase to _____

		Severe	Substantial	Moderate	Mild	None	
OUTCOME OVERALL RATING		**1**	**2**	**3**	**4**	**5**	
Indicators:							
230601	Weight gain between treatments	1	2	3	4	5	NA
230602	Nausea	1	2	3	4	5	NA
230603	Vomiting	1	2	3	4	5	NA
230604	Weakness	1	2	3	4	5	NA
230605	Fatigue	1	2	3	4	5	NA

Continued

H

Hemodialysis: Disruptive Effects—cont'd

		Severe	Substantial	Moderate	Mild	None	
230606	Malaise	1	2	3	4	5	NA
230607	Lethargy	1	2	3	4	5	NA
230608	Confusion	1	2	3	4	5	NA
230609	Anorexia	1	2	3	4	5	NA
230610	Constipation	1	2	3	4	5	NA
230611	Insomnia	1	2	3	4	5	NA
230612	Edema	1	2	3	4	5	NA
230613	Ascites	1	2	3	4	5	NA
230614	Dizziness	1	2	3	4	5	NA
230615	Pruritus	1	2	3	4	5	NA
230616	Bleeding	1	2	3	4	5	NA
230617	Bruising at fistula site	1	2	3	4	5	NA
230618	Muscle cramps	1	2	3	4	5	NA
230619	Anemia	1	2	3	4	5	NA
230620	Impaired concentration	1	2	3	4	5	NA
230621	Restless leg syndrome	1	2	3	4	5	NA
230622	Drop in blood pressure during dialysis	1	2	3	4	5	NA

Domain-*Physiologic Health (II)* **Class**-*Therapeutic Response (AA)* 7th edition 2024

OUTCOME CONTENT REFERENCES:

Bossola, M., Di Stasio, E., Monteburini, T., Parodi, E., Ippoliti, F., Bonomini, M., Santarelli, S., Eugenio Nebiolo, P., Sirolli, V., & Cenerelli, S. (2020). Intensity, duration, and frequency of post-dialysis fatigue in patients on chronic hemodialysis. *Journal of Renal Care, 46*(2), 115–123. https://doi.org/10.1111/jorc.12315

Cheng, Y., Li, Y., Zhang, F., Zhu, J., Wang, T., Wei, M., Mo, L., & Li, Y. (2020). Interdialytic blood pressure variability and the risk of stroke in maintenance hemodialysis patients. *Medicine, 99*(29), e21232. https://doi.org/10.1097/MD.0000000000021232

Fleishman, T. T., Dreiher, J., & Shvartzman, P. (2020). Patient-reported outcomes in maintenance hemodialysis: A cross-sectional, multicenter study. *Quality of Life Research, 29*(9), 2345–2354. https://doi.org/10.1007/s11136-020-02508-3

Kong, J. H., Davies, M. R. P., & Mount, P. F. (2021). Relationship between residual kidney function and symptom burden in haemodialysis patients. *Internal Medicine Journal, 51*(1), 52–61. https://doi.org/10.1111/imj.14775

National Kidney Foundation (2015). KDOQI clinical practice guideline for hemodialysis adequacy: 2015 update. *American Journal of Kidney Diseases: The official journal of the National Kidney Foundation, 66*(5), 884–930. https://doi.org/10.1053/j.ajkd.2015.07.015

Renz Pretto, C., Winkelmann, E. R., Hildebrandt, L. M., Aparecida Barbosa, D., de Fátima Colet, C., & Fernandes Stumm, E. M. (2020). Quality of life of chronic kidney patients on hemodialysis and related factors. *Revista Latino-Americana de Enfermagem (RLAE), 28*, 1–11. https://doi.org/10.1590/1518-8345.3641.3327

Hoarding Behavior Severity 1222

Definition: Severity of a persistent drive to acquire items with difficulty discarding or parting with possessions that may have little value leading to clutter that disrupts the use of living or workspaces.

OUTCOME TARGET RATING: Maintain at_____ Increase to_____

		Severe	Substantial	Moderate	Mild	None	
OUTCOME OVERALL RATING		1	2	3	4	5	
Indicators:							
122201	Emotional drive to buy items	1	2	3	4	5	NA
122202	Emotional drive to acquire free items	1	2	3	4	5	NA
122203	Lack of space to store possessions	1	2	3	4	5	NA

Hoarding Behavior Severity—cont'd

		Severe	Substantial	Moderate	Mild	None	
122204	Difficulty throwing items away	1	2	3	4	5	NA
122205	Degree of emotional distress with discarding items	1	2	3	4	5	NA
122206	Degree of emotional connection to possessions	1	2	3	4	5	NA
122207	Amount of clutter in living spaces	1	2	3	4	5	NA
122208	Desire to retains items that are not needed	1	2	3	4	5	NA
122209	Desire to keep items even when space is limited	1	2	3	4	5	NA
122210	Lack of livable space in home because of clutter	1	2	3	4	5	NA
122211	Inability to invite others to home because of clutter	1	2	3	4	5	NA
122212	Inability to work because of lack of useable space	1	2	3	4	5	NA
122213	Inability to easily walk-through home because of clutter	1	2	3	4	5	NA
122214	Anxiety from thoughts of throwing away unneeded items	1	2	3	4	5	NA
122215	Emotional distress with living environment	1	2	3	4	5	NA
122216	Conflict with family because of hoarding behaviors	1	2	3	4	5	NA
122217	Safety issues related to hoarding environment	1	2	3	4	5	NA
122218	Sanitation issues related to hoarding environment	1	2	3	4	5	NA
122219	Social isolation related to hoarding	1	2	3	4	5	NA
122220	Depression level associated with hoarding	1	2	3	4	5	NA
122221	Financial burden of hoarding	1	2	3	4	5	NA
122222	Risk of eviction from home	1	2	3	4	5	NA

Domain--*Psychosocial Health (III)*   **Class-**-*Psychological Well-Being (M)*   *7th edition 2024*

OUTCOME CONTENT REFERENCES:
Bodryzlova, Y., Audet, J. S., Bergeron, K., & O'Connor, K. (2019). Group cognitive-behavioural therapy for hoarding disorder: Systematic review and meta-analysis. *Health & Social Care in the Community, 27*, 517– 530. https://doi.org/10.1111/hsc.12598
Carey, E. A., de Bolger, A. D. P., & Wootton, B. M. (2019). Psychometric properties of the hoarding disorder-dimensional scale. *Journal of Obsessive-Compulsive and Related Disorders, 21*, 91–96.
Dozier, M. E., Davidson, E. J., Pittman, J. O., & Ayers, C. R. (2020). Personality traits in adults with hoarding disorder. *Journal of Affective Disorders, 276*, 191–196.
Frost, R. O., Steketee, G., & Grisham, J. (2004). Measurement of compulsive hoarding: Saving inventory- revised. *Behaviour Research and Therapy, 42*(10), 1163–1182. https://doi.org/10.1016/j.brat.2003.07.006
McCabe-Bennett, H., Lachman, R., Girard, T. A., & Antony, M. M. (2020). A virtual reality study of the relationships between hoarding, clutter, and claustrophobia. *CyberPsychology, Behavior & Social Networking, 23*(2), 83–89. https://doi.org/10.1089/cyber.2019.0320
Roane, D. M., Landers, A., Sherratt, J., & Wilson, G. S. (2017). Hoarding in the elderly: A critical review of the recent literature. *International Psychogeriatrics, 29*(7), 1077–1084. https://doi.org/10.1017/S1041610216002465
Robertson, L., Paparo, J., & Wootton, B. M. (2020). Understanding barriers to treatment and treatment delivery preferences for individuals with symptoms of hoarding disorder: A preliminary study. *Journal of Obsessive-Compulsive and Related Disorders, 26*, 100560.
+Tolin, D. F., Frost, R. O., & Steketee, G. (2010). A brief interview for assessing compulsive hoarding: The Hoarding Rating Scale-Interview. *Psychiatry Research, 178*(1), 147–152. https://doi.org/10.1016/j.psychres.2009.05.001
Varcarolis, E. M., & Fosbre, C. D. (2021). *Essential of psychiatric-mental health nursing: A communication approach to evidence-based practice* (4th ed.). Elsevier.

Hoarding Cessation Behavior

1413

Definition: Personal actions to minimize the drive to acquire items and the difficulty associated with discarding or parting with household possessions that may have little value

OUTCOME TARGET RATING: Maintain at_____ Increase to_____

		Never Demonstrated	Rarely Demonstrated	Sometimes Demonstrated	Often Demonstrated	Consistently Demonstrated	
OUTCOME OVERALL RATING		1	2	3	4	5	
Indicators:							
141301	Monitors emotional drive to buy items	1	2	3	4	5	NA
141302	Monitors emotional drive to acquire free items	1	2	3	4	5	NA
141303	Evaluates space available to store possessions	1	2	3	4	5	NA
141304	Categorizes items into keep or discard	1	2	3	4	5	NA
141305	Handles items only once when sorting	1	2	3	4	5	NA
141306	Recognizes emotional distress level with discarding items	1	2	3	4	5	NA
141307	Recognizes emotional connection to possessions	1	2	3	4	5	NA
141308	Uses strategies to reduce emotional attachment to possessions	1	2	3	4	5	NA
141309	Recognizes desire to retain items that are not needed	1	2	3	4	5	NA
141310	Evaluates lack of livable space in home due to clutter	1	2	3	4	5	NA
141311	Removes trash from home	1	2	3	4	5	NA
141312	Recognizes inability to invite others to home because of clutter	1	2	3	4	5	NA
141313	Acknowledges inability to work because of lack of useable space	1	2	3	4	5	NA
141314	Acknowledges inability to easily walk-through home because of clutter	1	2	3	4	5	NA
141315	Recognizes anxiety level from thoughts of throwing away items	1	2	3	4	5	NA
141316	Acknowledges distress with living environment	1	2	3	4	5	NA
141317	Reduces amount of clutter in living spaces	1	2	3	4	5	NA
141318	Removes clutter from walkways	1	2	3	4	5	NA
141319	Removes clutter from beds and furniture	1	2	3	4	5	NA
141320	Reduces conflict with family because of hoarding behaviors	1	2	3	4	5	NA
141321	Removes safety issues related to hoarding environment	1	2	3	4	5	NA
141322	Reduces sanitation issues related to hoarding environment	1	2	3	4	5	NA
141323	Reduces social isolation related to hoarding	1	2	3	4	5	NA
141324	Monitors depression level associated with hoarding	1	2	3	4	5	NA
141325	Uses strategies to reinforce new behaviors	1	2	3	4	5	NA
141326	Reduces financial burden of hoarding	1	2	3	4	5	NA
141327	Reduces risk of eviction from home	1	2	3	4	5	NA

Domain-Health Knowledge & Behavior (IV) *Class*- Health Behavior (Q) *7th edition 2024*

OUTCOME CONTENT REFERENCES:
Bodryzlova, Y., Audet, J. S., Bergeron, K., & O'Connor, K. (2019). Group cognitive-behavioural therapy for hoarding disorder: Systematic review and meta-analysis. *Health & Social Care in the Community, 27*, 517–530. https://doi.org/10.1111/hsc.12598
Bratiotis, C., Sorrentino-Schmalisch, C., & Steketee, G. (2011). *The hoarding handbook.* Oxford University Press.
Carey, E. A., de Bolger, A. D. P., & Wootton, B. M. (2019). Psychometric properties of the hoarding disorder-dimensional scale. *Journal of Obsessive-Compulsive and Related Disorders, 21*, 91–96. https://doi.org/10.1016/j.jocrd.2018.01.003
Chater, C., Shaw, J., & McKay, S. M. (2013). Hoarding in the home, *Home Healthcare Nurse, 31*(3), 144–154. https://doi.org/10.1097/NHH.0b013e3182838847
Dacey, E. (2020). *Reclaim your life from hoarding: Practical strategies for decluttering your home, organizing your space, and freeing yourself.* Rockridge Press.
Dozier, M. E., Davidson, E. J., Pittman, J. O., & Ayers, C. R. (2020). Personality traits in adults with hoarding disorder. *Journal of Affective Disorders, 276*, 191–196. https://doi.org/10.1016/j.jad.2020.07.033
+Frost, R. O., Steketee, G., & Grisham, J. (2004). Measurement of compulsive hoarding: Saving Inventory- revised. *Behaviour Research and Therapy, 42*(10), 1163–1182. https://doi.org/10.1016/j.brat.2003.07.006
McCabe-Bennett, H., Lachman, R., Girard, T. A., & Antony, M. M. (2020). A virtual reality study of the relationships between hoarding, clutter, and claustrophobia. *CyberPsychology, Behavior & Social Networking, 23*(2), 83–89. https://doi.org/10.1089/cyber.2019.0320
Roane, D. M., Landers, A., Sherratt, J., & Wilson, G. S. (2017). Hoarding in the elderly: A critical review of the recent literature. *International Psychogeriatrics, 29*(7), 1077–1084. https://doi.org/10.1017/S1041610216002465
Robertson, L., Paparo, J., & Wootton, B. M. (2020). Understanding barriers to treatment and treatment delivery preferences for individuals with symptoms of hoarding disorder: A preliminary study. *Journal of Obsessive-Compulsive and Related Disorders, 26*, 100560.
+Tolin, D. F., Frost, R. O., & Steketee, G. (2010). A brief interview for assessing compulsive hoarding: The Hoarding Rating Scale-Interview. *Psychiatry Research, 178*(1), 147–152. https://doi.org/10.1016/j.psychres.2009.05.001
Varcarolis, E. M., & Fosbre, C.D. (2021). *Essentials of psychiatric-mental health nursing: A communication approach to evidence-based practice* (4th ed.). Elsevier.
Yap, K., & Grisham, J. R. (2020). Object attachment and emotions in hoarding disorder. *Comprehensive Psychiatry, 100*, 152179. https://doi.org/10.1016/j.comppsych.2020.152179

H

Hope   1201

Definition: Optimism that is personally satisfying and life-supporting

OUTCOME TARGET RATING: Maintain at_____ Increase to_____

		Never Demonstrated	Rarely Demonstrated	Sometimes Demonstrated	Often Demonstrated	Consistently Demonstrated	
OUTCOME OVERALL RATING		1	2	3	4	5	
Indicators:							
120101	Expresses expectation of a positive future	1	2	3	4	5	NA
120102	Expresses faith	1	2	3	4	5	NA
120103	Expresses will to live	1	2	3	4	5	NA
120104	Expresses reasons to live	1	2	3	4	5	NA
120105	Expresses meaning and purpose in life	1	2	3	4	5	NA
120106	Expresses optimism	1	2	3	4	5	NA
120107	Expresses belief in self	1	2	3	4	5	NA
120108	Expresses belief in others	1	2	3	4	5	NA
120109	Expresses inner peace	1	2	3	4	5	NA
120110	Expresses sense of self-control	1	2	3	4	5	NA
120111	Exhibits enthusiasm for life	1	2	3	4	5	NA
120114	Uses social support	1	2	3	4	5	NA
120112	Sets goals for the future	1	2	3	4	5	NA

Domain-*Psychosocial Health (III)*   **Class**-*Psychological Well-Being (M)*   *1st edition 1997; revised 2004, 2018*

OUTCOME CONTENT REFERENCES:
+Beckman, E. E., Leber, W. R., Watkins, J. T., Boyer, J. L., & Cook, J. B. (1986). Development of an instrument to measure Beck's cognitive triad: The Cognitive Triad Inventory. *Journal of Consulting and Clinical Psychology, 54*(4), 566–567.
Beck, A., Weissman, A., Lester, D., & Trexler, L. (1974). The measurement of pessimism: The Hopelessness Scale. *Journal of Consulting and Clinical Psychology, 42*(6), 861–865.
Duggleby, W., Hicks, D., Nekolaichuk, C., Holtslander, L., Williams, A., Chambers, T., & Eby, J. (2012). Hope, older adults, and chronic illness: A metasynthesis of qualitative research. *Journal of Advanced Nursing, 68*(6), 1211–1223. https://doi.org/10.1111/j.1365-2648.2011.05919.x
Griggs, S., & Walker, R. (2016). The role of hope for adolescents with a chronic illness: An integrative review. *Journal of Pediatric Nursing, 31*(4), 404–421. https://doi.org/10.1016/j.pedn.2016.02.011

Hydration   **0602**

Definition: Adequate water in the intracellular and extracellular compartments of the body

OUTCOME TARGET RATING: Maintain at_____ Increase to_____

		Severely Compromised	Substantially Compromised	Moderately Compromised	Mildly Compromised	Not Compromised	
OUTCOME OVERALL RATING		1	2	3	4	5	
Indicators:							
060228	Body weight fluctuations	1	2	3	4	5	NA
060229	Sensation of thirst	1	2	3	4	5	NA
060201	Skin turgor	1	2	3	4	5	NA
060230	Skin moisture	1	2	3	4	5	NA
060202	Moist mucous membranes	1	2	3	4	5	NA
060231	Perspiration with exercise	1	2	3	4	5	NA
060215	Fluid intake in recommended levels	1	2	3	4	5	NA
060211	Urine output 5 to 8 times per day	1	2	3	4	5	NA
060232	Urine osmolality	1	2	3	4	5	NA
060233	Urine specific gravity	1	2	3	4	5	NA
060234	Urine color	1	2	3	4	5	NA
060216	Serum sodium	1	2	3	4	5	NA
060235	Serum osmolality	1	2	3	4	5	NA
060236	Vital signs	1	2	3	4	5	NA
060217	Tissue perfusion	1	2	3	4	5	NA
060218	Cognitive function	1	2	3	4	5	NA

Domain-*Physiologic Health (II)*   **Class**-*Fluid & Electrolytes (G)*   *1st edition 1997; revised 2004, 2013, 2024*

OUTCOME CONTENT REFERENCES:

Ashraf, M. M., & Rea, R. (2017). Effect of dehydration on blood tests. *Practical Diabetes, 34*(5), 169–171. https://doi.org/10.1002/pdi.2111

Bahouth, M. N., Gottesman, R. F., & Szanton, S. L. (2018). Primary 'dehydration' and acute stroke: A systematic research review. *Journal of Neurology, 265*(10), 2167–2181. https://doi.org/10.1007/s00415-018-8799-6

Barrado, M. Y., Hatter, L., Moore, K. J., Sampson, E. L., Rait, G., Manthorpe, J., Smith, C. H., Nair, P., & Davies, N. (2021). Nutrition and hydration for people living with dementia near the end of life: A qualitative systematic review. *Journal of Advanced Nursing, 77*(2), 664–680. https://doi.org/10.1111/jan.14654

Huether, S. E., McCance, K. L., & Brashers, V. L. (2020). *Understanding pathophysiology* (7th ed.). Elsevier.

Ignatavicius, D. D., Workman, M. L., Rebar, C. R., & Heimgartner, N. M. (2021). *Medical-surgical nursing: Concepts for interprofessional care* (10th ed.). Elsevier.

Kavouras, S. A. (2002). Assessing hydration status. *Current Opinion in Clinical Nutrition and Metabolic Care, 5*(5), 519–524.

Kear, T. M. (2017). Fluid and electrolyte management across the age continuum. *Nephrology Nursing Journal, 44*(6), 491–497.

Potter, P. A., & Perry, A. G. (2021). *Fundamentals of nursing* (10th ed.). Elsevier.

Perrier, E. T., Armstrong, L. E., Bottin, J. H., Clark, W. F., Dolci, A., Guelinckx, I., Iroz, A., Kavouras, S. A., Lang, F., Lieberman, H. R., Melander, O., Morin, C., Seksek, I., Stookey, J. D., Tack, I., Vanhaecke, T., Vecchio, M., & Péronnet, F. (2021). Hydration for health hypothesis: A narrative review of supporting evidence. *European Journal of Nutrition, 60*(3), 1167–1180. https://doi.org/10.1007/s00394-020-02296-z

Reddi, A. S. (2018). *Fluid, electrolyte, and acid-base disorders: Clinical evaluation and management* (2nd ed.). Springer.

Hyperactivity Level   **0915**

Definition: Severity of persistent patterns of impulsivity in a child

OUTCOME TARGET RATING: Maintain at_____ Increase to_____

		Severe	Substantial	Moderate	Mild	None	
OUTCOME OVERALL RATING		1	2	3	4	5	
Indicators:							
091511	Impulsivity	1	2	3	4	5	NA
091528	Excessive fidgeting of hands or feet	1	2	3	4	5	NA
091529	Squirms in seat	1	2	3	4	5	NA

Hyperactivity Level—cont'd

		Severe	Substantial	Moderate	Mild	None	
091513	Inability to remain seated	1	2	3	4	5	NA
091526	Excessive running	1	2	3	4	5	NA
091527	Excessive climbing	1	2	3	4	5	NA
091515	Excessive motor behavior	1	2	3	4	5	NA
091516	Difficulty playing quietly	1	2	3	4	5	NA
091530	Always "on the go" as if driven by a motor	1	2	3	4	5	NA
091517	Excessive talking	1	2	3	4	5	NA
091518	Blurts out answers before the question is completed	1	2	3	4	5	NA
091519	Difficulty waiting turn	1	2	3	4	5	NA
091520	Excessive interrupting of others	1	2	3	4	5	NA
091521	Intrusive, abrasive, loud, interpersonal interactions	1	2	3	4	5	NA
091522	Inappropriate aggressive behavior	1	2	3	4	5	NA
091523	Difficulty keeping hands to self	1	2	3	4	5	NA
091531	Uses other person's things without permission	1	2	3	4	5	NA
091532	Takes over what others are doing	1	2	3	4	5	NA
091533	Inappropriate social skills	1	2	3	4	5	NA
091534	Immaturity relative to chronological age	1	2	3	4	5	NA

Domain-*Physiologic Health (II)*   **Class**-*Neurocognitive (J)*   *3rd edition 2004; revised 2008, 2024*

OUTCOME CONTENT REFERENCES:
American Psychiatric Association. (2022). *Diagnostic and statistical manual of mental disorders* (5th ed., text rev.) https://doi.org/10.1176/appi.books.9780890425787
Balázs, J., & Keresztény, Á. (2014). Subthreshold attention deficit hyperactivity in children and adolescents: A systematic review. *European Child & Adolescent Psychiatry, 23*(6), 393–408. https://doi.org/10.1007/s00787-013-0514-7
Caldwell, C. L., Wasson, D., Anderson, M. A., Brighton, V., & Dixon, L. (2005). Development of the nursing outcome (NOC) label: Hyperactivity Level. *Journal of Child and Adolescent Psychiatric Nursing, 18*(3), 95–102. https://doi.org/10.1111/j.1744-6171.2005.00004.x
Hechtman, L. (2000). Assessment and diagnosis of attention deficit/hyperactive disorder. *Child and Adolescent Psychiatric Clinics of North America, 9*(3), 481–498.
Hockenberry, M. J., Wilson, D., & Rodgers, C. C. (Eds.). (2019). *Wong's nursing care of infants and children* (11th ed.). Elsevier.
+Øvergaard, K. R., Oerbeck, B., Friis, S., Pripp, A. H., Biele, G., Aase, H., & Zeiner, P. (2018). Attention-deficit/hyperactivity disorder in preschoolers: The accuracy of a short screener. *Journal of the American Academy of Child & Adolescent Psychiatry, 57*(6), 428–435. https://doi.org/10.1016/j.jaac.2018.03.008
Tandon, M., & Pergjika, A. (2017). Attention deficit hyperactivity disorder in preschool-age children. *Child and Adolescent Psychiatric Clinics, 26*(3). 523–538.

Hypercalcemia Severity   0607

Definition: Severity of signs and symptoms of increased serum calcium

OUTCOME TARGET RATING: Maintain at_____ Increase to_____

		Severe	Substantial	Moderate	Mild	None	
OUTCOME OVERALL RATING		1	2	3	4	5	
Indicators:							
060701	Increase in serum calcium	1	2	3	4	5	NA
060702	Electrocardiogram changes	1	2	3	4	5	NA
060703	Decreased heart rate	1	2	3	4	5	NA
060704	Increased blood pressure	1	2	3	4	5	NA
060705	Muscle weakness	1	2	3	4	5	NA
060706	Muscle pain	1	2	3	4	5	NA
060707	Decreased coordination	1	2	3	4	5	NA

Continued

Hypercalcemia Severity—cont'd

		Severe	Substantial	Moderate	Mild	None	
060708	Constipation	1	2	3	4	5	NA
060709	Anorexia	1	2	3	4	5	NA
060710	Nausea	1	2	3	4	5	NA
060711	Vomiting	1	2	3	4	5	NA
060712	Abdominal pain	1	2	3	4	5	NA
060713	Bone pain	1	2	3	4	5	NA
060714	Increased urine output	1	2	3	4	5	NA
060715	Thirst	1	2	3	4	5	NA
060716	Dehydration	1	2	3	4	5	NA
060717	Hypoactive deep tendon reflexes	1	2	3	4	5	NA
060718	Pathological fractures	1	2	3	4	5	NA
060719	Urinary tract stones	1	2	3	4	5	NA
060720	Impaired memory	1	2	3	4	5	NA
060721	Confusion	1	2	3	4	5	NA
060722	Headaches	1	2	3	4	5	NA
060723	Depression	1	2	3	4	5	NA
060724	Lethargy	1	2	3	4	5	NA
060725	Acute psychosis	1	2	3	4	5	NA
060726	Coma	1	2	3	4	5	NA

Domain-Physiologic Health (II)   *Class*-Fluid & Electrolytes (G)   *5th edition 2013; reviewed 2024*

OUTCOME CONTENT REFERENCES:
Bauldoff, G., Gubrud, P., & Carno, M. (2019). *Medical-surgical nursing: Critical thinking in patient care* (7th ed.). Pearson.
Hinkle, J. L., & Cheever, K. H. (2018). *Brunner & Suddarth's textbook of medical-surgical nursing* (14th ed.). Wolter Kluwer.
Hockenberry, M. J., Wilson, D., & Rodgers, C. C. (Eds.). (2019). *Wong's nursing care of infants and children* (11th ed.). Elsevier.
Huether, S. E., McCance, K. L., & Brashers, V. L. (2020). *Understanding pathophysiology* (7th ed.). Elsevier.
Ignatavicius, D. D., Workman, M. L., Rebar, C. R., & Heimgartner, N. M. (2021). *Medical-surgical nursing: Concepts for interprofessional care* (10th ed.). Elsevier.
Kear, T. M. (2017). Fluid and electrolyte management across the age continuum. *Nephrology Nursing Journal, 44*(6), 491–497.
Potter, P. A., & Perry, A. G. (2021). *Fundamentals of nursing* (10th ed.). Elsevier.
Reddi, A. S. (2018). *Fluid, electrolyte, and acid-base disorders: Clinical evaluation and management* (2nd ed.). Springer.

Hyperchloremia Severity   0608

Definition: Severity of signs and symptoms of increased serum chloride

OUTCOME TARGET RATING: Maintain at_____ Increase to_____

		Severe	Substantial	Moderate	Mild	None	
OUTCOME OVERALL RATING		1	2	3	4	5	
Indicators:							
060801	Increase in serum chloride	1	2	3	4	5	NA
060802	Increase in serum sodium	1	2	3	4	5	NA
060803	Decrease in serum pH	1	2	3	4	5	NA
060804	Decrease in serum bicarbonate	1	2	3	4	5	NA
060805	Increase in urine chloride	1	2	3	4	5	NA
060806	Increased respiratory rate	1	2	3	4	5	NA
060807	Increased depth of respirations	1	2	3	4	5	NA

Hyperchloremia Severity—cont'd

		Severe	Substantial	Moderate	Mild	None	
060808	Hypertension	1	2	3	4	5	NA
060809	Dyspnea	1	2	3	4	5	NA
060810	Lethargy	1	2	3	4	5	NA
060811	Weakness	1	2	3	4	5	NA
060812	Impaired cognition	1	2	3	4	5	NA
060813	Increased heart rate	1	2	3	4	5	NA
060814	Arrhythmias	1	2	3	4	5	NA
060815	Pitting edema	1	2	3	4	5	NA
060816	Coma	1	2	3	4	5	NA

Domain-*Physiologic Health (II)*   **Class**-*Fluid & Electrolytes (G)*   *5th edition 2013; reviewed 2024*

OUTCOME CONTENT REFERENCES:

Hinkle, J. L., & Cheever, K. H. (2018). *Brunner & Suddarth's textbook of medical-surgical nursing* (14th ed.). Wolter Kluwer.
Huether, S. E., McCance, K. L., & Brashers, V. L. (2020). *Understanding pathophysiology* (7th ed.). Elsevier.
Ignatavicius, D. D., Workman, M. L., Rebar, C. R., & Heimgartner, N. M. (2021). *Medical-surgical nursing: Concepts for interprofessional care* (10th ed.). Elsevier.
Martínez, R. M., Viñas, T., Manrique, G., & López-Herce, J. (2020). Hyperchloremia and hypernatremia in critically ill children. *Medicina Intensiva, 45*(9), e59–e61. https://doi.org/10.1016/j.medin.2020.10.002
Potter, P. A., & Perry, A. G. (2021). *Fundamentals of nursing* (10th ed.). Elsevier.
Reddi, A. S. (2018). *Fluid, electrolyte, and acid-base disorders: Clinical evaluation and management* (2nd ed.). Springer.

H

Hyperglycemia Severity   **2111**

Definition: Severity of signs and symptoms of elevated blood glucose levels

OUTCOME TARGET RATING: Maintain at_____ Increase to_____

		Severe	Substantial	Moderate	Mild	None	
OUTCOME OVERALL RATING		1	2	3	4	5	
Indicators:							
211123	Flushed appearance	1	2	3	4	5	NA
211101	Increased urine output	1	2	3	4	5	NA
211102	Increased thirst	1	2	3	4	5	NA
211103	Excessive hunger	1	2	3	4	5	NA
211104	Malaise	1	2	3	4	5	NA
211119	Weakness	1	2	3	4	5	NA
211105	Fatigue	1	2	3	4	5	NA
211106	Headaches	1	2	3	4	5	NA
211107	Blurred vision	1	2	3	4	5	NA
211108	Unexplained weight loss	1	2	3	4	5	NA
211109	Loss of appetite	1	2	3	4	5	NA
211110	Nausea	1	2	3	4	5	NA
211120	Dehydration	1	2	3	4	5	NA
211111	Dry mouth	1	2	3	4	5	NA
211112	Fruity breath	1	2	3	4	5	NA
211121	Weak pulse	1	2	3	4	5	NA
211113	Yeast infections	1	2	3	4	5	NA

Continued

Hyperglycemia Severity—cont'd

		Severe	Substantial	Moderate	Mild	None	
211114	Electrolyte disturbances	1	2	3	4	5	NA
211115	Impaired concentration	1	2	3	4	5	NA
211116	Mental status changes	1	2	3	4	5	NA
211122	Elevated urine ketones	1	2	3	4	5	NA
211117	Elevated blood glucose	1	2	3	4	5	NA
211118	Elevated A1C (glycated hemoglobin)	1	2	3	4	5	NA

Domain-Health & Life Quality (V)   **Class**-Symptom Status (V)   5th edition 2013; revised 2024

OUTCOME CONTENT REFERENCES:

American Diabetes Association. (2021). 6 Glycemic Targets: Standards of medical care in diabetes—2021. *Diabetes Care, 44*(Suppl 1), S73–S84. https://doi.org/10.2337/dc21-S006

Hockenberry, M. J., Rodgers, C. C., & Wilson, D. (Eds.). (2022). *Wong's essentials of pediatric nursing* (11th ed.). Elsevier.

Huether, S. E., McCance, K .L., & Brashers, V .L. (2020). *Understanding pathophysiology* (7th ed.). Elsevier.

Ignatavicius, D. D., Workman, M. L., Rebar, C. R., & Heimgartner, N. M. (2021). *Medical-surgical nursing: Concepts for interprofessional care* (10th ed.). Elsevier.

Lee, P. G., & Halter, J. B. (2017). The pathophysiology of hyperglycemia in older adults: Clinical considerations. *Diabetes Care, 40*(4), 444–452. https://doi.org/10.2337/dc16-1732

Wilson, W. E. (2021). *Handbook of diagnostic endocrinology* (3rd ed.). Elsevier.

Hyperkalemia Severity

0609

Definition: Severity of signs and symptoms of increased serum potassium

OUTCOME TARGET RATING: Maintain at_____ Increase to_____

		Severe	Substantial	Moderate	Mild	None	
OUTCOME OVERALL RATING		1	2	3	4	5	
Indicators:							
060901	Increase in serum potassium	1	2	3	4	5	NA
060902	Electrocardiogram changes	1	2	3	4	5	NA
060903	Increased heart rate	1	2	3	4	5	NA
060904	Decreased blood pressure	1	2	3	4	5	NA
060905	Arrhythmias	1	2	3	4	5	NA
060906	Anxiety	1	2	3	4	5	NA
060907	Muscle weakness	1	2	3	4	5	NA
060908	Flaccid paralysis	1	2	3	4	5	NA
060909	Paresthesias	1	2	3	4	5	NA
060910	Nausea	1	2	3	4	5	NA
060911	Intestinal colic	1	2	3	4	5	NA
060912	Abdominal cramps	1	2	3	4	5	NA
060913	Diarrhea	1	2	3	4	5	NA
060914	Neuromuscular irritability	1	2	3	4	5	NA
060915	Restlessness	1	2	3	4	5	NA
060916	Headache	1	2	3	4	5	NA
060917	Seizures	1	2	3	4	5	NA
060918	Coma	1	2	3	4	5	NA

Domain-Physiologic Health (II)   **Class**-Fluid & Electrolytes (G)   5th edition 2013; reviewed 2024

OUTCOME CONTENT REFERENCES:

Hinkle, J. L., & Cheever, K. H. (2018). *Brunner & Suddarth's textbook of medical-surgical nursing* (14th ed.). Wolter Kluwer.

Hockenberry, M. J., Wilson, D., & Rodgers, C. C. (Eds.). (2019). *Wong's nursing care of infants and children* (11th ed.). Elsevier.

Huether, S. E., McCance, K. L., & Brashers, V. L. (2020). *Understanding pathophysiology* (7th ed.). Elsevier.

Ignatavicius, D. D., Workman, M. L., Rebar, C. R., & Heimgartner, N. M. (2021). *Medical-surgical nursing: Concepts for interprofessional care* (10th ed.). Elsevier.

Kear, T. M. (2017). Fluid and electrolyte management across the age continuum. *Nephrology Nursing Journal, 44*(6), 491–497.

Potter, P. A., & Perry, A. G. (2021). *Fundamentals of nursing* (10th ed.). Elsevier.

Reddi, A. S. (2018). *Fluid, electrolyte, and acid-base disorders: Clinical evaluation and management* (2nd ed.). Springer.

Wetmore, J. B., Yan, H., Peng, Y., Gilbertson, D. T., & Herzog, C. A. (2021). Development and outcomes of hyperkalemia in hospitalized patients: Potential implications for care. *American Heart Journal, 241,* 59–67. https://doi.org/10.1016/j.ahj.2021.07.006

Hypermagnesemia Severity

0610

Definition: Severity of signs and symptoms of increased serum magnesium

OUTCOME TARGET RATING: Maintain at_____ Increase to_____

		Severe	Substantial	Moderate	Mild	None	
OUTCOME OVERALL RATING		**1**	**2**	**3**	**4**	**5**	
Indicators:							
061001	Increase in serum magnesium	1	2	3	4	5	NA
061002	Decreased blood pressure	1	2	3	4	5	NA
061003	Electrocardiogram changes	1	2	3	4	5	NA
061004	Decreased heart rate	1	2	3	4	5	NA
061005	Decreased respiratory rate	1	2	3	4	5	NA
061018	Respiratory distress	1	2	3	4	5	NA
061006	Hypoactive deep tendon reflexes	1	2	3	4	5	NA
061007	Soft tissue calcifications	1	2	3	4	5	NA
061008	Clumping of platelets	1	2	3	4	5	NA
061009	Delayed thrombin formation	1	2	3	4	5	NA
061010	Nausea	1	2	3	4	5	NA
061011	Vomiting	1	2	3	4	5	NA
061012	Weakness	1	2	3	4	5	NA
061013	Flushing	1	2	3.	4	5	NA
061014	Diaphoresis	1	2	3	4	5	NA
061015	Drowsiness	1	2	3	4	5	NA
061016	Cardiac arrest	1	2	3	4	5	NA
061017	Coma	1	2	3	4	5	NA

Domain-*Physiologic Health (II)*   **Class**-*Fluid & Electrolytes (G)*   *5th edition 2013; revised 2024*

OUTCOME CONTENT REFERENCES:

Elsevier. (2021). *Mosby's dictionary of medicine, nursing, and health professions* (11th ed.).

Hinkle, J. L., & Cheever, K. H. (2018). *Brunner & Suddarth's textbook of medical-surgical nursing* (14th ed.). Wolter Kluwer.

Hockenberry, M. J., Wilson, D., & Rodgers, C. C. (Eds.). (2019). *Wong's nursing care of infants and children* (11th ed.). Elsevier.

Huether, S. E., McCance, K. L., & Brashers, V. L. (2020). *Understanding pathophysiology* (7th ed.). Elsevier.

Ignatavicius, D. D., Workman, M. L., Rebar, C. R., & Heimgartner, N. M. (2021). *Medical-surgical nursing: Concepts for interprofessional care* (10th ed.). Elsevier.

Potter, P. A., & Perry, A. G. (2021). *Fundamentals of nursing* (10th ed.). Elsevier.

Reddi, A. S. (2018). *Fluid, electrolyte, and acid-base disorders: Clinical evaluation and management* (2nd ed.). Springer.

H

Hypernatremia Severity 0611

Definition: Severity of signs and symptoms of increased serum sodium

OUTCOME TARGET RATING: Maintain at_____ Increase to_____

		Severe	Substantial	Moderate	Mild	None	
OUTCOME OVERALL RATING		1	2	3	4	5	
Indicators:							
061101	Increase in serum sodium	1	2	3	4	5	NA
061102	Increased urine output	1	2	3	4	5	NA
061103	Decrease in urine sodium	1	2	3	4	5	NA
061104	Increase in urine specific gravity	1	2	3	4	5	NA
061105	Increased blood pressure	1	2	3	4	5	NA
061106	Increased heart rate	1	2	3	4	5	NA
061122	Dry skin	1	2	3	4	5	NA
061123	Dry mucous membranes	1	2	3	4	5	NA
061108	Thirst	1	2	3	4	5	NA
061124	Sweating	1	2	3	4	5	NA
061109	Anorexia	1	2	3	4	5	NA
061110	Nausea	1	2	3	4	5	NA
061111	Vomiting	1	2	3	4	5	NA
061112	Headache	1	2	3	4	5	NA
061113	Restlessness	1	2	3	4	5	NA
061114	Dizziness	1	2	3	4	5	NA
061115	Confusion	1	2	3	4	5	NA
061125	Weakness	1	2	3	4	5	NA
061126	Lethargy	1	2	3	4	5	NA
061127	Agitation	1	2	3	4	5	NA
061128	Peripheral edema	1	2	3	4	5	NA
061116	Muscle twitching	1	2	3	4	5	NA
061117	Seizures	1	2	3	4	5	NA
061118	Pulmonary edema	1	2	3	4	5	NA
061119	Weight gain	1	2	3	4	5	NA
061120	Papilledema	1	2	3	4	5	NA
061121	Coma	1	2	3	4	5	NA

Domain-*Physiologic Health (II)*   **Class**-*Fluid & Electrolytes (G)*   *5th edition 2013; revised 2024*

OUTCOME CONTENT REFERENCES:

Bertschi, L. A. (2020). Concentration and volume: Understanding sodium and water in the body: The etiology of dysnatremia can be complex. *AJN, American Journal of Nursing, 120*(1), 51–56. https://doi.org/10.1097/01.naj.0000652120.20393.19

Elsevier. (2021). *Mosby's dictionary of medicine, nursing, and health professions* (11th ed.).

Hinkle, J. L., & Cheever, K. H. (2018). *Brunner & Suddarth's textbook of medical-surgical nursing* (14th ed.). Wolter Kluwer.

Hockenberry, M. J., Wilson, D., & Rodgers, C. C. (Eds.). (2019). *Wong's nursing care of infants and children* (11th ed.). Elsevier.

Huether, S. E., McCance, K. L., & Brashers, V. L. (2020). *Understanding pathophysiology* (7th ed.). Elsevier.

Ignatavicius, D. D., Workman, M. L., Rebar, C. R., & Heimgartner, N. M. (2021). *Medical-surgical nursing: Concepts for interprofessional care* (10th ed.). Elsevier.

Kear, T. M. (2017). Fluid and electrolyte management across the age continuum. *Nephrology Nursing Journal, 44*(6), 491–497.

Metheny, N. A., & Krieger, M. M. (2020). Salt toxicity: A systematic review and case reports. *JEN: Journal of Emergency Nursing, 46*(4), 428–439. https://doi.org/10.1016/j.jen.2020.02.011

Potter, P. A., & Perry, A. G. (2021). *Fundamentals of nursing* (10th ed.). Elsevier.

Reddi, A. S. (2018). *Fluid, electrolyte, and acid-base disorders: Clinical evaluation and management* (2nd ed.). Springer.

Seay, N. W., Lehrich, R. W., & Greenberg, A. (2020). Diagnosis and management of disorders of body tonicity-hyponatremia and hypernatremia: Core curriculum. *American Journal of Kidney Diseases, 75*(2), 272–286. https://doi.org/10.1053/j.ajkd.2019.07.014

Hyperphosphatemia Severity   0612

Definition: Severity of signs and symptoms of increased serum phosphorus

OUTCOME TARGET RATING: Maintain at_____ Increase to_____

		Severe	Substantial	Moderate	Mild	None	
OUTCOME OVERALL RATING		1	2	3	4	5	
Indicators:							
061201	Increase in serum phosphorus	1	2	3	4	5	NA
061219	Decrease in serum calcium	1	2	3	4	5	NA
061202	Decreased blood pressure	1	2	3	4	5	NA
061203	Arrhythmias	1	2	3	4	5	NA
061204	Increased heart rate	1	2	3	4	5	NA
061222	Palpitations	1	2	3	4	5	NA
061205	Numbness	1	2	3	4	5	NA
061206	Tingling of fingers and hands	1	2	3	4	5	NA
061207	Tingling around mouth	1	2	3	4	5	NA
061208	Muscle cramps	1	2	3	4	5	NA
061209	Muscle spasms	1	2	3	4	5	NA
061210	Muscle weakness	1	2	3	4	5	NA
061211	Hyperactive deep tendon reflexes	1	2	3	4	5	NA
061212	Anorexia	1	2	3	4	5	NA
061213	Nausea	1	2	3	4	5	NA
061214	Vomiting	1	2	3	4	5	NA
061220	Decreased urine output	1	2	3	4	5	NA
061221	Impaired vision	1	2	3	4	5	NA
061215	Tetany	1	2	3	4	5	NA
061216	Seizures	1	2	3	4	5	NA
061217	Vascular calcifications	1	2	3	4	5	NA
061218	Soft tissue calcifications	1	2	3	4	5	NA

Domain-*Physiologic Health (II)*   **Class**-*Fluid & Electrolytes (G)*   *5th edition 2013; revised 2024*

OUTCOME CONTENT REFERENCES:
Hinkle, J. L., & Cheever, K. H. (2018). *Brunner & Suddarth's textbook of medical-surgical nursing* (14th ed.). Wolter Kluwer.
Huether, S. E., McCance, K. L., & Brashers, V. L. (2020). *Understanding pathophysiology* (7th ed.). Elsevier.
Koumakis, E., Cormier, C., Roux, C., & Briot, K. (2020). The causes of hypo- and hyperphosphatemia in humans. *Calcified Tissue International, 108*(1),41–73. https://doi.org/10.1007/s00223-020-00664-9
Martín, A. G., Varsavsky, M., Berdonces, M. C., Rubio, V. A., Exposito, M. R. A., Rodríguez, C. N., Moreno, P. R., Muñoz, M. R., Gimeno, E. J., Ortega, P. R., & Torres, M. M. (2020). Phosphate disorders and the clinical management of hypophosphatemia and hyperphosphatemia. *Endocrinology, Diabetes and Nutrition* (English ed.), *67*(3), 205–215. https://doi.org/10.1016/j.endinu.2019.06.004
Reddi, A. S. (2018). *Fluid, electrolyte, and acid-base disorders: Clinical evaluation and management* (2nd ed.). Springer.

H

Hypertension Severity

2112

Definition: Severity of signs and symptoms of chronic elevated blood pressure

OUTCOME TARGET RATING: Maintain at_____ Increase to_____

OUTCOME OVERALL RATING		Severe	Substantial	Moderate	Mild	None	
		1	2	3	4	5	
Indicators:							
211201	Fatigue	1	2	3	4	5	NA
211202	Nosebleeds	1	2	3	4	5	NA
211203	Irregular heartbeat	1	2	3	4	5	NA
211204	Blurred vision	1	2	3	4	5	NA
211205	Temporary paralysis	1	2	3	4	5	NA
211206	Alterations in speech	1	2	3	4	5	NA
211207	Headaches	1	2	3	4	5	NA
211208	Dizziness	1	2	3	4	5	NA
211209	Breathlessness	1	2	3	4	5	NA
211210	Excessive sweating	1	2	3	4	5	NA
211211	Nocturia	1	2	3	4	5	NA
211212	Tinnitus	1	2	3	4	5	NA
211213	Confusion	1	2	3	4	5	NA
211214	Convulsions	1	2	3	4	5	NA
211215	Nausea	1	2	3	4	5	NA
211216	Elevation of systolic blood pressure	1	2	3	4	5	NA
211217	Elevation of diastolic blood pressure	1	2	3	4	5	NA

Domain-*Health & Life Quality (V)*   **Class**-*Symptom Status (V)*   *5th edition 2013*

OUTCOME CONTENT REFERENCES:

Chummun, H. (2009). Hypertension-a contemporary approach to nursing care. *British Journal of Nursing, 18*(13), 784–789.

DeSimone, M. E., & Crowe, A. (2009). Nonpharmacological approaches in the management of hypertension. *Journal of the American Academy of Nurse Practitioners, 21*(4), 189–196. https://doi.org/10.1111/j.1745-7599.2009.00395.x

Good, L. B. (2010). Hypertension highlights: Blood pressure targets, global risk factors, and diabetes: The latest data are not encouraging. *Medscape Cardiology.* Retrieved from www.medscape.com/viewarticle/715584

Guidelines and Protocols Advisory Committee. (2008). *Hypertension-detection, diagnosis and management.* http://www.bcguidelines.ca/gpac/guideline_hypertension.html

National Heart, Lung, and Blood Institute (NHLBI). (2003). JNC 7 express: The seventh report of the Joint National Committee on Prevention, Detection, Evaluation, and Treatment of High Blood Pressure.

Hypocalcemia Severity

0613

Definition: Severity of signs and symptoms of decreased serum calcium

OUTCOME TARGET RATING: Maintain at_____ Increase to_____

OUTCOME OVERALL RATING		Severe	Substantial	Moderate	Mild	None	
		1	2	3	4	5	
Indicators:							
061301	Decrease in serum calcium	1	2	3	4	5	NA
061330	Decrease in serum magnesium	1	2	3	4	5	NA
061302	Decreased clotting time	1	2	3	4	5	NA
061331	Decreased blood pressure	1	2	3	4	5	NA

Hypocalcemia Severity—cont'd

		Severe	Substantial	Moderate	Mild	None	
061303	Decreased heart rate	1	2	3	4	5	NA
061304	Electrocardiogram changes	1	2	3	4	5	NA
061305	Hypotension	1	2	3	4	5	NA
061306	Anxiety	1	2	3	4	5	NA
061332	Irritability	1	2	3	4	5	NA
061307	Pain	1	2	3	4	5	NA
061308	Numbness of extremities	1	2	3	4	5	NA
061309	Tingling of fingers and toes	1	2	3	4	5	NA
061310	Tingling around mouth	1	2	3	4	5	NA
061311	Hyperactive deep tendon reflexes	1	2	3	4	5	NA
061313	Bone pain	1	2	3	4	5	NA
061314	Bone fracture	1	2	3	4	5	NA
061315	Positive Trousseau's sign	1	2	3	4	5	NA
061316	Positive Chvostek's sign	1	2	3	4	5	NA
061317	Muscle cramps	1	2	3	4	5	NA
061318	Carpopedal spasms	1	2	3	4	5	NA
061319	Laryngeal spasms	1	2	3	4	5	NA
061320	Bronchospasm	1	2	3	4	5	NA
061321	Neuromuscular irritability	1	2	3	4	5	NA
061322	Depression	1	2	3	4	5	NA
061323	Confusion	1	2	3	4	5	NA
061324	Impaired memory	1	2	3	4	5	NA
061325	Delirium	1	2	3	4	5	NA
061326	Hallucinations	1	2	3	4	5	NA
061333	Diarrhea	1	2	3	4	5	NA
061327	Tetany	1	2	3	4	5	NA
061328	Seizures	1	2	3	4	5	NA
061329	Increased urine output	1	2	3	4	5	NA

Domain-*Physiologic Health (II)*   **Class**-*Fluid & Electrolytes (G)*   *5th edition 2013; revised 2024*

OUTCOME CONTENT REFERENCES:

Bakon, S., Craft, J., & Christensen, M. (2019). Hypocalcaemia-induced tetany secondary to total thyroidectomy: A nursing case review. *Nursing in Critical Care*, *24*(6), 349–354. https://doi.org/10.1111/nicc.12309

Elsevier. (2021). *Mosby's dictionary of medicine, nursing, and health professions* (11th ed.).

Hinkle, J. L., & Cheever, K. H. (2018). *Brunner & Suddarth's textbook of medical-surgical nursing* (14th ed.). Wolter Kluwer.

Hockenberry, M. J., Wilson, D., & Rodgers, C. C. (Eds.). (2019). *Wong's nursing care of infants and children* (11th ed.). Elsevier.

Huether, S. E., McCance, K. L., & Brashers, V. L. (2020). *Understanding pathophysiology* (7th ed.). Elsevier.

Ignatavicius, D. D., Workman, M. L., Rebar, C. R., & Heimgartner, N. M. (2021). *Medical-surgical nursing: Concepts for interprofessional care* (10th ed.). Elsevier.

Kear, T. M. (2017). Fluid and electrolyte management across the age continuum. *Nephrology Nursing Journal, 44*(6), 491–497.

McMurran, A. E. L., Blundell, R., & Kim, V. (2020). Predictors of post-thyroidectomy hypocalcemia: A systematic and narrative review. *Journal of Laryngology & Otology, 134*(6), 541–552. https://doi.org/10.1017/S0022215120001024

Potter, P. A., & Perry, A. G. (2021). *Fundamentals of nursing* (10th ed.). Elsevier.

Vasudeva, M., Mathew, J. K., Groombridge, C., Tee, J. W., Johnny, C. S., Maini, A., & Fitzgerald, M. C. (2021). Hypocalcemia in trauma patients: A systematic review. *Journal of Trauma and Acute Care Surgery, 90*(2), 396–402. https://doi.org/10.1097/TA.0000000000003027

Hypochloremia Severity   0614

Definition: Severity of signs and symptoms of decreased serum chloride

OUTCOME TARGET RATING: Maintain at_____ Increase to_____

		Severe	Substantial	Moderate	Mild	None	
OUTCOME OVERALL RATING		1	2	3	4	5	
Indicators:							
061401	Decrease in serum chloride	1	2	3	4	5	NA
061402	Decrease in serum sodium	1	2	3	4	5	NA
061418	Decrease in serum potassium	1	2	3	4	5	NA
061403	Increase in serum pH	1	2	3	4	5	NA
061404	Increase in serum bicarbonate	1	2	3	4	5	NA
061405	Increase in serum carbon dioxide	1	2	3	4	5	NA
061406	Decrease in urine chloride	1	2	3	4	5	NA
061407	Agitation	1	2	3	4	5	NA
061418	Irritability	1	2	3	4	5	NA
061420	Arrhythmias	1	2	3	4	5	NA
061408	Neuromuscular irritability	1	2	3	4	5	NA
061409	Tremors	1	2	3	4	5	NA
061410	Muscle cramps	1	2	3	4	5	NA
061411	Hyperactive deep tendon reflexes	1	2	3	4	5	NA
061412	Tetany	1	2	3	4	5	NA
061413	Decreased respiratory rate	1	2	3	4	5	NA
061414	Shallow respirations	1	2	3	4	5	NA
061415	Arrhythmias	1	2	3	4	5	NA
061416	Seizures	1	2	3	4	5	NA
061417	Coma	1	2	3	4	5	NA

Domain-*Physiologic Health (II)*   **Class**-*Fluid & Electrolytes (G)*   5th edition 2013; revised 2024

OUTCOME CONTENT REFERENCES:
Cuthbert, J. J., Bhandari, S., & Clark, A. L. (2020). Hypochloraemia in patients with heart failure: Causes and consequences. *Cardiology Therapy, 9*(2), 333–347. https://doi.org/10.1007/s40119-020-00194-3
Hinkle, J. L., & Cheever, K. H. (2018). *Brunner & Suddarth's textbook of medical-surgical nursing* (14th ed.). Wolter Kluwer.
Huether, S. E. McCance, K. L., & Brashers, V. L. (2020). *Understanding pathophysiology* (7th ed.). Elsevier.
Ignatavicius, D. D., Workman, M. L., Rebar, C. R., & Heimgartner, N. M. (2021). *Medical-surgical nursing: Concepts for interprofessional care* (10th ed.). Elsevier.
Potter, P. A., & Perry, A. G. (2021). *Fundamentals of nursing* (10th ed.). Elsevier.
Reddi, A. S. (2018). *Fluid, electrolyte, and acid-base disorders: Clinical evaluation and management* (2nd ed.). Springer.

Hypoglycemia Severity   2113

Definition: Severity of signs and symptoms of decreased blood glucose levels

OUTCOME TARGET RATING: Maintain at_____ Increase to_____

		Severe	Substantial	Moderate	Mild	None	
OUTCOME OVERALL RATING		1	2	3	4	5	
Indicators:							
211323	Pallor	1	2	3	4	5	NA
211301	Shakiness	1	2	3	4	5	NA
211302	Sweating	1	2	3	4	5	NA

Hypoglycemia Severity—cont'd

		Severe	Substantial	Moderate	Mild	None	
211303	Nervousness	1	2	3	4	5	NA
211327	Chills	1	2	3	4	5	NA
211324	Anxiety	1	2	3	4	5	NA
211325	Tachycardia	1	2	3	4	5	NA
211304	Heart palpitations	1	2	3	4	5	NA
211305	Light-headedness	1	2	3	4	5	NA
211306	Hunger	1	2	3	4	5	NA
211326	Diaphoresis	1	2	3	4	5	NA
211307	Weakness	1	2	3	4	5	NA
211308	Dizziness	1	2	3	4	5	NA
211309	Sleepiness	1	2	3	4	5	NA
211310	Impaired vision	1	2	3	4	5	NA
211311	Nightmares	1	2	3	4	5	NA
211312	Irritability	1	2	3	4	5	NA
211313	Fatigue	1	2	3	4	5	NA
211314	Headaches	1	2	3	4	5	NA
211315	Paresthesia	1	2	3	4	5	NA
211316	Slurred speech	1	2	3	4	5	NA
211317	Impaired concentration	1	2	3	4	5	NA
211328	Poor judgement	1	2	3	4	5	NA
211318	Abnormal behavior	1	2	3	4	5	NA
211319	Confusion	1	2	3	4	5	NA
211320	Seizure	1	2	3	4	5	NA
211321	Coma	1	2	3	4	5	NA
211322	Decreased blood glucose levels	1	2	3	4	5	NA

Domain-*Health & Life Quality (V)*   **Class**-*Symptom Status (V)*   5th edition 2013; revised 2024

OUTCOME CONTENT REFERENCES:

American Diabetes Association. (2021). 6 Glycemic Targets: Standards of medical care in diabetes-2021. *Diabetes Care, 44*(Suppl 1), S73–S84. https://doi.org/10.2337/dc21-S006.

Fanelli, C. G., Lucidi, P., Bolli, G. B., Porcellati, F. (2020). Hypoglycemia. In Bonora E., & DeFronzo R. (Eds*). Diabetes complications, comorbidities and related disorders. endocrinology* (pp. 615–952). Springer. https://doi.org/10.1007/978-3-030-36694-0_22

Gómez, A. M., Imitola, A., Henao, D., García-Jaramillo, M., Giménez, M., Viñals, C., Grassi, B., Torres, M., Zuluaga, I., Muñoz, O. M., Rondón, M., León-Vargas, F., & Conget, I. (2021). Factors associated with clinically significant hypoglycemia in patients with type 1 diabetes using sensor-augmented pump therapy with predictive low-glucose management: A multicentric study on Iberoamerica. *Diabetes & Metabolic Syndrome: Clinical Research & Reviews, 15*(1), 267–272. https://doi.org/10.1016/j.dsx.2021.01.002

Hockenberry, M. J., Rodgers, C. C., & Wilson, D. (Eds.). (2022). *Wong's essentials of pediatric nursing* (11th ed.). Elsevier.

Huether, S. E., McCance, K. L., & Brashers, V.L. (2020). *Understanding pathophysiology* (7th ed.). Elsevier.

Ignatavicius, D. D., Workman, M. L., Rebar, C. R., & Heimgartner, N. M. (2021). *Medical-surgical nursing: Concepts for interprofessional care* (10th ed.). Elsevier.

Vijayakumar, P., Liu, S., McCoy, R. G., Karter, A. J., & Lipska, K. J. (2020). Changes in management of type 2 diabetes before and after severe hypoglycemia. *Diabetes Care, 43*(11), e188–e189. https://doi.org/10.2337/dc20-0458

Wilson, W. E. (2021). *Handbook of diagnostic endocrinology* (3rd ed.). Elsevier.

H

Hypokalemia Severity

0615

Definition: Severity of signs and symptoms of decreased serum potassium

OUTCOME TARGET RATING: Maintain at_____ Increase to_____

OUTCOME OVERALL RATING		Severe	Substantial	Moderate	Mild	None	
		1	2	3	4	5	
Indicators:							
061501	Decrease in serum potassium	1	2	3	4	5	NA
061502	Orthostatic hypotension	1	2	3	4	5	NA
061503	Decreased blood pressure	1	2	3	4	5	NA
061504	Arrhythmias	1	2	3	4	5	NA
061505	Changes in electrocardiogram	1	2	3	4	5	NA
061506	Fatigue	1	2	3	4	5	NA
061507	Lethargy	1	2	3	4	5	NA
061508	Apathy	1	2	3	4	5	NA
061509	Mental depression	1	2	3	4	5	NA
061510	Confusion	1	2	3	4	5	NA
061511	Anorexia	1	2	3	4	5	NA
061512	Nausea	1	2	3	4	5	NA
061513	Vomiting	1	2	3	4	5	NA
061514	Decreased bowel motility	1	2	3	4	5	NA
061515	Constipation	1	2	3	4	5	NA
061516	Polyuria	1	2	3	4	5	NA
061517	Abdominal distention	1	2	3	4	5	NA
061518	Muscle weakness	1	2	3	4	5	NA
061519	Decreased muscle tone	1	2	3	4	5	NA
061520	Flaccid paralysis	1	2	3	4	5	NA
061521	Paresthesias	1	2	3	4	5	NA
061522	Leg cramps	1	2	3	4	5	NA
061523	Hypoactive deep tendon reflexes	1	2	3	4	5	NA
061524	Coma	1	2	3	4	5	NA

Domain-*Physiologic Health (II)* **Class**-*Fluid & Electrolytes (G)* *5th edition 2013; reviewed 2024*

OUTCOME CONTENT REFERENCES:

Hinkle, J. L., & Cheever, K. H. (2018). *Brunner & Suddarth's textbook of medical-surgical nursing* (14th ed.). Wolter Kluwer.

Hirsch, T. M., & Braun, D. (2021). Hypokalemia. *JAAPA: Journal of the American Academy of Physician Assistants, 34*(1), 50–51. https://doi.org/10.1097/01.JAA.0000723960.54308.e9

Hockenberry, M. J., Wilson, D., & Rodgers, C. C. (Eds.). (2019). *Wong's nursing care of infants and children* (11th ed.). Elsevier.

Hoorn, E. J., Bovée, D. M., Geerse, D. A., Visser, W. J., & Geerse, D. (2020). Diet-exercise-induced hypokalemic metabolic alkalosis. *American Journal of Medicine, 133*(11), e667–e669. https://doi.org/10.1016/j.amjmed.2020.04.019

Huether, S. E., McCance, K. L., & Brashers, V. L. (2020). *Understanding pathophysiology* (7th ed.). Elsevier.

Ignatavicius, D. D., Workman, M. L., Rebar, C. R., & Heimgartner, N. M. (2021). *Medical-surgical nursing: Concepts for interprofessional care* (10th ed.). Elsevier.

Kear, T. M. (2017). Fluid and electrolyte management across the age continuum. *Nephrology Nursing Journal, 44*(6), 491–497.

Kwon, Y. E., Oh, D.-J., & Choi, H. M. (2020). Severe asymptomatic hypokalemia associated with prolonged licorice ingestion: A case report. *Medicine, 99*(30), 1–4. https://doi.org/10.1097/MD.0000000000021094

Potter, P. A., & Perry, A. G. (2021). *Fundamentals of nursing* (10th ed.). Elsevier.

Reddi, A. S. (2018). *Fluid, electrolyte, and acid-base disorders: Clinical evaluation and management* (2nd ed.). Springer.

H

Hypomagnesemia Severity 0616

Definition: Severity of signs and symptoms of decreased serum magnesium

OUTCOME TARGET RATING: Maintain at_____ Increase to_____

		Severe	Substantial	Moderate	Mild	None	
OUTCOME OVERALL RATING		1	2	3	4	5	
Indicators:							
061601	Decrease in serum magnesium	1	2	3	4	5	NA
061602	Increased blood pressure	1	2	3	4	5	NA
061603	Electrocardiogram changes	1	2	3	4	5	NA
061604	Neuromuscular irritability	1	2	3	4	5	NA
061605	Positive Babinski	1	2	3	4	5	NA
061606	Positive Trousseau's sign	1	2	3	4	5	NA
061607	Positive Chvostek's sign	1	2	3	4	5	NA
061608	Hyperactive deep tendon reflexes	1	2	3	4	5	NA
061609	Leg cramps	1	2	3	4	5	NA
061610	Nausea	1	2	3	4	5	NA
061611	Vomiting	1	2	3	4	5	NA
061622	Dysphagia	1	2	3	4	5	NA
061612	Mood changes	1	2	3	4	5	NA
061613	Vertigo	1	2	3	4	5	NA
061614	Depression	1	2	3	4	5	NA
061615	Agitation	1	2	3	4	5	NA
061616	Apprehension	1	2	3	4	5	NA
061623	Anorexia	1	2	3	4	5	NA
061617	Delirium	1	2	3	4	5	NA
061618	Confusion	1	2	3	4	5	NA
061619	Psychosis	1	2	3	4	5	NA
061620	Insomnia	1	2	3	4	5	NA
061621	Combativeness	1	2	3	4	5	NA

Domain-*Physiologic Health (II)*   **Class**-*Fluid & Electrolytes (G)*   *5th edition 2013; revised 2024*

OUTCOME CONTENT REFERENCES:
Elsevier. (2021). *Mosby's dictionary of medicine, nursing, and health professions* (11th ed.).
Hinkle, J. L., & Cheever, K. H. (2018). *Brunner & Suddarth's textbook of medical-surgical nursing* (14th ed.). Wolter Kluwer.
Hockenberry, M. J., Wilson, D., & Rodgers, C. C. (Eds.). (2019). *Wong's nursing care of infants and children* (11th ed.). Elsevier.
Huether, S. E., McCance, K. L., & Brashers, V. L. (2020). *Understanding pathophysiology* (7th ed.). Elsevier.
Ignatavicius, D. D., Workman, M. L., Rebar, C. R., & Heimgartner, N. M. (2021). *Medical-surgical nursing: Concepts for interprofessional care* (10th ed.). Elsevier.
Potter, P. A., & Perry, A. G. (2021). *Fundamentals of nursing* (10th ed.). Elsevier.
Reddi, A. S. (2018). *Fluid, electrolyte, and acid-base disorders: Clinical evaluation and management* (2nd ed.). Springer.

Hyponatremia Severity   0617

Definition: Severity of signs and symptoms of decreased serum sodium

OUTCOME TARGET RATING: Maintain at_____ Increase to_____

		Severe	Substantial	Moderate	Mild	None	
OUTCOME OVERALL RATING		1	2	3	4	5	
Indicators:							
061701	Decrease in serum sodium	1	2	3	4	5	NA
061702	Decrease in urine sodium	1	2	3	4	5	NA
061703	Decrease in urine specific gravity	1	2	3	4	5	NA
061704	Orthostatic hypotension	1	2	3	4	5	NA
061705	Decreased blood pressure	1	2	3	4	5	NA
061706	Increased heart rate	1	2	3	4	5	NA
061724	Dry skin	1	2	3	4	5	NA
061725	Dry mucous membranes	1	2	3	4	5	NA
061708	Anorexia	1	2	3	4	5	NA
061709	Nausea	1	2	3	4	5	NA
061710	Vomiting	1	2	3	4	5	NA
061711	Headache	1	2	3	4	5	NA
061712	Apathy	1	2	3	4	5	NA
061713	Impaired concentration	1	2	3	4	5	NA
061714	Lethargy	1	2	3	4	5	NA
061715	Fatigue	1	2	3	4	5	NA
061716	Dizziness	1	2	3	4	5	NA
061717	Confusion	1	2	3	4	5	NA
061718	Muscle cramps	1	2	3	4	5	NA
061719	Muscle weakness	1	2	3	4	5	NA
061720	Muscle twitching	1	2	3	4	5	NA
061726	Gait disturbances	1	2	3	4	5	NA
061727	Falls	1	2	3	4	5	NA
061728	Osteoporosis	1	2	3	4	5	NA
061729	Fractures	1	2	3	4	5	NA
061721	Seizures	1	2	3	4	5	NA
061722	Edema	1	2	3	4	5	NA
061723	Weight gain	1	2	3	4	5	NA

Domain-*Physiologic Health (II)*   **Class**-*Fluid & Electrolytes (G)*   *5th edition 2013; revised 2024*

OUTCOME CONTENT REFERENCES:

Bertschi, L. A. (2020). Concentration and volume: Understanding sodium and water in the body: The etiology of dysnatremia can be complex. *AJN, American Journal of Nursing, 120*(1), 51–56. https://doi.org/10.1097/01.naj.0000652120.20393.19

Felver, L. (2018). Fluid and electrolyte homeostasis and imbalances. In Banasik, J. L., & Copstead, L. E. C. (Eds.), *Pathophysiology* (6th ed., pp. 521–540). Elsevier.

Gankam Kengne, F., & Decaux, G. (2017). Hyponatremia and the brain. *Kidney International Reports, 3*(1), 24–35. https://doi.org/10.1016/j.ekir.2017.08.015

Hinkle, J. L., & Cheever, K. H. (2018). *Brunner & Suddarth's textbook of medical-surgical nursing* (14th ed.). Wolter Kluwer.

Hockenberry, M. J., Wilson, D., & Rodgers, C. C. (Eds.). (2019). *Wong's nursing care of infants and children* (11th ed.). Elsevier.

Huether, S. E., McCance, K. L., & Brashers, V. L. (2020). *Understanding pathophysiology* (7th ed.). Elsevier.

Ignatavicius, D. D., Workman, M. L., Rebar, C. R., & Heimgartner, N. M. (2021). *Medical-surgical nursing: Concepts for interprofessional care* (10th ed.). Elsevier.

Kear, T. M. (2017). Fluid and electrolyte management across the age continuum. *Nephrology Nursing Journal, 44*(6), 491–497.

Potter, P. A., & Perry, A. G. (2021). *Fundamentals of nursing* (10th ed.). Elsevier.

Seay, N. W., Lehrich, R. W., & Greenberg, A. (2020). Diagnosis and management of disorders of body tonicity-hyponatremia and hypernatremia: Core curriculum. *American Journal of Kidney Diseases, 75*(2), 272–286. https://doi.org/10.1053/j.ajkd.2019.07.014

Reddi, A. S. (2018). *Fluid, electrolyte, and acid-base disorders: Clinical evaluation and management* (2nd ed.). Springer.

Hypophosphatemia Severity   0618

Definition: Severity of signs and symptoms of decreased serum phosphorus

OUTCOME TARGET RATING: Maintain at_____ Increase to_____

		Severe	Substantial	Moderate	Mild	None	
OUTCOME OVERALL RATING		1	2	3	4	5	
Indicators:							
061801	Decrease in serum phosphorus	1	2	3	4	5	NA
061802	Paresthesias	1	2	3	4	5	NA
061803	Muscle weakness	1	2	3	4	5	NA
061804	Impaired swallowing	1	2	3	4	5	NA
061805	Bone pain	1	2	3	4	5	NA
061806	Chest pain	1	2	3	4	5	NA
061807	Cardiomyopathy	1	2	3	4	5	NA
061808	Confusion	1	2	3	4	5	NA
061809	Irritability	1	2	3	4	5	NA
061810	Fatigue	1	2	3	4	5	NA
061811	Seizures	1	2	3	4	5	NA
061812	Respiratory failure	1	2	3	4	5	NA
061813	Tissue hypoxia	1	2	3	4	5	NA
061814	Susceptibility to infections	1	2	3	4	5	NA
061819	Nystagmus	1	2	3	4	5	NA
061815	Double vision	1	2	3	4	5	NA
061816	Joint stiffness	1	2	3	4	5	NA
061817	Bleeding disorders	1	2	3	4	5	NA
061818	Impaired white blood cell function	1	2	3	4	5	NA

Domain-*Physiologic Health (II)*   **Class**-*Fluid & Electrolytes (G)*   *5th edition 2013; revised 2024*

OUTCOME CONTENT REFERENCES:
Hinkle, J. L., & Cheever, K. H. (2018). *Brunner & Suddarth's textbook of medical-surgical nursing* (14th ed.). Wolter Kluwer.
Hockenberry, M. J., Wilson, D., & Rodgers, C. C. (Eds.). (2019). *Wong's nursing care of infants and children* (11th ed.). Elsevier.
Huether, S. E., McCance, K. L., & Brashers, V. L. (2020). *Understanding pathophysiology* (7th ed.). Elsevier.
Ignatavicius, D. D., Workman, M. L., Rebar, C. R., & Heimgartner, N. M. (2021). *Medical-surgical nursing: Concepts for interprofessional care* (10th ed.). Elsevier.
Koumakis, E., Cormier, C., Roux, C., & Briot, K. (2020). The causes of hypo- and hyperphosphatemia in humans. *Calcified Tissue International*, 108(1),41–73. https://doi.org/10.1007/s00223-020-00664-9
Martín, A. G., Varsavsky, M., Berdonces, M. C., Rubio, V. A., Exposito, M. R. A., Rodríguez, C. N., Moreno, P. R., Muñoz, M. R., Gimeno, E. J., Ortega, P. R., & Torres, M. M. (2020). Phosphate disorders and the clinical management of hypophosphatemia and hyperphosphatemia. *Endocrinology, Diabetes and Nutrition* (English ed.), *67*(3), 205–215. https://doi.org/10.1016/j.endinu.2019.06.004
Potter, P. A., & Perry, A. G. (2021). *Fundamentals of nursing* (10th ed.). Elsevier.
Reddi, A. S. (2018). *Fluid, electrolyte, and acid-base disorders: Clinical evaluation and management* (2nd ed.). Springer.

Hypotension Severity

Definition: Severity of signs and symptoms of episodic low blood pressure

OUTCOME TARGET RATING: Maintain at_____ Increase to_____

	Severe	Substantial	Moderate	Mild	None	
OUTCOME OVERALL RATING	1	2	3	4	5	
Indicators:						
211401 Pallor	1	2	3	4	5	NA
211402 Clammy skin	1	2	3	4	5	NA
211403 Chronic cold extremities	1	2	3	4	5	NA
211404 Rapid respirations	1	2	3	4	5	NA
211405 Shallow respirations	1	2	3	4	5	NA
211406 Thready pulse	1	2	3	4	5	NA
211407 Irregular heart rate	1	2	3	4	5	NA
211408 Syncope	1	2	3	4	5	NA
211409 Blurred vision	1	2	3	4	5	NA
211410 Seizure activity	1	2	3	4	5	NA
211411 Anxiety	1	2	3	4	5	NA
211412 Dizziness	1	2	3	4	5	NA
211413 Lightheadedness on standing abruptly	1	2	3	4	5	NA
211414 Orthostatic hypotension	1	2	3	4	5	NA
211415 Obstructive sleep apnea	1	2	3	4	5	NA
211416 Mouth breathing	1	2	3	4	5	NA
211417 Nocturnal asthma	1	2	3	4	5	NA
211418 Snoring	1	2	3	4	5	NA
211419 Fatigue	1	2	3	4	5	NA
211420 Delirium	1	2	3	4	5	NA
211421 Low systolic blood pressure	1	2	3	4	5	NA
211422 Low diastolic blood pressure	1	2	3	4	5	NA

Domain-Health & Life Quality (V)   *Class*-Symptom Status (V)   5th edition 2013

OUTCOME CONTENT REFERENCES:

Arbogast, S., Alshekhlee, A., Hussain, Z., McNeeley, K., & Chelimksy, T. (2009). Hypotension unawareness in profound orthostatic hypotension. *The American Journal of Medicine, 122*(6), 574–580.

Dabrowski, G. P., Steinberg, S. M., Ferrara, J. J., & Flint, L. M. (2000). A critical assessment of endpoints of shock resuscitation. *Surgical Clinics of North America, 80*(3), 825–844.

Guilleminault, C., Faul, J., & Stoohs, R. (2001). Sleep-disordered breathing and hypotension. *American Journal of Respiratory and Critical Care Medicine, 164*(7), 1242–1247.

Guilleminault, C., Khramsov, A., Stoohs, R. A., Kushida, C., Pelayo, R., Kreutzer, M. L., & Chowdhuri, S. (2004). Abnormal blood pressure in prepubertal children with sleep-disordered breathing. *Pediatric Research, 55*(1), 76–84.

Lipsky, A. M., Gausche-Hill, M., Henneman, P. L., Loffredo, A. J., Eckhardt, P. B., Cryer, H. G., deVirgilio, C., Klein, S. L., Bongard, F. S., & Lewis, R. J. (2006). Prehospital hypotension is a predictor of the need for an emergent, therapeutic operation in trauma patients with normal systolic blood pressure in the emergency department. *Journal of Trauma, Injury, Infection and Critical Care, 61*(5), 1228–1233.

Mathew, T. P., Menown, I. B., McCarty, D., Gracey, H., Hill, L., & Adgey, A.A. (2003). Impact of pre-hospital care in patients with acute myocardial infarction compared with those first managed in-hospital. *European Heart Journal, 24*(2), 161–171.

Shapiro, N. I., Kociszewski, C., Harrison, T., Chang, Y., Wedel, S. K., & Thomas, S. H. (2003). Isolated prehospital hypotension after traumatic injuries: A predictor of mortality? *Journal of Emergency Medicine, 25*(2), 175–179.

Stell, A., Sinnott, R., Jiang, J., Donald, R., Chambers, I., Citerio, G., Enblad, P., Gregson, B., Howells, T., Kiening, K., Nilsson, P., Ragauskas, A., Sahuquillo, J., & Piper, I. (2009). Federating distributed clinical data for the prediction of adverse hypotensive events. *Philosophical Transactions. Series A, Mathematical, physical, and Engineering Sciences, 367*(1898), 2679–2690.

Weiss, A., Chagnac, A., Beloosesky, Y., Weinstein, T., Grinblat, J., & Grossman, E. (2004). Orthostatic hypotension in the elderly: Are the diagnostic criteria adequate? *Journal of Human Hypertension, 18*(5), 301–305.

Immobility Consequences: Physiological   0204

Definition: Severity of compromise in physical functioning due to impaired physical mobility

OUTCOME TARGET RATING: Maintain at_____ Increase to_____

		Severe	Substantial	Moderate	Mild	None	
OUTCOME OVERALL RATING		1	2	3	4	5	
Indicators:							
020401	Pressure injury	1	2	3	4	5	NA
020425	Loss of appetite	1	2	3	4	5	NA
020402	Constipation	1	2	3	4	5	NA
020403	Stool impaction	1	2	3	4	5	NA
020405	Hypoactive bowel	1	2	3	4	5	NA
020406	Paralytic ileus	1	2	3	4	5	NA
020407	Urinary calculi	1	2	3	4	5	NA
020408	Urinary retention	1	2	3	4	5	NA
020409	Fever	1	2	3	4	5	NA
020410	Urinary tract infection	1	2	3	4	5	NA
020426	Loss of muscle strength	1	2	3	4	5	NA
020427	Loss of muscle tone	1	2	3	4	5	NA
020428	Loss of range of motion (ROM)	1	2	3	4	5	NA
020413	Bone fracture	1	2	3	4	5	NA
020415	Contracted joints	1	2	3	4	5	NA
020416	Ankylosed joints	1	2	3	4	5	NA
020417	Orthostatic hypotension	1	2	3	4	5	NA
020418	Venous thrombosis	1	2	3	4	5	NA
020429	Decreased vital capacity	1	2	3	4	5	NA
020419	Lung congestion	1	2	3	4	5	NA
020422	Pneumonia	1	2	3	4	5	NA
020424	Venous stasis	1	2	3	4	5	NA
020430	Pain	1	2	3	4	5	NA

Domain-*Functional Health (I)*   **Class**-*Mobility (C)*   *1st edition 1997; revised 2000, 2004, 2013, 2024*

OUTCOME CONTENT REFERENCES:
Antunes, M. D., Oliveira, K. C. C. de, Acencio, F. R., Oliveira, D. V. de, Garcez, D. A. G., & Bennemann, R. M. (2019). Intestinal constipation in elderly and the relationship with physical activity, food and cognition: A systematic review. *Revista De Medicina, 98*(3), 202–207. https://doi.org/10.11606/issn.1679-9836.v98i3p202-207
Borklund-Lima, L., Müller-Staub, M., Michelle Cardozo, M. C., Bernardes, D. S., & Rabelo-Silva, E. R. (2019). Clinical indicators of Nursing Outcomes Classification for patient with risk for perioperative positioning injury: A cohort study. *Journal of Clinical Nursing, 28*, 4367–4378.
Crawford, A., & Harris, H. (2016). Caring for adults with impaired physical mobility. *Nursing. 46*(12), 36–41. https://doi.org/10.1097/01.NURSE.0000504674.19099.1d
Ferreira, R. C., & Duran, E. C. M. (2019). Clinical validation of nursing diagnosis "00085 Impaired Physical Mobility" in multiple traumas victims. *Revista Latino-Americana de Enfermagem, 27*, e3190. https://doi.org/10.1590/1518-8345.2859.3190
Joseph, I., & McCauley, R. (2019). Impact of early mobilization in the Intensive Care Unit on psychological issues. *Critical Care Nursing Clinics, 31*(4), 501–505. https://doi.org/10.1016/j.cnc.2019.07.005
Kalisch, B. J., Lee, S., & Dabney, B. W. (2014). Outcomes of inpatient mobilization: A literature review. *Journal of Clinical Nursing, 23*(11-12), 1486–501. https://doi.org/10.1111/jocn.12315
Koukourikos, K., Tsaloglidou, A., & Kourkouta, L. (2014). Muscle atrophy in intensive care unit patients. *Acta Informatica Medica. 22*(6), 406–10. https://doi.org/10.5455/aim.2014.22.406–410
Li, Z., Zhou, X., Cao, J., Li, Z., Wan, X., Li, J., Jiao, J., Liu, G., Liu, Y., Li, F., Song, B., Jin, J., Liu, Y., Wen, X., Cheng, S., & Wu, X. (2018). Nurses' knowledge and attitudes regarding major immobility complications among bedridden patients: A prospective multicentre study. *Journal of Clinical Nursing. 27*(9-10), 1969–1980. https://doi.org/10.1111/jocn.14339
Lucena, A. F., Argenta, C., Almeida, M. A., Moorhead, S., & Swanson, E. (2019). Validation of nursing outcomes and interventions to older adults care with Risk or Frail Elderly Syndrome: Proposal of linkages among NOC, NIC, and NANDA-I to clinical practice. *International Journal of Nursing Knowledge, 30*, 147–153. https://doi.org/10.1111/2047-3095.12225

Lucena, A. F., Argenta, C., Luzia, M. F., Almeida, M. A., Barreto, L. N. M., & Swanson, E. (2020). Multidimensional model of successful aging and nursing terminologies: similarities for use in the clinical practice. *Revista Gaúcha de Enfermagem (UFRGS), 41*, 1–16. https://doi.org/10.1590/1983-1447.2020.20190148

Musich, S., Wang, S. S., Ruiz, J., Hawkins, K., & Wicker, E. (2018). The impact of mobility limitations on health outcomes among older adults. *Geriatric Nursing, 39*(2), 162–169. https://doi.org/10.1016/j.gerinurse.2017.08.002

Parry, S. M., & Puthucheary, Z. A. (2015). The impact of extended bed rest on the musculoskeletal system in the critical care environment. *Extreme Physiology & Medicine, 4*(1), 1–8. https://doi.org/10.1186/s13728-015-0036-7

Plapler, P. G., Souza, D. R., Kaziyama, H. H. S., Battistella, L. R., & Barros-Filho, T. E. P. (2021). Relationship between the coronavirus disease 2019 pandemic and immobilization syndrome. *Clinics, 5*(76), e2652. https://doi.org/10.6061/clinics/2021/e2652

Potter, P. A., Perry, A. G., Stockert, P. A., & Hall, A. M. (2021). *Fundamentals of nursing* (10th ed.). Mosby.

Sartori, M., Favaretto, E., & Cosmi, B. (2021). Relevance of immobility as a risk factor for symptomatic proximal and isolated distal deep vein thrombosis in acutely ill medical inpatients. *Vascular Medicine, 26*(5), 542–548. https://doi.org/10.1177/1358863X21996825

Sobrado, C. W., Corrêa Neto, I. J. F., Pinto, R. A., Sobrado, L. F., Nahas, S. C., & Cecconello, I. (2018). Diagnosis and treatment of constipation: A clinical update based on the Rome IV criteria. *Journal of Coloproctology, 38*(02), 137–144. https://doi.org/10.1016/j.jcol.2018.02.003

Immobility Consequences: Psycho-Cognitive   0205

Definition: Severity of compromise in psychological and cognitive functioning due impaired mobility

OUTCOME TARGET RATING: Maintain at_____ Increase to_____

		Severe	Substantial	Moderate	Mild	None	
OUTCOME OVERALL RATING		1	2	3	4	5	
Indicators:							
020504	Perceptual distortions	1	2	3	4	5	NA
020515	Impaired concentration	1	2	3	4	5	NA
020507	Exaggerated emotions	1	2	3	4	5	NA
020508	Sleep disturbance	1	2	3	4	5	NA
020516	Negative self-esteem	1	2	3	4	5	NA
020510	Negative body image	1	2	3	4	5	NA
020513	Depression	1	2	3	4	5	NA
020514	Apathy	1	2	3	4	5	NA
020517	Decreased kinesthetic sense	1	2	3	4	5	NA
020518	Fear of falling	1	2	3	4	5	NA
020519	Feelings of dependency	1	2	3	4	5	NA

Domain-Functional Health (I)   **Class**-Mobility (C)   *1st edition 1997; revised 2004, 2024*

OUTCOME CONTENT REFERENCES:

Chen, L.-J., Fox, K. R., Sun, W.-J., Tsai, P.-S., Ku, P.-W., & Chu, D. (2018). Associations between walking parameters and subsequent sleep difficulty in older adults: A 2-year follow-up study. *Journal of Sport and Health Science, 7*(1), 95–101. https://doi.org/10.1016/j.jshs.2017.01.007

Domenech-Cebrían, P., Martinez-Martinez, M., & Cauli, O. (2019). Relationship between mobility and cognitive impairment in patients with Alzheimer's disease. *Clinical Neurology and Neurosurgery. 179*, 23–29. https://doi.org/10.1016/j.clineuro.2019.02.015

Edwards, K. A., Alschuler, K. A., Ehde, D. M., Battalio, S. L., & Jensen, M. P. (2017). Changes in resilience predict function in adults with physical disabilities: A longitudinal study. *Archives of Physical Medicine and Rehabilitation, 98*(2), 329–336. https://doi.org/10.1016/j.apmr.2016.09.123

Joseph, I., & McCauley, R. (2019). Impact of early mobilization in the Intensive Care Unit on psychological issues. *Critical Care Nursing Clinic of North America, 31*(4), 501–505. https://doi.org/10.1016/j.cnc.2019,07.005

Kalisch, B. J., Lee, S., & Dabney, B. W. (2014). Outcomes of inpatient mobilization: A literature review. *Journal of Clinical Nursing, 23*(11-12), 1486–501. https://doi.org/10.1111/jocn.12315

Karp, J. F., Zhang, J., Wahed, A. S., Anderson, S., Dew, M. A., Fitzgerald, G. K., Weiner, D. K., Albert, S., Gildengers, A., Butters, M., & Reynolds, C. F. (2019). Improving patient reported outcomes and preventing depression and anxiety in older adults with knee osteoarthritis: Results of a sequenced multiple assignment randomized trial (SMART) study. *American Journal of Geriatric Psychiatry, 27*(10), 1035–1045. https://doi.org/10.1016/j.jagp.2019.03.011

Lucena, A. F., Argenta, C., Almeida, M. A, Moorhead, S., & Swanson, E. (2019). Validation of nursing outcomes and interventions to older adults care with Risk or Frail Elderly Syndrome: Proposal of linkages among NOC, NIC, and NANDA-I to clinical practice. *International Journal of Nursing Knowledge, 30*(3), 147–153. https://doi.org/10.1111/2047-3095.12225

Lucena, A. F., Argenta, C., Luzia, M. F., Almeida, M. A., Barreto, L. N. M., & Swanson, E. (2020). Multidimensional Model of Successful Aging and nursing terminologies: Similarities for use in the clinical practice. *Revista Gaúcha de Enfermagem (UFRGS), 41*, 1–16. https://doi.org/10.1590/1983-1447.2020.20190148

Musich, S., Wang, S. S., Ruiz, J., Hawkins, K., & Wicker, E. (2018). The impact of mobility limitations on health outcomes among older adults. *Geriatric Nursing, 39*(2), 162–169. https://doi.org/10.1016/j.gerinurse.2017.08.002

Plapler, P. G., Souza, D. R., Kaziyama, H. H. S., Battistella, L. R., & Barros-Filho, T. E. P. (2021). Relationship between the coronavirus disease 2019 pandemic and immobilization syndrome. *Clinics, 5*(76), e2652. https://doi.org/10.6061/clinics/2021/e2652

Immune Hypersensitivity Response   0707

Definition: Severity of exaggerated immune responses resulting in harmful tissue damage or changes in laboratory values

OUTCOME TARGET RATING: Maintain at_____ Increase to_____

		Severe	Substantial	Moderate	Mild	None	
OUTCOME OVERALL RATING		1	2	3	4	5	
Indicators:							
070701	Alterations in skin	1	2	3	4	5	NA
070702	Alterations in mucosa	1	2	3	4	5	NA
070703	Allergic reactions	1	2	3	4	5	NA
070704	Localized inflammatory responses	1	2	3	4	5	NA
070705	Autoimmune events	1	2	3	4	5	NA
070706	Vasculitis	1	2	3	4	5	NA
070707	Transplant rejection	1	2	3	4	5	NA
070708	Graft-versus-host response	1	2	3	4	5	NA
070709	Itching	1	2	3	4	5	NA
070710	Jaundice	1	2	3	4	5	NA
070711	Level of auto-antibodies or auto-antigens	1	2	3	4	5	NA
070712	Increased bilirubin level	1	2	3	4	5	NA
070713	Alterations in complete blood count	1	2	3	4	5	NA
070714	Alterations in differential white blood count	1	2	3	4	5	NA
070715	Alterations in complement levels	1	2	3	4	5	NA
070716	Alterations in T4-cell level	1	2	3	4	5	NA
070717	Alterations in T8-cell level	1	2	3	4	5	NA
070724	Reactions to air pollution	1	2	3	4	5	NA
070725	Alterations in thermoregulation	1	2	3	4	5	NA
070726	Alterations in respiratory function	1	2	3	4	5	NA
070727	Alterations in cardiac function	1	2	3	4	5	NA
070728	Alterations in gastrointestinal function	1	2	3	4	5	NA
070729	Alterations in renal function	1	2	3	4	5	NA
070730	Alterations in liver function	1	2	3	4	5	NA
070731	Alterations in neurological function	1	2	3	4	5	NA
070732	Alterations in joint mobility	1	2	3	4	5	NA

Domain-*Physiologic Health (II)*   **Class**-*Immune Response (H)*   *3rd edition 2004; revised 2024*

OUTCOME CONTENT REFERENCES:

Downey, M. (2021). Refuel your immune system. *Life Extension, 27*(9), 46–52.
Glencross, D. A., Ho, T. R., Camiña, N., Hawrylowicz, C. M., & Pfeffer, P. E. (2020). Air pollution and its effects on the immune system. *Free Radical Biology & Medicine, 151,* 56–68. https://doi.org/10.1016/j.freeradbiomed.2020.01.179
Guttman-Yassky, E., Zhou, L., & Krueger, J. G. (2019). The skin as an immune organ: Tolerance versus effector responses and applications to food allergy and hypersensitivity reactions. *The Journal of Allergy and Clinical Immunology, 144*(2), 362–374. https://doi.org/10.1016/j.jaci.2019.03.021
Huether, S. E., McCance, K. L., & Brashers, V. L. (2020). *Understanding pathophysiology* (7th ed.). Elsevier.
Ignatavicius, D. D., Workman, M. L., Rebar, C. R., & Heimgartner, N. M. (2021). *Medical-surgical nursing: Concepts for interprofessional care* (10th ed.). Elsevier.
Marshall, J. S., Warrington, R., Watson, W., & Kim, H. L. (2018). An introduction to immunology and immunopathology. *Allergy, Asthma, and Clinical Immunology: Official Journal of the Canadian Society of Allergy and Clinical Immunology, 14*(Suppl 2), 49. https://doi.org/10.1186/s13223-018-0278-1

Immune Status

Definition: Natural and acquired appropriately targeted resistance to internal and external antigens

OUTCOME TARGET RATING: Maintain at_____ Increase to_____

		Severely Compromised	Substantially Compromised	Moderately Compromised	Mildly Compromised	Not Compromised	
OUTCOME OVERALL RATING		1	2	3	4	5	
Indicators:							
070203	Gastrointestinal function	1	2	3	4	5	NA
070204	Respiratory function	1	2	3	4	5	NA
070205	Genitourinary function	1	2	3	4	5	NA
070207	Body temperature	1	2	3	4	5	NA
070208	Skin integrity	1	2	3	4	5	NA
070209	Mucosa integrity	1	2	3	4	5	NA
070222	Adherence to recommended vaccinations	1	2	3	4	5	NA
070221	Screenings for infections	1	2	3	4	5	NA
070212	Antibody titers	1	2	3	4	5	NA
070213	Skin test reaction with exposure	1	2	3	4	5	NA
070214	Absolute white blood count	1	2	3	4	5	NA
070215	Differential white blood count	1	2	3	4	5	NA
070216	T4-cell level	1	2	3	4	5	NA
070217	T8-cell level	1	2	3	4	5	NA
070218	Complement levels	1	2	3	4	5	NA
070219	Thymus x-ray findings	1	2	3	4	5	NA
070223	Resistance to infections	1	2	3	4	5	NA
070224	Nutrient intake	1	2	3	4	5	NA
070225	Energy level	1	2	3	4	5	NA

Domain-*Physiologic Health (II)*   **Class**-*Immune Response (H)*   *1st edition 1997; revised 2004, 2008, 2024*

OUTCOME CONTENT REFERENCES:

Childs, C. E., Calder, P. C., & Miles, E. A. (2019). Diet and immune function. *Nutrients, 11*(8), 1933. https://doi.org/10.3390/nu11081933

Christ, A., Lauterbach, M., & Latz, E. (2019). Western diet and the immune system: An inflammatory connection. *Immunity, 51*(5), 794–811. https://doi.org/10.1016/j.immuni.2019.09.020

Huether, S. E., McCance, K. L., & Brashers, V. L. (2020). *Understanding pathophysiology* (7th ed.). Elsevier.

Ignatavicius, D. D., Workman, M. L., Rebar, C. R., & Heimgartner, N. M. (2021). *Medical-surgical nursing: Concepts for interprofessional care* (10th ed.). Elsevier.

Lee, G. Y., & Han, S. N. (2018). The role of vitamin E in immunity. *Nutrients, 10*(11), 1614. https://doi.org/10.3390/nu10111614

Lewis, E. D., Meydani, S. N., & Wu, D. (2019), Regulatory role of vitamin E in the immune system and inflammation. *IUBMB Life, 71*, 487–494. https://doi.org/10.1002/iub.1976

Maggini, S., Pierre, A., & Calder, P. C. (2018). Immune function and micronutrient requirements change over the life course. *Nutrients, 10*, 1531. https://doi.org/10.3390/nu10101531

Immunization Behavior   **1900**

Definition: Personal actions to obtain immunization to prevent a communicable disease

OUTCOME TARGET RATING: Maintain at_____ Increase to_____

		Never Demonstrated	Rarely Demonstrated	Sometimes Demonstrated	Often Demonstrated	Consistently Demonstrated	
OUTCOME OVERALL RATING		1	2	3	4	5	
Indicators:							
190001	Acknowledges disease risk without immunization	1	2	3	4	5	NA
190002	Describes risks associated with specific immunization	1	2	3	4	5	NA
190003	Describes contraindications to specific immunization	1	2	3	4	5	NA
190015	Obtains reputable information about age-specific immunization requirements	1	2	3	4	5	NA
190016	Maintains personal immunization record	1	2	3	4	5	NA
190017	Discusses concerns about specific immunization with health professional	1	2	3	4	5	NA
190004	Brings updated vaccination card to each visit	1	2	3	4	5	NA
190018	Reports health conditions to health professional before immunization	1	2	3	4	5	NA
190005	Obtains immunizations recommended for age	1	2	3	4	5	NA
190006	Describes relief measures for vaccine side effects	1	2	3	4	5	NA
190007	Reports any adverse reactions	1	2	3	4	5	NA
190009	Confirms date of next immunization	1	2	3	4	5	NA
190010	Obtains immunizations recommended with chronic illness	1	2	3	4	5	NA
190011	Obtains immunizations recommended for occupational risk	1	2	3	4	5	NA
190012	Obtains immunizations recommended for travel	1	2	3	4	5	NA
190019	Obtains financial assistance for immunization	1	2	3	4	5	NA
190013	Identifies community resources for immunization	1	2	3	4	5	NA

Domain-Health Knowledge & Behavior (IV)   *Class*-Safety (HH)   1st edition 1997; revised 2000, 2004, 2018

OUTCOME CONTENT REFERENCES:

Clift, K., & Rizzolo, D. (2014). Vaccine myths and misconceptions. *Journal of the American Academy of Physician Assistants, 27*(8), 21–25. https://doi.org/10.1097/01.JAA.0000451873.94189.56

Hamborsky, J., Kroger, A., & Wolfe, C. (Eds.). (2015). *Epidemiology and prevention of vaccine-preventable diseases*. Public Health Foundation.

Kim, D., Riley, L., Harriman, K., Hunter, P., & Bridges, C. (2017). Advisory committee on immunization practices recommended immunization schedule for adults aged 19 years or older—United States, 2017. *Morbidity and Mortality Weekly Report (MMWR), 66*(5), 136–138. https://doi.org/10.15585/mmwr.mm6605e2

National Center for Immunization and Respiratory Diseases. (2011). General recommendations on immunization—Recommendations of the Advisory Committee on Immunization Practices (ACIP). *Morbidity and Mortality Weekly Report (MMWR), 60*(2), 1–64.

Sevin, A., Romeo, C., Gagne, B., Brown, N., & Rodis, J. (2016). Factors influencing adults' immunization practices: A pilot survey study of a diverse, urban community in central Ohio. *BMC Public Health, 16*, 424. https://doi.org/10.1186/s12889-016-3107-9

Impulse Self-Control

Definition: Self-restraint of compulsive or impulsive behaviors

OUTCOME TARGET RATING: Maintain at_____   Increase to_____

OUTCOME OVERALL RATING	Never Demonstrated 1	Rarely Demonstrated 2	Sometimes Demonstrated 3	Often Demonstrated 4	Consistently Demonstrated 5	
Indicators:						
140501 Identifies harmful impulsive behaviors	1	2	3	4	5	NA
140502 Identifies feelings that lead to impulsive actions	1	2	3	4	5	NA
140503 Identifies behaviors that lead to impulsive actions	1	2	3	4	5	NA
140504 Identifies consequences of impulsive actions	1	2	3	4	5	NA
140518 Recognizes impact of decision-making	1	2	3	4	5	NA
140519 Recognizes impact of alcohol on impulsive behavior	1	2	3	4	5	NA
140520 Recognizes impact of drugs on impulsive behavior	1	2	3	4	5	NA
140521 Recognizes value of control	1	2	3	4	5	NA
140522 Uses tension reduction strategies	1	2	3	4	5	NA
140523 Uses stress reduction strategies	1	2	3	4	5	NA
140524 Maintains emotional stability	1	2	3	4	5	NA
140505 Recognizes risks in environment	1	2	3	4	5	NA
140514 Avoids high-risk environments	1	2	3	4	5	NA
140515 Avoids high-risk situations	1	2	3	4	5	NA
140507 Controls impulses	1	2	3	4	5	NA
140516 Obtains assistance when experiencing impulses	1	2	3	4	5	NA
140525 Uses recommended psychotherapy	1	2	3	4	5	NA
140509 Uses available social support	1	2	3	4	5	NA
140526 Follows medication regimen	1	2	3	4	5	NA
140517 Keeps referral appointments	1	2	3	4	5	NA
140527 Recognizes need for follow-up	1	2	3	4	5	NA
140511 Upholds contract to control behavior	1	2	3	4	5	NA
140528 Maintains reward system for controlling impulses	1	2	3	4	5	NA
140512 Maintains self-control without supervision	1	2	3	4	5	NA

Domain-Psychosocial Health (III)   **Class**-Self-Control (O)   *1st edition 1997; revised 2000, 2004, 2008, 2024*

OUTCOME CONTENT REFERENCES:

American Psychiatric Association (APA). (2022). *Diagnostic and statistical manual of mental disorders* (5th ed., text rev.). https://doi.org/10.1176/appi. books.9780890425787

Harvanko, A. M., Strickland, J. C., Slone, S. A., Shelton, B. J., & Reynolds, B. A. (2019). Dimensions of impulsive behavior: Predicting contingency management treatment outcomes for adolescent smokers. *Addictive Behaviors, 90*, 334–340. https://doi.org/10.1016/j.addbeh.2018.11.031

Kräplin, A., Höfler, M., Pooseh, S., Wolff, M., Krönke, K. M., Goschke, T., Bühringer, G., & Smolka, M. N. (2020). Impulsive decision-making predicts the course of substance-related and addictive disorders. *Psychopharmacology, 237*, 2709–2724. https://doi.org/10.1007/s00213-020-05567-z

+Lazzaro, T. A., Beggs, D. L., & McNeil, K. A. (1969). The development and validation of the Self-Report Test of Impulse Control. *Journal of Clinical Psychology, 25*(4), 434–438.

Peters, E. M., Bowen, R., & Balbuena, L. (2019). Mood instability contributes to impulsivity, non suicidal self-injury, and binge eating/purging in people with anxiety disorders. *Psychology and Psychotherapy: Theory, Research and Practice, 92*(3), 422–438. https://doi.org/10.1111/papt.12192

Staubitz, J. L., Lloyd, B. P., & Reed, D. D. (2020). Effects of self-control training for elementary students with emotional and behavioral disorders. *Journal of Applied Behavior Analysis, 53*(2), 857–874. https://doi.org/10.1002/jaba.634

Varcarolis, E. M., & Fosbre, C.D. (2021). Essentials of psychiatric-mental health nursing: A communication approach to evidence-based practice (4th ed.). Elsevier.

Infant Nutritional Status 1020

Definition: Adequacy of nutrients ingested and absorbed to meet metabolic needs and foster growth of an infant

OUTCOME TARGET RATING: Maintain at_____ Increase to_____

		Severe Deviation from Normal Range	Substantial Deviation from Normal Range	Moderate Deviation from Normal Range	Mild Deviation from Normal Range	No Deviation from Normal Range	
OUTCOME OVERALL RATING		1	2	3	4	5	
Indicators:							
102024	Nutrient intake	1	2	3	4	5	NA
102025	Oral food intake	1	2	3	4	5	NA
102026	Oral fluid intake	1	2	3	4	5	NA
102027	Food tolerance	1	2	3	4	5	NA
102028	Weight/height ratio	1	2	3	4	5	NA
102029	Hydration	1	2	3	4	5	NA
102030	Blood glucose	1	2	3	4	5	NA
102031	Hemoglobin	1	2	3	4	5	NA
102032	Total iron binding capacity	1	2	3	4	5	NA
102033	Serum albumin	1	2	3	4	5	NA
102034	Caloric intake	1	2	3	4	5	NA
102035	Protein intake	1	2	3	4	5	NA
102036	Fat intake	1	2	3	4	5	NA
102037	Carbohydrate intake	1	2	3	4	5	NA
102038	Vitamin intake	1	2	3	4	5	NA
102039	Mineral intake	1	2	3	4	5	NA
102040	Iron intake	1	2	3	4	5	NA
102041	Calcium intake	1	2	3	4	5	NA
102042	Sodium intake	1	2	3	4	5	NA
102043	Tube feeding intake	1	2	3	4	5	NA
102044	Intravenous fluid intake	1	2	3	4	5	NA
102045	Parenteral fluid intake	1	2	3	4	5	NA
102046	Growth	1	2	3	4	5	NA
102047	Head circumference	1	2	3	4	5	NA

Domain-*Physiologic Health (II)*   **Class**-*Digestion & Nutrition (K)*   *5th edition 2013; revised 2024*

OUTCOME CONTENT REFERENCES:

Atef, H., Abdel-Raouf, R., Zeid, A. S., Elsebaie, E. H., Abdalaleem, S., Amin, A. A., & Aboulghar, H. (2021). Development of a simple and valid nutrition screening tool for pediatric hospitalized patients with acute illness. *F1000Research, 10*, 173. https://doi.org/10.12688/f1000research.51186.1

Brugaletta, C., Le Roch, K., Saxton, J., Bizouerne, C., McGrath, M., & Kerac, M. (2020). Breastfeeding assessment tools for at-risk and malnourished infants aged under 6 months old: A systematic review. *F1000Research, 9*, 1310. https://f1000research.com/articles/9-1310/v2

Dudek, S. G. (2022). *Nutrition essentials for nursing practice* (9th ed.). Wolters Kluwer.

Elshafie, A. M., El-Lahony, D. M., Omar, Z. A., Bahbah, W. A., & Ghetas, H. R. (2019). Nutrition in critically ill pediatric patients: A systemic review. *Menoufia Medical Journal, 32*, 812–817. https://doi.org/10.1007/s00134-019-05922-5

Katz, D. L., Friedman, R. S. C., Joshi, S., Levitt, J., & Ye, M.-C. (2022). *Nutrition in clinical practice.* Wolters Kluwer.

Obbagy, J. E., English, L. K., Psota, T. L., Wong, Y. P., Butte, N. F., Dewey, K. G., Fox, M. K., Greer, F. R., Krebs, N. F., Scanlon, K. S., & Stoody, E. E. (2019). Complementary feeding and micronutrient status: A systematic review. *American Journal of Clinical Nutrition, 109*(Suppl. 7), 852S–871S. https://doi.org/10.1093/ajcn/nqy266

Ottolini, K. M., Andescavage, N., Keller, S., & Limperopoulos, C. (2020). Nutrition and the developing brain: The road to optimizing early neurodevelopment: A systematic review. *Pediatric Research, 87*(2),194–201. https://doi.org/10.1038/s41390-019-0508-3

Rana, R., McGrath, M., Gupta, P., Thakur, E., & Kerac, M. (2020). Feeding interventions for infants with growth failure in the first six months of life: A systematic review. *Nutrients, 12*(7), 2044. https://doi.org/10.3390/nu12072044

Scott, N., Delport, D., Hainsworth, S., Pearson, R., Morgan, C., Huang, S., Akuoku, J. K., Piwoz, E., Shekar, M., Levin, C., Toole, M., & Homer, C.S. (2020). Ending malnutrition in all its forms requires scaling up proven nutrition interventions and much more: A 129-country analysis. *BMC Medicine, 18*(1), 356. https://doi.org/10.1186/s12916-020-01786-5

Vaivada, T., Gaffey, M. F., & Bhutta, Z. A. (2017). Promoting early child development with interventions in health and nutrition: A systematic review. *Pediatrics, 140*(2), e20164308. https://doi.org/10.1542/peds.2016-4308

Wong, D. L., Hockenberry, M. J., & Marylin, J. (2018). *Wong's nursing care of infants and children* (11th ed.). Elsevier.

Infection Severity

Definition: Severity of signs and symptoms of infection

OUTCOME TARGET RATING: Maintain at_____ Increase to_____

		Severe	Substantial	Moderate	Mild	None	
OUTCOME OVERALL RATING		1	2	3	4	5	
Indicators:							
070301	Rash	1	2	3	4	5	NA
070302	Uncrusted vesicles	1	2	3	4	5	NA
070303	Foul-smelling discharge	1	2	3	4	5	NA
070304	Purulent sputum	1	2	3	4	5	NA
070305	Purulent drainage	1	2	3	4	5	NA
070336	Conjunctivitis	1	2	3	4	5	NA
070306	Pyuria	1	2	3	4	5	NA
070307	Fever	1	2	3	4	5	NA
070329	Hypothermia	1	2	3	4	5	NA
070330	Temperature instability	1	2	3	4	5	NA
070333	Pain	1	2	3	4	5	NA
070337	Joint pain	1	2	3	4	5	NA
070338	Muscle pain	1	2	3	4	5	NA
070339	Headache	1	2	3	4	5	NA
070334	Tenderness	1	2	3	4	5	NA
070309	Gastrointestinal symptoms	1	2	3	4	5	NA
070310	Lymphadenopathy	1	2	3	4	5	NA
070311	Malaise	1	2	3	4	5	NA
070312	Chilling	1	2	3	4	5	NA
070313	Unexplained cognitive impairment	1	2	3	4	5	NA
070331	Lethargy	1	2	3	4	5	NA
070332	Loss of appetite	1	2	3	4	5	NA
070340	Coughing	1	2	3	4	5	NA
070319	Chest x-ray infiltration	1	2	3	4	5	NA
070320	Blood culture colonization	1	2	3	4	5	NA
070335	Vascular access device colonization	1	2	3	4	5	NA
070321	Sputum culture colonization	1	2	3	4	5	NA
070322	Cerebrospinal fluid culture colonization	1	2	3	4	5	NA
070323	Wound site culture colonization	1	2	3	4	5	NA
070324	Urine culture colonization	1	2	3	4	5	NA
070325	Stool culture colonization	1	2	3	4	5	NA
070326	White blood count elevation	1	2	3	4	5	NA
070327	White blood count depression	1	2	3	4	5	NA

Site of infection_____

Domain-*Physiologic Health (II)*   **Class**-*Immune Response (H)*   *1st edition 1997; revised 2004, 2008, 2013, 2018*

OUTCOME CONTENT REFERENCES:

Arslan, S., Ucar, R., Caliskaner, A., Reisli, I., Guner, S., Sayer, E., & Baloglu, I. (2016). How effective are the 6 European Society of Immunodeficiency warning signs for primary immunodeficiency disease? *Annals of Allergy, Asthma & Immunology, 116*(2), 151–155. https://doi.org/10.1016/j.anai.2015.12.001

+Blodgett, T., Gardner, S., Blodgett, N., Peterson, L., & Pietraszak, M. (2015). A tool to assess the signs and symptoms of catheter-associated urinary tract infection: Development and reliability. *Clinical Nursing Research, 24*(4), 341–356. https://doi.org/10.1177/1054773814550506

Dasgupta, S., Reagan-Steiner, S., Goodenough, D., Russell, K., Tanner, M., Lewis, L., Petersen, E. E., Powers, A. M., Kniss, K., Meaney-Delman, D., Oduyebo, T., O'Leary, D., Chiu, S., Talley, P., Hennessey, M., Hills, S., Cohn, A., Gregory, C., & The Zika Virus Response Epidemiology and Laboratory Team. (2016). Patterns in Zika virus testing and infection, by report of symptoms and pregnancy status—United States, January 3–March 5, 2016. *Morbidity and Mortality Weekly Report, 65*(15), 395–399.

Deville, J., Equils, O., Huang, D., & Ang, J. (2011). The impact of linezolid and vancomycin treatment on local signs and symptoms of inflammation among pediatric patients with complicated skin and skin structure infections. *Clinical Pediatrics, 50*(11), 1064–1067. https://doi.org/10.1177/0009922810385107

Dut, R., & Kocagöz, S. (2016). Clinical signs and diagnostic tests in acute respiratory infections. *Indian Journal of Pediatrics, 83*(5), 380–385. https://doi.org/10.1007/s12098-015-1943-8

Gould, D. (2012). Causes, prevention and management of surgical site infection. *Nursing Standard, 26*(47), 47–56.

Hosseini, S., Zawawi, F., & Young, J. (2015). Atypical presentation of a common disease: Shingles of the larynx. *Journal of Voice, 29*(5), 600–602. https://doi.org/10.1016/j.jvoice.2014.10.010

Lindgren, C., Neuman, M., Monuteaux, M., Mandl, K., & Fine, A. (2016). Patient and parent-reported signs and symptoms for group A streptococcal pharyngitis. *Pediatrics, 138*(1), 1–7. https://doi.org/10.1542/peds.2016-0317

Infection Severity: Newborn   0708

Definition: Severity of signs and symptoms of infection during the first 28 days of life

OUTCOME TARGET RATING: Maintain at_____ Increase to_____

		Severe	Substantial	Moderate	Mild	None	
OUTCOME OVERALL RATING		1	2	3	4	5	
Indicators:							
070801	Temperature instability	1	2	3	4	5	NA
070802	Hypothermia	1	2	3	4	5	NA
070803	Tachypnea	1	2	3	4	5	NA
070804	Tachycardia	1	2	3	4	5	NA
070805	Bradycardia	1	2	3	4	5	NA
070806	Arrhythmias	1	2	3	4	5	NA
070807	Hypotension	1	2	3	4	5	NA
070808	Hypertension	1	2	3	4	5	NA
070809	Pale	1	2	3	4	5	NA
070810	Mottled skin	1	2	3	4	5	NA
070811	Cyanosis	1	2	3	4	5	NA
070812	Cold, clammy skin	1	2	3	4	5	NA
070813	Vomiting	1	2	3	4	5	NA
070814	Diarrhea	1	2	3	4	5	NA
070815	Abdominal distension	1	2	3	4	5	NA
070816	Feeding intolerance	1	2	3	4	5	NA
070817	Lethargy	1	2	3	4	5	NA
070818	Irritability	1	2	3	4	5	NA
070819	Seizures	1	2	3	4	5	NA
070820	Jitteriness	1	2	3	4	5	NA
070821	High-pitched cry	1	2	3	4	5	NA
070822	Rash	1	2	3	4	5	NA
070823	Uncrusted vesicles	1	2	3	4	5	NA
070824	Foul-smelling discharge	1	2	3	4	5	NA
070825	Purulent drainage	1	2	3	4	5	NA
070826	Conjunctivitis	1	2	3	4	5	NA
070827	Infected umbilicus	1	2	3	4	5	NA
070828	Blood culture colonization	1	2	3	4	5	NA
070829	Wound site culture colonization	1	2	3	4	5	NA
070830	Urine culture colonization	1	2	3	4	5	NA
070831	Stool culture colonization	1	2	3	4	5	NA

I

Continued

Infection Severity: Newborn—cont'd

		Severe	Substantial	Moderate	Mild	None	
070832	Chest x-ray infiltration	1	2	3	4	5	NA
070833	Cerebrospinal fluid culture colonization	1	2	3	4	5	NA
070834	White blood count elevation	1	2	3	4	5	NA
070835	White blood count depression	1	2	3	4	5	NA

Site of infection_____

Domain-*Physiologic Health (II)*   **Class**-*Immune Response (H)*   *3rd edition 2004; revised 2013*

OUTCOME CONTENT REFERENCES:

Albrutyn, E., & Talbot, G. H. (1987). Surveillance strategies: A primer. *Infection Control, 8*(11), 459–464.

Antonow, J. A., Smout, R. J., Gassaway, J., Horn, S. D., & Wilson, D. F. (2001). Variation among 10 pediatric hospitals: Sepsis evaluations for infants with bronchiolitis. *Journal of Nursing Care Quality, 15*(3), 39–49. https://doi.org/10.1097/00001786-200104000-00007

Deacon, J., & O'Neill, P. (Eds.). (1999). *Core curriculum for neonatal intensive care nursing* (2nd ed.). W.B. Saunders.

Griffin, M. P., & Moorman, J. R. (2001). Toward the early diagnosis of neonatal sepsis and sepsis-like illness using novel heart rate analysis. *Pediatrics, 107*(1), 97–104. https://doi.org/10.1542/peds.107.1.97

Mattson, S., & Smith, J. E. (Eds.). (2000). *Core curriculum for maternal-newborn nursing* (2nd ed.). W.B. Saunders.

Mullany, L. C., Darmstadt, G. L., Katz, J., Khatry, S. K., LeClerq, S. C., Adhikari, R. K., & Tielsch, J. M. (2006). Development of clinical sign based algorithms for community based assessment of omphalitis. *Archives of Disease in Childhood—Fetal & Neonatal Edition, 91*(2), F99–F104. https://doi.org/10.1136/adc.2005.080093

J

Information Processing   **0907**

Definition: Ability to acquire, organize, and use information

OUTCOME TARGET RATING: Maintain at_____ Increase to_____

		Never Demonstrated	Rarely Demonstrated	Sometimes Demonstrated	Often Demonstrated	Consistently Demonstrated	
OUTCOME OVERALL RATING		1	2	3	4	5	
Indicators:							
090717	Identifies common objects	1	2	3	4	5	NA
090718	Interprets the meaning of a sentence	1	2	3	4	5	NA
090719	Interprets the meaning of a paragraph	1	2	3	4	5	NA
090720	Interprets the meaning of a story	1	2	3	4	5	NA
090721	Comprehends universal symbols	1	2	3	4	5	NA
090722	Verbalizes a coherent message	1	2	3	4	5	NA
090723	Exhibits organization of thoughts	1	2	3	4	5	NA
090724	Exhibits logical order of thought processes	1	2	3	4	5	NA
090725	Explains similarity between two items	1	2	3	4	5	NA
090726	Explains dissimilarity between two items	1	2	3	4	5	NA
090727	Adds several numbers	1	2	3	4	5	NA
090728	Subtracts several numbers	1	2	3	4	5	NA
090729	Counts backward from 100	1	2	3	4	5	NA

Domain-*Physiologic Health (II)*   **Class**-*Neurocognitive (J)*   *1st edition 1997; revised 2004, 2008, 2024*

OUTCOME CONTENT REFERENCES:

Andersen. S. L., Sweigart, B., Glynn, N. W., Wojczynski, M. K., Thyagarajan, B., Mengel-From, J., Thielke, S., Perls, T. T., Libon, D. J., Au, R., Cosentino, S., & Sebastiani, P. (2021). Digital technology differentiates graphomotor and information processing speed patterns of behavior. *Journal of Alzheimer's Disease, 82*(1), 17–32. https://doi.org/10.3233/JAD-201119

+Folstein, M. F., Folstein, S. E., & McHugh, P. R. (1975). "Mini-Mental State"- A practical method for grading the cognitive state of patients for the clinician. *Journal of Psychiatric Research, 12*(3), 189–198.

Hogan-Quigley, B., Palm, M. L., & Bickley, L. (2021). *Bates nursing guide to physical examination and history taking* (3rd ed.). Wolters Kluwer.

Reed, S. K. (2016). A taxonomic analysis of abstraction. *Perspectives on Psychological Science, 11*(6), 817–837. https://doi.org/10.1177/1745691616646304

Scholl, A., Bloechle, J., Sassenberg, K., & Moeller, K. (2019). The power to adapt: How sense of power predicts number processing. *Canadian Journal of Experimental Psychology, 73*(3), 157–166. https://doi.org/10.1037/cep0000166

Joint Movement 0206

Definition: Active range of motion of all joints with self-initiated movement

OUTCOME TARGET RATING: Maintain at_____ Increase to_____

	Severe Deviation from Normal Range	Substantial Deviation from Normal Range	Moderate Deviation from Normal Range	Mild Deviation from Normal Range	No Deviation from Normal Range	
OUTCOME OVERALL RATING	1	2	3	4	5	
Indicators:						
020601 Jaw	1	2	3	4	5	NA
020602 Neck	1	2	3	4	5	NA
020620 Spine	1	2	3	4	5	NA
020603 Fingers (right)	1	2	3	4	5	NA
020604 Fingers (left)	1	2	3	4	5	NA
020605 Thumb (right)	1	2	3	4	5	NA
020606 Thumb (left)	1	2	3	4	5	NA
020607 Wrist (right)	1	2	3	4	5	NA
020608 Wrist (left)	1	2	3	4	5	NA
020609 Elbow (right)	1	2	3	4	5	NA
020610 Elbow (left)	1	2	3	4	5	NA
020611 Shoulder (right)	1	2	3	4	5	NA
020612 Shoulder (left)	1	2	3	4	5	NA
020613 Ankle (right)	1	2	3	4	5	NA
020614 Ankle (left)	1	2	3	4	5	NA
020615 Knee (right)	1	2	3	4	5	NA
020616 Knee (left	1	2	3	4	5	NA
020617 Hip (right)	1	2	3	4	5	NA
020618 Hip (left)	1	2	3	4	5	NA

Domain-Functional Health (I)   **Class**-Mobility (C)   *1st edition 1997; revised 2008; reviewed 2018*

OUTCOME CONTENT REFERENCES:

Ball, J., Dains, J., Flynn, J., Solomon, B., & Stewart, R. (2015). *Seidel's guide to physical examination* (8th ed.). Elsevier Mosby.
Bickley, L. (2017). *Bates' guide to physical examination and history taking* (12th ed.). Wolters Kluwer.
Cleland, J., Koppenhaver, S., & Su, J. (2016). *Netter's orthopaedic clinical examination: An evidenced-based approach* (3rd ed.). Elsevier.

Joint Movement: Ankle 0213

Definition: Active range of motion of the ankle with self-initiated movement

OUTCOME TARGET RATING: Maintain at_____ Increase to_____

	Severe Deviation from Normal Range	Substantial Deviation from Normal Range	Moderate Deviation from Normal Range	Mild Deviation from Normal Range	No Deviation from Normal Range	
OUTCOME OVERALL RATING	1	2	3	4	5	
Indicators:						
021301 Dorsal flexion 20 degrees (R)	1	2	3	4	5	NA
021302 Plantar flexion 45 degrees (R)	1	2	3	4	5	NA
021303 Inversion 30 degrees (R)	1	2	3	4	5	NA

Continued

Joint Movement: Ankle—cont'd

		Severe Deviation from Normal Range	Substantial Deviation from Normal Range	Moderate Deviation from Normal Range	Mild Deviation from Normal Range	No Deviation from Normal Range	
021304	Eversion 20 degrees (R)	1	2	3	4	5	NA
021305	Rotation (R)	1	2	3	4	5	NA
021306	Dorsal flexion 20 degrees (L)	1	2	3	4	5	NA
021307	Plantar flexion 45 degrees (L)	1	2	3	4	5	NA
021308	Inversion 30 degrees (L)	1	2	3	4	5	NA
021309	Eversion 20 degrees (L)	1	2	3	4	5	NA
021310	Rotation (L)	1	2	3	4	5	NA

Specify: Right (R)____ Left (L)____ Both____

Domain-Functional Health (I)   **Class**-Mobility (C)   *3rd edition 2004; reviewed 2018*

OUTCOME CONTENT REFERENCES:

Ball, J., Dains, J., Flynn, J., Solomon, B., & Stewart, R. (2015). *Seidel's guide to physical examination* (8th ed.). Elsevier Mosby.

Bickley, L. (2017). *Bates' guide to physical examination and history taking* (12th ed.). Wolters Kluwer.

Cleland, J., Koppenhaver, S., & Su, J. (2016). *Netter's orthopaedic clinical examination: An evidenced-based approach* (3rd ed.). Elsevier.

Joint Movement: Elbow   0214

Definition: Active range of motion of the elbow with self-initiated movement

OUTCOME TARGET RATING: Maintain at_____ Increase to_____

		Severe Deviation from Normal Range	Substantial Deviation from Normal Range	Moderate Deviation from Normal Range	Mild Deviation from Normal Range	No Deviation from Normal Range	
OUTCOME OVERALL RATING		1	2	3	4	5	
Indicators:							
021401	Extension 0 degrees (R)	1	2	3	4	5	NA
021402	Flexion 160 degrees (R)	1	2	3	4	5	NA
021403	Supination 90 degrees (R)	1	2	3	4	5	NA
021404	Pronation 90 degrees (R)	1	2	3	4	5	NA
021405	Extension 0 degrees (L)	1	2	3	4	5	NA
021406	Flexion 160 degrees (L)	1	2	3	4	5	NA
021407	Supination 90 degrees (L)	1	2	3	4	5	NA
021408	Pronation 90 degrees (L)	1	2	3	4	5	NA

Specify: Right (R)____ Left (L)____ Both____

Domain-Functional Health (I)   **Class**-Mobility (C)   *3rd edition 2004; reviewed 2018*

OUTCOME CONTENT REFERENCES:

Ball, J., Dains, J., Flynn, J., Solomon, B., & Stewart, R. (2015). *Seidel's guide to physical examination* (8th ed.). Elsevier Mosby.

Bickley, L. (2017). *Bates' guide to physical examination and history taking* (12th ed.). Wolters Kluwer.

Cleland, J., Koppenhaver, S., & Su, J. (2016). *Netter's orthopaedic clinical examination: An evidenced-based approach* (3rd ed.). Elsevier.

Joint Movement: Fingers   **0215**

Definition: Active range of motion of the fingers with self-initiated movement

OUTCOME TARGET RATING: Maintain at_____ Increase to_____

		Severe Deviation from Normal Range	Substantial Deviation from Normal Range	Moderate Deviation from Normal Range	Mild Deviation from Normal Range	No Deviation from Normal Range	
OUTCOME OVERALL RATING		1	2	3	4	5	
Indicators:							
021501	Metacarpophalangeal extension 0 degrees (R)	1	2	3	4	5	NA
021502	Metacarpophalangeal flexion 90 degrees (R)	1	2	3	4	5	NA
021503	Metacarpophalangeal hyperflexion 30 degrees (R)	1	2	3	4	5	NA
021504	Proximal interphalangeal extension 0 degrees (R)	1	2	3	4	5	NA
021505	Proximal interphalangeal flexion 100–120 degrees (R)	1	2	3	4	5	NA
021506	Distal interphalangeal extension 0 degrees (R)	1	2	3	4	5	NA
021507	Distal interphalangeal flexion 45–80 degrees (R)	1	2	3	4	5	NA
021508	Metacarpophalangeal extension 0 degrees (L)	1	2	3	4	5	NA
021509	Metacarpophalangeal flexion 90 degrees (L)	1	2	3	4	5	NA
021510	Metacarpophalangeal hyperflexion 30 degrees (L)	1	2	3	4	5	NA
021511	Proximal interphalangeal extension 0 degrees (L)	1	2	3	4	5	NA
021512	Proximal interphalangeal flexion 100–120 degrees (L)	1	2	3	4	5	NA
021513	Distal interphalangeal extension 0 degrees (L)	1	2	3	4	5	NA
021514	Distal interphalangeal flexion 45–80 degrees (L)	1	2	3	4	5	NA

Specify: Right hand (R)_____ Left hand (L)_____ Both_____

Domain-*Functional Health (I)*   **Class**-*Mobility (C)*   *3rd edition 2004; reviewed 2018*

OUTCOME CONTENT REFERENCES:
Ball, J., Dains, J., Flynn, J., Solomon, B., & Stewart, R. (2015). *Seidel's guide to physical examination* (8th ed.). Elsevier Mosby.
Bickley, L. (2017). *Bates' guide to physical examination and history taki*ng (12th ed.). Wolters Kluwer.
Cleland, J., Koppenhaver, S., & Su, J. (2016). *Netter's orthopaedic clinical examination: An evidenced-based approach* (3rd ed.). Elsevier.

Joint Movement: Hip

0216

Definition: Active range of motion of the hip with self-initiated movement

OUTCOME TARGET RATING: Maintain at_____ Increase to_____

		Severe Deviation from Normal Range	Substantial Deviation from Normal Range	Moderate Deviation from Normal Range	Mild Deviation from Normal Range	No Deviation from Normal Range	
OUTCOME OVERALL RATING		1	2	3	4	5	
Indicators:							
021601	Flexion knee straight 90 degrees (R)	1	2	3	4	5	NA
021602	Extension knee straight 0 degrees (R)	1	2	3	4	5	NA
021603	Hyperextension knee straight 15 degrees (R)	1	2	3	4	5	NA
021604	Flexion knee bent 120 degrees (R)	1	2	3	4	5	NA
021605	Abduction 45 degrees (R)	1	2	3	4	5	NA
021606	Adduction 30 degrees (R)	1	2	3	4	5	NA
021607	Internal rotation 40 degrees (R)	1	2	3	4	5	NA
021608	External rotation 45 degrees (R)	1	2	3	4	5	NA
021609	Flexion knee straight 90 degrees (L)	1	2	3	4	5	NA
021610	Extension knee straight 0 degrees (L)	1	2	3	4	5	NA
021611	Hyperextension knee straight 15 degrees (L)	1	2	3	4	5	NA
021612	Flexion knee bent 120 degrees (L)	1	2	3	4	5	NA
021613	Abduction 45 degrees (L)	1	2	3	4	5	NA
021614	Adduction 30 degrees (L)	1	2	3	4	5	NA
021615	Internal rotation 40 degrees (L)	1	2	3	4	5	NA
021616	External rotation 45 degrees (L)	1	2	3	4	5	NA

Specify: Right (R)_____ Left (L)_____ Both_____

Domain-*Functional Health (I)*   **Class**-*Mobility (C)*   *3rd edition 2004; reviewed 2018*

OUTCOME CONTENT REFERENCES:
Ball, J., Dains, J., Flynn, J., Solomon, B., & Stewart, R. (2015). *Seidel's guide to physical examination* (8th ed.). Elsevier Mosby.
Bickley, L. (2017). *Bates' guide to physical examination and history taking* (12th ed.). Wolters Kluwer.
Cleland, J., Koppenhaver, S., & Su, J. (2016). *Netter's orthopaedic clinical examination: An evidenced-based approach* (3rd ed.). Elsevier.

Joint Movement: Knee

0217

Definition: Active range of motion of the knee with self-initiated movement

OUTCOME TARGET RATING: Maintain at_____ Increase to_____

		Severe Deviation from Normal Range	Substantial Deviation from Normal Range	Moderate Deviation from Normal Range	Mild Deviation from Normal Range	No Deviation from Normal Range	
OUTCOME OVERALL RATING		1	2	3	4	5	
Indicators:							
021701	Extension 0 degrees (R)	1	2	3	4	5	NA
021702	Flexion 130 degrees (R)	1	2	3	4	5	NA
021703	Hyperextension 15 degrees (R)	1	2	3	4	5	NA

Joint Movement: Knee—cont'd

		Severe Deviation from Normal Range	Substantial Deviation from Normal Range	Moderate Deviation from Normal Range	Mild Deviation from Normal Range	No Deviation from Normal Range	
021704	Extension 0 degrees (L)	1	2	3	4	5	NA
021705	Flexion 130 degrees (L)	1	2	3	4	5	NA
021706	Hyperextension 15 degrees (L)	1	2	3	4	5	NA

Specify: Right (R)____ Left (L)____
Both____

Domain-*Functional Health (I)*   **Class**-*Mobility (C)*   *3rd edition 2004; reviewed 2018*

OUTCOME CONTENT REFERENCES:
Ball, J., Dains, J., Flynn, J., Solomon, B., & Stewart, R. (2015). *Seidel's guide to physical examination* (8th ed.). Elsevier Mosby.
Bickley, L. (2017). *Bates' guide to physical examination and history taking* (12th ed.). Wolters Kluwer.
Cleland, J., Koppenhaver, S., & Su, J. (2016). *Netter's orthopaedic clinical examination: An evidenced-based approach* (3rd ed.). Elsevier.

Joint Movement: Neck   **0218**

Definition: Active range of motion of the neck with self-initiated movement

OUTCOME TARGET RATING: Maintain at_____ Increase to_____

		Severe Deviation from Normal Range	Substantial Deviation from Normal Range	Moderate Deviation from Normal Range	Mild Deviation from Normal Range	No Deviation from Normal Range	
OUTCOME OVERALL RATING		1	2	3	4	5	
Indicators:							
021801	Flexion 45 degrees	1	2	3	4	5	NA
021802	Extension 55 degrees	1	2	3	4	5	NA
021803	Lateral bending 40 degrees (R)	1	2	3	4	5	NA
021804	Lateral bending 40 degrees (L)	1	2	3	4	5	NA
021805	Rotation	1	2	3	4	5	NA

Domain-*Functional Health (I)*   **Class**-*Mobility (C)*   *3rd edition 2004; reviewed 2018*

OUTCOME CONTENT REFERENCES:
Ball, J., Dains, J., Flynn, J., Solomon, B., & Stewart, R. (2015). *Seidel's guide to physical examination* (8th ed.). Elsevier Mosby.
Bickley, L. (2017). *Bates' guide to physical examination and history taking* (12th ed.). Wolters Kluwer.
Cleland, J., Koppenhaver, S., & Su, J. (2016). *Netter's orthopaedic clinical examination: An evidenced-based approach* (3rd ed.). Elsevier.

Joint Movement: Passive

Definition: Joint movement with assistance

OUTCOME TARGET RATING: Maintain at_____ Increase to_____

		Severe Deviation from Normal Range	Substantial Deviation from Normal Range	Moderate Deviation from Normal Range	Mild Deviation from Normal Range	No Deviation from Normal Range	
OUTCOME OVERALL RATING		1	2	3	4	5	
Indicators:							
020702	Neck	1	2	3	4	5	NA
020703	Fingers (right)	1	2	3	4	5	NA
020705	Thumb (right)	1	2	3	4	5	NA
020707	Wrist (right)	1	2	3	4	5	NA
020709	Elbow (right)	1	2	3	4	5	NA
020711	Shoulder (right)	1	2	3	4	5	NA
020713	Ankle (right)	1	2	3	4	5	NA
020715	Knee (right)	1	2	3	4	5	NA
020717	Hip (right)	1	2	3	4	5	NA
020704	Fingers (left)	1	2	3	4	5	NA
020706	Thumb (left)	1	2	3	4	5	NA
020708	Wrist (left)	1	2	3	4	5	NA
020710	Elbow (left)	1	2	3	4	5	NA
020712	Shoulder (left)	1	2	3	4	5	NA
020714	Ankle (left)	1	2	3	4	5	NA
020716	Knee (left)	1	2	3	4	5	NA
020718	Hip (left)	1	2	3	4	5	NA

Domain-*Functional Health (I)*   **Class**-*Mobility (C)*   *1st edition 1997; revised 2004; reviewed 2018*

OUTCOME CONTENT REFERENCES:
Ball, J., Dains, J., Flynn, J., Solomon, B., & Stewart, R. (2015). *Seidel's guide to physical examination* (8th ed.). Elsevier Mosby.
Bickley, L. (2017). *Bates' guide to physical examination and history taking* (12th ed.). Wolters Kluwer.
Cleland, J., Koppenhaver, S., & Su, J. (2016). *Netter's orthopaedic clinical examination: An evidenced-based approach* (3rd ed.). Elsevier.

Joint Movement: Shoulder

Definition: Active range of motion of the shoulder with self-initiated movement

OUTCOME TARGET RATING: Maintain at_____ Increase to_____

		Severe Deviation from Normal Range	Substantial Deviation from Normal Range	Moderate Deviation from Normal Range	Mild Deviation from Normal Range	No Deviation from Normal Range	
OUTCOME OVERALL RATING		1	2	3	4	5	
Indicators:							
021901	Forward flexion 180 degrees (R)	1	2	3	4	5	NA
021902	Extension 50 degrees (R)	1	2	3	4	5	NA
021903	External rotation 90 degrees (R)	1	2	3	4	5	NA

Joint Movement: Shoulder—cont'd

		Severe Deviation from Normal Range	Substantial Deviation from Normal Range	Moderate Deviation from Normal Range	Mild Deviation from Normal Range	No Deviation from Normal Range	
021904	Internal rotation 90 degrees (R)	1	2	3	4	5	NA
021905	Abduction 180 degrees (R)	1	2	3	4	5	NA
021906	Adduction 50 degrees (R)	1	2	3	4	5	NA
021907	Forward flexion 180 degrees (L)	1	2	3	4	5	NA
021908	Extension 50 degrees (L)	1	2	3	4	5	NA
021909	External rotation 90 degrees (L)	1	2	3	4	5	NA
021910	Internal rotation 90 degrees (L)	1	2	3	4	5	NA
021911	Abduction 180 degrees (L)	1	2	3	4	5	NA
021912	Adduction 50 degrees (L)	1	2	3	4	5	NA

Specify: Right (R)_____ Left (L)_____
Both_____

Domain-Functional Health (I)   **Class**-Mobility (C)   *3rd edition 2004; reviewed 2018*

OUTCOME CONTENT REFERENCES:
Ball, J., Dains, J., Flynn, J., Solomon, B., & Stewart, R. (2015). *Seidel's guide to physical examination* (8th ed.). Elsevier Mosby.
Bickley, L. (2017). *Bates' guide to physical examination and history taking* (12th ed.). Wolters Kluwer.
Cleland, J., Koppenhaver, S., & Su, J. (2016). *Netter's orthopaedic clinical examination: An evidenced-based approach* (3rd ed.). Elsevier.

Joint Movement: Spine   **0220**

Definition: Active range of motion of the spine with self-initiated movement

OUTCOME TARGET RATING: Maintain at_____ Increase to_____

		Severe Deviation from Normal Range	Substantial Deviation from Normal Range	Moderate Deviation from Normal Range	Mild Deviation from Normal Range	No Deviation from Normal Range	
OUTCOME OVERALL RATING		1	2	3	4	5	
Indicators:							
022001	Extension 30 degrees	1	2	3	4	5	NA
022002	Flexion 90 degrees	1	2	3	4	5	NA
022003	Lateral bending 35 degrees (R)	1	2	3	4	5	NA
022004	Rotation (R)	1	2	3	4	5	NA
022005	Lateral bending 35 degrees (L)	1	2	3	4	5	NA
022006	Rotation (L)	1	2	3	4	5	NA

Domain-Functional Health (I)   **Class**-Mobility (C)   *3rd edition 2004; reviewed 2018*

OUTCOME CONTENT REFERENCES:
Ball, J., Dains, J., Flynn, J., Solomon, B., & Stewart, R. (2015). *Seidel's guide to physical examination* (8th ed.). Elsevier Mosby.
Bickley, L. (2017). *Bates' guide to physical examination and history taking* (12th ed.). Wolters Kluwer.
Cleland, J., Koppenhaver, S., & Su, J. (2016). *Netter's orthopaedic clinical examination: An evidenced-based approach* (3rd ed.). Elsevier.

J

Joint Movement: Wrist

0221

Definition: Active range of motion of the wrist with self-initiated movement

OUTCOME TARGET RATING: Maintain at_____ Increase to_____

		Severe Deviation from Normal Range	Substantial Deviation from Normal Range	Moderate Deviation from Normal Range	Mild Deviation from Normal Range	No Deviation from Normal Range	
OUTCOME OVERALL RATING		1	2	3	4	5	
Indicators:							
022101	Radial deviation 20 degrees (R)	1	2	3	4	5	NA
022102	Ulnar deviation 55 degrees (R)	1	2	3	4	5	NA
022103	Flexion 90 degrees (R)	1	2	3	4	5	NA
022104	Extension 70 degrees (R)	1	2	3	4	5	NA
022105	Radial deviation 20 degrees (L)	1	2	3	4	5	NA
022106	Ulnar deviation 55 degrees (L)	1	2	3	4	5	NA
022107	Flexion 90 degrees (L)	1	2	3	4	5	NA
022108	Extension 70 degrees (L)	1	2	3	4	5	NA

Specify: Right (R)____ Left (L)____
Both____

Domain-Functional Health (I)　　**Class**-Mobility (C)　　*3rd edition 2004; reviewed 2018*

OUTCOME CONTENT REFERENCES:

Ball, J., Dains, J., Flynn, J., Solomon, B., & Stewart, R. (2015). *Seidel's guide to physical examination* (8th ed.). Elsevier Mosby.

Bickley, L. (2017). *Bates' guide to physical examination and history taking* (12th ed.). Wolters Kluwer.

Cleland, J., Koppenhaver, S., & Su, J. (2016). *Netter's orthopaedic clinical examination: An evidenced-based approach* (3rd ed.). Elsevier

Kidney Function   0504

Definition: Ability of the kidneys to regulate body fluids, filter blood, and eliminate waste products through the formation of urine

OUTCOME TARGET RATING: Maintain at_____ Increase to_____

		Severely Compromised	Substantially Compromised	Moderately Compromised	Mildly Compromised	Not Compromised	
OUTCOME OVERALL RATING		1	2	3	4	5	
Indicators:							
050424	8-hour urine output	1	2	3	4	5	NA
050402	24-hour intake and output balance	1	2	3	4	5	NA
050425	Skin turgor	1	2	3	4	5	NA
050405	Urine specific gravity	1	2	3	4	5	NA
050406	Urine color	1	2	3	4	5	NA
050408	Urine pH	1	2	3	4	5	NA
050409	Urine electrolytes	1	2	3	4	5	NA
050410	Arterial bicarbonate (HCO_3)	1	2	3	4	5	NA
050411	Arterial pH	1	2	3	4	5	NA
		Severe	**Substantial**	**Moderate**	**Mild**	**None**	
050426	Increased blood urea nitrogen	1	2	3	4	5	NA
050427	Increased serum creatinine	1	2	3	4	5	NA
050428	Increased serum potassium	1	2	3	4	5	NA
050429	Increased urine glucose	1	2	3	4	5	NA
050430	Increased urine protein	1	2	3	4	5	NA
050431	Increased white blood cells	1	2	3	4	5	NA
050414	Hematuria	1	2	3	4	5	NA
050415	Urine ketones	1	2	3	4	5	NA
050416	Urine abnormal microscopic findings	1	2	3	4	5	NA
050417	Kidney stone formation	1	2	3	4	5	NA
050418	Weight gain	1	2	3	4	5	NA
050419	Hypertension	1	2	3	4	5	NA
050420	Nausea	1	2	3	4	5	NA
050421	Fatigue	1	2	3	4	5	NA
050422	Malaise	1	2	3	4	5	NA
050423	Anemia	1	2	3	4	5	NA
050432	Edema	1	2	3	4	5	NA

Domain-*Physiologic Health (II)*   **Class**-*Elimination (F)*   *3rd edition 2004; revised 2013*

OUTCOME CONTENT REFERENCES:
Broscious, S. K., & Castagnola, J. (2006). Chronic kidney disease: Acute manifestations and role of critical care nurses. *Critical Care Nurse, 26*(4), 17–28.
Guyton, A. C., Hall, J. E., & Schmitt, W. (1997). *Human physiology and mechanisms of disease* (6th ed.). W.B. Saunders.
LeMone, P., Burke, K., & Bauldoff, G. (2011). *Medical-surgical nursing: Critical thinking in patient care* (5th ed., pp. 768–782). Pearson Education.
Potter, P., Perry, A., Stockert, P., & Hall, A. (2013). *Fundamentals of nursing* (8th ed.). Mosby Elsevier.
Roth, C., & Culp, K. (2001). Renal osteodystrophy in elderly patients with end-stage renal disease. *Journal of Gerontological Nursing, 27*(7), 46–51.
    https://doi.org/10.3928/0098-9134-20010701-12
Smeltzer, S., Bare, B., Hinkle, J., & Cheever, K. (2008). *Brunner & Suddarth's textbook of medical-surgical nursing* (11th ed., pp. 1492–1513). Lippincott Williams & Wilkins.

K

Knowledge: Acute Illness Management

1844

Definition: Extent of understanding conveyed about a reversible illness, its treatment, and the prevention of complications

OUTCOME TARGET RATING: Maintain at_____ Increase to_____

		No Knowledge	Limited Knowledge	Moderate Knowledge	Substantial Knowledge	Extensive Knowledge	
OUTCOME OVERALL RATING		1	2	3	4	5	
Indicators:							
184401	Cause and contributing factors	1	2	3	4	5	NA
184402	Usual course of illness	1	2	3	4	5	NA
184403	Benefits of illness management	1	2	3	4	5	NA
184404	Signs and symptoms of illness	1	2	3	4	5	NA
184405	Signs and symptoms of complications	1	2	3	4	5	NA
184406	Strategies to prevent complications	1	2	3	4	5	NA
184407	Strategies to prevent exposing others to illness	1	2	3	4	5	NA
184408	Strategies to manage comfort	1	2	3	4	5	NA
184409	Available treatment options	1	2	3	4	5	NA
184410	Correct use of non-prescription medication	1	2	3	4	5	NA
184411	Correct use of prescribed medication	1	2	3	4	5	NA
184412	Medication therapeutic effects	1	2	3	4	5	NA
184413	Medication side effects	1	2	3	4	5	NA
184414	Medication adverse effects	1	2	3	4	5	NA
184415	Potential medication interactions	1	2	3	4	5	NA
184416	Treatment regimen	1	2	3	4	5	NA
184417	Personal responsibilities for treatment regimen	1	2	3	4	5	NA
184425	Importance of monitoring temperature	1	2	3	4	5	NA
184426	Importance of adequate fluid intake	1	2	3	4	5	NA
184418	Importance of adherence to treatment regimen	1	2	3	4	5	NA
184419	Cultural influences on adherence with treatment regimen	1	2	3	4	5	NA
184420	Importance of adequate rest	1	2	3	4	5	NA
184421	Diet modifications	1	2	3	4	5	NA
184422	Strategies to cope with adverse effects of illness	1	2	3	4	5	NA
184423	Reputable sources of acute illness information related to illness	1	2	3	4	5	NA
184424	When to obtain assistance from a health professional	1	2	3	4	5	NA

Domain-Health Knowledge & Behavior (IV)   *Class*-Knowledge Health Condition (GG)   *5th edition 2013; revised 2024*

OUTCOME CONTENT REFERENCES:
Jones, R., Armstrong, D., Ashworth, M., & Peters, M. (2010). *Managing acute illness.* The King's Fund.
Ostermann, M., Liu, K., & Kashani, K. (2019). Fluid management in acute kidney injury. *Chest, 156*(3), 594–603. https://doi.org/10.1016/j.chest.2019.04.004
Potter, P., Perry, A., Stockert, P., & Hall, A. (2021). *Fundamentals of nursing* (10th ed.). Elsevier.

K

Knowledge: Allergy Management   3200

Definition: Extent of understanding conveyed about allergy and the prevention of an immune hypersensitivity response to a specific antigen

OUTCOME TARGET RATING: Maintain at_____ Increase to_____

		No Knowledge	Limited Knowledge	Moderate Knowledge	Substantial Knowledge	Extensive Knowledge	
OUTCOME OVERALL RATING		1	2	3	4	5	
Indicators:							
320001	Allergens that trigger an allergic response	1	2	3	4	5	NA
320002	Environmental triggering elements	1	2	3	4	5	NA
320003	Strategies to manage environmental triggers	1	2	3	4	5	NA
320004	Products with triggering allergens	1	2	3	4	5	NA
320005	Foods with triggering allergens	1	2	3	4	5	NA
320006	Interpretation of information on food labels	1	2	3	4	5	NA
320007	Potential threat of cross-contamination	1	2	3	4	5	NA
320008	Reputable sources of information about allergic response	1	2	3	4	5	NA
320009	Benefits of preventing an allergic response	1	2	3	4	5	NA
320010	Medication therapeutic effects	1	2	3	4	5	NA
320011	Medication side effects	1	2	3	4	5	NA
320012	Medication adverse effects	1	2	3	4	5	NA
320013	Proper administration of epinephrine auto-injection	1	2	3	4	5	NA
320014	Proper use of rescue inhaler	1	2	3	4	5	NA
320015	Importance of continual access to emergency medication	1	2	3	4	5	NA
320016	Replacement of emergency medication	1	2	3	4	5	NA
320017	Non-prescription therapies that are safe to use	1	2	3	4	5	NA
320018	Signs and symptoms of allergic response	1	2	3	4	5	NA
320019	Actions to take if an allergic response occurs	1	2	3	4	5	NA
320020	When to obtain assistance from a health professional	1	2	3	4	5	NA
320021	When to seek emergency care	1	2	3	4	5	NA
320022	Importance of informing all health professionals of allergy	1	2	3	4	5	NA
320023	Importance of identifying individuals to inform about risk of allergic response	1	2	3	4	5	NA
320024	Importance of informing individuals of actions to be taken with an allergic response	1	2	3	4	5	NA

Domain-*Health Knowledge & Behavior (IV)*   **Class**-*Knowledge Health Condition (GG)*   *6th edition 2018*

OUTCOME CONTENT REFERENCES:

+Klinnert, M., McQuaid, E., Fedele, D., Faino, A., Strand, M., Robinson, J., Atkins, D., Fleischer D. M., Hourihane, J. O'B., Chohen, S., & Fransen, H. (2015). Children's food allergies: Development of the food allergy management and adaption scale. *Journal of Pediatric Psychology, 40*(6), 572–580. https://doi.org/10.1093/jpepsy/jsv009

Nickolls, C., & Campbell, D. (2015). Top 10 food allergy myths. *Journal of Paediatrics and Child Health, 51*(9), 852–856. https://doi.org/10.1111/jpc.12902

Watson, R. (2013). Managing allergens from a food retailer perspective including an update on allergen labelling regulation. *Nutrition Bulletin, 38*(4), 405–409. https://doi.org/10.1111/nbu.12060

K

Knowledge: Anticoagulation Therapy Management   1845

Definition: Extent of understanding conveyed about the therapeutic purposes, actions, and risks of chemical agents that lengthen blood clotting time

OUTCOME TARGET RATING: Maintain at_____ Increase to_____

		No Knowledge	Limited Knowledge	Moderate Knowledge	Substantial Knowledge	Extensive Knowledge	
OUTCOME OVERALL RATING		1	2	3	4	5	
Indicators:							
184501	Specific thromboembolic disorder	1	2	3	4	5	NA
184502	Benefits of anticoagulation therapy	1	2	3	4	5	NA
184503	Correct use of prescribed medication	1	2	3	4	5	NA
184504	Adverse health effects of skipping medication	1	2	3	4	5	NA
184505	Importance of maintaining medication regimen	1	2	3	4	5	NA
184506	Medication therapeutic effects	1	2	3	4	5	NA
184507	Medication adverse effects	1	2	3	4	5	NA
184508	Medication side effects	1	2	3	4	5	NA
184509	Potential prescribed medication interactions with other agents	1	2	3	4	5	NA
184510	Potential non-prescription medication interactions with other agents	1	2	3	4	5	NA
184511	Herbal interactions	1	2	3	4	5	NA
184512	Prescribed diet	1	2	3	4	5	NA
184513	Food interactions	1	2	3	4	5	NA
184514	Importance of vitamin K restrictions	1	2	3	4	5	NA
184515	Therapeutic range of blood clotting time	1	2	3	4	5	NA
184516	Importance of required laboratory tests	1	2	3	4	5	NA
184517	Importance of regular blood clotting tests	1	2	3	4	5	NA
184518	Risk of bleeding	1	2	3	4	5	NA
184519	Risk of clotting	1	2	3	4	5	NA
184520	Importance of coordinated management with health professional	1	2	3	4	5	NA
184521	Importance of informing health professional of anticoagulation therapy	1	2	3	4	5	NA
184522	Strategies to reduce venous stasis	1	2	3	4	5	NA
184523	Strategies to reduce internal bleeding	1	2	3	4	5	NA
184540	Strategies to manage anticoagulation therapy prior to surgery	1	2	3	4	5	NA
184524	Strategies to prevent physical injury	1	2	3	4	5	NA
184525	Signs and symptoms of internal bleeding	1	2	3	4	5	NA
184526	Signs of external bleeding	1	2	3	4	5	NA
184527	Signs and symptoms of embolism	1	2	3	4	5	NA
184528	Signs and symptoms of atrial fibrillation	1	2	3	4	5	NA
184529	Signs and symptoms of stroke	1	2	3	4	5	NA
184530	Signs and symptoms of transient ischemic attack	1	2	3	4	5	NA
184531	Importance of monitoring vital signs	1	2	3	4	5	NA
184532	Benefits of activity restrictions	1	2	3	4	5	NA
184533	High-risk activities	1	2	3	4	5	NA
184534	Importance of alcohol abstinence	1	2	3	4	5	NA
184535	Importance of tobacco abstinence	1	2	3	4	5	NA
184536	When to obtain assistance from a health professional	1	2	3	4	5	NA
184537	Caregiver's role in treatment plan	1	2	3	4	5	NA
184538	Reputable sources of anticoagulation therapy information	1	2	3	4	5	NA
184539	Plan for obtaining immediate treatment if adverse signs and symptoms occur	1	2	3	4	5	NA

***Domain**-Health Knowledge & Behavior (IV)*   ***Class**-Knowledge Health Condition (GG)*   *5th edition 2013; revised 2024*

OUTCOME CONTENT REFERENCES:

Findlay, J., Keogh, M., & Cooper, L. (2010). Venous thromboembolism prophylaxis: The role of the nurse. *British Journal of Nursing, 19*(16), 1028–1032. https://doi.org/10.12968/bjon.2010.19.16.78190

Lancaster, S. L., Owens, A., Bryant, A. S., Ramey, L. S., Nicholson, J., Gossett, K., Forni, J. T., & Padgett, T. M. (2010). Emergency: Upper-extremity deep vein thrombosis. *AJN, American Journal of Nursing, 110*(5), 48–52. https://doi.org/10.1097/01.NAJ.0000372072.24134.a5

O'Hanlon, S. (2021). Anticoagulation therapy and fall reduction. *JAMA Internal Medicine, 181*(1), 142. https://doi.org/10.1001/jamainternmed.2020.5418

Potter, P. A., Perry, A. G., Stockert, P. A., & Hall, A. (2021). *Fundamentals of nursing* (10th ed.). Elsevier.

Smelser, W. W., & Jones, C. P. (2021). Management of anticoagulation and antiplatelet agents in the radical cystectomy patient. *Urologic Oncology, 39,* 691–697. https://doi.org/10.1016/j.urolonc.2019.12.011

Thelle, D. S. (2021). Bipolar disorder, schizophrenia, and uptake of oral anticoagulation therapy in patients with atrial fibrillation. *JAMA Network Open, 4*(5), 1–2. https://doi.org/10.1001/jamanetworkopen.2021.10116

Truong, L., Whitfield, K., Nickerson-Troy, J., & Francoforte, K. (2021). Drive-thru anticoagulation clinic: Can we supersize your care today? *Journal of the American Pharmacists Association, 61,* e65–e67. https://doi.org/10.1016/j.japh.2020.10.016

Van Damme, S., Van Deyk, K., Budts, W., Verhamme, P., & Moons, P. (2011). Patient knowledge of and adherence to oral anticoagulation therapy after mechanical heart-valve replacement for congenital or acquired valve defects. *Heart & Lung, 40*(2), 139–146. https://doi.org/10.1016/j.hrtlng.2009.11.005

Knowledge: Anxiety Management   1868

Definition: Extent of understanding conveyed about anxiety and interrelationships among causes, effects, and treatments on health

OUTCOME TARGET RATING: Maintain at_____   Increase to_____

		No Knowledge	Limited Knowledge	Moderate Knowledge	Substantial Knowledge	Extensive Knowledge	
OUTCOME OVERALL RATING		1	2	3	4	5	
Indicators:							
186801	Physical signs and symptoms of anxiety	1	2	3	4	5	NA
186802	Emotional signs and symptoms of anxiety	1	2	3	4	5	NA
186803	Behavioral responses to anxiety	1	2	3	4	5	NA
186804	Situations that increase risk for feeling anxious	1	2	3	4	5	NA
186805	Impact of anxiety on ability to concentrate	1	2	3	4	5	NA
186806	Benefits of controlling anxiety	1	2	3	4	5	NA
186807	Available non-pharmacological treatment options	1	2	3	4	5	NA
186808	Available medication	1	2	3	4	5	NA
186809	Medication therapeutic effects	1	2	3	4	5	NA
186810	Medication side effects	1	2	3	4	5	NA
186811	Medication adverse effects	1	2	3	4	5	NA
186812	Potential medication interactions	1	2	3	4	5	NA
186813	Importance of medication reconciliation with health professional	1	2	3	4	5	NA
186811	Methods to monitor anxiety level	1	2	3	4	5	NA
186812	Personal treatment options	1	2	3	4	5	NA
186813	Strategies to enhance coping	1	2	3	4	5	NA
186814	Importance of social relationships	1	2	3	4	5	NA
186815	Importance of sharing feelings with others	1	2	3	4	5	NA
186816	Available support groups	1	2	3	4	5	NA
186817	When to seek assistance from a health professional	1	2	3	4	5	NA

Domain-Health Knowledge & Behavior (IV)   *Class*-Knowledge Health Condition (GG)   7th edition 2024

OUTCOME CONTENT REFERENCES:

Ahmad, M., Bani Mohammad, E., & Anshasi, H. A. (2020). Virtual reality technology for pain and anxiety management among patients with cancer: A systematic review. *Pain Management Nursing, 21*(6), 601–607. https://doi.org/10.1016/j.pmn.2020.04.002

Andreescu, C., & Lee, S. (2020). Anxiety disorders in the elderly. *Advances in Experimental Medicine and Biology, 1191,* 561–576. https://doi.org/10.1007/978-981-32-9705-0_28

Boyd, M., & Luebbert, R. (2020). *Essentials of psychiatric nursing* (2nd ed.). Wolters Kluwer.

Drugs to treat anxiety disorders and obsessive compulsive disorders (OCD). (2021). *Journal of Psychosocial Nursing & Mental Health Services, 59*(5), 7–8. https://doi.org/10.3928/02793695-20210414-79

Edraki, M., Rambod, M., & Molazem, Z. (2018). The effect of coping skills training on depression, anxiety, stress, and self-efficacy in adolescents with diabetes: A randomized controlled trial. *International Journal of Community Based Nursing & Midwifery, 6*(4), 324–333.

Oberoi, S., Yang, J., Woodgate, R. L., Niraula, S., Banerji, S., Israels, S. J., Altman, G., Beattie, S., Rabbani, R., Askïn, N., Gupta, A., Sung, L., Abou-Setta, A. M., & Zarychanski, R. (2020). Association of mindfulness-based interventions with anxiety severity in adults with cancer: A systematic review and meta-analysis. *JAMA Network Open, 3*(8), e2012598. https://doi.org/10.1001/jamanetworkopen.2020.12598

Varcarolis, E. M., & Fosbre, C. D. (2021). *Essentials of psychiatric-mental health nursing* (4th ed.). Elsevier.

Knowledge: Arthritis Management   1831

Definition: Extent of understanding conveyed about arthritis, its treatment, and the prevention of disease progression and complications

OUTCOME TARGET RATING: Maintain at_____ Increase to_____

		No Knowledge	Limited Knowledge	Moderate Knowledge	Substantial Knowledge	Extensive Knowledge	
OUTCOME OVERALL RATING		1	2	3	4	5	
Indicators:							
183101	Cause and contributing factors	1	2	3	4	5	NA
183102	Usual course of disease	1	2	3	4	5	NA
183103	Signs and symptoms of early disease	1	2	3	4	5	NA
183104	Signs and symptoms of worsening disease	1	2	3	4	5	NA
183129	Potential comorbidities	1	2	3	4	5	NA
183105	Potential body changes due to disease	1	2	3	4	5	NA
183106	Benefits of disease management	1	2	3	4	5	NA
183107	Strategies to balance activity and rest	1	2	3	4	5	NA
183108	Energy conservation techniques	1	2	3	4	5	NA
183109	Benefits of regular exercise	1	2	3	4	5	NA
183110	Modification of daily activities	1	2	3	4	5	NA
183111	Factors that decrease the ability to perform physical activity	1	2	3	4	5	NA
183112	Effective exercise routine	1	2	3	4	5	NA
183130	Strategies to manage fatigue	1	2	3	4	5	NA
183113	Strategies to protect joints	1	2	3	4	5	NA
183114	Strategies to manage pain	1	2	3	4	5	NA
183115	Surgical treatment options	1	2	3	4	5	NA
183116	Medical treatment options	1	2	3	4	5	NA
183117	Medication therapeutic effects	1	2	3	4	5	NA
183118	Medication side effects	1	2	3	4	5	NA
183119	Medication adverse effects	1	2	3	4	5	NA
183120	When to obtain assistance from a health professional	1	2	3	4	5	NA
183121	Health beliefs that affect adherence to treatment	1	2	3	4	5	NA
183122	Adverse health effects of being overweight	1	2	3	4	5	NA
183123	Diet modifications	1	2	3	4	5	NA
183124	Correct use of assistive devices	1	2	3	4	5	NA
183125	Home safety measures	1	2	3	4	5	NA
183126	Fall prevention strategies	1	2	3	4	5	NA
183129	Psychosocial impact of physical limitations	1	2	3	4	5	NA
183127	Available support groups	1	2	3	4	5	NA
183128	Reputable sources of arthritis information	1	2	3	4	5	NA

Domain-Health Knowledge & Behavior (IV)   **Class**-Knowledge Health Condition (GG)   4th edition 2008; revised 2013, 2024

K

OUTCOME CONTENT REFERENCES:

Avrech Bar, M., Dao, T. T., DeBlock Vlodarchyk, L. R., & Backman, C. L. (2021). Fatherhood experiences of men with inflammatory arthritis: A preliminary grounded theory. *Arthritis Care & Research*, 73(6), 885–892. https://doi.org/10.1002/acr.24189

Beauvais, C., Rodère, M., Pereira, B., Legoupil, N., Piperno, M., Pallot Prades, B., Castaing, P., Wendling, D., Grange, L., Costantino, F., Carton, L., Soubrier, M., Coquerelle, P., Pham, T., Poivret, D., Cohen, J. D., Tavares, I., Nataf, H., Pouplin, S., Sordet, C., & Gossec, L. (2019). Essential knowledge for patients with rheumatoid arthritis or spondyloarthritis: Results of a multicentric survey in France among health professionals and patients. *Joint Bone Spine*, 86(6), 747–752. https://doi.org/10.1016/j.jbspin.2019.06.006

Davies, K., Dures, E., & Ng, W.-F. (2021). Fatigue in inflammatory rheumatic diseases: Current knowledge and areas for future research. *Nature Reviews Rheumatology*, 17(11), 651–664. https://doi.org/10.1038/s41584-021-00692-1

+Edworthy, S. M., Devins, G. M., & Watson, M. M. (1995). The Arthritis Knowledge Questionnaire. *Arthritis and Rheumatism*, 38(5), 590–600. https://doi.org/10.1002/art.1780380503

+Hammond, A., & Lincoln, N. (1999). The Joint Protection Knowledge Assessment (JPKA): Reliability and validity. *British Journal of Occupational Therapy*, 62(3), 117–122. https://doi.org/10.1177/030802269906200307

Hill, J., & Bird, H. (2007). Patient knowledge and misconceptions of osteoarthritis assessed by a validated self-completed knowledge questionnaire (PKQ-OA). *Rheumatology*, 46(5), 796–800. https://doi.org/10.1093/rheumatology/kel407

Huckleby, J., Williams, F., Ramos, R., & Nápoles, A. M. (2021). The effects of race/ethnicity and physician recommendation for physical activity on physical activity levels and arthritis symptoms among adults with arthritis. *BMC Public Health*, 21(1), 1–10. https://doi.org/10.1186/s12889-021-11570-6

Ke, C., Qiao, Y., Liu, S., Rui, Y., & Wu, Y. (2021). Longitudinal research on the bidirectional association between depression and arthritis. *Social Psychiatry & Psychiatric Epidemiology*, 56(7), 1241–1247. https://doi.org/10.1007/s00127-020-01994-7

Muir, J., Hegarty, R. S. M., Stebbings, S., & Treharne, G. J. (2020). Exploring the role of online health information and social media in the illness experience of arthritis-related fatigue: A focus group study. *Musculoskeletal Care*, 18(4), 501–509. https://doi.org/10.1002/msc.1494

Murphy, L. B., Theis, K. A., Brady, T. J., & Sacks, J. J. (2021). Supporting self-management education for arthritis: Evidence from the Arthritis Conditions and Health Effects Survey on the influential role of health care providers. *Chronic Illness*, 17(3), 217–231. https://doi.org/10.1177/1742395319869431

Zhang, W., Radhakrishnan, K., Becker, H., Acton, G. J., & Holahan, C. K. (2021). Self-regulation strategies among community-dwelling people aging with arthritis and multimorbidity. *Journal of Gerontological Nursing*, 47(1), 35–45. https://doi.org/10.3928/00989134-20201209-03

Knowledge: Asthma Management   1832

K

Definition: Extent of understanding conveyed about asthma, its treatment, and the prevention of complications

OUTCOME TARGET RATING: Maintain at_____ Increase to_____

		No Knowledge	Limited Knowledge	Moderate Knowledge	Substantial Knowledge	Extensive Knowledge	
OUTCOME OVERALL RATING		1	2	3	4	5	
Indicators:							
183201	Signs and symptoms of asthma	1	2	3	4	5	NA
183233	Reputable sources of asthma information	1	2	3	4	5	NA
183202	Benefits of disease management	1	2	3	4	5	NA
183203	Cause and contributing factors	1	2	3	4	5	NA
183204	Usual course of disease	1	2	3	4	5	NA
183234	Health beliefs that impact treatment	1	2	3	4	5	NA
183205	Potential complications of asthma	1	2	3	4	5	NA
183206	Strategies to manage asthma	1	2	3	4	5	NA
183207	Asthma management goals	1	2	3	4	5	NA
183208	Importance of continual access to inhaler	1	2	3	4	5	NA
183209	Effects on lifestyle	1	2	3	4	5	NA
183235	Relationship of physical stress to condition	1	2	3	4	5	NA
183236	Relationship of emotional stress to condition	1	2	3	4	5	NA
183211	Importance of adherence with treatment regimen	1	2	3	4	5	NA
183212	Importance of adherence with medication regimen	1	2	3	4	5	NA
183213	Actions to take in an emergency	1	2	3	4	5	NA
183214	Options for assistance with medical emergencies	1	2	3	4	5	NA
183215	Proper technique to measure peak expiratory flow	1	2	3	4	5	NA
183216	When to use peak flow meter	1	2	3	4	5	NA
183217	Conditions that trigger asthma	1	2	3	4	5	NA
183218	Strategies to manage controllable environmental risk factors	1	2	3	4	5	NA

Continued

Knowledge: Asthma Management—cont'd

		No Knowledge	Limited Knowledge	Moderate Knowledge	Substantial Knowledge	Extensive Knowledge	
183237	Strategies to manage controllable risk factors in the home	1	2	3	4	5	NA
183238	Strategies to manage controllable risk factors at work or school	1	2	3	4	5	NA
183239	Importance of smoking cessation	1	2	3	4	5	NA
183219	Benefits of ongoing self-monitoring	1	2	3	4	5	NA
183240	How to use a diary or app to monitor symptoms	1	2	3	4	5	NA
183220	Effective breathing techniques	1	2	3	4	5	NA
183221	Recommended physical activity	1	2	3	4	5	NA
183222	Activity restrictions	1	2	3	4	5	NA
183223	Leisure activity recommendations	1	2	3	4	5	NA
183225	Strategies to balance activity and rest	1	2	3	4	5	NA
183241	Strategies to enhance sleep	1	2	3	4	5	NA
183224	Medication used for asthma	1	2	3	4	5	NA
183242	Importance of keeping adequate supply of medication	1	2	3	4	5	NA
183243	How to use an inhaler or nebulizer correctly	1	2	3	4	5	NA
183226	Medication therapeutic effects	1	2	3	4	5	NA
183227	Medication side effects	1	2	3	4	5	NA
183228	Medication adverse effects	1	2	3	4	5	NA
183244	Importance of recommended immunizations	1	2	3	4	5	NA
183229	When to obtain assistance from a health professional	1	2	3	4	5	NA
183245	Importance of keeping appointments with health professional	1	2	3	4	5	NA
183230	When to obtain emergency treatment	1	2	3	4	5	NA
183231	Available support groups	1	2	3	4	5	NA
183232	Available community resources	1	2	3	4	5	NA

Domain-Health Knowledge & Behavior (IV)   **Class-**Knowledge Health Condition (GG)   4th edition 2008; revised 2013, 2024

OUTCOME CONTENT REFERENCES:

Cloutier, M. M., Dixon, A. E., Krishnan, J. A., Lemanske, R. F., Pace, W., & Schatz, M. (2020). Managing asthma in adolescents and adults: 2020 asthma guideline update from the National Asthma Education and Prevention Program. *Journal of American Medical Association, 324*(22), 2301–2317. https://doi.org/10.1001/jama.2020.21974

Curto, E., Crespo-Lessmann, A., González-Gutiérrez, M. V., Bardagí, S., Cañete, C., Pellicer, C., Bazús, T., del Carmen Vennera, M., Martínez, C., & Plaza, V. (2019). Is asthma in the elderly different? Functional and clinical characteristics of asthma in individuals aged 65 years and older. *Asthma Research and Practice, 5*(2), 2. https://doi.org/10.1186/s40733-019-0049-x

Dilber, O. M., Selma, F., Kurtuluş, A., Funda, A., & Şahin, D. S. (2021). Obstructive sleep apnea is a determinant of asthma control independent of smoking, reflux, and rhinitis. *Allergy and Asthma Proceedings, 42*(1), e25–e29. https://doi.org/10.2500/aap.2021.42.200098

Expert Panel Working Group of the National Heart, Lung, and Blood Institute (NHLBI) administered and coordinated National Asthma Education and Prevention Program Coordinating Committee (NAEPPCC), Cloutier, M. M., Baptist, A. P., Blake, K. V., Brooks, E. G., Bryant-Stephens, T., DiMango, E., Dixon, A. E., Elward, K. S., Hartert, T., Krishnan, J. A., Lemanske, R. F. Jr., Ouellette, D. R., Pace, W. D., Schatz, M., Skolnik, N. S., Stout, J. W., Teach, S. J., Umscheid, C. A., & Walsh, C. G. (2020). 2020 Focused Updates to the Asthma Management Guidelines: A Report from the National Asthma Education and Prevention Program Coordinating Committee Expert Panel Working Group. *The Journal of Allergy and Clinical Immunology, 146*(6), 1217–1270. https://doi.org/10.1016/j.jaci.2020.10.003

Gruffydd-Jones, K., & Hansen, K. (2019). Working for better asthma control: How can we improve the dialogue between patients and healthcare professionals? *Advanced Therapy, 37*(1), 1–9. https://doi.org/10.6084/m9.figshare.9994856.v2

Lovinsky-Desir, S., & O'Connor, G. T. (2020). Evolving strategies for long-term asthma management. *Journal of American Medical Association, 324*(22), 2265–2267. https://doi.org/10.1001/jama.2020.16895

Nanda, A., & Wasan, A. N. (2020). Asthma in adults. *Medical Clinics of North America, 104*(1), 95–108. https://doi.org/10.1016/j.mcna.2019.08.013

Knowledge: Attention Deficit Hyperactivity Disorder (ADHD) Management   **1869**

Definition: Extent of understanding conveyed about the dimensions, treatment, and behavioral support needed for a child with ADHD

OUTCOME TARGET RATING: Maintain at_____ Increase to_____

		No Knowledge	Limited Knowledge	Moderate Knowledge	Substantial Knowledge	Extensive Knowledge	
OUTCOME OVERALL RATING		1	2	3	4	5	
Indicators:							
186901	Current causative theories of ADHD	1	2	3	4	5	NA
186902	Signs and symptoms of ADHD	1	2	3	4	5	NA
186903	Usual symptoms of inattention	1	2	3	4	5	NA
186904	Usual symptoms of impulsivity	1	2	3	4	5	NA
186905	Usual symptoms of hyperactivity	1	2	3	4	5	NA
186906	Potential impact on family dynamics	1	2	3	4	5	NA
186907	Potential impact on social relationships	1	2	3	4	5	NA
186908	Associated risk for substance abuse	1	2	3	4	5	NA
186909	Associated risk for conduct disorders	1	2	3	4	5	NA
186910	Associated risk for anxiety	1	2	3	4	5	NA
186911	Associated risk for depression	1	2	3	4	5	NA
186912	Associated risk for learning disabilities	1	2	3	4	5	NA
186913	Associated risk for poor school performance	1	2	3	4	5	NA
186914	Options for recording symptoms of hyperactivity	1	2	3	4	5	NA
186915	Behavioral therapy as first treatment option	1	2	3	4	5	NA
186916	Types of multi-model treatment options	1	2	3	4	5	NA
186917	Medication used for ADHD	1	2	3	4	5	NA
186918	Importance of compliance with medication regimen	1	2	3	4	5	NA
186919	Medication therapeutic effects	1	2	3	4	5	NA
186920	Medication side effects	1	2	3	4	5	NA
186921	Potential for abuse of prescribed medication	1	2	3	4	5	NA
186922	Importance of providing positive reinforcement	1	2	3	4	5	NA
186923	Strategies to reduce environmental stimuli	1	2	3	4	5	NA
186924	Strategies on how to set appropriate consequences for undesirable behaviors	1	2	3	4	5	NA
186925	Strategies to help child take responsibility for behavior	1	2	3	4	5	NA
186926	Strategies to help child make better choices	1	2	3	4	5	NA
186927	Family role in ADHD	1	2	3	4	5	NA
186928	Importance of regularly scheduled reevaluation	1	2	3	4	5	NA
186929	Reputable sources of information on ADHD	1	2	3	4	5	NA
186930	Importance of coordinated management with teachers	1	2	3	4	5	NA
186931	Importance of coordinated management with health professionals	1	2	3	4	5	NA
186932	Available support groups	1	2	3	4	5	NA
186933	Available community resources	1	2	3	4	5	NA

*Domain-*Health Knowledge & Behavior (VI)   *Class-* Knowledge Health Condition (GG)   *7th edition 2024*

OUTCOME CONTENT REFERENCES:

Aduen, P., Day, A. T., Kofler, M. J., Harmon, S. L., Wells, E. L., & Sarver, D. E. (2018). Social problems in ADHD: Is it a skills acquisition or performance problem? *Journal of Psychopathology and Behavioral Assessment, 40*(3), 440–451. https://doi.org/10.1007/s10862-018-9649-7

Antai-Otong, D., & Zimmerman, M. L. (2016). Treatment approaches to attention deficit hyperactivity disorder. *The Nursing Clinics of North America, 51*(2), 199–211. https://doi.org/10.1016/j.cnur.2016.01.005

Center for Disease Control and Prevention (2021, September 28). Attention-Deficit/Hyperactivity Disorder (ADHD). https://www.cdc.gov/ncbddd/adhd/index.html

Hockenberry, M. J., Wilson, D., & Rodgers, C. C. (Eds.). (2019). *Wong's nursing care of infants and children* (11th ed.). Elsevier.

McQuade, J. D., Breaux, R., Mordy, A. E., & Taubin, D. (2021). Childhood ADHD symptoms, parent emotion socialization, and adolescent peer problems: Indirect effects through emotion dysregulation. *Journal of Youth & Adolescence, 50*(12), 2519–2532. https://doi.org/10.1007/s10964-021-01510-3

Paidipati, C. P., & Deatrick, J. A. (2015). The role of family phenomena in children and adolescents with attention deficit hyperactivity disorder. *Journal of Child and Adolescent Psychiatric Nursing, 28*(1), 3–13. https://doi.org/10.1111/jcap.12097

Pan, P.-Y., Jonsson, U., Şahpazoğlu Çakmak, S. S., Häge, A., Hohmann, S., Nobel Norrman, H., Buitelaar, J. K., Banaschewski, T., Cortese, S., Coghill, D., & Bölte, S. (2022). Headache in ADHD as comorbidity and a side effect of medications: A systematic review and meta-analysis. *Psychological Medicine, 52*(1), 14–25. https://doi.org/10.1017/S0033291721004141

Parsons, C. (2021). The Chronic Care Model and attention-deficit/hyperactivity disorder: A novel approach to improving the transition to postsecondary education. *The Journal for Nurse Practitioners, 17*(4). 412–417. https://doi.org/10.1016/j.nurpra.2020.11.024

Knowledge: Autism Spectrum Disorder Management   3201

Definition: Extent of understanding conveyed about types of autism, treatment, and the prevention of complications

OUTCOME TARGET RATING: Maintain at_____ Increase to_____

	No Knowledge	Limited Knowledge	Moderate Knowledge	Substantial Knowledge	Extensive Knowledge	
OUTCOME OVERALL RATING	**1**	**2**	**3**	**4**	**5**	
Indicators:						
320101 Signs and symptoms of autism	1	2	3	4	5	NA
320102 Types of autism	1	2	3	4	5	NA
320103 Specific type of autism diagnosis	1	2	3	4	5	NA
320104 Cause and contributing factors	1	2	3	4	5	NA
320105 Signs and symptoms of complications	1	2	3	4	5	NA
320106 Strategies to prevent complications	1	2	3	4	5	NA
320107 Importance of early treatment	1	2	3	4	5	NA
320108 Available treatment options	1	2	3	4	5	NA
320109 Evidence-based biomedical treatment	1	2	3	4	5	NA
320110 Strategies to implement applied behavioral analysis	1	2	3	4	5	NA
320111 Treatment therapeutic effects	1	2	3	4	5	NA
320112 Importance of adapting behaviors to meet treatment requirements	1	2	3	4	5	NA
320113 Correct use of prescribed medication	1	2	3	4	5	NA
320114 Medication therapeutic effects	1	2	3	4	5	NA
320115 Medication side effects	1	2	3	4	5	NA
320116 Available assistance for activities of daily living	1	2	3	4	5	NA
320117 Available assistance for instrumental activities of daily living	1	2	3	4	5	NA
320118 Strategies to cope with effects of autism	1	2	3	4	5	NA
320119 Strategies to reduce anxiety	1	2	3	4	5	NA
320120 Strategies to reduce stress	1	2	3	4	5	NA
320121 Strategies to minimize the impact of change	1	2	3	4	5	NA
320122 Effective relaxation techniques	1	2	3	4	5	NA
320123 Strategies to reduce environmental stimuli	1	2	3	4	5	NA
320124 Strategies for effective communication	1	2	3	4	5	NA
320125 Strategies to adapt to social environment	1	2	3	4	5	NA
320126 Adaptations for role performance	1	2	3	4	5	NA
320127 Strategies to maintain family routine	1	2	3	4	5	NA
320128 Family role in autism management	1	2	3	4	5	NA
320129 Psychosocial effects on family	1	2	3	4	5	NA
320130 Reputable sources of autism information	1	2	3	4	5	NA
320131 Importance of coordinated management with other health professionals	1	2	3	4	5	NA
320132 Available support group	1	2	3	4	5	NA
320133 Available community resources	1	2	3	4	5	NA

Domain-Health Knowledge & Behavior (IV)   **Class**-Knowledge Health Condition (GG)   6th edition 2018

K

OUTCOME CONTENT REFERENCES:

Carlsson, E., Miniscalco, C., Kadesjö, B., & Laakso, K. (2016). Negotiating knowledge: Parent's experience of the neuropsychiatric diagnostic process for children with autism. *International Journal of Language and Communication Disorders, 51*(3), 328–338. https://doi.org/10.1111/1460-6984.12210

Christensen, D., Baio, J., Braun, K., Bilder, D., Charles, J., Constantino, J., Daniels, J., Durkin, M. S., Fitzgerald, R. T., Kurzius-Spemcer, M., Lee, L.-C., Pettygrove, S., Robinson, C., Schulz, E., Wells. C., Wingate, M. S., Zohorrodny, W., & Yeargin-Allsopp, M. (2016). Prevalence and characteristics of autism spectrum disorder among children aged 8 years—autism and developmental disabilities monitoring network, 11 sites, United States, 2012. *Morbidity and Mortality Weekly Report, 65*(3), 1–23. https://doi.org/10.15585/mmwr.ss6503a1

Jo, H., Schieve, L., Rice, C., Yeargin-Allsopp, M., Tian, L., Blumberg, S., Kogan, M. D., & Boyle, C. (2015). Age at autism spectrum disorder (ASD) diagnosis by race, ethnicity, and primary household language among children with special health care needs, United States, 2009–2010. *Maternal and Child Health Journal, 19*(8), 1687–1697. https://doi.org/10.1007/s10995-015-1683-4

Rice, C., Zablotsky, B., Avila, R., Colpe, L., Schieve, L., Pringle, B, & Blumberg, S. (2016). Reported wandering behavior among children with autism spectrum disorder and/or intellectual disability. *Journal of Pediatrics, 174*, 232–239. https://doi.org/10.1016/j.jpeds.2016.03.047

Soke, G., Rosenberg, S., Hamman, R., Fingerlin, T., Robinson, C., Carpenter, L., Giarelli, E., Lee, L.-C., Wiggins, L. D., Durkin, M. S., DiGuiseppi, C. (2016). Brief report: Prevalence of self-injurious behaviors among children with autism spectrum disorder-a population-based study. *Journal of Autism and Developmental Disorders, 46*(11), 3607–3614. https://doi.org/10.1007/s10803-016-2879-1

Solomon, A. H., & Chung, B. (2012). Understanding autism: How family therapists can support parents of children with autism spectrum disorders. *Family Process, 51*(2), 250–264. https://doi.org/10.1111/j.1545-5300.2012.01399.x

Yang, D., Pelphrey, K., Sukhodolsky, D., Crowley, M., Dayan, E., Dvornek, N., Venkataraman, A., Duncan, J., Staib, L., & Ventola, P. (2016). Brain responses to biological motion predict treatment outcome in young children with autism. *Translational Psychiatry, 6*(11), e948. https://doi.org/10.1038/tp.2016.213

Knowledge: Body Mechanics   1827

Definition: Extent of understanding conveyed about proper body alignment, balance, and coordinated movement

OUTCOME TARGET RATING: Maintain at_____ Increase to_____

K

		No Knowledge	Limited Knowledge	Moderate Knowledge	Substantial Knowledge	Extensive Knowledge	
OUTCOME OVERALL RATING		1	2	3	4	5	
Indicators:							
182701	Natural spinal curves	1	2	3	4	5	NA
182702	Proper standing posture	1	2	3	4	5	NA
182703	Proper sitting posture	1	2	3	4	5	NA
182704	Proper lying posture	1	2	3	4	5	NA
182705	Proper lifting techniques	1	2	3	4	5	NA
182716	How to maintain a stable center of gravity	1	2	3	4	5	NA
182717	How to maintain a wide base of support	1	2	3	4	5	NA
182718	How to maintain proper body alignment	1	2	3	4	5	NA
182719	Importance of carrying items close to body	1	2	3	4	5	NA
182720	Importance of wearing proper shoes	1	2	3	4	5	NA
182721	Importance of avoiding sudden position changes	1	2	3	4	5	NA
182722	Importance of avoiding twisting or stretching motions	1	2	3	4	5	NA
182723	Importance of bending knees when lifting	1	2	3	4	5	NA
182724	Importance of changing feet positions frequently when standing	1	2	3	4	5	NA
182706	Exercises to improve posture	1	2	3	4	5	NA
182707	Exercises to improve muscle flexibility	1	2	3	4	5	NA
182708	Exercises to improve joint mobility	1	2	3	4	5	NA
182709	Exercises to improve muscle strength	1	2	3	4	5	NA
182710	Exercises to strengthen lower abdominal muscles	1	2	3	4	5	NA
182711	Positional causes of muscle or joint pain from sitting	1	2	3	4	5	NA
182712	Positional causes of muscle or joint pain from lying	1	2	3	4	5	NA
182713	Positional causes of muscle or joint pain from lifting	1	2	3	4	5	NA
182725	Importance of seeking assistance when needed	1	2	3	4	5	NA
182726	Common causes of back injury	1	2	3	4	5	NA
182714	Common symptoms of back injury	1	2	3	4	5	NA
182715	Personal risk activities	1	2	3	4	5	NA

Domain-*Health Knowledge & Behavior (IV)*   *Class*-*Knowledge Health Promotion (S)*   *3rd edition 2004; revised 2008, 2024*

OUTCOME CONTENT REFERENCES:

Kang, S. W. (2017). The use of body mechanics principle, clinical-practice fatigue, and practice satisfaction of nursing students, *NursingPlus Open, 3*, 6–10. https://doi.org/10.1016/j.npls.2017.03.001

Potter, P. A., Perry, A. G., Stockert, P. A., & Hall, A. (2021). *Fundamentals of nursing* (10th ed.). Elsevier.

Sorrentino, S. A., & Remmert, L. A. (2021). *Mosby's textbook for nursing assistants* (10th ed.). Elsevier.

Topcu, S. Y. (2017). Do Turkish patients with lumbar disc herniation know body mechanics? *Journal of Back and Musculoskeletal Rehabilitation, 30*(4), 835–840. https://doi.org/10.3233/BMR-160542

Yusoff, S. M., Firdaus, M. K. Z. H., Jamaludin, F. I. C., & Hasan, M. K. C. H. (2019). The need for educating healthcare professionals regarding good musculoskeletal health practice. *Enfermeria Clinica, 29*(2), 579–584. https://doi.org/10.1016/j.enfcli.2019.04.089

Knowledge: Bottle Feeding — 1846

Definition: Extent of understanding conveyed about providing fluids to an infant using a bottle

OUTCOME TARGET RATING: Maintain at_____ Increase to_____

		No Knowledge	Limited Knowledge	Moderate Knowledge	Substantial Knowledge	Extensive Knowledge	
OUTCOME OVERALL RATING		1	2	3	4	5	
Indicators:							
184601	Infant hunger cues	1	2	3	4	5	NA
184602	Safety of different types of bottles	1	2	3	4	5	NA
184603	Proper nipple type and hole size	1	2	3	4	5	NA
184604	Importance of hand sanitation	1	2	3	4	5	NA
184605	Preparation of infant formula	1	2	3	4	5	NA
184606	Methods to clean bottles and nipples	1	2	3	4	5	NA
184607	Proper storage of milk	1	2	3	4	5	NA
184608	Proper storage of mixed formula	1	2	3	4	5	NA
184609	Importance of checking expiration date of formula	1	2	3	4	5	NA
184610	Proper methods to warm bottle	1	2	3	4	5	NA
184611	Importance of testing temperature of fluid prior to feeding infant	1	2	3	4	5	NA
184612	Proper infant positioning while feeding	1	2	3	4	5	NA
184613	Proper bottle position while feeding	1	2	3	4	5	NA
184616	Infant cues to stop feeding	1	2	3	4	5	NA
184617	Reasons for avoidance of water for newborn	1	2	3	4	5	NA
184618	Proper technique to respond to choking	1	2	3	4	5	NA
184619	Signs of well-nourished infant	1	2	3	4	5	NA

Domain-*Health Knowledge & Behavior (IV)*   **Class**-*Knowledge Health Promotion (S)*   *5th edition 2013; revised 2024*

OUTCOME CONTENT REFERENCES:

Beal, J. A. (2018). Baby bottles and bisphenol A (BPA): Still a parental concern. *MCN: The American Journal of Maternal Child Nursing, 43*(6), 349. https://doi.org/10.1097/NMC.0000000000000477

Borghese-Lang, T., Morrison, L., Ogle, A., & Wright, A. (2003). Successful bottle feeding of the young infant. *Journal of Pediatric Health Care, 17*(2), 94–101.

Hockenberry, M. J., Wilson, D., & Rodgers, C. C. (Eds.). (2019). *Wong's nursing care of infants and children* (11th ed.). Elsevier.

Perry, S. E., Hockenberry, M. J., Lowdermilk, D. J., Wilson, D., Cashion, K., Rodgers, C. C., & Alden, K. R. (2018). *Maternal child nursing care* (6th ed.). Elsevier.

Thomas, J. (2007). A parent's guide to bottle feeding your premature baby. *Advances in Neonatal Care, 7*(6), 319–320. https://doi.org/10.1097/01.ANC.0000304972.69578.2c

Knowledge: Breastfeeding   1800

Definition: Extent of understanding conveyed about lactation and nourishment of an infant through breastfeeding

OUTCOME TARGET RATING: Maintain at_____ Increase to_____

		No Knowledge	Limited Knowledge	Moderate Knowledge	Substantial Knowledge	Extensive Knowledge	
OUTCOME OVERALL RATING		1	2	3	4	5	
Indicators:							
180001	Benefits of breastfeeding	1	2	3	4	5	NA
180002	Physiology of lactation	1	2	3	4	5	NA
180020	Fluid intake requirements for mother	1	2	3	4	5	NA
180003	Breastmilk composition, letdown process, foremilk versus hindmilk	1	2	3	4	5	NA
180004	Infant hunger cues	1	2	3	4	5	NA
180005	Proper technique for attaching infant to the breast	1	2	3	4	5	NA
180006	Proper infant positioning while nursing	1	2	3	4	5	NA
180007	Nutritive versus non-nutritive sucking	1	2	3	4	5	NA
180008	Evaluation of infant swallowing	1	2	3	4	5	NA
180009	Proper technique to break infant suction	1	2	3	4	5	NA
180010	Signs of adequate milk supply	1	2	3	4	5	NA
180011	Signs of well-nourished infant	1	2	3	4	5	NA
180012	Nipple evaluation	1	2	3	4	5	NA
180013	Signs of mastitis, blocked ducts, nipple trauma	1	2	3	4	5	NA
180014	Reasons for early avoidance of artificial nipples	1	2	3	4	5	NA
180021	Reasons for avoidance of water and supplements for infant	1	2	3	4	5	NA
180015	Proper breastmilk expression and storage techniques	1	2	3	4	5	NA
180016	Substances that transfer from mother to infant through breastmilk	1	2	3	4	5	NA
180022	Relationship between breastfeeding and infant immunity	1	2	3	4	5	NA
180017	Signs of weaning readiness	1	2	3	4	5	NA
180018	Strategies to access health care services	1	2	3	4	5	NA
180023	Available support groups	1	2	3	4	5	NA

Domain-Health Knowledge & Behavior (IV)   ***Class-****Knowledge Health Promotion (S)*   *1st edition 1997; revised 2004, 2008, 2013, 2024*

OUTCOME CONTENT REFERENCES:

Barbosa, G. E. F., Silva, V. B., Pereira, J. M., Soares, M. S., Medeiros, R. A., Filho, P. L. B., Pereira, L. B., de Pinho, L., & Caldeira, A. P. (2017). Initial breastfeeding difficulties and association with breast disorders among postpartum women. *Revista Paulista de Pediatria. 35*(3), 265–272. https://doi.org/10.1590/1984-0462/;2017;35;3;00004

Dias Emidio, S. C., Barbosa Dias, F. de S., Moorhead, S., Deberg, J., de Souza Oliveira-Kumakura, A. R., & Valentim Carmona, E. (2020). Conceptual and operational definition of nursing outcomes regarding the breastfeeding establishment. *Revista Latino-Americana de Enfermagem (RLAE), 28*, 1–12. https://doi.org/10.1590/1518-8345.3007.3259

Dias Emidio, S. C., Moorhead, S., Oliveira, H. C., Herdman, T. H., Oliveira-Kumakura, A. R. D. S., & Carmona, E. V. (2020). Validation of nursing outcomes related to breastfeeding establishment. *International Journal of Nursing Knowledge, 31*(2), 134–144. https://doi.org/10.1111/2047-3095.12256

Esterik, V. P. (2012). *Core curriculum for lactation consultant practice* (3rd ed.). Jones & Bartlett Learning.

Giglia, R., & Binns, C. (2006). Alcohol and lactation: A systematic review. *Nutrition & Dietetics, 63*(2), 103–116. https://doi.org/10.1111/bcpt.12149

Henderson, A. M., Pincombe, J., & Stamp, G. E. (2000). Assisting women to establish breastfeeding: Exploring midwives' practices. *Breastfeeding Review, 8*(3), 11–17.

McCarter-Spaulding, D. E. (2005). Medications in pregnancy and lactation. *MCN: American Journal of Maternal Child Nursing, 30*(1), 24–29.

Spahn, J. M., Callahan, E. H., Spill, M. K., Wong, Y. P., Benjamin-Neelon, S. E., Birch, L., Black, M. M., Cook, J. T., Faith, M. S., Mennella, J. A., & Casavale, K. O. (2019). Influence of maternal diet on flavor transfer to amniotic fluid and breast milk and children's responses: A systematic review. *The American Journal of Clinical Nutrition, 109*(Suppl. 7), 1003S–1026S. https://doi.org/10.1093/ajcn/nqy240

Wambach, K., & Riordan, J. (2015). *Breastfeeding and human lactation* (5th ed.). Jones & Bartlett Learning.

K

Knowledge: Cancer Management

1833

Definition: Extent of understanding conveyed about cancer, its treatment, and the prevention of disease progression and complications

OUTCOME TARGET RATING: Maintain at_____ Increase to_____

OUTCOME OVERALL RATING		No Knowledge 1	Limited Knowledge 2	Moderate Knowledge 3	Substantial Knowledge 4	Extensive Knowledge 5	
Indicators:							
183301	Abnormal screening results	1	2	3	4	5	NA
183302	Signs and symptoms of cancer	1	2	3	4	5	NA
183303	Specific cancer diagnosis	1	2	3	4	5	NA
183304	Cause and contributing factors	1	2	3	4	5	NA
183305	Usual course of disease	1	2	3	4	5	NA
183306	Stages of cancer	1	2	3	4	5	NA
183307	Signs and symptoms of recurrence	1	2	3	4	5	NA
183308	Available treatment options	1	2	3	4	5	NA
183309	Alternative treatments	1	2	3	4	5	NA
183310	Purpose of different treatment options	1	2	3	4	5	NA
183311	Benefits of different treatment options	1	2	3	4	5	NA
183312	Tests and procedures involved in treatment regimen	1	2	3	4	5	NA
183313	Steps in treatment regimen	1	2	3	4	5	NA
183314	Medication therapeutic effects	1	2	3	4	5	NA
183315	Medication adverse effects	1	2	3	4	5	NA
183316	Medication side effects	1	2	3	4	5	NA
183317	Potential complications of treatment	1	2	3	4	5	NA
183318	Signs and symptoms of complications	1	2	3	4	5	NA
183319	Precautions to prevent complications of treatment	1	2	3	4	5	NA
183320	Self-care responsibilities for ongoing treatment	1	2	3	4	5	NA
183321	Physical effects of cancer treatment	1	2	3	4	5	NA
183322	Effects on lifestyle	1	2	3	4	5	NA
183323	Effects on employment	1	2	3	4	5	NA
183324	Effects on sexuality	1	2	3	4	5	NA
183325	Strategies to cope with adverse effects of disease	1	2	3	4	5	NA
183326	Survival rate	1	2	3	4	5	NA
183327	Self-care issues during recovery	1	2	3	4	5	NA
183328	Importance of positive attitude for coping with cancer	1	2	3	4	5	NA
183335	Importance of informing genetic risk to family members	1	2	3	4	5	NA
183336	Importance of immune-mediated therapies	1	2	3	4	5	NA
183337	Importance of timely treatment	1	2	3	4	5	NA
183329	Reputable sources of cancer information	1	2	3	4	5	NA
183330	Available community resources	1	2	3	4	5	NA
183331	Available support groups	1	2	3	4	5	NA
183332	Financial resources for assistance	1	2	3	4	5	NA
183333	Health beliefs that affect adherence to treatment	1	2	3	4	5	NA
183334	Benefits of disease management	1	2	3	4	5	NA

Specify cancer_____

Domain-*Health Knowledge & Behavior (IV)*   **Class**-*Knowledge Health Condition (GG)*   *4th edition 2008; reviewed 2013; revised 2024*

OUTCOME CONTENT REFERENCES:

Al-Harithy, F. M., & Wazqar, D.Y. (2020). Factors associated with self-management practices and self-efficacy among adults with cancer under treatment in Saudi Arabia. *Journal of Clinical Nursing, 30*, 3301–3313. https://doi.org/10.1111/jocn.15843

Durnin, R., Shepherd, P., & Gilleece, T. (2021). An evaluation of the information needs of radiotherapy patients and their families. *Journal of Radiotherapy in Practice, 20*, 473–479. https://doi.org/10.1017/S1460396920000497

Heiter, E. (2020). Circulating tumor DNA for modern cancer management. *Clinical Chemistry, 66*(1), 143–145. https://doi.org/10.1373/clinchem.2019.304774

Khodabakhshi, A., Mahmoudi, M., Majd, H. M., & Davoodi, S. H. (2021). Possible nutrition-related mechanisms of metabolic management in cancer treatment. *International Journal of Cancer Management, 14*(1), 1–6. https://doi.org/10.5812/ijcm.107678

Largey, G., Briggs, P., Davies, H., Underhill, C., Ross, C., Harvey, K., Blum, R., Parker, C., Guthrie, C., Parente, P., Trevorah, B., Torres, J., Mott, C., Lancaster, C., Brand, M., Earnest, A., Pellegrini, B., Reed, M., Zalcberg, J., & Stirling, R. (2021). Victorian lung cancer service redesign project: Impacts of a quality improvement collaborative on timeliness and management in lung cancer. *Internal Medicine Journal, 51,* 2061–2068. https://doi.org/10.1111/imj.15043

Magnoni, F., Alessandrini, S., Alberti, L., Polizzi, A., Rotili, A., Veronesi, P., & Corso, G. (2021). Breast cancer surgery: New issues. *Current Oncology. 28,* 4053–066. https://doi.org/10.3390/curroncol28050344

Martin, J. C. (2020). Genetic biomarkers. *Clinical Journal of Oncology Nursing, 24*(6), 648–656. https://doi.org/10.1188/20.CJON.648-656

Plouvier, S. D., Bonnal, J.-L., Machuron, F., Colin, P., Vankemmel, O., Leroy, X., Duhamel, A., Villers, A., Saint, F., & Pasquier, D. Impact of age on bladder cancer management practices: A general population study. *Acta Oncologica, 59*(4), 462–466. https://doi.org/10.1080/0284186X.2020.1723164

Porro, B., de Boer, A. G. E. M., Frings-Dresen, M. H. W., & Roquelaure, Y. (2020). Self-efficacy and return to work in cancer survivors: Current knowledge and future prospects. *European Journal of Cancer Care, 29,* e13304. https://doi.org/10.1111/ecc.13304

Knowledge: Cancer Threat Reduction

1834

Definition: Extent of understanding conveyed about causes, prevention, and early detection of cancer

OUTCOME TARGET RATING: Maintain at_____ Increase to_____

		No Knowledge	Limited Knowledge	Moderate Knowledge	Substantial Knowledge	Extensive Knowledge	
OUTCOME OVERALL RATING		1	2	3	4	5	
Indicators:							
183401	Warning signs of cancer	1	2	3	4	5	NA
183402	Cause and contributing factors	1	2	3	4	5	NA
183421	Genetic risk factors	1	2	3	4	5	NA
183403	Genetic testing	1	2	3	4	5	NA
183404	Recommended cancer screenings	1	2	3	4	5	NA
183405	Cancer screening procedures	1	2	3	4	5	NA
183406	Recommended self-screenings for cancer detection	1	2	3	4	5	NA
183407	Benefits of adequate sleep	1	2	3	4	5	NA
183408	Benefits of regular exercise	1	2	3	4	5	NA
183409	Importance of oral screening	1	2	3	4	5	NA
183410	Diet recommendations for reducing risk	1	2	3	4	5	NA
183411	Correct use of nutritional supplements	1	2	3	4	5	NA
183412	Correct use of prescribed medication	1	2	3	4	5	NA
183413	Strategies to avoid exposure to carcinogens	1	2	3	4	5	NA
183414	Strategies to protect skin from sun exposure	1	2	3	4	5	NA
183415	Strategies to prevent cervical cancer	1	2	3	4	5	NA
183416	Strategies to manage controllable environmental risk factors	1	2	3	4	5	NA
183417	Adverse health effects of tobacco use	1	2	3	4	5	NA
183418	Safe sexual practices	1	2	3	4	5	NA
183419	When to obtain assistance from a health professional	1	2	3	4	5	NA
183420	Reputable sources of cancer prevention information	1	2	3	4	5	NA

Domain-Health Knowledge & Behavior (IV)   *Class-Knowledge Health Promotion (S)*   *4th edition 2008; revised 2013; reviewed 2024*

OUTCOME CONTENT REFERENCES:
Mayer, B., Joshweseoma, L., & Sehongva, G. (2019). Environmental risk perceptions and community health: Arsenic, air pollution, and threats to traditional values of the Hopi tribe. *Journal of Community Health, 44,* 896–902. https://doi.org/10.1007/s10900-019-00627-8

Neugut, A. L., El-Sadr, W. M., & Ruff, P. (2021). The looming threat: Cancer in Sub-Saharan Africa. *The Oncologist, 26,* e2099–e2101. https://doi.org/10.1002/onco.13963

Potter, P., Perry, A., Stockert, P., & Hall, A. (2021). *Fundamentals of nursing* (10th ed.). Elsevier.

van Zandwijk, N., Reid, G., & Frank, A. L. (2020). Asbestos-related cancers: The 'hidden killer' remains a global threat. *Expert Review of Anticancer Therapy, 20*(4), 271–278. https://doi.org/10.1080/14737140.2020.1745067

K

Knowledge: Cardiac Disease Management 1830

Definition: Extent of understanding conveyed about heart disease, its treatment, and the prevention of disease progression and complications

OUTCOME TARGET RATING: Maintain at_____ Increase to_____

		No Knowledge	Limited Knowledge	Moderate Knowledge	Substantial Knowledge	Extensive Knowledge	
OUTCOME OVERALL RATING		1	2	3	4	5	
Indicators:							
183001	Usual course of disease	1	2	3	4	5	NA
183002	Signs and symptoms of early disease	1	2	3	4	5	NA
183003	Signs and symptoms of worsening disease	1	2	3	4	5	NA
183040	Signs and symptoms of complications	1	2	3	4	5	NA
183041	Signs and symptoms of anxiety	1	2	3	4	5	NA
183042	Signs and symptoms of depression	1	2	3	4	5	NA
183004	Benefits of disease management	1	2	3	4	5	NA
183005	Strategies to reduce risk factors	1	2	3	4	5	NA
183028	Strategies to decrease treatment side effects	1	2	3	4	5	NA
183006	Importance of completing cardiac rehabilitation	1	2	3	4	5	NA
183007	Family's role in treatment plan	1	2	3	4	5	NA
183008	Methods to measure blood pressure	1	2	3	4	5	NA
183029	Methods to monitor heart rate	1	2	3	4	5	NA
183009	Strategies to limit sodium intake	1	2	3	4	5	NA
183010	Benefits of following a low-fat, low-cholesterol diet	1	2	3	4	5	NA
183011	Strategies to increase diet adherence	1	2	3	4	5	NA
183012	Strategies to limit fluid intake	1	2	3	4	5	NA
183013	Importance of monitoring weight	1	2	3	4	5	NA
183014	Importance of alcohol restrictions	1	2	3	4	5	NA
183015	Importance of tobacco abstinence	1	2	3	4	5	NA
183030	Recommended work activity	1	2	3	4	5	NA
183031	Recommended physical activity	1	2	3	4	5	NA
183032	Recommended leisure activity	1	2	3	4	5	NA
183017	Benefits of regular exercise	1	2	3	4	5	NA
183018	Energy conservation techniques	1	2	3	4	5	NA
183043	Adaptations for sexual performance	1	2	3	4	5	NA
183044	Effects on sexuality	1	2	3	4	5	NA
183021	Medication therapeutic effects	1	2	3	4	5	NA
183033	Medication side effects	1	2	3	4	5	NA
183034	Medication adverse effects	1	2	3	4	5	NA
183022	Strategies to manage stress	1	2	3	4	5	NA
183045	Recommended vaccines	1	2	3	4	5	NA
183046	What to do when symptoms occur	1	2	3	4	5	NA
183035	When to obtain assistance from a health professional	1	2	3	4	5	NA
183047	Importance of keeping scheduled appointments	1	2	3	4	5	NA
183025	Care options for assistance with medical emergencies	1	2	3	4	5	NA
183026	Importance of family learning cardiopulmonary resuscitation	1	2	3	4	5	NA
183027	Cultural influences on adherence to treatment regimen	1	2	3	4	5	NA
183036	Available support groups	1	2	3	4	5	NA
183037	Reputable sources of cardiac disease information	1	2	3	4	5	NA

Domain-*Health Knowledge & Behavior (IV)*   **Class**-*Knowledge Health Condition (GG)*   *3rd edition 2004; revised 2008, 2013, 2024*

K

OUTCOME CONTENT REFERENCES:

Hendriks, J., Andreae, C., Ågren, S., Eriksson, H., Hjelm, C., Walfridsson, U., Ski, C. F., Thylén, I., & Jaarsma, T. (2020). Cardiac disease and stroke: Practical implications for personalized care in cardiac-stroke patients. A state-of-the-art review supported by the Association of Cardiovascular Nursing and Allied Professions. *European Journal of Cardiovascular Nursing: Journal of the Working Group on Cardiovascular Nursing of the European Society of Cardiology,* *19*(6), 495–504. https://doi.org/10.1177/1474515119895734

Huang, Z., Yap, Q. V., Chan, Y. H., Ho, J. S., Tan, S. Y., Koh, W. P., Chua, T., & Yoon, S. (2021). Knowledge of heart disease, preventive behavior and source of information in a multi-ethnic Asian population: A population-based survey. *Journal of Community Health, 46*(1), 31–40. https://doi.org/10.1007/s10900-020-00838-4

Ignatavicius, D. D., Workman, M. L., Rebar, C. R., & Heimgartner, N. M. (2021). *Medical-surgical nursing: Concepts for interprofessional care* (10th ed.). Elsevier.

Thomas, R. J., Beatty, A. L., Beckie, T. M., Brewer, L. C., Brown, T. M., Forman, D. E., Franklin, B. A., Keteyian, S. J., Kitzman, D. W., Regensteiner, J. G., Sanderson, B. K., & Whooley, M. A. (2019). Home-based cardiac rehabilitation: A scientific statement from the American Association of Cardiovascular and Pulmonary Rehabilitation, the American Heart Association, and the American College of Cardiology. *Journal of the American College of Cardiology, 74*(1), 133–153. https://doi.org/10.1016/j.jacc.2019.03.008

Zhou, Y., Liao, J., Feng, F., Ji, M., Zhao, C., & Wang, X. (2018). Effects of a nurse-led phone follow-up education program based on the self-efficacy among patients with cardiovascular disease. *The Journal of Cardiovascular Nursing, 33*(1), E15–E23. https://doi.org/10.1097/JCN.0000000000000414

Knowledge: Cardiac Rehabilitation   3202

Definition: Extent of understanding conveyed about prescribed exercise, nutritional, and behavioral therapy to reduce risk factors after a cardiac event

OUTCOME TARGET RATING: Maintain at_____ Increase to_____

OUTCOME OVERALL RATING	No Knowledge 1	Limited Knowledge 2	Moderate Knowledge 3	Substantial Knowledge 4	Extensive Knowledge 5	
Indicators:						
320201 Individualized exercise plan	1	2	3	4	5	NA
320202 Heart healthy diet options	1	2	3	4	5	NA
320203 Importance of gradually increasing physical activity throughout the rehabilitation period	1	2	3	4	5	NA
320204 Barriers to implementing heart healthy behaviors	1	2	3	4	5	NA
320205 Strategies to find transportation to cardiac rehabilitation sessions	1	2	3	4	5	NA
320206 Importance of changing unhealthy behaviors	1	2	3	4	5	NA
320207 Smoking cessation resources and strategies	1	2	3	4	5	NA
320208 A normal blood pressure reading	1	2	3	4	5	NA
320209 A normal heart rate	1	2	3	4	5	NA
320210 Management of symptoms related to heart condition	1	2	3	4	5	NA
320211 Strategies to manage stress	1	2	3	4	5	NA
320212 Benefits of cardiac rehabilitation in conjunction with pharmacologic treatment	1	2	3	4	5	NA
320213 Importance of monitoring cholesterol levels	1	2	3	4	5	NA
320214 Interpretation of cholesterol levels	1	2	3	4	5	NA
320215 Weight loss strategies	1	2	3	4	5	NA
320216 Importance of completing cardiac rehabilitation	1	2	3	4	5	NA

Domain-Health Knowledge & Behavior (IV)   *Class*-Knowledge Health Condition (GG)   6th edition 2018

OUTCOME CONTENT REFERENCES:

Balady, G., Ades, P., Bittner, V., Franklin, B., Gordon, N., Thomas, R., Tomaselli, G. F., & Yancy, C. W. (2011). Referral, enrollment, and delivery of cardiac rehabilitation/secondary prevention programs at clinical centers and beyond: A presidential advisory from the American Heart Association. *Circulation, 124*(25), 2951–2960. https://doi.org/10.1161/CIR.0b013e31823b21e2

Dalal, H. M., Doherty, P., & Taylor, R. S. (2015). Cardiac rehabilitation. *British Medical Journal, 351*. https://doi.org/10.1136/bmj.h5000

Gaalema, D., Cutler, A., Higgins, S., & Ades, P. (2015). Smoking and cardiac rehabilitation participation: Associations with referral, attendance, and adherence. *Preventive Medicine, 80*, 67–74. https://doi.org/10.1016/j.ypmed.2015.04.009

Gaalema, D. E., Savage, P. D., Rengo, J. L., Cutler, A. Y., Higgins, S. T., & Ades, P. A. (2016). Financial incentives to promote cardiac rehabilitation participation and adherence among Medicaid patients. *Preventive Medicine, 92*, 47–50. https://doi.org/10.1016/j.ypmed.2015.11.032

Sandesara, P., Lambert, C., Gordon, N., Fletcher, G., Franklin, B., Wenger, N., & Sperling, L. (2015). Cardiac rehabilitation and risk reduction: Time to "rebrand and reinvigorate." *Journal of the American College of Cardiology, 65*(4), 389–395. https://doi.org/10.1016/j.jacc.2014.10.059

Knowledge: Celiac Disease Management

3203

Definition: Extent of understanding conveyed about celiac disease, its treatment, and the prevention of disease progression and complications

OUTCOME TARGET RATING: Maintain at_____ Increase to_____

		No Knowledge	Limited Knowledge	Moderate Knowledge	Substantial Knowledge	Extensive Knowledge	
OUTCOME OVERALL RATING		**1**	**2**	**3**	**4**	**5**	
Indicators:							
320301	Cause and contributing factors	1	2	3	4	5	NA
320302	Usual course of disease	1	2	3	4	5	NA
320303	Benefits of disease management	1	2	3	4	5	NA
320304	Signs and symptoms of gluten intolerance	1	2	3	4	5	NA
320305	Relationship between diet and signs and symptoms	1	2	3	4	5	NA
320306	Long-term consequences of untreated celiac disease	1	2	3	4	5	NA
320307	Importance of strict adherence to gluten-free diet	1	2	3	4	5	NA
320308	Importance of supplemental vitamins	1	2	3	4	5	NA
320309	Food retailers selling gluten-free foods	1	2	3	4	5	NA
320310	Interpretation of information on food labels	1	2	3	4	5	NA
320311	Food consistent with cultural beliefs	1	2	3	4	5	NA
320312	Potential threat of cross contamination	1	2	3	4	5	NA
320313	Non-food gluten sources	1	2	3	4	5	NA
320314	Plan for eating out	1	2	3	4	5	NA
320315	Plan for social situations	1	2	3	4	5	NA
320316	Effects on lifestyle	1	2	3	4	5	NA
320317	Importance of participation in educational program	1	2	3	4	5	NA
320318	Importance of follow-up appointments	1	2	3	4	5	NA
320319	Importance of coordinated management with other health professionals	1	2	3	4	5	NA
320320	Available support group	1	2	3	4	5	NA
320321	Financial resources for assistance	1	2	3	4	5	NA
320322	Reputable sources of information	1	2	3	4	5	NA
320323	When to obtain assistance from a health professional	1	2	3	4	5	NA

Domain-Health Knowledge & Behavior (IV)   **Class**-Knowledge Health Condition (GG)   6th edition 2018

OUTCOME CONTENT REFERENCES:

Dowd, A., Jung, M., Chen, M., & Beauchamp, M. (2016). Prediction of adherence to a gluten-free diet using protection motivation theory among adults with celiac disease. *Journal of Human Nutrition & Dietetics, 29*(3), 391–398. https://doi.org/10.1111/jhn.12321

Jacobsson, L., Milberg, A., Hjelm, K., & Friedrichsen, M. (2016). Gaining perspective on own illness—the lived experiences of a patient education programme for women with treated coeliac disease. *Journal of Clinical Nursing, 25*(9-10), 1229–1237. https://doi.org/10.1111/jocn.13123

Silvester, J., Weiten, D., Graff, L., Walker, J., & Duerksen, D. (2016). Living gluten-free: Adherence, knowledge, lifestyle adaptations and feelings towards a gluten-free diet. *Journal of Human Nutrition & Dietetics, 29*(3), 374–382. https://doi.org/10.1111/jhn.12316

Zarkadas, M., Dubois, S., Maclsaac, K., Cantin, I., Rashid, M., Roberts, K. C., La Vielle, S., Godefroy, S., & Pulido, O. M. (2013). Living with coeliac disease and a gluten-free diet: A Canadian perspective. *Journal of Human Nutrition and Dietetics, 26*(1), 10–23. https://doi.org/10.1111/j.1365-277X.2012.01288.x

Knowledge: Child Physical Safety   1801

Definition: Extent of understanding conveyed about safely caring for a child from 1 year through 17 years of age

OUTCOME TARGET RATING: Maintain at_____ Increase to_____

		No Knowledge	Limited Knowledge	Moderate Knowledge	Substantial Knowledge	Extensive Knowledge	
OUTCOME OVERALL RATING		1	2	3	4	5	
Indicators:							
180101	Appropriate activities for child's developmental level	1	2	3	4	5	NA
180132	Vaccination requirements for age	1	2	3	4	5	NA
180133	Safe food preparation and storage	1	2	3	4	5	NA
180119	Diving hazards	1	2	3	4	5	NA
180103	Strategies to prevent drowning	1	2	3	4	5	NA
180104	Strategies to prevent electrical shock	1	2	3	4	5	NA
180105	Benefits of protective helmet	1	2	3	4	5	NA
180120	First-aid techniques	1	2	3	4	5	NA
180108	Correct use of safety seats and seat belts	1	2	3	4	5	NA
180121	Age-appropriate cardiopulmonary resuscitation techniques	1	2	3	4	5	NA
180122	Heimlich maneuver	1	2	3	4	5	NA
180106	Strategies to prevent choking	1	2	3	4	5	NA
180111	Strategies to prevent farm accidents	1	2	3	4	5	NA
180123	Strategies to prevent motor vehicle accidents	1	2	3	4	5	NA
180134	Benefits of protective gear for high-risk activities	1	2	3	4	5	NA
180135	Strategies to prevent baby circle walker accidents	1	2	3	4	5	NA
180124	Strategies to prevent cycle accidents	1	2	3	4	5	NA
180136	Strategies to prevent skateboard accidents	1	2	3	4	5	NA
180112	Strategies to prevent falls	1	2	3	4	5	NA
180113	Strategies to prevent playground accidents	1	2	3	4	5	NA
180137	Strategies to secure household cleaners and poisons	1	2	3	4	5	NA
180114	Strategies to prevent burns	1	2	3	4	5	NA
180115	Correct use of smoke detectors	1	2	3	4	5	NA
180138	Correct use of carbon monoxide detectors	1	2	3	4	5	NA
180139	Importance of developing a home fire evacuation plan	1	2	3	4	5	NA
180116	Proper surveillance of outdoor play	1	2	3	4	5	NA
180140	Strategies to prevent sunburn	1	2	3	4	5	NA
180141	Strategies to prevent frostbite or hypothermia	1	2	3	4	5	NA
180142	Strategies to prevent animal bites	1	2	3	4	5	NA
180117	Importance of teaching stranger awareness	1	2	3	4	5	NA
180143	Strategies to prevent abduction	1	2	3	4	5	NA
180125	Strategies to prevent tobacco use	1	2	3	4	5	NA
180126	Strategies to prevent alcohol use	1	2	3	4	5	NA
180144	Strategies to prevent vaping	1	2	3	4	5	NA
180127	Strategies to prevent recreational drug use	1	2	3	4	5	NA
180145	Strategies to monitor internet contacts	1	2	3	4	5	NA
180128	Strategies to prevent firearm injuries	1	2	3	4	5	NA
180146	Strategies to prevent gang participation	1	2	3	4	5	NA
180129	Strategies to prevent participation in violence	1	2	3	4	5	NA
180130	Strategies to prevent medication misuse	1	2	3	4	5	NA
180131	Strategies to prevent exposure to toxic chemicals	1	2	3	4	5	NA

K

Domain-Health Knowledge & Behavior (IV)   *Class*-Knowledge Health Promotion (S)   *1st edition 1997; revised 2004, 2008, 2024*

OUTCOME CONTENT REFERENCES:
Ahern, N. R., Kemppainen, J., & Thacker, P. (2016). Awareness and knowledge of child and adolescent risky behaviors: A parent's perspective. *Journal of Child and Adolescent Psychiatric Nursing, 29*(1), 6–14. https://doi.org/10.1111/jcap.12129
Bright, M. A., Sayedul Huq, M., Patel, S., Miller, M. D., & Finkelhor, D. (2022). Child safety matters: Randomized control trial of a school-based, child victimization prevention curriculum. *Journal of Interpersonal Violence, 37*(1/2), 538–556. https://doi.org/10.1177/0886260520909185
Hagan, J. F., Shaw, J. S., & Duncan, P. M. (Eds.). (2017). *Bright futures: Guidelines for health supervision of infants, children, and adolescents* (4th ed.). American Academy of Pediatrics.
Hockenberry, M. J., Wilson, D., & Rodgers, C. C. (Eds.). (2019). *Wong's nursing care of infants and children* (11th ed.). Elsevier.
Kennya, M. C., & Wurteleb, S. K. (2016). Teaching preschoolers safety rules: A pilot study of injury prevention. *Children's Health Care, 45*(4), 428–440. https://doi.org/10.1080/02739615.2015.1065743
Perry, S. E., Hockenberry, M. J., Lowdermilk, D. J., Wilson, D., Cashion, K., Rodgers, C. C., & Alden, K. R. (2018). *Maternal child nursing care* (6th ed.). Elsevier.

Knowledge: Chronic Anemia Management   3204

Definition: Extent of understanding conveyed about persistent anemia, its causes, treatment, and the prevention of complications

OUTCOME TARGET RATING: Maintain at_____ Increase to_____

OUTCOME OVERALL RATING	No Knowledge 1	Limited Knowledge 2	Moderate Knowledge 3	Substantial Knowledge 4	Extensive Knowledge 5	
Indicators:						
320401 Contributing factors	1	2	3	4	5	NA
320402 Signs and symptoms of anemia	1	2	3	4	5	NA
320403 Importance of well-balanced diet	1	2	3	4	5	NA
320423 Importance of hydration	1	2	3	4	5	NA
320424 Importance of iron-fortified food	1	2	3	4	5	NA
320404 Importance of nutritional supplements	1	2	3	4	5	NA
320405 Importance of iron supplements	1	2	3	4	5	NA
320406 Factors that impact the ability to perform activity	1	2	3	4	5	NA
320407 Energy conservation techniques	1	2	3	4	5	NA
320408 Modification of daily activities	1	2	3	4	5	N/A
320409 Strategies to perform activity safely	1	2	3	4	5	N/A
320410 Medical treatment options	1	2	3	4	5	NA
320411 Medication therapeutic effects	1	2	3	4	5	NA
320412 Medication side effects	1	2	3	4	5	NA
320413 Medication adverse effects	1	2	3	4	5	NA
320414 Benefits of symptom management	1	2	3	4	5	N/A
320415 Signs and symptoms of cardiac complications	1	2	3	4	5	N/A
320416 Tests and procedures involved in treatment regimen	1	2	3	4	5	NA
320417 When to obtain assistance from a health professional	1	2	3	4	5	N/A
320418 Importance of follow-up care	1	2	3	4	5	N/A
320425 Importance of obtaining recommended vaccines	1	2	3	4	5	N/A
320421 Psychosocial effects of anemia	1	2	3	4	5	N/A
320422 Reputable sources of anemia-specific information	1	2	3	4	5	N/A

Domain-Health Knowledge & Behavior (IV)   *Class*-Knowledge Health Condition (GG)   6th edition 2018; revised 2024

OUTCOME CONTENT REFERENCES:
Benson, C. S., Shah, A., Stanworth, S. J., Frise, C. J., Spiby, H., Lax, S. J., Murray, J., & Klein, A. A. (2021). The effect of iron deficiency and anaemia on women's health. *Anaesthesia, 76*(Suppl. 4), 84–95. https://doi.org/10.1111/anac.15405
Cappellini, M. D., Musallam, K. M., & Taher, A. T. (2020). Iron deficiency anaemia revisited. *Journal of Internal Medicine, 287*(2), 153–170. https://doi.org/10.1111/joim.13004
de Miranda, F. R., Ivo, M. L., Teston, E. F., Lino, I. G. T., Mandetto, M. A., & Marcheti, M. A. (2020). Families' experiences in managing children with sickle cell anemia: Implications for care. *Revista Enfermagem UERJ, 28*, e51594. https://doi.org/10.12957/reuerj.2020.S1594
Elstrott, B., Khan, L., Olson, S., Raghunathan, V., DeLoughery, T., & Shatzel, J. J. (2020). The role of iron repletion in adult iron deficiency anemia and other diseases. *European Journal of Haematology, 104*(3), 153–161. https://doi.org/10.1111/ejh.13345
Hockenberry, M. J., Rodgers, C. C., & Wilson, D. (2022). *Wong's essential of pediatric nursing* (11th ed.). Elsevier.
Wiciński, M., Liczner, G., Cadelski, K., Kolnierzk, T., Nowaczewska, M., & Malinowski, B. (2020). Anemia of chronic diseases: Wider diagnostics—better treatment? *Nutrients, 12*(6), 121–217. https://doi.org/10.3390/nu12061784

Knowledge: Chronic Disease Management   1847

Definition: Extent of understanding conveyed about a specific chronic disease, its treatment, and the prevention of disease progression and complications

OUTCOME TARGET RATING: Maintain at_____ Increase to_____

		No Knowledge	Limited Knowledge	Moderate Knowledge	Substantial Knowledge	Extensive Knowledge	
OUTCOME OVERALL RATING		1	2	3	4	5	
Indicators:							
184701	Cause and contributing factors	1	2	3	4	5	NA
184702	Usual course of disease	1	2	3	4	5	NA
184703	Benefits of disease management	1	2	3	4	5	NA
184704	Signs and symptoms of chronic disease	1	2	3	4	5	NA
184731	Pattern of signs and symptoms	1	2	3	4	5	NA
184705	Signs and symptoms of disease progression	1	2	3	4	5	NA
184732	Strategies to manage signs and symptoms	1	2	3	4	5	NA
184706	Signs and symptoms of complications	1	2	3	4	5	NA
184707	Strategies to prevent complications	1	2	3	4	5	NA
184733	Strategies to adapt lifestyle	1	2	3	4	5	NA
184708	Strategies to balance activity and rest	1	2	3	4	5	NA
184709	Strategies to manage pain	1	2	3	4	5	NA
184710	Available treatment options	1	2	3	4	5	NA
184711	Correct use of prescribed medication	1	2	3	4	5	NA
184712	Medication therapeutic effects	1	2	3	4	5	NA
184713	Medication side effects	1	2	3	4	5	NA
184714	Medication adverse effects	1	2	3	4	5	NA
184715	Potential medication interactions	1	2	3	4	5	NA
184734	Importance of medication reconciliation with health professional	1	2	3	4	5	NA
184716	Required laboratory tests	1	2	3	4	5	NA
184717	Procedures involved in treatment regimen	1	2	3	4	5	NA
184735	Strategies to manage continuous care needs	1	2	3	4	5	NA
184718	Personal responsibilities for treatment regimen	1	2	3	4	5	NA
184719	Importance of adherence with treatment regimen	1	2	3	4	5	NA
184736	Strategies for follow-up treatment	1	2	3	4	5	NA
184720	Recommended immunizations	1	2	3	4	5	NA
184721	Cultural influences on adherence to treatment regimen	1	2	3	4	5	NA
184722	Prescribed diet	1	2	3	4	5	NA
184723	Strategies for tobacco cessation	1	2	3	4	5	NA
184724	Strategies to cope with adverse effects of disease	1	2	3	4	5	NA
184725	Financial resources for assistance	1	2	3	4	5	NA
184737	Available educational opportunities	1	2	3	4	5	NA
184726	Available support groups	1	2	3	4	5	NA
184727	Available community resources	1	2	3	4	5	NA
184728	Reputable sources of chronic disease information	1	2	3	4	5	NA
184729	When to obtain assistance from a health professional	1	2	3	4	5	NA
184730	Actions to take in an emergency	1	2	3	4	5	NA

Domain-Health Knowledge & Behavior (IV)   *Class*-Knowledge Health Condition (GG)   *5th edition 2013; revised 2024*

OUTCOME CONTENT REFERENCES:

Bauer, M. S., Weaver, K., Kim, B., Miller, C., Lew, R., Stolzmann, K., Sullivan, J. L., Riendeau, R., Connolly, S., Pitcock, J., Ludvigsen, S. M., & Elwy, A. R. (2019). The Collaborative Chronic Care Model for mental health conditions. *Medical Care, 57,* S221–S227. https://doi.org/10.1097/MLR.0000000000001145

Crespo, R., Christiansen, M., Tieman, K., & Wittberg, R. (2020). An emerging model for community health worker-based chronic care management for patients with high health care costs in rural Appalachia. *Prevention of Chronic Disease, 17,* 190316. https://doi.org/10.58888/pcd17.190316

Francesconi, P., Ballo, P., Profili, F., Policardo, L., Roti, L., & Zuppiroli, A. (2019). Chronic Care Model for the management of patients with heart failure in primary care. *Health Services Insights, 12,* 1–2. https://doi.org/10.1177/1178632919866200

K

Llewellyn, S. (2019). The Chronic Care Model, kidney disease, and primary care: A scoping review. *Nephrology Nursing Journal, 46*(3), 301–313.

Osmarin, V. M., Bavaresco, T., de Fátima Lucena, A., & Echer, I. C. (2018). Clinical indicators for knowledge assessment of venous ulcer patients. *Acta Paulista de Enfermagem, 31*(4), 391–398. https://doi.org/10.1590/1982-0194201800055

Parsons, C. (2021). The Chronic Care Model and attention-deficit/hyperactivity disorder: A novel approach to improving the transition to postsecondary education. *The Journal for Nurse Practitioners, 17*(4). 412–417. https://doi.org/10.1016/j.nurpra.2020.11.024

Tillman, P. (2020). Applying the Chronic Care Model in a free clinic. *The Journal for Nurse Practitioners, 16*(8), e117–e121. https://doi.org/10.1016/j.nurpra.2020.05.016

Wagner, E. H. (2021). Organizing care for patients with chronic illness revisited. *The Milbank Quarterly, 97*(3),1–5. https://doi.org/10.1111/1468-0009.12416

Knowledge: Chronic Obstructive Pulmonary Disease Management   1848

Definition: Extent of understanding conveyed about chronic obstructive pulmonary disease, its treatment, and the prevention of disease progression and complications

OUTCOME TARGET RATING: Maintain at_____ Increase to_____

	No Knowledge	Limited Knowledge	Moderate Knowledge	Substantial Knowledge	Extensive Knowledge	
OUTCOME OVERALL RATING	1	2	3	4	5	
Indicators:						
184801 Cause and contributing factors	1	2	3	4	5	NA
184802 Specific disease process	1	2	3	4	5	NA
184803 Risk factors for disease progression	1	2	3	4	5	NA
184804 Signs and symptoms of chronic obstructive pulmonary disease	1	2	3	4	5	NA
184805 Signs and symptoms of disease relapse	1	2	3	4	5	NA
184806 Benefits of disease management	1	2	3	4	5	NA
184807 Signs and symptoms of complications	1	2	3	4	5	NA
184808 Strategies to prevent complications	1	2	3	4	5	NA
184809 Strategies to adapt lifestyle to energy level	1	2	3	4	5	NA
184810 Strategies to balance activity and rest	1	2	3	4	5	NA
184838 Strategies to manage exacerbations	1	2	3	4	5	NA
184811 Energy conservation techniques	1	2	3	4	5	NA
184812 Medication therapeutic effects	1	2	3	4	5	NA
184813 Medication side effects	1	2	3	4	5	NA
184814 Medication adverse effects	1	2	3	4	5	NA
184815 Correct use of prescribed medication	1	2	3	4	5	NA
184839 Importance of medication reconciliation with health professional	1	2	3	4	5	NA
184816 Importance of completing prescribed antibiotics	1	2	3	4	5	NA
184817 Correct use of inhaler	1	2	3	4	5	NA
184818 Safety issues related to oxygen use	1	2	3	4	5	NA
184819 Actions to take in an emergency	1	2	3	4	5	NA
184820 Importance of adherence with treatment regimen	1	2	3	4	5	NA
184821 Importance of adherence with medication regimen	1	2	3	4	5	NA
184840 Importance of dietary influences	1	2	3	4	5	NA
184841 Importance of weight control	1	2	3	4	5	NA
184822 Prescribed procedures	1	2	3	4	5	NA
184823 Adequate fluid intake	1	2	3	4	5	NA
184824 Strategies to manage chronic obstructive pulmonary disease	1	2	3	4	5	NA
184825 Strategies for smoking cessation	1	2	3	4	5	NA
184826 Strategies to prevent disease progression	1	2	3	4	5	NA
184827 Strategies to manage controllable environmental risk factors	1	2	3	4	5	NA
184828 Effective breathing techniques	1	2	3	4	5	NA
184829 Effects on lifestyle	1	2	3	4	5	NA

K

Knowledge: Chronic Obstructive Pulmonary Disease Management—cont'd

		No Knowledge	Limited Knowledge	Moderate Knowledge	Substantial Knowledge	Extensive Knowledge	
184830	When to obtain assistance from a health professional	1	2	3	4	5	NA
184831	When to obtain emergency treatment	1	2	3	4	5	NA
184842	Importance of obtaining recommended immunizations	1	2	3	4	5	NA
184834	Importance of follow-up care	1	2	3	4	5	NA
184835	Benefits of pulmonary rehabilitation program	1	2	3	4	5	NA
184843	Reputable e-health resources	1	2	3	4	5	NA
184836	Available support groups	1	2	3	4	5	NA
184837	Available community resources	1	2	3	4	5	NA

Domain-Health Knowledge & Behavior (IV)   **Class**-Knowledge Health Condition (GG)   5th edition 2013; revised 2024

OUTCOME CONTENT REFERENCES:

Baker, E., & Fatoye, F. (2019). Patient perceived impact of nurse-led self-management interventions for COPD: A systematic review of qualitative research. *International Journal of Nursing Studies, 91*, 22–34. https://doi.org/10.1016/j.ijnurstu.2018.12.004

Scoditti, E., Massaro, M., Garbarino, S., & Toraldo, D. M. (2019). Role of diet in chronic obstructive pulmonary disease prevention and treatment. *Nutrients, 11*(6), 1357. https://doi.org/10.3390/nu11061357

Sönnerfors, P., Roaldsen, K. S., Ståhle, A., Wadell, K., & Halvarsson, A. (2021). Access to, use, knowledge, and preferences for information technology and technical equipment among people with chronic obstructive pulmonary disease (COPD) in Sweden. A cross-sectional survey study. *BMC Medical Informatics and Decision Making, 21*(1), 1–10. https://doi.org/10.1186/s12911-021-01544-4

Usmani, O. S. (2019). Choosing the right inhaler for your asthma or COPD patient. *Therapeutics and Clinical Risk Management, 15*, 461–472. https://doi.org/10.2147/TCRM.S160365

Yang, H., Wang, H., Du, L., Wang, Y., Wang, X., & Zhang, R. (2019). Disease knowledge and self-management behavior of COPD patients in China. *Medicine, 98*(8), e14460. https://doi.org/10.1097/MD.0000000000014460

K

Knowledge: Community Health Resources   1870

Definition: Extent of understanding conveyed about available public and private health care resources

OUTCOME TARGET RATING: Maintain at_____ Increase to_____

		No Knowledge	Limited Knowledge	Moderate Knowledge	Substantial Knowledge	Extensive Knowledge	
OUTCOME OVERALL RATING		1	2	3	4	5	
Indicators:							
187001	Reputable health care resources	1	2	3	4	5	NA
187002	Recommended internet resources	1	2	3	4	5	NA
187003	Strategies to access health care services	1	2	3	4	5	NA
187004	Sources of financial support	1	2	3	4	5	NA
187005	Available social support from family	1	2	3	4	5	NA
187006	Available social support from friends	1	2	3	4	5	NA
187007	Available social support from neighborhood	1	2	3	4	5	NA
187008	Available community resources	1	2	3	4	5	NA
187009	Available community support groups	1	2	3	4	5	NA
187010	Available religious support groups	1	2	3	4	5	NA
187011	Available hospital services	1	2	3	4	5	NA
187012	Available rehabilitation services	1	2	3	4	5	NA
187013	Available home care services	1	2	3	4	5	NA
187014	Available long-term care services	1	2	3	4	5	NA
187015	Available mental health services	1	2	3	4	5	NA
187016	Available hospice care services	1	2	3	4	5	NA
187017	Available suicide hotlines	1	2	3	4	5	NA
187018	Available poison control center hotlines	1	2	3	4	5	NA
187019	Available health care hotlines	1	2	3	4	5	NA

Continued

Knowledge: Community Health Resources—cont'd

		No Knowledge	Limited Knowledge	Moderate Knowledge	Substantial Knowledge	Extensive Knowledge	
187020	Available service organizations	1	2	3	4	5	NA
187021	Available respite care services	1	2	3	4	5	NA
187022	Available specialists for diagnosis	1	2	3	4	5	NA
187023	Available research trials for diagnosis	1	2	3	4	5	NA
187024	Available veterans' services	1	2	3	4	5	NA
187025	Available government support programs	1	2	3	4	5	NA
187026	Available care coordination services	1	2	3	4	5	NA
187027	Available transportation services	1	2	3	4	5	NA

Domain-Health Knowledge & Behavior (IV)   **Class**-Knowledge Health Promotion (S)   7th edition 2024

OUTCOME CONTENT REFERENCES:

Bradley, C. J., Yabroft, K. R., Zafar, S. A., & Shih, Y. T. (2021). Time to add screening for financial hardships as a quality measure? *CA: A Cancer Journal for Clinicians, 71*(2), 100–106. https://doi.org/10.3322/caac.21653

Coughlin, S. S. (2008). Surviving cancer or other serious illness: A review of individual and community resources. *CA: A Cancer Journal for Clinicians, 58*(1), 60–64. https://doi.org/10.3322/CA.2007.0001

Henning-Smith, C., Shippee, T., & Capistrant, B. (2018). Later-life disability in environmental context: Why living arrangements matter. *The Gerontologist, 58*(5), 853–862. https://doi.org/10.1093/geront/gnx019

Ruths, S., Baste, V., Bakken, M. S., Engesæter, L. B., Lie, S. A., & Haugland, S. (2017). Municipal resources and patient outcomes through the first year after a hip fracture. *BMC Health Services Research, 17*(1), 144. https://doi.org/10.1186/s12913-017-2087-5

Schroeder, S. D. (2017). Utilization of community resources. *South Dakota Medicine: The Journal of the South Dakota State Medical Association, Spec,* 59–61.

Stanhope, M., & Lancaster, J. (2020). *Public health nursing: Population-centered health care in the community* (10th ed.). Elsevier.

Weaver, R. H., & Roberto, K. A. (2017). Home and community-based service use by vulnerable older adults. *The Gerontologist, 57*(3), 540–551. https://doi.org/10.1093/geront/gnv149

K

Knowledge: Conception Prevention

1821

Definition: Extent of understanding conveyed about prevention of unintended pregnancy

OUTCOME TARGET RATING: Maintain at_____ Increase to_____

		No Knowledge	Limited Knowledge	Moderate Knowledge	Substantial Knowledge	Extensive Knowledge	
OUTCOME OVERALL RATING		1	2	3	4	5	
Indicators:							
182105	How conception occurs	1	2	3	4	5	NA
182116	Advantages of having a child	1	2	3	4	5	NA
182117	Disadvantages of having a child	1	2	3	4	5	NA
182107	Influence of personal values on chosen contraceptive method	1	2	3	4	5	NA
182108	Periodic rhythm method	1	2	3	4	5	NA
182109	Chemical barrier methods	1	2	3	4	5	NA
182110	Hormonal therapy methods	1	2	3	4	5	NA
182111	Mechanical barrier methods	1	2	3	4	5	NA
182118	Long-acting reversible contraception methods	1	2	3	4	5	NA
182112	Surgical treatment options	1	2	3	4	5	NA
182101	How chosen contraceptive method works	1	2	3	4	5	NA
182119	Side effects of chosen method	1	2	3	4	5	NA
182120	Costs associated with chosen contraceptive method	1	2	3	4	5	NA
182121	How to obtain preferred contraceptive	1	2	3	4	5	NA
182102	Correct use of chosen contraceptive method	1	2	3	4	5	NA
182103	Effectiveness of chosen contraceptive method	1	2	3	4	5	NA
182104	Effects of chosen contraceptive on sexually transmitted disease transmission	1	2	3	4	5	NA

Domain-Health Knowledge & Behavior (IV)   **Class**-Knowledge Health Promotion (S)   2nd edition 2000; revised 2004, 2008, 2013, 2024

OUTCOME CONTENT REFERENCES:

Ayorinde, A. A., Boardman, F., McGranahan, M., Porter, L., Eze, N. A., Sallis, A., Buck, R., Hadley, A., Ludeke, M., Mann, S., & Oyebode, O. (2021). Enabling women to access preferred methods of contraception: A rapid review and behavioural analysis. *BMC Public Health, 21*(1), 1–13. https://doi.org/10.1186/s12889-021-12212-7

Boog, K. (2021). Managing the side effects of contraception. *Practice Nursing, 32*(6), 226–231. https://doi.org/10.12968/pnur.2021.32.6.226

Colquitt, C. W., & Martin, T. S. (2017). Contraceptive methods. *Journal of Pharmacy Practice, 30*(1), 130–135.https://doi.org/10.1177/0897190015585751

Lin, C. J., Maier, J., Nwankwo, C., Burley, C., de Borja, L., Aaraj, Y. A., Lewis, E., Rhem, M., Nowalk, M. P., & South-Paul, J. (2021). Awareness and use of contraceptive methods and perceptions of long-acting reversible contraception among white and non-white women. *Journal of Women's Health, 30*(9), 1313–1320. https://doi.org/10.1089/jwh.2020.8642

Woodhams, E. J., & Gilliam, M. (2019). Contraception. *Annals of Internal Medicine, 170*(3), ITC18–ITC32. https://doi.org/10.7326/AITC201902050

Yarger, J., Schroeder, R., Blum, M., Cabral, M. A., Brindis, C. D., Perelli, B., & Harper, C. C. (2021). Concerns about the cost of contraception among young women attending community college. *Women's Health Issues, 31*(5), 420–425. https://doi.org/10.1016/j.whi.2021.03.006

Knowledge: Coronary Artery Disease Management   **1849**

Definition: Extent of understanding conveyed about coronary heart disease, its treatment, and the prevention of disease progression and complications

OUTCOME TARGET RATING: Maintain at_____ Increase to_____

		No Knowledge	Limited Knowledge	Moderate Knowledge	Substantial Knowledge	Extensive Knowledge	
OUTCOME OVERALL RATING		**1**	**2**	**3**	**4**	**5**	
Indicators:							
184901	Usual course of disease	1	2	3	4	5	NA
184902	Cause and contributing factors	1	2	3	4	5	NA
184903	Signs and symptoms of early disease	1	2	3	4	5	NA
184904	Signs and symptoms of worsening disease	1	2	3	4	5	NA
184905	Types of pain associated with disease	1	2	3	4	5	NA
184906	Strategies to reduce risk factors	1	2	3	4	5	NA
184907	Importance of completing cardiac rehabilitation	1	2	3	4	5	NA
184908	Methods to monitor blood pressure	1	2	3	4	5	NA
184909	Methods to monitor heart rate	1	2	3	4	5	NA
184910	Methods to monitor heart rhythm	1	2	3	4	5	NA
184911	Benefits of disease management	1	2	3	4	5	NA
184943	Treatment options	1	2	3	4	5	NA
184912	Medication schedule	1	2	3	4	5	NA
184913	Medication therapeutic effects	1	2	3	4	5	NA
184914	Medication side effects	1	2	3	4	5	NA
184915	Medication adverse effects	1	2	3	4	5	NA
184944	Importance of cardiac rehabilitation	1	2	3	4	5	NA
184916	Importance of limiting sodium intake	1	2	3	4	5	NA
184917	Benefits of following a low-fat, low-cholesterol diet	1	2	3	4	5	NA
184918	Strategies to increase diet adherence	1	2	3	4	5	NA
184919	Strategies to maintain optimal weight	1	2	3	4	5	NA
184920	Benefits of maintaining optimal weight	1	2	3	4	5	NA
184921	Importance of alcohol restrictions	1	2	3	4	5	NA
184922	Importance of tobacco abstinence	1	2	3	4	5	NA
184923	Rationale for regular exercise	1	2	3	4	5	NA
184924	Guidelines for activity level	1	2	3	4	5	NA
184925	Guidelines for sexual activity	1	2	3	4	5	NA
184926	Strategies to prevent blood clots	1	2	3	4	5	NA
184927	Adverse health effects of stress on coronary artery disease	1	2	3	4	5	NA
184928	Adverse health effects of anger on coronary artery disease	1	2	3	4	5	NA
184929	Strategies to manage stress	1	2	3	4	5	NA
184930	Strategies to manage anger	1	2	3	4	5	NA

K

Continued

Knowledge: Coronary Artery Disease Management—cont'd

	No Knowledge	Limited Knowledge	Moderate Knowledge	Substantial Knowledge	Extensive Knowledge	
184945 Strategies to manage depression	1	2	3	4	5	NA
184946 Importance of obtaining recommended vaccines	1	2	3	4	5	NA
184933 Importance of periodic screening of cholesterol level	1	2	3	4	5	NA
184934 Importance of periodic screening of blood glucose level	1	2	3	4	5	NA
184935 Rationale for controlling blood glucose level	1	2	3	4	5	NA
184936 When to obtain assistance from a health professional	1	2	3	4	5	NA
184937 Care options for assistance with medical emergencies	1	2	3	4	5	NA
184938 Family's role in treatment plan	1	2	3	4	5	NA
184939 Importance of family learning cardiopulmonary resuscitation	1	2	3	4	5	NA
184940 Cultural influences on compliance to treatment regimen	1	2	3	4	5	NA
184941 Available support groups	1	2	3	4	5	NA
184942 Reputable sources of cardiac disease information	1	2	3	4	5	NA

Domain-Health Knowledge & Behavior (IV) **Class**-Knowledge Health Condition (GG) 5th edition 2013; revised 2024

OUTCOME CONTENT REFERENCES:

Akten, I. M., Akin, S., Kurbun, H., & Erbatu, B. (2021). Assessment of Turkish patients' knowledge about management of cardiac risk factors. *International Journal of Caring Sciences, 14*(1), 410–421.

Galougahi, K. K., Petrossian, G., Stone, G. W., & Ali, Z. A. (2020). The year in review: Advances in interventional cardiology in 2019. *Current Opinion in Cardiology, 35*(4), 325–331. https://doi.org/10.1097/HCO.0000000000000752

Jia, S., Liu, Y., & Yuan, J. (2020). Evidence in guidelines for treatment of coronary artery disease. *Advances in Experimental Medicine and Biology, 1177*, 37–73. https://doi.org/10.1007/978-981-15-2517-9_2

Jung, H. G., & Yang, Y. K. (2021). Factors influencing health behavior practice in patients with coronary artery diseases. *Health and Quality of Life Outcomes, 19*(3), 1–9. https://doi.org/10.1186/s12955-020-01635-2

Lu, M., Hravnak, M., Ma, J., Lin, Y., Zhang, X., Shen, Y., & Xia, H. (2020). Prediction of changes in adherence to secondary prevention among patients with coronary artery disease. *Nursing Research, 69*(5), E199–E207. https://doi.org/10.1097/NNR.0000000000000433

Lu, M., Xia, H., Ma, J., Lin, Y., Zhang, X., Shen, Y., & Hravnak, M. (2020). Relationship between adherence to secondary prevention and health literacy, self-efficacy and disease knowledge among patients with coronary artery disease in China. *European Journal of Cardiovascular Nursing, 19*(3), 230–237. https://doi.org/10.1177/1474515119880059

Wójcicki, K., Krycińska, R., Tokarek, T., Siudak, Z., Dziewierz, A., Rajtar-Salwa, R., Januszek, R., Siwiec, A., Reczek, L., & Dudek, D. (2019). Knowledge and prevalence of risk factors for coronary artery disease in patients after the first and repeated percutaneous coronary intervention. *Kardiologia Pollska (Polish Heart Journal), 78*(2), 147–153. https://doi.org/10.33963/KP.15070

Knowledge: Cup Feeding · 1850

Definition: Extent of understanding conveyed about providing fluids to an infant using a small cup

OUTCOME TARGET RATING: Maintain at_____ Increase to_____

	No Knowledge	Limited Knowledge	Moderate Knowledge	Substantial Knowledge	Extensive Knowledge	
OUTCOME OVERALL RATING	1	2	3	4	5	
Indicators:						
185001 Infant hunger cues	1	2	3	4	5	NA
185017 Importance of hand sanitation	1	2	3	4	5	NA
185003 Importance of cup sanitation	1	2	3	4	5	NA
185004 Proper storage of milk	1	2	3	4	5	NA
185018 Preparation of formula	1	2	3	4	5	NA
185019 Importance of checking temperature of milk or formula	1	2	3	4	5	NA
185002 Proper infant positioning while feeding	1	2	3	4	5	NA
185005 Proper placement of cup brim	1	2	3	4	5	NA
185006 Proper placement of tongue	1	2	3	4	5	NA
185007 Regulation of milk flow	1	2	3	4	5	NA
185009 Methods to monitor infant swallowing	1	2	3	4	5	NA

K

Knowledge: Cup Feeding—cont'd

		No Knowledge	Limited Knowledge	Moderate Knowledge	Substantial Knowledge	Extensive Knowledge	
185010	Proper technique to respond to choking	1	2	3	4	5	NA
185011	Methods to allow infant to pace feeding	1	2	3	4	5	NA
185008	Time required for feeding	1	2	3	4	5	NA
185014	Infant cues to stop feeding	1	2	3	4	5	NA
185015	Reasons for avoidance of water for newborn	1	2	3	4	5	NA
185016	Signs of well-nourished infant	1	2	3	4	5	NA

Domain-Health Knowledge & Behavior (IV)   **Class**-Knowledge Health Promotion (S)   5th edition 2013; revised 2024

OUTCOME CONTENT REFERENCES:

Dowling, D. A., Meier, P. P., DiFiore, J. M., Blatz, M., & Martin, R. J. (2002). Cup feeding for preterm infants: Mechanics and safety. *Journal of Human Lactation*, 18(1), 13–20. https://doi.org/10.1177/089033440201800103

Flint, A., New, K., & Davies, M. W. (2016). Cup feeding versus other forms of supplemental enteral feeding for newborn infants unable to fully breastfeed. *The Cochrane Database of Systematic Reviews*. https://doi.org/10.1002/14651858.CD005092

Lang, S., Lawrence, C., & Orme, R. (1994). Cup feeding: An alternative method of infant feeding. *Archives of Disease in Childhood, 71*(4), 365–369. https://doi.org/10.1136/adc.71.4.365

McKinney, C. M., Robin, P., Glass, R. P., Coffey, P., Rue, T., Vaughn, M. G., & Cunningham, M. (2016). Feeding neonates by cup: A systematic review of the literature. *Maternal Child Health Journal 20*(8), 1620–1633. https://doi.org/10.1007/s10995-016-1961-9

Penny, F., Judge, M., Brownell, E., & McGrath, J. M. (2018). Cup feeding as a supplemental, alternative feeding method for preterm breastfed infants: An integrative review. *Maternal and Child Health Journal, 22*(11), 1568–1579. https://doi.org/10.1007/s10995-018-2632-9

Vollrath, K., Rosenberg, A., Gabrielski, L., Deacon, J., Marshall, S., Rihn, A., & Grover, T. (2019). NICU discharge feeding bundle improves accuracy of post-discharge feeding preparation and potentially prevents readmission. *Advances in Neonatal Care, 19*(2), 90–96. https://doi.org/10.1097/ANC.0000000000000571

Yilmaz, G., Caylan, N., Karacan, C. D., Bodur, I., & Gokcay, G. (2014). Effect of cup feeding and bottle feeding on breastfeeding in late preterm infants: A randomized controlled study. *Journal of Human Lactation, 30*(2), 174–179. https://doi.org/10.1177/0890334413517940

K

Knowledge: Dementia Management   1851

Definition: Extent of understanding conveyed about progressive dementia, its course over an extended period of time, and plan for supportive care as the disease progresses

OUTCOME TARGET RATING: Maintain at_____   Increase to_____

		No Knowledge	Limited Knowledge	Moderate Knowledge	Substantial Knowledge	Extensive Knowledge	
OUTCOME OVERALL RATING		1	2	3	4	5	
Indicators:							
185102	Type of dementia	1	2	3	4	5	NA
185103	Stages of dementia	1	2	3	4	5	NA
185104	Usual course of neurological losses	1	2	3	4	5	NA
185105	Signs and symptoms of neurological losses	1	2	3	4	5	NA
185106	Usual progression of functional losses	1	2	3	4	5	NA
185107	Signs and symptoms of functional losses	1	2	3	4	5	NA
185108	Importance of sharing feelings about losses	1	2	3	4	5	NA
185109	Importance of stimulating remaining mental functions	1	2	3	4	5	NA
185119	Family's role in disease management	1	2	3	4	5	NA
185120	Signs and symptoms of behavioral changes	1	2	3	4	5	NA
185121	Signs and symptoms of psychiatric changes	1	2	3	4	5	NA
185122	Factors that decrease the ability to perform activities of daily living	1	2	3	4	5	NA
185123	Factors that decrease the ability to perform instrumental activities of daily living	1	2	3	4	5	NA
185124	Treatment options	1	2	3	4	5	NA
185133	Strategies to orient to person, place, and time	1	2	3	4	5	NA

Continued

Knowledge: Dementia Management—cont'd

		No Knowledge	Limited Knowledge	Moderate Knowledge	Substantial Knowledge	Extensive Knowledge	
185125	Strategies for medication adherence	1	2	3	4	5	NA
185126	Strategies to reduce environmental stimuli	1	2	3	4	5	NA
185134	Strategies to promote sleep	1	2	3	4	5	NA
185127	Strategies to balance activity and rest	1	2	3	4	5	NA
185110	Compensatory strategies for memory losses	1	2	3	4	5	NA
185111	Compensatory strategies for losses in judgment	1	2	3	4	5	NA
185135	Compensatory strategies for sensory losses	1	2	3	4	5	NA
185112	Compensatory strategies to remember names	1	2	3	4	5	NA
185113	Compensatory strategies to remember instructions	1	2	3	4	5	NA
185114	Compensatory strategies to remember locations	1	2	3	4	5	NA
185115	Compensatory strategies to maintain personal safety	1	2	3	4	5	NA
185128	Importance of tobacco abstinence	1	2	3	4	5	NA
185129	Relationship between progression and remaining abilities	1	2	3	4	5	NA
185130	Reputable sources of dementia information	1	2	3	4	5	NA
185131	When to obtain assistance from a health professional	1	2	3	4	5	NA
185132	Available community resources	1	2	3	4	5	NA
185116	Strategies to maintain safety of others	1	2	3	4	5	NA
185117	Plan for care in later stages of dementia	1	2	3	4	5	NA
185136	Identification of specialized dementia unit	1	2	3	4	5	NA
185118	Plan for end-of-life care	1	2	3	4	5	NA

Domain-Health Knowledge & Behavior (IV) **Class**-Knowledge Health Condition (GG) 5th edition 2013; revised 2018, 2024

OUTCOME CONTENT REFERENCES:

Balli, F. N., Unsal, P., Halil, M. G., Dogu, B. B., Cankurtaran, M., & Demirkan, K. (2021). Effect of clinical pharmacists' interventions on dementia treatment adherence and caregivers' knowledge. *Geriatrics & Gerontology International, 21*(6), 506–511. https://doi.org/10.1111/ggi.14170

Moore, K. J., Lee, C. Y., Sampson, E. L., & Candy, B. (2020). Do interventions that include education on dementia progression improve knowledge, mental health and burden of family carers? A systematic review. *Dementia, 19*(8), 2555–2581. https://doi.org/10.1177/1471301219831530

Pettigrew, C., Brichko, R., Black, B., O'Connor, M. K., Austrom, M. G., Robinson, M. T., Lindauer, A., Shah, R. C., Peavy, G. M., Meyer, K., Schmitt, F. A., Lingler, J. H., Domoto-Reilly, K., Farrar-Edwards, D., & Albert, M. (2020). Attitudes toward advance care planning among persons with dementia and their caregivers. *International Psychogeriatrics, 32*(5), 585–599. https://doi.org/10.1017/S1041610219000784

Tan, G. T. H., Yuan, Q., Devi, F., Wang, P., Ng, L. L., Goveas, R., Chong, S. A., & Subramaniam, M. (2021). Dementia knowledge and its demographic correlates amongst informal dementia caregivers in Singapore, *Aging & Mental Health, 25*(5), 864–872. https://doi.org/10.1080/13607863.2020.1740914

Varcarolis, E. M., & Fosbre, C. D. (2021). *Essentials of psychiatric-mental health nursing* (4th ed.). Elsevier.

Vrijsen, J., Matulessij, T. F., Joxhorst, T., de Rooij, S. E., & Smidt, N. (2021). Knowledge, health beliefs and attitudes towards dementia and dementia risk reduction among the Dutch general population: A cross-sectional study. *BMC Public Health, 21*(1), 857–868. https://doi.org/10.1186/s12889-021-10913-7

Williams, P. (2020). *Basic geriatric nursing* (7th ed.). Elsevier.

Knowledge: Depression Management

1836

Definition: Extent of understanding conveyed about depression and interrelationships among causes, effects, and treatments

OUTCOME TARGET RATING: Maintain at_____ Increase to_____

		No Knowledge	Limited Knowledge	Moderate Knowledge	Substantial Knowledge	Extensive Knowledge	
OUTCOME OVERALL RATING		1	2	3	4	5	
Indicators:							
183601	Physical signs and symptoms of depression	1	2	3	4	5	NA
183602	Emotional signs and symptoms of depression	1	2	3	4	5	NA
183603	Chronic conditions that increase risk for depression	1	2	3	4	5	NA
183604	Benefits of disease management	1	2	3	4	5	NA

K

Knowledge: Depression Management—cont'd

		No Knowledge	Limited Knowledge	Moderate Knowledge	Substantial Knowledge	Extensive Knowledge	
183605	Available treatment options	1	2	3	4	5	NA
183626	Available treatment options using telehealth	1	2	3	4	5	NA
183606	Personal treatment regimen	1	2	3	4	5	NA
183607	Relationship of treatment regimen to goals	1	2	3	4	5	NA
183608	Importance of completing treatment regimen	1	2	3	4	5	NA
183609	Personal treatment therapeutic effects	1	2	3	4	5	NA
183610	Importance of adherence with treatment regimen	1	2	3	4	5	NA
183611	Importance of adherence with medication regimen	1	2	3	4	5	NA
183612	Factors contributing to depression	1	2	3	4	5	NA
183613	Factors that alleviate depression	1	2	3	4	5	NA
183614	Strategies to reduce precursors of depression	1	2	3	4	5	NA
183615	Strategies to facilitate recovery	1	2	3	4	5	NA
183616	Adverse health effects of depression on daily functioning	1	2	3	4	5	NA
183617	Interrelationship of self-esteem and body image to depression	1	2	3	4	5	NA
183618	Relationship of substance use to depression	1	2	3	4	5	NA
183619	Medication therapeutic effects	1	2	3	4	5	NA
183620	Medication side effects	1	2	3	4	5	NA
183621	Medication adverse effects	1	2	3	4	5	NA
183622	Potential medication interactions	1	2	3	4	5	NA
183627	How to select a health professional	1	2	3	4	5	NA
183628	Importance of social support	1	2	3	4	5	NA
183623	Available support groups	1	2	3	4	5	NA
183624	Available community resources	1	2	3	4	5	NA
183625	When to obtain assistance from a health professional	1	2	3	4	5	NA

Domain-Health Knowledge & Behavior (IV)   **Class**-Knowledge Health Condition (GG)   4th edition 2008; revised 2013, 2024

OUTCOME CONTENT REFERENCES:

Berman, J., Pardasani, M., & Powell, M. (2020). The impact of Age-Tastic! on health literacy about depression among older adults: A pilot study. *Educational Gerontology, 46*(3), 117–128. https://doi.org/10.1080/03601277.2020.1714832

Coles, M. E., Ravid, A., Gibb, B., George-Denn, D. B., Bronstien, L. R., & McLead, S. (2016). Adolescent mental health literacy: Young people's knowledge of depression and social anxiety disorder. *Journal of Adolescent Health, 58*(1), 57–62. https://doi.org/10.1016/j.jadohealth.2015.09.017

El-Den, S., O'Reilly, C. L., Gardner, D. M., Murphy, A. L., & Chen, T. F. (2019). Content validation of a questionnaire measuring basic perinatal depression knowledge. *Women & Health, 59*(6), 615–630. https://doi.org/10.1080/03630242.2018.1539431

McCoy, K. T., Costa, C. B., Pancione, K., & Hammonds, L. S. (2019). Anticipating changes for depression management in primary care. *Nursing Clinics of North America, 54*(4), 457–471. https://doi.org/10.1016/j.cnur.2019.07.001

Marinucci, A., Grové, C., & Allen, K.-A. (2022) A scoping review and analysis of mental health literacy interventions for children and youth. *School Psychology Review*. [Online ahead of print] https://doi.org/10.1080/2372966X.2021.2018918

+Mirsalimi, F., Ghofranipour, F., Noroozi, A., & Montazeri, A. (2020). The Postpartum Depression Literacy Scale (PoDLiS): Development and psychometric properties. *BMC Pregnancy & Childbirth, 20*(1), 1–13. https://doi.org/10.1186/s12884-019-2705-9

National Institute of Mental Health. (2017). Transforming the understanding and treatment of mental illnesses: Major depression. https://www.nimh.nih.gov/health/statistics/majordepression.shtml

Ng, S. H., Tan, N. J. H., Luo, Y., Goh, W. S., Ho, R., & Ho, C. S. H. (2021). A systematic review of youth and teen mental health first aid: Improving adolescent mental health. *Journal of Adolescent Health, 69*(2), 199–210. https://doi.org/10.1016/j.jadohealth.2020.10.018

Singh, S., Zaki, R. A., & Farid, N. D. N. (2019). A systematic review of depression literacy: Knowledge, help-seeking and stigmatizing attitudes among adolescents. *Journal of Adolescence, 74*, 154–172. https://doi.org/10.1016/j.adolescence.2019.06.004

Townsend, L., Musci, R., Stuart, E., Ruble, A., Beaudry, M. B., Schweizer, B., Owen, M., Goode, C., Johnson, S. L., Bradshaw, C., Wilcox, H., & Swartz, K. (2017). The association of school climate, depression literacy, and mental health stigma among high school students. *Journal of School Health, 87*(8), 567–574. https://doi.org/10.1111/josh.12527

K

Knowledge: Diabetes Management 1820

Definition: Extent of understanding conveyed about diabetes, its treatment, and the prevention of complications

OUTCOME TARGET RATING: Maintain at_____ Increase to_____

	No Knowledge	Limited Knowledge	Moderate Knowledge	Substantial Knowledge	Extensive Knowledge	
OUTCOME OVERALL RATING	1	2	3	4	5	
Indicators:						
182030 Cause and contributing factors	1	2	3	4	5	NA
182031 Signs and symptoms of early disease	1	2	3	4	5	NA
182002 Role of diet in blood glucose control	1	2	3	4	5	NA
182003 Prescribed meal plan	1	2	3	4	5	NA
182004 Strategies to increase diet adherence	1	2	3	4	5	NA
182005 Role of exercise in blood glucose control	1	2	3	4	5	NA
182032 Role of sleep in blood glucose control	1	2	3	4	5	NA
182006 Hyperglycemia and related symptoms	1	2	3	4	5	NA
182007 Hyperglycemia prevention	1	2	3	4	5	NA
182008 Procedures to be followed in treating hyperglycemia	1	2	3	4	5	NA
182009 Hypoglycemia and related symptoms	1	2	3	4	5	NA
182010 Hypoglycemia prevention	1	2	3	4	5	NA
182011 Procedures to be followed in treating hypoglycemia	1	2	3	4	5	NA
182012 Importance of maintaining blood glucose level within target range	1	2	3	4	5	NA
182013 Impact of acute illness on blood glucose level	1	2	3	4	5	NA
182033 How to use a monitoring device	1	2	3	4	5	NA
182044 How to use a glucose log or app to record blood glucose test results	1	2	3	4	5	NA
182015 Actions to take in response to blood glucose levels	1	2	3	4	5	NA
182016 Prescribed insulin regimen	1	2	3	4	5	NA
182034 Correct use of insulin	1	2	3	4	5	NA
182027 Proper technique to draw up and administer insulin	1	2	3	4	5	NA
182018 Plan for rotation of injection sites	1	2	3	4	5	NA
182019 Onset, peak, and duration of prescribed insulin	1	2	3	4	5	NA
182035 Proper disposal of syringes and needles	1	2	3	4	5	NA
182020 Prescribed oral medication regimen	1	2	3	4	5	NA
182036 Correct use of prescribed medication	1	2	3	4	5	NA
182037 Correct use of non-prescription medication	1	2	3	4	5	NA
182045 Importance of medication reconciliation with health provider	1	2	3	4	5	NA
182038 Proper medication storage	1	2	3	4	5	NA
182039 Medication therapeutic effects	1	2	3	4	5	NA
182040 Medication side effects	1	2	3	4	5	NA
182041 Medication adverse effects	1	2	3	4	5	NA
182042 When to obtain assistance from a health professional	1	2	3	4	5	NA
182046 Importance of partnering with health care provider	1	2	3	4	5	NA
182047 Develops plan for emergencies	1	2	3	4	5	NA
182028 Correct procedure for urine ketone testing	1	2	3	4	5	NA
182029 Importance of dilated eye exam and vision testing by an ophthalmologist	1	2	3	4	5	NA
182023 Preventive foot care practices	1	2	3	4	5	NA
182048 Importance of inspecting skin for breakdown or pressure	1	2	3	4	5	NA
182049 Importance of smoking cessation	1	2	3	4	5	NA
182050 Importance of monitoring for signs and symptoms of depression	1	2	3	4	5	NA

K

Knowledge: Diabetes Management—cont'd

		No Knowledge	Limited Knowledge	Moderate Knowledge	Substantial Knowledge	Extensive Knowledge	
182051	Importance of keeping vaccinations current	1	2	3	4	5	NA
182043	Reputable sources of diabetes information	1	2	3	4	5	NA
182024	Benefits of disease management	1	2	3	4	5	NA
180252	Importance of social support	1	2	3	4	5	NA

Domain-*Health Knowledge & Behavior (IV)*   **Class**-*Knowledge Health Condition (GG)*   *2nd edition 2000; revised 2004, 2008, 2013, 2024*

OUTCOME CONTENT REFERENCES:

American Diabetes Association. (2019). Lifestyle management: Standards of medical care in diabetes. *Diabetes Care, 42*(Suppl. 1), S46–S60. https://doi.org/10.2337/dc19-S005

Brito-Brito, P. R., Martín-García, Á., Oter-Quintana, C., Paloma-Castro, O., Romero-Sánchez, J. M., & Group, CoNOCidiet-Diabetes Research. (2020). Development and content validation of a NOC-based instrument for measuring dietary knowledge in patients with diabetes: CoNOCidiet diabetes. *International Journal of Nursing Knowledge, 31*(1), 59–73. https://doi.org/10.1111/2047-3095.12243

Chasens, A. R., Imes, C. C., Kariuki, J. K., Luyster, F. S., Morris, J. L., DiNardo, M. M., Godzik, C. M., Jeon, B., & Yang, K. (2021). Sleep and metabolic syndrome. *Nursing Clinics of North America, 56*(2), 203–217. https://doi.org/10.1016/j.cnur.2020.10.012

Cradock, K. A., ÓLaighin, G., Finucane, F. M., McKay, R., Quinlan, L. R., Martin Ginis, K. A., & Gainforth, H. L. (2017). Diet behavior change techniques in type 2 diabetes: A systematic review and meta-analysis. *Diabetes Care, 40*(12), 1800–1810. https://doi.org/10.2337/dc17-0462

Cruz-Cobo, C., & Santi-Cano, M. J. (2020). Efficacy of diabetes education in adults with diabetes mellitus type 2 in primary care: A systematic review. *Journal of Nursing Scholarship,52*(2), 155–163. https://doi.org/10.1111/jnu.12539

Davis, J., Fischl, A. H., Beck, J., Browning, L., Carter, A., Condon, J. E., Dennison, M., Francis, T., Hughes, P. J., Jaime, S., Lau, K. H. K., McArthur, T., McAvoy, K., Magee, M., Newby, O., Ponder, S. W., Quraishi, U., Rawlings, K., Socke, J., & Stancil, M. (2022). 2022 National standards for diabetes self-management, education and support. *Diabetes Care, 45*(2), 484–494. https://doi.org/10.2337/dc21-2396

García, A. A., Bose, E., Zuñiga, J. A., & Zhang, W. (2019). Mexican Americans' diabetes symptom prevalence, burden, and clusters. *Applied Nursing Research, 46*, 37–42. https://doi.org/10.1016/j.apnr.2019.02.002

Hernandez, L., Leutwyler, H., Cataldo, J., Kanaya, A., Swislocki, A., & Chesla, C. (2019). Symptom experience of older adults with type 2 diabetes and diabetes-related distress. *Nursing Research, 68*(5), 374–382. https://doi.org/10.1097/NNR.0000000000000370

Ismail, L., Materwala, H., & Al Kaabi, J. (2021). Association of risk factors with type 2 diabetes: A systematic review. *Computational and Structural Biotechnology Journal, 19*, 1759–1785. https://doi.org/10.1016/j.csbj.2021.03.003

Lavdaniti, M. (2020). The impact of smoking on individuals with diabetes type 2. *International Journal of Caring Sciences, 13*(3), e2304.

Levesque, C. (2017). Therapeutic lifestyle changes for diabetes mellitus. *Nursing Clinics of North America, 52*(4), 679–692. https://doi.org/10.1016/j.cnur.2017.07.012

Oh, H., & Moorhead, S. (2019). Validation of the knowledge and self-management Nursing Outcomes Classification for adults with diabetes. *CIN: Computers, Informatics, Nursing, 37*(4), 222–228. https://doi.org/10.1097/CIN.0000000000000495

Romero, S. J. M., Brito, B. P. R., Martínez, A. C. E., Martín, G. Á., Rodríguez, Á. M., Group, C., & Paloma, C. O. (2021). A new instrument for measuring dietary knowledge in patients with diabetes: Psychometric testing of the CoNOCidiet-Diabetes. *International Journal of Nursing Knowledge, 32*(1), 20–28. https://doi.org/10.1111/2047-3095.12288

K

Knowledge: Diagnostic & Therapeutic Procedures   **1867**

Definition: Extent of understanding conveyed about diagnostic and therapeutic procedures used to diagnose, monitor, or treat a clinical condition

OUTCOME TARGET RATING: Maintain at_____ Increase to_____

		No Knowledge	Limited Knowledge	Moderate Knowledge	Substantial Knowledge	Extensive Knowledge	
OUTCOME OVERALL RATING		1	2	3	4	5	
Indicators:							
186701	Type of procedure	1	2	3	4	5	NA
186702	Purpose of the procedure	1	2	3	4	5	NA
186703	Time frames required for the procedure	1	2	3	4	5	NA
186704	Required tissue biopsies	1	2	3	4	5	NA
186705	Preparation required prior to the procedure	1	2	3	4	5	NA
186706	Frequently asked questions about the procedure	1	2	3	4	5	NA
186707	Food restrictions prior to the procedure	1	2	3	4	5	NA
186708	Fluid restrictions prior to the procedure	1	2	3	4	5	NA

Continued

Knowledge: Diagnostic & Therapeutic Procedures—cont'd

		No Knowledge	Limited Knowledge	Moderate Knowledge	Substantial Knowledge	Extensive Knowledge	
186709	Medication restrictions prior to the procedure	1	2	3	4	5	NA
186710	Type of bowel preparation required	1	2	3	4	5	NA
186711	Importance of following instructions for the procedure	1	2	3	4	5	NA
186712	Consent requirements	1	2	3	4	5	NA
186713	Sedation requirements	1	2	3	4	5	NA
186714	Anesthesia requirements	1	2	3	4	5	NA
186715	Use of immobilizations devices	1	2	3	4	5	NA
186716	Positions required during the procedure	1	2	3	4	5	NA
186717	Expected sensations during the procedure	1	2	3	4	5	NA
186718	Vital sign monitoring requirements	1	2	3	4	5	NA
186719	Potential complications of the procedure	1	2	3	4	5	NA
186720	Postprocedure recovery routine	1	2	3	4	5	NA
186721	When to expect results	1	2	3	4	5	NA

Domain-*Health Knowledge & Behavior (IV)*   **Class**-*Knowledge Health Promotion (S)*   *6th edition 2018*

OUTCOME CONTENT REFERENCES:

Coté, C., Wilson, S., & American Academy of Pediatrics & American Academy of Pediatric Dentistry. (2016). Guidelines for monitoring and management of pediatric patients before, during, and after sedation for diagnostic and therapeutic procedures: Update 2016. *Pediatrics, 138*(1), e20161212. https://doi.org/10.1542/peds.2016-1212

Devcich, D., Ellis, C., Waltham, N., Broadbent, E., & Petrie, K. (2014). Seeing what's happening on the inside: Patients' views of the value of diagnostic cardiac computed tomography angiography. *British Journal of Health Psychology, 19*(4), 810–822. https://doi.org/10.1111/bjhp.12080

Gibb, L. (2014). Procedure. *Bioethical Inquiry, 11*(3), 279–282. https://doi.org/10.1007/s11673-014-9540-5

Mathus-Vliegen, E., Pellisé, M., Heresbach, D., Fischbach, W., Dixon, T., Belsey, J., Parente, F., Rio-Tinto, R., Brown, A., Toth, E., Crosta, C., Layer, P., Epstein, O., & Boustiere, C. (2013). Consensus guidelines for the use of bowel preparation prior to colonic diagnostic procedures: Colonoscopy and small bowel video capsule endoscopy. *Current Medical Research and Opinion, 29*(8), 931–945. https://doi.org/10.1185/03007995.2013.803055

Zieleskiewicz, L., Muller, L., Lakhal, K., Meresse, Z., Arbelot, C., Bertrand, P.-M., Bouhemad, B., Cholley, B., Demory, D., Duperret, S., Duranteau, J., Guervilly, C., Hammad, E., Ichai, C., Jaber, S., Langeron, O., Lefrant, J.-Y., Mahjoub, Y., Maury, E., Meaudre, E., Fabrice, M., Muller, M., Nafati, C., Perbeert, S., Quintard, H., Rui, B., Vigne, C., Chaumorte, K., Allaouchiche, B., Martin. C., Constantin, J.-M., De Backer, D., & Leone, M. (2015). Point-of-care ultrasound in intensive care units: Assessment of 1073 procedures in a multicentric, prospective, observational study. *Intensive Care Medicine, 41*(9), 1638–1647. https://doi.org/10.1007/s00134-015-3952-5

Knowledge: Disease Management   **1803**

Definition: Extent of understanding conveyed about a specific disease process, its treatment, and the prevention of disease progression and potential complications

OUTCOME TARGET RATING: Maintain at_____ Increase to_____

		No Knowledge	Limited Knowledge	Moderate Knowledge	Substantial Knowledge	Extensive Knowledge	
OUTCOME OVERALL RATING		1	2	3	4	5	
Indicators:							
180302	Characteristics of specific disease	1	2	3	4	5	NA
180303	Cause and contributing factors	1	2	3	4	5	NA
180304	Risk factors	1	2	3	4	5	NA
180305	Physiological effects of disease	1	2	3	4	5	NA
180306	Signs and symptoms of disease	1	2	3	4	5	NA
180318	Treatment options	1	2	3	4	5	NA
180319	Required laboratory tests	1	2	3	4	5	NA
180320	Medication available for disease management	1	2	3	4	5	NA

Knowledge: Disease Management—cont'd

		No Knowledge	Limited Knowledge	Moderate Knowledge	Substantial Knowledge	Extensive Knowledge	
180321	Personal responsibilities for treatment regimen	1	2	3	4	5	NA
180307	Usual course of disease process	1	2	3	4	5	NA
180308	Strategies to minimize disease progression	1	2	3	4	5	NA
180322	Strategies to manage signs and symptoms	1	2	3	4	5	NA
180309	Potential complications of disease	1	2	3	4	5	NA
180310	Signs and symptoms of disease complications	1	2	3	4	5	NA
180313	Psychosocial effects of disease on self	1	2	3	4	5	NA
180314	Psychosocial effects of disease on family	1	2	3	4	5	NA
180323	Strategies to adapt lifestyle	1	2	3	4	5	NA
180315	Benefits of disease management	1	2	3	4	5	NA
180316	Available support groups	1	2	3	4	5	NA
180324	Available educational opportunities	1	2	3	4	5	NA
180317	Reputable sources of disease-specific information	1	2	3	4	5	NA
180325	When to seek help from a health professional	1	2	3	4	5	NA

Specify disease_____

Domain-*Health Knowledge & Behavior (IV)*   **Class**-*Knowledge Health Condition (GG)*   *1st edition 1997; revised 2004, 2008, 2013, 2024*

OUTCOME CONTENT REFERENCES:

de Araújo Ferreira, J. K., Costa Pessoa, N. R., Pereira Pôrto, N., Mendes Santos, L. N., de Carvalho Lira, A. L. B., & de Queiroz Frazão, C. M. F. (2018). Knowledge: Disease Process in patients undergoing hemodialysis. *Investigacion & Educacion En Enfermeria, 36*(2), 26–35. https://doi.org/10.17533/udea.iee.v36n2e04

García Fernandez, F. P., & Carrascosa García, M. I. (2008). Nursing outcomes in pluripathology process to improve clinical practice. *Gerokomos, 19*(4), 18–24.

Heine, M., Lategan, F., Erasmus, M., Lombaard, C., Mc Carthy, N., Olivier, J., van Niekerk, M., & Hanekom, S. (2021). Health education interventions to promote health literacy in adults with selected non-communicable diseases living in low-to-middle income countries: A systematic review and meta-analysis. *Journal of Evaluation in Clinical Practice, 27*(6), 1417–1428. https://doi.org/10.1111/jep.13554

Nutbeam, D. (2021). From health education to digital health literacy—Building on the past to shape the future. *Global Health Promotion, 28*(4), 51–55. https://doi.org/10.1177/17579759211044079

Porfírio Ferreira, P. B., Sententa Porto, I., do Espirito Santo, F. H., Almeida de Figueiredo, N. M., Cruz Enders, B., Eiras Cameron, L., & Carvalho de Araújo, S. T. (2022). Health education for hospitalized patient in nursing care: A conceptual analysis. *Revista Brasileira de Enfermagem, 75*(2), 1–9. https://doi.org/10.1590/0034-7167-2020-0459

Souza Carneiro, C., Dias de Oliveira, A. P., Lima Lopes, J., Bachion, M. M., Herdman, T. H., Moorhead, S. A., & Bottura Leite de Barros, A. L. (2016). Outpatient clinic for health education: Contribution to self-management and self-care for people with heart failure. *International Journal of Nursing Knowledge, 27*(1), 49–55. https://doi.org/10.1111/2047-3095.12071

K

Knowledge: Dysrhythmia Management   **1852**

Definition: Extent of understanding conveyed about cardiac conduction irregularity, its treatment, and the prevention of disease progression and complications

OUTCOME TARGET RATING: Maintain at_____ Increase to_____

		No Knowledge	Limited Knowledge	Moderate Knowledge	Substantial Knowledge	Extensive Knowledge	
OUTCOME OVERALL RATING		1	2	3	4	5	
Indicators:							
185201	Type of dysrhythmia	1	2	3	4	5	NA
185202	Methods to monitor blood pressure	1	2	3	4	5	NA
185203	Methods to monitor heart rate	1	2	3	4	5	NA
185204	Methods to monitor heart rhythm	1	2	3	4	5	NA
185205	Signs and symptoms of dysrhythmia	1	2	3	4	5	NA
185206	Relationship of lightheadedness to dysrhythmia	1	2	3	4	5	NA
185207	Relationship of dizziness to dysrhythmia	1	2	3	4	5	NA

Continued

Knowledge: Dysrhythmia Management—cont'd

		No Knowledge	Limited Knowledge	Moderate Knowledge	Substantial Knowledge	Extensive Knowledge	
185234	Effects of fatigue on heart rhythm	1	2	3	4	5	NA
185208	Effects of exercise on heart rhythm	1	2	3	4	5	NA
185209	Effects of fever on heart rhythm	1	2	3	4	5	NA
185210	Effects of anxiety on heart rhythm	1	2	3	4	5	NA
185211	Effects of caffeine on heart rhythm	1	2	3	4	5	NA
185235	Effects of alcohol on heart rhythm	1	2	3	4	5	NA
185236	Effects of tobacco on heart rhythm	1	2	3	4	5	NA
185212	Effects of other stimulants on heart rhythm	1	2	3	4	5	NA
185213	Signs and symptoms of overexertion	1	2	3	4	5	NA
185214	Strategies to control anxiety	1	2	3	4	5	NA
185215	Factors that precede dysrhythmia onset	1	2	3	4	5	NA
185216	Strategies to eliminate causative factors	1	2	3	4	5	NA
185217	Effects on lifestyle	1	2	3	4	5	NA
185218	Strategies to cope with lifestyle changes	1	2	3	4	5	NA
185219	Adaptations for role performance	1	2	3	4	5	NA
185220	Guidelines for sexual activity	1	2	3	4	5	NA
185237	Treatment options	1	2	3	4	5	NA
185221	Benefits of prescribed medication	1	2	3	4	5	NA
185222	Importance of adherence with prescribed medication schedule	1	2	3	4	5	NA
185223	Medication schedule	1	2	3	4	5	NA
185224	Importance of maintaining medication blood levels	1	2	3	4	5	NA
185225	Medication therapeutic effects	1	2	3	4	5	NA
185226	Medication side effects	1	2	3	4	5	NA
185227	Medication adverse effects	1	2	3	4	5	NA
185238	Importance of medication reconciliation with health professional	1	2	3	4	5	NA
185239	Importance of comorbid conditions impact on treatment plan	1	2	3	4	5	NA
185228	Actions to take in an emergency	1	2	3	4	5	NA
185229	Importance of family learning cardiopulmonary resuscitation	1	2	3	4	5	NA
185230	Cultural influences on adherence to treatment regimen	1	2	3	4	5	NA
185231	Available support groups	1	2	3	4	5	NA
185232	Reputable sources of cardiac disease information	1	2	3	4	5	NA
185233	When to obtain assistance from a health professional	1	2	3	4	5	NA

Domain-*Health Knowledge & Behavior (IV)*   **Class**-*Knowledge Health Condition (GG)*   *5th edition 2013; revised 2024*

OUTCOME CONTENT REFERENCES:

Bond, C., Morgenstern, J., Heitz, C., & Milne, W. K. (2020). Hot off the press: Chemical versus electrical cardioversion for atrial fibrillation. *Academic Emergency Medicine, 27*(4), 333–335. https://doi.org/10.1111/acem13874

Gammone, M. A., & D'orazio, N. (2021). Cocoa overconsumption and cardiac rhythm: Potential arrhythmogenic trigger or beneficial pleasure? *Current Research in Nutrition and Food Science, 9*(1), 40–51. https://doi.org/10.12944/CRNFSJ.9.1.05

Methangkool, E., Howard-Quijano, K., & Mahajan, A. (2018). Cardiac dysrhythmias: Understanding mechanisms, drug treatments, and novel therapies. *Advances in Anesthesia, 36*(1), 181–199. https://doi.org/10.1016/j.aan.2018.07.008

Normand, C., Kaye, D. M., Povsic, T. J., & Dickstein, K. (2019). Beyond pharmacological treatment: An insight into therapies that target specific aspects of heart failure pathophysiology. *Lancet, 393*(10175), 1045–1055. https://doi.org/10.1016/S0140-6736(18)32216-5

Potter, P. A., Perry, A. G., Stockert. P. A., & Hall, A. M. (2021). *Fundamentals of nursing* (10th ed.). Elsevier.

Ravid, J. D., Kamel, M. H., & Chitalia, V. C. (2021). Uraemic solutes as therapeutic targets in CKD-associated cardiovascular disease. *Nature, 17*(6), 402–416. https://doi.org/10.1038/s41581-021-00408-4

Xu, W., Sun, G., Lin, Z., Chen, M., Yang, B., Chen, H., & Cao, K. (2010). Knowledge, attitude, and behavior in patients with atrial fibrillation undergoing radiofrequency catheter ablation. *Journal of Interventional Cardiac Electrophysiology, 28*(3), 199–207. https://doi.org/10.1007/s10840-010-9496-2

Knowledge: Eating Disorder Management   1853

Definition: Extent of understanding conveyed about an eating disorder, its treatment, and the prevention of disease progression and complications

OUTCOME TARGET RATING: Maintain at_____ Increase to_____

		No Knowledge	Limited Knowledge	Moderate Knowledge	Substantial Knowledge	Extensive Knowledge	
OUTCOME OVERALL RATING		**1**	**2**	**3**	**4**	**5**	
Indicators:							
185301	Healthy target weight	1	2	3	4	5	NA
185302	Healthy nutritional practices	1	2	3	4	5	NA
185303	Relationship among diet, exercise, and weight	1	2	3	4	5	NA
185304	Achievable weight gain goals	1	2	3	4	5	NA
185305	Achievable weight loss goals	1	2	3	4	5	NA
185306	Adverse health effects of emotional states on food and fluid intake	1	2	3	4	5	NA
185307	Effects of social situations on food and fluid intake	1	2	3	4	5	NA
185308	Strategies for situations that affect food and fluid intake	1	2	3	4	5	NA
185309	Maladaptive eating responses	1	2	3	4	5	NA
185310	Daily fluid intake that meets body needs	1	2	3	4	5	NA
185311	Caloric intake appropriate for metabolic needs	1	2	3	4	5	NA
185312	Nutrient intake appropriate for individual needs	1	2	3	4	5	NA
185313	Signs and symptoms of nutritional deficits	1	2	3	4	5	NA
185314	Strategies to create a healthy attitude about food	1	2	3	4	5	NA
185315	Realistic exercise routine	1	2	3	4	5	NA
185316	Strategies to manage stress	1	2	3	4	5	NA
185317	Strategies to gain sense of personal control	1	2	3	4	5	NA
185318	Strategies to decrease preoccupation with food	1	2	3	4	5	NA
185319	Strategies to avoid purging behaviors	1	2	3	4	5	NA
185320	Strategies to avoid binging behaviors	1	2	3	4	5	NA
185321	Strategies to promote an accurate perception of body image	1	2	3	4	5	NA
185322	Strategies to promote satisfaction with body image	1	2	3	4	5	NA
185323	Strategies to promote self-esteem	1	2	3	4	5	NA
185324	Factors that trigger relapse	1	2	3	4	5	NA
185325	Strategies to prevent relapses	1	2	3	4	5	NA
185326	Signs and symptoms of depression	1	2	3	4	5	NA
185327	Strategies to reduce depression	1	2	3	4	5	NA
185334	Strategies to control comorbidities	1	2	3	4	5	NA
185335	Characteristics of positive family relationships	1	2	3	4	5	NA
185328	Characteristics of supportive relationships	1	2	3	4	5	NA
185329	Prescribed medication regimen	1	2	3	4	5	NA
185330	Potential dangers of non-prescription medication	1	2	3	4	5	NA
185331	Available support groups	1	2	3	4	5	NA
185332	Available community resources	1	2	3	4	5	NA
185333	When to obtain assistance from a health professional	1	2	3	4	5	NA

Domain-*Health Knowledge & Behavior (IV)*   **Class**-*Knowledge Health Condition (GG)*   *5th edition 2013; revised 2024*

OUTCOME CONTENT REFERENCES:

Baudinet, J., Eisler, I., Dawson, L., & Simic, M. (2021). Multi-family therapy for eating disorders: A systematic scoping review of the quantitative and qualitative findings. *International Journal of Eating Disorders, 54*, 2095–2120. https://doi.org/10.1002/eat.23616

Kenny, B., Orellana, L., Fuller-Tyszkiewicz, M., Moodie, M., Brown, V., & Williams, J. (2021). Depression and eating disorders in early adolescence: A network analysis approach. *International Journal of Eating Disorders, 54*, 2143–2154. https://doi.org/10.1002/eat.23627

Potter, P., Perry, A., Stockert, P., & Hall, A. (2021). *Fundamentals of nursing* (10th ed.). Elsevier.

Rosenbaum, D. L., White, K. S., & Artime, T. M. (2021). Coping with childhood maltreatment: Avoidance and eating disorder symptoms. *Journal of Health Psychology, 26*(14), 2832–2840. https://doi.org/10.1177/1359105320937068

Sollid, C., Clausen, L., & Maimburg, R. D. (2021). The first 20 weeks of pregnancy is a high-risk period for eating disorder relapse. *International Journal of Eating Disorders, 54*, 2132–2142. https://doi.org/10.1002/eat.23620

Varcarolis, E. M., & Fosbre, C. D. (2021). *Essentials of psychiatric-mental health nursing* (4th ed.). Elsevier.

Knowledge: Energy Conservation

1804

Definition: Extent of understanding conveyed about energy conservation techniques

OUTCOME TARGET RATING: Maintain at_____ Increase to_____

		No Knowledge	Limited Knowledge	Moderate Knowledge	Substantial Knowledge	Extensive Knowledge	
OUTCOME OVERALL RATING		**1**	**2**	**3**	**4**	**5**	
Indicators:							
180401	Recommended physical activity	1	2	3	4	5	NA
180402	Activity restrictions	1	2	3	4	5	NA
180403	Appropriate activities	1	2	3	4	5	NA
180404	Factors that increase energy expenditure	1	2	3	4	5	NA
180405	Factors that decrease energy expenditure	1	2	3	4	5	NA
180406	Energy limitations	1	2	3	4	5	NA
180424	Methods to identify activities of importance	1	2	3	4	5	NA
180425	Strategies to modify living environment	1	2	3	4	5	NA
180407	Strategies to balance activity and rest	1	2	3	4	5	NA
180426	Strategies to control stress	1	2	3	4	5	NA
180416	Energy conservation techniques	1	2	3	4	5	NA
180422	Methods to monitor heart rate	1	2	3	4	5	NA
180423	Effective breathing techniques	1	2	3	4	5	NA
180419	Proper body mechanics	1	2	3	4	5	NA
180420	Work simplification techniques	1	2	3	4	5	NA
180421	Correct use of assistive devices	1	2	3	4	5	NA
180427	Community resources to assist with conserving energy	1	2	3	4	5	NA

Domain-*Health Knowledge & Behavior (IV)*   **Class**-*Knowledge Health Promotion (S)*   *1st edition 1997; revised 2004, 2008, 2013, 2024*

OUTCOME CONTENT REFERENCES:

Gwin, J. A., Church, D. D., Hatch-McChesney, A., Howard, E. E., Carrigan, C. T., Murphy, N. E., Wilson, M. A., Margolis, L. M., Carbone, J. W., Wolfe, R. R., Ferrando, A. A., & Pasiakos, S. M. (2021). Effects of high versus standard essential amino acid intakes on whole-body protein turnover and mixed muscle protein synthesis during energy deficit: A randomized, crossover study. *Clinical Nutrition, 40,* 767–777. https://doi.org/10.1016/j.clnu.2020.07.019

Potter, P. A, Perry, A. G., Stockert, P. A., & Hall, A. M. (2021). *Fundamentals of nursing* (10th ed.). Elsevier.

Williams, P. (2020). *Basic geriatric nursing* (7th ed.). Elsevier.

Knowledge: Epilepsy Management

3205

Definition: Extent of understanding conveyed about epilepsy, its treatment, and the prevention of complications

OUTCOME TARGET RATING: Maintain at_____ Increase to_____

		No Knowledge	Limited Knowledge	Moderate Knowledge	Substantial Knowledge	Extensive Knowledge	
OUTCOME OVERALL RATING		**1**	**2**	**3**	**4**	**5**	
Indicators:							
320501	Cause and contributing factors	1	2	3	4	5	NA
320502	Types of epilepsy	1	2	3	4	5	NA
320503	Signs and symptoms of epilepsy	1	2	3	4	5	NA
320504	Usual course of disease	1	2	3	4	5	NA
320505	Disease prognosis	1	2	3	4	5	NA
320506	Diagnostic tests	1	2	3	4	5	NA
320507	Risk factors for seizure	1	2	3	4	5	NA
320508	Triggers of seizure	1	2	3	4	5	NA

K

Knowledge: Epilepsy Management—cont'd

		No Knowledge	Limited Knowledge	Moderate Knowledge	Substantial Knowledge	Extensive Knowledge	
320509	Available treatment options	1	2	3	4	5	NA
320510	Alternative treatment options	1	2	3	4	5	NA
320511	Importance of reporting therapeutic effects to health professional	1	2	3	4	5	NA
320512	Specific treatment regimen	1	2	3	4	5	NA
320513	Medication side effects	1	2	3	4	5	NA
320514	Medication adverse effect	1	2	3	4	5	NA
320515	Potential medication interactions	1	2	3	4	5	NA
320516	Adverse health effects of skipping medication	1	2	3	4	5	NA
320517	Importance of maintaining a diary of seizure activity	1	2	3	4	5	NA
320518	Strategies to maintain effective respiratory pattern during a seizure	1	2	3	4	5	NA
320519	Strategies to prevent injury during a seizure	1	2	3	4	5	NA
320520	Course of action when a seizure occurs	1	2	3	4	5	NA
320521	Importance of assistance from others during a seizure	1	2	3	4	5	NA
320522	Importance of informing individuals of actions to be taken when a seizure occurs	1	2	3	4	5	NA
320523	When to obtain emergency treatment	1	2	3	4	5	NA
320524	Driving restrictions	1	2	3	4	5	NA
320525	Strategies to provide safety during physical activity	1	2	3	4	5	NA
320526	Importance of adequate sleep-wake pattern	1	2	3	4	5	NA
320527	Recommended diet	1	2	3	4	5	NA
320528	Importance of alcohol restrictions	1	2	3	4	5	NA
320529	Importance of avoiding drug misuse	1	2	3	4	5	NA
320530	Safety issues related to epilepsy	1	2	3	4	5	NA
320531	Strategies to manage stress	1	2	3	4	5	NA
320532	Importance of coordinated management with health professional	1	2	3	4	5	NA
320533	Importance of follow-up care	1	2	3	4	5	NA
320534	Benefits of social support	1	2	3	4	5	NA
320535	Effects of disease on family	1	2	3	4	5	NA
320536	Available community resources	1	2	3	4	5	NA

Domain-*Health Knowledge & Behavior (IV)*   **Class**-*Knowledge Health Condition (GG)*   *6th edition 2018*

K

OUTCOME CONTENT REFERENCES:

Coker, M., Bhargava, S., Fitzgerald, M., & Doherty, C. (2011). What do people with epilepsy know about their condition? Evaluation of a subspecialty clinic population. *Seizure, 20*(1), 55–59. https://doi.org/10.1016/j.seizure.2010.10.007

+Dilorio, C., Faherty, B., & Manteuffel, B. (1992). The development and testing of an instrument to measure self-efficacy in persons with epilepsy. *Journal of Neuroscience Nursing, 24*(1), 9–13. https://doi.org/10.1097/01376517-199202000-00004

Dilorio, C., Faherty, B., & Manteuffel, B. (1993). Learning needs of persons with epilepsy: A comparison of perceptions of persons with epilepsy, nurses and physicians. *Journal of Neuroscience Nursing, 25*(1), 22–29. https://doi.org/10.1097/01376517-199302000-00006

England, M. J., Liverman, C. T., Schultz, A. M., & Strawbridge, L. M. (Eds.). (2012). *Epilepsy across the spectrum: Promoting health and understanding*. The National Academies Press.

+Escoffery, C., Bamps, Y., LaFrance, W. C. Jr., Stoll, S., Shegog, R., Buelow, J., Shafer, P., Thompson, N. J., McGee, R. E., & Hatfield, K. (2015). Development of the Adult Epilepsy Self-Management Measurement Instrument (AESMMI). *Epilepsy & Behavior, 50*, 172–183. https://doi.org/10.1016/j.yebeh.2015.07.025

Goldstein, L. H., Minchin, L., Stubbs, P., & Fenwick, P. B. (1997). Are what people know about their epilepsy and what they want to from an epilepsy service related? *Seizure, 6*(6), 435–442. https://doi.org/10.1016/s1059-1311(97)80017-9

Granelli, S., & McGrath, J. (2004). Neonatal seizures: Diagnosis, pharmacologic interventions, and outcomes. *Journal of Perinatal & Neonatal Nursing, 18*(3), 275–287. https://doi.org/10.1097/00005237-200407000-00009

Hanscomb, A., & Smithson, W. H. (2012). Living with epilepsy—Information, support and self-management. In W. H. Smithson & M. C. Walker (Eds.), *ABC of epilepsy* (pp. 30–33). Wiley-Blackwell.

May, T. W., & Pfäfflin, M. (2002). The efficacy of an educational treatment program for patients with epilepsy (MOSES): Results of a controlled, randomized study. *Epilepsia, 43*(5), 539–549. https://doi.org/10.1046/j.1528-1157.2002.23801.x

Knowledge: Fall Prevention

1828

Definition: Extent of understanding conveyed about prevention of falls

OUTCOME TARGET RATING: Maintain at_____ Increase to_____

		No Knowledge	Limited Knowledge	Moderate Knowledge	Substantial Knowledge	Extensive Knowledge	
OUTCOME OVERALL RATING		**1**	**2**	**3**	**4**	**5**	
Indicators:							
182801	Correct use of assistive devices	1	2	3	4	5	NA
182802	Correct use of safety devices	1	2	3	4	5	NA
182803	Appropriate footwear	1	2	3	4	5	NA
182804	Correct use of grab bars	1	2	3	4	5	NA
182805	Correct use of safety gates	1	2	3	4	5	NA
182806	Correct use of window guards	1	2	3	4	5	NA
182807	Correct use of environmental lighting	1	2	3	4	5	NA
182808	When to ask for personal assistance	1	2	3	4	5	NA
182822	Familiarity with surroundings	1	2	3	4	5	NA
182823	Importance of steady gait	1	2	3	4	5	NA
182809	Use of safe transfer procedure	1	2	3	4	5	NA
182810	Reasons for restraints	1	2	3	4	5	NA
182811	Exercises to reduce risk for falls	1	2	3	4	5	NA
182824	Importance of movement	1	2	3	4	5	NA
182812	Prescribed medication that increase risk for falls	1	2	3	4	5	NA
182813	Chronic conditions that increase risk for falls	1	2	3	4	5	NA
182814	Acute illnesses that increase risk for falls	1	2	3	4	5	NA
182815	Blood pressure changes that increase risk for falls	1	2	3	4	5	NA
182816	Non-prescription medication that increase risk for falls	1	2	3	4	5	NA
182817	Strategies to safely ambulate	1	2	3	4	5	NA
182825	Strategies to maneuver stairs	1	2	3	4	5	NA
182826	Strategies for snow-ice removal	1	2	3	4	5	NA
182827	Importance of attention to varying surface heights	1	2	3	4	5	NA
182828	Importance of completing fall risk assessment	1	2	3	4	5	NA
182829	Strategies to modify home environment	1	2	3	4	5	NA
182830	Fall prevention plan	1	2	3	4	5	NA
182818	Importance of maintaining clear walkway	1	2	3	4	5	NA
182819	Safe use of step stools and ladders	1	2	3	4	5	NA
182820	Importance of using non-skid mats	1	2	3	4	5	NA
182821	Strategies to keep floor surfaces safe	1	2	3	4	5	NA

Domain-*Health Knowledge & Behavior (IV)*   **Class**-*Knowledge Health Promotion (S)*   *3rd edition 2004; revised 2008, 2024*

OUTCOME CONTENT REFERENCES:

de Freitas Luzia, M., Argenta, C., de Abreu Almeida, M., & de Fátima Lucena, A. (2018). Conceptual definitions of indicators for the nursing outcome "Knowledge: Fall Prevention." *Revista Brasileira de Enfermagem, 71*(2), 431–439. https://doi.org/10.1590/0034-7167-2016-0686

de Freitas Luzia, M., Vidor, I. D., da Silva, A. C. F. E., & de Fátima Lucena, A. (2020). Fall prevention in hospitalized patients: Evaluation through the Nursing Outcomes Classification/NOC. *Applied Nursing Research, 54*, 151273. https://doi.org/10.1016/j.apnr.2020.151273

Flint, J., Morris, M., Nguyen, A. T., Keglovits, M., Somerville, E. K., Hu, Y.-L., & Stark, S. L. (2020). Fall prevention bingo: Effects of a novel community-based education tool on older adults' knowledge and readiness to reduce risks for falls. *American Journal of Health Education, 51*(6), 406–412. https://doi.org/10.1080/19325037.2020.1822236

Hunter, S. W., Higa, J., Frengopoulos, C., Viana, R., & Payne, M. P. C. (2020). Evaluating knowledge of falls risk factors and falls prevention strategies among lower extremity amputees after inpatient prosthetic rehabilitation: A prospective study. *Disability and Rehabilitation, 42*(16), 2252–2261. https://doi.org/10.1080/09638288.2018.1555721

Kuljeerung, O., & Lach, H. W. (2021). Extrinsic and behavioral fall risk factors in people with Parkinson's disease: An integrative review. *Rehabilitation Nursing, 46*(1), 3–10. https://doi.org/10.1097/rnj.0000000000000265

Lee, E. (2019). Use of the Nursing Outcomes Classification for falls and fall prevention by nurses in South Korea. *International Journal of Nursing Knowledge, 30*(1), 28–33. https://doi.org/10.1111/2047-3095.12201

Naseri, C., McPhail, S. M., Haines, T. P., Morris, M. E., Shorr, R., Etherton-Beer, C., Netto, J., Flicker, L., Bulsara, M., Lee, D.-C. A., Francis-Coad, J., Waldron, N., Boudville, A., & Hill, A.-M. (2020). Perspectives of older adults regarding barriers and enablers to engaging in fall prevention activities after hospital discharge. *Health and Social Care in the Community, 28*(5), 1710–1722. https://doi.org/10.1111/hsc.12996

Twibell, K. R., Siela, D., Delaney, L., Avila, P., Spradlin, A. M., & Coers, G. (2020). Perspectives of inpatients with cancer on engagement in fall prevention. *Oncology Nursing Forum, 47*(4), 457–468. https://doi.org/10.1188/20.ONF.457-468

Zhang, W., Low, L. F., Schwenk, M., Mills, N., Gwynn, J. D., & Clemson, L. (2019). Review of gait, cognition, and fall risks with implications for fall prevention in older adults with dementia. *Dementia and Geriatric Cognitive Disorders, 48*(1/2), 17–29. https://doi.org/10.1159/000504340

Knowledge: Fertility Promotion   1816

Definition: Extent of understanding conveyed about fertility testing and the conditions that affect conception

OUTCOME TARGET RATING: Maintain at_____ Increase to_____

		No Knowledge	Limited Knowledge	Moderate Knowledge	Substantial Knowledge	Extensive Knowledge	
OUTCOME OVERALL RATING		**1**	**2**	**3**	**4**	**5**	
Indicators:							
181601	Effect of age	1	2	3	4	5	NA
181602	Effect of coital frequency	1	2	3	4	5	NA
181603	Effect of nutrition	1	2	3	4	5	NA
181604	Adverse health effects	1	2	3	4	5	NA
181606	Effect of heat on sperm count	1	2	3	4	5	NA
181607	Effect of tight clothes on sperm count	1	2	3	4	5	NA
181608	Effect of physical anomalies	1	2	3	4	5	NA
181609	Effect of pelvic surgery	1	2	3	4	5	NA
181610	Effect of pelvic infections	1	2	3	4	5	NA
181611	Influence of vaginal/uterine environment	1	2	3	4	5	NA
181612	Effect of hormone levels	1	2	3	4	5	NA
181613	Effect of thyroid function	1	2	3	4	5	NA
181614	Use of basal body temperature to predict ovulation	1	2	3	4	5	NA
181615	Symptothermal method	1	2	3	4	5	NA
181616	Ultrasonography	1	2	3	4	5	NA
181617	Influence of semen characteristics	1	2	3	4	5	NA
181618	Influence of sperm count	1	2	3	4	5	NA
181619	Postcoital test	1	2	3	4	5	NA
181620	Fertility monitoring devices	1	2	3	4	5	NA
181621	Options to reverse sterilization	1	2	3	4	5	NA
181622	Methods for semen collection	1	2	3	4	5	NA
181624	Egg freezing methods	1	2	3	4	5	NA
181625	Fertilization methods	1	2	3	4	5	NA

K

Domain-Health Knowledge & Behavior (IV)   **Class**-Knowledge Health Promotion (S)   *2nd edition 2000; revised 2004, 2008, 2013, 2024*

OUTCOME CONTENT REFERENCES:

Bellver, J., & Donnez, J. (2019). Introduction: Infertility etiology and offspring health. *Fertility and Sterility, 111*(6), 1033–1035. https://doi.org/10.1016/j.fertnstert.2019.04.043

Grieger, J. A. (2020). Preconception diet, fertility, and later health in pregnancy. *Current Opinion in Obstetrics & Gynecology, 32*(3), 227–232. https://doi.org/10.1097/GCO.0000000000000629

Jensen, A., & Wrede, J. (2020). Fertility awareness-based methods for family planning: A literature review. *Journal of Christian Nursing, 37*(4), 212–220. https://doi.org/10.1097/CNJ.0000000000000758

Obelenienė, B., Narbekovas, A., & Juškevičius, J. (2021). Anthropological and methodical differences of natural family planning and fertility awareness-based methods. *The Linacre Quarterly, 88*(1), 14–23. https://doi.org/10.1177/0024363919886517

Pedro, J., Brandão, T., Schmidt, L., Costa, M. E., & Martins, M. V. (2018). What do people know about fertility? A systematic review on fertility awareness and its associated factors. *Upsala Journal of Medical Sciences, 123*(2), 71–81. https://doi.org/10.1080/03009734.2018.1480186

Sung, S., & Abramovitz, A. (2021, July 26). Natural family planning. In *Statpearls*. StatPearls Publishing. https://www.ncbi.nlm.nih.gov/books/NBK546661

Vander Borght, M., & Wyns, C. (2018). Fertility and infertility: Definition and epidemiology. *Clinical Biochemistry, 62*, 2–10. https://doi.org/10.1016/j.clinbiochem.2018.03.012

Knowledge: Foot Care   1871

Definition: Extent of understanding conveyed about how to maintain healthy feet and prevent complications

OUTCOME TARGET RATING: Maintain at_____ Increase to_____

		No Knowledge	Limited Knowledge	Moderate Knowledge	Substantial Knowledge	Extensive Knowledge	
OUTCOME OVERALL RATING		1	2	3	4	5	
Indicators:							
187101	Importance of maintaining healthy feet	1	2	3	4	5	NA
187102	Importance of washing feet daily	1	2	3	4	5	NA
187103	Importance of drying feet thoroughly	1	2	3	4	5	NA
187104	Importance of testing bath water temperature	1	2	3	4	5	NA
187105	Importance of proper care of nails	1	2	3	4	5	NA
187106	Importance of applying moisturizers to dry areas of feet	1	2	3	4	5	NA
187107	Importance of wearing clean socks	1	2	3	4	5	NA
187108	Importance of proper fitting shoes	1	2	3	4	5	NA
187109	Importance of inspecting feet for marks from socks or shoes	1	2	3	4	5	NA
187110	Importance of inspecting feet for injuries	1	2	3	4	5	NA
187111	Importance of inspecting soles of feet using a mirror	1	2	3	4	5	NA
187112	Benefits of foot exams by health professional	1	2	3	4	5	NA
187113	Importance of prompt actions to address new lesions identified	1	2	3	4	5	NA
187114	Benefits of proper fitting shoes and slippers	1	2	3	4	5	NA
187115	Importance of avoiding going barefoot	1	2	3	4	5	NA
187116	Signs and symptoms of infection	1	2	3	4	5	NA
187117	Signs and symptoms of nail fungus	1	2	3	4	5	NA
187118	Signs and symptoms of athletes' foot	1	2	3	4	5	NA
187119	Signs and symptoms of ingrown nails	1	2	3	4	5	NA
187120	Signs and symptoms of edema	1	2	3	4	5	NA
187121	Signs and symptoms of poor circulation	1	2	3	4	5	NA
187122	Signs and symptoms of skin breakdown	1	2	3	4	5	NA
187123	Signs and symptoms of necrosis	1	2	3	4	5	NA
187124	Importance of having changes in bone structure evaluated by a health professional	1	2	3	4	5	NA
187125	Risk factors for complications	1	2	3	4	5	NA

Domain-*Health Knowledge & Behavior (IV)*   **Class**- *Knowledge Health Promotion (S)*   *7th edition 2024*

K

OUTCOME CONTENT REFERENCES:

Hanley, G., Chiou, P. Y., Liu, C. Y., Chen, H. M., & Pfeiffer, S. (2020). Foot care knowledge, attitudes and practices among patients with diabetic foot and amputation in St. Kitts and Nevis. *International Wound Journal, 17*(5), 1142–1152. https://doi.org/10.1111/iwj.13446

Hodgson, L., Growcott, C., Williams, A., Nester, C., & Morrison, S. (2020). First steps: Parent health behaviours related to children's foot health. *Journal of Child Health Care, 24*(2), 221–232. https://doi.org/10.1177/1367493519864752

Morrison, S. C., Barrett, L., & Haines, D. (2020). Foot care needs for children and young people with intellectual and developmental disabilities. *British Journal of Learning Disabilities, 48*(1), 4–9. https://doi.org/10.1111/bld.12291

Pérez-Panero, A. J., Ruiz-Muñoz, M., Cuesta-Vargas, A. I., & Gónzalez-Sánchez, M. (2019). Prevention, assessment, diagnosis and management of diabetic foot based on clinical practice guidelines: A systematic review. *Medicine, 98*(35), e16877. https://doi.org/10.1097/MD.0000000000016877

Ramirez-Perdomo, C., Perdomo-Romero, A., Rodríguez-Vélez, M. (2019). Knowledge and practices for diabetic foot prevention. *Revista Gaúcha de Enfermagem, 40*, e20180161. https://doi.org/10.1590/1983-1447.2019.20180161

Rice, J., Handley, M., & Jolley, J. (2015). Comprehensive foot care education in home-based settings. *Home Healthcare Now, 33*(5), 275–280. https://doi.org/10.1097/NHH.0000000000000237

Yılmaz Karadağ, F., Saltoğlu, N., Ak, Ö., Çınar Aydın, G., Şenbayrak, S., Erol, S., Mıstanoğlu Özatağ, D., Kadanalı, A., Küçükardalı, Y., Çomoğlu, Ş., Yörük, G., Akkoyunlu, Y., Meriç Koç, M., & Altunçekiç Yıldırım, A. (2019). Foot self-care in diabetes mellitus: Evaluation of patient awareness. *Primary Care Diabetes, 13*(6), 515–520. https://doi.org/10.1016/j.pcd.2019.06.003

Knowledge: Health Behavior   1805

Definition: Extent of understanding conveyed about the promotion and protection of health

OUTCOME TARGET RATING: Maintain at_____ Increase to_____

		No Knowledge	Limited Knowledge	Moderate Knowledge	Substantial Knowledge	Extensive Knowledge	
OUTCOME OVERALL RATING		**1**	**2**	**3**	**4**	**5**	
Indicators:							
180501	Healthy nutritional practices	1	2	3	4	5	NA
180520	Recommended fluid intake	1	2	3	4	5	NA
180521	Effective weight management strategies	1	2	3	4	5	NA
180502	Benefits of regular exercise	1	2	3	4	5	NA
180522	Methods to monitor vital signs	1	2	3	4	5	NA
180503	Strategies to manage stress	1	2	3	4	5	NA
180504	Normal sleep-wake patterns	1	2	3	4	5	NA
180505	Methods of family planning	1	2	3	4	5	NA
180506	Adverse health effects of tobacco use	1	2	3	4	5	NA
180507	Adverse health effects of alcohol use	1	2	3	4	5	NA
180508	Adverse health effects of recreational drug use	1	2	3	4	5	NA
180509	Safe use of prescribed medication	1	2	3	4	5	NA
180510	Safe use of non-prescription medication	1	2	3	4	5	NA
180511	Effects of caffeine use	1	2	3	4	5	NA
180523	Importance of social support	1	2	3	4	5	NA
180512	Strategies to reduce the risk of accidental injury	1	2	3	4	5	NA
180513	Strategies to avoid exposure to environmental hazards	1	2	3	4	5	NA
180514	Strategies to prevent transmission of infectious disease	1	2	3	4	5	NA
180524	Recommended immunizations	1	2	3	4	5	NA
180518	Health promotion services	1	2	3	4	5	NA
180519	Health protection services	1	2	3	4	5	NA
180525	Strategies to manage acute illness	1	2	3	4	5	NA
180526	Strategies to manage chronic conditions	1	2	3	4	5	NA
180527	Strategies to manage mental health problems	1	2	3	4	5	NA
180516	Self-screening techniques	1	2	3	4	5	NA
180528	Sources of reliable health information	1	2	3	4	5	NA

Domain-Health Knowledge & Behavior (IV)   *Class-Knowledge Health Promotion (S)*   *1st edition 1997; revised 2004, 2008, 2013, 2024*

K

OUTCOME CONTENT REFERENCES:

Chen, J., Fowler, K. J., & Grams, M. E. (2020). Knowledge is power: Patient education as a tool for patient activation. *American Journal of Kidney Diseases*, *76*(2), 163–165. https://doi.org/10.1053/j.ajkd.2020.03.012

Head, B. J., Maas, M., & Johnson, M. (2003). Validity and community-health-nursing sensitivity of six outcomes for community health nursing with older clients. *Public Health Nursing, 20*(5), 385–398. https://doi.org/10.1046/j.1525-1446.2003.20507.x

Korkmaz Aslan, G., Kartal, A., Turan, T., Taşdemir Yiğitoğlu, G., & Kocakabak, C. (2021). Association of electronic health literacy with health-promoting behaviours in adolescents. *International Journal of Nursing Practice, 27*(2), 1–9. https://doi.org/10.1111/ijn.12921

Muralidharan, A., Peeples, A., & Lucksted, A. (2021). Health behavior change processes among adults with serious mental illness engaged in illness self-management. *Qualitative Health Research, 31*(6), 1155–1168. https://doi.org/10.1177/1049732321992049

Odzakovic, E., Hellström, I., Nedlund, A.-C., & Kullberg, A. (2021). Health promotion initiative: A dementia-friendly local community in Sweden. *Dementia* (London), *20*(6), 1971–1987. https://doi.org/10.1177/1471301220977736

Sheffield, D., & Irons, J. Y. (2021). Songs for health education and promotion: A systematic review with recommendations. *Public Health, 198*, 280–289. https://doi.org/10.1016/j.puhe.2021.07.020

Siaki, L., Hasslen, S., Hoffecker, L., & Trego, L. L. (2021). Sleep health in U.S. military women: A scoping review of the literature, 2000–2019. *Women's Health Issues, 31*, S22–S32. https://doi.org/10.1016/j.whi.2021.03.001

Thatthong, N., Sranacharoenpong, K., Praditsorn, P., Churak, P., Ponprachanuvut, P., Srisangwan, N., & Keeratichamroen, A. (2020). Innovative tool for health promotion for at-risk Thai people with hypertension. *Journal of Public Health, 28*(4), 437–443. https://doi.org/10.1007/s10389-019-01028-w

Weiss, L., Quint, E., Leto, C., Vaughn, I., Redrovan, A., Fernandes, M., Lamourt, K., Edgar, C., & Reso, A. (2021). Evaluation of an integrated health promotion program for a low-income urban population: Findings and lessons learned. *Public Health Nursing, 38*(4), 571–578. https://doi.org/10.1111/phn.12839

Wilson, J., Heinsch, M., Betts, D., Booth, D., & Kay-Lambkin, F. (2021). Barriers and facilitators to the use of e-health by older adults: A scoping review. *BMC Public Health, 21*(1), 1–12. https://doi.org/10.1186/s12889-021-11623-w

Knowledge: Health Resources 1806

Definition: Extent of understanding conveyed about relevant health care resources to support individual or family health care needs

OUTCOME TARGET RATING: Maintain at_____ Increase to_____

		No Knowledge	Limited Knowledge	Moderate Knowledge	Substantial Knowledge	Extensive Knowledge	
OUTCOME OVERALL RATING		1	2	3	4	5	
Indicators:							
180601	Reputable health care resources	1	2	3	4	5	NA
180610	Available patient educational programs	1	2	3	4	5	NA
180611	Available health care services	1	2	3	4	5	NA
180612	Benefits of case management	1	2	3	4	5	NA
180608	Strategies to access health care services	1	2	3	4	5	NA
180602	When to obtain assistance from a health professional	1	2	3	4	5	NA
180603	Emergency measures	1	2	3	4	5	NA
180604	Emergency care resources	1	2	3	4	5	NA
180605	Importance of follow-up care after discharge	1	2	3	4	5	NA
180606	Plan for follow-up care needs	1	2	3	4	5	NA
180607	Available community resources to support care needs	1	2	3	4	5	NA
180613	Available care providers to support care in the home	1	2	3	4	5	NA
180614	Available transportation services for appointments	1	2	3	4	5	NA
180615	Available medical equipment to support care	1	2	3	4	5	NA
180616	Available sources of health care supplies	1	2	3	4	5	NA
180617	Available sources of financial support for health care needs	1	2	3	4	5	NA
180618	Available benefits of insurance coverage	1	2	3	4	5	NA

Domain-Health Knowledge & Behavior (IV)   **Class**-Knowledge Health Promotion (S)   *1st edition 1997; revised 2004, 2008, 2024*

OUTCOME CONTENT REFERENCES:

Coughlin, S. S. (2008). Surviving cancer or other serious illness: A review of individual and community resources. *CA: A Cancer Journal for Clinicians*, 58(1), 60–64. https://doi.org/10.3322/CA.2007.0001

Henning-Smith, C., Shippee, T., & Capistrant, B. (2018). Later-life disability in environmental context: Why living arrangements matter. *The Gerontologist*, 58(5), 853–862. https://doi.org/10.1093/geront/gnx019

Stanhope, M., & Lancaster, J. (2020). *Public health nursing: Population-centered health care in the community* (10th ed.). Elsevier.

Weaver, R. H., & Roberto, K. A. (2017). Home and community-based service use by vulnerable older adults. *The Gerontologist*, 57(3), 540–551. https://doi.org/10.1093/geront/gnv149

Knowledge: Healthy Diet 1854

Definition: Extent of understanding conveyed about a balanced nutritious diet

OUTCOME TARGET RATING: Maintain at_____ Increase to_____

		No Knowledge	Limited Knowledge	Moderate Knowledge	Substantial Knowledge	Extensive Knowledge	
OUTCOME OVERALL RATING		1	2	3	4	5	
Indicators:							
185401	Achievable dietary goals	1	2	3	4	5	NA
185402	Optimal personal weight range	1	2	3	4	5	NA
185403	Relationship among diet, exercise, and weight	1	2	3	4	5	NA
185404	Fluid intake appropriate for metabolic needs	1	2	3	4	5	NA

Knowledge: Healthy Diet—cont'd

		No Knowledge	Limited Knowledge	Moderate Knowledge	Substantial Knowledge	Extensive Knowledge	
185405	Caloric intake appropriate for metabolic needs	1	2	3	4	5	NA
185406	Nutrient intake appropriate for individual needs	1	2	3	4	5	NA
185407	Recommended nutritional guidelines	1	2	3	4	5	NA
185408	Foods consistent with nutritional guidelines	1	2	3	4	5	NA
185409	Recommended daily vitamin intake	1	2	3	4	5	NA
185410	Recommended daily mineral intake	1	2	3	4	5	NA
185411	Dietary recommendations for healthy fats, proteins, and carbohydrates	1	2	3	4	5	NA
185412	Dietary recommendations for sodium	1	2	3	4	5	NA
185413	Guidelines for food portions	1	2	3	4	5	NA
185414	Interpretation of nutritional information on food labels	1	2	3	4	5	NA
185415	Nutritional value of whole-grain versus refined-grain products	1	2	3	4	5	NA
185416	Recommended daily protein servings	1	2	3	4	5	NA
185417	Recommended daily fruit servings	1	2	3	4	5	NA
185418	Recommended daily vegetable servings	1	2	3	4	5	NA
185419	Recommended daily dairy servings	1	2	3	4	5	NA
185420	Importance of eating breakfast	1	2	3	4	5	NA
185421	Importance of distributing food intake throughout the day	1	2	3	4	5	NA
185422	Strategies to increase diet adherence	1	2	3	4	5	NA
185423	Strategies to avoid saturated fats	1	2	3	4	5	NA
185424	Strategies to avoid foods with high caloric value and low nutritional value	1	2	3	4	5	NA
185425	Safety recommendations for food storage	1	2	3	4	5	NA
185426	Safety recommendations for food preparation	1	2	3	4	5	NA
185427	Guidelines for nutritional supplements	1	2	3	4	5	NA
185428	Potential food and medication interactions	1	2	3	4	5	NA
185429	Potential food and herbal supplement interactions	1	2	3	4	5	NA

Domain-Health Knowledge & Behavior (IV)   **Class**-Knowledge Health Promotion (S)   5th edition 2013; reviewed 2024

K

OUTCOME CONTENT REFERENCES:

Bernstein, M. (2017). Nutritional needs of the older adult. *Physical Medicine Rehabilitation Clinics of North America, 28*(4), 747–766. https://doi.org/10.1016/j.pmr.2017.06.008

Bigand, T. L., Dietz, J., Gubitz, H. N., & Wilson, M. (2021). Barriers and facilitators to healthy eating among adult food bank users. *Western Journal of Nursing Research, 43*(7), 660–667. https://doi.org/10.1177/0193945920969689

Hockenberry, M. J., Wilson, D., & Rodgers, C. C. (Eds.). (2019). *Wong's nursing care of infants and children* (11th ed.). Elsevier.

Jeffs, E., Williman, J., Brunton, C., Gullam, J., & Walls, T. (2020). Pregnant women's knowledge of, and adherence to, New Zealand Food Safety in Pregnancy guidelines. *New Zealand Medical Journal, 133*(1525), 41–52. https://doi.org/10.1111/ajo.12523

Konek, S. H., & Becker, P. J. (2019). *Samour and King's pediatric nutrition in clinical care.* Jones & Bartlett.

Matwiejczyk, L., Mehta, K., Scott, J., Tonkin, E., & Coveney, J. (2018). Characteristics of effective interventions promoting healthy eating for preschoolers in childcare settings: An umbrella review. *Nutrients, 10*(3), 293. https://doi.org/10.3390/nu10030293

Rust, N. A., Ridding, L., Ward, C., Clark, B., Kehoe, L., Dora, M., Whittingham, M. J., McGowan, P., Chaudhary, A., Reynolds, C. J., Trivedy, C., & West, N. (2020). How to transition to reduced-meat diets that benefit people and the planet. *The Science of the Total Environment, 718*, 137208. https://doi.org/10.1016/j.scitotenv.2020.137208

Shorey, S., & Chan, V. (2021). Effectiveness of healthy eating interventions among children: A quantitative systematic review. *Journal of Advanced Nursing, 77*(2), 583–594. https://doi.org/10.1111/jan.14606

U.S. Department of Agriculture & U.S. Department of Health and Human Services. (2020). *Dietary guidelines for Americans, 2020–2025* (9th ed.). https://www.dietaryguidelines.gov

Vecchio, R., & Cavallo, C. (2019). Increasing healthy food choices through nudges: A systematic review. *Food Quality and Preference, 78*, 103714. https://doi.org/10.1016/j.foodqual.2019.05.014

Vermeulen, S. J., Park, T., Khoury, C. K., & Bene, C. (2020). Changing diets and the transformation of the global food system. *Annals of the New York Academy of Science, 1478*, 3–17. https://doi.org/10.1111/nyas.14446

Knowledge: Healthy Lifestyle

1855

Definition: Extent of understanding conveyed about a healthy balanced lifestyle consistent with one's values, strengths, and interests

OUTCOME TARGET RATING: Maintain at_____ Increase to_____

		No Knowledge	Limited Knowledge	Moderate Knowledge	Substantial Knowledge	Extensive Knowledge	
OUTCOME OVERALL RATING		**1**	**2**	**3**	**4**	**5**	
Indicators:							
185501	Optimal personal weight range	1	2	3	4	5	NA
185502	Optimal body mass index range	1	2	3	4	5	NA
185503	Optimal body fat percentage	1	2	3	4	5	NA
185504	Strategies to maintain healthy diet	1	2	3	4	5	NA
185505	Importance of water for adequate hydration	1	2	3	4	5	NA
185506	Recommended daily fruit servings	1	2	3	4	5	NA
185507	Recommended daily vegetable servings	1	2	3	4	5	NA
185508	Strategies to limit saturated fat and cholesterol intake	1	2	3	4	5	NA
185509	Strategies to limit sodium intake	1	2	3	4	5	NA
185510	Importance of food portions	1	2	3	4	5	NA
185511	Recommended vitamin supplements	1	2	3	4	5	NA
185512	Recommended mineral supplements	1	2	3	4	5	NA
185513	Strategies to avoid second-hand smoke	1	2	3	4	5	NA
185514	Strategies for tobacco cessation	1	2	3	4	5	NA
185515	Importance of alcohol use in moderation	1	2	3	4	5	NA
185537	Adverse health effects of tobacco use	1	2	3	4	5	NA
185538	Adverse health effects of alcohol use	1	2	3	4	5	NA
185539	Adverse health effects of drug use	1	2	3	4	5	NA
185516	Benefits of regular exercise	1	2	3	4	5	NA
185517	Importance of being physically active	1	2	3	4	5	NA
185518	Strategies to limit use of electronic devices	1	2	3	4	5	NA
185519	Personal factors affecting health behaviors	1	2	3	4	5	NA
185520	Environmental factors affecting health behaviors	1	2	3	4	5	NA
185540	Strategies to avoid exposure to environmental hazards	1	2	3	4	5	NA
185548	Importance of testing for radon	1	2	3	4	5	NA
185549	Importance of testing private well water	1	2	3	4	5	NA
185550	Importance of using a carbon monoxide detector	1	2	3	4	5	NA
185551	Importance of fire alarms	1	2	3	4	5	NA
185521	Barriers to maintain healthy behaviors	1	2	3	4	5	NA
185541	Risk for hereditary disease	1	2	3	4	5	NA
185522	Strategies to prevent disease	1	2	3	4	5	NA
185523	Strategies to prevent infection	1	2	3	4	5	NA
185524	Strategies to prevent accidents	1	2	3	4	5	NA
185552	Importance of obtaining recommended vaccines	1	2	3	4	5	NA
185525	Benefits of social support	1	2	3	4	5	NA
185553	Importance of lifelong learning	1	2	3	4	5	NA
185526	Importance of sharing thoughts, feelings, and beliefs	1	2	3	4	5	NA
185544	Importance of purposeful life	1	2	3	4	5	NA
185527	Importance of preventive screenings	1	2	3	4	5	NA
185545	Recommended health screenings	1	2	3	4	5	NA
185546	Recommended self-screenings for cancer detection	1	2	3	4	5	NA
185528	Importance of oral health care	1	2	3	4	5	NA
185529	Importance of protection against ultraviolet radiation	1	2	3	4	5	NA
185530	Adverse health effects of being overweight	1	2	3	4	5	NA
185531	Strategies to enhance self-esteem	1	2	3	4	5	NA
185532	Strategies to reduce stress	1	2	3	4	5	NA

K

Knowledge: Healthy Lifestyle—cont'd

		No Knowledge	Limited Knowledge	Moderate Knowledge	Substantial Knowledge	Extensive Knowledge	
185554	Importance of sleep	1	2	3	4	5	NA
185533	Importance of maintaining optimism	1	2	3	4	5	NA
185534	Importance of mental stimulation	1	2	3	4	5	NA
185535	Strategies to promote life balance	1	2	3	4	5	NA
185536	When to obtain assistance from a health professional	1	2	3	4	5	NA
185547	Reputable health care resources	1	2	3	4	5	NA

Domain-*Health Knowledge & Behavior (IV)*   **Class**-*Knowledge Health Promotion (S)*   *5th edition 2013; revised 2018, 2024*

OUTCOME CONTENT REFERENCES:

Arena, R., Myers, J., Kaminsky, L. A., Williams, M., Sabbahi, A., Popovic, D., Axtell, R., Faghy, M. A., Hills, A. P., Olivares, S. L. O., Lopez, M., Pronk, N. P., Laddu, D., Babu, A. S., Josephson, R., Whitsel, L. P., Severin, R., Christle, J. W., Dourado, V. Z., Niebauer, J., Savage, P., Ausford, L. D., & Lavie, C. J. (2021). Current activities centered on healthy living and recommendations for the future: A position statement for the HL-PIVOT Network. *Current Problems in Cardiology, 46*(6), 1–45. https://doi.org/10.1016/j.cpcardiol.2021.100823

Browne, J., Cather, C., Zvonar, V., Thayer, K., Skiest, H., Arntz, D., Kritikos, K., Schnitzer, K., Brown, H., Evins, A. E., & Donovan, A. (2021). Developing a sound body: Open trial results of a group healthy lifestyle intervention for young adults with psychosis. *Community Mental Health Journal, 57*(5), 864–871. https://doi.org/10.1007/s10597-020-00655-y

Catchings, S., Steinberg, D., Fruth, J., & Sabol, V. K. (2021). The treatment of obesity in the multidisciplinary setting. *The Journal for Nurse Practitioners, 17*(6), 707–711. https://doi.org/10.1016/j.nurpra.2021.02.007

Cristiani, V., Kumbamu, A., Asiedu, G. B., Johnson, S. K., O'Brien, J. R. G., Ziebart, G., Mogen, M. R., Lynch, B., & Kumar, S. (2021). Use of community based participatory research to design interventions for healthy lifestyle in an alternative learning environment. *Journal of Primary Care & Community Health, 12*, 1–8. https://doi.org/10.1177/21501327211014749

Gleason, J. A., Taggert, E., & Goun, B. (2021). Characteristics and behaviors among a representative sample of New Jersey adults practicing environmental risk-reduction behaviors. *Journal of Public Health Management & Practice, 27*(6), 588–597. https://doi.org/10.1097/PHH.0000000000001106

Saxena, S., Vo, J., Millage, J., Wong, D., Bélanger, P., Fournier, A., Bodiam, L., Allison, A., & Longmuir, P. E. (2021). Developing patient resources to enable the exchange of healthy lifestyle information between clinicians and families of children with complex heart problems. *Child: Care, Health and Development, 47*(3), 357–366. https://doi.org/10.1111/cch.12848

Valatka, R., Krizo, J., & Mallat, A. (2021). A survey-based assessment of "matter of balance" participant fall-related experience. *Journal of Trauma Nursing, 28*(5), 304–309. https://doi.org/10.1097/JTN.0000000000000602

K

Knowledge: Heart Failure Management   1835

Definition: Extent of understanding conveyed about heart failure, its treatment, and the prevention of disease progression and complications

OUTCOME TARGET RATING: Maintain at_____ Increase to_____

		No Knowledge	Limited Knowledge	Moderate Knowledge	Substantial Knowledge	Extensive Knowledge	
OUTCOME OVERALL RATING		1	2	3	4	5	NA
Indicators:							
183501	Cause and contributing factors	1	2	3	4	5	NA
183502	Signs and symptoms of early disease	1	2	3	4	5	NA
183503	Benefits of disease management	1	2	3	4	5	NA
183560	Usual course of disease	1	2	3	4	5	NA
183530	Role of diagnostic tests for disease management	1	2	3	4	5	NA
183504	Basic actions of the heart	1	2	3	4	5	NA
183505	Signs and symptoms of progressive heart failure	1	2	3	4	5	NA
183538	Signs and symptoms of complications	1	2	3	4	5	NA
183507	Signs and symptoms of anemia	1	2	3	4	5	NA
183539	Barriers to self-care	1	2	3	4	5	NA
183540	Strategies to manage dyspnea	1	2	3	4	5	NA
183561	Strategies to manage fatigue	1	2	3	4	5	NA
183541	Strategies to manage tachycardia	1	2	3	4	5	NA
183542	Strategies to manage edema	1	2	3	4	5	NA

Continued

Knowledge: Heart Failure Management—cont'd

		No Knowledge	Limited Knowledge	Moderate Knowledge	Substantial Knowledge	Extensive Knowledge	
183512	Relationship of physical and emotional stress to condition	1	2	3	4	5	NA
183513	Psychosocial effects of heart failure	1	2	3	4	5	NA
183562	Signs and symptoms of anxiety	1	2	3	4	5	NA
183515	Strategies to control anxiety	1	2	3	4	5	NA
183563	Strategies to control depression	1	2	3	4	5	NA
183543	Signs and symptoms of depression	1	2	3	4	5	NA
183544	Counseling available for depression	1	2	3	4	5	NA
183516	Treatments to improve cardiac performance	1	2	3	4	5	NA
183545	Health behaviors to promote physiologic stability	1	2	3	4	5	NA
183517	Strategies to promote peripheral circulation	1	2	3	4	5	NA
183546	Benefits of adequate rest	1	2	3	4	5	NA
183547	Benefits of regular exercise	1	2	3	4	5	NA
183548	Recommended physical activity	1	2	3	4	5	NA
183511	Signs and symptoms of overexertion	1	2	3	4	5	NA
183549	Strategies to prevent overexertion	1	2	3	4	5	NA
183519	Strategies to balance activity and rest	1	2	3	4	5	NA
183521	Strategies to increase resistance to infection	1	2	3	4	5	NA
183550	Recommended immunizations	1	2	3	4	5	NA
183524	Factors contributing to weight changes	1	2	3	4	5	NA
183525	Strategies to manage weight	1	2	3	4	5	NA
183551	Prescribed diet	1	2	3	4	5	NA
183526	Strategies to increase diet compliance	1	2	3	4	5	NA
183552	Recommended fluid intake	1	2	3	4	5	NA
183564	Strategies to manage thirst	1	2	3	4	5	NA
183553	Importance of tobacco abstinence	1	2	3	4	5	NA
183554	Strategies for smoking cessation	1	2	3	4	5	NA
183555	Importance of alcohol restrictions	1	2	3	4	5	NA
183565	Correct name of prescribed medication	1	2	3	4	5	NA
183566	Correct use of prescribed medication	1	2	3	4	5	NA
183527	Medication therapeutic effects	1	2	3	4	5	NA
183528	Medication side effects	1	2	3	4	5	NA
183529	Medication adverse effects	1	2	3	4	5	NA
183531	Self-monitoring techniques	1	2	3	4	5	NA
183556	Correct use of a pulse oximeter	1	2	3	4	5	NA
183557	Correct use of oxygen	1	2	3	4	5	NA
183532	Effects on lifestyle	1	2	3	4	5	NA
183533	Adaptations for role performance	1	2	3	4	5	NA
183558	Risks associated with travel	1	2	3	4	5	NA
183559	Adaptations for travel	1	2	3	4	5	NA
183534	Effects on sexuality	1	2	3	4	5	NA
183535	Adaptations for sexual performance	1	2	3	4	5	NA
183536	Available support groups	1	2	3	4	5	NA
183567	Actions to promote dignified death	1	2	3	4	5	NA
183537	When to obtain assistance from a health professional	1	2	3	4	5	NA

Domain-Health Knowledge & Behavior (IV) **Class**-Knowledge Health Condition (GG) 4th edition 2008; revised 2013, 2024

OUTCOME CONTENT REFERENCES:

Allida, S. M., Hayward, C. S., & Newton, P. J. (2018). Thirst in heart failure: What do we know so far? *Current Opinion in Supportive and Palliative Care, 12*(1), 4–9. https://doi.org/10.1097/SPC.0000000000000314

Awoke, M. S., Baptiste, D. L., Davidson, P., Roberts, A., & Dennison-Himmelfarb, C. (2019). A quasi-experimental study examining a nurse-led education program to improve knowledge, self-care, and reduce readmission for individuals with heart failure. *Contemporary Nurse, 55*(1), 15–26. https://doi.org/10.1080/10376178.2019.1568198

Boyde, M., Peters, R., Hwang, R., Korczyk, D., Ha, T., & New, N. (2017). The self-care educational intervention for patients with heart failure: A study protocol. *The Journal of Cardiovascular Nursing, 32*(2), 165–170. https://doi.org/10.1097/JCN.0000000000000318

da Costa Ferreira, N., Takao Lopes, C., Moorhead, S., Gengo e Silva Butcher, R. de C. (2021). Content validation of the nursing outcome Knowledge Heart Failure Management: Brazilian nurses' opinions. *International Journal of Nursing Knowledge, 32*(3), 206–214. https://doi.org/10.1111/2047-3095.12312

Ignatavicius, D. D., Workman, M. L., Rebar, C. R., & Heimgartner, N. M. (2021). *Medical-surgical nursing: Concepts for interprofessional care* (10th ed.). Elsevier.

Tripoliti, E. E., Karanasiou, G. S., Kalatzis, F. G., Bechlioulis, A., Goletsis, Y., Naka, K., & Fotiadis, D. I. (2019). HEARTEN KMS—A knowledge management system targeting the management of patients with heart failure. *Journal of Biomedical Informatics, 94*, 103203. https://doi.org/10.1016/j.jbi.2019.103203

Zhao, Q., Chen, C., Zhang, J., Ye, Y., & Fan, X. (2020). Effects of self-management interventions on heart failure: Systematic review and meta-analysis of randomized controlled trials. *International Journal of Nursing Studies, 110*, 103689. https://doi.org/10.1016/j.ijnurstu.2020.103689

Knowledge: Human Immunodeficiency Virus Management   3206

Definition: Extent of understanding conveyed about human immunodeficiency virus (HIV), its treatment, and prevention of progression and complications

OUTCOME TARGET RATING: Maintain at_____ Increase to_____

	No Knowledge	Limited Knowledge	Moderate Knowledge	Substantial Knowledge	Extensive Knowledge	
OUTCOME OVERALL RATING	1	2	3	4	5	
Indicators						
320601 Personal meaning of diagnosis	1	2	3	4	5	NA
320602 Usual course of disease	1	2	3	4	5	NA
320603 Signs and symptoms of disease	1	2	3	4	5	NA
320604 Prevention of disease transmission	1	2	3	4	5	NA
320605 Plan of care agreed upon with health professional	1	2	3	4	5	NA
320606 Importance of disclosing human immunodeficiency virus positive status to intimate partners	1	2	3	4	5	NA
320607 Importance of taking antiretroviral medication	1	2	3	4	5	NA
320608 Medication therapeutic effects	1	2	3	4	5	NA
320609 Medication side effects	1	2	3	4	5	NA
320610 Medication adverse effects	1	2	3	4	5	NA
320640 Importance of monitoring signs and symptoms	1	2	3	4	5	NA
320611 Importance of obtaining required laboratory tests	1	2	3	4	5	NA
320612 Importance of monitoring CD4 T lymphocyte count	1	2	3	4	5	NA
320613 Interpretation of laboratory tests	1	2	3	4	5	NA
320614 Importance of monitoring viral load	1	2	3	4	5	NA
320615 Safe disposal of contaminated materials	1	2	3	4	5	NA
320616 Importance of lifelong vigilance	1	2	3	4	5	NA
320617 Importance of modifying unhealthy behaviors	1	2	3	4	5	NA
320618 Importance of exercise	1	2	3	4	5	NA
320641 Importance of strategies to manage fatigue	1	2	3	4	5	NA
320619 Importance of Healthy diet	1	2	3	4	5	NA
320620 Importance of refraining from intravenous drug use	1	2	3	4	5	NA
320621 Safe sex practices	1	2	3	4	5	NA
320642 Importance of smoking cessation	1	2	3	4	5	NA
320622 Infection prevention strategies	1	2	3	4	5	NA
320623 Impact of social inequities	1	2	3	4	5	NA
320624 Stigma associated with human immunodeficiency virus	1	2	3	4	5	NA
320625 Coping strategies	1	2	3	4	5	NA
320626 Trajectory of change in self-image	1	2	3	4	5	NA
320627 Importance of forgiving self for life circumstances	1	2	3	4	5	NA
320628 Importance of forgiving others for life circumstances	1	2	3	4	5	NA
320643 Importance of seeking assistance with activities of disease management when needed	1	2	3	4	5	NA
320629 Strategies to manage stress	1	2	3	4	5	NA
320630 Importance of reporting depressive symptoms to provider	1	2	3	4	5	NA

K

Continued

Knowledge: Human Immunodeficiency Virus Management—cont'd

		No Knowledge	Limited Knowledge	Moderate Knowledge	Substantial Knowledge	Extensive Knowledge	
320644	Importance of obtaining recommended vaccines	1	2	3	4	5	NA
320633	Benefits of attending peer support groups	1	2	3	4	5	NA
320634	Benefits of disease management	1	2	3	4	5	NA
320635	Importance of sharing information about human immunodeficiency virus with others	1	2	3	4	5	NA
320645	Impact of treatment burden	1	2	3	4	5	NA
320636	Importance of obtaining support from family	1	2	3	4	5	NA
320637	Importance of obtaining support from friends	1	2	3	4	5	NA
320638	Importance of keeping appointments with health provider	1	2	3	4	5	NA
320639	Available community resources	1	2	3	4	5	NA

Domain-Health Knowledge & Behavior (IV)   **Class**-Knowledge Health Condition (GG)   6th edition 2018; revised 2024

OUTCOME CONTENT REFERENCES:

Boucher, L. M., O'Brien, K. K., Baxter, L. N., Fitzgerald, M. L., Liddy, C. E., & Kendall, C. E. (2019). Healthy aging with HIV: The role of self-management support. *Patient Education and Counseling, 102*(8), 1565–1569 https://doi.org/10.1016/j.pec.2019.02.019

Cook, L. (2021). HIV stigma reduction and health literacy education program with a cross-generational population in an African American faith-based church. *Journal of Public Health: From Theory to Practice, 29*(5), 1089–1106. https://doi.org/10.1007/s10389-020-01203-4

Harkness, A., Satyanarayana, S., Mayo, D., Smith-Alvarez, R., Rogers, B. G., Prado, G., & Safren, S. (2021). Scaling up and out HIV prevention and behavioral health services to Latino sexual minority men in South Florida: Multi-level implementation barriers, facilitators, and strategies. *AIDS Patient Care and STDs, 35*(5), 167–179. https://doi.org/10.1089/apc.2021.0018

Ignatavicius, D. D., Workman, M. L., Rebar, C. R., & Heimgartner, N. M. (2021). *Medical-surgical nursing: Concepts for interprofessional collaborative care*. Elsevier.

Rodriguez, C. A., Winnett, A., Wong, M., Krishnam, N., Martínez, N. O., Perez, L. J., Kolevic, L., Lecca, L., & Franke, M. F. (2021). Feasibility and acceptability of an adolescent-friendly rap video to improve health literacy among HIV-positive youth in urban Peru. *AIDS and Behavior, 25*(4), 1290–1298. https://doi.org/10.1007/s10461-020-03098-4

Schreiner, N., Perazzo, J, Digennaro, S., Burant, C., Daly, B., & Webel, A. (2020). Associations between symptom severity and treatment burden in people living with HIV. *Journal of Advanced Nursing, 76*, 2348–2358. https://doi.org/10.1111/jan.14461

Schreiner, N., Perazzo, J., Digennaro, S., Currie, J., Daly, B., & Webel, A. (2019). A descriptive, cross-sectional study examining treatment burden in people living with HIV. *Applied Nursing Research, 46*, 31–36. https://doi.org/10.1016/j.apnr.2019.02.009

Schreiner, N., Perazzo, J., Digennaro, S., Currie, J., Daly, B., & Webel, A. (2020). Examining the association between item specific treatment burden and adherence in people living with HIV. *Western Journal of Nursing Research, 42*(7), 495–502. https://doi.org/10.1177/01939-45919880317

K

Knowledge: Hypertension Management

1837

Definition: Extent of understanding conveyed about high blood pressure, its treatment, and the prevention of complications

OUTCOME TARGET RATING: Maintain at_____ Increase to_____

		No Knowledge	Limited Knowledge	Moderate Knowledge	Substantial Knowledge	Extensive Knowledge	
OUTCOME OVERALL RATING		1	2	3	4	5	
Indicators:							
183701	Normal range for systolic blood pressure	1	2	3	4	5	NA
183702	Normal range for diastolic blood pressure	1	2	3	4	5	NA
183703	Target blood pressure	1	2	3	4	5	NA
183704	Methods to measure blood pressure	1	2	3	4	5	NA
183705	Potential complications of hypertension	1	2	3	4	5	NA
183706	Available treatment options	1	2	3	4	5	NA
183707	Benefits of long-term treatment	1	2	3	4	5	NA
183708	Signs and symptoms of exacerbation of hypertension	1	2	3	4	5	NA
183709	Correct use of prescribed medication	1	2	3	4	5	NA

Knowledge: Hypertension Management—cont'd

	No Knowledge	Limited Knowledge	Moderate Knowledge	Substantial Knowledge	Extensive Knowledge	
183710	Medication therapeutic effects	1	2	3	4	5	NA
183711	Medication side effects	1	2	3	4	5	NA
183712	Medication adverse effects	1	2	3	4	5	NA
183713	Importance of adherence to treatment	1	2	3	4	5	NA
183714	Importance of informing health professional of all current medication	1	2	3	4	5	NA
183715	Importance of keeping follow-up appointments	1	2	3	4	5	NA
183716	Benefits of ongoing self-monitoring	1	2	3	4	5	NA
183717	Recommended schedule for monitoring blood pressure	1	2	3	4	5	NA
183718	Benefits of weight loss	1	2	3	4	5	NA
183719	Benefits of lifestyle modifications	1	2	3	4	5	NA
183720	Strategies to manage stress	1	2	3	4	5	NA
183721	Prescribed diet	1	2	3	4	5	NA
183722	Strategies to change dietary habits	1	2	3	4	5	NA
183723	Strategies to limit sodium intake	1	2	3	4	5	NA
183724	Strategies to increase diet adherence	1	2	3	4	5	NA
183725	Adverse health effects of alcohol use	1	2	3	4	5	NA
183726	Importance of tobacco abstinence	1	2	3	4	5	NA
183727	Benefits of regular exercise	1	2	3	4	5	NA
183728	Reputable sources of hypertension information	1	2	3	4	5	NA
183729	Available support groups	1	2	3	4	5	NA
183730	When to obtain assistance from a health professional	1	2	3	4	5	NA
183732	Importance of partnering with health care provider	1	2	3	4	5	NA
183731	Benefits of disease management	1	2	3	4	5	NA

Domain-*Health Knowledge & Behavior (IV)*   **Class**-*Knowledge Health Condition (GG)*   *4th edition 2008; revised 2013, 2024*

OUTCOME CONTENT REFERENCES:

Abegaz, T. M., Shehab, A., Gebreyohannes, E. A., Bhagavathula, A. S., & Elnour, A. A. (2017). Nonadherence to antihypertensive drugs: A systematic review and meta-analysis. *Medicine, 96*(4), e5641. https://doi.org/10.1097/MD.0000000000005641

+Baliz Erkoc, S., Isikli, B., Metintas, S., & Kalyoncu, C. (2012). Hypertension Knowledge-Level Scale (HK-LS): A study on development, validity and reliability. *International Journal of Environmental Research and Public Health, 9*(3), 1018–1029. https://doi.org/10.3390/ijerph9031018

+Hereibi, M. J., Arthur, J. P., Mantovani, M. F., Mattei, A. T., & Bortolato-Major, C. (2021). Construct validity and reliability of the Brazilian version of Hypertension Knowledge-Level Scale. *Revista Gaucha de Enfermagem, 42*, e20190429. https://doi.org/10.1590/1983-1447.2021.20190429

Jankowska-Polańska, B., Uchmanowicz, I., Dudek, K., & Mazur, G. (2016). Relationship between patients' knowledge and medication adherence among patients with hypertension. *Patient Preference and Adherence, 10*, 2437–2447. https://doi.org/10.2147/PPA.S117269

Kario, K. (2020). Management of hypertension in the digital era. *Hypertension, 76*(3), 640–650. https://doi.org/10.1161/HYPERTENSIONAHA.120.14742

Li, R., Liang, N., Bu, F., & Hesketh, T. (2020). The effectiveness of self-management of hypertension in adults using mobile health: Systematic review and meta-analysis. *JMIR mHealth and uHealth, 8*(3), e17776. https://doi.org/10.2196/17776

Oh, H., & Moorhead, S. (2020). Validation of the knowledge and self-management Nursing Outcomes Classification outcomes for adults with hypertension and lipid disorder. *Online Journal of Nursing Informatics, 24*(2), 1. https://doi.org/10.1097/CIN.0000000000000495

Peacock, E., & Krousel-Wood, M. (2017). Adherence to antihypertensive therapy. *The Medical Clinics of North America, 101*(1), 229–245. https://doi.org/10.1016/j.mcna.2016.08.005

Swaminathan, R., Cohen, E., Philley, M., Hokanson, J., & Young, K. (2020). Impact of self-measured blood pressure monitoring on hypertension management. *Blood Pressure Monitoring, 25*(5), 259–262. https://doi.org/10.1097/MBP.0000000000000455

Warren-Findlow, J., Krinner, L. M., Vinoski Thomas, E., Coffman, M. J., Gordon, B., & Howden, R. (2020). Relative and cumulative effects of hypertension self-care behaviors on blood pressure. *Western Journal of Nursing Research, 42*(3), 157–164. https://doi.org/10.1177/0193945919851111

Whelton, P. K., Carey, R. M., Aronow, W. S., Casey, D. E., Collins, K. J., Dennison Himmelfarb, C., & Wright, J. T. (2018). 2017 ACC/AHA/AAPA/ABC/ACPM/AGS/APHA/ASH/ASPC/NMA/PCNA guideline for the prevention, detection, evaluation, and management of high blood pressure in adults: A report of the American College of Cardiology/American Heart Association Task Force on Clinical Practice Guidelines. *Journal of the American College of Cardiology, 71*(19), e127–e248. https://doi.org/10.1016/j.jacc.2017.11.006

Wright, K. D., Still, C. H., Jones, L. M., & Moss, K. O. (2018). Designing a cocreated intervention with African American older adults for hypertension. *International Journal of Hypertension, 2018*, 7591289. https://doi.org/10.1155/2018/7591289

K

Knowledge: Infant Care | 1819

Definition: Extent of understanding conveyed about caring for a baby from birth to first birthday

OUTCOME TARGET RATING: Maintain at_____ Increase to_____

		No Knowledge	Limited Knowledge	Moderate Knowledge	Substantial Knowledge	Extensive Knowledge	
OUTCOME OVERALL RATING		**1**	**2**	**3**	**4**	**5**	
Indicators:							
181901	Normal infant characteristics	1	2	3	4	5	NA
181902	Normal growth and development	1	2	3	4	5	NA
181903	Proper holding of infant	1	2	3	4	5	NA
181904	Proper infant positioning	1	2	3	4	5	NA
181905	Infant safety practices and accidents prevention	1	2	3	4	5	NA
181928	Age-appropriate cardiopulmonary resuscitation techniques	1	2	3	4	5	NA
181908	Nutritive versus non-nutritive sucking	1	2	3	4	5	NA
181909	Pros and cons of infant feeding choices	1	2	3	4	5	NA
181910	Infant feeding techniques	1	2	3	4	5	NA
181930	Introduction of healthy foods at 6 months	1	2	3	4	5	NA
181931	Skin to skin contact	1	2	3	4	5	NA
181911	Signs and symptoms of dehydration	1	2	3	4	5	NA
181912	Signs and symptoms of jaundice	1	2	3	4	5	NA
181913	Infant bathing	1	2	3	4	5	NA
181914	Umbilical cord care	1	2	3	4	5	NA
181915	Infant diapering	1	2	3	4	5	NA
181916	Appropriate clothing for environment	1	2	3	4	5	NA
181917	Methods to measure body temperature	1	2	3	4	5	NA
181918	Infant sleep-wake patterns	1	2	3	4	5	NA
181919	Infant communication cues	1	2	3	4	5	NA
181920	Infant stimulation methods	1	2	3	4	5	NA
181921	Infant relaxation techniques	1	2	3	4	5	NA
181922	Strategies to adjust to addition of infant	1	2	3	4	5	NA
181923	Special care needs	1	2	3	4	5	NA
181924	Considerations when choosing a childcare provider	1	2	3	4	5	NA
181926	Precautions when pets are in the household	1	2	3	4	5	NA
181925	Available community resources	1	2	3	4	5	NA
181929	Available support groups	1	2	3	4	5	NA

K

Domain-Health Knowledge & Behavior (IV)   *Class*-Knowledge Health Promotion (S)   *2nd edition 2000; revised 2004, 2008, 2013, 2024*

OUTCOME CONTENT REFERENCES:

Dao, A., & McMullin, J. (2019). Unintentional injury, supervision, and discourses on childproofing devices. *Medical Anthropology, 38*(1), 15–29. https://doi.org/10.1080/01459740.2018.1482548

Hagan, J. F., Shaw, J. S., & Duncan, P. M. (Eds.). (2017). *Bright futures: Guidelines for health supervision of infants, children, and adolescents* (4th ed.). American Academy of Pediatrics.

Hockenberry, M. J., Wilson, D., & Rodgers, C. C. (Eds.). (2019). *Wong's nursing care of infants and children* (11th ed.). Elsevier.

Hwang, S. S., & Corwin, M. J. (2017). Safe infant sleep practices: Parental engagement, education, and behavior change. *Pediatric Annals, 46*(8), e291–e296. https://doi.org/10.3928/19382359-20170719-02

Johnson, E., & Hunt, R. (2019). Infant skin care: Updates and recommendations. *Current Opinion in Pediatrics. 31*(4), 476–481. https://doi.org/10.1097/MOP.0000000000000791

Kotowski, J., Fowler, C., Hourigan, C., & Orr, F. (2020). Bottle-feeding an infant feeding modality: An integrative literature review. *Maternal & Child Nutrition, 16*(2), e12939. https://doi.org/10.1111/mcn.12939

Sayres, S., & Visentin, L. (2018). Breastfeeding: Uncovering barriers and offering solutions. *Current Opinion Pediatrics, 30*(4), 591–596. https://doi.org/10.1097/MOP.0000000000000647

Knowledge: Infection Management   1842

Definition: Extent of understanding conveyed about infection, its treatment, and the prevention of disease progression and complications

OUTCOME TARGET RATING: Maintain at_____ Increase to_____

	No Knowledge	Limited Knowledge	Moderate Knowledge	Substantial Knowledge	Extensive Knowledge	
OUTCOME OVERALL RATING	1	2	3	4	5	
Indicators:						
184201 Mode of transmission	1	2	3	4	5	NA
184202 Factors contributing to infection transmission	1	2	3	4	5	NA
184203 Practices that reduce transmission	1	2	3	4	5	NA
184204 Signs and symptoms of infection	1	2	3	4	5	NA
184206 Monitoring procedures for infection	1	2	3	4	5	NA
184207 Importance of hand sanitation	1	2	3	4	5	NA
184208 Actions to increase resistance to infection	1	2	3	4	5	NA
184209 Treatment for diagnosed infection	1	2	3	4	5	NA
184210 Follow-up for diagnosed infection	1	2	3	4	5	NA
184211 Signs and symptoms of exacerbation of infection	1	2	3	4	5	NA
184212 Correct name of medication	1	2	3	4	5	NA
184213 Medication side effects	1	2	3	4	5	NA
184214 Medication therapeutic effects	1	2	3	4	5	NA
184215 Medication adverse effects	1	2	3	4	5	NA
184216 Potential medication interactions	1	2	3	4	5	NA
184217 Importance of adherence to treatment	1	2	3	4	5	NA
184218 Use of probiotics in the treatment of infection	1	2	3	4	5	NA
184219 Risk of drug resistance	1	2	3	4	5	NA
184220 Importance of completing medication regimen	1	2	3	4	5	NA
184221 Influences of nutrition on infection	1	2	3	4	5	NA
184222 Strategies to manage stress	1	2	3	4	5	NA
184223 Factors that affect immune response	1	2	3	4	5	NA
184224 Available support groups	1	2	3	4	5	NA
184225 Available community resources	1	2	3	4	5	NA
184226 When to obtain assistance from a health professional	1	2	3	4	5	NA

Domain-*Health Knowledge & Behavior (IV)*   **Class**-*Knowledge Health Condition (GG)*   *4th edition 2008; revised 2013; reviewed 2024*

OUTCOME CONTENT REFERENCES:

Kim, J., & Jang, E. (2021). Factors influencing healthcare-associated infection control of caregivers. *Journal of Korean Critical Care Nursing, 14*(1), 63-75. https://doi.org/10.34250/jkccn.2021.14.1.63

Johnson, S., Lavergne, V., Skinner, A., Gonzales-Luna, A. J., Garey, K. W., Kelly, C. P., & Wilcox, M. H. (2021). Clinical practice guideline by the Infectious Disease Society of America (IDSA) and Society for Healthcare Epidemiology of America (SHEA): 2021 Focused update guidelines on management of *Clostridioides difficile* infection in adults. *Clinical Infectious Diseases, 73*(5), e1029-44. https://doi.org/10.1093/cid/ciab549

Joseph, A. (2006). *The impact of the environment on infections in healthcare facilities.* Robert Wood Johnson Foundation.

Potter, P., Perry, A., Stockert, P., & Hall, A. (2021). *Fundamentals of nursing* (10th ed.). Elsevier.

K

Knowledge: *Inflammatory Bowel Disease Management* 1856

Definition: Extent of understanding conveyed about the inflammatory bowel disease process, its treatment, and the prevention of relapses or complications

OUTCOME TARGET RATING: Maintain at_____ Increase to_____

	No Knowledge	Limited Knowledge	Moderate Knowledge	Substantial Knowledge	Extensive Knowledge	
OUTCOME OVERALL RATING	1	2	3	4	5	
Indicators:						
185601 Cause and contributing factors	1	2	3	4	5	NA
185602 Risk factors for disease progression	1	2	3	4	5	NA
185603 Usual course of disease	1	2	3	4	5	NA
185604 Signs and symptoms of inflammatory bowel disease	1	2	3	4	5	NA
185605 Area of bowel affected by disease	1	2	3	4	5	NA
185606 Signs and symptoms of disease relapse	1	2	3	4	5	NA
185635 Potential effects of comorbidities on disease	1	2	3	4	5	NA
185607 Benefits of disease management	1	2	3	4	5	NA
185608 Strategies to balance activity and rest	1	2	3	4	5	NA
185609 Energy conservation techniques	1	2	3	4	5	NA
185610 Medication therapeutic effects	1	2	3	4	5	NA
185611 Medication side effects	1	2	3	4	5	NA
185612 Medication adverse effects	1	2	3	4	5	NA
185613 Medical treatment options	1	2	3	4	5	NA
185614 Surgical treatment options	1	2	3	4	5	NA
185615 Psychosocial effects of disease	1	2	3	4	5	NA
185616 Relationship of physical and emotional stress to condition	1	2	3	4	5	NA
185636 Importance of sources of social support	1	2	3	4	5	NA
185617 Role of diagnostic tests for disease management	1	2	3	4	5	NA
185637 Role of bloodwork for disease management	1	2	3	4	5	NA
185638 Importance of monitoring bone density	1	2	3	4	5	NA
185618 Potential complications of disease	1	2	3	4	5	NA
185619 Strategies to minimize disease progression	1	2	3	4	5	NA
185639 Importance of regular exercise	1	2	3	4	5	NA
185620 Prescribed diet	1	2	3	4	5	NA
185640 Importance of fluids	1	2	3	4	5	NA
185621 Trigger foods	1	2	3	4	5	NA
185622 Strategies to modify nutritional requirements	1	2	3	4	5	NA
185641 Importance of weight control	1	2	3	4	5	NA
185623 Strategies to enhance bowel function	1	2	3	4	5	NA
185624 Factors that trigger relapse	1	2	3	4	5	NA
185625 Strategies to manage pain	1	2	3	4	5	NA
185626 Effects on lifestyle	1	2	3	4	5	NA
185627 Strategies to adapt lifestyle to energy level	1	2	3	4	5	NA
185642 Strategies to promote well-being	1	2	3	4	5	NA
185628 Effects on sexuality	1	2	3	4	5	NA
185629 Potential effects of pregnancy	1	2	3	4	5	NA
185630 Activity restrictions during a relapse	1	2	3	4	5	NA
185631 Importance of tobacco abstinence	1	2	3	4	5	NA
185632 Impact of disease on growth and development	1	2	3	4	5	NA
185642 Available community resources	1	2	3	4	5	NA
185633 Available support groups	1	2	3	4	5	NA
185634 When to obtain assistance from a health professional	1	2	3	4	5	NA

***Domain*-**Health Knowledge & Behavior (IV) ***Class*-**Knowledge Health Condition (GG) *5th edition 2013; revised 2024*

OUTCOME CONTENT REFERENCES:

Conley, S., & Redeker, N. (2016). A systematic review of self-management interventions for inflammatory bowel disease. *Journal of Nursing Scholarship, 48*(2), 118–127. https://doi.org/10.1111/jnu.12189

Crosby, S., Schuh, M. J., Cladera, F., & Farraye, F. A. (2021). Vaccination of patients with inflammatory bowel disease during the COVID-19 pandemic. *Gastroenterology & Hepatology, 17*(1), 18–30.

El Ouali, S., Rubin, D. T., Cohen, B. L., Regueiro, M. D., & Rieder, F. (2021). Optimal inflammatory bowel disease management during the global coronavirus disease 2019 pandemic. *Current Opinion in Gastroenterology, 37*(4), 313–319. https://doi.org/10.1097/MOG.0000000000000741

Grover, Z., & Alex, A. (2019). Management of inflammatory bowel disease in children: It is time for an individualized approach. *Journal of Paediatrics and Child Health, 56*, 1677–1684. https://doi.org/10.1111/jpc.14652

Kamp. K. J., West, P., Holmstrom, A., Luo, Z., Wyatt, G., & Given, B. (2019). Systematic review of social support on psychological symptoms and self-management behaviors among adults with inflammatory bowel disease. *Journal of Nursing Scholarship, 51*(4), 380–389. https://doi.org/10.1111/jnu.12487

Tran, L., & Mulligan, K. (2019). A systematic review of self-management interventions for children and adolescents with inflammatory bowel disease. *Inflammatory Bowel Disease, 25*(4), 685–698. https://doi.org/10.1093/ibd/izy299

Trindade, I. A., Ferreira, C., & Pinto-Gouveia, J. (2020). Shame and emotion regulation in inflammatory bowel disease: Effects on psychosocial functioning. *Journal of Health Psychology, 25*(4), 511–521. https://doi.org/10.1177/1359105317718925

Tun, G. S. Z., Cripps, S., & Lobo, A. J. (2018). Crohn's disease: Management in adults, children and young people—Concise guidance. *Clinical Medicine, 18*(3), 1–8. https://doi.org/10.7861/clinmedicine.18-3-231

Knowledge: Kidney Disease Management   1857

Definition: Extent of understanding conveyed about kidney disease, its treatment, and the prevention of disease progression and complications

OUTCOME TARGET RATING: Maintain at_____ Increase to_____

		No Knowledge	Limited Knowledge	Moderate Knowledge	Substantial Knowledge	Extensive Knowledge	
OUTCOME OVERALL RATING		**1**	**2**	**3**	**4**	**5**	
Indicators:							
185701	Specific kidney disease	1	2	3	4	5	NA
185702	Signs and symptoms of kidney disease	1	2	3	4	5	NA
185738	Signs and symptoms of kidney infection	1	2	3	4	5	NA
185739	Signs and symptoms of kidney stones	1	2	3	4	5	NA
185703	Usual course of disease	1	2	3	4	5	NA
185704	Cause and contributing factors	1	2	3	4	5	NA
185740	Treatment options	1	2	3	4	5	NA
185705	Risk factors for complications	1	2	3	4	5	NA
185706	Signs and symptoms of complications	1	2	3	4	5	NA
185707	Strategies to prevent complications	1	2	3	4	5	NA
185708	Strategies to minimize disease progression	1	2	3	4	5	NA
185709	Relationship of kidney disease to hypertension	1	2	3	4	5	NA
185710	Signs and symptoms of fluid volume excess	1	2	3	4	5	NA
185711	Strategies to reduce risk of bleeding	1	2	3	4	5	NA
185712	Activity precautions	1	2	3	4	5	NA
185713	Strategies to increase resistance to infection	1	2	3	4	5	NA
185741	Strategies to cope with pain	1	2	3	4	5	NA
185714	Strategies to maintain adequate nutrition	1	2	3	4	5	NA
185715	Dietary restrictions	1	2	3	4	5	NA
185716	Fluid restrictions	1	2	3	4	5	NA
185717	Relationship of fluid intake and weight	1	2	3	4	5	NA
185718	Importance of monitoring intake and output	1	2	3	4	5	NA
185742	Importance of catheter care	1	2	3	4	5	NA
185719	Required laboratory tests	1	2	3	4	5	NA
185720	Role of laboratory tests for disease management	1	2	3	4	5	NA
185721	Recommended schedule for monitoring blood pressure	1	2	3	4	5	NA
185722	Importance of maintaining blood glucose level within target range	1	2	3	4	5	NA

Continued

Knowledge: Kidney Disease Management—cont'd

		No Knowledge	Limited Knowledge	Moderate Knowledge	Substantial Knowledge	Extensive Knowledge	
185723	Medication used for kidney disease	1	2	3	4	5	NA
185724	Medication therapeutic effects	1	2	3	4	5	NA
185725	Medication side effects	1	2	3	4	5	NA
185726	Medication adverse effects	1	2	3	4	5	NA
185743	Importance of medication reconciliation with health professional	1	2	3	4	5	NA
185727	Potential dangers of taking non-prescription medication	1	2	3	4	5	NA
185728	Importance of adherence with treatment regimen	1	2	3	4	5	NA
185729	Importance of adequate sleep	1	2	3	4	5	NA
185730	Strategies to cope with adverse effects of disease	1	2	3	4	5	NA
185744	Strategies to cope with lifestyle changes	1	2	3	4	5	NA
185731	Strategies to cope with changes in body image	1	2	3	4	5	NA
185733	Strategies to decrease nausea	1	2	3	4	5	NA
185734	When to obtain assistance from a health professional	1	2	3	4	5	NA
185735	Available support groups	1	2	3	4	5	NA
185736	Available community resources	1	2	3	4	5	NA
185737	Benefits of disease management	1	2	3	4	5	NA

Domain-Health Knowledge & Behavior (IV)   **Class**-Knowledge Health Condition (GG)   5th edition 2013; revised 2024

K

OUTCOME CONTENT REFERENCES:

Almutary, H. H. (2020). Assessment of kidney disease knowledge among chronic kidney disease patients in the Kingdom of Saudi Arabia. *Journal of Renal Care, 47*(2), 96–102. https://doi.org/10.1111/jorc.12363

Dannewitz, B., Sommerer, C., Stölzel, P., Baid-Agrawal, S., Nadal, J., Bärthlein, B., Wanner, C., Eckhardt, K. U., Zeier, M., Schlagenhauf, U., Kranc, V., & Jockel-Schneider, Y. (2019). Status of periodontal health in German patients suffering from chronic kidney disease—Data from the GCKD study. *Journal of Clinical Periodontology, 47*(1), 19–29. https://doi.org/10.1111/jcpe.13208

Ignatavicius, D. D, Workman, M. L., Rebar, C. R., & Heimgartner, N. M. (2021). *Medical-surgical nursing: Concepts for interprofessional collaborative care* (10th ed.). Elsevier.

Phillips, R., McLaughlin, L., Williams, D., Williams, H., Noyes, J., Jones, C., Oleary, C., Mallett, C., & Griffin, S. (2020). Engaging and supporting women with chronic kidney disease with pre-conception decision-making (including their experiences during COVID 19): A mixed methods study protocol. *Journal of Advanced Nursing, 77*, 2887–2897. https://doi.org/10.1111/jan.14803

Rainey, H., Hussain, S., & Thomas, N. (2020). Innovative education for people with chronic kidney disease: An evaluation study. *Journal of Renal Care, 46*(4), 197–205. https://doi.org/10.1111/jorc.12325

Siew, E. D., Parr, S. K., Wild, M. G., Levea, S. L., Mehta, K. G., Umeukeje, E. M., Silver, S. A., Ikizler, T. A., & Cavanaugh, K. L. (2019). Kidney disease awareness and knowledge among survivors of acute kidney injury. *American Journal of Nephrology, 49*, 449–459. https://doi.org/10.1159/000499862

Smith Brown, J., & Elliott, R. W. (2021). Social determinants of health: Understanding the basics and their impact on chronic kidney disease. *Nephrology Nursing Journal, 48*(2), 131–135. https://doi.org/10.37526/1526-744X

+Wembenyui, C., Douglas, C., & Bonner, A. (2021). Validation of the Australian version of the Chronic Kidney Disease Self-Management Instrument. *International Journal of Nursing Practice, 27*(2), 1–9. https://doi.org/10.1111/ijn.12857

Knowledge: Kidney Failure Management

1872

Definition: Extent of understanding conveyed about chronic kidney disease, its treatment, and the prevention of disease progression and complications

OUTCOME TARGET RATING: Maintain at_____ Increase to_____

		No Knowledge	Limited Knowledge	Moderate Knowledge	Substantial Knowledge	Extensive Knowledge	
OUTCOME OVERALL RATING		1	2	3	4	5	
Indicators:							
187201	Usual course of disease	1	2	3	4	5	NA
187202	Signs and symptoms of early-stage disease	1	2	3	4	5	NA
187203	Signs and symptoms of worsening disease	1	2	3	4	5	NA

Knowledge: Kidney Failure Management—cont'd

		No Knowledge	Limited Knowledge	Moderate Knowledge	Substantial Knowledge	Extensive Knowledge	
187204	Benefits of disease management	1	2	3	4	5	NA
187205	Systemic effects of kidney disease on body systems	1	2	3	4	5	NA
187206	Strategies to reduce risk factors	1	2	3	4	5	NA
187207	Kidney replacement treatment options	1	2	3	4	5	NA
187208	Potential options for kidney transplantation	1	2	3	4	5	NA
187209	Importance of routine laboratory testing	1	2	3	4	5	NA
187210	Implications of biochemical test results	1	2	3	4	5	NA
187211	Importance of adhering to treatment schedule	1	2	3	4	5	NA
187212	Strategies to decrease treatment side effects	1	2	3	4	5	NA
187213	Routine care of dialysis vascular access site	1	2	3	4	5	NA
187214	Protection strategies for vascular access site	1	2	3	4	5	NA
187215	Emergency care for access site problems	1	2	3	4	5	NA
187216	Methods to measure daily fluid intake	1	2	3	4	5	NA
187217	Methods to measure daily urinary output	1	2	3	4	5	NA
187218	Methods to measure blood pressure	1	2	3	4	5	NA
187219	Methods to monitor heart rate	1	2	3	4	5	NA
187220	Methods to monitor respiratory rate	1	2	3	4	5	NA
187221	Importance of dietary restrictions for protein, potassium, sodium, and phosphorus	1	2	3	4	5	NA
187222	Strategies to follow prescribed diet	1	2	3	4	5	NA
187223	Strategies to increase diet compliance	1	2	3	4	5	NA
187224	Recommended fluid intake per day	1	2	3	4	5	NA
187225	Strategies to limit fluid intake	1	2	3	4	5	NA
187226	Strategies to spread fluid intake over 24-hour day	1	2	3	4	5	NA
187227	Importance of monitoring weight daily	1	2	3	4	5	NA
187228	Importance of establishing dry weight	1	2	3	4	5	NA
187229	Importance of monitoring for fluid overload	1	2	3	4	5	NA
187230	Importance of alcohol restrictions	1	2	3	4	5	NA
187231	Importance of tobacco abstinence	1	2	3	4	5	NA
187232	Strategies to manage fatigue	1	2	3	4	5	NA
187233	Energy conservation techniques	1	2	3	4	5	NA
187234	Recommended work activity	1	2	3	4	5	NA
187235	Recommended physical activity	1	2	3	4	5	NA
187236	Recommended leisure activity	1	2	3	4	5	NA
187237	Benefits of regular exercise	1	2	3	4	5	NA
187238	Adaptations for sexual performance	1	2	3	4	5	NA
187239	Effects on sexuality	1	2	3	4	5	NA
187240	Importance of medication reconciliation with health provider	1	2	3	4	5	NA
187241	Medication therapeutic effects	1	2	3	4	5	NA
187242	Medication side effects	1	2	3	4	5	NA
187243	Medication adverse effects	1	2	3	4	5	NA
187244	Use of anticoagulants during hemodialysis	1	2	3	4	5	NA
187245	Signs and symptoms of anxiety	1	2	3	4	5	NA
187246	Signs and symptoms of depression	1	2	3	4	5	NA
187247	Strategies to manage stress	1	2	3	4	5	NA

K

Continued

Knowledge: Kidney Failure Management—cont'd

		No Knowledge	Limited Knowledge	Moderate Knowledge	Substantial Knowledge	Extensive Knowledge	
187248	Strategies to modify lifestyle	1	2	3	4	5	NA
187249	Recommended immunizations	1	2	3	4	5	NA
187250	Strategies to prevent infections	1	2	3	4	5	NA
187251	What to do when unusual or new symptoms occur	1	2	3	4	5	NA
187252	When to obtain assistance from a health professional	1	2	3	4	5	NA
187253	Importance of keeping scheduled appointments	1	2	3	4	5	NA
187254	Care options for assistance with medical emergencies	1	2	3	4	5	NA
187255	Cultural influences on compliance to treatment regimen	1	2	3	4	5	NA
187256	Importance of evaluating and reframing life goals	1	2	3	4	5	NA
187257	Strategies for managing symptom burden	1	2	3	4	5	NA
187258	Available support groups	1	2	3	4	5	NA
187259	Reputable sources of kidney disease information	1	2	3	4	5	NA

Domain-*Health Knowledge & Behavior (IV)*   **Class**-*Knowledge Health Condition (GG)*   7th edition 2024

OUTCOME CONTENT REFERENCES:

Bertschi, L. A. (2020). Abnormal basic metabolic panel findings: Implications for nursing. *AJN, American Journal of Nursing, 120*(6), 58–66. https://doi.org/10.1097/01.naj.0000668764.99872.89

Chen, J., Fowler, K. J., & Grams, M.E. (2020). Knowledge is power: Patient education as a tool for patient activation. *American Journal of Kidney Diseases, 76*(2), 163–165. https://doi.org/10.1053/j.ajkd.2020.03.012

Chen, T. K., Knicely, D. H., & Grams, M. E. (2020). Chronic kidney disease diagnosis and management: A review. *Journal of American Medical Association, 322,* 1294–1304. https://doi.org/10.1001/jama.2019.14745

Correia, B. R., Brandão, M. A. G., Lopes, R. O. P., Silva, P. C. G., Zaccaro, K. R. L., Benevides, A. B., Duarte, S. C. M., & Silva, R. C. (2021). Arteriovenous fistula maturation clinical assessment for hemodialysis: A scoping review. *Acta Paulista de Enfermagen, 34,* eAPE00232. https://doi.org/10.37689/acta-ape/2021AR00232

El Monem, M. M. A., & Salim, H. M. (2020). Nursing guidelines to improve sexual function and quality of life among women undergoing hemodialysis. *Central European Journal of Nursing & Midwifery, 11*(4), 171–179. https://doi.org/10.15452/CEJNM.2020.11.0029

Frament, J., Hall, R. K., & Manley, H. J. (2020). Medication reconciliation: The foundation of medication safety for patients requiring dialysis. *American Journal of Kidney Diseases, 76*(6), 868–876. https://doi.org/10.1053/j.ajkd.2020.07.021

González, A. M., Gutman, T., Lopez-Vargas, P., Anumudu, S., Arce, C. M., Craig, J. C., Eckardt, K. U., Harris, T., Levey, A. S., Lightstone, L., Scholes-Robertson, N., Shen, J. I., Teixeira-Pinto, A., Wheeler, D. C., White, D., Wilkie, M., Jadoul, M., Winkelmayer, W. C., & Tong, A. (2020). Patient and caregiver priorities for outcomes in CKD: A multinational nominal group technique study. *American Journal of Kidney Diseases, 76*(5), 679–689. https://doi.org/10.1053/j.ajkd.2016.02.037

Guerra-Guerrero, V., Camargo Plazas, P., Cameron, B. L., Santos Salas, A. V., & Cofre González, C. G. (2020). Understanding the life experience of people on hemodialysis: Adherence to treatment and quality of life. *CANNT Journal, 30*(4), 24–32.

Huether, S. E., McCance, K. L., & Brashers, V. L. (2020). *Understanding pathophysiology* (7th ed.). Elsevier.

Ignatavicius, D. D., Workman, M. L., Rebar, C. R., & Heimgartner, N. M. (2021). *Medical-surgical nursing: Concepts for interprofessional care* (10th ed.). Elsevier.

Ikizler, T. A., Burrowes, J. D., Byham-Gray, L. D., Campbell, K. L., Carrero, J., Chan, W., Denis Fouque, D., Friedman, A. N., Ghaddar, S. D., Goldstein-Fuchs, J., Kaysen, G. A., Kopple, J. D., Teta, D., Yee-Moon Wang, A., & Cuppari, L. (2020). KDOQI clinical practice guideline for nutrition in CKD: 2020 update. *American Journal of Kidney Diseases, 76*(3, Suppl. 1), S1–S107. https://doi.org/10.1053/j.ajkd.2020.05.006

Murali, K. M., Mullan, J., Roodenrys, S., Hassan, H. C., Lambert, K., & Lonergan, M. (2019). Strategies to improve dietary, fluid, dialysis or medication adherence in patients with end stage kidney disease on dialysis: A systematic review and meta-analysis of randomized intervention trials. *PLOS One, 14*(1), e0211479. https://doi.org/10.1371/journal.pone.0211479

Ng, M. S. N., Wong, C. L., Ho, E. H. S., Hui, Y. H., Miaskowski, C., & So, W. K. W. (2020). Burden of living with multiple concurrent symptoms in patients with end-stage renal disease. *Journal of Clinical Nursing, 29*(13/14), 2589–2601. https://doi.org/10.1111/jocn.15282

Perl, J., Fuller, D. S., Bieber, B. A., Boudville, N., Kanjanabuch, T., Ito, Y., Nessim, S. J., Piraino, B. M., Pisoni, R. L., Robinson, B. M., Schaubel, D. E., Schreiber, M. J., Teitelbaum, I., Woodrow, G., Zhao, J., & Johnson, D. W. (2020). Peritoneal dialysis-related infection rates and outcomes: Results from the peritoneal dialysis outcomes and practice patterns study (PDOPPS). *American Journal of Kidney Diseases, 76*(1), 42–53. https://doi.org/10.1053/j.ajkd.2019.09.016

Sousa, H., Ribeiro, O., Paúl, C., Costa, E., Miranda, V., Ribeiro, F., & Figueiredo, D. (2019). Social support and treatment adherence in patients with end-stage renal disease: A systematic review. *Seminars in Dialysis, 32*(6), 562–574. https://doi.org/10.1111/sdi.12831

K

Knowledge: Labor & Delivery   1817

Definition: Extent of understanding conveyed about labor and delivery

OUTCOME TARGET RATING: Maintain at_____ Increase to_____

		No Knowledge	Limited Knowledge	Moderate Knowledge	Substantial Knowledge	Extensive Knowledge	
OUTCOME OVERALL RATING		1	2	3	4	5	
Indicators:							
181701	Delivery options	1	2	3	4	5	NA
181702	Role of the labor coach	1	2	3	4	5	NA
181703	Signs and symptoms of labor	1	2	3	4	5	NA
181704	Stages of labor and delivery	1	2	3	4	5	NA
181705	Strategies to control pain	1	2	3	4	5	NA
181706	Effective breathing techniques	1	2	3	4	5	NA
181707	Effective relaxation techniques	1	2	3	4	5	NA
181708	Effective positioning techniques	1	2	3	4	5	NA
181709	Potential medical procedures	1	2	3	4	5	NA
181710	Potential delivery complications	1	2	3	4	5	NA
181711	Effective pushing techniques	1	2	3	4	5	NA
181714	Delivery of infant	1	2	3	4	5	NA
181712	Delivery of placenta	1	2	3	4	5	NA

Domain-*Health Knowledge & Behavior (IV)*   **Class**-*Knowledge Health Promotion (S)*   *2nd edition 2000; revised 2004, 2008, 2024*

K

OUTCOME CONTENT REFERENCES:

Amiri, P., Mirghafourvand, M., Esmaeilpour, K., Kamalifard, M., & Ivanbagha, R. (2019), The effect of distraction techniques on pain and stress during labor: A randomized controlled clinical trial. *BMC Pregnancy Childbirth, 19*(1), 534. http//doi.org/10.1186/s12884-019-2683-y

Desseauve, D., Fradet, L., Lacouture, P., & Pierre, F. (2017). Position for labor and birth: State of knowledge and biomechanical perspectives. *European Journal of Obstetrics & Gynecology and Reproductive Biology, 208*, 46–54. http//doi.org/10.1016/j.ejogrb.2016.11.006

Henrique, A. J., Gabrielloni, M. C., Rodney, P., & Barbieri, M. (2018). Non-pharmacological interventions during childbirth for pain relief, anxiety, and neuroendocrine stress parameters: A randomized controlled trial. *International Journal of Nursing Practice, 24*(3), 12642. http//doi.org/10.1111/ijn.12642

Jones, L., Othman, M., Dowswell, T., Alfirevic, Z., Gates, S., Newburn, M., Jordan, S., Lavender, T., & Neilson, J. P. (2012). Pain management for women in labour: An overview of systematic reviews. *Cochrane Database of Systematic Reviews.* http//doi.org/10.1002/14651858.CD009234.pub2

Karaduman, S., & Akköz Çevik, S. (2020). The effect of sacral massage on labor pain and anxiety: A randomized controlled trial. *Japan Journal of Nursing Science, 17*(1), 12272. http//doi.org/10.1111/jjns.12272

Mattson, S. (Ed.). (2015). *Core curriculum for maternal-newborn nursing* (5th ed.). W.B. Saunders.

Smith, C. A., Levett, K. M., Collins, C. T., Armour, M., Dahlen, H. G., & Suganuma, M. (2018). Relaxation techniques for pain management in labour. *Cochrane Database of Systematic Reviews.* http//doi.org/10.1002/14651858.CD009514.pub2

Teixeira, L. A., Nakano, A. R., & Nucci, M. F. (2018). Labor and birth: Knowledge, reflection, and different perspectives. *História, Ciências, Saúde-Manguinhos, 25*(4), 913–915. http//doi.org/10.1590/S0104-59702018000500002

Knowledge: Lipid Disorder Management   1858

Definition: Extent of understanding conveyed about hyperlipidemia, its treatment, and the prevention of complications

OUTCOME TARGET RATING: Maintain at_____ Increase to_____

		No Knowledge	Limited Knowledge	Moderate Knowledge	Substantial Knowledge	Extensive Knowledge	
OUTCOME OVERALL RATING		1	2	3	4	5	
Indicators:							
185801	Cause and contributing factors	1	2	3	4	5	NA
185822	Relationship of lipidemia to heart disease	1	2	3	4	5	NA
185823	Relationship of lipidemia to endocrine diseases	1	2	3	4	5	NA
185824	Increased risk for women at menopause	1	2	3	4	5	NA
185802	Signs and symptoms of complications	1	2	3	4	5	NA

Continued

Knowledge: Lipid Disorder Management—cont'd

		No Knowledge	Limited Knowledge	Moderate Knowledge	Substantial Knowledge	Extensive Knowledge	
185803	Required laboratory tests for monitoring lipid levels	1	2	3	4	5	NA
185804	Target lipid levels	1	2	3	4	5	NA
185825	Available treatment options	1	2	3	4	5	NA
185805	Benefits of lifestyle modifications	1	2	3	4	5	NA
185806	Benefits of weight loss	1	2	3	4	5	NA
185807	Benefits of aerobic exercise	1	2	3	4	5	NA
185808	Prescribed diet	1	2	3	4	5	NA
185126	Importance of vitamin D intake	1	2	3	4	5	NA
185809	Strategies to change dietary habits	1	2	3	4	5	NA
185810	Correct use of prescribed medication	1	2	3	4	5	NA
185811	Potential medication interactions with food	1	2	3	4	5	NA
185812	Medication therapeutic effects	1	2	3	4	5	NA
185813	Medication side effects	1	2	3	4	5	NA
185814	Medication adverse effects	1	2	3	4	5	NA
185815	Importance of adherence to treatment	1	2	3	4	5	NA
185816	Recommendations for alcohol use	1	2	3	4	5	NA
185817	Importance of tobacco abstinence	1	2	3	4	5	NA
185818	Reputable sources of hyperlipidemia information	1	2	3	4	5	NA
185819	Available support groups	1	2	3	4	5	NA
185820	When to obtain assistance from a health professional	1	2	3	4	5	NA
185821	Benefits of hyperlipidemia management	1	2	3	4	5	NA

Domain-Health Knowledge & Behavior (IV)   **Class**-Knowledge Health Condition (GG)   5th edition 2013; revised 2024

OUTCOME CONTENT REFERENCES:

Berman, A. N., & Blankstein, R. (2019). Optimizing dyslipidemia management for the prevention of cardiovascular disease: A focus on risk assessment and therapeutic options. *Current Cardiology Reports, 21*(9), 110. https://doi.org/10.1007/s11886-019-1175-z

Dombalis, S., & Nash, A. (2021). The effect of statins in children and adolescents with familial hypercholesterolemia: A systematic review. *Journal of Pediatric Healthcare, 35*(3), 292–303. https://doi.org/10.1016/j.pedhc.2020.11.007

Ko, S. H., & Kim, H. S. (2020). Menopause-associated lipid metabolic disorders and foods beneficial for postmenopausal women. *Nutrients, 12*(1), 202. https://doi.org/10.3390/nu12010202

Liang, T., Wu, L., Xi, Y., Li, Y., Xie, X., Fan, C., Yang, L., Yang, S., Chen, X., Zhang, J., & Wu, Q. (2021). Probiotics supplementation improves hyperglycemia, hypercholesterolemia, and hypertension in type 2 diabetes mellitus: An update of meta-analysis. *Critical Reviews in Food Science & Nutrition, 61*(10), 1670–1688. https://doi.org/10.1080/10408398.2020.176448

Lowenstein, C. J., & Cameron, S. J. (2010). High-density lipoprotein metabolism and endothelial function. *Current Opinion in Endocrinology, Diabetes & Obesity, 17*(2), 166–170. https://doi.org/10.1097/MED.0b013e32833727ee

Newman, C. B., Blaha, M. J., Boord, J. B., Cariou, B., Chait, A., Fein, H. G., Ginsberg, H. N., Goldberg, I. J., Murad, M. H., Subramanian, S., & Tannock, L. R. (2020). Lipid management in patients with endocrine disorders: An Endocrine Society Clinical Practice Guideline. *The Journal of Clinical Endocrinology and Metabolism, 105*(12), dgaa674. https://doi.org/10.1210/clinem/dgaa674

Oh, H., & Moorhead, S. (2020). Validation of the knowledge and self-management Nursing Outcomes Classification outcomes for adults with hypertension and lipid disorder. *Online Journal of Nursing Informatics, 24*(2), 1. https://doi.org/10.1097/CIN.0000000000000495

Silverman, M. G., Ference, B. A., Im, K., Wiviott, S. D., Giugliano, R. P., Grundy, S. M., Baunwald, E., & Sabatine, M. S. (2016). Association between lowering LDL-C and cardiovascular risk reduction among different therapeutic interventions: A systematic review and meta-analysis. *Journal of the American Medical Association, 316*(12), 1289–1297. https://doi.org/10.1001/jama.2016.13985

Vázquez-Manjarrez, N., Guevara-Cruz, M., Flores-López, A., Pichardo-Ontiveros, E., Tovar, A. R., & Torres, N. (2021). Effect of a dietary intervention with functional foods on LDL-C concentrations and lipoprotein subclasses in overweight subjects with hypercholesterolemia: Results of a controlled trial. *Clinical Nutrition, 40*(5), 2527–2534. https://doi.org/10.1016/j.clnu.2021.02.048

K

Knowledge: Liver Disease Management   1873

Definition: Extent of understanding conveyed about liver disease, its treatment, and the prevention of disease progression and complications

OUTCOME TARGET RATING: Maintain at_____ Increase to_____

		No Knowledge	Limited Knowledge	Moderate Knowledge	Substantial Knowledge	Extensive Knowledge	
OUTCOME OVERALL RATING		**1**	**2**	**3**	**4**	**5**	
Indicators:							
187301	Usual course of disease	1	2	3	4	5	NA
187302	Signs and symptoms	1	2	3	4	5	NA
187303	Cause and contributing factors	1	2	3	4	5	NA
187304	Benefits of disease management	1	2	3	4	5	NA
187305	Available treatment options	1	2	3	4	5	NA
187306	Risk factors for disease progression	1	2	3	4	5	NA
187307	Strategies for managing symptoms	1	2	3	4	5	NA
187308	Signs and symptoms of complications	1	2	3	4	5	NA
187309	Strategies to prevent complications	1	2	3	4	5	NA
187310	Strategies to prevent relapses	1	2	3	4	5	NA
187311	Cultural influences on adherence with treatment regimen	1	2	3	4	5	NA
187312	Treatment impact on comorbid conditions	1	2	3	4	5	NA
187313	Personal responsibilities for treatment regimen	1	2	3	4	5	NA
187314	Strategies to manage pain	1	2	3	4	5	NA
187315	Strategies to manage diet	1	2	3	4	5	NA
187316	Strategies to manage fatigue	1	2	3	4	5	NA
187317	Strategies to manage depression	1	2	3	4	5	NA
187318	Strategies to eliminate smoking	1	2	3	4	5	NA
187319	Required laboratory tests and scans	1	2	3	4	5	NA
187320	Importance of hepatitis screening	1	2	3	4	5	NA
187321	Importance of health screening	1	2	3	4	5	NA
187322	Strategies to adapt treatment to lifestyle	1	2	3	4	5	NA
187323	Therapeutic treatment effects	1	2	3	4	5	NA
187324	Treatment side effects	1	2	3	4	5	NA
187325	Medication therapeutic effects	1	2	3	4	5	NA
187326	Medication side effects	1	2	3	4	5	NA
187327	Medication adverse effects	1	2	3	4	5	NA
187328	Impact of alcohol	1	2	3	4	5	NA
187329	Impact of illegal substances	1	2	3	4	5	NA
187330	Information about hepatoxic medications	1	2	3	4	5	NA
187331	Recommended vaccinations	1	2	3	4	5	NA
187332	Reputable sources of information	1	2	3	4	5	NA
187333	Reputable e-health sources of information	1	2	3	4	5	NA
187334	Plans for medical emergencies	1	2	3	4	5	NA
187335	Importance of follow-up care	1	2	3	4	5	NA
187336	When to obtain assistance from a health professional	1	2	3	4	5	NA
187337	When to obtain emergency treatment	1	2	3	4	5	NA
187338	Options for liver transplant	1	2	3	4	5	NA
187339	Available support groups	1	2	3	4	5	NA
187340	Available community resources	1	2	3	4	5	NA

K

Domain-Health Knowledge & Behavior (IV)   *Class- Knowledge Health Condition (GG)*   *7th edition 2024*

OUTCOME CONTENT REFERENCES:

Beg, S., Curtis, S., & Shariff, M. (2016). Patient education and its effect on self-management in cirrhosis: A pilot study. *European Journal of Gastroenterology & Hepatology, 28*(5), 582–587. https://doi.org/10.1097/MEG.0000000000000579

Boundreault, S., Chen, J., Wu, K. Y., Plüddemann, A., & Heneghan, C. (2020). Self-management programmes for cirrhosis: A systematic review. *Journal of Clinical Nursing, 29*, 3625–3637. https://doi.org/10.1111/jocn.15416

Brewer, C. (2019). Hepatitis A and B: Updates for general practice nurses. *Practice Nursing, 30*(4), 120–125. https://doi.org/10.129681/pnur.2019.30.4.172

Hansen, L., Leo, M. C., Chang, M. F., Zucker, B. L., & Sasaki, A. (2014). Pain and self-care behaviours in adult patients with end-stage liver disease. *Journal of Palliative Care, 30*(1), 32–40.

Hayward, K. L., Horsfall, L. U., Ruffin, B. J., Cottrell, W. N., Chachay, V. S., Irvine, K. M., Martin, J. H., Powell, E. E., & Valery, P. C. (2017). Optimising care of patients with chronic disease: Patient-oriented education may improve disease knowledge and self-management. *Internal Medicine Journal, 47*, 952–955. https://doi.org/10.1111/imj.13505

Lau-Walker, M., Presky, J., Webzell, I., Murrells, T., & Heaton, N. (2015). Patients with alcohol-related liver disease—Beliefs about their illness and factors that influence their self-management. *Journal of Advanced Nursing, 72*(1), 173–185. https://doi.org/10.1111/jan.12826

Lin, W.-S., Lee, T.-T., Yang, Y.-H., & Mills, M. E. (2019). Environmental factors affecting self-management of chronic hepatis B from the patients' perspective. *Journal of Clinical Nursing, 28*, 4128–4138. https://doi.org/10.1111/jocn.14973

Robinson, L., Newton, J. L., Jones, D., & Dawson, P. (2014). Promoting self-management and adherence with strength and balance training for older people with long-term conditions: A mixed methods study. *Journal of Evaluation in Clinical Practice, 20*, 318–326. https://doi.org/10.1111/jep.12128

Knowledge: Lymphedema Management   3207

Definition: Extent of understanding conveyed about lymphedema, its treatment, and the prevention of disease progression and complications

OUTCOME TARGET RATING: Maintain at_____ Increase to_____

		No Knowledge	Limited Knowledge	Moderate Knowledge	Substantial Knowledge	Extensive Knowledge	
OUTCOME OVERALL RATING		**1**	**2**	**3**	**4**	**5**	
Indicators:							
320701	Signs and symptoms	1	2	3	4	5	NA
320702	Cause and contributing factors	1	2	3	4	5	NA
320703	Signs and symptoms of complications	1	2	3	4	5	NA
320704	Components of combined decongestive therapy	1	2	3	4	5	NA
320705	Purpose of combined decongestive therapy	1	2	3	4	5	NA
320706	Types of pressure wraps	1	2	3	4	5	NA
320707	Methods of bandaging	1	2	3	4	5	NA
320708	Manual lymphatic therapy	1	2	3	4	5	NA
320709	Correct use of intermittent pneumatic compression pump	1	2	3	4	5	NA
320733	Non-surgical treatment options	1	2	3	4	5	NA
320734	Surgical treatment options	1	2	3	4	5	NA
320711	Importance of adherence to treatment regimen	1	2	3	4	5	NA
320712	Risk-reduction strategies	1	2	3	4	5	NA
320713	Treatment burden	1	2	3	4	5	NA
320714	Medication therapeutic effects	1	2	3	4	5	NA
320715	Medication side effects	1	2	3	4	5	NA
320716	Medication adverse effects	1	2	3	4	5	NA
320717	Physical effects of progression	1	2	3	4	5	NA
320718	Psychosocial impact	1	2	3	4	5	NA
320719	Physiologic impact	1	2	3	4	5	NA
320720	Adaptations of role performance	1	2	3	4	5	NA
320721	Family's role in treatment regimen	1	2	3	4	5	NA
320722	Perception of body image	1	2	3	4	5	NA
320723	Perceived diminished sexuality	1	2	3	4	5	NA
320724	Effects on lifestyle	1	2	3	4	5	NA
320725	Effects on employment	1	2	3	4	5	NA
320726	Effects on perceptions of self-efficacy	1	2	3	4	5	NA
320727	Effects on self-regulation	1	2	3	4	5	NA

Knowledge: Lymphedema Management—cont'd

	No Knowledge	Limited Knowledge	Moderate Knowledge	Substantial Knowledge	Extensive Knowledge	
320728	Financial resources for assistance	1	2	3	4	5	NA
320729	Cultural influences on adherence to treatment regimen	1	2	3	4	5	NA
320730	Available community support resources	1	2	3	4	5	NA
320731	Available support groups	1	2	3	4	5	NA
320732	Benefits of disease management	1	2	3	4	5	NA

Domain-Health Knowledge & Behavior (IV)   **Class**-Knowledge Health Condition (GG)   6th edition 2018; revised 2024

OUTCOME CONTENT REFERENCES:

Bittar, S., Simman, R., & Lurie, F. (2020). Lymphedema: A practical approach and clinical update. *Wounds, 32*(3), 86–92.

Fish, M. L., Grover, R., & Schwarz, G. S. (2020). Quality-of-life outcomes in surgical vs nonsurgical treatment of breast cancer-related lymphedema: A systematic review. *JAMA Surgery, 155*(6), 513–519. https://doi.org/10.1001/jamasurg.2020.0230

Iyer, D., Jannaway, M., Yang, Y., & Scallan, J. P. (2020). Lymphatic valves and lymph flow in cancer-related lymphedema. *Cancers, 12*(8), 1–18. https://doi.org/10.3390/cancers12082297

Kristiansen, M., Halle, M., Pignatti, M., & Skogh, A.-C. D. (2020). Evaluation and selection of lower limb lymphedema patients for lymphaticovenular anastomosis: A prospective study. *Injury, 9*, S108–S113. https://doi.org/10.1016/j.injury.2020.02.110

Kutlay, S., Ozdemir, E. C., Pala, Z., Ozen, S., & Sanli, H. (2019). Complete decongestive therapy is an option for the treatment of rosacea lymphedema (Morbihan disease): Two cases. *Physical Therapy, 99*(4), 406–410. https://doi.org/10.1093/ptj/pzy155

Ostby, P. L., & Armer, J. M. (2015). Complexities of adherence and post-cancer lymphedema management. *Journal of Personalized Medicine, 5*(4), 370–388. https://doi.org/10.3390/jpm5040370

Wanchai, A., & Armer, J. M. (2021). Manual lymphedema drainage for reducing risk for and managing breast cancer-related lymphedema after breast surgery: A systematic review. *Nursing for Women's Health, 25*(5), 377–383. https://doi.org/10.1016/j.nwh.2021.07.005

K

Knowledge: Medication   **1808**

Definition: Extent of understanding conveyed about the safe use of medication

OUTCOME TARGET RATING: Maintain at_____ Increase to_____

		No Knowledge	Limited Knowledge	Moderate Knowledge	Substantial Knowledge	Extensive Knowledge	
OUTCOME OVERALL RATING		1	2	3	4	5	
Indicators:							
180801	Importance of informing health professional of all current medication	1	2	3	4	5	NA
180802	Correct name of medication	1	2	3	4	5	NA
180803	Appearance of medication	1	2	3	4	5	NA
180819	Medication therapeutic effects	1	2	3	4	5	NA
180805	Medication side effects	1	2	3	4	5	NA
180820	Medication adverse effects	1	2	3	4	5	NA
180807	Use of memory aids	1	2	3	4	5	NA
180808	Potential medication interactions	1	2	3	4	5	NA
180809	Potential medication interactions with other agents	1	2	3	4	5	NA
180810	Correct use of prescribed medication	1	2	3	4	5	NA
180821	Correct use of non-prescription medication	1	2	3	4	5	NA
180822	Proper technique for self-injection	1	2	3	4	5	NA
180827	Proper technique for using an inhaler	1	2	3	4	5	NA
180811	Self-monitoring techniques	1	2	3	4	5	NA
180812	Proper medication storage	1	2	3	4	5	NA
180815	Proper disposal of medication	1	2	3	4	5	NA
180813	Proper care of administration devices	1	2	3	4	5	NA
180823	Proper disposal of syringes and needles	1	2	3	4	5	NA

Continued

Knowledge: Medication—cont'd

		No Knowledge	Limited Knowledge	Moderate Knowledge	Substantial Knowledge	Extensive Knowledge	
180824	Strategies to obtain required medication	1	2	3	4	5	NA
180825	Strategies to obtain required supplies	1	2	3	4	5	NA
180828	Importance of medication reconciliation with health professional	1	2	3	4	5	NA
180826	Available financial support	1	2	3	4	5	NA
180816	Required laboratory tests for monitoring medication	1	2	3	4	5	NA
180817	Importance of using medical alert identification	1	2	3	4	5	NA

Specify medication(s)_____

Domain-Health Knowledge & Behavior (IV)   **Class**-Knowledge Health Promotion (S)   *1st edition 1997; revised 2004, 2008, 2013, 2024*

OUTCOME CONTENT REFERENCES:

Abolhassani, N., Castioni, J., Santschi, V., Waeber, G., & Marques-Vidal, P. (2021). Trends and determinants of polypharmacy and potential drug-drug interactions at discharge from hospital between 2009–2015. *Journal of Patient Safety, 21*(6), e1171–e1178. https://doi.org/10.1097/PTS.0000000000000482

Gidey, M. T., Birhanu, A. H., Tsadik, A. G., Welie, A. G., & Assefa, B. T. (2020). Knowledge, attitude, and practice of unused and expired medication disposal among patients visiting Ayder Comprehensive Specialized Hospital. *BioMed Research International, 8*(3), 1–7. https://doi.org/10.1155/2020/9538127

Guirguis, L. M., Singh, R. L., Fox, L. L., Neufeld, S. M., & Bond, I. (2020). Medication education provided to school-aged children: A systematic scoping review. *Journal of School Health, 90*(11), 887–897. https://doi.org/10.1111/josh.12953

Hemenway, A. N., Kandil, M. M., & MacDowell, M. (2021). The association of medication knowledge and adherence scores with hospital readmission. *Hospital Pharmacy, 56*(4), 205–209. https://doi.org/10.1177/0018578719883808

Jester, D. J., Molinari, V., Zgibor, J. C., & Volicer, L. (2021). Prevalence of psychotropic polypharmacy in nursing home residents with dementia: A meta-analysis. *International Psychogeriatrics, 33*(10), 1083–1098. https://doi.org/10.1017/S1041610220004032

Lester, P. E., Sahansra, S., Shen, M., Becker, M., & Islam, S. (2019). Medication reconciliation: An educational module. *MedEdPORTAL: The Journal of Teaching and Learning Resources, 15*, 10852. https://doi.org/10.15766/mep_2374-8265.10852

Ozavci, G., Bucknall, T., Woodward-Kron, R., Hughes, C., Jorm, C., Joseph, K., & Manias, E. (2021). Knowledge and power relations in older patients' communication about medications across transitions of care. *Qualitative Health Research, 31*(14), 2678–2691. https://doi.org/10.1177/10497323211043494

Puspitasari, A. D., Prabawati, B. M., & Rosyid, A. N. (2021). Community knowledge and attitude in recognizing asthma symptoms and using medication for asthma attacks: A cross-sectional study. *Journal of Basic & Clinical Physiology & Pharmacology, 32*(4), 467–472. https://doi.org/10.1515/jbcpp-2020-0466

Zhang, X., Jiao, J., Guo, N., Bo, H., Xu, T., & Wu, X. (2021). Association of polypharmacy with falls among older Chinese inpatients: A nationwide cohort study. *Geriatrics & Gerontology International, 21*(9), 810–817. https://doi.org/10.1111/ggi.14245

K

Knowledge: Multiple Sclerosis Management   1838

Definition: Extent of understanding conveyed about multiple sclerosis, its treatment, and the prevention of relapses or complications

OUTCOME TARGET RATING: Maintain at_____ Increase to_____

		No Knowledge	Limited Knowledge	Moderate Knowledge	Substantial Knowledge	Extensive Knowledge	
OUTCOME OVERALL RATING		**1**	**2**	**3**	**4**	**5**	
Indicators:							
183801	Signs and symptoms of multiple sclerosis	1	2	3	4	5	NA
183836	Course of disease for progressive multiple sclerosis	1	2	3	4	5	NA
183837	Course of disease for relapsing-remitting multiple sclerosis	1	2	3	4	5	NA
183803	Therapeutic effects of personal treatment regimen	1	2	3	4	5	NA
183838	Strategies to individualize plan of care	1	2	3	4	5	NA
183839	Relationship of comorbid conditions to disease	1	2	3	4	5	NA
183840	Benefits of optimism	1	2	3	4	5	NA
183841	Strategies to manage anxiety	1	2	3	4	5	NA
183842	Strategies to manage depression	1	2	3	4	5	NA
183832	Adaptations to performing roles	1	2	3	4	5	NA
183843	Relationship of sleep quality to disease	1	2	3	4	5	NA

Knowledge: Multiple Sclerosis Management—cont'd

		No Knowledge	Limited Knowledge	Moderate Knowledge	Substantial Knowledge	Extensive Knowledge	
183804	Benefits of adequate rest	1	2	3	4	5	NA
183805	Relationship of fatigue to disease	1	2	3	4	5	NA
183806	Strategies to control fatigue	1	2	3	4	5	NA
183807	Factors that decrease energy expenditure	1	2	3	4	5	NA
183808	Energy conservation techniques	1	2	3	4	5	NA
183826	Strategies to balance activity and rest	1	2	3	4	5	NA
183809	Strategies to manage stress	1	2	3	4	5	NA
183810	Factors that trigger relapse	1	2	3	4	5	NA
183812	Strategies to control symptoms	1	2	3	4	5	NA
183813	Benefits of disease management	1	2	3	4	5	NA
183814	When to obtain assistance from a health professional	1	2	3	4	5	NA
183815	Medication therapeutic effects	1	2	3	4	5	NA
183816	Medication side effects	1	2	3	4	5	NA
183817	Medication adverse effects	1	2	3	4	5	NA
183818	Strategies to decrease treatment regimen side effects	1	2	3	4	5	NA
183819	Proper technique for self-injection	1	2	3	4	5	NA
183820	Potential prescribed medication interactions with other medication	1	2	3	4	5	NA
183821	Alternative complementary treatments	1	2	3	4	5	NA
183844	Strategies to define stigma-related experiences	1	2	3	4	5	NA
183845	Strategies to deal with impact of stigmatized experiences	1	2	3	4	5	NA
183846	Strategies to promote wellness	1	2	3	4	5	NA
183847	Strategies to promote well-being	1	2	3	4	5	NA
183822	Strategies to manage cognitive limitations	1	2	3	4	5	NA
183848	Strategies to address mobility limitations	1	2	3	4	5	NA
183849	Strategies to prevent falls	1	2	3	4	5	NA
183850	Importance of oral health checkups	1	2	3	4	5	NA
183851	Strategies to achieve a well-balanced diet	1	2	3	4	5	NA
183825	Strategies to increase resistance to infection	1	2	3	4	5	NA
183827	Strategies to cope with unpredictability of disease	1	2	3	4	5	NA
183852	Strategies to adapt to functional limitations	1	2	3	4	5	NA
183834	Strategies to enhance bladder function	1	2	3	4	5	NA
183835	Strategies to enhance bowel function	1	2	3	4	5	NA
183829	Surgical treatment options	1	2	3	4	5	NA
183853	Reputable e-health resources	1	2	3	4	5	NA
183830	Available support groups	1	2	3	4	5	NA
183854	Available mental health resources	1	2	3	4	5	NA
183855	Available resources for rehabilitation	1	2	3	4	5	NA
183833	Reputable sources of multiple sclerosis information	1	2	3	4	5	NA

Domain-Health Knowledge & Behavior (IV)   **Class**-Knowledge Health Condition (GG)   4th edition 2008; revised 2013, 2024

OUTCOME CONTENT REFERENCES:

Bromley, L., Horvath, P. J., Bennett, S. E., Weinstock-Guttman, B., & Ray, A. D. (2019). Impact of nutritional intake on function in people with mild-to-moderate multiple sclerosis. *International Journal of MS Care, 21*, 1–9. https://doi.org/10.7224/1537-2073.2017-039

Camilleri, M. (2021). Gastrointestinal motility disorders in neurologic disease. *The Journal of Clinical Investigation, 131*(4), 1–13. https://doi.org/10.1172/JCI143771

Carletto, S., Cavalera, C., Sadowski, I., Rovaris, M., Borghi, M., Khoury, B., Ostacoli, L., & Pagnini, F. (2020). Mindfulness-based interventions for the improvement of well-being in people with multiple sclerosis: A systematic review. *Psychosomatic Medicine, 82*(6), 600–613. https://doi.org/10.1097/PSY.0000000000000819

Coote, S., Comber, L., Quinn, G., Santoyo-Medina, C., Kalron, A., & Gunn, H. (2020). Falls in people with multiple sclerosis. *International Journal of MS Care, 22*, 247–255. https://doi.org/10.7224/1537-2073.2020-014

Eldridge-Smith, E. D., Loew, M., & Stepleman, L. M. (2019). The adaptation and validation of a stigma measure for individuals with multiple sclerosis. *Disability and Rehabilitation, 43*(2), 262–269. https://doi.org/10.1080/096338288.2019.1617793

Matthews, P. M., Block, V. J., & Leocani, L. (2020). E-health and multiple sclerosis. *Current Opinion in Neurology, 33*(3), 271–276. https://doi.org/10.1097/WCO.0000000000000823

Maurino, J., Sotoca, J., Sempere, A. P., Brieva, L., López de Silanes, C., Caminero, A. B., Terzaghi, M., Gracia-Gil, J., & Saposnik, G. (2021). High-efficacy disease-modifying therapies in people with relapsing multiple sclerosis: The role of risk attitude in treatment decisions. *The Patient—Patient-Centered Outcomes Research, 14*, 241–248. https://doi.org/10.1007/s40271-020-00454-3

Moiola, L., Rommer, P. S., & Zettl, U. K. (2020). Prevention and management of adverse effects of disease modifying treatments in multiple sclerosis. *Current Opinion in Neurology, 33*(3), 286–294. https://doi.org/10.1097/WCO.0000000000000824

Nelson, L. M., & Bourdette, D. (2020). Two decades of research. Time to incorporate comorbidity management into the care of MS? *Neurology, 95*(5), 193–194. https://doi.org/10.1212/WNL.0000000000010036

Rahn, A. C., Solari, A., Beckerman, H., Nicholas, R., Wilkie, D., Heesen, C., & Giordano, A. (2020). "I will respect the autonomy of my patient" A scoping review of shared decision making in multiple sclerosis. *International Journal of MS Care, 22*(6), 285–293. https://doi.org/10.7224/1537-2073.2020-027

Salter, A., Kowalec, K., Fitzgerald, K. C., Cutter, G., & Marrie, R. A. Comorbidity is associated with disease activity in MS. *Neurology, 95*, e446–e456. https://doi.org/10.1212/WNL.0000000000010024

Thakolwiboon, S., Zhao-Fleming, H., Pan, J., Scott, J. K., Shoji, E., Sohn, G., & Avila, M. (2020). Disease-modifying therapies during the COVID-19 outbreak. *International Journal of MS Care, 22*(4), 151–157. https://doi.org/10.7224/1537-2073.2020-037

White, E. K., Sullivan, A. B., & Drerup, M. (2019). Impact of sleep disorders on depression and patient-perceived health-related quality of life in multiple sclerosis. *International Journal of MS Care, 21*(1), 10–14. https://doi.org/10.7224/1537-2073.2017-068

Knowledge: Musculoskeletal Rehabilitation   3208

Definition: Extent of understanding conveyed about a prescribed rehabilitation therapy to restore and enhance musculo-skeletal function and prevent complications from disease, trauma, or surgery

OUTCOME TARGET RATING: Maintain at_____ Increase to_____

OUTCOME OVERALL RATING	No Knowledge	Limited Knowledge	Moderate Knowledge	Substantial Knowledge	Extensive Knowledge	
	1	2	3	4	5	
Indicators:						
320801 Usual course of recovery	1	2	3	4	5	NA
320802 Individualized rehabilitation plan	1	2	3	4	5	NA
320803 Phases of rehabilitation plan	1	2	3	4	5	NA
320804 Goals of each rehabilitation phase	1	2	3	4	5	NA
320805 Benefits of rehabilitation therapy	1	2	3	4	5	NA
320806 Expected discomfort of affected area	1	2	3	4	5	NA
320807 Strategies to reduce pain after therapy session	1	2	3	4	5	NA
320808 Strategies to maintain motivation for rehabilitation therapy	1	2	3	4	5	NA
320809 Prescribed exercises	1	2	3	4	5	NA
320810 Strategies to include prescribed exercise in daily routine	1	2	3	4	5	NA
320811 Importance to communicate progress	1	2	3	4	5	NA
320812 Proper body alignment	1	2	3	4	5	NA
320813 Correct use of assistive device	1	2	3	4	5	NA
320814 Strategies to manage pain	1	2	3	4	5	NA
320815 Strategies to protect affected area	1	2	3	4	5	NA
320816 Activity restrictions	1	2	3	4	5	NA
320817 Range of motion restrictions	1	2	3	4	5	NA
320818 Modification of activities of daily living	1	2	3	4	5	NA
320819 Benefits of frequent ambulation	1	2	3	4	5	NA
320820 Methods to measure activity tolerance	1	2	3	4	5	NA
320821 Methods to measure active range of motion	1	2	3	4	5	NA
320822 Methods to measure flexibility	1	2	3	4	5	NA
320823 Methods to measure muscle strength	1	2	3	4	5	NA
320824 Methods to change body positions safely	1	2	3	4	5	NA
320825 Methods to monitor affected area for edema	1	2	3	4	5	NA
320826 Benefits of adequate rest	1	2	3	4	5	NA
320827 Benefits of adequate sleep	1	2	3	4	5	NA
320828 Benefits of a healthy diet	1	2	3	4	5	NA

K

Knowledge: Musculoskeletal Rehabilitation—cont'd

	No Knowledge	Limited Knowledge	Moderate Knowledge	Substantial Knowledge	Extensive Knowledge	
320829	Strategies to reduce stress	1	2	3	4	5	NA
320830	Effective coping strategies	1	2	3	4	5	NA
320831	Importance of follow-up appointments	1	2	3	4	5	NA
320832	Risk of injury	1	2	3	4	5	NA
320833	Strategies to prevent complications	1	2	3	4	5	NA
320834	Strategies to prevent falls	1	2	3	4	5	NA
320835	Strategies to prevent repeated injury	1	2	3	4	5	NA

Domain-*Health Knowledge & Behavior (IV)*   **Class**-*Knowledge Health Condition (GG)*   *6th edition 2018*

OUTCOME CONTENT REFERENCES:

Clarke, S., & Santy-Tomlinson, J. (2014). *Orthopaedic and trauma nursing: An evidence-based approach to musculoskeletal care*. Wiley Blackwell.

Enseki, K. R., & Berliner, M. (2013). Rehabilitation following total hip arthroplasty surgery. *Topics in Geriatric Rehabilitation, 29*(4), 260–267. https://doi.org/10.1682/JRRD.2014.05.0132

Taylor, N., Peiris, C., Kennedy, G., & Shields, N. (2016). Walking tolerance of patients recovering from hip fracture: A phase I trial. *Disability and Rehabilitation, 38*(19), 1900–1908. https://doi.org/10.3109/09638288.2015.1107776

Westby, M. D., & Backman, C. L. (2010). Patient and health professional views on rehabilitation practices and outcomes following total hip and knee arthroplasty for osteoarthritis: A focus group study. *BMC Health Service Research, 10*(1), 1–15. https://doi.org/10.1186/1472-6963-10-119

Knowledge: Osteoporosis Management   1859

K

Definition: Extent of understanding conveyed about osteoporosis, its treatment, and the prevention of disease progression and complications

OUTCOME TARGET RATING: Maintain at_____ Increase to_____

	No Knowledge	Limited Knowledge	Moderate Knowledge	Substantial Knowledge	Extensive Knowledge	
OUTCOME OVERALL RATING	**1**	**2**	**3**	**4**	**5**	
Indicators:						
185901	Cause and contributing factors	1	2	3	4	5	NA
185902	Signs and symptoms of osteoporosis	1	2	3	4	5	NA
185903	Relationship of bone metabolism and osteoporosis	1	2	3	4	5	NA
185904	Relationship of testosterone and estrogen levels and osteoporosis	1	2	3	4	5	NA
185905	Risk of fracture	1	2	3	4	5	NA
185906	Recommended daily calcium supplements	1	2	3	4	5	NA
185907	Recommended daily vitamin D supplements	1	2	3	4	5	NA
185908	Benefits of sunlight exposure for source of vitamin D	1	2	3	4	5	NA
185909	Prescribed diet	1	2	3	4	5	NA
185910	Strategies to change dietary habits	1	2	3	4	5	NA
185911	Benefits of weight-bearing exercise	1	2	3	4	5	NA
185912	Benefits of muscle strengthening exercise	1	2	3	4	5	NA
185913	Benefits of lifestyle modifications	1	2	3	4	5	NA
185928	Importance of seeking available treatment options	1	2	3	4	5	NA
185914	Medication that reduces bone density	1	2	3	4	5	NA
185915	Prescribed medication	1	2	3	4	5	NA
185916	Strategies to take prescribed medication as scheduled	1	2	3	4	5	NA
185917	Medication therapeutic effects	1	2	3	4	5	NA
185918	Medication side effects	1	2	3	4	5	NA
185919	Medication adverse effects	1	2	3	4	5	NA
185920	Usual course of treatment	1	2	3	4	5	NA

Continued

Knowledge: Osteoporosis Management—cont'd

	No Knowledge	Limited Knowledge	Moderate Knowledge	Substantial Knowledge	Extensive Knowledge	
185921 Importance of adherence to treatment	1	2	3	4	5	NA
185922 Recommended bone mineral density testing	1	2	3	4	5	NA
185923 Importance of alcohol restrictions	1	2	3	4	5	NA
185924 Importance of tobacco abstinence	1	2	3	4	5	NA
185925 Strategies to prevent falls	1	2	3	4	5	NA
185926 Available social support	1	2	3	4	5	NA
185927 Available community resources	1	2	3	4	5	NA

Domain-Health Knowledge & Behavior (IV)   **Class**-Knowledge Health Condition (GG)   5th edition 2013; revised 2024

OUTCOME CONTENT REFERENCES:

Chandran, M., Mitchell, P. J., Amphansap, T., Bhadada, S. K., Chadha, M., Chan, D.-C., Chung, Y.-S., Ebeling, P., Gilchrist, N., Khan, A. H., Halbout, P., Hew, F. L., Lan., H.-P. T., Lau, T. C., Lee, J. K., Lekamwasam, S., Lyubomirsky, G., Mercado-Asis, L. B., Mithal, A., Nguyen, T. V., Pandey, D., Reid, I. R., Suzuki, A., Chit, T. T., Tiu, K. L., Valleenukul, T., Young, C. K., & Zhao Y. L. on behalf of the Asia Pacific Consortium on Osteoporosis (APCO). (2021). Development of the Asia Pacific Consortium on Osteoporosis (APCO) framework: Clinical standards of care for the screening, diagnosis, and management of osteoporosis in the Asia-Pacific region. *Osteoporosis International, 32*, 1249–1275. https://doi.org/10.1007/s00198-020-05742-0

Chaplin, S. (2021). SIGN on managing osteoporosis and fragility fracture prevention. *Prescriber, 32*(2), 29–32. https://doi.org/10.1002/psb.1896

Farrah, Z., & Jawad, A. S. M. (2020). Optimising the management of osteoporosis. *Clinical Medicine, 20*(5), e196-201. https://doi.org/10.7861/clinmed.2020-0131

Fritz, R., Edwards, L., & Jaocb, R. (2021). Osteoporosis in adult patients with intellectual and developmental disabilities: Special considerations for diagnosis, prevention, and management. *The Southern Medical Association, 114*(4), 246-251. https://doi.org/10.14423/SMJ.0000000000001231

McClung, M. R. (2021). Role of bone-forming agents in the management of osteoporosis. *Aging and Clinical Experimental Research, 33*, 775–791. https://doi.org/10.1007/s40520-020-01708-8

NAMS Position Statement. (2021). Management of osteoporosis in postmenopausal women: The 2021 position statement of the North American Menopause Society. *Menopause, 28*(9), 973–997. https://doi.org/10.1097/GME.0000000000001831

Potter, P., Perry, A., Stockert, P., & Hall, A. (2021). *Fundamentals of nursing* (10th ed.). Elsevier.

Rozenberg, S., Bruyère, O., Bergmann, P., Cavalier, E., Gielen, E., Goemaere, S., Kaufman, J. M., Lapauw, B., Laurent, M. R., De Schepper, J., & Body, J. J. (2020). How to manage osteoporosis before the age of 50. *Maturitas, 138*, 14–25. https://doi.org/10.1016/j.maturitas.2020.05.004

Schousboe, J. T., Shepherd, J. A., & Baim, S. (2013). Executive summary of the 2013 International Society for Clinical Densitometry position development conference on bone densitometry. *Journal of Clinical Densitometry, 16*(4), 455–466. https://doi.org/10.1016/j.jocd.2013.08.004

Knowledge: Ostomy Care

1829

Definition: Extent of understanding conveyed about maintenance of an ostomy for elimination

OUTCOME TARGET RATING: Maintain at_____ Increase to_____

	No Knowledge	Limited Knowledge	Moderate Knowledge	Substantial Knowledge	Extensive Knowledge	
OUTCOME OVERALL RATING	1	2	3	4	5	
Indicators:						
182902 Purpose of ostomy	1	2	3	4	5	NA
182901 Function of ostomy	1	2	3	4	5	NA
182918 Characteristics of stool	1	2	3	4	5	NA
182909 Supplies required to care for ostomy	1	2	3	4	5	NA
182919 Proper storage of supplies	1	2	3	4	5	NA
182915 Procedure to change ostomy bag	1	2	3	4	5	NA
182916 Procedure to empty ostomy bag	1	2	3	4	5	NA
182908 Schedule for changing ostomy bag	1	2	3	4	5	NA
182905 How to measure stoma	1	2	3	4	5	NA
182907 Complications related to stoma	1	2	3	4	5	NA
182920 Complications related to intestinal function	1	2	3	4	5	NA
182903 Skin care needs around ostomy	1	2	3	4	5	NA
182904 Irrigation techniques	1	2	3	4	5	NA

Knowledge: Ostomy Care—cont'd

		No Knowledge	Limited Knowledge	Moderate Knowledge	Substantial Knowledge	Extensive Knowledge	
182910	Flatus-producing foods	1	2	3	4	5	NA
182911	Recommended diet modifications	1	2	3	4	5	NA
182912	Fluid intake requirements	1	2	3	4	5	NA
182913	Odor control mechanisms	1	2	3	4	5	NA
182921	Modification of medications	1	2	3	4	5	NA
182914	Modification of daily activities	1	2	3	4	5	NA
182922	When to obtain assistance from health professional	1	2	3	4	5	NA
182917	Available support groups	1	2	3	4	5	NA

Domain-*Health Knowledge & Behavior (IV)*   **Class**-*Knowledge Health Promotion (S)*   *3rd edition 2004; revised 2008, 2013, 2024*

OUTCOME CONTENT REFERENCES:

Chabal, L. O., Prentice, J. L., & Ayello, E. A. (2021). Practice implications from the WCET* international ostomy guideline 2020. *World Council of Enterostomal Therapists, 41*(2), 10–21. https://doi.org/10.33235/wcet.41.2.10-21

Ignatavicius, D. D., Workman, M. L., Rebar, C. R., & Heimgartner, N. M. (2021). *Medical-surgical nursing, concepts for interprofessional collaborative care* (10th ed.). Elsevier.

Lataillade, L., & Chabal, L. (2021). Therapeutic patient education: A multifaceted approach to ostomy care. *Advanced Skin & Wound Care, 34*, 36–42. https://doi.org/10.1097/01.ASW.0000722756.35017.02

Potter, P. A., Perry, A. G., Stockert, P. A., & Hall, A. M. (2021). *Fundamentals of nursing* (10th ed.). Elsevier.

Stetzer, M. N. (2021). Essential ostomy knowledge for nurses: Promoting adaptation in children with new ostomy and their caregivers. *Pediatric Nursing, 47*(2), 71–78.

K

Knowledge: Pain Management   1843

Definition: Extent of understanding conveyed about causes, symptoms, and treatment of pain

OUTCOME TARGET RATING: Maintain at_____ Increase to_____

		No Knowledge	Limited Knowledge	Moderate Knowledge	Substantial Knowledge	Extensive Knowledge	
OUTCOME OVERALL RATING		1	2	3	4	5	
Indicators:							
184342	Pain as a warning signal	1	2	3	4	5	NA
184301	Cause and contributing factors	1	2	3	4	5	NA
184302	Signs and symptoms of pain	1	2	3	4	5	NA
184303	Strategies to control pain	1	2	3	4	5	NA
184304	Strategies to manage chronic pain	1	2	3	4	5	NA
184305	Prescribed medication regimen	1	2	3	4	5	NA
184306	Correct use of prescribed medication	1	2	3	4	5	NA
184307	Correct use of non-prescription medication	1	2	3	4	5	NA
184308	Safe use of prescribed medication	1	2	3	4	5	NA
184309	Safe use of non-prescription medication	1	2	3	4	5	NA
184310	Medication therapeutic effects	1	2	3	4	5	NA
184311	Medication side effects	1	2	3	4	5	NA
184312	Medication adverse effects	1	2	3	4	5	NA
184313	Potential medication interactions	1	2	3	4	5	NA
184314	Potential medication interactions with other agents	1	2	3	4	5	NA
184315	Safety issues related to medication	1	2	3	4	5	NA
184316	Proper medication storage	1	2	3	4	5	NA
184317	Proper disposal of medication	1	2	3	4	5	NA
184318	Importance of adherence with medication regimen	1	2	3	4	5	NA
184343	Importance of adherence with exercise regimen	1	2	3	4	5	NA

Continued

Knowledge: Pain Management—cont'd

		No Knowledge	Limited Knowledge	Moderate Knowledge	Substantial Knowledge	Extensive Knowledge	
184319	Importance of informing health professional of all current medication	1	2	3	4	5	NA
184320	Activity restrictions	1	2	3	4	5	NA
184321	Activity precautions	1	2	3	4	5	NA
184322	Effective positioning techniques	1	2	3	4	5	NA
184323	Effective relaxation techniques	1	2	3	4	5	NA
184324	Effective guided imagery	1	2	3	4	5	NA
184325	Effective distraction	1	2	3	4	5	NA
184326	Effective heat/cold application	1	2	3	4	5	NA
184327	Effective electrical stimulation	1	2	3	4	5	NA
184328	Effective meditation techniques	1	2	3	4	5	NA
184329	Benefits of transcutaneous electrical nerve stimulation	1	2	3	4	5	NA
184330	Benefits of hypnosis	1	2	3	4	5	NA
184344	Benefits of music therapy	1	2	3	4	5	NA
184331	Benefits of acupuncture	1	2	3	4	5	NA
184332	Benefits of biofeedback	1	2	3	4	5	NA
184333	Benefits of massage	1	2	3	4	5	NA
184334	Benefits of ongoing self-monitoring	1	2	3	4	5	NA
184335	Benefits of lifestyle modifications	1	2	3	4	5	NA
184336	Benefits of weight loss	1	2	3	4	5	NA
184337	Strategies for pain prevention	1	2	3	4	5	NA
184345	Cultural influences on pain	1	2	3	4	5	NA
184338	When to obtain assistance from a health professional	1	2	3	4	5	NA
184339	Available support groups	1	2	3	4	5	NA
184340	Available community resources	1	2	3	4	5	NA
184341	Reputable sources of pain control information	1	2	3	4	5	NA

Domain-Health Knowledge & Behavior (IV)   **Class**-Knowledge Health Promotion (S)   4th edition 2008; revised 2013, 2024

OUTCOME CONTENT REFERENCES:

Dagg, B., Forgerson, P., Macartney, G., & Chartrand, J. (2020). Adolescent patients' management of postoperative pain after discharge: A qualitative study. *Pain Management Nursing 21*(6), 565–571. https://doi.org/10.1016/j.pmn.2020.04.003

Ekstedt, M., & Rustøen, T. (2019). Factors that hinder and facilitate cancer patients' knowledge of pain management. *Journal of Pain and Symptom Management, 57*(4), 753–760. https://doi.org/10.1016/j.jpainsymman.2018.12.334

Kongsted, A., Ris, I., Kjaer, P., & Hartvigsen, J. (2021). Self-management at the core of back pain care: 10 key points for clinicians. *Brazilian Journal of Physical Therapy, 25*(4), 396–406. https://doi.org/10.1016/j.bjpt.2021.05.002

Ledingham, A., Cohn, E. S., Baker, K. R., & Keysor, J. J. (2020). Exercise adherence: Belief of adults with knee osteoarthritis over 2 years. *Physiotherapy theory and Practice, 36*(12), 1363–1378. https://doi.org/10.1080/09593985.2019.1566943

Pancorbo-Hidalgo, P. L., & Bellido-Vallejo, J. C. (2019). Psychometric evaluation of the nursing outcome Knowledge: Pain Management in people with chronic pain. *International Journal of Environmental Research and Public Health, 16*(23), 4604. https://doi.org/10.3390/ijerph16234604

Pate, J. W., Veage, S., Lee, S., Hancock, M. J., Hush, J. M., & Pacey, V. (2019). Which patients with chronic pain are more likely to improve pain biology knowledge following education? *Pain Practice, 19*(4), 363–369. https://doi.org/10.1111/papr.12748

Warren, C., Jaisankar, P., Saneski, E., Tenberg, A., & Scala, E. (2020). Understanding barriers and facilitators to nonpharmacological pain management on adult inpatient units. *Pain Management Nursing, 21*(6), 480–487. https://doi.org/10.1016/j.pmn.2020.06.006

Knowledge: Parenting   1826

Definition: Extent of understanding conveyed about provision of a nurturing and constructive environment for a child from 1 year through 17 years of age

OUTCOME TARGET RATING: Maintain at_____ Increase to_____

		No Knowledge	Limited Knowledge	Moderate Knowledge	Substantial Knowledge	Extensive Knowledge	
OUTCOME OVERALL RATING		1	2	3	4	5	
Indicators:							
182601	Normal growth and development for age	1	2	3	4	5	NA
182602	Normal child behavior for age	1	2	3	4	5	NA
182629	Importance of health exams	1	2	3	4	5	NA
182630	Importance of dental exams	1	2	3	4	5	NA
182638	Importance of eye exams	1	2	3	4	5	NA
182631	Immunization recommendations	1	2	3	4	5	NA
182603	Safety needs	1	2	3	4	5	NA
182632	Importance of exercise	1	2	3	4	5	NA
182633	Age-appropriate toys	1	2	3	4	5	NA
182604	Injury prevention strategies	1	2	3	4	5	NA
182605	Nutritional needs	1	2	3	4	5	NA
182606	Physical care needs	1	2	3	4	5	NA
182607	Psychological needs	1	2	3	4	5	NA
182608	Emotional needs	1	2	3	4	5	NA
182634	Self-esteem needs	1	2	3	4	5	NA
182609	Stimulation needs	1	2	3	4	5	NA
182610	Socialization needs	1	2	3	4	5	NA
182611	Spiritual needs	1	2	3	4	5	NA
182612	Moral guidance needs	1	2	3	4	5	NA
182613	Health supervision needs	1	2	3	4	5	NA
182614	Illness prevention strategies	1	2	3	4	5	NA
182615	Management of common health problems	1	2	3	4	5	NA
182616	Age-appropriate expectations	1	2	3	4	5	NA
182620	Methods of discipline appropriate for developmental age	1	2	3	4	5	NA
182621	Methods of discipline appropriate for unacceptable behavior	1	2	3	4	5	NA
182618	Basic care needs	1	2	3	4	5	NA
182635	Importance of educational needs	1	2	3	4	5	NA
182619	Effective communication strategies	1	2	3	4	5	NA
182622	Motor vehicle safety measures	1	2	3	4	5	NA
182636	Maintenance of a clean home	1	2	3	4	5	NA
182623	Strategies to manage controllable environmental risk factors	1	2	3	4	5	NA
182624	Strategies to prevent tobacco use	1	2	3	4	5	NA
182625	Strategies to prevent alcohol use	1	2	3	4	5	NA
182626	Strategies to prevent recreational drug use	1	2	3	4	5	NA
182627	Strategies to prevent exposure to toxic chemicals	1	2	3	4	5	NA
182637	Strategies to prevent abduction	1	2	3	4	5	NA
182628	Available support groups	1	2	3	4	5	NA

K

Domain-Health Knowledge & Behavior (IV)   *Class*-Knowledge Health Promotion (S)   *3rd edition 2004; revised 2008, 2013, 2024*

OUTCOME CONTENT REFERENCES:

Bornstein, M. H. (2019). *Handbook of parenting* (3rd ed.). Routledge.

Hagan, J. F., Shaw, J. S., & Duncan, P. M. (Eds.). (2017). *Bright futures: Guidelines for health supervision of infants, children, and adolescents* (4th ed.). American Academy of Pediatrics.

Hockenberry, M. J., Wilson, D., & Rodgers, C. C. (Eds.). (2019). *Wong's nursing care of infants and children* (11th ed.). Elsevier.

National Institute on Drug Abuse. (2019). *Family checkup: Positive parenting prevents drug abuse.* https://archives.drugabuse.gov/publications/family-checkup

Perry, S. E., Hockenberry, M. J., Lowdermilk, D. J., Wilson, D., Cashion, K., Rodgers, C. C., & Alden, K. R. (2018). *Maternal child nursing care* (6th ed.). Elsevier.

Sanders, M. R., & Morawska, A. (2018). *Handbook of parenting and child development across the lifespan.* Springer

Sebire, S. J., Jago, R., Wood, L., Thompson, J. L., Zahra, J., & Lawlor, D. A. (2016). Examining a conceptual model of parental nurturance, parenting practices and physical activity among 5 - 6-year-olds. *Social Science & Medicine, 148*, 18–24. https://doi.org/10.1016/j.socscimed.2015.11.022

Knowledge: Parkinson Disease Management 1874

Definition: Extent of understanding conveyed about Parkinson disease, its treatment, and the prevention of complications

OUTCOME TARGET RATING: Maintain at_____ Increase to_____

		No Knowledge	Limited Knowledge	Moderate Knowledge	Substantial Knowledge	Extensive Knowledge	
OUTCOME OVERALL RATING		1	2	3	4	5	
Indicators:							
187401	Reputable sources of information	1	2	3	4	5	NA
187402	Cause and contributing factors	1	2	3	4	5	NA
187403	Stages of disease progression	1	2	3	4	5	NA
187404	Signs and symptoms of early disease	1	2	3	4	5	NA
187405	Signs and symptoms of disease progression	1	2	3	4	5	NA
187406	Available treatment options	1	2	3	4	5	NA
187407	Postural changes that affect gait	1	2	3	4	5	NA
187408	Impact of motor function on balance	1	2	3	4	5	NA
187409	Fall prevention strategies	1	2	3	4	5	NA
187410	Home safety measures	1	2	3	4	5	NA
187411	Use of mobility aides	1	2	3	4	5	NA
187412	Benefits of regular exercise	1	2	3	4	5	NA
187413	Activity modifications to reduce fatigue	1	2	3	4	5	NA
187414	Use of yoga to increase body awareness	1	2	3	4	5	NA
187415	Importance of physical therapy	1	2	3	4	5	NA
187416	Importance of occupational therapy	1	2	3	4	5	NA
187417	Importance of speech therapy	1	2	3	4	5	NA
187418	Typical medication prescribed for motor symptoms	1	2	3	4	5	NA
187419	Importance of medication adherence	1	2	3	4	5	NA
187420	Medication therapeutic effects	1	2	3	4	5	NA
187421	Medication side effects	1	2	3	4	5	NA
187422	Medication adverse effects	1	2	3	4	5	NA
187423	Potential medication and food interactions	1	2	3	4	5	NA
187424	Impact of disease progression on self-care activities	1	2	3	4	5	NA
187425	Pressure injury prevention strategies	1	2	3	4	5	NA
187426	Importance of monitoring risk for constipation	1	2	3	4	5	NA
187427	Importance of monitoring risk for urinary retention	1	2	3	4	5	NA
187428	Importance of monitoring for orthostatic hypotension	1	2	3	4	5	NA
187429	Importance of monitoring sleep pattern	1	2	3	4	5	NA
187430	Importance of monitoring daytime sleepiness	1	2	3	4	5	NA
187431	Importance of monitoring nutrition	1	2	3	4	5	NA
187432	Importance of nutritional supplements	1	2	3	4	5	NA
187433	Importance of evaluating swallowing ability	1	2	3	4	5	NA
187434	Strategies to enhance communication	1	2	3	4	5	NA
187435	Strategies to evaluate cognition	1	2	3	4	5	NA

K

Knowledge: Parkinson Disease Management—cont'd

		No Knowledge	Limited Knowledge	Moderate Knowledge	Substantial Knowledge	Extensive Knowledge	
187436	Psychosocial effects of disease on self-concept	1	2	3	4	5	NA
187437	Psychosocial effects of disease on family	1	2	3	4	5	NA
187438	Family role in treatment plan	1	2	3	4	5	NA
187439	Family role in providing care	1	2	3	4	5	NA
187440	When to seek help from a health professional	1	2	3	4	5	NA
187441	Available support groups	1	2	3	4	5	NA

Domain- *Health Knowledge & Behavior (IV)*   **Class-** *Knowledge Health Condition (GG)*   *7th edition 2024*

OUTCOME CONTENT REFERENCES:

Armstrong, M. J., & Okun, M. S. (2020). Diagnosis and treatment of Parkinson disease: A review. *JAMA, 323*(6), 548–560. https://doi.org/10.1001/jama.2019.22360

Hawkins, B. L., Van Puymbroeck, M., Walter, A., Sharp, J., Woshkolup, K., Urrea-Mendoza, E., Revilla, F., & Schmid, A. A. (2018). Perceived activities and participation outcomes of a yoga intervention for individuals with Parkinson's disease: A mixed methods study. *International Journal of Yoga Therapy, 28*(1), 51–61. https://doi.org/10.17761/2018-00018R2

Hellqvist, C., Berterö, C., Dizdar, N., Sund-Levander, M., & Hagell, P. (2020). Self-management education for persons with Parkinson's disease and their care partners: A quasi-experimental case-control study in clinical practice. *Parkinson's Disease, 6920943.* https://doi.org/10.1155/2020/6920943

Hill, H. M., Swink, L. A., Atler, K. E., Anderson, A. K., Fling, B. W., & Schmid, A. A. (2021). Merging yoga and occupational therapy for Parkinson's disease improves fatigue management and activity and participation measures. *British Journal of Occupational Therapy, 84*(4), 230–239. https://doi.org/10.1177/0308022620909086

Huether, S. E., McCance, K. L., & Brashers, V. L. (2020). *Understanding pathophysiology* (7th ed.). Elsevier.

Ignatavicius, D. D., Workman, M. L., Rebar, C. R., & Heimgartner, N. M. (2021). *Medical-surgical nursing: Concepts for interprofessional care* (10th ed.). Elsevier.

Kimber, T. E. (2021), Approach to the patient with early Parkinson disease: Diagnosis and management. *Internal Medicine Journal, 51*, 20–26. https://doi.org/10.1111/imj.15148

Martignon, C., Pedrinolla, A., Ruzzante, F., Giuriato, G., Laginestra, F. G., Bouça-Machado, R., Ferreira, J. J., Tinazzi, M., Schena, F., & Venturelli, M. (2021). Guidelines on exercise testing and prescription for patients at different stages of Parkinson's disease. *Aging Clinical & Experimental Research, 33*(2), 221–246. https://doi.org/10.1007/s40520-020-01612-1

Mouchaileh, N., & Hughes, A. J. (2020). Pharmacological management of Parkinson's disease in older people. *Journal of Pharmacy Practice & Research, 50*, 445–454. https://doi.org/10.1002/jppr.1683

Pang, M. Y. (2021). Physiotherapy management of Parkinson's disease. *Journal of Physiotherapy, 67*(3), 163–176. https://doi.org/10.1016/j.jphys.2021.06.004

Sin, M., & Khemani, P. (2020). Neurogenic orthostatic hypotension: An underrecognized complication of Parkinson's disease. *Journal of Neuroscience Nursing, 52*(5), 230–233. https://doi.org/10.1097/JNN.0000000000000528

K

Knowledge: Peripheral Artery Disease Management   1860

Definition: Extent of understanding conveyed about peripheral artery disease, its treatment, and the prevention of disease progression and complications

OUTCOME TARGET RATING: Maintain at_____ Increase to_____ Specify extremity_____

		No Knowledge	Limited Knowledge	Moderate Knowledge	Substantial Knowledge	Extensive Knowledge	
OUTCOME OVERALL RATING		1	2	3	4	5	
Indicators:							
186001	Cause and contributing factors	1	2	3	4	5	NA
186002	Signs and symptoms of peripheral artery disease	1	2	3	4	5	NA
186003	Benefits of disease management	1	2	3	4	5	NA
186004	Relationship of claudication to peripheral artery disease	1	2	3	4	5	NA
186005	Signs and symptoms of intermittent claudication	1	2	3	4	5	NA
186006	Signs and symptoms of worsening disease	1	2	3	4	5	NA
186007	Stages of peripheral artery disease	1	2	3	4	5	NA
186008	Signs and symptoms of heart disease	1	2	3	4	5	NA
186009	Signs and symptoms of stroke	1	2	3	4	5	NA
186010	Adverse health effects of ischemia if untreated	1	2	3	4	5	NA

Continued

Knowledge: Peripheral Artery Disease Management—cont'd

		No Knowledge	Limited Knowledge	Moderate Knowledge	Substantial Knowledge	Extensive Knowledge	
186011	Role of blood cholesterol in atherosclerosis	1	2	3	4	5	NA
186012	Importance of controlling blood cholesterol level	1	2	3	4	5	NA
186013	Medications that reduce risk of heart attack and stroke	1	2	3	4	5	NA
186014	Importance of tobacco abstinence	1	2	3	4	5	NA
186015	Importance of monitoring lower extremities skin color	1	2	3	4	5	NA
186016	Importance of monitoring lower extremities temperature	1	2	3	4	5	NA
186017	Importance of monitoring lower extremities sensation	1	2	3	4	5	NA
186018	Importance of monitoring lower extremities muscle strength	1	2	3	4	5	NA
186019	Benefits of prescribed exercise	1	2	3	4	5	NA
186020	Strategies to relieve discomfort	1	2	3	4	5	NA
186021	Strategies to comply with exercise program	1	2	3	4	5	NA
186022	Strategies to increase walking tolerance	1	2	3	4	5	NA
186023	Importance of monitoring blood pressure	1	2	3	4	5	NA
186024	Benefits of a healthy diet	1	2	3	4	5	NA
186025	Importance of weight control	1	2	3	4	5	NA
186026	Importance of controlling blood glucose level	1	2	3	4	5	NA
186027	Surgical treatment options	1	2	3	4	5	NA

Domain-*Health Knowledge & Behavior (IV)* **Class**-*Knowledge Health Condition (GG)*   *5th edition 2013; reviewed 2024*

K

OUTCOME CONTENT REFERENCES:

Bauersachs, R., Debus, S., Nehler, M., Huelsebeck, M., Balradj, J., Bowrin, K., & Briere, J.-B. (2020). A targeted literature review of the disease burden in patients with symptomatic peripheral artery disease. *Angiology, 7*(4), 303–314. https://doi.org/10.1177/0003319719896477

Brunelle, C., & Mulgrew, J. (2011). Exercise for intermittent claudication. *Physical Therapy, 91*(7), 991–1001. https://doi.org/10.1002/14651858.CD000990.pub4

Hess, C. N., Cannon, C. P., Beckman, J. A., Goodney, P. P., Patel, M. R., Hiatt, W. R., Mues, K. E., Orroth, K. K., Shannon, E., & Bonaca, M. P. (2021). Effectiveness of blood lipid management in patients with peripheral artery disease. *Journal of the American College of Cardiology, 77*(24), 3016–3027. https://doi.org/10.1016/j.jacc.2021.04.060

Potter, P., Perry, A., Stockert, P., & Hall, A. (2021). *Fundamentals of nursing* (10th ed.). Elsevier.

Sagris, M., Kokkinidis, D. G., Lempesis, I. G., Giannopoulos, S., Rallidis, L., Mena-Hurtado, C., & Bakoyiannis, C. (2020). Nutrition, dietary habits, and weight management to prevent and treat patients with peripheral artery disease. *Review of Cardiovascular Medicine, 21*(4), 565–575. https://doi.org/10.31083/j.rcm.2020.04.202

Selvin, E., Wattanakit, K., Steffes, M., Coresh, J., & Sharrett, A. (2006). HbA1c and peripheral arterial disease in diabetes: The atherosclerosis risk in communities study. *Diabetes Care, 29*(4), 877–882. https://doi.org/10.2337/diacare.29.04.06.dc05-2018

Weissler, E. H., Narcisse, D. I., Rymer, J. A., Armstrong, E. J., Secernsky, E., Gray, W. A., Mustapha, J. A., Adams, G. L., Ansel, G. M., Patel, M. R., & Jones, W. S. (2021). Characteristics and outcomes of patients with diabetes mellitus undergoing peripheral vascular intervention for infralingual symptomatic peripheral artery disease. *Vascular and Endovascular Surgery, 55*(2), 124–134. https://doi.org/10.1177/1538574420968671

Whipple, M. O., Schorr, E. N., Talley, K. M. C., Wolfson, J., Lindquist, R., Bronas, U. G., & Treat-Jacobson, D. (2021). Individuals differences in response to supervised exercise therapy for peripheral artery disease. *Western Journal of Nursing Research, 43*(8), 770–784. https://doi.org/10.1177/0193945920977479

Knowledge: Personal Safety

1809

Definition: Extent of understanding conveyed about risk reduction and prevention of unintentional injuries to self

OUTCOME TARGET RATING: Maintain at_____ Increase to_____

		No Knowledge	Limited Knowledge	Moderate Knowledge	Substantial Knowledge	Extensive Knowledge	
OUTCOME OVERALL RATING		1	2	3	4	5	
Indicators:							
180917	Age-specific safety risks	1	2	3	4	5	NA
180918	Personal high-risk behaviors	1	2	3	4	5	NA
180922	Leisure activities that increase risk for injury	1	2	3	4	5	NA
180923	Health conditions that increase risk	1	2	3	4	5	NA

Knowledge: Personal Safety—cont'd

		No Knowledge	Limited Knowledge	Moderate Knowledge	Substantial Knowledge	Extensive Knowledge	
180934	Recommended vaccinations for age	1	2	3	4	5	NA
180919	Work safety risks	1	2	3	4	5	NA
180920	Community safety risks	1	2	3	4	5	NA
180901	Suffocation prevention	1	2	3	4	5	NA
180924	Aspiration precautions	1	2	3	4	5	NA
180935	Risks associated with tobacco use	1	2	3	4	5	NA
180936	Risks associated with alcohol use	1	2	3	4	5	NA
180937	Risks associated with drug use	1	2	3	4	5	NA
180925	Safe food preparation	1	2	3	4	5	NA
180926	Safe food storage	1	2	3	4	5	NA
180902	Fall prevention strategies	1	2	3	4	5	NA
180903	Risk reduction strategies	1	2	3	4	5	NA
180904	Home safety measures	1	2	3	4	5	NA
180938	Home security measures	1	2	3	4	5	NA
180939	Internet safety	1	2	3	4	5	NA
180940	Weather safety procedures	1	2	3	4	5	NA
180905	Water safety	1	2	3	4	5	NA
180906	Fire safety	1	2	3	4	5	NA
180907	Burn prevention	1	2	3	4	5	NA
180908	Electrocution prevention	1	2	3	4	5	NA
180927	Strategies to avoid known allergens	1	2	3	4	5	NA
180928	Strategies to avoid environmental contaminants	1	2	3	4	5	NA
180909	Poison prevention	1	2	3	4	5	NA
180931	Safe sexual practices	1	2	3	4	5	NA
180941	Strategies to prevent intimate partner violence	1	2	3	4	5	NA
180942	Strategies to prevent stranger violence	1	2	3	4	5	NA
180910	Bicycle safety guidelines	1	2	3	4	5	NA
180942	Motorcycle safety guidelines	1	2	3	4	5	NA
180911	Pedestrian safety measures	1	2	3	4	5	NA
180912	Benefits of protective helmet	1	2	3	4	5	NA
180913	Firearm safety measures	1	2	3	4	5	NA
180915	Motor vehicle safety measures	1	2	3	4	5	NA
180916	Emergency procedures	1	2	3	4	5	NA
180943	Safe use of cell phones when walking or driving	1	2	3	4	5	NA
180929	Safe use of prescribed medication	1	2	3	4	5	NA
180930	Correct use of assistive devices	1	2	3	4	5	NA
180932	Appropriate clothing for activity	1	2	3	4	5	NA
180933	Safety devices appropriate for activity	1	2	3	4	5	NA

Domain-Health Knowledge & Behavior (IV)   **Class**-Knowledge Health Promotion (S)   1st edition 1997; revised 2004, 2008, 2013, 2024

K

OUTCOME CONTENT REFERENCES:

Brown, T., & Moran, M. (2019). Pediatric sports-related injuries. *Clinical Pediatrics*, 58(2), 199–212. https://doi.org/10.1177/0009922818810879

Emery, C. A., & Pasanen, K. (2019). Current trends in sport injury prevention. Best practice & research. *Clinical Rheumatology*, 33(1), 3–15. https://doi.org/10.1016/j.berh.2019.02.009

Maxwell, L., Skues, J., Wise, L., Theiler, S., & Pfeifer, J. (2021). Public stranger violence—What makes you vulnerable? A comparison of perspectives from young adults and industry experts. *Journal of Interpersonal Violence*, 36(11/12), 5277–5296. https://doi.org/10.1177/0886260518804836

Piccirillo, M. L., Taylor Dryman, M., & Heimberg, R. G. (2016). Safety behaviors in adults with social anxiety: Review and future directions. *Behavior Therapy*, 47(5), 675–687. https://doi.org/10.1016/j.beth.2015.11.005

Potter, P. A., Perry, A. G., Stockert, P. A., & Hall, A. M. (2021). *Fundamentals of nursing* (10th ed.). Elsevier.

Ropaka, M., Nikolaou, D., & Yannis, G. (2020). Investigation of traffic and safety behavior of pedestrians while texting or web-surfing. *Traffic Injury Prevention*, 21(6), 389–394. https://doi.org/10.1080/15389588.2020.1770741

Wang, H., Shi, L., & Schwebel, D. C. (2019). Relations between adolescent sensation seeking and traffic injury: Multiple-mediating effects of road safety attitudes, intentions and behaviors. *Traffic Injury Prevention*, 20(8), 789–795. https://doi.org/10.1080/15389588.2019.1666982

Williams, P. (2020). *Basic geriatric nursing* (7th ed.). Elsevier.

Knowledge: Pneumonia Management   1861

Definition: Extent of understanding conveyed about pneumonia, its treatment, and the prevention of complications

OUTCOME TARGET RATING: Maintain at_____ Increase to_____

	No Knowledge	Limited Knowledge	Moderate knowledge	Substantial knowledge	Extensive knowledge	
OUTCOME OVERALL RATING	1	2	3	4	5	
Indicators:						
186101 Cause and contributing factors	1	2	3	4	5	NA
186102 Specific disease process	1	2	3	4	5	NA
186103 Risk factors for reoccurrence	1	2	3	4	5	NA
186104 Signs and symptoms of disease progression	1	2	3	4	5	NA
186105 Signs and symptoms of disease relapse	1	2	3	4	5	NA
186106 Benefits of disease management	1	2	3	4	5	NA
186107 Signs and symptoms of complications	1	2	3	4	5	NA
186108 Strategies to prevent complications	1	2	3	4	5	NA
186109 Strategies to balance activity and rest	1	2	3	4	5	NA
186134 Strategies to deal with fatigue	1	2	3	4	5	NA
186110 Energy conservation techniques	1	2	3	4	5	NA
186111 Medication therapeutic effects	1	2	3	4	5	NA
186112 Medication side effects	1	2	3	4	5	NA
186113 Medication adverse effects	1	2	3	4	5	NA
186114 Potential medication interactions with other agents	1	2	3	4	5	NA
186115 Potential prescribed medication interactions with other medication	1	2	3	4	5	NA
186116 Safety issues related to medication	1	2	3	4	5	NA
186117 Correct use of prescribed medication	1	2	3	4	5	NA
186118 Importance of completing prescribed antibiotics	1	2	3	4	5	NA
186135 Importance of steroids in treatment	1	2	3	4	5	NA
186119 Diagnostic tests	1	2	3	4	5	NA
186120 Expected effects of treatment	1	2	3	4	5	NA
186121 Prescribed procedures	1	2	3	4	5	NA
186122 Correct use of bulb syringe to clear nasal airway	1	2	3	4	5	NA
186123 Correct procedure to administer nebulizer treatments at home	1	2	3	4	5	NA
186137 Coughing techniques to clear secretions	1	2	3	4	5	NA
186124 Correct method for performing chest percussion	1	2	3	4	5	NA
186125 Correct method for performing postural drainage	1	2	3	4	5	NA
186126 Adequate fluid intake	1	2	3	4	5	NA
186127 Strategies for smoking cessation	1	2	3	4	5	NA
186128 Strategies to avoid exposure to smoke	1	2	3	4	5	NA
186136 Importance of obtaining recommended vaccines	1	2	3	4	5	NA
186131 Follow-up care	1	2	3	4	5	NA
186132 Potential effects of other disease conditions	1	2	3	4	5	NA
186133 Potential effects of age on treatment	1	2	3	4	5	NA

Domain-Health Knowledge & Behavior (IV)   *Class*-Knowledge Health Condition (GG)   *5th edition 2013; revised 2024*

OUTCOME CONTENT REFERENCES:

Carnahan, J. L., Shearn, A. J., Lieb, K. M., & Unroe, K. T. (2021). Pneumonia management in nursing homes: Findings from a CMS Demonstration Project. *JGIM: Journal of General Internal Medicine, 36*(2), 570–572. https://doi.org/10.1007/s11606-020-05885-0

Crame, E., Shields, M. D., & McCrossan, P. (2021). Paediatric pneumonia: A guide to diagnosis, investigation and treatment. *Personal Practice, 31*(6), 250–257. https://doi.org/10.1016/j.paed.2021.03.005

Ignatavicius, D. D., Workman, M. L., Rebar, C. J., & Heimgartner N. M. (2021). *Medical-surgical nursing: Concepts for interprofessional collaborative care.* (10th ed.). Elsevier.

Liu, C., Cao, Y., Lin, J., Ng, L., Needleman, I., Walsh, T., & Li, C. (2018). Oral care measures for preventing nursing home-acquired pneumonia. *The Cochrane Database of Systematic Reviews, 9*(9), CD012416. https://doi.org/10.1002/14651858.CD012416.pub2

K

Martin-Loeches, I., & Torres, A. (2021). New guidelines for severe community-acquired pneumonia. *Current Opinion Pulmonary Medicine, 27*, 210–215. https://doi.org/10.1097/MCP.0000000000000760

Waterer, G. W. (2021). Applying the lessons learned from coronavirus disease 2019 to improve pneumonia management. *Current Opinion in Infectious Diseases, 34*(2), 175–179. https://doi.org/10.1097/QCO.0000000000000710

Williams, P. (2020). *Basic geriatric nursing* (7th ed.). Elsevier.

Knowledge: Postpartum Maternal Health   1818

Definition: Extent of understanding conveyed about maternal health in the period following birth of infant

OUTCOME TARGET RATING: Maintain at_____ Increase to_____

		No Knowledge	Limited Knowledge	Moderate Knowledge	Substantial Knowledge	Extensive Knowledge	
OUTCOME OVERALL RATING		**1**	**2**	**3**	**4**	**5**	
Indicators:							
181801	Normal physical sensations following delivery	1	2	3	4	5	NA
181802	Routine monitoring	1	2	3	4	5	NA
181803	Normal vaginal discharge	1	2	3	4	5	NA
181804	Breast changes	1	2	3	4	5	NA
181805	Uterine involution patterns	1	2	3	4	5	NA
181806	Fundal massage	1	2	3	4	5	NA
181807	Perineal care	1	2	3	4	5	NA
181808	Episiotomy care	1	2	3	4	5	NA
181809	Cesarean section care	1	2	3	4	5	NA
181810	Coughing techniques following surgery	1	2	3	4	5	NA
181820	Recommended nutrient intake	1	2	3	4	5	NA
181821	Recommended fluid intake	1	2	3	4	5	NA
181822	Energy level changes	1	2	3	4	5	NA
181812	Strategies to balance activity and rest	1	2	3	4	5	NA
181813	Recommended exercise	1	2	3	4	5	NA
181814	Time frame for resumption of sexual activity	1	2	3	4	5	NA
181815	Contraceptive options	1	2	3	4	5	NA
181816	Psychological changes	1	2	3	4	5	NA
181823	Postpartum body changes	1	2	3	4	5	NA
181824	Maternal role performance	1	2	3	4	5	NA
181829	Breastfeeding management	1	2	3	4	5	NA
181825	Strategies to manage postpartum depression	1	2	3	4	5	NA
181826	Strategies to manage stress	1	2	3	4	5	NA
181827	Strategies to bond with infant	1	2	3	4	5	NA
181818	Available social support	1	2	3	4	5	NA
181828	When to obtain assistance from a health professional	1	2	3	4	5	NA

Domain-Health Knowledge & Behavior (IV)   **Class**-*Knowledge Health Promotion (S)*   *2nd edition 2000; revised 2004, 2008, 2024*

OUTCOME CONTENT REFERENCES:

Baratieri, T., & Natal, S. (2019). Postpartum program actions in primary health care: An integrative review. *Ciencia & Saude Coletiva, 24*(11), 4227–4238. http//doi.org/10.1590/1413-812320182411.28112017

De Maria, A. L., Delay, C., Sundstrom, B., Wakefield, A. L., Avina, A., & Meier, S. (2019). Understanding women's postpartum sexual experiences. *Culture, Health & Sexuality, 21*(10), 1162–1176. https://doi.org/10.1080/13691058.2018.1543802

Dunn, K., Bayer, L. L., & Mody, S. K. (2016). Postpartum contraception: An exploratory study of lactation consultants' knowledge and practices. *Contraception, 94*(1), 87–92. http//doi.org/10.1016/j.contraception.2016.03.007

Gomez, H. B., & Hoffman, M. K. (2021). Text messaging as a means to engage patients in the postpartum period. *Clinical Obstetrics and Gynecology, 64*(2), 366–374. https://doi.org/10.1097/GRF.0000000000000609

Lambrinou, C. P., Karaglani, E., & Manios, Y. (2019). Breastfeeding and postpartum weight loss. *Current Opinion in Clinical Nutrition and Metabolic Care, 22*(6), 413–417. https://doi.org/10.1097/MCO.0000000000000597

Martínez-Galiano, J. M., Hernández-Martínez, A., Rodríguez-Almagro, J., Delgado-Rodríguez, M., & Gómez-Salgado, J. (2019). Relationship between parity and the problems that appear in the postpartum period. *Scientific Reports, 9*(1), 11763. https://doi.org/10.1038/s41598-019-47881-3

K

Mattson, S. (Ed.). (2015). *Core curriculum for maternal-newborn nursing* (5th ed.). W.B. Saunders.

+Mirsalimi, F., Ghofranipour, F., Noroozi, A., & Montazeri, A. (2020). The Postpartum Depression Literacy Scale (PoDLiS): Development and psychometric properties. *BMC Pregnancy Childbirth, 20*(1), 13. https://doi.org/10.1186/s12884-019-2705-9

Mokhtari, F., Bahadoran, P., & Baghersad, Z. (2018). Effectiveness of postpartum homecare program as a new method on mothers' knowledge about the health of the mother and the infant. *Iran Journal of Nursing Midwifery Research, 23*(4), 316–321. http//doi.org/10.4103/Ijnmr.ijnmr

Murray, S. S., & McKinney, E. S. (2018). *Foundations of maternal-newborn and women's health nursing* (7th ed.). Elsevier.

Ricci, S. (2017). *Essentials of maternity, newborn, and women's health nursing* (4th ed.). Wolters Kluwer.

Suplee, P. D., Bingham, D., & Kleppel, L. (2017). Nurses' knowledge and teaching of possible postpartum complications. *MCN, The American Journal of Maternal/Child Nursing, 42*(6), 338–344. https://doi.org/10.1097/NMC.0000000000000371

Knowledge: Preconception Maternal Health   1822

Definition: Extent of understanding conveyed about maternal health prior to conception to insure a healthy pregnancy

OUTCOME TARGET RATING: Maintain at_____ Increase to_____

		No Knowledge	Limited Knowledge	Moderate Knowledge	Substantial Knowledge	Extensive Knowledge	
OUTCOME OVERALL RATING		**1**	**2**	**3**	**4**	**5**	
Indicators:							
182201	Factors to consider when deciding to become a parent	1	2	3	4	5	NA
182213	Usual course of pregnancy	1	2	3	4	5	NA
182203	Recommended diet	1	2	3	4	5	NA
182218	Recommended vitamin supplements	1	2	3	4	5	NA
182204	Strategies to balance activity and rest	1	2	3	4	5	NA
182214	Adverse health effects of alcohol use	1	2	3	4	5	NA
182215	Adverse health effects of tobacco use	1	2	3	4	5	NA
182216	Adverse health effects of drug use	1	2	3	4	5	NA
182206	Maternal risk factors	1	2	3	4	5	NA
182207	Environmental hazards at home that affect fetal development	1	2	3	4	5	NA
182211	Environmental hazards at work that affect fetal development	1	2	3	4	5	NA
182208	Risk for hereditary disease	1	2	3	4	5	NA
182217	Anatomic and physiological changes of pregnancy	1	2	3	4	5	NA
182219	Psychological changes associated with pregnancy	1	2	3	4	5	NA

Domain-Health Knowledge & Behavior (IV)   *Class*-Knowledge Health Promotion (S)   *2nd edition 2000; revised 2004, 2008, 2013, 2024*

OUTCOME CONTENT REFERENCES:

Barker, M., Dombrowski, S. U., Colbourn, T., Fall, C. H. D., Kriznik, N. M., Lawrence, W. T., Norris, S. A., Ngaiza, G., Patel, D., Skordis-Worrall, J., Sniehotta, F. F., Steegers-Theunissen, R., Vogel, C., Woods-Townsend, K., & Stephenson, J. (2018). Intervention strategies to improve nutrition and health behaviours before conception. *Lancet, 391*(10132), 1853–1864. https://doi.org/10.1016/S0140-6736(18)30313-1

Jensen, A., & Wrede, J. (2020). Fertility awareness-based methods for family planning: A literature review. *Journal of Christian Nursing, 37*(4), 212–220. https://doi.org/10.1097/CNJ.0000000000000758

Mensch, B. S., Chuang, E. K., Melnikas, A. J., & Psaki, S. R. (2019). Evidence for causal links between education and maternal and child health: Systematic review. *Tropical Medicine in International Health, 24*(5), 504–522. https://doi.org/10.1111/tmi.13218

Obelenienė, B., Narbekovas, A., & Juškevičius, J. (2021). Anthropological and methodical differences of natural family planning and fertility awareness-based methods. *Linacre Quarterly, 88*(1), 14–23. https://doi.org/10.1177/0024363919886517

Sung, S., & Abramovitz, A. (2021). Natural family planning. In *StatPearls*. StatPearls Publishing. https://pubmed.ncbi.nlm.nih.gov/31536267/

Knowledge: Pregnancy   1810

Definition: Extent of understanding conveyed about promotion of a healthy pregnancy and prevention of complications

OUTCOME TARGET RATING: Maintain at_____ Increase to_____

		No Knowledge	Limited Knowledge	Moderate Knowledge	Substantial Knowledge	Extensive Knowledge	
OUTCOME OVERALL RATING		1	2	3	4	5	
Indicators:							
181026	Importance of frequent prenatal care	1	2	3	4	5	NA
181027	Importance of prenatal education	1	2	3	4	5	NA
181003	Warning signs of pregnancy complications	1	2	3	4	5	NA
181004	Major fetal developmental milestones	1	2	3	4	5	NA
181029	Fetal movement pattern	1	2	3	4	5	NA
181005	Anatomic and physiologic changes of pregnancy	1	2	3	4	5	NA
181006	Psychological changes associated with pregnancy	1	2	3	4	5	NA
181030	Emotional changes associated with pregnancy	1	2	3	4	5	NA
181007	Strategies to balance activity and rest	1	2	3	4	5	NA
181008	Proper body mechanics	1	2	3	4	5	NA
181009	Benefits of regular exercise	1	2	3	4	5	NA
181010	Healthy nutritional practices	1	2	3	4	5	NA
181011	Healthy weight gain pattern	1	2	3	4	5	NA
181031	Correct use of nutritional supplements	1	2	3	4	5	NA
181032	Correct use of medication	1	2	3	4	5	NA
181033	Correct use of non-prescription medication	1	2	3	4	5	NA
181013	Importance of dental care	1	2	3	4	5	NA
181039	Breastfeeding techniques	1	2	3	4	5	NA
181040	Puerperal modifications	1	2	3	4	5	NA
181014	Appropriate self-care for discomforts of pregnancy	1	2	3	4	5	NA
181015	Safe sexual practices	1	2	3	4	5	NA
181016	Correct use of motor vehicle safety devices	1	2	3	4	5	NA
181034	Birthing options	1	2	3	4	5	NA
181018	Signs and symptoms of labor	1	2	3	4	5	NA
181019	Effective labor techniques	1	2	3	4	5	NA
181020	Strategies to prevent infection	1	2	3	4	5	NA
181035	Signs of potential domestic abuse	1	2	3	4	5	NA
181021	Strategies to escape domestic abuse	1	2	3	4	5	NA
181022	Strategies to adjust to addition of infant	1	2	3	4	5	NA
181023	Environmental hazards	1	2	3	4	5	NA
181024	Teratogenic agents	1	2	3	4	5	NA
181036	Adverse health effects of tobacco use	1	2	3	4	5	NA
181037	Adverse health effects of alcohol use on fetus	1	2	3	4	5	NA
181038	Adverse health effects of illicit drug use on fetus	1	2	3	4	5	NA

K

Domain-Health Knowledge & Behavior (IV)   *Class*-Knowledge Health Promotion (S)   *2nd edition 2000; revised 2004, 2008, 2013, 2024*

OUTCOME CONTENT REFERENCES:

Association of Women's Health, Obstetric, and Neonatal Nurses. (2016). *Core curriculum for maternal-newborn nursing* (5th ed.).

Ferreira, C. L. M., Guerra, C. M. L., Silva, A. I. T. J., do Rosário, H. R. V., & Pereira, M. B. F. L. O. (2019). Exercise in pregnancy: The impact of an intervention program in the duration of labor and mode of delivery. *Revista Brasileira de Ginecologia e Obstetrícia, 41*(2). 68–75. https://doi.org/10.1055/s-0038-1675613

Holness, N. (2018). High-risk pregnancy. *The Nursing Clinics of North America, 53*(2), 241–251. https://doi.org/10.1016/j.cnur.2018.01.010

Lowdermilk, D. L., & Perry, S. E. (2019). *Maternity & women's health care* (12th ed.). Mosby.

Mate, A., Reyes-Goya, C., Santana-Garrido, Á., & Vázquez, C. M. (2021). Lifestyle, maternal nutrition and healthy pregnancy. *Current Vascular Pharmacology. 19*(2), 132–140. https://doi.org/10.2174/1570161118666200401112955

O'Shaughnessy, E., O'Donoghue, K., & Leitao, S. (2021). Termination of pregnancy: Staff knowledge and training. *Sexual Reproductive Healthcare, 28*, 100613. https://doi.org/10.1016/j.srhc.2021.100613

Sammaritano, L. R., & Bermas, B. L. (2018). Management of pregnancy and lactation. *Best Practice & Research Clinical Rheumatology, 32*(6), 750–766. https://doi.org/10.1016/j.berh.2019.03.007

Uslu Yuvaci, H., Cinar, N., Yalnizoglu Caka, S., Topal, S., Peksen, S., Saglam, N., & Cevrioglu, A. S. (2021). Effects of antepartum education on worries about labor and mode of delivery. *Journal of Psychosomantic Obstetrics & Gynaecology, 42*(3), 228–234. https://doi.org/10.1080/0167482X.2020.1725465

Knowledge: Pregnancy & Postpartum Sexual Function   1839

Definition: Extent of understanding conveyed about sexual function during pregnancy and postpartum

OUTCOME TARGET RATING: Maintain at_____ Increase to_____

OUTCOME OVERALL RATING	No Knowledge	Limited Knowledge	Moderate Knowledge	Substantial Knowledge	Extensive Knowledge	
	1	2	3	4	5	
Indicators:						
183901 Non-pregnant anatomy	1	2	3	4	5	NA
183902 Normal changes in body image	1	2	3	4	5	NA
183903 Physiology of female sexual functioning	1	2	3	4	5	NA
183904 Anatomic and physiological changes of pregnancy	1	2	3	4	5	NA
183905 Psychological changes associated with pregnancy	1	2	3	4	5	NA
183906 Emotional changes associated with pregnancy	1	2	3	4	5	NA
183907 Anatomic and physiological changes of postpartum	1	2	3	4	5	NA
183908 Psychological changes associated with postpartum	1	2	3	4	5	NA
183909 Emotional changes associated with postpartum	1	2	3	4	5	NA
183910 Potential changes in sexual desire and response	1	2	3	4	5	NA
183911 Intercourse restrictions during pregnancy	1	2	3	4	5	NA
183912 Intercourse restrictions during postpartum	1	2	3	4	5	NA
183913 Modification of coital position to prevent injury	1	2	3	4	5	NA
183914 Modification of coital position to prevent discomfort	1	2	3	4	5	NA
183915 Modification of sexual activity for mutual satisfaction	1	2	3	4	5	NA
183916 Use of vaginal water-based lubricant	1	2	3	4	5	NA
183917 Safe sexual practices	1	2	3	4	5	NA
183918 Strategies to prevent sexually transmitted diseases	1	2	3	4	5	NA
183919 Importance of contraception during early postpartum	1	2	3	4	5	NA
183920 Societal influences on personal sexual behavior	1	2	3	4	5	NA
183921 Cultural influences on personal sexual behavior	1	2	3	4	5	NA

Domain-*Health Knowledge & Behavior (IV)*   **Class**-*Knowledge Health Promotion (S)*   *4th edition 2008; revised 2013, 2024*

OUTCOME CONTENT REFERENCES:

Cassis, C., Mukhopadhyay, S., Morris, E., & Giarenis, I. (2021). What happens to female sexual function during pregnancy? *European Journal of Obstetrics & Gynecology and Reproductive Biology, 258*, 265–268. https://doi.org/10.1016/j.ejogrb.2021.01.003

Dahlgren, H., Jansson, M. H., Franzén, K., Hiyoshi, A., & Nilsson, K. (2022). Sexual function in primiparous women: A prospective study. *International Urogynecology Journal, 33*, 1567–1582. https://doi.org/10.1007/s00192-021-05029-w

Daud, S., Zahid, A. Z. M., Mohamad, M., Abdullah, B., & Mohamad, N. A. N. (2019). Prevalence of sexual dysfunction in pregnancy. *Archives of Gynecology and Obstetrics, 300*(5), 1279–1285. https://doi.org/10.1007/s00404-019-05273-y

Davari-Tanha, F., A'lam, Z. R., Shirazi, M., Askari, F., & Ghajarzadeh, M. (2020). Comparison of sexual function in pregnant women with different gestational age. *Maedica (Bucur), 15*(3), 335–338. https://doi.org/10.26574/maedica.2020.15.3.335

Doke, P. P., Vaidya, V. M., Narula, A., Patil, A. V., Panchanadikar, T. M., & Wagh, G. N. (2021). Risk of non-resumption of vaginal sex and dyspareunia among cesarean-delivered women. *Journal of Family Medicine and Primary Care, 10*(7), 2600–2607. https://doi.org/10.4103/jfmpc.jfmpc_2482_20

Gommesen, D., Nøhr, E., Qvist, N., & Rasch, V. (2019). Obstetric perineal tears, sexual function and dyspareunia among primiparous women 12 months postpartum: A prospective cohort study. *BMJ Open, 9*(12), e032368. https://doi.org/10.1136/bmjopen-2019-032368

Gutzeit, O., Levy, G., & Lowenstein, L. (2019). Postpartum female sexual function: Risk factors for postpartum sexual dysfunction. *Sexual Medicine, 8*(1), 8–13. https://doi.org/10.1016/j.esxm.2019.10.005

Khalesi, Z. B., Bokaie, M., & Attari, S. M. (2018). Effect of pregnancy on sexual function of couples. *African Health Science, 18*(2), 227–234. https://doi.org/10.4314/ahs.v18i2.5

Lowdermilk, D. L., Cashion, C. M., Perry, S., Alden, K., & Olshansky, E. (2019). *Maternity & women's health care* (12th ed.). Elsevier.

Ninivaggio, C., Rogers, R. G., Leeman, L., Migliaccio, L., Teaf, D., & Qualls, C. (2017). Sexual function changes during pregnancy. *International Urogynecology Journal, 28*(6), 923–929. https://doi.org/10.1007/s00192-016-3200-8

Sheikhi, Z. P., Navidian, A., & Rigi, M. (2020). Effect of sexual health education on sexual function and resumption of sexual intercourse after childbirth in primiparous women. *Journal of Education and Health Promotion, 9*, 87. https://doi.org/10.4103/jehp.jehp_591_19

Knowledge: Prescribed Activity 1811

Definition: Extent of understanding conveyed about physical activity recommended by a health professional for a specific condition

OUTCOME TARGET RATING: Maintain at_____ Increase to_____

OUTCOME OVERALL RATING	No Knowledge	Limited Knowledge	Moderate Knowledge	Substantial Knowledge	Extensive Knowledge	
	1	**2**	**3**	**4**	**5**	
Indicators:						
181101 Prescribed activity	1	2	3	4	5	NA
181102 Purpose of prescribed activity	1	2	3	4	5	NA
181103 Expected effects of prescribed activity	1	2	3	4	5	NA
181104 Prescribed activity restrictions	1	2	3	4	5	NA
181105 Prescribed activity precautions	1	2	3	4	5	NA
181121 Realistic goals about prescribed activity	1	2	3	4	5	NA
181116 Strategies to safely ambulate	1	2	3	4	5	NA
181122 Strategies to avoid injury	1	2	3	4	5	NA
181125 Strategies to prevent falls	1	2	3	4	5	NA
181117 Appropriate footwear	1	2	3	4	5	NA
181106 Factors that decrease the ability to perform prescribed activity	1	2	3	4	5	NA
181107 Strategies to gradually increase prescribed activity	1	2	3	4	5	NA
181123 Strategies to incorporate physical activity into life routine	1	2	3	4	5	NA
181124 Strategies to monitor progress in prescribed physical activity	1	2	3	4	5	NA
181118 Methods to monitor heart rate	1		3	4	5	NA
181119 Methods to monitor respiratory rate	1	2	3	4	5	NA
181111 Realistic prescribed activity routine	1	2	3	4	5	NA
181110 Barriers to implementing prescribed activity routine	1	2	3	4	5	NA
181112 Proper performance of prescribed activity	1	2	3	4	5	NA
181120 Benefits of prescribed activity	1	2	3	4	5	NA
181126 Impact of social support for exercise participation	1	2	3	4	5	NA
181127 Use of app to monitor the number of steps per day	1	2	3	4	5	NA

Domain-Health Knowledge & Behavior (IV)   **Class**-Knowledge Health Condition (GG)   *1st edition 1997; revised 2004, 2008, 2013, 2024*

OUTCOME CONTENT REFERENCES:

Barker, K., & Eickmeyer, S. (2020). Therapeutic exercise. *The Medical Clinics of North America, 104*(2), 189–198. https://doi.org/10.1016/j.mcna.2019.10.003

Capozzi, L. C., Daun, J. T., Ester, M., Mosca, S., Langelier, D., Francis, G. J., Chang, E., Mina, D. S., Fu, J. B., & Culos-Reed, S. N. (2021). Physical activity for individuals living with advanced cancer: Evidence and recommendations. *Seminars in Oncology Nursing, 37*(4), 151170. https://doi.org/10.1016/j.soncn.2021.151170

Cattadori, G., Segurini, C., Picozzi, A., Padeletti, L., & Anzà, C. (2018). Exercise and heart failure: An update. *ESC Heart Failure, 5*(2), 222–232. https://doi.org/10.1002/ehf2.12225

Chavez, A., Scales, R., & Kling, J. M. (2021). Promoting physical activity in older women to maximize health. *Cleveland Clinic Journal of Medicine, 88*(7), 405–415. https://doi.org/10.3949/ccjm.88a.20170

Dibben, G. O., Dalal, H. M., Taylor, R. S., Doherty, P., Tang, L. H., & Hillsdon, M. (2018). Cardiac rehabilitation and physical activity: Systematic review and meta-analysis. *Heart* (British Cardiac Society), *104*(17), 1394–1402. https://doi.org/10.1136/heartjnl-2017-312832

Garber C. E. (2019). The health benefits of exercise in overweight and obese patients. *Current Sports Medicine Reports, 18*(8), 287–291. https://doi.org/10.1249/JSR.0000000000000619

Jia, R. X., Liang, J. H., Xu, Y., & Wang, Y. Q. (2019). Effects of physical activity and exercise on the cognitive function of patients with Alzheimer disease: A meta-analysis. *BMC Geriatrics, 19*(1), 181. https://doi.org/10.1186/s12877-019-1175-2

Jimeno-Almazán, A., Pallarés, J. G., Buendía-Romero, Á., Martínez-Cava, A., Franco-López, F., Sánchez-Alcaraz Martínez, B. J., Bernal-Morel, E., & Courel-Ibáñez, J. (2021). Post-COVID-19 syndrome and the potential benefits of exercise. *International Journal of Environmental Research and Public Health, 18*(10), 5329. https://doi.org/10.3390/ijerph18105329

Kim, Y., Lai, B., Mehta, T., Thirumalai, M., Padalabalanarayanan, S., Rimmer, J. H., & Motl, R. W. (2019). Exercise training guidelines for multiple sclerosis, stroke, and Parkinson disease: Rapid review and synthesis. *American Journal of Physical Medicine & Rehabilitation, 98*(7), 613–621. https://doi.org/10.1097/PHM.0000000000001174

Schujmann, D. S., Lunardi, A. C., & Fu, C. (2018). Progressive mobility program and technology to increase the level of physical activity and its benefits in respiratory, muscular system, and functionality of ICU patients: Study protocol for a randomized controlled trial. *Trials, 19*(1), 274. https://doi.org/10.1186/s13063-018-2641-4

Valenzuela, P. L., Castillo-García, A., Morales, J. S., de la Villa, P., Hampel, H., Emanuele, E., Lista, S., & Lucia, A. (2020). Exercise benefits on Alzheimer's disease: State-of-the-science. *Ageing Research Reviews, 62*, 101108. https://doi.org/10.1016/j.arr.2020.101108

K

Knowledge: Prescribed Diet   1802

Definition: Extent of understanding conveyed about a nutritional regimen recommended by a health professional for a specific health condition

OUTCOME TARGET RATING: Maintain at_____ Increase to_____

		No Knowledge	Limited Knowledge	Moderate Knowledge	Substantial Knowledge	Extensive Knowledge	
OUTCOME OVERALL RATING		**1**	**2**	**3**	**4**	**5**	
Indicators:							
180201	Prescribed diet	1	2	3	4	5	NA
180202	Rationale for prescribed diet	1	2	3	4	5	NA
180203	Benefits of prescribed diet	1	2	3	4	5	NA
180204	Dietary goals	1	2	3	4	5	NA
180205	Relationship among diet, exercise, and weight	1	2	3	4	5	NA
180227	Importance of fresh fruit and vegetables	1	2	3	4	5	NA
180206	Foods allowed	1	2	3	4	5	NA
180218	Fluids allowed	1	2	3	4	5	NA
180207	Foods to avoid	1	2	3	4	5	NA
180219	Fluids to avoid	1	2	3	4	5	NA
180221	Food consistent with cultural beliefs	1	2	3	4	5	NA
180222	Recommended food intake distribution throughout the day	1	2	3	4	5	NA
180223	Recommended food portions	1	2	3	4	5	NA
180208	Interpretation of nutritional information on food labels	1	2	3	4	5	NA
180209	Guidelines for food preparation	1	2	3	4	5	NA
180211	Menu planning based on prescribed diet	1	2	3	4	5	NA
180212	Strategies to change dietary habits	1	2	3	4	5	NA
180227	Food intake plans for social situations	1	2	3	4	5	NA
180224	Strategies for situations that affect food and fluid intake	1	2	3	4	5	NA
180217	Self-monitoring techniques	1	2	3	4	5	NA
180215	Potential food and medication interactions	1	2	3	4	5	NA
180225	Potential food and herbal supplement interactions	1	2	3	4	5	NA
180226	Strategies to increase adherence	1	2	3	4	5	NA

Specify diet_____

Domain-Health Knowledge & Behavior (IV)   **Class**-Knowledge Health Condition (GG)   *1st edition 1997; revised 2004, 2008, 2013, 2024*

OUTCOME CONTENT REFERENCES:

Abu-Janb, N., & Jaana, M. (2020). Facilitators and barriers to adherence to gluten-free diet among adults with celiac disease: A systematic review. *Journal of Human Nutrition and Diet, 33*, 786–810. https://doi.org/10.1111/jhn.12754

+Bottcher, M. R., Marincic, P. Z., Nahay, K. L., Baerlocher, B. E., Willis, A. W., Park, J., Gaillard, P., & Greene, M. W. (2017). Nutrition knowledge and Mediterranean diet adherence in the southeast United States: Validation of a field-based survey instrument. *Appetite, 111*, 166–176. https://doi.org/10.1016/j.appet.2016.12.029

Brito, B. P. R., Martín, G. Á., Oter, Q. C., Paloma, C. O., & Romero, S. J. M. (2020). Development and content validation of a NOC-based instrument for measuring dietary knowledge in patients with diabetes: CoNOCidiet-Diabetes. *International Journal of Nursing Knowledge, 31*(1), 59–73. https://doi.org/10.1111/2047-3095.12243

Jeffs, E., Williman, J., Brunton, C., Gullam, J., & Walls, T. (2020). Pregnant women's knowledge of, and adherence to, New Zealand Food Safety in Pregnancy guidelines. *New Zealand Medical Journal, 133*(1525), 41–52. https://doi.org/10.1111/ajo.12523

Kim, R. J., Lopez, R., Snair, M., & Tang, A. (2021). Mediterranean diet adherence and metabolic syndrome in U.S. adolescents. *International Journal of Food Sciences and Nutrition, 72*(4), 537–547. https://doi.org/10.1080/09637486.2020.1840533

Lazarou, C., Panagiotakos, D., & Matalas, A. L. (2021). The role of diet in prevention and management of type 2 diabetes: Implications for public health. *Critical Reviews in Food Science and Nutrition, 52*(5), 382–389, https://doi.org/10.1080/10408398.2010.500258

Ling, R. Z. Q., Jiao, N., Hassan, N. B., He, H., & Wang, W. (2020). Adherence to diet and medication and the associated factors among patient with chronic heart failure in a multi-ethnic society. *Heart & Lung, 49*(2), 144–150. https://doi.org/10.1016/j.hrtlng.2019.11.003

Magnoni, M., Scarano, P., Vergani, V., Berteotti, M., Gallone, G., Cristell, N., Maseri, A., & Cianflone, D. (2020). Impact of adherence to a Mediterranean diet pattern on patients with first acute myocardial infarction. *Nutrition, Metabolism & Cardiovascular Diseases, 30*(4), 574–580. https://doi.org/10.1016/j.numecd.2019.11.014

Silvester, J. A., Weiten, D., Graff, L. A., Walker, J. R., & Duerksen, D. R. (2016). Living gluten-free: Adherence, knowledge, lifestyle adaptations and feelings towards a gluten-free diet. *Journal of Human Nutrition and Diet, 29*, 374–382. https://doi.org/10.1111/jhn.12316

Knowledge: Preterm Infant Care   1840

Definition: Extent of understanding conveyed about the care of a premature infant born 24 to 37 weeks (term) gestation

OUTCOME TARGET RATING: Maintain at_____ Increase to_____

		No Knowledge	Limited Knowledge	Moderate Knowledge	Substantial Knowledge	Extensive Knowledge	
OUTCOME OVERALL RATING		1	2	3	4	5	
Indicators:							
184001	Cause and contributing factors for prematurity	1	2	3	4	5	NA
184002	Premature infant characteristics	1	2	3	4	5	NA
184003	Major developmental milestones	1	2	3	4	5	NA
184004	Proper infant positioning	1	2	3	4	5	NA
184005	Infant sleep-wake pattern	1	2	3	4	5	NA
184006	Respiratory needs	1	2	3	4	5	NA
184007	Thermoregulation needs	1	2	3	4	5	NA
184008	Skin care needs	1	2	3	4	5	NA
184009	Physiologic monitoring needs	1	2	3	4	5	NA
184010	Hydration monitoring needs	1	2	3	4	5	NA
184011	Glucose monitoring needs	1	2	3	4	5	NA
184012	Pain management strategies	1	2	3	4	5	NA
184013	Prescribed medication	1	2	3	4	5	NA
184014	Diagnostic imaging tests	1	2	3	4	5	NA
184015	Laboratory tests	1	2	3	4	5	NA
184016	Nutritional needs	1	2	3	4	5	NA
184028	Premature infant feeding strategies	1	2	3	4	5	NA
184017	Importance of environmental control	1	2	3	4	5	NA
184018	Benefits of kangaroo care	1	2	3	4	5	NA
184019	Neonatal intensive care routine	1	2	3	4	5	NA
184020	Parenting strategies in the hospital	1	2	3	4	5	NA
184021	Strategies to enhance bonding with infant	1	2	3	4	5	NA
184022	Strategies to adjust to addition of infant	1	2	3	4	5	NA
184023	Strategies to enhance sibling support	1	2	3	4	5	NA
184024	Available support groups	1	2	3	4	5	NA
184025	Reputable sources of preterm infant care information	1	2	3	4	5	NA
184026	Financial resources for assistance	1	2	3	4	5	NA
184027	Discharge planning	1	2	3	4	5	NA

Domain-Health Knowledge & Behavior (IV)   **Class**-Knowledge Health Promotion (S)   *4th edition 2008; revised 2013, 2024*

K

OUTCOME CONTENT REFERENCES:

Aragona, E., & Conroy, R. (2017). Newborn care curriculum: The late preterm infant in the Level II Neonatal Intensive Care Unit. *MedEdPORTAL, 13*, 10657. https://doi.org/10.15766/mep_2374-8265.10657

Asadi, S., Bloomfield, F. H., & Harding, J. E. (2019). Nutrition in late preterm infants. *Seminars in Perinatology, 43*(7), 151160. https://doi.org/10.1053/j.semperi.2019.06.008

Bellù, R., & Condò, M. (2017). Breastfeeding promotion: Evidence and problems. *La Pediatria Medica e Chirurgica, 39*(2), 156. https://doi.org/10.4081/pmc.2017.156

DeMauro, S. B., & Jensen, E. A. (2021). Evolving respiratory care of the preterm infant. *JAMA Pediatrics, 175*(10), 1004–1005. https://doi.org/10.1001/jamapediatrics.2021.1918

Hay, W. W. (2017). Optimizing nutrition of the preterm infant. *Chinese Journal of Contemporary Pediatric, 19*(1), 1–21. https://doi.org/10.7499/j.issn.1008-8830.2017.01.001

McPherson, C., Miller, S. P., El-Dib, M., Massaro, A. N., & Inder, T. E. (2020). The influence of pain, agitation, and their management on the immature brain. *Pediatric Research, 88*(2), 168–175. https://doi.org/10.1038/s41390-019-0744-6

Merenstein, G. B. (2020). *Handbook of neonatal intensive care* (9th ed.). Mosby.

Nunes, C. R. D. N., Campos, L. G., Lucena, A. M., Pereira, J. M., Costa, P. R. D., Lima, F. A. F., & Azevedo, V. M. G. O. (2017). Relationship between the use of kangaroo position on preterm babies and mother-child interaction upon discharge. *Revista Paulista de Pediatria, 35*(2), 136–143. https://doi.org/10.1590/1984-0462/;2017;35;2;00006

Segar J. L. (2020). A physiological approach to fluid and electrolyte management of the preterm infant: Review. *Journal of Neonatal-Perinatal Medicine, 13*(1), 11–19. https://doi.org/10.3233/NPM-190309

Knowledge: School Age Child Psychosocial Safety 1875

Definition: Extent of understanding conveyed about protecting the psychosocial safety of a child from 6 to 18 years old

OUTCOME TARGET RATING: Maintain at_____ Increase to_____

		No Knowledge	Limited Knowledge	Moderate Knowledge	Substantial Knowledge	Extensive Knowledge	
OUTCOME OVERALL RATING		1	2	3	4	5	
Indicators:							
187501	Importance of daily routine	1	2	3	4	5	NA
187502	Importance of age-appropriate expectations	1	2	3	4	5	NA
187503	Importance of structure in child's life	1	2	3	4	5	NA
187504	Strategies to monitor playmate interactions	1	2	3	4	5	NA
187505	Strategies to monitor schoolmate interactions	1	2	3	4	5	NA
187506	Strategies to monitor siblings' interactions	1	2	3	4	5	NA
187507	Strategies to monitor adult contacts	1	2	3	4	5	NA
187508	Strategies to foster open communication	1	2	3	4	5	NA
187509	Strategies to discourage secrets	1	2	3	4	5	NA
187510	Importance of setting clear rules for behavior	1	2	3	4	5	NA
187511	Methods of discipline appropriate for developmental age	1	2	3	4	5	NA
187512	Benefits of positive social relationships	1	2	3	4	5	NA
187513	Impact of peer pressure	1	2	3	4	5	NA
187514	Situations considered as stressful by child	1	2	3	4	5	NA
187515	Strategies to help child cope with stressful situations	1	2	3	4	5	NA
187516	Benefits of stress management	1	2	3	4	5	NA
187517	Strategies to evaluate potential caregivers	1	2	3	4	5	NA
187518	Strategies to identify sex offenders in neighborhood	1	2	3	4	5	NA
187519	Strategies to provide close supervision of outdoor activities	1	2	3	4	5	NA
187520	Importance of being aware of potential lures used to approach child	1	2	3	4	5	NA
187521	Strategies to teach about bad strangers	1	2	3	4	5	NA
187522	Strategies to prevent abduction	1	2	3	4	5	NA
187523	Strategies to prevent neglect	1	2	3	4	5	NA
187524	Strategies to prevent physical abuse	1	2	3	4	5	NA
187525	Strategies to prevent sexual abuse	1	2	3	4	5	NA
187526	Strategies to prevent emotional abuse	1	2	3	4	5	NA
187527	Strategies to identify bullying	1	2	3	4	5	NA
187528	Strategies to monitor internet use	1	2	3	4	5	NA
187529	Strategies to monitor social media	1	2	3	4	5	NA
187530	Identification of high-risk behaviors for age group	1	2	3	4	5	NA
187531	Signs and symptoms of depression	1	2	3	4	5	NA
187532	Signs and symptoms of loneliness	1	2	3	4	5	NA
187533	Signs and symptoms of anxiety	1	2	3	4	5	NA

Domain-Health Knowledge & Behavior (IV)   **Class**-Knowledge Health Promotion (S)   7th edition 2024

OUTCOME CONTENT REFERENCES:

Ahern, N. R., Kemppainen, J., & Thacker, P. (2016). Awareness and knowledge of child and adolescent risky behaviors: A parent's perspective. *Journal of Child and Adolescent Psychiatric Nursing, 29*(1), 6–14. https://doi.org/10.1111/jcap.12129

Byrne, A., Hagen, M. G., & Thompson, L. (2021). Gun safety for children. *JAMA Pediatrics, 175*(3), 332. https://doi.org/10.1001/jamapediatrics.2020.5989

Hagan, J. F., Shaw, J. S., & Duncan, P. M. (Eds.). (2017). *Bright futures: Guidelines for health supervision of infants, children, and adolescents* (4th ed.). American Academy of Pediatrics.

Hockenberry, M. J., Wilson, D., & Rodgers, C. C. (Eds.). (2019). *Wong's nursing care of infants and children* (11th ed.). Elsevier.

Miltenberger, R. G., Sanchez, S., & Valbuena, D. (2020). Pediatric prevention: Teaching safety skills. *Pediatric Clinics of North America, 67*(3), 573–584. https://doi.org/10.1016/j.pcl.2020.02.011

Perry, S. E., Hockenberry, M. J., Lowdermilk, D. J., Wilson, D., Cashion, K., Rodgers, C. C., & Alden, K. R. (2018). *Maternal child nursing care* (6th ed.). Elsevier.

Knowledge: Sexual Function

1815

Definition: Extent of understanding conveyed about sexual development, phases of sexual response, and responsible sexual practices

OUTCOME TARGET RATING: Maintain at_____ Increase to_____

		No Knowledge	Limited Knowledge	Moderate Knowledge	Substantial Knowledge	Extensive Knowledge	
OUTCOME OVERALL RATING		**1**	**2**	**3**	**4**	**5**	
Indicators:							
181517	Male sexual anatomy	1	2	3	4	5	NA
181518	Female sexual anatomy	1	2	3	4	5	NA
181502	Function of sexual anatomy	1	2	3	4	5	NA
181519	Phases of sexual response	1	2	3	4	5	NA
181520	Impact of stress on sexual function	1	2	3	4	5	NA
181521	Impact of chronic illness on sexual function	1	2	3	4	5	NA
181522	Impact of alcohol on sexual function	1	2	3	4	5	NA
181523	Impact of medication on sexual function	1	2	3	4	5	NA
181524	Impact of drug use on sexual function	1	2	3	4	5	NA
181525	Medication to improve sexual performance	1	2	3	4	5	NA
181503	Physical changes with puberty	1	2	3	4	5	NA
181504	Emotional changes with puberty	1	2	3	4	5	NA
181505	Reproduction	1	2	3	4	5	NA
181506	Physical changes with aging	1	2	3	4	5	NA
181507	Emotional changes with aging	1	2	3	4	5	NA
181508	Societal influences on personal sexual behavior	1	2	3	4	5	NA
181509	Safe sexual practices	1	2	3	4	5	NA
181513	Strategies for safe sex	1	2	3	4	5	NA
181510	Effective contraceptive methods	1	2	3	4	5	NA
181511	Strategies to prevent sexually transmitted diseases	1	2	3	4	5	NA
181514	Risks associated with multiple sexual partners	1	2	3	4	5	NA
181515	Potential consequences of sexual activity	1	2	3	4	5	NA
181516	Benefits of delaying sexual activity in adolescence	1	2	3	4	5	NA

Domain-Health Knowledge & Behavior (IV)   **Class**-Knowledge Health Promotion (S)   2nd edition 2000; revised 2004, 2008, 2013, 2024

K

OUTCOME CONTENT REFERENCES:

Aepfelbacher, J. A., Chaudhury, C. S., Mee, T., Purdy, J. B., Hawkins, K., Curl, K. A., Dee, N., & Hadigan, C. (2020). Reproductive and sexual health knowledge, experiences, and milestones in young adults with life-long HIV. *AIDS Care, 32*(3), 354–361. https://doi.org/10.1080/09540121.2019.1679711

Athey, R. A., Kershaw, V., & Radley, S. (2021). Systematic review of sexual function in older women. *European Journal of Obstetrics, Gynecology, and Reproductive Biology, 267*, 198–204. https://doi.org/10.1016/j.ejogrb.2021.11.011

Ayalon, L., Gewirtz-Meydan, A., Levkovich, I., & Karkabi, K. (2021). Older men and women reflect on changes in sexual functioning in later life. *Sexual & Relationship Therapy, 36*(4), 347–367. https://doi.org/10.1080/14681994.2019.1633576

Byers, E. S., O'Sullivan, L. F., & Hughes, K. (2021). Sexual functioning of late adolescents and young adults in relationships: Association with individual characteristics and relationship factors. *Sexual & Relationship Therapy, 36*(2/3), 178–197. https://doi.org/10.1080/14681994.2019.1626982

Gunasekara, K., & Dupesh Khan, S. (2019). *Sexual medicine.* Springer.

Rantell, A. (2021). *Sexual function and pelvic floor dysfunction: A guide for nurses and allied health professionals.* Springer.

Sierra, J. C., Gómez-Carranza, J., Álvarez-Muelas, A., & Cervilla, O. (2021). Association of sexual attitudes with sexual function: General vs. specific attitudes. *International Journal of Environmental Research and Public Health, 18*(19), 10390. https://doi.org/10.3390/ijerph181910390

Tavares, I. M., Moura, C. V., & Nobre, P. J. (2020). The role of cognitive processing factors in sexual function and dysfunction in women and men: A systematic review. *Sexual Medicine Reviews, 8*(3), 403–430. https://doi.org/10.1016/j.sxmr.2020.03.002

Knowledge: Stress Management   1862

Definition: Extent of understanding conveyed about the stress process and strategies to reduce or cope with stress

OUTCOME TARGET RATING: Maintain at_____ Increase to_____

		No Knowledge	Limited Knowledge	Moderate Knowledge	Substantial Knowledge	Extensive Knowledge	
OUTCOME OVERALL RATING		1	2	3	4	5	
Indicators:							
186201	Factors that cause stress	1	2	3	4	5	NA
186202	Factors that increase stress	1	2	3	4	5	NA
186203	Physical stress response	1	2	3	4	5	NA
186204	Cognitive stress response	1	2	3	4	5	NA
186205	Affective stress response	1	2	3	4	5	NA
186206	Behavioral stress response	1	2	3	4	5	NA
186207	Spiritual stress response	1	2	3	4	5	NA
186208	Role of stress in illness	1	2	3	4	5	NA
186209	Benefits of stress management	1	2	3	4	5	NA
186210	Cognitive therapy techniques	1	2	3	4	5	NA
186211	Stress inoculation techniques	1	2	3	4	5	NA
186212	Problem-solving approaches	1	2	3	4	5	NA
186213	Effective meditation techniques	1	2	3	4	5	NA
186214	Effective relaxation techniques	1	2	3	4	5	NA
186215	Effective stress reduction techniques	1	2	3	4	5	NA
186216	Effective communication techniques	1	2	3	4	5	NA
186217	Benefits of adequate sleep	1	2	3	4	5	NA
186218	Benefits of healthy diet	1	2	3	4	5	NA
186219	Benefits of regular exercise	1	2	3	4	5	NA
186220	Benefits of massage	1	2	3	4	5	NA
186221	Benefits of prayer	1	2	3	4	5	NA
186222	Benefits of hypnosis	1	2	3	4	5	NA
186223	Benefits of music	1	2	3	4	5	NA
186224	Effects on lifestyle	1	2	3	4	5	NA
186225	Benefits of lifestyle modifications	1	2	3	4	5	NA
186229	Benefits of spending time outdoors	1	2	3	4	5	NA
186230	Benefits of pet therapy	1	2	3	4	5	NA
186226	Strategies to replace negative and irrational thoughts	1	2	3	4	5	NA
186227	Available support groups	1	2	3	4	5	NA
186228	Strategies to increase social support	1	2	3	4	5	NA

Domain-Health Knowledge & Behavior (IV)   **Class**-Knowledge Health Promotion (S)   5th edition 2013; revised 2024

OUTCOME CONTENT REFERENCES:

Carlson, L. E., Toivonen, K., & Subnis, U. (2019). Integrative approaches to stress management. *Cancer Journal* (Sudbury, Mass.), *25*(5), 329–336. https://doi.org/10.1097/PPO.0000000000000395

Dusek, J. A., Hibberd, P. L., Buczynski, B., Chang, B., Dusek, K. C., Johnston, J. M., Wohlhueter, A. L., Benson, H., & Zusman, R. M. (2008). Stress management versus lifestyle modification on systolic hypertension and medication elimination: A randomized trial. *Journal of Alternative & Complementary Medicine, 14*(2), 129–138.

Koertge, J., Janszky, I., Sundin, Ö., Blom, M., Georgiades, A., Lászl, K. D., Alinaghizadeh, H., & Ahnve, S. (2008). Effects of a stress management program on vital exhaustion and depression in women with coronary heart disease: A randomized controlled intervention study. *Journal of Internal Medicine, 263*(3), 281–293. https://doi.org/10.1111/j.1365-2796.2007.01887.x

McCance, K., & Huether, S. (2009). *Pathophysiology: The biological basis for disease in adults and children* (6th ed.). Mosby.

Macía, P., Barranco, M., Gorbeña, S., Álvarez-Fuentes, E., & Iraurgi, I. (2021). Resilience and coping strategies in relation to mental health outcomes in people with cancer. *PLOS One, 16*(5), e0252075. https://doi.org/10.1371/journal.pone.0252075

Monteiro, A., Santos, R. L., Kimura, N., Baptista, M., & Dourado, M. (2018). Coping strategies among caregivers of people with Alzheimer disease: A systematic review. *Trends in Psychiatry and Psychotherapy, 40*(3), 258–268. https://doi.org/10.1590/2237-6089-2017-0065

Overholser, J. C., & Fisher, L. B. (2009). Contemporary perspectives on stress management: Medication, meditation or mitigation. *Journal of Contemporary Psychotherapy, 39*(3), 147–155. https://doi.org/10.1007/s10879-009-9114-8

Stanley, B., Martínez-Alés, G., Gratch, I., Rizk, M., Galfalvy, H., Choo, T. H., & Mann, J. J. (2021). Coping strategies that reduce suicidal ideation: An ecological momentary assessment study. *Journal of Psychiatric Research, 133*, 32–37. https://doi.org/10.1016/j.jpsychires.2020.12.012

Knowledge: Stroke Management 1863

Definition: Extent of understanding conveyed about stroke, its treatment, and the prevention of disease progression and complications

OUTCOME TARGET RATING: Maintain at_____ Increase to_____

		No Knowledge	Limited Knowledge	Moderate Knowledge	Substantial Knowledge	Extensive Knowledge	
OUTCOME OVERALL RATING		**1**	**2**	**3**	**4**	**5**	
Indicators:							
186301	Specific type of stroke	1	2	3	4	5	NA
186302	Cause and contributing factors	1	2	3	4	5	NA
186303	Usual course of ischemic disease	1	2	3	4	5	NA
186304	Signs and symptoms of ischemic disease	1	2	3	4	5	NA
186305	Usual course of hemorrhagic disease	1	2	3	4	5	NA
186306	Signs and symptoms of hemorrhagic disease	1	2	3	4	5	NA
186307	Psychosocial effects of disease	1	2	3	4	5	NA
186331	Relationship of comorbidities to condition	1	2	3	4	5	NA
186332	Relationship of diet to condition	1	2	3	4	5	NA
186333	Relationship of physical stress to condition	1	2	3	4	5	NA
186334	Relationship of emotional stress to condition	1	2	3	4	5	NA
186309	Surgical treatment options	1	2	3	4	5	NA
186310	Available treatment options	1	2	3	4	5	NA
186311	Alternative treatment options	1	2	3	4	5	NA
186312	Medication therapeutic effects	1	2	3	4	5	NA
186313	Medication side effects	1	2	3	4	5	NA
186314	Medication adverse effects	1	2	3	4	5	NA
186315	When to obtain emergency treatment	1	2	3	4	5	NA
186316	Complications of stroke	1	2	3	4	5	NA
186317	Effects on lifestyle	1	2	3	4	5	NA
186318	Guidelines for sexual activity	1	2	3	4	5	NA
186319	Energy conservation techniques	1	2	3	4	5	NA
186320	Strategies to minimize disease progression	1	2	3	4	5	NA
186321	Strategies for smoking cessation	1	2	3	4	5	NA
186322	Strategies to manage hypertension	1	2	3	4	5	NA
186323	Strategies to adapt to sensory losses	1	2	3	4	5	NA
186324	Strategies to maintain skin integrity	1	2	3	4	5	NA
186325	Strategies to adapt to cognitive changes	1	2	3	4	5	NA
186326	Strategies to prevent aspiration	1	2	3	4	5	NA
186327	Importance of completing rehabilitation	1	2	3	4	5	NA
186328	Available support groups	1	2	3	4	5	NA
186329	Risk factors for complications	1	2	3	4	5	NA
186330	Reputable sources of stroke prevention information	1	2	3	4	5	NA

Domain-Health Knowledge & Behavior (IV) **Class-**Knowledge Health Condition (GG) 5th edition 2013; revised 2024

OUTCOME CONTENT REFERENCES:

Fournier, J., Finestone, H., Lauzon, J., & Campbell, M. (2021). Prevalence, impact, and treatment of co-occurring osteoarthritis in patients with stroke undergoing rehabilitation. *Stroke, 52*, e618–e621. https://doi.org/10.1161/STROKEAHA.121.034270

Gorelick, P. B., Whelton, P. K., Sorond, F., & Carey R. M. (2020). Blood pressure management in stroke. *Hypertension, 76*, 1688–1695. https://doi.org/10.1161/HYPERTENSIONAHA.120.14653

Kleindorfer D. O., Towfighi, A., Chaturvedi, S., Cockroft, K. M., Gutierrez, J., Lombardi-Hill, D., Kamel, H., Kernan, W. N., Kittner, S. J., Leira, E .C., Lennon, O., Meschia, J. F., Nguyen, T. N., Pollak, P. M., Santangeli, P., Sharrief, A. Z., Smith, S. C., Turan, T. N., & Williams, L .S. (2021). 2021 guideline for the prevention of stroke in patients with stroke and transient ischemic attack. *Stroke, 52*, e364–e464. https://doi.org/10.1161/STR.0000000000000375

Johnson, M., Moorhead, S., Bulechek, G., Butcher, H., Maas, M., & Swanson, E. (2012). Stroke. In *NOC and NIC linkages to NANDA-I and clinical conditions: Supporting critical reasoning and quality care* (3rd ed., pp. 352–355). Elsevier Mosby.

Potter, P., Perry, A., Stockert, P., & Hall, A. (2021). *Fundamentals of nursing* (10th ed.). Elsevier

Tiedeman, C., Suthers, B., Julien, B., Hackett, A., & Oakley, P. (2019). Management of stroke in the Australian indigenous population: From hospitals to communities. *Internal Medicine Journal, 49*, 962–968. https://doi.org/10.1111/imj.14303

Knowledge: Stroke Threat Reduction 1864

Definition: Extent of understanding conveyed about the causes and the prevention of stroke

OUTCOME TARGET RATING: Maintain at_____ Increase to_____

OUTCOME OVERALL RATING		No Knowledge 1	Limited Knowledge 2	Moderate Knowledge 3	Substantial Knowledge 4	Extensive Knowledge 5	
Indicators:							
186401	Signs and symptoms of stroke	1	2	3	4	5	NA
186402	Types of stroke and related syndromes	1	2	3	4	5	NA
186403	Cause and contributing factors	1	2	3	4	5	NA
186404	Therapies that increase risk	1	2	3	4	5	NA
186405	Lifestyle risk factors	1	2	3	4	5	NA
186406	Genetic risk factors	1	2	3	4	5	NA
186407	Tests to assess risk factors	1	2	3	4	5	NA
186408	Benefits of reducing risk factors	1	2	3	4	5	NA
186409	Stroke prevention guidelines	1	2	3	4	5	NA
186410	Strategies for smoking cessation	1	2	3	4	5	NA
186411	Strategies to manage hypertension	1	2	3	4	5	NA
186412	Importance of alcohol restrictions	1	2	3	4	5	NA
186413	Strategies to manage weight	1	2	3	4	5	NA
186414	Strategies to manage diabetes	1	2	3	4	5	NA
186415	Strategies to manage carotid artery disease	1	2	3	4	5	NA
186416	Strategies to manage atrial fibrillation	1	2	3	4	5	NA
186417	Strategies to manage high cholesterol	1	2	3	4	5	NA
186418	Strategies to promote exercise	1	2	3	4	5	NA
186419	Strategies to manage previous stroke events	1	2	3	4	5	NA
186420	Strategies to manage chronic bacterial infections	1	2	3	4	5	NA
186421	Prescribed diet	1	2	3	4	5	NA
186422	Strategies to maintain hydration	1	2	3	4	5	NA
186423	Anticoagulant preventive therapy	1	2	3	4	5	NA
186424	Alternative preventive therapies	1	2	3	4	5	NA
186425	When to obtain assistance from a health professional	1	2	3	4	5	NA
186426	Plan for obtaining immediate treatment if adverse signs and symptoms occur	1	2	3	4	5	NA

Domain-Health Knowledge & Behavior (IV) *Class*-Knowledge Health Promotion (S) 5th edition 2013; revised 2018

OUTCOME CONTENT REFERENCES:

Bay, J., Spiroski, A.-M., Fogg-Rogers, L., McCann, C., Faull, R., & Barber, P. (2015). Stroke awareness and knowledge in an urban New Zealand population. *Journal of Stroke and Cerebrovascular Diseases, 24*(6), 1153–1162. https://doi.org/10.1016/j.jstrokecerebrovasdis.2015.01.003

Christian, A. H., Rosamond, W., White, A. R., & Mosca, L. (2007). Nine-year trends and racial and ethnic disparities in women's awareness of heart disease and stroke: An American Heart Association national study. *Journal of Women's Health, 16*(1), 68–81. https://doi.org/10.1089/jwh.2006.M072

Johnson, M., Moorhead, S., Bulechek, G., Butcher, H., Maas, M., & Swanson, E. (2012). Stroke. In *NOC and NIC linkages to NANDA-I and clinical conditions: Supporting critical reasoning and quality care* (3rd ed., pp. 352–355). Elsevier Mosby.

National Stroke Association. (2008). *Stroke facts.*

National Stroke Association. (2008). *Stroke prevention guidelines.*

Williams, L., Franklin, B., Evans, M., Jackson, C., Hill, A., & Minor, M. (2015). Turn the beat around: A stroke prevention program for African-American churches. *Public Health Nursing, 33*(1), 11–20. https://doi.org/10.1111/phn.12234

World Health Organization. (2005). *Avoiding heart attacks and strokes: Don't be a victim—protect yourself.*

K

Knowledge: Substance Use Control   1812

Definition: Extent of understanding conveyed about controlling the use of addictive drugs, toxic chemicals, tobacco, or alcohol

OUTCOME TARGET RATING: Maintain at_____ Increase to_____

		No Knowledge	Limited Knowledge	Moderate Knowledge	Substantial Knowledge	Extensive Knowledge	
OUTCOME OVERALL RATING		1	2	3	4	5	
Indicators:							
181201	Personal risk for substance misuse	1	2	3	4	5	NA
181218	Negative effects of use on self	1	2	3	4	5	NA
181219	Negative effects of use on others	1	2	3	4	5	NA
181206	Personal responsibility to manage substance misuse	1	2	3	4	5	NA
181220	Importance of willingness to eliminate use	1	2	3	4	5	NA
181221	Barriers to elimination of substance use	1	2	3	4	5	NA
181222	Lifestyle modifications to eliminate use	1	2	3	4	5	NA
181203	Benefits of eliminating substance use	1	2	3	4	5	NA
181205	Social consequences of substance use	1	2	3	4	5	NA
181207	Threats to substance use control	1	2	3	4	5	NA
181208	Social support for substance use control	1	2	3	4	5	NA
181223	Available treatment options	1	2	3	4	5	NA
181224	Medication helpful with substance control	1	2	3	4	5	NA
181225	Behavioral modification strategies	1	2	3	4	5	NA
181226	Effective coping strategies	1	2	3	4	5	NA
181227	Strategies to address depression	1	2	3	4	5	NA
181228	Strategies to address anxiety	1	2	3	4	5	NA
181209	Strategies to prevent substance use	1	2	3	4	5	NA
181210	Strategies to manage substance use	1	2	3	4	5	NA
181211	Benefits of ongoing self-monitoring	1	2	3	4	5	NA
181229	Benefits of alternative therapies	1	2	3	4	5	NA
181230	Benefits of complementary therapies	1	2	3	4	5	NA
181212	Potential for relapse in efforts to control substance use	1	2	3	4	5	NA
181231	Warnings of impending relapse	1	2	3	4	5	NA
181213	Strategies to prevent relapses in substance use	1	2	3	4	5	NA
181232	Strategies to cope with withdrawal symptoms	1	2	3	4	5	NA
181214	Signs of dependence during substance withdrawal	1	2	3	4	5	NA
181216	Signs and symptoms of substance withdrawal	1	2	3	4	5	NA
181233	Importance of health professional resources	1	2	3	4	5	NA
181234	Importance of limited contact with risk-taking peers	1	2	3	4	5	NA
181235	Available community resources	1	2	3	4	5	NA
181217	Available support groups	1	2	3	4	5	NA
181236	Importance of harm reduction programs	1	2	3	4	5	NA
181237	Reputable sources of information	1	2	3	4	5	NA
181238	Reputable sources of e-health information	1	2	3	4	5	NA

Specify substance_____

Domain-*Health Knowledge & Behavior (IV)*   **Class**-*Knowledge Health Promotion (S)*   *1st edition 1997; revised 2004, 2008, 2024*

OUTCOME CONTENT REFERENCES:
American Society of Addiction Medicine. (2020). The ASAM national practice guideline for the treatment of opioid use disorder: 2020 focused update. *Journal of Addiction Medicine, 14*(2S, Suppl. 1), 1–91. https://doi.org/10.1097/ADM.0000000000000633
Blackwell, C. W., & Castillo, H. L. (2020). Use of electronic nicotine delivery systems (ENDS) in lesbian, gay, bisexual, transgender and queer persons: Implications for public health nursing. *Public Health Nursing, 37*, 569–580. https://doi.org/10.1111/phn.12746
Bold, K. W., Rosen, R. L., Steinberg, M. L., Epstein, E. E., McCrady, B. S., & Williams, J. M. (2020). Smoking characteristics and alcohol use among women in treatment for alcohol use disorder. *Addictive Behaviors, 101*, 1–8. https://doi.org/10.1016/j.addbeh.2019.106137
Case, K. R., Hinds, J. T., Creamer, M. R., Loukas, A., & Perry, C. L. (2020). Who is JUULing and why? An examination of young adult electronic nicotine delivery systems users. *Journal of Adolescent Health, 6*, 48–55. https://doi.org/10.1016/j.jadohealth.2019.05.030
DiSilvio, B., Baqdunes, M., Alhajbusain, A., & Cheema, T. (2021). Smoking addiction and strategies for cessation. *Critical Care Nursing Quarterly, 44*(1), 33–48. https://doi.org/10.1097/CNQ.0000000000000338

K

Haass-Koffler, C. L., Souza, R. D., Wilmott, J. P., Aston, E. R., & Song, J. H. (2021). A combined alcohol and smoking cue-reactivity paradigm in people who drink heavily and smoke cigarettes: Preliminary findings. *Alcohol and Alcoholism, 56*(1), 47–56. https://doi.org/10.1093/alcalc/agaa089

Hughes, J. R. (2020). An update on hardening: A qualitative review. *Nicotine &Tobacco Research, 22*(6), 867–871. https://doi.org/10.1093/ntr/ntz042

Knapp, A. A., Allan, N. P., Cloutier, R., Blumenthal, H., Moradi, S., Budney, A. J., & Lord, S. E. (2021). Effects of anxiety sensitivity on cannabis, alcohol, and nicotine use among adolescents: Evaluating pathways through anxiety, withdrawal symptoms, and coping motives. *Journal of Behavioral Medicine, 44,* 187–201. https://doi.org/10.1007/s10865-020-00182-x

Kurti, A. N. (2020). Reducing tobacco use among women of childbearing age: Contributions of tobacco regulatory science and tobacco control. *Experimental and Clinical Psychopharmacology, 28*(5), 501–516. https://doi.org/10.1037/pha0000342

Li, C., Li, Y., Ma, M., Zhang, Y., Bao, J., Ge, W., Liu, Y., Peng, C., & He, L. (2021). The impact of COVID-19 pandemic on headache symptoms and drug withdrawal among patients with medication overuse headache: A cross-sectional study. *The Journal of Headache and Pain, 22,* 41 1–11. https://doi.org/10.1186/s10194-021-01256-0

Manning, V., Arunogiri, S., Frei, M., Ridley, K., Mroz, K., Campbell, S., & Lubman, D. (2018). *Alcohol and other drug withdrawal: practice guidelines* (3rd ed.). Turning Point.

Nguyen, T. A., & Lam, S. W. (2020). Phenobarbital and symptom-triggered lorazepam versus lorazepam alone for severe alcohol withdrawal in the intensive care unit. *Alcohol, 82,* 23–27. https://doi.org/10.1016/j.alcohol.2019.07.004

Pergolizzi, J. V., Raffa, R. B., & Rosenblatt, M. H. (2019). Opioid withdrawal symptoms, a consequence of chronic opioid use and opioid use disorder: Current understanding and approaches to management. *Journal of Clinical Pharmacy and Therapeutics, 45,* 892–903. https://doi.org/10.1111/jcpt.13114

Robinson, J. D., Li, L., Chen, M., Lerman, C., Tyndale, R. F., Schnoll, R. A., Hawk, L. W. Jr., George, T. P., Benowitz, N. L., & Cinciripini, P. M. (2019). Evaluating the temporal relationship between withdrawal symptoms and smoking relapse. *Psychology of Addictive Behaviors, 33*(2), 105–116. https://doi.org/10.1037/adb0000434

Sharifpour, A., Taghizadeh, F., Zarghami, M., & Alipour, A. (2021). The effectiveness of individual interventions on smoking cessation of chronic obstructive pulmonary disease patients. *Journal of Nursing and Midwifery Science, 7,* 13–21. https://doi.org/10.4103/JNMS.JMNS_38_19

Srivastava, A. B., Mariani, J. J., & Levin, F. R. (2020). New directions in the treatment of opioid withdrawal. *Lancet, 395*(10241), 1938–1948. https://doi.org/10.1016/S0140-6736(20)30852-7

Tonkin, S. S., Williams, T. F., Simms, L. J., Tiffany, S. T., Mahoney, M. C., Schnoll, R. A., Cinciripini, P. M., & Hawk, L. W. Jr. (2020). Withdrawal symptom, treatment mechanism, and/or side effect? Developing an explicit measurement model for smoking cessation research. *Nicotine & Tobacco Research, 22*(4), 482–491. https://doi.org/10.1093/ntr/nty262

U.S. Preventive Services Task Force. (2021). Interventions for tobacco smoking cessation in adults, including pregnant persons: U.S. Preventive Services Task Force Recommendation Statement. *JAMA, 325*(3), 265–279. https://doi.org/10.1001/jama.2020.25019

Wootton, R. E., Greenstone, H. S. R., Abdellaoui, A., Denys, D., Verweij, K. J. H., Munafò, M. R., & Treur, J. L. (2020). Bidirectional effects between loneliness, smoking, and alcohol use: Evidence from a Mendelian randomization study. *Addiction, 116,* 400–406. https://doi.org/10.1111/add.15142

K

Knowledge: Thrombus Threat Reduction   1865

Definition: Extent of understanding conveyed about causes, prevention, and early detection of blood clots within the circulatory system

OUTCOME TARGET RATING: Maintain at_____ Increase to_____

	No Knowledge	Limited Knowledge	Moderate Knowledge	Substantial Knowledge	Extensive Knowledge	
OUTCOME OVERALL RATING	1	2	3	4	5	
Indicators:						
186501 Risk factors for venous stasis	1	2	3	4	5	NA
186502 Risk factors for intimal injury	1	2	3	4	5	NA
186503 Risk factors for hypercoagulation	1	2	3	4	5	NA
186504 Importance of lifelong vigilance for risk factors	1	2	3	4	5	NA
186505 Strategies to reduce venous stasis	1	2	3	4	5	NA
186506 Strategies to reduce intimal injury	1	2	3	4	5	NA
186507 Strategies to reduce hypercoagulation	1	2	3	4	5	NA
186508 Signs and symptoms of thrombi	1	2	3	4	5	NA
186509 Benefits of maintaining optimal weight	1	2	3	4	5	NA
186510 Importance of monitoring blood pressure	1	2	3	4	5	NA
186511 Benefits of activity restrictions	1	2	3	4	5	NA
186512 High-risk activities	1	2	3	4	5	NA
186513 Importance of alcohol restrictions	1	2	3	4	5	NA
186514 Importance of tobacco abstinence	1	2	3	4	5	NA
186515 Benefits of regular exercise	1	2	3	4	5	NA
186516 Medication therapeutic effects	1	2	3	4	5	NA

Knowledge: Thrombus Threat Reduction—cont'd

		No Knowledge	Limited Knowledge	Moderate Knowledge	Substantial Knowledge	Extensive Knowledge	
186517	Medication side effects	1	2	3	4	5	NA
186518	Medication adverse effects	1	2	3	4	5	NA
186519	Potential non-prescription medication interactions	1	2	3	4	5	NA
186520	Herbal interactions	1	2	3	4	5	NA
186521	Importance of maintaining medication regimen	1	2	3	4	5	NA
186522	When to obtain assistance from a health professional	1	2	3	4	5	NA
186523	Caregiver's role in treatment plan	1	2	3	4	5	NA
186524	Available support groups	1	2	3	4	5	NA
186525	Reputable sources of thrombus prevention information	1	2	3	4	5	NA
186526	Plan for obtaining immediate treatment if adverse signs and symptoms occur	1	2	3	4	5	NA

Domain-Health Knowledge & Behavior (IV)   **Class**-Knowledge Health Promotion (S)   5th edition 2013; revised 2018

OUTCOME CONTENT REFERENCES:

Agnelli, G., & Becattini, C. (2008). Treatment of DVT: How long is enough and how do you predict recurrence. *Journal of Thrombosis and Thrombolysis, 25*(1), 37–44. https://doi.org/10.1007/s11239-007-0103-z

Alphonsa, A., Sharma, K., Sharma, G., & Bhatia, R. (2015). Knowledge regarding oral anticoagulation therapy among patients with stroke and those at high risk of thromboembolic events. *Journal of Stroke and Cerebrovascular Diseases, 24*(3), 668–672. https://doi.org/10.1016/j.jstrokecerebrovasdis.2014.11.007

Fekrazad, M. H., Lopes, R. D., Stashenko, G. J., Alexander, J. H., & Garcia, D. (2009). Treatment of venous thromboembolism: Guidelines translated for the clinician. *Journal of Thrombosis and Thrombolysis, 28*(3), 270–275. https://doi.org/10.1007/s11239-009-0374-7

Fitzgerald, J. (2010). Venous thromboembolism: Have we made headway? *Orthopaedic Nursing, 29*(4), 226–234. https://doi.org/10.1097/NOR.0b013e3181e517af

Headley, C.M., & Melander, S. (2011). When it may be a pulmonary embolism. *Nephrology Nursing Journal, 38*(2), 127–152.

Kearon, C., Kahn, S., Agnelli, G., Goldhaber, S., Raskob, G., Comerota, A., & American College of Chest Physicians. (2008). Antithrombotic therapy for venous thromboembolic disease: American College of Chest Physicians evidence-based clinical practice guidelines (8th ed.). *Chest, 133*(Suppl. 6), 454S-545S.

Lancaster, S. L., Owens, A., Bryant, A. S., Ramey, L. S., Nicholson, J., Gossett, K., Forni, J. T., & Padgett, T. M. (2010). Emergency: Upper-extremity deep vein thrombosis. *AJN, American Journal of Nursing, 110*(5), 48–52. https://doi.org/10.1097/01.NAJ.0000372072.24134.a5

Lankshear, A., Harden, J., & Simms, J. (2010). Safe practice for patients receiving anticoagulant therapy. *Nursing Standard, 24*(20), 47–56. https://doi.org/10.7748/ns2010.01.24.20.47.c8157

Meetoo, D. (2010). In too deep: Understanding, detecting and managing DVT. *British Journal of Nursing (BJN), 19*(16), 1021–1022, 1024–1027. https://doi.org/10.12968/bjon.2010.19.16.78188

Shaughnessy, K. (2007). Massive pulmonary embolism. *Critical Care Nurse, 27*(1), 39–40, 42–51.

Yee, C. A. (2010). Conquering pulmonary embolism. *OR Nurse, 4*(5), 18–24.

K

Knowledge: Time Management   1866

Definition: Extent of understanding conveyed about strategies to complete commitments within an expected time frame with minimum stress

OUTCOME TARGET RATING: Maintain at_____ Increase to_____

		No Knowledge	Limited Knowledge	Moderate Knowledge	Substantial Knowledge	Extensive Knowledge	
OUTCOME OVERALL RATING		1	2	3	4	5	
Indicators:							
186601	Importance to prioritizing commitments	1	2	3	4	5	NA
186602	Importance of setting short-term goals	1	2	3	4	5	NA
186603	Importance of setting long-term goals	1	2	3	4	5	NA
186604	Strategies to prioritize commitments	1	2	3	4	5	NA
186605	Realistic timeframe for each activity	1	2	3	4	5	NA
186606	Personal limitations that affect time management	1	2	3	4	5	NA

Continued

Knowledge: Time Management—cont'd

		No Knowledge	Limited Knowledge	Moderate Knowledge	Substantial Knowledge	Extensive Knowledge	
186607	Strategies to organize personal space	1	2	3	4	5	NA
186608	Strategies to structure commitments	1	2	3	4	5	NA
186609	Strategies to manage commitments within timeframe	1	2	3	4	5	NA
186610	Strategies to balance competing demands	1	2	3	4	5	NA
186611	Strategies to track progress toward completion of commitments	1	2	3	4	5	NA
186612	Strategies for delegating activities	1	2	3	4	5	NA
186613	Strategies to minimize interruptions	1	2	3	4	5	NA
186614	Strategies to reassess commitment priorities	1	2	3	4	5	NA
186615	Strategies to prevent feeling overwhelmed	1	2	3	4	5	NA
186617	Strategies for managing social media	1	2	3	4	5	NA
186618	Strategies for managing online meetings	1	2	3	4	5	NA
186616	Benefits of time management	1	2	3	4	5	NA

Domain-*Health Knowledge & Behavior (IV)*   **Class**-*Knowledge Health Promotion (S)*   *5th edition 2013; revised 2024*

OUTCOME CONTENT REFERENCES:
Codina, N., & Pestana, J. V. (2019). Time matters differently in leisure experience for men and women: Leisure dedication and time perspective. *International Journal of Environmental Research and Public Health, 16*(14), 2513. https://doi.org/10.3390/ijerph16142513

Janeslätt, G. K., Holmqvist, K. L., White, S., & Holmefur, M. (2018). Assessment of time management skills: Psychometric properties of the Swedish version. *Scandinavian Journal of Occupational Therapy, 25*(3), 153–161. https://doi.org/10.1080/11038128.2017.1375009

Kelly, J. D., (2019). Your best life: Unlock more time in your day for rest and relaxation-that's an order. *Clinical Orthopaedics and Related Research, 477*(12), 2644–2646. https://doi.org/10.1097/CORR.0000000000001013

Wang, W. C. (2019). Exploring the relationship among free-time management, leisure boredom, and internet addiction in undergraduates in Taiwan. *Psychological Reports, 122*(5), 1651–1665. https://doi.org/10.1177/0033294118789034

+White, S. M., Riley, A., & Flom, P. (2013). Assessment of Time Management Skills (ATMS): A practice-based outcome questionnaire, *Occupational Therapy in Mental Health, 29*(3), 215-231, https://doi.org/10.1080/0164212X.2013.819481

Knowledge: Treatment Procedure   1814

Definition: Extent of understanding conveyed about a procedure required as part of a treatment regimen and carried out by a patient or caregiver

OUTCOME TARGET RATING: Maintain at_____ Increase to_____

		No Knowledge	Limited Knowledge	Moderate Knowledge	Substantial Knowledge	Extensive Knowledge	
OUTCOME OVERALL RATING		**1**	**2**	**3**	**4**	**5**	
Indicators:							
181413	Self-care responsibilities for procedure	1	2	3	4	5	NA
181401	Treatment procedure	1	2	3	4	5	NA
181402	Purpose of procedure	1	2	3	4	5	NA
181414	Frequency of procedure	1	2	3	4	5	NA
181403	Steps in procedure	1	2	3	4	5	NA
181415	Benefits related to procedure	1	2	3	4	5	NA
181405	Precautions related to procedure	1	2	3	4	5	NA
181406	Restrictions related to procedure	1	2	3	4	5	NA
181404	Correct use of equipment	1	2	3	4	5	NA
181407	Proper care of equipment	1	2	3	4	5	NA

Knowledge: Treatment Procedure—cont'd

		No Knowledge	Limited Knowledge	Moderate Knowledge	Substantial Knowledge	Extensive Knowledge	
181416	Supplies needed for the procedure	1	2	3	4	5	NA
181417	Treatment effects	1	2	3	4	5	NA
181410	Treatment side effects	1	2	3	4	5	NA
181418	Impact of procedure on lifestyle	1	2	3	4	5	NA
181409	Appropriate action for complications	1	2	3	4	5	NA
181412	Contraindications for procedure	1	2	3	4	5	NA
181419	When to obtain assistance from health professional	1	2	3	4	5	NA

Specify procedure _____

Domain-Health Knowledge & Behavior (IV)   **Class**-Knowledge Health Condition (GG)   *1st edition 1997; revised 2004, 2008, 2024*

OUTCOME CONTENT REFERENCES:

Bruno, E., Biondi, A., Thorpe, S., & Richardson, M. P., on behalf of the RADAR-CNS Consortium. (2020). *Seizure: European Journal of Epilepsy, 81*, 230–240. https://doi.org/10.1016/j.aeizure.2020.08.023

McConville, H., Harvey, M., Callahan, C., Motley, L., Difilippo, H., & White, C. (2017). CAR T-Cell therapy Effects. Review of procedures and patient education. *Clinical Journal of Oncology Nursing, 21*(3), E79–E86. https://doi.org/10.1188/17.CJON.E79-E86

McDonald, J., McKinlay, E., Keeling, S., & Levack, W. (2017). The 'wayfinding' experience of family carers who learn to manage technical health procedures at home: A grounded theory study. *Scandinavian Journal of Caring Sciences, 31*, 850–858. https://doi.org/10.1111/scs.12406

Van Halsema, E. E., Hoen, C. A., de Koning, P. S., Rosmolen, W. D., van Hooft, J. E., & Bergman, J. J. (2018). Self-dilation for therapy-resistant benign esophageal strictures. *Surgical Endoscopy, 3*, 3200–3207. https://doi.org/10.1007//s00464-018-6037-z

Walter, E., Avgush, S., Daly, C., & Crump, C. (2020). The impact of the great recession on diabetes management in a high-risk population. *Journal of Health Care for the Poor and Underserved, 31*(2), 1007–1017. https://doi.org/10.1353/hpu.2020.0074

K

Knowledge: Treatment Regimen   1813

Definition: Extent of understanding conveyed about a specific treatment regimen

OUTCOME TARGET RATING: Maintain at_____ Increase to_____

		No Knowledge	Limited Knowledge	Moderate Knowledge	Substantial Knowledge	Extensive Knowledge	
OUTCOME OVERALL RATING		1	2	3	4	5	
Indicators:							
181310	Specific disease process	1	2	3	4	5	NA
181316	Benefits of disease management	1	2	3	4	5	NA
181301	Benefits of treatment regimen	1	2	3	4	5	NA
181302	Self-care responsibilities for ongoing treatment	1	2	3	4	5	NA
181303	Self-care responsibilities for emergency situations	1	2	3	4	5	NA
181315	Self-monitoring techniques	1	2	3	4	5	NA
181304	Expected effects of treatment	1	2	3	4	5	NA
181317	Potential side effects of regimen	1	2	3	4	5	NA
181305	Prescribed diet	1	2	3	4	5	NA
181306	Prescribed medication regimen	1	2	3	4	5	NA
181307	Prescribed physical activity	1	2	3	4	5	NA
181308	Prescribed exercise	1	2	3	4	5	NA
181309	Prescribed procedure	1	2	3	4	5	NA

Continued

Knowledge: Treatment Procedure—cont'd

		No Knowledge	Limited Knowledge	Moderate Knowledge	Substantial Knowledge	Extensive Knowledge	
181318	Regimen restrictions	1	2	3	4	5	NA
181319	Type of equipment needed	1	2	3	4	5	NA
181320	Equipment maintenance	1	2	3	4	5	NA
181321	Proper disposal of equipment	1	2	3	4	5	NA
181322	Proper disposal of contaminated materials	1	2	3	4	5	NA
181323	Impact of regimen on lifestyle	1	2	3	4	5	NA
181324	Use of mobile app to increase adherence	1	2	3	4	5	NA
181324	Specific lifestyle choices for treatment	1	2	3	4	5	NA
181325	When to obtain regimen changes from health professional	1	2	3	4	5	NA

Domain-Health Knowledge & Behavior (IV)   **Class**-Knowledge Health Condition (GG)   *1st edition 1997; revised 2004, 2008, 2013, 2024*

OUTCOME CONTENT REFERENCES:

Despins, L. A., & Wakefield, B. J. (2020). Making sense of blood glucose data and self-management in individuals with type 2 diabetes mellitus: A qualitative study. *Journal of Clinical Nursing, 29*(13-14), 2572–2588. https://doi.org/10.1111/jocn.15280

Ibrahim Abu-El-Noor, N., Ibrahim Aljeesh, Y., Bottcher, B., & Khalil Abu-El-Noor, M. (2021). Impact of a mobile phone app on adherence to treatment regimens among hypertensive patients: A randomized clinical trial study. *European Journal of Cardiovascular Nursing, 20*(5), 428–435. https://doi.org/10.1177/1474515120938235

McConville, H., Harvey, M., Callahan, C., Motley, L., Difilippo, H., & White, C. (2017). CAR T-Cell therapy effects. Review of procedures and patient education. *Clinical Journal of Oncology Nursing, 21*(3), E79–E86. https://doi.org/10.1188/17.CJON.E79-E86

Pietrzykowski, Ł., Kasprzak, M., Michalski, P., Kosobucka, A., Fabiszak, T., & Kubica, A. (2022). The influence of patient expectations on adherence to treatment regimen after myocardial infarction. *Patient Education & Counseling, 105*(2), 426–431. https://doi.org/10.1016/j.pec.2021.05.030

Knowledge: Weight Management   **1841**

Definition: Extent of understanding conveyed about the promotion and maintenance of optimal body weight and fat percentage congruent with height, frame, gender, and age

OUTCOME TARGET RATING: Maintain at_____ Increase to_____

		No Knowledge	Limited Knowledge	Moderate Knowledge	Substantial Knowledge	Extensive Knowledge	
OUTCOME OVERALL RATING		1	2	3	4	5	
Indicators:							
184101	Optimal personal weight range	1	2	3	4	5	NA
184102	Optimal body mass index	1	2	3	4	5	NA
184103	Strategies to reach optimal weight	1	2	3	4	5	NA
184104	Strategies to maintain optimal weight	1	2	3	4	5	NA
184105	Relationship among diet, exercise, and weight	1	2	3	4	5	NA
184106	Health risks related to overweight	1	2	3	4	5	NA
184107	Health risks related to underweight	1	2	3	4	5	NA
184108	Appetite versus hunger	1	2	3	4	5	NA
184109	Healthy nutritional practices	1	2	3	4	5	NA
184110	Adequate fluid intake	1	2	3	4	5	NA
184111	Strategies to modify food intake	1	2	3	4	5	NA
184112	Food cravings that trigger unhealthy eating	1	2	3	4	5	NA
184113	Emotional states that trigger unhealthy eating	1	2	3	4	5	NA
184114	Benefits of regular exercise	1	2	3	4	5	NA
184115	Exercises to maintain optimal weight	1	2	3	4	5	NA
184116	Barriers to implementing exercise routine	1	2	3	4	5	NA

K

Knowledge: Weight Management—cont'd

		No Knowledge	Limited Knowledge	Moderate Knowledge	Substantial Knowledge	Extensive Knowledge	
184117	Strategies to modify behavior	1	2	3	4	5	NA
184118	Lifestyle changes to promote optimal weight	1	2	3	4	5	NA
184119	Benefits of prescribed weight loss medication	1	2	3	4	5	NA
184120	Potential dangers of non-prescription medication	1	2	3	4	5	NA
184121	Surgical treatment options for weight loss	1	2	3	4	5	NA
184131	Benefits of regular sleep	1	2	3	4	5	NA
184122	Benefits of hypnosis	1	2	3	4	5	NA
184123	Benefits of alternative therapies	1	2	3	4	5	NA
184124	Benefits of social support	1	2	3	4	5	NA
184125	Risks associated with treatment options	1	2	3	4	5	NA
184126	Available support groups	1	2	3	4	5	NA
184127	Available community resources	1	2	3	4	5	NA
184128	Reputable sources of weight management information	1	2	3	4	5	NA
184129	Self-monitoring techniques	1	2	3	4	5	NA
184130	When to obtain assistance from a health professional	1	2	3	4	5	NA

Domain-*Health Knowledge & Behavior (IV)*   **Class**-*Knowledge Health Promotion (S)*   *4th edition 2008; revised 2013, 2024*

OUTCOME CONTENT REFERENCES:

Cheng, F. W., Garay, J. L., & Handu, D. (2021). Weight management interventions for adults with overweight or obesity: An evidence analysis center scoping review. *Journal of the Academy of Nutrition and Dietetics, 121*(9), 1855–1865. https://doi.org/10.1016/j.jand.2020.07.022

Ensign, A., & Couch, K. (2021). Improving effective weight management in a university health center. *The Journal for Nurse Practitioners, 17,* 1183–1188. https://doi.org/10.1016/j.nurpra.2021.09.023

House, E. T., Gow, M. L., Lister, N. B., Baur, L. A., Garnett, S. P., Paxton, S. J., & Jebeile, H. (2021). Pediatric weight management, dietary restraint, dieting, and eating disorder risk: A systematic review. *Nutrition Reviews, 79*(10), 1114–1133. https://doi.org/10.1093/nutrit/nuaa127

Killian, H. J., Pallotto, I. K., Sweeney, B. R., & Gillette, M. L. D. (2022). Weight management outcomes of youth with autism spectrum disorder seeking treatment from a multidisciplinary team. *Journal of Autism and Developmental Disorders, 52,* 791–799. https://doi.org/10.1007/s10803-021-04982-1

Kuk, J. L., Christensen, R. A. G., Samani, E. K., & Wharton, S. (2021). Predictors of weight loss and weight gain in weight management patients during the COVID-19 pandemic. *Journal of Obesity, 2021,* 1–8. https://doi.org/10.1155/2021/4881430

LaVela, S. L., Jones, K., Heienmann, A. W., Bartle, B., & Ehrlich-Jones, L. S. (2021). Motivators, goal setting and helpful feedback for weight management among individuals with spinal cord injury. *Rehabilitation Psychology, 66*(3), 257–264. https://doi.org/10.1037/rep0000385

Leslie, J. L., Stough, C. O., Lee, S.-Y., Mitchell, M. L., & Kalarchian, M. (2021). Healthy measures: Feasibility study of a moderate carbohydrate weight management intervention. *Public Health Nursing, 38,* 1126–1130. https://doi.org/10.1111/phn.12937

Potter, P., Perry, A., Stockert, P., & Hall, A. (2021). *Fundamentals of nursing* (10th ed.). Elsevier.

Suire, K. B., Kavookjian, J., Feiss, R., & Wadsworth, D. D. (2021). Motivational interviewing for weight management among women: A meta-analysis and systemic review of RCTs. *International Journal of Behavioral Medicine, 28,* 403–416. https://doi.org/10.1007/s12529-020-09934-0

Tee, L. P., Brandreth, R. A., Sauven, N., Clarke, L., & Frampton, I. (2021). Successful outcomes in children's specialist weight management: Impact assessment of a novel early year's weight management programme. *Journal of Human Nutrition and Diet, 34,* 819-826. https://doi.org/10.1111/jhn.12872

K

Knowledge: Wound Management

3209

Definition: Extent of understanding conveyed about caring for a surgical incision, puncture, ulcer, or open wound following tissue injury

OUTCOME TARGET RATING: Maintain at_____   Increase to_____

		No Knowledge	Limited Knowledge	Moderate Knowledge	Substantial Knowledge	Extensive Knowledge	
OUTCOME OVERALL RATING		1	2	3	4	5	
Indicators:							
320901	Type of wound	1	2	3	4	5	NA
320902	Type of closure	1	2	3	4	5	NA
320903	Risks associated with wound type	1	2	3	4	5	NA

Continued

Knowledge: Wound Management—cont'd

		No Knowledge	Limited Knowledge	Moderate Knowledge	Substantial Knowledge	Extensive Knowledge	
320904	Bathing restrictions	1	2	3	4	5	NA
320905	Modification of daily activity	1	2	3	4	5	NA
320906	Signs and symptoms of infection	1	2	3	4	5	NA
320907	Importance of completing antibiotic therapy	1	2	3	4	5	NA
320908	Pain control strategies for dressing changes	1	2	3	4	5	NA
320909	Supplies required to care for wound	1	2	3	4	5	NA
320910	Where to obtain supplies	1	2	3	4	5	NA
320911	When to ask for personal assistance	1	2	3	4	5	NA
320912	History of sensitivity to tape	1	2	3	4	5	NA
320913	History of sensitivity to cleansing solution	1	2	3	4	5	NA
320914	Importance of hand washing	1	2	3	4	5	NA
320915	Self-care activities for cleaning wound	1	2	3	4	5	NA
320916	Characteristics of wound healing	1	2	3	4	5	NA
320917	Use of ointments	1	2	3	4	5	NA
320918	Self-care activities for dressing change	1	2	3	4	5	NA
320919	Self-care activities for wound irrigation	1	2	3	4	5	NA
320920	Self-care activities for wound drainage system	1	2	3	4	5	NA
320921	Types of drainage expected	1	2	3	4	5	NA
320922	Self-care activities for packing open wound	1	2	3	4	5	NA
320923	Signs of wound dehiscence	1	2	3	4	5	NA
320924	Disposal of contaminated materials	1	2	3	4	5	NA
320925	Evidence of tissue granulation	1	2	3	4	5	NA
320926	Importance of tetanus immunization	1	2	3	4	5	NA
320927	Benefits of a healthy diet	1	2	3	4	5	NA
320928	Importance of reporting increased bleeding to health professional	1	2	3	4	5	NA
320929	Importance of reporting increased drainage to health professional	1	2	3	4	5	NA
320930	Importance of reporting fever to health professional	1	2	3	4	5	NA
320931	Importance of keeping appointments with health professional	1	2	3	4	5	NA
320932	Importance of using sunscreen once healing occurs	1	2	3	4	5	NA

Domain-Health Knowledge & Behavior (IV)   **Class**-Knowledge Health Condition (GG)   6th edition 2018

OUTCOME CONTENT REFERENCES:

Black, K., Cico, S., & Caglar, D. (2015). Wound management. *Pediatrics in Review, 36*(5), 207–216. https://doi.org/10.1542/pir.36-5-207

Chen, Y.-C., Wang, Y.-C., Chen, W.-K., Smith, M., Huang, H.-M., & Huang, L.-C. (2012). The effectiveness of a health education intervention on self-care of traumatic wounds. *Journal of Clinical Nursing, 22*(17/18), 2499–2508. https://doi.org/10.1111/j.1365-2702.2012.04295.x

Cousins, Y. (2014). Wound care considerations in neonates. *Nursing Standards, 28*(46), 61–70. https://doi.org/10.7748/ns.28.46.61.e8402

Zarchi, K., Martinussen, T., & Jemec, G. (2015). Wound healing and all-cause mortality in 958 wound patients treated in home care. *Wound Repair and Regeneration, 23*(5), 753–758. https://doi.org/10.1111/wrr.12335

Leisure Participation   **1604**

Definition: Use of relaxing, interesting, and enjoyable activities to promote well-being

OUTCOME TARGET RATING: Maintain at_____ Increase to_____

		Never Demonstrated	Rarely Demonstrated	Sometimes Demonstrated	Often Demonstrated	Consistently Demonstrated	
OUTCOME OVERALL RATING		1	2	3	4	5	
Indicators:							
160401	Participates in activities other than regular work	1	2	3	4	5	NA
160410	Participates in high physical demand leisure activities	1	2	3	4	5	NA
160411	Participates in low physical demand leisure activities	1	2	3	4	5	NA
160414	Participates in social activities with others	1	2	3	4	5	NA
160415	Participates in hobbies	1	2	3	4	5	NA
160416	Participates in volunteer activities	1	2	3	4	5	NA
160412	Selects leisure activities of interest	1	2	3	4	5	NA
160402	Expresses satisfaction with leisure activities	1	2	3	4	5	NA
160404	Feels relaxed after leisure activities	1	2	3	4	5	NA
160413	Enjoys leisure activities	1	2	3	4	5	NA
160405	Exhibits creativity through leisure activities	1	2	3	4	5	NA
160407	Identifies recreational options	1	2	3	4	5	NA
160417	Explores new leisure activities	1	2	3	4	5	NA

Domain-*Health Knowledge & Behavior (IV)*   **Class**-*Health Behavior (Q)*   *1st edition 1997; revised 2004, 2008, 2024*

OUTCOME CONTENT REFERENCES:
Boot, W. R., Andringa, R., Harrell, E. H., Dieciuc, M. A., & Roque, N. A. (2020). Older adults and video gaming for leisure: Lessons from the Center for Research and Education on Aging and Technology Enhancement (CREATE). *Gerontechnology, 19*(2), 138–146. https://doi.org/10.4017/gt.2020.19.2.006.00
+Drummond, A. E. R., & Walker, M. F. (1994). The Nottingham Leisure Questionnaire for stroke patients. *British Journal of Occupational Therapy, 57*(11), 414–418.
+Drummond, A. E. R., Parker, C. J., Gladman, J. R., & Logan, P. A. (2001). Development and validation of the Nottingham Leisure Questionnaire (NLQ). *Clinical Rehabilitation, 15*(6), 647–56. https://doi.org/10.1191/0269215501cr438oa
Merims, D., Natan, M. B., & Seleznev, I. (2018). The effect of leisure activities, purpose in life, and spirituality on short-term outcomes of geriatric rehabilitation. *Topics in Geriatric Rehabilitation, 34*(3), 207–212. https://doi.org/10.1097/TGR.0000000000000196
Nastasi, J. A. (2020). Occupational therapy interventions supporting leisure and social participation for older adults with low vision: A systematic review. *American Journal of Occupational Therapy, 74*, 7401185020. https://doi.org/10.5014/ajot.2020.038521
Smallfield, S., & Molitor, W. L. (2018). Occupational therapy interventions supporting social participation and leisure engagement for community dwelling older adults: A systematic review. *American Journal of Occupational Therapy, 72*, 7204190020. https://doi.org/10.5014/ajot.2018.030627

Lifestyle Balance   **2013**

Definition: Personal actions to live a healthy, balanced lifestyle consistent with one's values, strengths, and interests through conscious adherence to daily health habits and efforts to reduce or minimize stress

OUTCOME TARGET RATING: Maintain at_____ Increase to_____

		Never Demonstrated	Rarely Demonstrated	Sometimes Demonstrated	Often Demonstrated	Consistently Demonstrated	
OUTCOME OVERALL RATING		1	2	3	4	5	
Indicators:							
201301	Recognizes need for balancing life activities	1	2	3	4	5	NA
201302	Seeks information about strategies to balance life activities	1	2	3	4	5	NA

Continued

L

Lifestyle Balance—cont'd

		Never Demonstrated	Rarely Demonstrated	Sometimes Demonstrated	Often Demonstrated	Consistently Demonstrated	
201303	Considers personal needs and values when choosing life activities	1	2	3	4	5	NA
201304	Identifies personal strengths	1	2	3	4	5	NA
201305	Identifies major sources of stress	1	2	3	4	5	NA
201306	Uses strategies to reduce stress	1	2	3	4	5	NA
201307	Evaluates areas of perceived imbalance in lifestyle	1	2	3	4	5	NA
201308	Limits activities that contribute to a sense of feeling burdened	1	2	3	4	5	NA
201309	Uses strategies to balance work activities and family roles	1	2	3	4	5	NA
201310	Uses time management in daily routine	1	2	3	4	5	NA
201311	Organizes time and energy to meet personal goals	1	2	3	4	5	NA
201312	Modifies role responsibilities within the family as needed	1	2	3	4	5	NA
201313	Uses strategies to adapt to multiple role responsibilities	1	2	3	4	5	NA
201314	Engages in activities that meet psychological needs	1	2	3	4	5	NA
201315	Synchronizes daily activities with biological rhythms	1	2	3	4	5	NA
201316	Engages in activities that promote personal growth	1	2	3	4	5	NA
201317	Engages in activities consistent with personal values	1	2	3	4	5	NA

Domain- *Health Knowledge & Behavior (IV)*   **Class-***Health Supporting Life Skills (II)*   *5th edition 2013*

OUTCOME CONTENT REFERENCES:

Christiansen, C. H., & Matuska, K. M. (2006). Lifestyle balance: A review of concepts and research. *Journal of Occupational Science, 13*(1), 49–61. https://doi.org/10.1080/14427591.200609686570

Grant, N., Wardle, J., & Steptoe, A. (2009). The relationship between life satisfaction and health behavior: A cross-cultural analysis of young adults. *International Journal of Behavioral Medicine, 16*(3), 259–268. https://doi.org/10.1007/s12529-009-9032-x

Hwang, J. E. (2010). Promoting healthy lifestyles with aging: Development and validation of the Health Enhancement Lifestyle Profile (HELP) using the Rasch measurement model. *American Journal of Occupational Therapy, 64*(5), 786–795. https://doi.org/10.5014/ajot.2010.09088

Kennedy, C., & Miller, M. (2005). The future of fitness: Is "lifestyle enhancement" the wellness balance we should help clients seek in the coming years? *IDEA Fitness Journal, 2*(7), 104–108.

Lawrence, W., & Sherrod, D. (2009). Are you successfully balancing your work and home life? *Nursing Management, 40*(5), 51, 53. https://doi.org/10.1097/01.NUMA.0000351538.49522.42

Matuska, K. M., & Christiansen, C. H. (2008). A proposed model of lifestyle balance. *Journal of Occupational Science, 15*(1), 9–19. https://doi.org/10.1080/14427591.2008.9686602

Teta, J., & Teta, K. (2005). The impact of lifestyle choices and hormonal balance on coping with stress. *Townsend Letter for Doctors & Patients, 269*, 8–91.

Liver Function   0803

Definition: Ability of the liver to manufacture, store, alter, and secrete substances essential for metabolism and other body functions

OUTCOME TARGET RATING: Maintain at_____ Increase to_____

		Severely Compromised	Substantially Compromised	Moderately Compromised	Mildly Compromised	Not Compromised	
OUTCOME OVERALL RATING		1	2	3	4	5	
Indicators:							
080301	Appetite	1	2	3	4	5	NA
080302	Color of stool	1	2	3	4	5	NA
080303	Sleep	1	2	3	4	5	NA
080304	Stamina	1	2	3	4	5	NA
080305	Albumin/globulin ratio	1	2	3	4	5	NA
080306	Skin turgor	1	2	3	4	5	NA
080307	Consciousness	1	2	3	4	5	NA
		Severe	**Substantial**	**Moderate**	**Mild**	**None**	
080308	Increased total serum bilirubin	1	2	3	4	5	NA
080309	Increased direct serum bilirubin	1	2	3	4	5	NA
080310	Prolonged prothrombin time	1	2	3	4	5	NA
080311	Serum ammonia level	1	2	3	4	5	NA
080312	Increased alanine transaminase (ALT) (SGPT)	1	2	3	4	5	NA
080313	Increased aspartate aminotransferase (AST) (SGOT)	1	2	3	4	5	NA
080314	Increased gamma-glutamyl transferase (GGT)	1	2	3	4	5	NA
080315	Jaundice	1	2	3	4	5	NA
080316	Pruritus	1	2	3	4	5	NA
080317	Spider angiomas	1	2	3	4	5	NA
080318	Petechiae	1	2	3	4	5	NA
080319	Palmar erythema	1	2	3	4	5	NA
080320	Tremor	1	2	3	4	5	NA
080321	Muscle atrophy	1	2	3	4	5	NA
080322	Ascites	1	2	3	4	5	NA
080323	Weight gain	1	2	3	4	5	NA
080324	Dilated abdominal wall veins	1	2	3	4	5	NA
080325	Increased abdominal girth	1	2	3	4	5	NA
080326	Abdominal pain	1	2	3	4	5	NA
080327	Liver tenderness	1	2	3	4	5	NA
080328	Bruising	1	2	3	4	5	NA
080329	Hematemesis	1	2	3	4	5	NA
080330	Blood in stools	1	2	3	4	5	NA
080331	Anorexia	1	2	3	4	5	NA
080332	Fatigue	1	2	3	4	5	NA
080333	Agitation	1	2	3	4	5	NA

Domain-*Physiologic Health (II)*   **Class**-*Metabolic Regulation (I)*   *5th edition 2013; reviewed 2024*

OUTCOME CONTENT REFERENCES:
Cheng, M. L., Nakib, D., Perciani, C. T., & MacParland, S. A. (2021). The immune niche of the liver. *Clinical Science* (London, England), *135*(20), 2445–2466. https://doi.org/10.1042/CS20190654
Huether, S. E., McCance, K. L., & Brashers, V. L. (2020). *Understanding pathophysiology* (7th ed.). Elsevier.
Ignatavicius, D. D., Workman, M. L., Rebar, C. R., & Heimgartner, N. M. (2021). *Medical-surgical nursing: Concepts for interprofessional care* (10th ed.). Elsevier.
Kortgen, A., Recknagel, P., & Bauer, M. (2010). How to assess liver function? *Current Opinion in Critical Care, 16*(2), 136–141. https://doi.org/10.1097/MCC.0b013e3283361813
Piantanida, E., Ippolito, S., Gallo, D., Masiello, E., Premoli, P., Cusini, C., Rosetti, S., Sabatino, J., Segato, S., Trimarchi, F., Bartalena, L., & Tanda, M. L. (2020). The interplay between thyroid and liver: Implications for clinical practice. *Journal of Endocrinological Investigation, 43*(7), 885–899. https://doi.org/10.1007/s40618-020-01208-6
Trefts, E., Gannon, M., & Wasserman, D. H. (2017). The liver. *Current Biology, 27*(21), R1147–R1151. https://doi.org/10.1016/j.cub.2017.09.019

Loneliness Severity 1203

Definition: Severity of emotional, social, or existential signs and symptoms of isolation

OUTCOME TARGET RATING: Maintain at_____ Increase to_____

		Severe	Substantial	Moderate	Mild	None	
OUTCOME OVERALL RATING		1	2	3	4	5	
Indicators:							
120301	Sense of unfounded dread	1	2	3	4	5	NA
120302	Sense of desperation	1	2	3	4	5	NA
120303	Sense of extreme restlessness	1	2	3	4	5	NA
120304	Sense of hopelessness	1	2	3	4	5	NA
120305	Sense of not belonging	1	2	3	4	5	NA
120306	Sense of loss due to separation from another	1	2	3	4	5	NA
120307	Sense of social isolation	1	2	3	4	5	NA
120308	Sense of not being understood	1	2	3	4	5	NA
120309	Sense of being excluded	1	2	3	4	5	NA
120310	Sense that time seems endless	1	2	3	4	5	NA
120311	Difficulty in planning	1	2	3	4	5	NA
120312	Difficulty in contacting others	1	2	3	4	5	NA
120313	Difficulty overcoming separateness	1	2	3	4	5	NA
120314	Difficulty in effecting a mutual relationship	1	2	3	4	5	NA
120315	Mood fluctuations	1	2	3	4	5	NA
120316	Impaired concentration	1	2	3	4	5	NA
120317	Non-assertiveness	1	2	3	4	5	NA
120318	Difficulty making decisions	1	2	3	4	5	NA
120328	Unhealthy eating pattern	1	2	3	4	5	NA
120320	Sleep disturbance	1	2	3	4	5	NA
120321	Headaches	1	2	3	4	5	NA
120322	Nausea	1	2	3	4	5	NA
120323	Decreased activity level	1	2	3	4	5	NA
120324	Pain	1	2	3	4	5	NA
120325	Spiritual discomfort	1	2	3	4	5	NA
120329	Sadness	1	2	3	4	5	NA
120327	Depression	1	2	3	4	5	NA
120330	Lack of purpose in life	1	2	3	4	5	NA

Domain-*Psychosocial Health (III)*   **Class**-*Psychological Well-Being (M)*   *1st edition 1997; revised 2004, 2008, 2013, 2024*

OUTCOME CONTENT REFERENCES:
+Hughes, M. E., Waite, L. J., Hawkley, L. C., & Cacioppo. J. T. (2004). A short scale for measuring loneliness in large surveys: Results from two population-based studies. *Research in Aging, 26*(6), 655–672. https://doi.org/10.1177/0164027504268574
+Lee, C., Cho, B., Yang, Q., Chang, S. J., Ryu, S.-I., Noh, E.-Y., & Park, Y.-H. (2021). A psychometric analysis of the 20-item Revised University of California Los Angeles Loneliness Scale among Korean older adults living alone. *Research in Gerontological Nursing, 14*(6), 306–316. https://doi.org/10.3928/19404921-20210924-03
Malhotra, R., Tareque, M. I., Saito, Y., Ma, S., Chiu, C., & Chan, A. (2021). Loneliness and health expectancy among older adults: A longitudinal population-based study. *Journal of the American Geriatrics Society, 69*(11), 3092–3102. https://doi.org/10.1111/jgs.17343
O'Shea, B. Q., Finlay, J. M., Kler, J., Joseph, C. A., & Kobayashi, L. C. (2021). Loneliness among U.S. adults aged ≥55 early in the COVID-19 pandemic: Findings from the COVID-19 coping study. *Public Health Reports, 136*(6), 754–764. https://doi.org/10.1177/00333549211029965

Peng, A., Tang, Y., He, S., Ji, S., Dong, B., & Chen, L. (2021). Association between loneliness, sleep behavior and quality: A propensity-score-matched case-control study. *Sleep Medicine, 86*, 19–24. https://doi.org/10.1016/j.sleep.2021.08.008

Shah, S., Nogueras, D., van Woerden, H. C., & Kiparoglou, V. (2020). The COVID-19 pandemic: A pandemic of lockdown loneliness and the role of digital technology. *Journal of Medical Internet Research, 22*(11), e22287. https://doi.org/10.2196/22287

van Tilburg, T. G. (2021). Social, emotional, and existential loneliness: A test of the multidimensional concept. *Gerontologist, 61*(7), e335–e344. https://doi.org/10.1093/geront/gnaa082

Vedder, A., Boerner, K., Stokes, J. E., Henk, A. W., Schut, A. W., Boelen, P. A., & Stroebe, M. S. (2022). A systematic review of loneliness in bereavement: Current research and future directions. *Current Opinion in Psychology, 43*, 48–64. https://doi.org/10.1016/j.copsyc.2021.06.003

Yanguas, J., Pinazo-Henandis, S., & Tarazona-Santabalbina, F. J. (2018). The complexity of loneliness. *Acta Bio-Medical: Atenei Parmensis, 89*(2), 302–314. https://doi.org/10.23750/abm.v89i2.7404

Lymphedema Severity   2117

Definition: Severity of adverse physical, emotional, and social responses due to lymphedema

OUTCOME TARGET RATING: Maintain at_____ Increase to_____

OUTCOME OVERALL RATING	Severe 1	Substantial 2	Moderate 3	Mild 4	None 5	
Indicators:						
211701 Edema of affected area	1	2	3	4	5	NA
211702 Pitting edema of affected area	1	2	3	4	5	NA
211703 Aching of affected area	1	2	3	4	5	NA
211704 Skin firmness of affected area	1	2	3	4	5	NA
211705 Skin tightness of affected area	1	2	3	4	5	NA
211706 Heaviness of affected area	1	2	3	4	5	NA
211707 Numbness of affected area	1	2	3	4	5	NA
211708 Limited physical function	1	2	3	4	5	NA
211709 Limited mobility	1	2	3	4	5	NA
211710 Stiffness of affected area	1	2	3	4	5	NA
211711 Development of pockets of fluid	1	2	3	4	5	NA
211712 Chest wall edema	1	2	3	4	5	NA
211713 Increased temperature of affected extremity	1	2	3	4	5	NA
211714 Redness of affected area	1	2	3	4	5	NA
211715 Blistering of affected area	1	2	3	4	5	NA
211716 Pain	1	2	3	4	5	NA
211717 Depression level	1	2	3	4	5	NA
211718 Anxiety level	1	2	3	4	5	NA
211719 Sense of hopelessness	1	2	3	4	5	NA
211720 Sense of helplessness	1	2	3	4	5	NA
211721 Sense of social exclusion	1	2	3	4	5	NA
211722 Sense of social isolation	1	2	3	4	5	NA
211723 Sense of abandonment	1	2	3	4	5	NA
211724 Emotional disturbance	1	2	3	4	5	NA
211725 Negative body image	1	2	3	4	5	NA
211726 Negative self-esteem	1	2	3	4	5	NA
211727 Symptom burden	1	2	3	4	5	NA
211728 Treatment burden	1	2	3	4	5	NA

Domain-*Health & Life Quality (V)*   **Class**-*Symptom Status (V)*   6th edition 2018

OUTCOME CONTENT REFERENCES:

Armer, J. M., Henggeler, M. H., Brooks, C. W., Zagar, E. A., Homan, S., & Stewart, B. R. (2008). The health deviation of post-breast cancer lymphedema: Symptom assessment and impact on self-care agency. *Self-Care, Dependent-Care & Nursing, 16*(1), 14–21.

Armer, J., Hulett, J., Bernas, M., Ostby, P., Stewart, B., & Cormier, J. (2013). Best practice guidelines in assessment, risk reduction, management, and surveillance for post-breast cancer lymphedema. *Current Breast Cancer Reports, 5*(2), 134–144. https://doi.org/10.1007/s12609-013-0105-0

Dominick, S. A., Madlensky, L., Natarajan, L., & Pierce, J. P. (2012). Risk factors associated with breast cancer-related lymphedema in the WHEL study. *Journal of Cancer Survivorship, 7*(1), 115–123. https://doi.org/10.1007/s11764-012-0251-9

Fu, M. R., Ridner, S. H., Hu, S. H., Stewart, B. R., Cormier, J. N., & Armer, J. M. (2013). Psychosocial impact of lymphedema: A systematic review of literature from 2004 to 2011. *Psycho-Oncology, 22*(7), 1466–1484. https://doi.org/10.1002/pon.3201

Ostby, P. L., & Armer, J. M. (2015). Complexities of adherence and post-cancer lymphedema management. *Journal of Personalized Medicine, 5*(4), 370–388. https://doi.org/10.3390/jpm5040370

Maternal Status: Antepartum 2509

Definition: Extent to which maternal well-being is within normal limits from conception to the onset of labor

OUTCOME TARGET RATING: Maintain at_____ Increase to_____

		Severe Deviation from Normal Range	Substantial Deviation from Normal Range	Moderate Deviation from Normal Range	Mild Deviation from Normal Range	No Deviation from Normal Range	
OUTCOME OVERALL RATING		**1**	**2**	**3**	**4**	**5**	
Indicators:							
250901	Emotional attachment to fetus	1	2	3	4	5	NA
250902	Coping with discomforts of pregnancy	1	2	3	4	5	NA
250903	Mood lability	1	2	3	4	5	NA
250904	Weight change	1	2	3	4	5	NA
250907	Cognitive status	1	2	3	4	5	NA
250908	Visual acuity	1	2	3	4	5	NA
250910	Neurological reflexes	1	2	3	4	5	NA
250916	Blood pressure	1	2	3	4	5	NA
250917	Radial pulse rate	1	2	3	4	5	NA
250926	Apical heart rate	1	2	3	4	5	NA
250929	Respiratory rate	1	2	3	4	5	NA
250918	Body temperature	1	2	3	4	5	NA
250919	Urine protein	1	2	3	4	5	NA
250920	Urine glucose	1	2	3	4	5	NA
250921	Blood glucose	1	2	3	4	5	NA
250922	Hemoglobin	1	2	3	4	5	NA
250923	Liver enzymes	1	2	3	4	5	NA
250924	Blood count	1	2	3	4	5	NA
250931	Fundus height	1	2	3	4	5	NA
		Severe	Substantial	Moderate	Mild	None	
250905	Edema	1	2	3	4	5	NA
250906	Headache	1	2	3	4	5	NA
250909	Seizure activity	1	2	3	4	5	NA
250911	Nausea	1	2	3	4	5	NA
250928	Vomiting	1	2	3	4	5	NA
250912	Abdominal pain	1	2	3	4	5	NA
250913	Epigastric pain	1	2	3	4	5	NA
250914	Vaginal bleeding	1	2	3	4	5	NA
250915	Vaginal discharge	1	2	3	4	5	NA
250927	Heartburn	1	2	3	4	5	NA
250930	Constipation	1	2	3	4	5	NA
250932	Backache	1	2	3	4	5	NA

Domain-*Health & Life Quality (V)*   **Class**- *Health Status (JJ)*   *2nd edition 2000; revised 2004, 2008, 2013, 2024*

OUTCOME CONTENT REFERENCES:

American College of Obstetricians and Gynecologists, Committee on Practice Bulletins—Obstetrics. (2018). ACOG Practice Bulletin No. 189: Nausea and vomiting of pregnancy. *Obstetrics & Gynecology, 131*(1), e15– e30. https://doi.org/10.1097/AOG.0000000000002456

Folk, D. M. (2018). Hypertensive disorders of pregnancy: Overview and current recommendations. *Journal of Midwifery & Women's Health, 63*(3), 289–300. https://doi.org/10.1111/jmwh.12725

Kominiarek, M. A., Gray, E. L., Vyhmeister, H., Grobman, W., & Simon, M. (2018). Association of gestational weight gain with prenatal care model. *Journal of Midwifery & Women's Health, 63,* 283–288. https://doi.org/10.1111/jmwh.12759

Lowdermilk, D. L., Cashion, M. C., Perry, S. E., Alden, K. R., & Olshansky, E. (2019). *Maternity and women's health care* (12th ed.). Mosby.

Maddahi, M. S., Dolatian, M., Khoramabadi, M., & Talebi, A. (2016). Correlation of maternal-fetal attachment and health practices during pregnancy with neonatal outcomes. *Electronic Physician Journal, 8*(7), 2639–2644. https://doi.org/10.19082/2639

O'Meara, A. (2019). *Maternity, newborn, and women's health nursing: A case-based approach* (1st ed.). Wolters Kluwer.

Saturno-Hernández, P. J., Martínez-Nicolás, I., Moreno-Zegbe, E., Fernández-Elorriaga, M., & Poblano-Verástegui, O. (2019). Indicators for monitoring maternal and neonatal quality care: A systematic review. *BMC Pregnancy Childbirth, 25*(19), 1–10. https://doi.org/10.1186/s12884-019-2173-2

Tunçalp, Ö., Pena-Rosas, J. P., Lawrie, T., Bucagu, M., Oladapo, O. T., Portela, A., & Metin Gülmezoglu, A. (2017). WHO recommendations on antenatal care for a positive pregnancy experience—Going beyond survival. *BJOG: An International Journal of Obstetrics and Gynecology, 124*(6), 60–862. https://doi.org/10.1111/1471-0528.14599

M

Maternal Status: Intrapartum 2510

Definition: Extent to which maternal well-being is within normal limits from onset of labor to delivery

OUTCOME TARGET RATING: Maintain at_____ Increase to_____

		Severe Deviation from Normal Range	Substantial Deviation from Normal Range	Moderate Deviation from Normal Range	Mild Deviation from Normal Range	No Deviation from Normal Range	
OUTCOME OVERALL RATING		**1**	**2**	**3**	**4**	**5**	
Indicators:							
251001	Coping with discomforts of labor	1	2	3	4	5	NA
251003	Use of techniques to facilitate labor	1	2	3	4	5	NA
251004	Uterine contraction frequency	1	2	3	4	5	NA
251005	Uterine contraction duration	1	2	3	4	5	NA
251006	Uterine contraction intensity	1	2	3	4	5	NA
251007	Progression of cervical dilation	1	2	3	4	5	NA
251009	Blood pressure	1	2	3	4	5	NA
251010	Radial pulse rate	1	2	3	4	5	NA
251021	Apical heart rate	1	2	3	4	5	NA
251011	Blood glucose	1	2	3	4	5	NA
251012	Body temperature	1	2	3	4	5	NA
251013	Urine output	1	2	3	4	5	NA
251014	Visual acuity	1	2	3	4	5	NA
251015	Cognitive status	1	2	3	4	5	NA
251016	Neurological reflexes	1	2	3	4	5	NA
251026	Partograph status	1	2	3	4	5	NA
251027	Hydration	1	2	3	4	5	NA
		Severe	**Substantial**	**Moderate**	**Mild**	**None**	
251008	Vaginal bleeding	1	2	3	4	5	NA
251017	Seizure activity	1	2	3	4	5	NA
251018	Headache	1	2	3	4	5	NA
251019	Epigastric pain	1	2	3	4	5	NA
251022	Pain with contractions	1	2	3	4	5	NA
251023	Back pain	1	2	3	4	5	NA
251024	Nausea	1	2	3	4	5	NA
251025	Vomiting	1	2	3	4	5	NA

M

Domain- *Health & Life Quality (V)* **Class-** *Health Status (JJ)* *2nd edition 2000; revised 2004, 2024*

OUTCOME CONTENT REFERENCES:

Ashwal, E., Livne, M. Y., Benichou, J. I. C., Unger, R., Hiersch, L., Aviram, A., Mani, A., & Yogev, Y. (2020). Contemporary patterns of labor in nulliparous and multiparous women. *American Journal of Obstetrics and Gynecology, 222*(3), 267.e1–267.e9. https://doi.org/10.1016/j.ajog.2019.09.035

Bohren, M. A., Hofmeyr, G. J., Sakala, C., Fukuzawa, R. K., & Cuthbert, A. (2017). Continuous support for women during childbirth. *Cochrane Database Systematic Review, 7*(7). https://doi.org/10.1002/14651858.CD003766.pub6

Lavender, T., & Bernitz, S. (2020). Use of the partograph—Current thinking. *Best Practice & Research Clinical Obstetrics & Gynecology, 67*, 33–43. https://doi.org/10.1016/j.bpobgyn.2020.03.01

Mattson, S. (Ed.). (2015). *Core curriculum for maternal-newborn nursing, core curriculum for maternal-newborn nursing* (5th ed.). Saunders.

Olza, I., Leahy-Warren, P., Benyamini, Y., Kazmierczak, M., Karlsdottir, S. I., Spyridou, A., Crespo-Mirasol, E., Takács, L., Hall, P. J., Murphy, M., Jonsdottir, S. S., Downe, S., & Nieuwenhuijze, M. J. (2018). Women's psychological experiences of physiological childbirth: A meta-synthesis. *BMJ Open, 8*(10), e020347. https://doi.org/10.1136/bmjopen-2017-020347

Wolf, M. F., Shnaider, O., Sharabi, L., Biderman, S. N., Elon, R., & Bornstein, J. (2019). Optimal continuous support accompanying labor—The midwives' and laboring women's point of view. *Israel Journal of Health Policy Research, 8*(1), 27. https://doi.org/10.1186/s13584-019-0299-3

Maternal Status: Postpartum 2511

Definition: Extent to which maternal well-being is within normal limits from delivery of placenta to completion of involution

OUTCOME TARGET RATING: Maintain at_____ Increase to_____

		Severe Deviation from Normal Range	Substantial Deviation from Normal Range	Moderate Deviation from Normal Range	Mild Deviation from Normal Range	No Deviation from Normal Range	
OUTCOME OVERALL RATING		1	2	3	4	5	
Indicators:							
251101	Mood equilibrium	1	2	3	4	5	NA
251102	Comfort	1	2	3	4	5	NA
251103	Blood pressure	1	2	3	4	5	NA
251104	Apical heart rate	1	2	3	4	5	NA
251123	Radial pulse rate	1	2	3	4	5	NA
251105	Peripheral circulation	1	2	3	4	5	NA
251106	Uterine fundal height	1	2	3	4	5	NA
251107	Lochia amount	1	2	3	4	5	NA
251124	Lochia color	1	2	3	4	5	NA
251108	Breast fullness	1	2	3	4	5	NA
251109	Breast comfort	1	2	3	4	5	NA
251110	Perineal healing	1	2	3	4	5	NA
251111	Incisional healing	1	2	3	4	5	NA
251112	Body temperature	1	2	3	4	5	NA
251114	Urinary elimination	1	2	3	4	5	NA
251115	Bowel elimination	1	2	3	4	5	NA
251116	Food and fluid intake	1	2	3	4	5	NA
251117	Physical activity	1	2	3	4	5	NA
251118	Endurance	1	2	3	4	5	NA
251119	Liver enzymes	1	2	3	4	5	NA
251120	Hemoglobin	1	2	3	4	5	NA
251121	White blood count	1	2	3	4	5	NA
251129	Blood glucose	1	2	3	4	5	NA
		Severe	**Substantial**	**Moderate**	**Mild**	**None**	
251113	Infection	1	2	3	4	5	NA
251125	Incisional pain	1	2	3	4	5	NA
251126	Fatigue	1	2	3	4	5	NA
251127	Vaginal bleeding	1	2	3	4	5	NA
251128	Depression	1	2	3	4	5	NA
251130	Lacerations	1	2	3	4	5	NA
251131	Perineal pain	1	2	3	4	5	NA

Domain- *Health & Life Quality (V)*   **Class-** *Health Status (JJ)*   *2nd edition 2000; revised 2004, 2013, 2024*

OUTCOME CONTENT REFERENCES:

American College of Obstetricians and Gynecologists, Committee on Practice Bulletins—Obstetrics. (2018). ACOG Practice Bulletin No. 189: Nausea and vomiting of pregnancy. *Obstetrics & Gynecology, 131*(5), e15–e30. https://doi.org/10.1097/AOG.0000000000002456

American College of Obstetricians and Gynecologists. (2018). ACOG Committee Opinion No. 736: Optimizing postpartum are. *Obstetrics & Gynecology, 131*(5), e140–e150. https://doi.org/10.1097/AOG.0000000000002633

Durmaz, A., & Komurcu, N. (2018). Relationship between maternal characteristics and postpartum hemorrhage: A meta-analysis study. *Journal of Nursing Research, 26*(5), 362–372. https://doi.org/10.1097/jnr.0000000000000245

Figueiredo, J. V., Fialho, A. V. M., Mendonça, G. M. M., Rodrigues, D. P., & Silva, L. F. D. (2018). Pain in the immediate puerperium: Nursing care contribution. *Revista Brasileira de Enfermagem, 71*(Suppl. 3), 1343–1350. https://doi.org/10.1590/0034-7167-2017-0345

Lowdermilk, D. L., Cashion, M. C., Perry, S. E., Alden, K. R., & Olshansky, E. (2019). *Maternity and women's health care* (12th ed.). Mosby.

O'Meara, A. (2019). *Maternity, newborn, and women's health nursing: A case-based approach* (1st ed.). Wolters Kluwer.

Walker, K. C., Arbour, M. W., & Wika, J. C. (2019). Consolidation of guidelines of postpartum care: Recommendations to address maternal morbidity and mortality. *Nursing for Women's Health, 23*(6), 508–517. https://doi.org/10.1016/j.nwh.2019.09.004

Mechanical Ventilation Response: Adult 0411

Definition: Alveolar exchange and tissue perfusion are effectively supported by mechanical ventilation

OUTCOME TARGET RATING: Maintain at_____ Increase to_____

		Severe Deviation from Normal Range	Substantial Deviation from Normal Range	Moderate Deviation from Normal Range	Mild Deviation from Normal Range	No Deviation from Normal Range	
OUTCOME OVERALL RATING		1	2	3	4	5	
Indicators:							
041102	Respiratory rate	1	2	3	4	5	NA
041103	Respiratory rhythm	1	2	3	4	5	NA
041104	Depth of inspiration	1	2	3	4	5	NA
041126	Inspiratory capacity	1	2	3	4	5	NA
041106	Tidal volume	1	2	3	4	5	NA
041107	Vital capacity	1	2	3	4	5	NA
041108	FiO_2 (fraction of inspired oxygen) meets oxygen demand	1	2	3	4	5	NA
041109	PaO_2 (partial pressure of oxygen in arterial blood)	1	2	3	4	5	NA
041110	$PaCO_2$ (partial pressure of carbon dioxide in arterial blood)	1	2	3	4	5	NA
041111	Arterial pH	1	2	3	4	5	NA
041112	Oxygen saturation	1	2	3	4	5	NA
041113	Peripheral tissue perfusion	1	2	3	4	5	NA
041114	End-tidal carbon dioxide	1	2	3	4	5	NA
041115	Pulmonary function tests	1	2	3	4	5	NA
041116	Chest x-ray findings	1	2	3	4	5	NA
041117	Ventilation-perfusion balance	1	2	3	4	5	NA
041135	Blood pressure	1	2	3	4	5	NA
041136	Arterial blood gas analysis (aBGA)	1	2	3	4	5	NA
041137	Cognition	1	2	3	4	5	NA
		Severe	Substantial	Moderate	Mild	None	
041122	Asymmetrical chest wall movement	1	2	3	4	5	NA
041123	Asymmetrical chest wall expansion	1	2	3	4	5	NA
041124	Difficulty breathing with ventilator	1	2	3	4	5	NA
041127	Adventitious breath sounds	1	2	3	4	5	NA
041134	Atelectasis	1	2	3	4	5	NA
041125	Anxiety	1	2	3	4	5	NA
041128	Restlessness	1	2	3	4	5	NA
041129	Impaired skin integrity at artificial airway site	1	2	3	4	5	NA
041130	Hypoxia	1	2	3	4	5	NA
041131	Pulmonary infection	1	2	3	4	5	NA
041138	Fever	1	2	3	4	5	NA
041132	Respiratory secretions	1	2	3	4	5	NA
041139	Discomfort	1	2	3	4	5	NA
041133	Difficulty communicating needs	1	2	3	4	5	NA
041140	Body mass index (BMI)	1	2	3	4	5	NA

Type and mode of ventilation_____

Domain-Physiologic Health (II)   *Class*-Cardiopulmonary (E)   *3rd edition 2004; revised 2008, 2024*

M

OUTCOME CONTENT REFERENCES:

Bassi, T. G., Rohrs, E. C., & Reynolds, S. C. (2021). Systematic review of cognitive impairment and brain insult after mechanical ventilation. *Critical Care, 25*(1), 1–12. https://doi.org/10.1186/s13054-021-03521-9

Bickley, L. S., Szilagyi, P. G., Hoffman, R. M., & Soriano, R. P. (2021). *Bates' guide to physical examination and history taking* (13th ed.). Wolters Kluwer.

Choron, R. L., Butts, C. A., Bargoud, C., Krumrei, N. J., Teichman, A. L., Schroeder, M. E., Bover Manderski, M. T., Cai, J., Song, C., Rodricks, M. B., Lissauer, M., & Gupta, R. (2021). Fever in the ICU: A predictor of mortality in mechanically ventilated COVID-19 patients. *Journal of Intensive Care Medicine, 36*(4), 484–493. https://doi.org/10.1177/0885066620979622

Huether, S. E., McCance, K. L., & Brashers, V. L. (2020). *Understanding pathophysiology* (7th ed.). Elsevier.

Ignatavicius, D. D., Workman, M. L., Rebar, C. R., & Heimgartner, N. M. (2021). *Medical-surgical nursing: Concepts for interprofessional care* (10th ed.). Elsevier.

+Kotfis, K., Strzelbicka, M., Zegan-Barańska, M., Safranow, K., Brykczyński, M., Żukowski, M., Ely, E. W., & POL-BPS Study Group. (2018). Validation of the Behavioral Pain Scale to assess pain intensity in adult, intubated postcardiac surgery patients: A cohort observational study. POL-BPS. *Medicine, 97*(38), e12443. https://doi.org/10.1097/MD.0000000000012443

Naghibi, T., Shafigh, N., & Mazloomzadeh, S. (2020). Role of omega-3 fatty acids in the prevention of delirium in mechanically ventilated patients. *Journal of Research in Medical Sciences, 25*, 10. https://doi.org/10.4103/jrms

Schavemaker, R., Schultz, M. J., Lagrand, W. K., van Slobbe-Bijlsma, E. R., Neto, A. S., Paulus, F. for the PRoVENT-COVID, & Collaborative Group. (2021). Associations of body mass index with ventilation management and clinical outcomes in invasively ventilated patients with ARDS related to COVID-19: Insights from the PRoVENT-COVID study. *Journal of Clinical Medicine, 10*(1176), 1176. https://doi.org/10.3390/jcm1006117

Shao, D., Straub, J., & Matrka, L. (2020). Obesity as a predictor of prolonged mechanical ventilation. *Otolaryngology-Head & Neck Surgery, 163*(4), 750–754. https://doi.org/10.1177/0194599820923601

Mechanical Ventilation Weaning Response: Adult 0412

Definition: Respiratory and psychological adjustment to progressive removal of mechanical ventilation

OUTCOME TARGET RATING: Maintain at_____ Increase to_____

	Severe Deviation from Normal Range	Substantial Deviation from Normal Range	Moderate Deviation from Normal Range	Mild Deviation from Normal Range	No Deviation from Normal Range	
OUTCOME OVERALL RATING	1	2	3	4	5	
Indicators:						
041202	Spontaneous respiratory rate	1	2	3	4	5	NA
041203	Spontaneous respiratory rhythm	1	2	3	4	5	NA
041204	Spontaneous respiratory depth	1	2	3	4	5	NA
041205	Apical heart rate	1	2	3	4	5	NA
041208	PaO_2 (partial pressure of oxygen in arterial blood)	1	2	3	4	5	NA
041209	$PaCO_2$ (partial pressure of carbon dioxide in arterial blood)	1	2	3	4	5	NA
041210	Arterial pH	1	2	3	4	5	NA
041237	Arterial blood gas analysis (ABGA)	1	2	3	4	5	NA
041211	Oxygen saturation	1	2	3	4	5	NA
041212	Vital capacity	1	2	3	4	5	NA
041213	Tidal volume	1	2	3	4	5	NA
041214	Minute ventilation <10 L/minute	1	2	3	4	5	NA
041215	Positive end-expiratory pressure	1	2	3	4	5	NA
041219	Chest x-ray findings	1	2	3	4	5	NA
041220	Ventilation-perfusion balance	1	2	3	4	5	NA

		Severe	Substantial	Moderate	Mild	None	
041223	Difficulty breathing on own	1	2	3	4	5	NA
041224	Respiratory secretions	1	2	3	4	5	NA
041225	Anxiety	1	2	3	4	5	NA
041226	Fear	1	2	3	4	5	NA
041227	Impaired gag reflex	1	2	3	4	5	NA
041228	Impaired cough reflex	1	2	3	4	5	NA
041229	Impaired drive to breath	1	2	3	4	5	NA
041230	Adventitious breath sounds	1	2	3	4	5	NA
041231	Asymmetrical chest wall movement	1	2	3	4	5	NA

M

Mechanical Ventilation Weaning Response: Adult—cont'd

		Severe	Substantial	Moderate	Mild	None	
041232	Asymmetrical chest wall expansion	1	2	3	4	5	NA
041233	Atelectasis	1	2	3	4	5	NA
041234	Restlessness	1	2	3	4	5	NA
041235	Discomfort	1	2	3	4	5	NA
041238	Sedation level	1	2	3	4	5	NA
041239	Body mass index (BMI)	1	2	3	4	5	NA
041236	Difficulty communicating needs	1	2	3	4	5	NA

Domain-*Physiologic Health (II)* **Class**-*Cardiopulmonary (E)* *3rd edition 2004; revised 2008, 2024*

OUTCOME CONTENT REFERENCES:

Ghiani, A., Paderewska, J., Sainis, A., Crispin, A., Walcher, S., & Neurohr, C. (2020). Variables predicting weaning outcome in prolonged mechanically ventilated tracheotomized patients: A retrospective study. *Journal of Intensive Care, 8*,19. https://doi.org/10.1186/s40560-020-00437-4

Huether, S. E., McCance, K. L., & Brashers, V. L. (2020). *Understanding pathophysiology* (7th ed.). Elsevier.

Ignatavicius, D. D., Workman, M. L., Rebar, C. R., & Heimgartner, N. M. (2021). *Medical-surgical nursing: Concepts for interprofessional care* (10th ed.). Elsevier.

Leonov, Y., Kisil, I., Perlov, A., Stoichev, V., Ginzburg, Y., Nazarenko, A., & Gimelfarb, Y. (2020). Predictors of successful weaning in patients requiring extremely prolonged mechanical ventilation. *Advances in Respiratory Medicine, 88*(6), 477–484. https://doi.org/10.5603/ARM.a2020.0151

Liu, W., Yang, Y., Jiao, Y., Zhang, K., Hai, Y., Li, H., Xing, H., Xu, B., Bai, H., Zhao, Y., Bao, H., Zhang, S., Ren, W., Yang, L., Yang, H., Tian, J., Wang, M., & Guoet, T. (2020). Evaluation of the effects of applying the Ventricular Care Bundle (VCB) method for reducing ventilator-associated pneumonia (VAP) in the intensive care unit of a general Chinese tertiary hospital. *Annals of Palliative Medicine, 9*(5), 2853–2861. https://doi.org/10.21037/apm-20-289

Schavemaker, R., Schultz, M. J., Lagrand, W. K., van Slobbe-Bijlsma, E. R., Neto, A. S., & Paulus, F. for the PRoVENT-COVID, & Collaborative Group. (2021). Associations of body mass index with ventilation management and clinical outcomes in invasively ventilated patients with ARDS related to COVID-19: Insights from the PRoVENT-COVID study. *Journal of Clinical Medicine, 10*(1176), 1176. https://doi.org/10.3390/jcm1006117

Medication Response 2301

M

Definition: Therapeutic and adverse effects of prescribed medication

OUTCOME TARGET RATING: Maintain at_____ Increase to_____

	Severely Compromised	Substantially Compromised	Moderately Compromised	Mildly Compromised	Not Compromised	
OUTCOME OVERALL RATING	1	2	3	4	5	
Indicators:						
230114 Medication regimen adherence	1	2	3	4	5	NA
230101 Expected therapeutic effects	1	2	3	4	5	NA
230115 Medication tolerance	1	2	3	4	5	NA
230102 Expected change in blood chemistries	1	2	3	4	5	NA
230103 Expected change in symptoms	1	2	3	4	5	NA
230111 Maintenance of expected blood levels	1	2	3	4	5	NA
230112 Expected behavioral response	1	2	3	4	5	NA

	Severe	Substantial	Moderate	Mild	None	
230105 Allergic reaction	1	2	3	4	5	NA
230116 Medication side effects	1	2	3	4	5	NA
230106 Medication adverse effects	1	2	3	4	5	NA
230107 Medication interactions	1	2	3	4	5	NA
230117 Change in gut microbiome composition and function	1	2	3	4	5	NA
230118 Change in structure of medication by gut microbiome	1	2	3	4	5	NA
230119 Interactions with over-the-counter medications	1	2	3	4	5	NA
230113 Adverse behavioral effects	1	2	3	4	5	NA

Specify medication_____

Domain-*Physiologic Health (II)* **Class**-*Therapeutic Response (AA)* *2nd edition 2000; revised 2004, 2008, 2024*

OUTCOME CONTENT REFERENCES:

Ayele, A. A., Tegegn, H. G., Ayele, T. A., & Ayalew, M. B. (2019). Medication regimen complexity and its impact on medication adherence and glycemic control among patients with type 2 diabetes mellitus in an Ethiopian general hospital. *BMJ Open Diabetes Research & Care, 7*(1), e000685. https://doi.org/10.1136/bmjdrc-2019-000685

Błeszyńska, E., Wierucki, Ł., Zdrojewski, T., & Renke, M. (2020). Pharmacological interactions in the elderly. *Medicina (Kaunas, Lithuania), 56*(7), 320. https://doi.org/10.3390/medicina56070320

Broyles, A. D., Banerji, A., Barmettler, S., Biggs, C. M., Blumenthal, K., Brennan, P. J., Breslow, R. G., Brockow, K., Buchheit, K. M., Cahill, K. N., Cernadas, J., Chiriac, A. M., Crestani, E., Demoly, P., Dewachter, P., Dilley, M., Farmer, J. R., Foer, D., Fried, A. J., Garon, S. L., Giannetti, M. P., Hepner, D. L., Hong, D. I., Hsu, J. T., Kothari, P. H., Kyin, T., Lax, T., Lee, M. J., Lee-Sarwar, K., Liu, A., Logsdon, S., Louisias, M., MacGinnitie, A., Maciag, M., Minnicozzi, S., Norton, A. E., Otani, I. M., Park, M., Patil, S., Phillips, E. J., Picard, M., Platt, C. D., Rachid, R., Rodriguez, T., Romano, A., Stone, C. A. Jr., Torres, M. J., Verdú, M., Wang, A. L., Wickner, P., Wolfson, A. R., Wong, J. T., Yee, C., Zhou, J., & Castells, M. (2021). Practical guidance for the evaluation and management of drug hypersensitivity: Specific drugs. *Journal of Allergy Clinical Immunology Practice, 8*(9), S16–S116. https://doi.org/10.1016/j.jaip.2020.08.006

Dykewicz, M. S., & Lam, J. K. (2020). Drug hypersensitivity reactions. *The Medical Clinics of North America, 104*(1), 109–128. https://doi.org/10.1016/j.mcna.2019.09.003

Gnjidic, D., Husband, A., & Todd, A. (2018). Challenges and innovations of delivering medicines to older adults. *Advanced Drug Delivery Reviews, 135*, 97–105. https://doi.org/10.1016/j.addr.2018.08.003

Katzung, B. G., & Trevor, A. J. (2020). *Basic and clinical pharmacology* (15th ed.). McGraw Hill.

Kim, J., & Parish, A. L. (2017). Polypharmacy and medication management in older adults. *The Nursing Clinics of North America, 52*(3), 457–468. https://doi.org/10.1016/j.cnur.2017.04.007

Kizior, R. J., & Hodgson, K. (2021). *Saunders nursing drug handbook 2021*. Saunders.

Waheed, A., Hill, T., & Dhawan, N. (2016). Drug allergy. *Primary Care, 43*(3), 393–400. https://doi.org/10.1016/j.pop.2016.04.005

Wakai, E., Ikemura, K., Kato, C., & Okuda, M. (2021). Effect of number of medications and complexity of regimens on medication adherence and blood pressure management in hospitalized patients with hypertension. *PLOS One, 16*(6), e0252944. https://doi.org/10.1371/journal.pone.0252944

Weersma, R. K., Zhernakova, A., & Fu, J. (2020). Interaction between drugs and the gut microbiome. *Gut, 69*(8), 1510–1519. https://doi.org/10.1136/gutjnl-2019-320204

Memory 0908

Definition: Ability to cognitively retrieve and report previously stored information

OUTCOME TARGET RATING: Maintain at_____ Increase to_____

		Never Demonstrated	Rarely Demonstrated	Sometimes Demonstrated	Often Demonstrated	Consistently Demonstrated	
OUTCOME OVERALL RATING		1	2	3	4	5	
Indicators:							
090801	Recalls immediate information accurately	1	2	3	4	5	NA
090802	Recalls recent information accurately	1	2	3	4	5	NA
090803	Recalls remote information accurately	1	2	3	4	5	NA

Domain-*Physiologic Health (II)* **Class**-*Neurocognitive (J)* *1st edition 1997; reviewed 2018; revised 2004, 2024*

OUTCOME CONTENT REFERENCES:

Cordell, C. B., Borson, S., Boustani, M., Chodosh, J., Reuben, D., Verghese, J., Thies, W., & Fried, L. B. (2013). Alzheimer's Association recommendations for operationalizing the detection of cognitive impairment during the Medicare Annual Wellness Visit in a primary care setting. *Alzheimer's & Dementia, 9*, 141–150. https://doi.org/10.1016/j.jalz.2012.09.011

Fletcher, K. A., Hicks, V. L., Johnson, R. H., Laverentz, D. M., Phillips, C. J., Pierce, L. N. B., Wilhoite, D. L., & Gay, J. E. (2019). A concept analysis of conceptual learning: A guide for educators. *Journal of Nursing Education, 58*(1), 7–15. https://doi.org/10.3928/01484834-201900103-03

Hogan-Quigley, B., Palm, M. L., & Bickley, L. (2021). *Bates nursing guide to physical examination and history taking* (3rd ed.). Wolters Kluwer.

Norris, D. (2017). Short-term memory and long-term memory are still different. *Psychological Bulletin, 143*(9), 992–1009. https://doi.org/10.1037/bul0000108

Shin, J. (2020). A meta-analysis of the relationship between working memory and second language reading comprehension: Does task type mater? *Applied Psycholinguistics, 41*, 873–900. https://doi.org/10.1017/S0142716420000272

Smith, T. O., Neal, S. R., Peryer, G., Sheehan, K. J., Tan, M. P., & Myint, P. K. (2019). Orientation and verbal fluency in the English longitudinal study of ageing: Modifiable risk factors for falls? *International Psychogeriatrics, 31*(10), 1491–1498. https://doi.org/10.1017/S1041610218002065

Metabolic Acidosis Severity   0619

Definition: Severity of signs and symptoms of decreased blood pH due to decreased bicarbonate and increased hydrogen ions

OUTCOME TARGET RATING: Maintain at_____ Increase to_____

		Severe	Substantial	Moderate	Mild	None	
OUTCOME OVERALL RATING		1	2	3	4	5	
Indicators:							
061901	Decreased blood plasma pH	1	2	3	4	5	NA
061902	Increased serum hydrogen ions	1	2	3	4	5	NA
061903	Decreased serum bicarbonate	1	2	3	4	5	NA
061904	Elevated anion gap	1	2	3	4	5	NA
061905	Increased serum potassium	1	2	3	4	5	NA
061906	Increased respiratory rate	1	2	3	4	5	NA
061907	Increased respiratory depth	1	2	3	4	5	NA
061922	Decreased blood pressure	1	2	3	4	5	NA
061908	Hypoxia	1	2	3	4	5	NA
061909	Kussmaul-Kien respiration	1	2	3	4	5	NA
061910	Arrhythmias	1	2	3	4	5	NA
061911	Peripheral vasodilation	1	2	3	4	5	NA
061912	Hypotension	1	2	3	4	5	NA
061913	Cold, clammy skin	1	2	3	4	5	NA
061914	Headache	1	2	3	4	5	NA
061915	Drowsiness	1	2	3	4	5	NA
061922	Decreased level of consciousness	1	2	3	4	5	NA
061916	Confusion	1	2	3	4	5	NA
061917	Abdominal pain	1	2	3	4	5	NA
061918	Anorexia	1	2	3	4	5	NA
061919	Nausea	1	2	3	4	5	NA
061920	Vomiting	1	2	3	4	5	NA
061921	Seizures	1	2	3	4	5	NA

Domain-*Physiologic Health (II)*   **Class**-*Fluid & Electrolytes (G)*   *5th edition 2013; revised 2024*

M

OUTCOME CONTENT REFERENCES:
Harding, M. M., Kwong, J., Roberts, D., Hagler, D., & Reinisch, C. (2020). *Lewis's medical-surgical nursing* (11th ed.). Elsevier.
Hinkle, J. L., & Cheever, K. H. (2018). *Brunner & Suddarth's textbook of medical-surgical nursing* (14th ed.). Wolter Kluwer.
Huether, S. E., McCance, K. L., & Brashers, V. L. (2020). *Understanding pathophysiology* (7th ed.). Elsevier.
Jones, M. B. (2010). Pediatric care: Basic interpretation of metabolic acidosis. *Critical Care Nurse, 30*(5), 63–70. https://doi.org/10.4037/ccn2010521
Kovacic, V., Roguljic, L., & Kovacic, V. (2003). Metabolic acidosis of chronically hemodialyzed patients. *American Journal of Nephrology, 23*(3), 158–164. https://doi.org/10.1159/000070205
Mohammed, H. M., & Abdallah Abdelatief, D., (2016). Easy blood gas analysis: Implications for nursing. *Egyptian Journal of Chest Diseases and Tuberculosis, 65*(1), 369–376. https://doi.org/10.1016/j.ejcdt.2015.11.009
Reddy, P., & Mooradian, A. (2009). Clinical utility of anion gap in deciphering acid-base disorders. *International Journal of Clinical Practice, 63*(10), 1516–1525. https://doi.org/10.1111/j.1742-1241.2009.02000.x

Metabolic Alkalosis Severity   0620

Definition: Severity of signs and symptoms of increased blood pH and bicarbonate due to conditions that cause excessive acid loss or increased bicarbonate retention

OUTCOME TARGET RATING: Maintain at_____ Increase to_____

	Severe	Substantial	Moderate	Mild	None	
OUTCOME OVERALL RATING	1	2	3	4	5	
Indicators:						
062001 Increased blood plasma pH	1	2	3	4	5	NA
062002 Decreased serum hydrogen ions	1	2	3	4	5	NA
062003 Increased serum bicarbonate	1	2	3	4	5	NA
062004 Decreased serum potassium	1	2	3	4	5	NA
062005 Decreased ionized serum calcium	1	2	3	4	5	NA
062006 Decreased respiratory rate	1	2	3	4	5	NA
062007 Decreased respiratory rhythm	1	2	3	4	5	NA
062008 Atrial tachycardia	1	2	3	4	5	NA
062009 Premature ventricular contractions	1	2	3	4	5	NA
062016 Decreased bowel motility	1	2	3	4	5	NA
062010 Dizziness	1	2	3	4	5	NA
062011 Seizures	1	2	3	4	5	NA
062012 Confusion	1	2	3	4	5	NA
062017 Paresthesia	1	2	3	4	5	NA
062014 Hyperactive reflexes	1	2	3	4	5	NA
062015 Hypertonic muscles	1	2	3	4	5	NA

Domain-*Physiologic Health (II)*   **Class**-*Fluid & Electrolytes (G)*   *5th edition 2013; revised 2024*

OUTCOME CONTENT REFERENCES:
Harding, M. M., Kwong, J., Roberts, D., Hagler, D., & Reinisch, C. (2020). *Lewis's medical-surgical nursing* (11th ed.). Elsevier
Hinkle, J. L., & Cheever, K. H. (2018). *Brunner & Suddarth's textbook of medical-surgical nursing* (14th ed.). Wolter Kluwer.
Huang, L. H., & Priestley, M. A. (2017, October 19). *Pediatric Metabolic Alkalosis.* https://emedicine.medscape.com/article/906819-overview
Huether, S. E., McCance, K. L., & Brashers, V. L. (2020). *Understanding pathophysiology* (7th ed.). Elsevier.
Mohammed, H. M., & Abdallah Abdelatief, D. (2016). Easy blood gas analysis: Implications for nursing. *Egyptian Journal of Chest Diseases and Tuberculosis,* *65*(1), 369–376. https://doi.org/10.1016/j.ejcdt.2015.11.009

Metabolic Function   0804

Definition: Ability of the metabolic system to regulate chemical transformations through anabolism and catabolism

OUTCOME TARGET RATING: Maintain at_____ Increase to_____

	Severe Deviation from Normal Range	Substantial Deviation from Normal Range	Moderate Deviation from Normal Range	Mild Deviation from Normal Range	No Deviation from Normal Range	
OUTCOME OVERALL RATING	1	2	3	4	5	
Indicators:						
080401 Fasting blood glucose	1	2	3	4	5	NA
080402 Glycosylated hemoglobin (HbA1c)	1	2	3	4	5	NA
080403 Total bilirubin	1	2	3	4	5	NA
080404 Direct bilirubin	1	2	3	4	5	NA
080405 Total protein	1	2	3	4	5	NA
080406 Albumin	1	2	3	4	5	NA

M

Metabolic Function—cont'd

		Severe Deviation from Normal Range	Substantial Deviation from Normal Range	Moderate Deviation from Normal Range	Mild Deviation from Normal Range	No Deviation from Normal Range	
080407	Sodium	1	2	3	4	5	NA
080408	Potassium	1	2	3	4	5	NA
080409	Chloride	1	2	3	4	5	NA
080410	Calcium	1	2	3	4	5	NA
080411	Total cholesterol	1	2	3	4	5	NA
080412	High-density lipoprotein (HDL) cholesterol	1	2	3	4	5	NA
080413	Low-density lipoprotein (LDL) cholesterol	1	2	3	4	5	NA
080414	Very low-density lipoprotein (VLDL) cholesterol	1	2	3	4	5	NA
080415	Triglycerides	1	2	3	4	5	NA
080416	Glutamic-oxalacetic transaminase (GOT)	1	2	3	4	5	NA
080417	Gamma-glutamyl transferase (GGT)	1	2	3	4	5	NA
080418	Glutamic-pyruvic transaminase (GPT)	1	2	3	4	5	NA
080419	Alanine transaminase (ALT)	1	2	3	4	5	NA
080420	Aspartate aminotransferase (AST)	1	2	3	4	5	NA
080421	Alkaline phosphatase	1	2	3	4	5	NA
080422	Creatinine	1	2	3	4	5	NA
080423	Blood urea nitrogen (BUN)	1	2	3	4	5	NA
080424	Uric acid	1	2	3	4	5	NA

Domain-*Physiologic Health (II)*   **Class**-*Metabolic Regulation (1)*   6th edition 2018

OUTCOME CONTENT REFERENCES:

Abete, I., Goyenechea, E., Zulet, M., & Martinez, J. (2011). Obesity and metabolic syndrome: Potential benefit from specific nutritional components. *Nutrition, Metabolism and Cardiovascular Diseases, 21*(Suppl. 2), B1–B15. https://doi.org/10.1016/j.numecd.2011.05.001

Choi, S. H., Yun, K. E., & Choi, H. J. (2013). Relationships between serum total bilirubin levels and metabolic syndrome in Korean adults. *Nutrition, Metabolism and Cardiovascular Diseases, 23*(1), 31–37. https://doi.org/10.1016/j.numecd.2011.03.001

Grundy, S. M. (2011). The metabolic syndrome. In *Atlas of atherosclerosis and metabolic syndrome* (5th ed., pp. 1–26). Springer.

Jenko-Pražnikar, Z., Petelin, A., Jurdana, M., & Žiberna, L. (2013). Serum bilirubin levels are lower in overweight asymptomatic middle-aged adults: An early indicator of metabolic syndrome? *Metabolism, 62*(7), 976–985. https://doi.org/10.1016/j.metabol.2013.01.011

Kastorini, C., Milionis, H., Esposito, K., Giugliano, D., Goudevenos, J., & Panagiotakos, D. (2011). The effect of mediterranean diet on metabolic syndrome and its components: A meta-analysis of 50 studies and 534,906 individuals. *Journal of the American College of Cardiology, 57*(11), 1299–1313. https://doi.org/10.1016/j.jacc.2010.09.073

Kim, S., & Kang, S. (2013). Serum albumin levels: A simple answer to a complex problem? Are we on the right track of assessing metabolic syndrome? *Endocrinology and Metabolism, 28*(1), 17–19. https://doi.org/10.3803/EnM.2013.28.1.17

Navaneethan, S. D., Schold, J. D., Kirwan, J. P., Arrigain, S., Jolly, S. E., Poggio, E. D., Beddhu, S., & Nally, J. V. (2013). Metabolic syndrome, ESRD, and death in CKD. *Clinical Journal of the American Society of Nephrology, 8*(6), 945–952. https://doi.org/10.2215/CJN.09870912

Park, E. Y., Lim, M. K., Oh, J.-K., Cho, H., Bae, M. J., Yun, E. H., Kim, D.-I., & Shin, H.-R. (2013). Independent and supra-additive effects of alcohol consumption, cigarette smoking, and metabolic syndrome on the elevation of serum liver enzyme levels. *PLOS One, 8*(5), e63439. https://doi.org/10.1371/journal.pone.0063439

Povel, C. M., Beulens, J. W., van der Schouw, Y. T., Dollé, M. E. T., Spijkerman, A. M. W., Verschuren, W. M. M., Feskens, E. J. M., & Boer, J. M. A. (2013). Metabolic syndrome model definitions predicting type 2 diabetes and cardiovascular disease. *Diabetes Care, 36*(2), 362–368. https://doi.org/10.2337/dc11-2546

Tang, M., Armstrong, C., Leidy, H., & Campbell, W. (2013). Normal vs. high-protein weight loss diets in men: Effects on body composition and indices of metabolic syndrome. *Obesity, 21*(3), E204–E210. https://doi.org/10.1002/oby.20078

Taverne, F., Richard, C., Couture, P., & Lamarche, B. (2013). Abdominal obesity, insulin resistance, metabolic syndrome and cholesterol homeostasis. *PharmaNutrition, 1*(4), 130–136. https://doi.org/10.1016/j.phanu.2013.07.003

Zapolski, T., Waciński, P., Kondracki, B., Rychta, E., Buraczyńska, M., & Wysokiński, A. (2011). Uric acid as a link between renal dysfunction and both pro-inflammatory and prothrombotic state in patients with metabolic syndrome and coronary artery disease. *Kardiologia Polska, 69*(4), 319–326.

M

Mobility 0208

Definition: Ability to move purposefully in own environment independently with or without assistive device

OUTCOME TARGET RATING: Maintain at_____ Increase to_____

		Severely Compromised	Substantially Compromised	Moderately Compromised	Mildly Compromised	Not Compromised	
OUTCOME OVERALL RATING		1	2	3	4	5	
Indicators:							
020801	Balance	1	2	3	4	5	NA
020809	Coordination	1	2	3	4	5	NA
020810	Gait	1	2	3	4	5	NA
020803	Muscle movement	1	2	3	4	5	NA
020804	Joint movement	1	2	3	4	5	NA
020816	Right leg strength	1	2	3	4	5	NA
020817	Left leg strength	1	2	3	4	5	NA
020818	Right ankle strength	1	2	3	4	5	NA
020819	Left ankle strength	1	2	3	4	5	NA
020820	Right foot strength	1	2	3	4	5	NA
020821	Left foot strength	1	2	3	4	5	NA
020802	Body positioning performance	1	2	3	4	5	NA
020805	Transfer performance	1	2	3	4	5	NA
020822	Ability to walk forward	1	2	3	4	5	NA
020823	Ability to walk backwards	1	2	3	4	5	NA
020824	Ability to run	1	2	3	4	5	NA
020825	Ability to jump	1	2	3	4	5	NA
020826	Ability to crawl	1	2	3	4	5	NA
020814	Moves with ease	1	2	3	4	5	NA

Domain-*Functional Health (I)* **Class**-*Mobility (C)* *1st edition 1997; revised 2004, 2018, 2024*

M

OUTCOME CONTENT REFERENCES:

Alcazar, J., Alegre, L. M., Suetta, C., Júdice, P. B., Van Roie, E., González-Gross, M., Rodríguez-Mañas, L., Casajús, J. A., Magalhães, J. P., Nielsen, B. R., García-García, F. J., Delecluse, C., Sardinha, L. B., & Ara, I. (2021). Threshold of relative muscle power required to rise from a chair and mobility limitations and disability in older adults. *Medicine & Science in Sports & Exercise, 53*(11), 2217–2224. https://doi.org/10.1249/MSS.0000000000002717

Costa, R. B., dos Santos, E. R., Lopes, C. T., & Bergamasco, E. C. (2016). Adequacy of the activities in the nursing intervention exercise therapy: Ambulation for medical-surgical patients with impaired physical mobility. *International Journal of Nursing Knowledge, 27*(4), 201–204. https://doi.org/10.1111/2047-3095.12114

de Jesus, I. T. M., Orlandi, F. de S., Gomes, G. A. de O., Say, K. G., Guarisco, L. P. C., Orlandi, A. A. dos S., Pott-Junior, H., & Zazzetta, M. S. (2021). Frailty state transitions among non-frail and vulnerable older adults: Does mobility performance really matter? *Geriatric Nursing, 42*(6), 1367–1372. https://doi.org/10.1016/j.gerinurse.2021.09.007

Ferreira, R. C., Moorhead, S. A., Zuchatti, B. V., Begnami, N. E. d. S., Ribeiro, E., Carvalho, L. A. C., & Duran, E. C. M. (2022). Nursing outcomes for patients with multiple traumas and impaired physical mobility: An integrative review. *International Journal of Nursing Knowledge*, Advance online publication. https://doi.org/10.1111/2047-3095.12384

Futrell, E. E., Roberts, D., & Toole, E. (2022). The effects of intrinsic foot muscle strengthening on functional mobility in older adults: A systematic review. *Journal of the American Geriatrics Society, 70*(2), 531–540. https://doi.org/10.1111/jgs.17541

Luoma-Halkola, H., & Häikiö, L. (2022). Independent living with mobility restrictions: Older people's perceptions of their out-of-home mobility. *Ageing & Society, 42*(2), 249–270. https://doi.org/10.1017/S0144686X20000823

Maritz, C. A., Pigman, J., Grävare Silbernagel, K., & Crenshaw, J. (2021). Effects of backward walking training on balance, mobility, and gait in community-dwelling older adults. *Activities, Adaptation & Aging, 45*(3), 202–216. https://doi.org/10.1080/01924788.2020.1757329

+Parikh, H., Kalariya, B., & Kachhadiya, H. (2021). Screening of stroke patients using Performance Oriented Mobility Assessment (POMA) Scale. *Indian Journal of Physiotherapy & Occupational Therapy, 15*(4), 26–31. https://doi.org/10.37506/ijpot.v15i4.16492

+Podsiadlo, D., & Richardson, S. (1991). The timed "Up & Go": A test of basic functional mobility for frail elderly persons. *Journal of the American Geriatrics Society, 39*(2), 142–148. https://doi.org/10.1111/j.1532-5415.1991.tb01616.x

Rincé, G., Couturier, C., Berrut, G., Dylis, A., Montero-Odasso, M., & Deschamps, T. (2021). Impact of an individual personalised rehabilitation program on mobility performance in older-old people. *Aging Clinical & Experimental Research, 33*(10), 2821–2830. https://doi.org/10.1007/s40520-021-01812-3

Sommers, J., Vredeveld, T., Lindeboom, R., Nollet, F., Engelbert, R. H., & van der Schaaf, M. (2016). The Morton Mobility Index is feasible, reliable, and valid in patients with critical illness. *Physical Therapy, 96*(10), 1658–1666. https://doi.org/10.2522/ptj.20150339

West, B. A., Bergen, G., & Moreland, B. (2021). Older adults' attitudes about future mobility changes and the usefulness of mobility assessment materials. *Journal of Applied Gerontology, 40*(10), 1356–1365. https://doi.org/10.1177/0733464820947927

Mood Equilibrium   1204

Definition: Appropriate adjustment of prevailing emotional tone and behaviors in response to life circumstances

OUTCOME TARGET RATING: Maintain at_____ Increase to_____

	Never Demonstrated	Rarely Demonstrated	Sometimes Demonstrated	Often Demonstrated	Consistently Demonstrated	
OUTCOME OVERALL RATING	1	2	3	4	5	
Indicators:						
120401 Exhibits affect that fits situation	1	2	3	4	5	NA
120402 Exhibits non-labile mood	1	2	3	4	5	NA
120403 Exhibits impulse control	1	2	3	4	5	NA
120404 Reports adequate sleep	1	2	3	4	5	NA
120405 Exhibits concentration	1	2	3	4	5	NA
120406 Speaks at moderate pace	1	2	3	4	5	NA
120423 Maintains personal grooming and hygiene	1	2	3	4	5	NA
120411 Wears appropriate clothing for situation	1	2	3	4	5	NA
120412 Maintains stable weight	1	2	3	4	5	NA
120413 Exhibits normal appetite	1	2	3	4	5	NA
120424 Reports adherence with medication regimen	1	2	3	4	5	NA
120425 Reports adherence with treatment regimen	1	2	3	4	5	NA
120415 Shows interest in surroundings	1	2	3	4	5	NA
120417 Exhibits stable energy level	1	2	3	4	5	NA
120418 Accomplishes daily tasks	1	2	3	4	5	NA

	Consistently Demonstrated	Often Demonstrated	Sometimes Demonstrated	Rarely Demonstrated	Never Demonstrated	
120407 Flight of ideas	1	2	3	4	5	NA
120408 Grandiosity	1	2	3	4	5	NA
120409 Euphoria	1	2	3	4	5	NA
120416 Suicide ideation	1	2	3	4	5	NA
120420 Depression	1	2	3	4	5	NA
120421 Lethargy	1	2	3	4	5	NA
120422 Hyperactivity	1	2	3	4	5	NA
120426 Difficulty making decisions	1	2	3	4	5	NA

Domain-*Psychosocial Health (III)*   **Class**-*Psychological Well-Being (M)*   *1st edition 1997; revised 2004, 2008, 2024*

OUTCOME CONTENT REFERENCES:

Boyd, M., & Luebbert, R. (2020). *Essentials of psychiatric nursing* (2nd ed.). Wolters Kluwer.

+de Souza, C. M., Carissimi, A., Costa, D., Francisco, A. P., Medeiros, M. S., Ilgenfritz, C. A., de Oliveira, M. A., Frey, B. N., & Hidalgo, M. P. (2016). The Mood Rhythm Instrument: Development and preliminary report. *Revista Brasileira de Psiquiatria, 38*(2), 148–153. https://doi.org/10.1590/1516-4446-2015-1763

Kuźnicki, P., Kempiński, R., & Neubauer, K. (2020). The emerging role of mood disorders in inflammatory bowel diseases. *Advances in Clinical Experimental Medicine, 29*(12), 1505–1510. https://doi.org/10.17219/acem/127676

Norris, T. L. (2019). *Porth's pathophysiology: Concepts of altered health states* (10th ed.). Wolters Kluwer.

+Oliveira, M. A. B., Epifano, K., Mathur, S., Carvalho, F. G., Scop, M., Carissimi, A., Francisco, A. P., Garay, L. L. S., Adan, A., Hidalgo, M. P., & Frey, B. N. (2020). Validation of the English version of the Mood Rhythm Instrument. *BMC Psychology, 8*(1), 35. https://doi.org/10.1186/s40359-020-00397-2

+Underwood, B., & Froming, W. J. (1980). The Mood Survey: A personality measure of happy and sad moods. *Journal of Personality Assessment, 44*(4), 404–413. https://doi.org/10.1207/s15327752jpa440411

Motivation 1209

Definition: Inner urge that moves or prompts an individual to positive action(s)

OUTCOME TARGET RATING: Maintain at_____ Increase to_____

OUTCOME OVERALL RATING	Never Demonstrated 1	Rarely Demonstrated 2	Sometimes Demonstrated 3	Often Demonstrated 4	Consistently Demonstrated 5	
Indicators:						
120901 Plans for the future	1	2	3	4	5	NA
120919 Evaluates need for behavior change	1	2	3	4	5	NA
120902 Develops an action plan	1	2	3	4	5	NA
120903 Obtains resources as needed	1	2	3	4	5	NA
120904 Obtains support as needed	1	2	3	4	5	NA
120905 Self-initiates goal directed behavior	1	2	3	4	5	NA
120906 Seeks new experiences to improve health	1	2	3	4	5	NA
120907 Maintains positive self-esteem	1	2	3	4	5	NA
120908 Welcomes opportunity to make contributions	1	2	3	4	5	NA
120916 Maintains flexibility	1	2	3	4	5	NA
120910 Expresses belief in ability to perform action	1	2	3	4	5	NA
120911 Expresses that performance will lead to desired outcome	1	2	3	4	5	NA
120920 Completes required tasks	1	2	3	4	5	NA
120913 Accepts responsibility for actions	1	2	3	4	5	NA
120917 Anticipates intrinsic reward	1	2	3	4	5	NA
120918 Anticipates extrinsic reward	1	2	3	4	5	NA
120915 Expresses intent to act	1	2	3	4	5	NA
120921 Visualizes future self	1	2	3	4	5	NA

Domain-*Psychosocial Health (III)* **Class**-*Psychological Well-Being (M)* *3rd edition 2004; revised 2008, 2024*

OUTCOME CONTENT REFERENCES:

Carter, K. F., & Kulbok, P. A. (2002). Motivation for health behaviours: A systematic review of the nursing literature. *Journal of Advanced Nursing, 40*, 316–330. https://doi.org/10.1046/j.1365-2648.2002.02373.x

Gillison, F. B., Rouse, P., Standage, M., Sebire, S. J., & Ryan, R. M. (2019). A meta-analysis of techniques to promote motivation for health behaviour change from a self-determination theory perspective. *Health Psychology Review, 13*(1), 110–130, https://doi.org/10.1080/17437199.2018.1534071

Helping patients find motivation to make changes. (2019). *Hospital Case Management. 27*(9). https://www.reliasmedia.com/articles/144860-helping-patients-find-motivation-to-make-changes

Lombardi, D. R., Button, M. L., Henny, A., & Westra, H. A. (2014). Measuring motivation: Change talk and counter-change talk in cognitive behavioral therapy for generalized anxiety. *Cognitive Behaviour Therapy, 43*(1), 12–21, https://doi.org/10.1080/16506073.2013.846400

+McEwen, M. (1993). The Health Motivation Assessment Inventory. *Western Journal of Nursing Research, 15*(6), 770–779. https://doi.org/10.1177/019394599301500608

Santos, T. S. S., Julián, C., Vincenzi, S. L., de Andrade, D. F., Slater, B., de Assis, M. A. A., Kafatos, A., de Henauw, S., Gottrand, F., Androutsos, O., Kersting, M., Sjöström, M., Forsner, M., & Moreno, L. A. (2021). A new measure of health motivation influencing food choices and its association with food intakes and nutritional biomarkers in European adolescents. *Public Health Nutrition, 24*(4), 685–695. https://doi.org/10.1017/S1368980019004658

+Thomas, S. D., Hathaway, D. K., & Arheart, K. L. (1990). Development of the General Health Motivation Scale. *Western Journal of Nursing Research, 12*(3), 318–335. https://doi.org/10.1177/019394599001200305

Vroom, V. (1964). *Work and motivation*. Wiley.

M

Musculoskeletal Rehabilitation Participation   1637

Definition: Personal actions to restore and enhance musculoskeletal function and prevent complications from disease, trauma, or surgery

OUTCOME TARGET RATING: Maintain at_____ Increase to_____

		Never Demonstrated	Rarely Demonstrated	Sometimes Demonstrated	Often Demonstrated	Consistently Demonstrated	
OUTCOME OVERALL RATING		1	2	3	4	5	
Indicators:							
163701	Collaborates with health provider to create an individualized rehabilitation plan	1	2	3	4	5	NA
163702	Participates in setting short-term goals	1	2	3	4	5	NA
163703	Participates in setting long-term goals	1	2	3	4	5	NA
163704	Expresses concerns related to rehabilitation	1	2	3	4	5	NA
163705	Uses pain medication before activity if needed	1	2	3	4	5	NA
163706	Performs prescribed exercises	1	2	3	4	5	NA
163707	Maintains body alignment	1	2	3	4	5	NA
163708	Uses strategies to manage pain	1	2	3	4	5	NA
163709	Uses assistive device correctly	1	2	3	4	5	NA
163710	Follows activity restrictions	1	2	3	4	5	NA
163711	Seeks assistance for mobility	1	2	3	4	5	NA
163712	Seeks assistance for self-care	1	2	3	4	5	NA
163713	Performs frequent ambulation	1	2	3	4	5	NA
163714	Monitors activity tolerance	1	2	3	4	5	NA
163715	Monitors active range of motion	1	2	3	4	5	NA
163716	Monitors flexibility	1	2	3	4	5	NA
163717	Monitors muscle strength	1	2	3	4	5	NA
163718	Uses strategies to change body positions safely	1	2	3	4	5	NA
163719	Monitors affected area for edema	1	2	3	4	5	NA
163720	Reports changes in symptoms	1	2	3	4	5	NA
163721	Keeps appointments with health professional	1	2	3	4	5	NA
163722	Uses strategies to prevent complications	1	2	3	4	5	NA
163723	Uses strategies to prevent falls	1	2	3	4	5	NA
163724	Reports progress in rehabilitation	1	2	3	4	5	NA

Domain-*Health Knowledge & Behavior (IV)*   **Class**-*Health Behavior (Q)*   *6th edition 2018*

M

OUTCOME CONTENT REFERENCES:
Clarke, S., & Santy-Tomlinson, J. (2014). *Orthopaedic and trauma nursing: An evidence-based approach to musculoskeletal care*. Wiley Blackwell.
Enseki, K. R., & Berliner, M. (2013). Rehabilitation following total hip arthroplasty surgery. *Topics in Geriatric Rehabilitation, 29*(4), 260–267. https://doi.org/10.1097/TGR.0b013e318292e8dc
Taylor, N., Peiris, C., Kennedy, G., & Shields, N. (2016). Walking tolerance of patients recovering from hip fracture: A phase I trial. *Disability and Rehabilitation, 38*(19), 1900–1908. https://doi.org/10.3109/09638288.2015.1107776
Westby, M. D., & Backman, C. L. (2010). Patient and health professional views on rehabilitation practices and outcomes following total hip and knee arthroplasty for osteoarthritis: A focus group study. *BMC Health Service Research, 10*(1), 1–15. https://doi.org/10.1186/1472-6963-10-119

Nausea & Vomiting Control 1618

Definition: Personal actions to control nausea, retching, and vomiting symptoms

OUTCOME TARGET RATING: Maintain at_____ Increase to_____

		Never Demonstrated	Rarely Demonstrated	Sometimes Demonstrated	Often Demonstrated	Consistently Demonstrated	
OUTCOME OVERALL RATING		1	2	3	4	5	
Indicators:							
161801	Recognizes onset of nausea	1	2	3	4	5	NA
161802	Describes causal factors	1	2	3	4	5	NA
161803	Recognizes precipitating stimuli	1	2	3	4	5	NA
161804	Uses diary to monitor symptoms over time	1	2	3	4	5	NA
161805	Uses preventive measures	1	2	3	4	5	NA
161813	Uses naps to restore energy	1	2	3	4	5	NA
161814	Uses acupressure points for early feelings of queasiness	1	2	3	4	5	NA
161815	Drinks small amounts of fluid	1	2	3	4	5	NA
161816	Consumes smaller meals	1	2	3	4	5	NA
161817	Chooses bland foods	1	2	3	4	5	NA
161818	Uses ginger as an alternative therapy	1	2	3	4	5	NA
161806	Avoids causal factors when possible	1	2	3	4	5	NA
161807	Avoids disagreeable odors	1	2	3	4	5	NA
161808	Uses antiemetic medication as recommended	1	2	3	4	5	NA
161809	Reports failure of antiemetic treatment	1	2	3	4	5	NA
161810	Reports bothersome side effects from antiemetics	1	2	3	4	5	NA
161811	Reports uncontrolled symptoms to health professional	1	2	3	4	5	NA
161819	Reports nausea controlled	1	2	3	4	5	NA
161820	Reports retching controlled	1	2	3	4	5	NA
161821	Reports vomiting controlled	1	2	3	4	5	NA

Domain-*Health Knowledge & Behavior (IV)* **Class**-*Health Behavior (Q)* *3rd edition 2004; revised 2018*

OUTCOME CONTENT REFERENCES:

Arslan, M., & Ozdemir, L. (2015). Oral intake of ginger for chemotherapy-induced nausea and vomiting among women with breast cancer. *Clinical Journal of Oncology Nursing, 19*(5), E92–E97. https://doi.org/10.1188/15.CJON.E92-E97

Collins, A. S. (2011). Postoperative nausea and vomiting in adults: Implications for critical care. *Critical Care Nurse, 31*(6), 36–45. https://doi.org/10.4037/ccn2011470

Nelson, L. (2016). Alterations in gastrointestinal function. In J. K. Itano (Ed.), *Core curriculum for oncology nursing* (5th ed., pp. 340–362). Elsevier.

Revell, M. A. (2017). Self-care of nausea and vomiting in the first trimester of pregnancy. *International Journal of Childbirth Education, 32*(1), 35–38.

N

Nausea & Vomiting: Disruptive Effects   2106

Definition: Severity of observed or reported disruptive effects of chronic nausea, retching, and vomiting on daily functioning

OUTCOME TARGET RATING: Maintain at_____ Increase to_____

	Severe	Substantial	Moderate	Mild	None	
OUTCOME OVERALL RATING	1	2	3	4	5	
Indicators:						
210601 Decreased fluid intake	1	2	3	4	5	NA
210602 Decreased food intake	1	2	3	4	5	NA
210603 Decreased urine output	1	2	3	4	5	NA
210604 Altered fluid balance	1	2	3	4	5	NA
210605 Altered serum electrolytes	1	2	3	4	5	NA
210606 Altered acid/base balance	1	2	3	4	5	NA
210625 Loss of appetite	1	2	3	4	5	NA
210626 Intolerance of odors	1	2	3	4	5	NA
210607 Altered nutritional status	1	2	3	4	5	NA
210608 Weight loss	1	2	3	4	5	NA
210609 Malaise	1	2	3	4	5	NA
210610 Lethargy	1	2	3	4	5	NA
210611 Intolerance of movement	1	2	3	4	5	NA
210612 Impaired physical activity	1	2	3	4	5	NA
210613 Interrupted sleep	1	2	3	4	5	NA
210614 Withdrawal from interpersonal relationships	1	2	3	4	5	NA
210615 Impaired role performance	1	2	3	4	5	NA
210616 Impaired work performance	1	2	3	4	5	NA
210627 Impaired school performance	1	2	3	4	5	NA
210617 Interference with leisure activities	1	2	3	4	5	NA
210618 Interference with activities of daily living (ADLs)	1	2	3	4	5	NA
210619 Anxiety	1	2	3	4	5	NA
210620 Depression	1	2	3	4	5	NA
210621 Emotional stress	1	2	3	4	5	NA
210622 Helplessness	1	2	3	4	5	NA
210623 Side effects from antiemetic medication	1	2	3	4	5	NA
210624 Treatment delays due to symptom severity	1	2	3	4	5	NA
210628 Delayed hospital discharge	1	2	3	4	5	NA

Domain-Health & Life Quality (V)   *Class*-Symptom Status (V)   *3rd edition 2004; revised 2013, 2024*

OUTCOME CONTENT REFERENCES:

Cangemi, D., & Kuo, B. (2019). Practical perspectives in the treatment of nausea and vomiting. *Journal of Clinical Gastroenterology, 53*(3), 170–178. https://doi.org/10.1097/MCG.0000000000001164

Heckroth, M., Luckett, R. T., Moser, C., Parajuli, D., & Abell, T. L. (2021). Nausea and vomiting in 2021: A comprehensive update. *Journal of Clinical Gastroenterology, 55*(4), 279–299. https://doi.org/10.1097/MCG.0000000000001485

Ignatavicius, D. D., Workman, M. L., Rebar, C. R., & Heimgartner, N. M. (2021). *Medical-surgical nursing: Concepts for interprofessional care* (10th ed.). Elsevier.

Kovac, A. L. (2021). Postoperative nausea and vomiting in pediatric patients. *Paediatric Drugs, 23*(1), 11–37. https://doi.org/10.1007/s40272-020-00424-0

Navari, R. M. (2020). Nausea and vomiting in advanced cancer. *Current Treatment Options in Oncology, 21*(2), 1–10. https://doi.org/10.1007/s11864-020-070

N

Nausea & Vomiting Severity

2107

Definition: Severity of signs and symptoms of nausea, retching, and vomiting

OUTCOME TARGET RATING: Maintain at_____ Increase to_____

		Severe	Substantial	Moderate	Mild	None	
OUTCOME OVERALL RATING		1	2	3	4	5	
Indicators:							
210701	Frequency of nausea	1	2	3	4	5	NA
210702	Intensity of nausea	1	2	3	4	5	NA
210703	Distress of nausea	1	2	3	4	5	NA
210704	Frequency of retching	1	2	3	4	5	NA
210705	Intensity of retching	1	2	3	4	5	NA
210706	Distress of retching	1	2	3	4	5	NA
210707	Frequency of vomiting	1	2	3	4	5	NA
210708	Intensity of vomiting	1	2	3	4	5	NA
210709	Distress of vomiting	1	2	3	4	5	NA
210710	Excessive secretion of saliva	1	2	3	4	5	NA
210711	Alteration in taste	1	2	3	4	5	NA
210712	Intolerance of odors	1	2	3	4	5	NA
210713	Weight loss	1	2	3	4	5	NA
210714	Heartburn	1	2	3	4	5	NA
210715	Gastric pain	1	2	3	4	5	NA
210716	Projectile vomiting	1	2	3	4	5	NA
210717	Blood in emesis	1	2	3	4	5	NA
210718	Coffee ground emesis	1	2	3	4	5	NA
210719	Fecal odor of emesis	1	2	3	4	5	NA
210721	Constipation	1	2	3	4	5	NA
210722	Dehydration	1	2	3	4	5	NA
210720	Electrolyte imbalance	1	2	3	4	5	NA

Duration of nausea: ____(hours) ____(days) ____(months)

Amount of emesis _____(cc)

Domain-Health & Life Quality (V)   *Class*-Symptom Status (V)   *3rd edition 2004; revised 2013, 2024*

OUTCOME CONTENT REFERENCES:

Cangemi, D., & Kuo, B. (2019). Practical perspectives in the treatment of nausea and vomiting. *Journal of Clinical Gastroenterology, 53*(3), 170–178. https://doi.org/10.1097/MCG.0000000000001164

Heckroth, M., Luckett, R. T., Moser, C., Parajuli, D., & Abell, T. L. (2021). Nausea and vomiting in 2021: A comprehensive update. *Journal of Clinical Gastroenterology, 55*(4), 279–299. https://doi.org/10.1097/MCG.0000000000001485

Ignatavicius, D. D., Workman, M. L., Rebar, C. R., & Heimgartner, N. M. (2021). *Medical-surgical nursing: Concepts for interprofessional care* (10th ed.). Elsevier.

Navari, R. M. (2020). Nausea and vomiting in advanced cancer. *Current Treatment Options in Oncology, 21*(2), 1–10. https://doi.org/10.1007/s11864-020-0704-8

Wickham, R. J. (2020). Nausea and vomiting: A palliative care imperative. *Current Oncology Reports, 22*(1), 1. https://doi.org/10.1007/s11912-020-0871-6

N

Neglect Cessation   2513

Definition: Evidence that a dependent adult or child is no longer experiencing substandard or omitted care

OUTCOME TARGET RATING: Maintain at_____ Increase to_____

		None	Limited	Moderate	Substantial	Extensive	
OUTCOME OVERALL RATING		1	2	3	4	5	
Indicators:							
251309	Evidence of meeting nutritional needs	1	2	3	4	5	NA
251310	Evidence of personal hygiene maintained	1	2	3	4	5	NA
251311	Evidence of wearing suitable clothing	1	2	3	4	5	NA
251312	Evidence of safe living environment	1	2	3	4	5	NA
251313	Evidence of emotional stability	1	2	3	4	5	NA
251314	Evidence of financial stability	1	2	3	4	5	NA
251315	Evidence of spiritual opportunities	1	2	3	4	5	NA
251316	Evidence of health care needs met	1	2	3	4	5	NA
251317	Evidence of school attendance	1	2	3	4	5	NA
251307	Protection from environmental hazards	1	2	3	4	5	NA
251318	Evidence of adequate supervision	1	2	3	4	5	NA

Domain-*Family Health (VI)*   **Class**-*Family Member Health Status (Z)*   *3rd edition 2004; revised 2018, 2024*

OUTCOME CONTENT REFERENCES:

Carr, A. (2018). Couple therapy, family therapy and systemic interventions for adult-focused problems: *Journal of Family Therapy, 40*(4), 492–536. https://doi.org/10.1111/1467-6427.12225

Carr, A. (2019). Family therapy and systemic interventions for child-focused problems: The current evidence base. *Journal of Family Therapy, 41*(2), 153–213. https://doi.org/10.1111/1467-6427.12226

Coluccia, A., Pozza, A., Ferretti, F., Carabellese, E., Masti, A., & Gualtieri, G. (2020). Online romance scams: Relational dynamics and psychological characteristics of the victims and scammers. A scoping review. *Clinical Practice and Epidemiology in Mental Health, 16*, 24–35. https://doi.org/10.2174/1745017902016010024

Cui, N., & Liu, J. (2020). Physical abuse, emotional abuse, and neglect and childhood behavior problems: A meta-analysis of studies in mainland China. *Trauma, Violence, & Abuse, 21*(1), 206–224. https://doi.org/10.1177/1524838018757750

Digman, C. (2020). Lost voices part 2: Modifying psychological therapies for two young men with complex learning disabilities following alleged sexual and physical abuse: A case study in trauma recovery. *British Journal of Learning Disabilities, 49*, 205–216. https://doi.org/10.1111/bld.12370

Flaherty, E., Legano, L., Idzerda, S., & Council on Child Abuse and Neglect. (2019). Ongoing pediatric health care for the child who has been maltreated. *Pediatrics, 143*, 8–16. https://doi.org/10.1542/peds.2019-0284

Lansford, J. E., Godwin, J., McMahon, R. J., Crowley, M., Pettit, G. S., Bates, J. E., Cole, J. D., & Dodge, K. A. (2021). Early physical abuse and adult outcomes. *Pediatrics, 147*(1), e20200873. https://doi.org/10.1542/peds.2020-0873

Lee, K., Tang, W., Jones, S., Xu, L., & Cong, Z. (2021). The money smart for older adults' program: A qualitative study of the participants' financial well-being. *Journal of Gerontological Social Work, 64*(2), 120–134. https://doi.org/10.1080/01634372.2020.1814477

+Lictenberg, P. A., Gross, E., & Ficker, L. J. (2020). Quantifying risk of financial incapacity and financial exploitation in community-dwelling older adults: Utility of a scoring system for the Lichtenberg Financial Decision-Making Rating Scale. *Clinical Gerontologist, 36*(2), 132–146. https://doi.org/10.1080/073171115.2018.1485812

Morgan, V. A., Di Prinzio, P., Valuri, G., Croft, M., McNeil, T., & Jablensky, J. (2019). Are familial liability for schizophrenia and obstetric complications associated with risk of psychotic illness, after adjusting for other environmental stressors in childhood? *Australian & New Zealand Journal of Psychiatry, 53*(11), 1105–1115. https://doi.org/10.1177/0004867419864427

Russo, A., Reginelli, A., Pignatiello, M., Cioce, F., Mazzei, G., Fabozzi, O., Parlato, V., Cappabianca, S., & Giovine, S. (2018). Imaging of violence against the elderly and the women. *Seminars in Ultrasound CT MRI, 40*, 18–24. https://doi.org/10.1053/j.sult.2018.10.004

Salimath, G., & Raddi, S. A. (2020). Correlation between physical abuse and depression among school going adolescents (10–16 years of age): A school-based study. *Online Journal of Health and Allied Sciences, 19*(2), 1–5.

Varcarolis, E. M., & Fosbre, C. D. (2021). *Essentials of psychiatric-mental health nursing* (4th ed.). Elsevier.

Widom, C. S. (2017). Long term impact of childhood abuse and neglect on crime and violence. *Clinical Psychology: Science and Practice, 24*(2), 186–202. https://doi.org/10.1111/cpsp.12194

Williams, P. (2020). *Basic geriatric nursing* (7th ed.). Elsevier.

Wilson, P. R., Thorpe, R. J. Jr., Sharps, P., & Laughon, K. (2019). The relationship between housing instability and intimate partner violence: A retrospective study. *Public Health Nursing, 38*, 32–39. https://doi.org/10.1111/phn.12819

Yoon, S., Cummings, S., Nugent, W. R., & Forrest-Bank, S. (2020). Protective factors against suicidal ideation among community-dwelling older adults with experience of spousal physical abuse: Focusing on direct and indirect protections. *Aging & Mental Health, 24*(11), 1854–1863. https://doi.org/10.1080/13607863.2019.1636208

N

Neglect: Disruptive Effects   2516

Definition: Severity of observed or reported disruptive effects due to experiencing substandard care

OUTCOME TARGET RATING: Maintain at_____ Increase to_____

	Severe	Substantial	Moderate	Mild	None	
OUTCOME OVERALL RATING	1	2	3	4	5	
Indicators:						
251601 Fatigue	1	2	3	4	5	NA
251602 Attention seeking behavior	1	2	3	4	5	NA
251603 Anxiety	1	2	3	4	5	NA
251604 Depression	1	2	3	4	5	NA
251605 Perceived stress	1	2	3	4	5	NA
251606 Irritability	1	2	3	4	5	NA
251607 Low self-esteem	1	2	3	4	5	NA
251608 Inappropriate social behavior	1	2	3	4	5	NA
251609 Inability to interact with others	1	2	3	4	5	NA
251610 Suicidal ideations	1	2	3	4	5	NA
251611 Substance abuse of opioids	1	2	3	4	5	NA
251612 Substance abuse of cocaine	1	2	3	4	5	NA
251613 Malnutrition	1	2	3	4	5	NA
251614 Unstable access to food	1	2	3	4	5	NA
251615 Personal hygiene deficit	1	2	3	4	5	NA
251616 Inappropriate clothing	1	2	3	4	5	NA
251617 Alcohol consumption	1	2	3	4	5	NA
251618 Absence from school	1	2	3	4	5	NA
251619 Impact on school performance	1	2	3	4	5	NA
251620 Housing instability	1	2	3	4	5	NA
251621 Financial hardship	1	2	3	4	5	NA
251622 Cognitive deficits	1	2	3	4	5	NA
251623 Communication deficits	1	2	3	4	5	NA
251624 Employment instability	1	2	3	4	5	NA

Domain-Health & Life Quality (V)   **Class**-Symptom Status (V)   7th edition 2024

OUTCOME CONTENT REFERENCES:

Cui, N., & Liu, J. (2020). Physical abuse, emotional abuse, and neglect and childhood behavior problems: A meta-analysis of studies in mainland China. *Trauma, Violence, & Abuse, 21*(1), 206–224. https://doi.org/10.1177/1524838018757750

De Bellis, M. D., Morey, R. A., Nooner, K. B., Woolley, D. P., Haswell, C. C., & Hooper, S. R. (2019). A pilot study of neurocognitive function and brains structures in adolescents with alcohol use disorders: Does maltreatment history matter? *Child Maltreatment, 24*(4), 374–388. https://doi.org/10.1177/1077559518810525

Flaherty, E., Legano, L., Idzerda, S., & Council on Child Abuse and Neglect. (2019). Ongoing pediatric health care for the child who has been maltreated. *Pediatrics, 143*, 8–16. https://doi.org/10.1542/peds.2019-0284

Hawkins, M., & Panzera, A. (2021). Food insecurity: A key determinant of health. *Archives of Psychiatric Nursing, 35*, 113–117. https://doi.org/10.1016/j.apnu.2020.10.01

Palazón-Carrión, E., & Sala-Roca, J. (2020). Communication and language in abused and institutionalized minors. A scoping review. *Children and Youth Services Review, 112*, 104904. https://doi.org/10.1016/j.childyouth.2020.104904

Palmer, C. J., Williams, Y., & Harrington, A. (2019). Explaining the effects of childhood trauma: The long and winding road. *Journal of Psychiatric and Mental Health Nursing, 27*(3), 205–210. https://doi.org/10.1111/jpm.12581

Sierau, S., Warmingham, J., White, L. O., Klein, A. M., & von Klitzing, K. (2020). Childhood emotional and conduct problems in childhood and adolescence differentially associated with intergenerational maltreatment continuity and parental internalizing symptoms. *Journal of Abnormal Child Psychology, 48*, 29–42. https://doi.org/10.1007/s10802-019-00575-w

van Delft, I., Finkenauer, C., de Schipper, J. C., & Lamers-Winkelman, F. (2021). Talking about feelings: Mother-child emotion dialogues among sexually abused children. *Journal of Interpersonal Violence, 36*(9–10), NP4941–NP4963. https://doi.org/10.1177/0886260518795176

Varcarolis, E. M., & Fosbre, C. D. (2021). *Essentials of psychiatric-mental health nursing* (4th ed.). Elsevier.

Widom, C. S. (2017). Long term impact of childhood abuse and neglect on crime and violence. *Clinical Psychology: Science and Practice. 24*(2), 186–202. https://doi.org/10.1111/cpsp.12194

Wilson, P. R., Thorpe, R. J. Jr., Sharps, P., & Laughon, K. (2021). The relationship between housing instability and intimate partner violence: A retrospective study. *Public Health Nursing, 38*, 32–39. https://doi.org/10.1111/phn.12819

Neglect Recovery   2512

Definition: Personal actions to show physical, emotional, and spiritual healing following the cessation of substandard care

OUTCOME TARGET RATING: Maintain at_____ Increase to_____

OUTCOME OVERALL RATING	Never Demonstrated 1	Rarely Demonstrated 2	Sometimes Demonstrated 3	Often Demonstrated 4	Consistently Demonstrated 5	
Indicators:						
251231 Maintains personal hygiene	1	2	3	4	5	NA
251232 Selects suitable clothing for weather	1	2	3	4	5	NA
251233 Maintains clean living environment	1	2	3	4	5	NA
251234 Maintains safe living environment	1	2	3	4	5	NA
251235 Communicates at appropriate age level	1	2	3	4	5	NA
251236 Shows interest in life	1	2	3	4	5	NA
251237 Trusts others	1	2	3	4	5	NA
251238 Expresses pride in self	1	2	3	4	5	NA
251239 Expresses hope	1	2	3	4	5	NA
251240 Emotional needs met	1	2	3	4	5	NA
251241 Discusses emotional experiences with others	1	2	3	4	5	NA
251242 Advocates for self	1	2	3	4	5	NA
251243 Interacts with others	1	2	3	4	5	NA
251244 Expands social network	1	2	3	4	5	NA
251245 Participates in treatment programs	1	2	3	4	5	NA
251246 Obtains appropriate health care	1	2	3	4	5	NA
251247 Eats nutritious meals	1	2	3	4	5	NA
251248 Maintains medication regimen	1	2	3	4	5	NA
251249 Uses appropriate equipment or appliance for care	1	2	3	4	5	NA
251250 Obtains cognitive stimulation	1	2	3	4	5	NA
251251 Achieves academic success	1	2	3	4	5	NA
251252 Achieves successful employment	1	2	3	4	5	NA
251253 Performs responsibilities reasonable for age	1	2	3	4	5	NA
251254 Behaves according to social norms	1	2	3	4	5	NA
251255 Abstinence from substance abuse	1	2	3	4	5	NA
251256 Seeks available community resources	1	2	3	4	5	NA
251257 Attends support groups	1	2	3	4	5	NA
251258 Participates in spiritual activities	1	2	3	4	5	NA

Domain-*Family Health (VI)*   **Class**-*Family Member Health Status (Z)*   *1st edition 1997; revised 2004, 2008, 2024*

N

OUTCOME CONTENT REFERENCES:

Bartlett, J. D., & Smith, S. (2019). The role of early care and education in addressing early childhood trauma. *American Journal of Community Psychology, 64*(3-4), 359–372. https://doi.org/10.1002/ajcp.12380

Beaton, J., & Thielking, M. (2019). Chronic mistrust and complex trauma: Australian psychologists' perspectives on the treatment of young women with a history of childhood maltreatment. *Australian Psychologist, 55*(3), 230–243. https://doi.org/10.1111/ap.12430

Carr, A. (2018). Couple therapy, family therapy and systematic interventions for adult-focused problems: The current evidence base. *Journal of Family Therapy, 41*(4), 492–526. https://doi.org/10.1111/1467-6427.12225

Carr, A. (2019). Family therapy and systematic interventions for child-focused problems: The current evidence base. *Journal of Family Therapy, 41*(2), 155–213. https://doi.org/10.1111/1467-6427.12226

De Bellis, M. D., Morey, R. A., Nooner, K. B., Woolley, D. P., Haswell, C. C., & Hooper, S. R. (2019). A pilot study of neurocognitive function and brain structures in adolescents with alcohol use disorders: Does maltreatment history matter? *Child Maltreatment, 24*(4), 374–388. https://doi.org/10.1177/1077559518810525

Flaherty, E., Legano, L., Idzerda, S., & Council on Child Abuse and Neglect. (2019). Ongoing pediatric health care for the child who has been maltreated. *Pediatrics, 143*(4), 8–16. https://doi.org/10.1542/peds.2019-0284

Palazón-Carrión, E., & Sala-Roca, J. (2020). Communication and language in abused and institutionalized minors. A scoping review. *Children And Youth Services Review, 112*, 104904. https://doi.org/10.1016/j.childyouth.2020.104904

van Delft, I., Finkenauer, C., De Schipper, J. C., & Lamers-Winkelman, F. (2021). Talking about feelings: Mother-child emotion dialogues among sexually abused children. *Journal of Interpersonal Violence, 36*(9-10), NP4941–NP4963. https://doi.org/10.1177/0886260518795176

Varcarolis, E. M., & Fosbre, C. D. (2021). *Essentials of psychiatric-mental health nursing* (4th ed.). Elsevier.

Williams, P. (2020). *Basic geriatric nursing* (7th ed.). Elsevier.

Neurological Function 0909

Definition: Ability of the peripheral and central nervous systems to receive, process, and respond to internal and external stimuli

OUTCOME TARGET RATING: Maintain at_____ Increase to_____

OUTCOME OVERALL RATING		Severely Compromised 1	Substantially Compromised 2	Moderately Compromised 3	Mildly Compromised 4	Not Compromised 5	
Indicators:							
090901	Consciousness	1	2	3	4	5	NA
090902	Central motor control	1	2	3	4	5	NA
090903	Cranial sensory and motor function	1	2	3	4	5	NA
090904	Spinal sensory and motor function	1	2	3	4	5	NA
090905	Autonomic function	1	2	3	4	5	NA
090906	Intracranial pressure	1	2	3	4	5	NA
090907	Communication appropriate to situation	1	2	3	4	5	NA
090908	Pupil size	1	2	3	4	5	NA
090909	Pupil reactivity	1	2	3	4	5	NA
090910	Eye movement pattern	1	2	3	4	5	NA
090911	Breathing pattern	1	2	3	4	5	NA
090913	Sleep-rest pattern	1	2	3	4	5	NA
090917	Blood pressure	1	2	3	4	5	NA
090918	Pulse pressure	1	2	3	4	5	NA
090919	Respiratory rate	1	2	3	4	5	NA
090920	Hyperthermia	1	2	3	4	5	NA
090921	Apical heart rate	1	2	3	4	5	NA
090922	Radial pulse rate	1	2	3	4	5	NA
090923	Cognitive orientation	1	2	3	4	5	NA
090924	Cognitive status	1	2	3	4	5	NA
		Severe	Substantial	Moderate	Mild	None	
090914	Seizure activity	1	2	3	4	5	NA
090915	Headaches	1	2	3	4	5	NA

Domain-*Physiologic Health (II)* **Class**-*Neurocognitive (J)*   *1st edition 1997; reviewed 2018; revised 2004, 2024*

OUTCOME CONTENT REFERENCES:
Hickey, J. V., & Strayer, A. L. (Eds.). (2019). *The clinical practice of neurological and neurosurgical nursing* (8th ed.). Wolters Kluwer.
Huether, S. E., McCance, K. L., & Brashers, V. L. (2020). *Understanding pathophysiology* (7th ed.). Elsevier.
Ignatavicius, D. D., Workman, M. L., Rebar, C. R., & Heimgartner, N. M. (2021). *Medical-surgical nursing: Concepts for interprofessional care* (10th ed.). Elsevier.
Louis, E. D., Mayer, S. A., & Noble, J. M. (2021). *Merritt's neurology* (14th ed.). Wolters Kluwer.
+Teasdale, G., & Jennett, B. (1974). Assessment of coma and impaired consciousness: A practical scale. *Lancet, 2*(7872), 81–84.
   https://doi.org/10.1016/s0140-6736(74)91639-0

Neurological Function: Autonomic   0910

Definition: Ability of the autonomic nervous system to coordinate visceral and homeostatic functions

OUTCOME TARGET RATING: Maintain at_____ Increase to_____

		Severely Compromised	Substantially Compromised	Moderately Compromised	Mildly Compromised	Not Compromised	
OUTCOME OVERALL RATING		1	2	3	4	5	
Indicators:							
091001	Apical heart rate	1	2	3	4	5	NA
091020	Radial pulse rate	1	2	3	4	5	NA
091002	Systolic blood pressure	1	2	3	4	5	NA
091003	Diastolic blood pressure	1	2	3	4	5	NA
091004	Cardiac pump effectiveness	1	2	3	4	5	NA
091005	Vasodilatation response	1	2	3	4	5	NA
091006	Vasoconstriction response	1	2	3	4	5	NA
091007	Perspiration response pattern	1	2	3	4	5	NA
091008	Goose bumps response pattern	1	2	3	4	5	NA
091009	Bowel elimination pattern	1	2	3	4	5	NA
091010	Intestinal motility	1	2	3	4	5	NA
091011	Urinary elimination pattern	1	2	3	4	5	NA
091021	Pupil reactivity	1	2	3	4	5	NA
091013	Thermoregulation	1	2	3	4	5	NA
091014	Peripheral tissue perfusion	1	2	3	4	5	NA
091015	Sexual organ response	1	2	3	4	5	NA
		Severe	**Substantial**	**Moderate**	**Mild**	**None**	
091016	Bronchospasms	1	2	3	4	5	NA
091017	Intestinal spasms	1	2	3	4	5	NA
091018	Bladder spasms	1	2	3	4	5	NA
091022	Headaches	1	2	3	4	5	NA
091023	Dilated pupils	1	2	3	4	5	NA
091024	Constricted pupils	1	2	3	4	5	NA
091025	Hyperthermia	1	2	3	4	5	NA
091026	Dysreflexia	1	2	3	4	5	NA

Domain-Physiologic Health (II)   **Class**-Neurocognitive (J)   *1st edition 1997; reviewed 2018; revised 2004, 2024*

OUTCOME CONTENT REFERENCES:
Hickey, J. V., & Strayer, A. L. (Eds.). (2019). *The clinical practice of neurological and neurosurgical nursing* (8th ed.). Wolters Kluwer.
Huether, S. E., McCance, K. L., & Brashers, V. L. (2020). *Understanding pathophysiology* (7th ed.). Elsevier.
Ignatavicius, D. D., Workman, M. L., Rebar, C. R., & Heimgartner, N. M. (2021). *Medical-surgical nursing: Concepts for interprofessional care* (10th ed.). Elsevier.
Louis, E. D., Mayer, S. A., & Noble, J. M. (2021). *Merritt's neurology* (14th ed.). Wolters Kluwer.
+Teasdale, G., & Jennett, B. (1974). Assessment of coma and impaired consciousness: A practical scale. *Lancet, 2*(7872), 81–84.
    https://doi.org/10.1016/s0140-6736(74)91639-0

N

Neurological Function: Central Motor Control   0911

Definition: Ability of the central nervous system to coordinate skeletal muscle activity for body movement

OUTCOME TARGET RATING: Maintain at_____ Increase to_____

	Severely Compromised	Substantially Compromised	Moderately Compromised	Mildly Compromised	Not Compromised	
OUTCOME OVERALL RATING	1	2	3	4	5	
Indicators:						
091101 Balance	1	2	3	4	5	NA
091103 Maintenance of posture	1	2	3	4	5	NA
091104 Infantile reflexes (automatisms)	1	2	3	4	5	NA
091105 Babinski's reflex	1	2	3	4	5	NA
091106 Deep tendon reflexes	1	2	3	4	5	NA
091112 Purposeful movement on command	1	2	3	4	5	NA
	Severe	**Substantial**	**Moderate**	**Mild**	**None**	
091113 Gait abnormalities	1	2	3	4	5	NA
091107 Spasticity	1	2	3	4	5	NA
091108 Involuntary movements	1	2	3	4	5	NA
091109 Nystagmus	1	2	3	4	5	NA
091110 Seizure activity	1	2	3	4	5	NA

Domain-*Physiologic Health (II)*   **Class**-*Neurocognitive (J)*   *1st edition 1997; reviewed 2018; revised 2004, 2024*

OUTCOME CONTENT REFERENCES:
Hickey, J. V., & Strayer, A. L. (Eds.). (2019). *The clinical practice of neurological and neurosurgical nursing* (8th ed.). Wolters Kluwer.
Huether, S. E., McCance, K. L., & Brashers, V. L. (2020). *Understanding pathophysiology* (7th ed.). Elsevier.
Ignatavicius, D. D., Workman, M. L., Rebar, C. R., & Heimgartner, N. M. (2021). *Medical-surgical nursing: Concepts for interprofessional care* (10th ed.). Elsevier.
Louis, E. D., Mayer, S. A., & Noble, J. M. (2021). *Merritt's neurology* (14th ed.). Wolters Kluwer.
Shahrokhi, M., & Asuncion, R. M. D. (2021, April 29). Neurologic Exam. In *StatPearls*. StatPearls Publishing. https://www.ncbi.nlm.nih.gov/books/NBK557589/

Neurological Function: Consciousness   0912

Definition: Ability of the central nervous system to maintain arousal, orientation, attention, and respond to the environment

OUTCOME TARGET RATING: Maintain at_____ Increase to_____

	Severely Compromised	Substantially Compromised	Moderately Compromised	Mildly Compromised	Not Compromised	
OUTCOME OVERALL RATING	1	2	3	4	5	
Indicators:						
091201 Opens eyes to external stimuli	1	2	3	4	5	NA
091215 Responds to auditory stimuli	1	2	3	4	5	NA
091202 Cognitive orientation	1	2	3	4	5	NA
091203 Communication appropriate to situation	1	2	3	4	5	NA
091204 Obeys commands	1	2	3	4	5	NA
091205 Motor responses to noxious stimuli	1	2	3	4	5	NA
091206 Attends to environmental stimuli	1	2	3	4	5	NA
	Severe	**Substantial**	**Moderate**	**Mild**	**None**	
091207 Seizure activity	1	2	3	4	5	NA
091209 Abnormal flexion	1	2	3	4	5	NA
091210 Abnormal extension	1	2	3	4	5	NA

Neurological Function: Consciousness—cont'd

		Severe	Substantial	Moderate	Mild	None	
091211	Stupor	1	2	3	4	5	NA
091212	Trance state	1	2	3	4	5	NA
091213	Delirium	1	2	3	4	5	NA
091214	Coma	1	2	3	4	5	NA

Glasgow Coma Scale score_____

Domain-Physiologic Health (II)   *Class*-Neurocognitive (J)   *1st edition 1997; reviewed 2018; revised 2004, 2008, 2024*

OUTCOME CONTENT REFERENCES:

Hickey, J. V., & Strayer, A. L. (Eds.). (2019). *The clinical practice of neurological and neurosurgical nursing* (8th ed.). Wolters Kluwer.

Huether, S. E., McCance, K. L., & Brashers, V. L. (2020). *Understanding pathophysiology* (7th ed.). Elsevier.

Ignatavicius, D. D., Workman, M. L., Rebar, C. R., & Heimgartner, N. M. (2021). *Medical-surgical nursing: Concepts for interprofessional care* (10th ed.). Elsevier.

Kostick, K. M., Halm, A., O'Brien, K., Kothari, S., & Blumenthal-Barby, J. S. (2021). Conceptualizations of consciousness and continuation of care among family members and health professionals caring for patients in a minimally conscious state. *Disability & Rehabilitation*, *43*(16), 2285–2294. https://doi.org/10.1080/09638288.2019.1697383

Louis, E. D., Mayer, S. A., & Noble, J. M. (2021). *Merritt's neurology* (14th ed.). Wolters Kluwer.

+Teasdale, G., & Jennett, B. (1974). Assessment of coma and impaired consciousness: A practical scale. *Lancet*, *2*(7872), 81–84. https://doi.org/10.1016/s0140-6736(74)91639-0

Neurological Function: Cranial Sensory/Motor   0913

Definition: Ability of the cranial nerves to convey sensory and motor impulses

OUTCOME TARGET RATING: Maintain at_____ Increase to_____

		Severely Compromised	Substantially Compromised	Moderately Compromised	Mildly Compromised	Not Compromised	
OUTCOME OVERALL RATING		**1**	**2**	**3**	**4**	**5**	
Indicators:							
091301	Olfaction	1	2	3	4	5	NA
091302	Vision	1	2	3	4	5	NA
091303	Corneal reflex	1	2	3	4	5	NA
091304	Taste	1	2	3	4	5	NA
091305	Hearing	1	2	3	4	5	NA
091317	Speech	1	2	3	4	5	NA
091306	Facial sensation	1	2	3	4	5	NA
091307	Facial muscle movement	1	2	3	4	5	NA
091318	Facial symmetry	1	2	3	4	5	NA
091319	Bilateral muscle strength	1	2	3	4	5	NA
091308	Swallowing	1	2	3	4	5	NA
091309	Gag reflex	1	2	3	4	5	NA
091310	Tongue movement	1	2	3	4	5	NA
091312	Purposeful head movement	1	2	3	4	5	NA
091320	Purposeful shoulder movement	1	2	3	4	5	NA

		Severe	Substantial	Moderate	Mild	None	
091314	Dizziness	1	2	3	4	5	NA
091315	Pronator drift	1	2	3	4	5	NA
091321	Involuntary head movement	1	2	3	4	5	NA
091322	Involuntary facial movement	1	2	3	4	5	NA
091323	Tics	1	2	3	4	5	NA
091324	Hoarseness	1	2	3	4	5	NA
091325	Nasal tone to voice	1	2	3	4	5	NA
091326	Unilateral facial paralysis	1	2	3	4	5	NA

Domain-Physiologic Health (II)   *Class*-Neurocognitive (J)   *1st edition 1997; reviewed 2018; revised 2004, 2024*

N

OUTCOME CONTENT REFERENCES:
Hickey, J. V., & Strayer, A. L. (Eds.). (2019). *The clinical practice of neurological and neurosurgical nursing* (8th ed.). Wolters Kluwer.
Huether, S. E., McCance, K. L., & Brashers, V. L. (2020). *Understanding pathophysiology* (7th ed.). Elsevier.
Ignatavicius, D. D., Workman, M. L., Rebar, C. R., & Heimgartner, N. M. (2021). *Medical-surgical nursing: Concepts for interprofessional care* (10th ed.). Elsevier.
Louis, E. D., Mayer, S. A., & Noble, J. M. (2021). *Merritt's neurology* (14th ed.). Wolters Kluwer.
+Teasdale, G., & Jennett, B. (1974). Assessment of coma and impaired consciousness: A practical scale. *Lancet, 2*(7872), 81–84.
  https://doi.org/10.1016/s0140-6736(74)91639-0

Neurological Function: Peripheral

0917

Definition: Ability of the peripheral nervous system to transmit impulses to and from the central nervous system

OUTCOME TARGET RATING: Maintain at_____ Increase to_____

		Severely Compromised	Substantially Compromised	Moderately Compromised	Mildly Compromised	Not Compromised	
OUTCOME OVERALL RATING		1	2	3	4	5	
Indicators:							
091701	Sensation in upper right extremity	1	2	3	4	5	NA
091702	Sensation in upper left extremity	1	2	3	4	5	NA
091703	Sensation in lower right extremity	1	2	3	4	5	NA
091704	Sensation in lower left extremity	1	2	3	4	5	NA
091705	Sensation equal bilaterally	1	2	3	4	5	NA
091706	Motor function in upper right extremity	1	2	3	4	5	NA
091707	Motor function in upper left extremity	1	2	3	4	5	NA
091708	Motor function in lower right extremity	1	2	3	4	5	NA
091709	Motor function in lower left extremity	1	2	3	4	5	NA
091710	Motor function equal bilaterally	1	2	3	4	5	NA
091711	Skin color in upper right extremity	1	2	3	4	5	NA
091712	Skin color in upper left extremity	1	2	3	4	5	NA
091713	Skin color in lower right extremity	1	2	3	4	5	NA
091714	Skin color in lower left extremity	1	2	3	4	5	NA
091715	Proprioception in upper right extremity	1	2	3	4	5	NA
091716	Proprioception in upper left extremity	1	2	3	4	5	NA
091717	Proprioception in lower right extremity	1	2	3	4	5	NA
091718	Proprioception in lower left extremity	1	2	3	4	5	NA
091719	Proprioception equal bilaterally	1	2	3	4	5	NA
091720	Hot/cold discrimination in upper right extremity	1	2	3	4	5	NA
091721	Hot/cold discrimination in upper left extremity	1	2	3	4	5	NA
091722	Hot/cold discrimination in lower right extremity	1	2	3	4	5	NA
091723	Hot/cold discrimination in lower left extremity	1	2	3	4	5	NA
091724	Hot/cold discrimination equal bilaterally	1	2	3	4	5	NA
091725	Muscle tone in upper right extremity	1	2	3	4	5	NA
091726	Muscle tone in upper left extremity	1	2	3	4	5	NA
091727	Muscle tone in lower right extremity	1	2	3	4	5	NA
091728	Muscle tone in lower left extremity	1	2	3	4	5	NA
091729	Muscle tone equal bilaterally	1	2	3	4	5	NA
		Severe	**Substantial**	**Moderate**	**Mild**	**None**	
091730	Hyperesthesia in upper right extremity	1	2	3	4	5	NA
091731	Hyperesthesia in upper left extremity	1	2	3	4	5	NA
091732	Hyperesthesia in lower right extremity	1	2	3	4	5	NA
091733	Hyperesthesia in lower left extremity	1	2	3	4	5	NA

Neurological Function: Peripheral—cont'd

		Severe	Substantial	Moderate	Mild	None	
091734	Hypoesthesia in upper right extremity	1	2	3	4	5	NA
091735	Hypoesthesia in upper left extremity	1	2	3	4	5	NA
091736	Hypoesthesia in lower right extremity	1	2	3	4	5	NA
091737	Hypoesthesia in lower left extremity	1	2	3	4	5	NA
091738	Pain in upper right extremity	1	2	3	4	5	NA
091739	Pain in upper left extremity	1	2	3	4	5	NA
091740	Pain in lower right extremity	1	2	3	4	5	NA
091741	Pain in lower left extremity	1	2	3	4	5	NA
091742	Paresthesia in upper right extremity	1	2	3	4	5	NA
091743	Paresthesia in upper left extremity	1	2	3	4	5	NA
091744	Paresthesia in lower right extremity	1	2	3	4	5	NA
091745	Paresthesia in lower left extremity	1	2	3	4	5	NA

Domain-*Physiologic Health (II)*   **Class**-*Neurocognitive (J)*   *4th edition 2008; revised 2024*

OUTCOME CONTENT REFERENCES:

Andalib, S., Biller, J., Di Napoli, M., Moghimi, N., McCullough, L. D., Rubinos, C. A., O'Hana Nobleza, C., Azarpazhooh, M. R., Catanese, L., Elicer, I., Jafari, M., Liberati, F., Camejo, C., Torbey, M., & Divani, A. A. (2021). Peripheral nervous system manifestations associated with COVID-19. *Current Neurology and Neuroscience Reports, 21*(3), 9. https://doi.org/10.1007/s11910-021-01102-5

Huether, S. E., McCance, K. L., & Brashers, V. L. (2020). *Understanding pathophysiology* (7th ed.). Elsevier.

Ignatavicius, D. D., Workman, M. L., Rebar, C. R., & Heimgartner, N. M. (2021). *Medical-surgical nursing: Concepts for interprofessional care* (10th ed.). Elsevier.

Louis, E. D., Mayer, S. A., & Noble, J. M. (2021). *Merritt's neurology* (14th ed.). Wolters Kluwer.

Neurological Function: Spinal Sensory/Motor   0914

Definition: Ability of the spinal nerves to convey sensory and motor impulses

OUTCOME TARGET RATING: Maintain at_____ Increase to_____

N

		Severely Compromised	Substantially Compromised	Moderately Compromised	Mildly Compromised	Not Compromised	
OUTCOME OVERALL RATING		1	2	3	4	5	
Indicators:							
091401	Head and shoulder movement	1	2	3	4	5	NA
091402	Autonomic function	1	2	3	4	5	NA
091403	Deep tendon reflexes	1	2	3	4	5	NA
091404	Upper body skin sensation	1	2	3	4	5	NA
091409	Lower body skin sensation	1	2	3	4	5	NA
091405	Upper body strength	1	2	3	4	5	NA
091410	Lower body strength	1	2	3	4	5	NA
		Severe	Substantial	Moderate	Mild	None	
091406	Flaccidity	1	2	3	4	5	NA
091407	Pronator drift	1	2	3	4	5	NA
091411	Involuntary movement	1	2	3	4	5	NA
091412	Fasciculation	1	2	3	4	5	NA

Domain-*Physiologic Health (II)*   **Class**-*Neurocognitive (J)*   *1st edition 1997; reviewed 2018; revised 2004, 2024*

OUTCOME CONTENT REFERENCES:

Hickey, J. V., & Strayer, A. L. (Eds.). (2019). *The clinical practice of neurological and neurosurgical nursing* (8th ed.). Wolters Kluwer.

Huether, S. E., McCance, K. L., & Brashers, V. L. (2020). *Understanding pathophysiology* (7th ed.). Elsevier.

Ignatavicius, D. D., Workman, M. L., Rebar, C. R., & Heimgartner, N. M. (2021). *Medical-surgical nursing: Concepts for interprofessional care* (10th ed.). Elsevier.

Louis, E. D., Mayer, S. A., & Noble, J. M. (2021). *Merritt's neurology* (14th ed.). Wolters Kluwer.

+Teasdale, G., & Jennett, B. (1974). Assessment of coma and impaired consciousness: A practical scale. *Lancet, 2*(7872), 81–84. https://doi.org/10.1016/s0140-6736(74)91639-0

Newborn Adaptation

Definition: Adaptive response to the extrauterine environment by a physiologically mature newborn during the first 28 days

OUTCOME TARGET RATING: Maintain at_____ Increase to_____

		Severe Deviation from Normal Range	Substantial Deviation from Normal Range	Moderate Deviation from Normal range	Mild Deviation from Normal Range	No Deviation from Normal Range	
OUTCOME OVERALL RATING		1	2	3	4	5	
Indicators:							
011801	Apgar score	1	2	3	4	5	NA
011802	Gestational age index	1	2	3	4	5	NA
011803	Apical heart rate (100–160 bpm)	1	2	3	4	5	NA
011804	Respiratory rate (30–60)	1	2	3	4	5	NA
011805	Blood pressure ratio of arm to leg	1	2	3	4	5	NA
011806	Oxygen saturation >90%	1	2	3	4	5	NA
011807	Thermoregulation	1	2	3	4	5	NA
011808	Skin color	1	2	3	4	5	NA
011809	Eyes clear	1	2	3	4	5	NA
011810	Cord drying	1	2	3	4	5	NA
011811	Weight	1	2	3	4	5	NA
011812	Feeding tolerance	1	2	3	4	5	NA
011813	Suck reflex	1	2	3	4	5	NA
011827	Coordinates suck, swallowing, and breathing pattern	1	2	3	4	5	NA
011814	Muscle tone	1	2	3	4	5	NA
011815	Smooth, synchronous movement	1	2	3	4	5	NA
011816	Attentiveness to stimuli	1	2	3	4	5	NA
011817	Response to stimuli	1	2	3	4	5	NA
011818	Sustained alertness during interaction	1	2	3	4	5	NA
011819	Interaction with caregiver	1	2	3	4	5	NA
011820	Self-consolability	1	2	3	4	5	NA
011821	Blood glucose	1	2	3	4	5	NA
011822	Coombs test	1	2	3	4	5	NA
011823	Bilirubin level	1	2	3	4	5	NA
011824	Bowel elimination	1	2	3	4	5	NA
011825	Urinary elimination	1	2	3	4	5	NA

Domain-Functional Health (I)   **Class**-Growth & Development (B)   2nd edition 2000; revised 2004, 2024

OUTCOME CONTENT REFERENCES:

Crovetto, F., Fumagalli, M., De Carli, A., Baffero, G. M., Nozza, S., Dessimone, F., Vergani, P., Fedele, L., Mosca, F., & Acaia, B. (2018). Obstetric risk factors for poor neonatal adaptation at birth. *Journal of Maternal-Fetal Neonatal Medicine, 31*(18), 2429–2435. https://doi.org/10.1080/14767058.2017.1344635

Gualdrón, L. M. V., & Villalobos, M. M. D. (2019). Effect of infant stimulation on the adaptation to birth: A randomized trial. *Revista Latin-Americana Enfermagem, 27.* https://doi.org/10.1590/1518-8345.2896.3176

Guimarães, M. A. P., Alves, C. R. L., Cardoso, A. A., & Magalhães, L. C. (2017). Observation of neonatal behavior: Cross-cultural adaptation of the newborn behavioral observations. *Revista Paulista de Pediatria, 36*(1), 8. https://doi.org/10.1590/1984-0462/;2018;36;1;00017

Kenner, C., Altimier, L., & Boykova, M. (2019). *Comprehensive neonatal nursing care* (6th ed.). Springer.

Morton, S. U., & Brodsky, D. (2016). Fetal physiology and the transition to extrauterine life. *Clinical Perinatology, 43*(3), 395–407. https://doi.org/10.1016/j.clp.2016.04.001

Murray, S. S., & McKinney, E. S. (2018). *Foundations of maternal-newborn and women's health nursing* (7th ed.). Elsevier.

Verklan, T., Walden, M., & Forest, S. (2021). *Core curriculum for neonatal intensive care nursing* (6th ed.). Elsevier.

Nutritional Status   1004

Definition: Adequacy of nutrients ingested and absorbed to meet metabolic needs

OUTCOME TARGET RATING: Maintain at_____ Increase to_____

	Severe Deviation from Normal Range	Substantial Deviation from Normal Range	Moderate Deviation from Normal Range	Mild Deviation from Normal Range	No Deviation from Normal Range	
OUTCOME OVERALL RATING	1	2	3	4	5	
Indicators:						
100401 Nutrient intake	1	2	3	4	5	NA
100402 Food intake	1	2	3	4	5	NA
100408 Fluid intake	1	2	3	4	5	NA
100403 Energy	1	2	3	4	5	NA
100405 Weight/height ratio	1	2	3	4	5	NA
100411 Hydration	1	2	3	4	5	NA

Domain-*Physiologic Health (II)*   **Class**-*Digestion & Nutrition (K)*   *1st edition 1997; revised 2004, 2013, 2024*

OUTCOME CONTENT REFERENCES:

Dudek, S. G. (2022). *Nutrition essentials for nursing practice* (9th ed.). Wolters Kluwer.

+Guigoz, Y., Vellas, B., & Garry, P. J. (1996). Mini Nutritional Assessment: A practical assessment tool for grading the nutritional state of elderly patients. *Facts and Research in Gerontology, 4*(Suppl. 2), 15–59. https://doi.org/10.1016/s0899-9007(98)00171-3

Katz, D. L., Friedman, R. S. C., Joshi, S., Levitt, J., & Ye, M.-C. (2022). *Nutrition in clinical practice*. Wolters Kluwer.

U.S. Department of Health and Human Services and U.S. Department of Agriculture. (2020). 2020–2025 *Dietary guidelines for Americans* (9th ed.).

Nutritional Status: Biochemical Measures   1005

Definition: Adequacy of chemical and mineral indices of nutritional status in blood and urine

OUTCOME TARGET RATING: Maintain at_____ Increase to_____

	Severe Deviation from Normal Range	Substantial Deviation from Normal Range	Moderate Deviation from Normal Range	Mild Deviation from Normal Range	No Deviation from Normal Range	
OUTCOME OVERALL RATING	1	2	3	4	5	
Indicators:						
100501 Serum albumin	1	2	3	4	5	NA
100502 Serum prealbumin	1	2	3	4	5	NA
100514 Serum creatinine	1	2	3	4	5	NA
100503 Hematocrit	1	2	3	4	5	NA
100504 Hemoglobin	1	2	3	4	5	NA
100510 Serum transferrin	1	2	3	4	5	NA
100505 Total iron binding capacity	1	2	3	4	5	NA
100506 Lymphocyte count	1	2	3	4	5	NA
100507 Blood glucose	1	2	3	4	5	NA
100508 Blood cholesterol	1	2	3	4	5	NA
100509 Blood triglycerides	1	2	3	4	5	NA
100511 24-hour urinary creatinine	1	2	3	4	5	NA
100512 Urinary urea nitrogen	1	2	3	4	5	NA
100515 C-reactive protein test	1	2	3	4	5	NA
100516 Zinc	1	2	3	4	5	NA
100517 Calcium	1	2	3	4	5	NA
100518 Folate	1	2	3	4	5	NA
100519 Potassium	1	2	3	4	5	NA

Continued

Nutritional Status: Biochemical Measures—cont'd

		Severe Deviation from Normal Range	Substantial Deviation from Normal Range	Moderate Deviation from Normal Range	Mild Deviation from Normal Range	No Deviation from Normal Range	
100520	Selenium	1	2	3	4	5	NA
100521	Vitamin A	1	2	3	4	5	NA
100522	Vitamin B	1	2	3	4	5	NA
100523	Vitamin B 6	1	2	3	4	5	NA
100524	Vitamin B 12	1	2	3	4	5	NA
100525	Vitamin C	1	2	3	4	5	NA
100526	Vitamin D	1	2	3	4	5	NA
100527	Vitamin E	1	2	3	4	5	NA

Domain-Physiologic Health (II)   **Class**-Digestion & Nutrition (K)   1st edition 1997; revised 2004, 2024

OUTCOME CONTENT REFERENCES:

Bailey, R. L., Miller, P. E., Mitchell, D. C., Hartman, T. J., Lawrence, F. R., Sempos, C. T., & Smiciklas-Wright, H. (2009). Dietary screening tool identifies nutritional risk in older adults. *The American Journal of Clinical Nutrition, 90*(1), 177–183. https://doi.org/10.3945/ajcn.2008.27268

Brazier, A., Lowe, N. M., Zaman, M., Shahzad, B., Ohly, H., McArdle, H. J., Ullah, U., Broadley, M. R., Bailey, E. H., Young, S. D., Tishkovskaya, S., & Khan, M. J. (2020). Micronutrient status and dietary diversity of women of reproductive age in rural Pakistan. *Nutrients, 12*(11), 3407. https://doi.org/10.3390/nu12113407

Dudek, S. G. (2022). *Nutrition essentials for nursing practice* (9th ed.). Wolters Kluwer.

Katz, D. L., Friedman, R. S. C., Joshi, S., Levitt, J., & Ye, M.-C. (2022). *Nutrition in clinical practice*. Wolters Kluwer.

Lázaro Cuesta, L., Rearte, A., Rodríguez, S., Niglia, M., Scipioni, H., Rodríguez, D., Salinas, R., Sosa, C., & Rasse, S. (2018). Anthropometric and biochemical assessment of nutritional status and dietary intake in school children aged 6–14 years, Province of Buenos Aires, Argentina. *Archivos Argentinos de Pediatria, 116*(1), e34–e46. https://doi.org/10.5546/aap.2018.eng.e34

Terán, G., Cuna, W., Brañez, F., Persson, K., Rottenberg, M. E., Nylén, S., & Rodriguez, C. (2018). Differences in nutritional and health status in school children from the highlands and lowlands of Bolivia. *The American Journal of Tropical Medicine and Hygiene, 98*(1), 326–333. https://doi.org/10.4269/ajtmh.17–0143

Truijen, S., Hayhoe, R., Hooper, L., Schoenmakers, I., Forbes, A., & Welch, A. A. (2021). Predicting malnutrition risk with data from routinely measured clinical biochemical diagnostic tests in free-living older populations. *Nutrients, 13*(6), 1883. https://doi.org/10.3390/nu13061883

+Zhang, X., Zhang, X., Zhu, Y., Tao, J., Zhang, Z., Zhang, Y., Wang, Y., Ke, Y., Ren, C., & Xu, J. (2020). Predictive value of Nutritional Risk Screening 2002 and Mini Nutritional Assessment Short Form in mortality in Chinese hospitalized geriatric patients. *Clinical Interventions in Aging, 15*, 441–449. https://doi.org/10.2147/CIA.S244910

N

Nutritional Status: Energy   1007

Definition: Adequacy of nutrient intake to provide cellular energy

OUTCOME TARGET RATING: Maintain at_____ Increase to_____

		Severe Deviation from Normal Range	Substantial Deviation from Normal Range	Moderate Deviation from Normal Range	Mild Deviation from Normal Range	No Deviation from Normal Range	
OUTCOME OVERALL RATING		**1**	**2**	**3**	**4**	**5**	
Indicators:							
100701	Stamina	1	2	3	4	5	NA
100702	Endurance	1	2	3	4	5	NA
100703	Hand grip strength	1	2	3	4	5	NA
100708	Muscle tone	1	2	3	4	5	NA
100704	Tissue healing	1	2	3	4	5	NA
100705	Infection resistance	1	2	3	4	5	NA
100706	Growth (children)	1	2	3	4	5	NA

Domain-Physiologic Health (II)   **Class**-Digestion & Nutrition (K)   1st edition 1997; revised 2004, 2013, 2024

OUTCOME CONTENT REFERENCES:
Bo, S., Fadda, M., Fedele, D., Pellegrini, M., Ghigo, E., & Pellegrini, N. (2020). A critical review on the role of food and nutrition in the energy balance. *Nutrients, 12*(4), 1161. https://doi.org/10.3390/nu12041161
Colaizzo-Anas, T., Smith, V., Tetewsky, S., & Wieczorek, W. F. (2016). Energy-related nutrition literacy. *Topics in Clinical Nutrition, 31*(1), 59–72. https://doi.org/10.1097/TIN.0000000000000058
Dudek, S. G. (2022). *Nutrition essentials for nursing practice* (9th ed.). Wolters Kluwer.
Katz, D. L., Friedman, R. S. C., Joshi, S., Levitt, J., & Ye, M.-C. (2022). *Nutrition in clinical practice*. Wolters Kluwer.
Rocks, T., Pelly, F., Slater, G., & Martin, L. A. (2016). The relationship between dietary intake and energy availability, eating attitudes and cognitive restraint in students enrolled in undergraduate nutrition degrees. *Appetite, 107*, 406–414. https://doi.org/10.1016/j.appet.2016.08.105
Viner, R. T., Harris, M., Berning, J. R., & Meyer, N. L. (2015). Energy availability and dietary patterns of adult male and female competitive cyclists with lower than expected bone mineral density. *International Journal of Sport Nutrition and Exercise Metabolism, 25*(6), 594–602. https://doi.org/10.1123/ijsnem.2015-0073

Nutritional Status: Food & Fluid Intake   1008

Definition: Adequacy of food and fluid intake and nutritional alternatives over a 24-hour period

OUTCOME TARGET RATING: Maintain at_____ Increase to_____

	Severe Deviation from Normal Range	Substantial Deviation from Normal Range	Moderate Deviation from Normal Range	Mild Deviation from Normal Range	No Deviation from Normal Range	
OUTCOME OVERALL RATING	1	2	3	4	5	
Indicators:						
100807 Oral food intake	1	2	3	4	5	NA
100808 Tube feeding intake	1	2	3	4	5	NA
100809 Oral fluid intake	1	2	3	4	5	NA
100810 Intravenous fluid intake	1	2	3	4	5	NA
100811 Parenteral nutrition intake	1	2	3	4	5	NA

Domain-*Physiologic Health (II)*   **Class**-*Digestion & Nutrition (K)*   *1st edition 1997; reviewed 2018; revised 2004, 2024*

OUTCOME CONTENT REFERENCES:
Bakewell, C., Corlett, C., Sharrard, A., Howarth, L. J., & Lee, A. C. (2021). Current trends in paediatric enteral tube feeding. *Paediatrics & Child Health, 31*(8), 308–315. https://doi.org/10.1016/j.paed.2021.05.002
Beck, A. M., Seemer, J., Knudsen, A. W., & Munk, T. (2021). Narrative review of low-intake dehydration in older adults. *Nutrients, 13*(9), 3142. https://doi.org/10.3390/nu13093142
Chouraqui, J.-P., Tavoularis, G., Simeoni, U., Ferry, C., & Turck, D. (2020). Food, water, energy, and macronutrient intake of non-breastfed infants and young children (0–3 years). *European Journal of Nutrition, 59*(1), 67–80. https://doi.org/10.1007/s00394-018-1883-y
Dudek, S. G. (2022). *Nutrition essentials for nursing practice* (9th ed.). Wolters Kluwer.
Engelheart, S., & Akner, G. (2015). Dietary intake of energy, nutrients and water in elderly people living at home or in nursing home. *Journal of Nutrition, Health & Aging, 19*(3), 265–272. https://doi.org/10.1007/s12603-015-0440-0
Ferreira-Pêgo, C., Guelinckx, I., Moreno, L. A., Kavouras, S. A., Gandy, J., Martinez, H., Bardosono, S., Abdpllahi, M., Nasseri, E., Jarosz, A., Bobio, N., & Salas-Salvadó, J. (2015). Total fluids intake and its determinants: Cross-sectional surveys among adults in 13 countries worldwide. *European Journal of Nutrition, 54*(Suppl. 2), S35–S43. https://doi.org/10.1007/s00394-015-0943-9
Giménez-Legarre, N., Flores-Barrantes, P., Miguel-Berges, M. L., Moreno, L. A., & Santaliestra-Pasías, A. M. (2020). Breakfast characteristics and their association with energy, macronutrients, and food intake in children and adolescents: A systematic review and meta-analysis. *Nutrients, 12*(8), 2460. https://doi.org/10.3390/nu12082460
Katz, D. L., Friedman, R. S. C., Joshi, S., Levitt, J., & Ye, M.-C. (2022). *Nutrition in clinical practice*. Wolters Kluwer.
Keller, H., Beck, A. M., & Namasivayam, A. (2015). Improving food and fluid intake for older adults living in long-term care: A research agenda. *Journal of the American Medical Directors Association, 16*(2), 93–100. https://doi.org/10.1016/j.jamda.2014.10.017
Waksmańska, W., Bobiński, R., Łukasik, R., & Pielesz, A. (2020). The consumption of milk, vegetables and fruits, fish, whole meal bread, and fast food meals among 15-year-old teenagers depending on the BMI value. *International Journal of Child & Adolescent Health, 13*(3), 279–287.

N

Nutritional Status: Nutrient Intake 1009

Definition: Adequacy of nutrient intake from food and fluids to meet metabolic needs

OUTCOME TARGET RATING: Maintain at_____ Increase to_____

		Severe Deviation from Normal Range	Substantial Deviation from Normal Range	Moderate Deviation from Normal Range	Mild Deviation from Normal Range	No Deviation from Normal Range	
OUTCOME OVERALL RATING		1	2	3	4	5	
Indicators:							
100901	Caloric intake	1	2	3	4	5	NA
100902	Protein intake	1	2	3	4	5	NA
100903	Fat intake	1	2	3	4	5	NA
100904	Carbohydrate intake	1	2	3	4	5	NA
100910	Fiber intake	1	2	3	4	5	NA
100905	Vitamin intake	1	2	3	4	5	NA
100906	Mineral intake	1	2	3	4	5	NA
100912	Iodine intake	1	2	3	4	5	NA
100907	Iron intake	1	2	3	4	5	NA
100908	Calcium intake	1	2	3	4	5	NA
100911	Sodium intake	1	2	3	4	5	NA
100913	Fluid intake	1	2	3	4	5	NA

Domain-*Physiologic Health (II)*   **Class**-*Digestion & Nutrition (K)*   1st edition 1997; revised 2004, 2008, 2024

OUTCOME CONTENT REFERENCES:

Dudek, S. G. (2022). *Nutrition essentials for nursing practice* (9th ed.). Wolters Kluwer.

European Food Safety Authority (EFSA). (2017). Dietary reference values for nutrients. Summary report. *EFSA Supporting Publication, 14*(12), e15121. https//doi.org/10.2903/sp.efsa.2017.e15121

Giménez-Legarre, N., Flores-Barrantes, P., Miguel-Berges, M. L., Moreno, L. A., & Santaliestra-Pasías, A. M. (2020). Breakfast characteristics and their association with energy, macronutrients, and food intake in children and adolescents: A systematic review and meta-analysis. *Nutrients, 12*(8), 2460. https://doi.org/10.3390/nu12082460

Katz, D. L., Friedman, R. S. C., Joshi, S., Levitt, J., & Ye, M.-C. (2022). *Nutrition in clinical practice.* Wolters Kluwer.

Singer, P., Blaser, A. R., Berger, M. M., Alhazzani, W., Calder, P. C., Casaer, M. P., Hiesmayr, M., Mayer, K., Montejo, J. C., Pichard, C., Preiser, J. C., van Zanten, A., Oczkowski, S., Szczeklik, W., & Bischoff, S. C. (2019). ESPEN guideline on clinical nutrition in the intensive care unit. *Clinical Nutrition, 38*(1), 48–79. https://doi.org/10.1016/j.clnu.2018.08.037

U.S. Department of Health and Human Services and U.S. Department of Agriculture. (2020). 2020–2025 *Dietary guidelines for Americans* (9th ed.). https://www.dietaryguidelines.gov/

Volkert, D., Beck, A. M., Cederholm, T., Cruz-Jentoft, A., Goisser, S., Hooper, L., Kiesswetter, E., Maggio, M., Raynaud-Simon, A., Sieber, C. C., Sobotka, L., van Asselt, D., Wirth, R., & Bischoff, S. C. (2019). ESPEN guideline on clinical nutrition and hydration in geriatrics. *Clinical Nutrition, 38*(1), 10–47. https://doi.org/10.1016/j.clnu.2018.05.024

O

Oral Health 1100

Definition: Condition of the mouth, teeth, gums, and tongue

OUTCOME TARGET RATING: Maintain at_____ Increase to_____

		Severely Compromised	Substantially Compromised	Moderately Compromised	Mildly Compromised	Not Compromised	
OUTCOME OVERALL RATING		1	2	3	4	5	
Indicators:							
110001	Cleanliness of mouth	1	2	3	4	5	NA
110002	Cleanliness of teeth	1	2	3	4	5	NA
110003	Cleanliness of gums	1	2	3	4	5	NA
110004	Cleanliness of tongue	1	2	3	4	5	NA

Oral Health—cont'd

		Severely Compromised	Substantially Compromised	Moderately Compromised	Mildly Compromised	Not Compromised	
110005	Cleanliness of dentures	1	2	3	4	5	NA
110006	Cleanliness of dental appliances	1	2	3	4	5	NA
110007	Fit of dentures	1	2	3	4	5	NA
110008	Fit of dental appliances	1	2	3	4	5	NA
110009	Moistness of lips	1	2	3	4	5	NA
110010	Moisture of oral mucosa and tongue	1	2	3	4	5	NA
110011	Color of mucosa membranes	1	2	3	4	5	NA
110012	Oral mucosa integrity	1	2	3	4	5	NA
110013	Tongue integrity	1	2	3	4	5	NA
110014	Gum integrity	1	2	3	4	5	NA
		Severe	Substantial	Moderate	Mild	None	
110026	Absence of teeth	1	2	3	4	5	NA
110027	Erosion of enamel	1	2	3	4	5	NA
110017	Halitosis	1	2	3	4	5	NA
110018	Bleeding	1	2	3	4	5	NA
110021	Pain	1	2	3	4	5	NA
110028	Toothache	1	2	3	4	5	NA
110029	Tooth fracture	1	2	3	4	5	NA
110022	Oral mucosa lesions	1	2	3	4	5	NA
110023	Dental caries	1	2	3	4	5	NA
110024	Gingivitis	1	2	3	4	5	NA
110025	Periodontal disease	1	2	3	4	5	NA

Dental Prosthesis YES / NO

Domain-Physiologic Health (II)　**Class**-Tissue Integrity (L)　1st edition 1997; revised 2004, 2008, 2013; reviewed 2024

OUTCOME CONTENT REFERENCES:

Bickley, L. S., Szilagyi, P. G., Hoffman, R. M., & Soriano, R. P. (2021). *Bates' guide to physical examination and history taking* (13th ed.). Wolters Kluwer.

Dholam, K. P., Sharma, M. R., Gurav, S. V., Singh, G. P., & Prabhash, K. (2021). Oral and dental health status in patients undergoing neoadjuvant chemotherapy for locally advanced head and neck cancer. *Oral Surgery, Oral Medicine, Oral Pathology & Oral Radiology, 132*(5), 539–548. https://doi.org/10.1016/j.oooo.2021.07.018

Everaars, B., Weening-Verbree, L. F., Jerković-Ćosić, K., Schoonmade, L., Bleijenberg, N., de Wit, N. J., & van der Heijden, G. (2020). Measurement properties of oral health assessments for non-dental healthcare professionals in older people: A systematic review. *BMC Geriatrics, 20*(1), 4. https://doi.org/10.1186/s12877-019-1349-y

Gandhi, J., Gurunathan, D., Doraikannan, S., Balasubramaniam, A., & Gandhi, J. M. (2021). Oral health status for primary dentition—A pilot study. *Journal of the Indian Society of Pedodontics & Preventive Dentistry, 39*(4), 369–372. https://doi.org/10.4103/jisppd.jisppd_155_21

+Kayser-Jones, J., Bird, W. F., Paul, S. M., Long, L., & Schell, E. S. (1995). An instrument to assess the oral health status of nursing home residents. *The Gerontologist, 35*(6), 814–824. https://doi.org/10.1093/geront/35.6.814

Moharrami, M., Perez, A., Mohebbi, S. Z., Bassir, S. H., & Amin, M. (2022). Oral health status of individuals with obsessive-compulsive disorder considering oral hygiene habits. *Special Care in Dentistry, 42*(1), 41–48. https://doi.org/10.1111/scd.12632

Pabbla, A., Duijster, D., Grasveld, A., Sekundo, C., Agyemang, C., & van der Heijden, G. (2021). Oral health status, oral health behaviours and oral health care utilisation among migrants residing in Europe: A systematic review. *Journal of Immigrant & Minority Health, 23*(2), 373–388. https://doi.org/10.1007/s10903-020-01056-9

Thapa, R., Chimoriya, R., & Arora, A. (2021). The development and psychometric properties of oral health assessment instruments used by non-dental professionals for nursing home residents: A systematic review. *BMC Geriatrics, 21*(1), 35. https://doi.org/10.1186/s12877-020-01989-8

P

Pain: Adverse Psychological Response   1306

Definition: Severity of observed or reported adverse cognitive, emotional, and fear responses to physical pain

OUTCOME TARGET RATING: Maintain at_____ Increase to_____

OUTCOME OVERALL RATING		Severe 1	Substantial 2	Moderate 3	Mild 4	None 5	
Indicators:							
130601	Slowing of thought processes	1	2	3	4	5	NA
130602	Memory impairment	1	2	3	4	5	NA
130603	Interference with concentration	1	2	3	4	5	NA
130604	Indecision	1	2	3	4	5	NA
130605	Pain distress	1	2	3	4	5	NA
130606	Concern about tolerating the pain	1	2	3	4	5	NA
130607	Concern about burdening others	1	2	3	4	5	NA
130608	Concern about abandonment	1	2	3	4	5	NA
130624	Pessimistic about the future	1	2	3	4	5	NA
130609	Depression	1	2	3	4	5	NA
130610	Anxiety	1	2	3	4	5	NA
130611	Sadness	1	2	3	4	5	NA
130612	Helplessness	1	2	3	4	5	NA
130613	Hopelessness	1	2	3	4	5	NA
130614	Worthlessness	1	2	3	4	5	NA
130625	Loneliness	1	2	3	4	5	NA
130615	Sense of isolation	1	2	3	4	5	NA
130626	Irritability	1	2	3	4	5	NA
130627	Restlessness	1	2	3	4	5	NA
130628	Fear of the cause that produces the pain	1	2	3	4	5	NA
130617	Fear of unbearable pain	1	2	3	4	5	NA
130616	Fear of procedures and equipment	1	2	3	4	5	NA
130629	Fear of work limitations	1	2	3	4	5	NA
130618	Annoyance with disruptive effects of pain	1	2	3	4	5	NA
130619	Suicidal thoughts	1	2	3	4	5	NA
130620	Pessimistic thoughts	1	2	3	4	5	NA
130621	Bitterness toward others	1	2	3	4	5	NA
130622	Anger over disabling effects of pain	1	2	3	4	5	NA

Domain-*Health & Life Quality (V)*   **Class**-*Symptom Status (V)*   *2nd edition 2000; revised 2004, 2018, 2024*

OUTCOME CONTENT REFERENCES:

Bair, M. J., Outcalt, S. D., Ang, D., Wu, J., & Yu, Z. (2020). Pain and psychological outcomes among Iraq and Afghanistan veterans with chronic pain and PTSD: ESCAPE trial longitudinal results. *Pain Medicine, 21*(7), 1369–1376. https://doi.org/10.1093/pm/pnaa007

Bellido-Vallejo, J. C., & Pancorbo-Hidalgo, P. L. (2020), Psychometric evaluation of the nursing outcome "Pain: Adverse Psychological Response" in patients with chronic pain. *International Journal of Nursing Knowledge, 31*(3), 164–172. https://doi.org/10.1111/2047-3095.12267

Burke, A. L., Mathias, J. L., & Denson, L. A. (2015). Psychological functioning of people living with chronic pain: A meta-analytic review. *British Journal of Clinical Psychology, 54*(3), 345–360. https://doi.org/10.1111/bjc.12078

Costa, E. C. V., Vale, S., Sobral, M., & Graça Pereira, M. (2016). Illness perceptions are the main predictors of depression and anxiety symptoms in patients with chronic pain. *Psychology, Health & Medicine, 21*(4), 483–495. https://doi.org/10.1080/13548506.2015.1109673

Frumkin, M. R., Haroutounian, S., & Rodebaugh, T. L. (2020). Examining emotional pain among individuals with chronic physical pain: Nomothetic and idiographic approaches. *Journal of Psychosomatic Research, 136*, 110172. https://doi.org/10.1016/j.jpsychores.2020.110172

Lerman, S. F., Rudich, Z., Brill, S., Shalev, H., & Shahar, G. (2015). Longitudinal associations between depression, anxiety, pain, and pain-related disability in chronic pain patients. *Psychosomatic Medicine, 77*(3), 333–341. https://doi.org/10.1097/PSY.0000000000000158

Oliveira, D. S., Mendonça, L. V. F., Sampaio, R. S. M., de Castro-Lopes, J. M. P. D., & de Azevedo, L. F. R. (2019). The impact of anxiety and depression on the outcomes of chronic low back pain multidisciplinary pain management—A multicenter prospective cohort study in pain clinics with one-year follow-up. *Pain Medicine, 20*(4), 736–746. https://doi.org/10.1093/pm/pny128

Pain Control   1605

Definition: Personal actions to eliminate or reduce pain

OUTCOME TARGET RATING: Maintain at_____ Increase to_____

		Never Demonstrated	Rarely Demonstrated	Sometimes Demonstrated	Often Demonstrated	Consistently Demonstrated	
OUTCOME OVERALL RATING		1	2	3	4	5	
Indicators:							
160502	Recognizes pain onset	1	2	3	4	5	NA
160501	Describes primary causal factors	1	2	3	4	5	NA
160514	Describes factors contributing to pain	1	2	3	4	5	NA
160515	Obtains information about pain control	1	2	3	4	5	NA
160516	Describes pain	1	2	3	4	5	NA
160517	Discusses pain treatment options with health professional	1	2	3	4	5	NA
160518	Sets pain relief goals with health professional	1	2	3	4	5	NA
160510	Uses diary to monitor symptoms over time	1	2	3	4	5	NA
160529	Monitors pain level with mHealth apps	1	2	3	4	5	NA
160503	Uses pain preventive measures	1	2	3	4	5	NA
160530	Uses topical non-steroidal medication	1	2	3	4	5	NA
160504	Uses non-analgesic relief measures	1	2	3	4	5	NA
160519	Monitors therapeutic effects of non-analgesic relief measures	1	2	3	4	5	NA
160520	Monitors adverse effects of non-analgesic relief measures	1	2	3	4	5	NA
160505	Uses analgesic as recommended	1	2	3	4	5	NA
160521	Monitors therapeutic effects of analgesic	1	2	3	4	5	NA
160522	Monitors adverse effects of analgesic	1	2	3	4	5	NA
160523	Avoids misuse of drugs	1	2	3	4	5	NA
160524	Avoids misuse of alcohol	1	2	3	4	5	NA
160531	Performs recommended exercises	1	2	3	4	5	NA
160532	Uses complementary therapies	1	2	3	4	5	NA
160525	Performs effective stress reduction techniques	1	2	3	4	5	NA
160526	Uses effective coping strategies	1	2	3	4	5	NA
160527	Perform effective relaxation techniques	1	2	3	4	5	NA
160513	Reports changes in pain symptoms to health professional	1	2	3	4	5	NA
160507	Reports uncontrolled pain symptoms to health professional	1	2	3	4	5	NA
160508	Uses available resources	1	2	3	4	5	NA
160509	Recognizes associated symptoms of pain	1	2	3	4	5	NA
160511	Reports pain controlled	1	2	3	4	5	NA
160528	Keeps appointments with health professional	1	2	3	4	5	NA

Domain-Health Knowledge & Behavior (IV)   **Class-**Health Behavior (Q)   *1st edition 1997; revised 2000, 2004, 2018, 2024*

OUTCOME CONTENT REFERENCES:
Bellido-Vallejo, J. C., & Pancorbo-Hidalgo, P. L. (2017). Cultural adaptation and psychometric evaluation of the Spanish version of the nursing outcome "Pain control" in primary care patients with chronic pain. *Pain Management Nursing, 18,* 337–350. https://doi.org/10.1016/j.pmn.2017.04.001
Fortune, S., & Frawley, J. (2021). Optimizing pain control and minimizing opioid use in trauma patients. *AACN Advanced Critical Care, 32*(1), 89–104. https://doi.org/10.4037/aacnacc2021519
Kissi, A., Hughes, S., Van Ryckeghem, D., De Houwer, J., & Crombez, G. (2021). When pain becomes uncontrolled: An experimental analysis of the impact of instruction on pain-control attempts. *Pain, 162,* 760–769. https://doi.org/10.1097/j.pain.0000000000002088
Leziak, K., Yee, L. M., Grobman, W. A., & Badreldin, N. (2021). Patient experience with postpartum pain management in the face of the opioid crisis. *Journal of Midwifery & Women's Health, 66*(2), 1–8. https://doi.org/10.1111/jmwh.13212
Marti, C. L., Bakker, C. J., Breth, M. S., Gao, G., Lee, K., Lee, M. A., Tiase, V. L., Tunby, L. J., Wyatt, T. H., & Janeway, L. M. (2021). The efficacy of mobile health interventions used to manage acute or chronic pain: A systematic review. *Research in Nursing & Health, 44*(1), 111–128. https://doi.org/10.1002/nur.22097

P

Nava-Bringas, T. I., Romero-Fierro, L. O., Trani-Chagoya, Y. P., Macías-Hernández, S. I., García-Guerrero, E., Hernández-López, M., Roberto, C. Z. (2021). Stabilization exercises versus flexion exercises in degenerative Spondylolisthesis: A randomized controlled trial. *PTJ: Physical Therapy & Rehabilitation Journal, 101*(8), 1–8. https://doi.org/10.1093/ptj/pzab108

Patton, L., Avsar, P., Nugent, L., O'Connor, T., Patton, D., & Moore, Z. (2021). What is the impact of specialist palliative care outpatient consultations on pain in adult patients with cancer? A systematic review. *European Journal of Oncology Nursing, 55*, 1–8. https://doi.org/10.1016/j.ejon.2021.102034

Renda, S., & Slater, T. (2021). Nonopioid management of chronic pain. *Journal of Radiology Nursing, 40*(1), 23–29. https://doi.org/10.1016/j.jradnu.2020.07.006

Sampaio, F. M. C., Araújo, O. S. S. L., Sequeira, C. A. D. C., Lluch Canut, M. T., & Martins, T. (2017). Evaluation of the psychometric properties of NOC outcomes "Anxiety Level" and "Anxiety Self-Control" in a Portuguese outpatient sample. *International Journal of Nursing Knowledge, 29*(3), 184–191. https://doi.org/10.1111/2047-3095.12169

Yu, C. W., Kirubarajan, A., Yau, M., Armstrong, D., & Johnson, D. E. (2021). Topical pain control for corneal abrasions: A systematic review and meta-analysis. *Academic Emergency Medicine, 28*(8), 890–908. https://doi.org/10.1111/acem.14222

Pain: Disruptive Effects   2101

Definition: Severity of observed or reported disruptive effects of chronic pain on daily functioning

OUTCOME TARGET RATING: Maintain at_____ Increase to_____

OUTCOME OVERALL RATING		Severe 1	Substantial 2	Moderate 3	Mild 4	None 5	
Indicators:							
210127	Discomfort	1	2	3	4	5	NA
210115	Loss of appetite	1	2	3	4	5	NA
210108	Impaired concentration	1	2	3	4	5	NA
210128	Disruption of sense of control	1	2	3	4	5	NA
210135	Anxiety	1	2	3	4	5	NA
210110	Impaired mood	1	2	3	4	5	NA
210111	Lack of patience	1	2	3	4	5	NA
210136	Frustration	1	2	3	4	5	NA
210112	Interrupted sleep	1	2	3	4	5	NA
210119	Disruption of routine	1	2	3	4	5	NA
210113	Impaired physical mobility	1	2	3	4	5	NA
210134	Impaired physical activity	1	2	3	4	5	NA
210129	Interference with activities of daily living	1	2	3	4	5	NA
210137	Interference with instrumental activities of daily living	1	2	3	4	5	NA
210102	Impaired role performance	1	2	3	4	5	NA
210138	Interference to social activities	1	2	3	4	5	NA
210101	Disruption of interpersonal relationships	1	2	3	4	5	NA
210132	Impaired life enjoyment	1	2	3	4	5	NA
210133	Hopelessness	1	2	3	4	5	NA
210117	Impaired urinary elimination	1	2	3	4	5	NA
210120	Impaired bowel elimination	1	2	3	4	5	NA
210123	Absenteeism from work	1	2	3	4	5	NA
210130	Impaired work performance	1	2	3	4	5	NA
210122	Difficulty maintaining employment	1	2	3	4	5	NA
210124	Absenteeism from school	1	2	3	4	5	NA
210131	Impaired school performance	1	2	3	4	5	NA
210139	Difficulty maintaining school enrollment	1	2	3	4	5	NA

Domain- Health & Life Quality (V)   **Class**-Symptom Status (V)   *1st edition 1997; revised 2004, 2008, 2013, 2024*

OUTCOME CONTENT REFERENCES:

Lindgren, I., Gard, G., & Brogårdh, C. (2018). Shoulder pain after stroke—Experiences, consequences in daily life and effects of interventions: A qualitative study. *Disability & Rehabilitation, 40*(10), 1176–1182. https://doi.org/10.1080/09638288.2017.1290699

Mun, C. J., Lemery-Chalfant, K., Wilson, M., & Shaw, D. S. (2021). Predictors and consequences of pediatric pain symptom trajectories: A 14-year longitudinal study. *Pain Medicine, 22*(10), 2162–2173. https://doi.org/10.1093/pm/pnab173

Nieto, R., Sora, B., Boixadós, M., & Ruiz, G. (2020). Understanding the experience of functional abdominal pain through written narratives by families. *Pain Medicine, 21*(6), 1093–1105. https://doi.org/10.1093/pm/pnz147

Pancorbo-Hidalgo, P. L., & Bellido-Vallejo, J. C. (2019). Clinical validation of the nursing outcome "Pain: Disruptive Effects" in people with chronic pain in Spain. *Journal of Nursing Measurement, 27*(3), 384–400. https://doi.org/10.1891/1061-3749.27.3.384

P

Pain Level 2102

Definition: Severity of reported pain intensity or observed physical or behavioral symptoms of pain

OUTCOME TARGET RATING: Maintain at_____ Increase to_____

	Severe	Substantial	Moderate	Mild	None	
OUTCOME OVERALL RATING	1	2	3	4	5	
Indicators:						
210201 Reported pain intensity	1	2	3	4	5	NA
210229 Negative vocalization	1	2	3	4	5	NA
210221 Rubbing affected area	1	2	3	4	5	NA
210230 Moaning	1	2	3	4	5	NA
210225 Tearing	1	2	3	4	5	NA
210231 Crying	1	2	3	4	5	NA
210206 Facial expressions of pain	1	2	3	4	5	NA
210224 Wincing	1	2	3	4	5	NA
210232 Dilation of pupils	1	2	3	4	5	NA
210208 Restlessness	1	2	3	4	5	NA
210222 Agitation	1	2	3	4	5	NA
210223 Irritability	1	2	3	4	5	NA
210233 Tossing and turning in bed	1	2	3	4	5	NA
210234 Thrashing of legs and arms	1	2	3	4	5	NA
210226 Diaphoresis	1	2	3	4	5	NA
210218 Pacing	1	2	3	4	5	NA
210219 Narrowed mental focus	1	2	3	4	5	NA
210235 Inconsolability	1	2	3	4	5	NA
210209 Muscle tension	1	2	3	4	5	NA
210227 Nausea	1	2	3	4	5	NA

Site of pain _____

Pain Description _____

Domain-Health & Life Quality (V) **Class**-*Symptom Status (V)* 1st edition 1997; revised 2004, 2008, 2024

OUTCOME CONTENT REFERENCES:

Bellido-Vallejo, J. C., Rodríguez-Torres, M. C., López-Medina, I. M., & Pancorbo-Hidalgo, P. L. (2013). Adaptación cultural y validación de contenido del resultado «Nivel del dolor» de la Clasificación de Resultados de Enfermería [Cultural adaptation and content validation of the «Pain level» outcome of the Nursing Outcomes Classification]. *Enfermeria Clinica, 23*(4), 154–159. https://doi.org/10.1016/j.enfcli.2013.06.004

Bellido-Vallejo, J. C., Rodríguez-Torres, M. C., López-Medina, I. M., & Pancorbo-Hidalgo, P. L. (2016). Psychometric testing of the Spanish version of the pain level outcome scale in hospitalized patients with acute pain. *International Journal of Nursing Knowledge, 27*(1), 10–16. https://doi.org/10.1111/2047-3095.12070

+Boitor, M., Fiola, J. L., & Gélinas, C. (2016). Validation of the Critical-Care Pain Observation Tool and vital signs in relation to the sensory and affective components of pain during mediastinal tube removal in postoperative cardiac surgery intensive care unit adults. *The Journal of Cardiovascular Nursing, 31*(5), 425–432. https://doi.org/10.1097/JCN.0000000000000250

Fedele, S., Strasser, S., & Roulin, M. (2020). Validation of the Critical Care Pain Observational Tool in palliative care. *Pain Management Nursing, 21*(4), 360–364. https://doi.org/10.1016/j.pmn.2019.12.003

Gélinas, C. (2016). Pain assessment in the critically ill adult: Recent evidence and new trends. *Intensive & Critical Care Nursing, 34*, 1–11. https://doi.org/10.1016/j.iccn.2016.03.001

Herr, K., Coyne, P. J., McCaffery, M., Manworren, R., & Merkel, S. (2011). Pain assessment in the patient unable to self-report: Position statement with clinical practice recommendations. *Pain Management Nursing, 12*(4), 230–250. https://doi.org/10.1016/j.pmn2011.10.002

Hockenberry, M. J., Wilson, D., & Rodgers, C. C. (Eds.). (2019). *Wong's nursing care of infants and children* (11th ed.). Elsevier.

Hogans, B. B., & Barrevald. A. M. (2020). *Pain care essentials*. Oxford University Press.

Ignatavicius, D. D., Workman, M. L., Rebar, C. R., & Heimgartner, N. M. (2021). *Medical-surgical nursing: Concepts for interprofessional care* (10th ed.). Elsevier.

Mello, B. S., Massutti, T. M., Longaray, V. K., Trevisan, D. F., & de Fátima Lucena, A. (2016). Applicability of the Nursing Outcomes Classification (NOC) to the evaluation of cancer patients with acute or chronic pain in palliative care. *Applied Nursing Research, 29*, 12–18. https://doi.org/10.1016/j.apnr.2015.04.001

+Melzack, R. (1975). The McGill Pain Questionnaire: Major properties and scoring methods. *Pain, 30*(1), 277–299. https://doi.org/10.1016/0304-3959(75)90044-5

+Merkel, S., Voepel-Lewis, T., & Malviya, S. (2002). Pain control: Pain assessment in infants and young children: The FLACC scale. *AJN, American Journal of Nursing, 102*(10), 55–58. https://doi.org/10.1016/j.jpain.2018.02.013

Potter, P. A., Perry, A. G., Stockert, P. A., & Hall, A. M. (2021). *Fundamentals of nursing* (10th ed.). Elsevier.

Scher, C., Petti, E., Meador, L., Van Cleave, J. H., Liang, E., & Reid, M.C. (2020). Multidimensional pain assessment tools for ambulatory and inpatient nursing practice. *Pain Management Nursing, 21*(5), 416–422. https://doi.org/10.1016/j.pmn.2020.03.007

P

Panic Level 1217

Definition: Severity of sudden, intense feelings of apprehension, fright, terror, or nervousness

OUTCOME TARGET RATING: Maintain at_____ Increase to_____

		Severe	Substantial	Moderate	Mild	None	
OUTCOME OVERALL RATING		1	2	3	4	5	
Indicators:							
121701	Intensity of panic attack	1	2	3	4	5	NA
121702	Feelings of distress	1	2	3	4	5	NA
121703	Increased pulse rate	1	2	3	4	5	NA
121704	Sweating	1	2	3	4	5	NA
121705	Trembling	1	2	3	4	5	NA
121706	Shortness of breath	1	2	3	4	5	NA
121707	Crying	1	2	3	4	5	NA
121708	Feelings of choking	1	2	3	4	5	NA
121709	Chest pain	1	2	3	4	5	NA
121710	Nausea	1	2	3	4	5	NA
121711	Dizziness	1	2	3	4	5	NA
121712	Feeling faint	1	2	3	4	5	NA
121713	Unsteady	1	2	3	4	5	NA
121714	Chills	1	2	3	4	5	NA
121715	Hot flashes	1	2	3	4	5	NA
121716	Numbness in extremities	1	2	3	4	5	NA
121717	Feelings of detachment from reality	1	2	3	4	5	NA
121718	Fear of losing control	1	2	3	4	5	NA
121719	Fear of dying	1	2	3	4	5	NA
121720	Fear of having another panic attack	1	2	3	4	5	NA
121721	Decreased productivity	1	2	3	4	5	NA
121722	Decreased school achievement	1	2	3	4	5	NA
121723	Interference with social activities	1	2	3	4	5	NA
121724	Interference with family function	1	2	3	4	5	NA

Domain-*Psychosocial Health (III)*   **Class**-*Psychological Well-Being (M)*   *6th edition 2018*

OUTCOME CONTENT REFERENCES:

American Psychiatric Association. (2013). *Diagnostic and statistical manual of mental disorders* (5th ed.). https://doi.org/10.1176/appi.books.9780890425596

American Psychiatric Association, Work Group on Panic Disorder. (2009). *Practice guideline for the treatment of patients with panic disorder* (2nd ed.). https://www.psychiatryonline.org/guidelines

Pincus, D., Ehrenreich, J., & Mattis, S. (2008). *Mastery of anxiety and panic for adolescents: Riding the wave: Therapist guide.* Oxford University Press.

+Shear, M. K., Brown, T. A., Barlow, D. H., Money, R., Sholomskas, D. E., Woods, S. W., Gorman, J. M., & Papp, L. A. (1997). Multicenter collaborative Panic Disorder Severity Scale. *American Journal of Psychiatry, 154*(11), 1571–1575. https://doi.org/10.1176/ajp.154.11.1571

+Shear, M., Rucci, P., Williams, J., Frank, E., Grochocinski, V., Bilt, J., Houck, P., & Wang, T. (2001). Reliability and validity of the Panic Disorder Severity Scale: Replication and extension. *Journal of Psychiatric Research, 35*(5), 293–296. https://doi.org/10.1016/s0022-3956(01)00028-0

P

Panic Self-Control 1412

Definition: Personal actions to eliminate or reduce sudden, intense feelings of apprehension, fright, terror, or nervousness

OUTCOME TARGET RATING: Maintain at_____ Increase to_____

		Never Demonstrated	Rarely Demonstrated	Sometimes Demonstrated	Often Demonstrated	Consistently Demonstrated	
OUTCOME OVERALL RATING		1	2	3	4	5	
Indicators:							
141201	Identifies signs and symptoms before panic attack	1	2	3	4	5	NA
141202	Identifies triggers of panic attack	1	2	3	4	5	NA
141203	Verbalizes concerns	1	2	3	4	5	NA
141204	Verbalizes feelings following panic attack	1	2	3	4	5	NA
141205	Seeks information to reduce panic episodes	1	2	3	4	5	NA
141206	Use effective coping strategies	1	2	3	4	5	NA
141207	Uses anxiety reduction techniques	1	2	3	4	5	NA
141208	Uses stress reduction technique	1	2	3	4	5	NA
141209	Performs calm deep breathing	1	2	3	4	5	NA
141210	Performs muscle relaxation	1	2	3	4	5	NA
141211	Performs exercise daily	1	2	3	4	5	NA
141212	Monitors anxiety escalation	1	2	3	4	5	NA
141213	Uses breathing control technique for hyperventilation	1	2	3	4	5	NA
141214	Eliminates tobacco use	1	2	3	4	5	NA
141215	Avoids caffeine	1	2	3	4	5	NA
141216	Avoids medication containing stimulants	1	2	3	4	5	NA
141217	Avoids drug misuse	1	2	3	4	5	NA
141218	Avoids alcohol misuse	1	2	3	4	5	NA
141219	Monitors length of time between episodes	1	2	3	4	5	NA
141220	Adheres to prescribed medication	1	2	3	4	5	NA
141221	Keeps appointments with health professional	1	2	3	4	5	NA
141222	Seeks social support	1	2	3	4	5	NA

Domain-Psychosocial Health (III)   *Class*-Self-Control (O)   6th edition 2018

OUTCOME CONTENT REFERENCES:
American Psychiatric Association. (2013). *Diagnostic and statistical manual of mental disorders: DSM 5* (5th ed.). https://doi.org/10.1176/appi.books.9780890425596
American Psychiatric Association, Work Group on Panic Disorder. (2010). *Practice guideline for the treatment of patients with panic disorder* (2nd ed.). https://www.psychiatryonline.org/guidelines
Townsend, M. (2015). *Psychiatric mental health nursing: Concepts of care in evidence-based practice* (8th ed.). F.A. Davis.
Tusaie, K. K., & Fitzpatrick, J. J. (Eds.). (2013). *Advanced practice psychiatric nursing: Integrating psychotherapy, psychopharmacology, and complementary and alternative approaches.* Springer.

P

Parent Adaptation to Infant Hospitalization   1316

Definition: Parental adaptive response to admission of an infant from birth to first birthday to an acute or intensive care unit for treatment

OUTCOME TARGET RATING: Maintain at_____ Increase to_____

		Never Demonstrated	Rarely Demonstrated	Sometimes Demonstrated	Often Demonstrated	Consistently Demonstrated	
OUTCOME OVERALL RATING		**1**	**2**	**3**	**4**	**5**	
Indicators:							
131601	Interacts with health care team	1	2	3	4	5	NA
131602	Adapts to complexity of the child's health diagnosis	1	2	3	4	5	NA
131603	Remains optimistic about infant's clinical condition	1	2	3	4	5	NA
131604	Provides infant health history	1	2	3	4	5	NA
131605	Adapts to being in hospital environment	1	2	3	4	5	NA
131606	Copes with the stress of infant's hospitalization	1	2	3	4	5	NA
131607	Participates in support groups	1	2	3	4	5	NA
131608	Maintains bond with infant	1	2	3	4	5	NA
131609	Provides comfort measures for infant	1	2	3	4	5	NA
131610	Provides diversional activities for infant	1	2	3	4	5	NA
131611	Participates in social interactions with infant	1	2	3	4	5	NA
131612	Participates in play therapy	1	2	3	4	5	NA
131613	Mother continues breastfeeding	1	2	3	4	5	NA
131614	Reports infant's feeding schedule	1	2	3	4	5	NA
131615	Reports infant's sleep routine	1	2	3	4	5	NA
131616	Participates in treatment decisions	1	2	3	4	5	NA
131617	Participates involved in treatment plan	1	2	3	4	5	NA
131618	Participates in physical care	1	2	3	4	5	NA
131619	Provides emotional support	1	2	3	4	5	NA
131620	Provides comfort items	1	2	3	4	5	NA
131621	Learns how to provide required treatments	1	2	3	4	5	NA
131622	Receives support from family members	1	2	3	4	5	NA
131623	Arranges care for siblings	1	2	3	4	5	NA
131624	Expresses satisfaction with nursing care	1	2	3	4	5	NA
131625	Considers need for palliative care	1	2	3	4	5	NA
131626	Finds meaning in the experience	1	2	3	4	5	NA
131627	Participates in discharge planning	1	2	3	4	5	NA

Domain-*Psychosocial Health (III)*   **Class**-*Psychosocial Adaptation (N)*   *7th edition 2024*

OUTCOME CONTENT REFERENCES:

Bradshaw, S., Bem, D., Shaw, K., Taylor, B., Chiswell, C., Salama, M., Bassett, E., Kaur, G., & Cummins, C. (2019). Improving health, well-being, and parenting skills in parents of children with special health care needs and medical complexity—A scoping review. *BMC Pediatrics, 19*(1), 301. https://doi.org/10.1186/s12887-019-1648-7

Boland, L., Graham, I. D., Légaré, F., Lewis, K., Jull, J., Shephard, A., Lawson, M. L., Davis, A., Yameogo, A., & Stacey, D. (2019). Barriers and facilitators of pediatric shared decision-making: A systematic review. *Implementation Science, 14*(1), 7. https://doi.org/10.1186/s13012-018-0851-5

de Man, M., Segers, E. W., Schappin, R., van der Leeden, K., Wösten-van Asperen, R. M., Breur, H., de Weerth, C., & van den Hoogen, A. (2021). Parental experiences of their infant's hospital admission undergoing cardiac surgery: A systematic review. *Acta Paediatric, 110*(6), 1730–1740. https://doi.org/10.1111/apa.15694

Hallman, M. L., & Bellury, L. M. (2020). Communication in pediatric critical care units: A review of the literature. *Critical Care Nurse, 40*(2), e1–e15. https://doi.org/10.4037/ccn2020751

Hames, J. L., Gasteiger, C., McKenzie, M. R., Rowley, S., Serlachius, A. S., Juth, V., & Petrie, K. J. (2021). Predictors of parental stress from admission to discharge in the neonatal special care unit. *Child Care, Health & Development, 47*(2), 243–251. https://doi.org/10.1111/cch.12829

Jerofke-Owen, T. A., McAndrew, N. S., Gralton, K. S., Totka, J. P., Weiss, M. E., Fial, A. V., & Sawin, K. J. (2022). Engagement of families in the care of hospitalized pediatric patients: A scoping review. *Journal of Family Nursing, 28*(2), 151–171. https://doi.org/10.1177/10748407211048894

P

Kasparian, N. A., Kan, J. M., Sood, E., Wray, J., Pincus, H. A., & Newburger, J. W. (2019). Mental health care for parents of babies with congenital heart disease during intensive care unit admission: Systematic review and statement of best practice. *Early Human Development, 139*, 104837. https://doi.org/10.1016/j.earlhumdev.2019.104837

Macho, P. (2017). Individualized developmental care in the NICU: A concept analysis. *Advances in Neonatal Care, 17*(3), 162–174. https://doi.org/10.1097/ANC.0000000000000374

Reid, S., Bredemeyer, S., & Chiarella, M. (2019). Integrative review of parents' perspectives of the nursing role in neonatal family-centered care. *Journal of Obstetric, Gynecologic, and Neonatal Nursing, 48*(4), 408–417. https://doi.org/10.1016/j.jogn.2019.05.001

Stragliotto Bazzan, J., Marten Milbrath, V., Bärtschi Gabatz, R. I., Cordeiro, F. R., Freitag, V. L., & Schwartz, E. (2020). The family's adaptation process to their child's hospitalization in an intensive care unit. *Revista Da Escola de Enfermagem Da USP, 54*, 1–8. https://doi.org/10.1590/S1980-220X2018056203614

Parent Adaptation to Toddler Hospitalization   1317

Definition: Parental adaptive response to admission of a toddler to an acute or intensive care unit for treatment

OUTCOME TARGET RATING: Maintain at_____ Increase to_____

		Never Demonstrated	Rarely Demonstrated	Sometimes Demonstrated	Often Demonstrated	Consistently Demonstrated	
OUTCOME OVERALL RATING		1	2	3	4	5	
Indicators:							
131701	Interacts with health care team	1	2	3	4	5	NA
131702	Adapts to complexity of the child's health diagnosis	1	2	3	4	5	NA
131703	Remains optimistic about toddler's clinical condition	1	2	3	4	5	NA
131704	Provides toddler's health history	1	2	3	4	5	NA
131705	Adapts to hospital environment	1	2	3	4	5	NA
131706	Uses effective coping strategies	1	2	3	4	5	NA
131707	Participates in support groups	1	2	3	4	5	NA
131708	Plans for care of siblings	1	2	3	4	5	NA
131709	Copes with the stress of toddler's hospitalization	1	2	3	4	5	NA
131710	Maintains bond with toddler	1	2	3	4	5	NA
131711	Provides comfort measures	1	2	3	4	5	NA
131712	Provides diversional activities	1	2	3	4	5	NA
131713	Participates in social interactions with toddler	1	2	3	4	5	NA
131714	Participates in play therapy	1	2	3	4	5	NA
131715	Reports toddler's skills with use of a cup	1	2	3	4	5	NA
131716	Reports toddler's food preferences	1	2	3	4	5	NA
131717	Reports toddler's nap routine	1	2	3	4	5	NA
131718	Reports toddler's sleep routine	1	2	3	4	5	NA
131719	Participates in treatment decisions	1	2	3	4	5	NA
131720	Participates in treatment plan	1	2	3	4	5	NA
131721	Participates in physical care	1	2	3	4	5	NA
131722	Provides emotional support	1	2	3	4	5	NA
131723	Provides comfort items	1	2	3	4	5	NA
131724	Provides favorite toys	1	2	3	4	5	NA
131725	Reads books with toddler	1	2	3	4	5	NA
131726	Learns how to provide required treatments	1	2	3	4	5	NA
131727	Provides treatments needed at home	1	2	3	4	5	NA

P

Continued

Parent Adaptation to Toddler Hospitalization—cont'd

		Never Demonstrated	Rarely Demonstrated	Sometimes Demonstrated	Often Demonstrated	Consistently Demonstrated	
131728	Learns about possible developmental delays from extended hospitalizations	1	2	3	4	5	NA
131729	Receives support from family members	1	2	3	4	5	NA
131730	Communicates with extended family	1	2	3	4	5	NA
131731	Expresses satisfaction with nursing care	1	2	3	4	5	NA
131732	Considers the need for palliative care	1	2	3	4	5	NA
131733	Finds meaning in the experience	1	2	3	4	5	NA
131734	Participates in discharge planning	1	2	3	4	5	NA

Domain-Psychosocial Health (III)   *Class*-Psychosocial Adaptation (N)   7th edition 2024

OUTCOME CONTENT REFERENCES:

Aarthun, A., Oymar, K. A., & Akerjordet, K. (2018). How health professionals facilitate parents' involvement in decision-making at the hospital: A parental perspective. *Journal of Child Health Care, 22*(1), 108–121. https://doi.org/10.1177/1367493517744279

Boland, L., Graham, I. D., Légaré, F., Lewis, K., Jull, J., Shephard, A., Lawson, M. L., Davis, A., Yameogo, A., & Stacey, D. (2019). Barriers and facilitators of pediatric shared decision-making: A systematic review. *Implementation Science: IS, 14*(1), 7. https://doi.org/10.1186/s13012-018-0851-5

Bradshaw, S., Bem, D., Shaw, K., Taylor, B., Chiswell, C., Salama, M., Bassett, E., Kaur, G., & Cummins, C. (2019). Improving health, well-being and parenting skills in parents of children with special health care needs and medical complexity—A scoping review. *BMC Pediatrics, 19*(1), 301. https://doi.org/10.1186/s12887-019-1648-7

Chien, C.-H., Lee, T.-Y., & Lin, M.-T. (2021). Factors affecting motor development of toddlers who received cardiac corrective procedures during infancy. *Early Human Development, 158*. https://doi.org/10.1016/j.earlhumdev.2021.105392

de Man, M., Segers, E. W., Schappin, R., van der Leeden, K., Wösten-van Asperen, R. M., Breur, H., de Weerth, C., & van den Hoogen, A. (2021). Parental experiences of their infant's hospital admission undergoing cardiac surgery: A systematic review. *Acta Paediatrica, 110*(6), 1730–1740. https://doi.org/10.1111/apa.15694

Hallman, M. L., & Bellury, L. M. (2020). Communication in pediatric critical care units: A review of the literature. *Critical Care Nurse, 40*(2), e1–e15. https://doi.org/10.4037/ccn2020751

Hockenberry, M. J., Wilson, D., & Rodgers, C. C. (Eds.). (2019). *Wong's nursing care of infants and children* (11th ed.). Elsevier.

Hye-Yul, H., Shin-Jeong, K., Wayne, E. K., & Kyung-Ah, K. (2018). Factors influencing the caregiving performance of mothers of hospitalized toddlers with acute respiratory diseases: A path analysis. *Journal of Child Health Care, 22*(4), 591–605. https://doi.org/10.1177/1367493518767064

Jerofke-Owen, T. A., McAndrew, N. S., Gralton, K. S., Totka, J. P., Weiss, M. E., Fial, A. V., & Sawin, K. J. (2021). Engagement of families in the care of hospitalized pediatric patients: A scoping review. *Journal of Family Nursing, 28*(2), 151–171. https://doi.org/10.1177/10748407211048894

Perry, S. E., Hockenberry, M. J., Lowdermilk, D. J., Wilson, D., Cashion, K., Rodgers, C. C., & Alden, K. R. (2018). *Maternal child nursing care* (6th ed.). Elsevier.

Stragliotto Bazzan, J., Marten Milbrath, V., Bärtschi Gabatz, R. I., Cordeiro, F. R., Freitag, V. L., & Schwartz, E. (2020). The family's adaptation process to their child's hospitalization in an intensive care unit. *Revista Da Escola de Enfermagem Da USP, 54*, 1–8. https://doi.org/10.1590/S1980-220X2018056203614

P

Parent-Infant Attachment   **1500**

Definition: Parent and infant behaviors that demonstrate an enduring affectionate bond

OUTCOME TARGET RATING: Maintain at_____ Increase to_____

		Never Demonstrated	Rarely Demonstrated	Sometimes Demonstrated	Often Demonstrated	Consistently Demonstrated	
OUTCOME OVERALL RATING		1	2	3	4	5	
Indicators:							
150001	Practices healthy behaviors during pregnancy	1	2	3	4	5	NA
150002	Assigns specific attributes to fetus	1	2	3	4	5	NA
150003	Prepares for infant prior to birth	1	2	3	4	5	NA
150004	Verbalizes positive feelings toward infant	1	2	3	4	5	NA
150005	Holds infant close	1	2	3	4	5	NA
150006	Touches, strokes, pats infant	1	2	3	4	5	NA

Parent-Infant Attachment—cont'd

	Never Demonstrated	Rarely Demonstrated	Sometimes Demonstrated	Often Demonstrated	Consistently Demonstrated	
150007	Kisses infant	1	2	3	4	5	NA
150008	Smiles at infant	1	2	3	4	5	NA
150009	Visits nursery	1	2	3	4	5	NA
150012	Uses eye contact	1	2	3	4	5	NA
150013	Vocalizes to infant	1	2	3	4	5	NA
150014	Plays with infant	1	2	3	4	5	NA
150015	Responds to infant cues	1	2	3	4	5	NA
150016	Consoles infant	1	2	3	4	5	NA
150024	Holds infant for feeding	1	2	3	4	5	NA
150018	Keeps infant dry, clean, and warm	1	2	3	4	5	NA
150019	Infant looks at parent	1	2	3	4	5	NA
150020	Infant responds to parent's cues	1	2	3	4	5	NA
150021	Infant seeks proximity with parent	1	2	3	4	5	NA

Specify parent _____

Domain-Psychosocial Health (III)   **Class**-Social Interaction (P)   1st edition 1997; revised 2004, 2008, 2024

OUTCOME CONTENT REFERENCES:

Cooke, J. E., Kochendorfer, L. B., Stuart-Parrigon, K. L., Koehn, A. J., & Kerns, K. A. (2019). Parent-child attachment and children's experience and regulation of emotion: A meta-analytic review. Emotion, 19(6), 1103–1126. https://doi.org/10.1037/emo0000504

Gibbs, B. G., Forste, R., & Lybbert, E. (2018). Breastfeeding, parenting, and infant attachment behaviors. Maternal Child Health Journal, 22(4), 579–588. https://doi.org/10.1007/s10995-018-2427-z

Gibson, R., & Kilcullen, M. (2020). The impact of web cameras on parent-infant attachment in the neonatal intensive care unit. Journal of Pediatric Nursing, 52, e77–e83. https://doi.org/10.1016/j.pedn.2020.01.009

Heo, Y. J., & Oh, W. O. (2019). The effectiveness of a parent participation improvement program for parents on partnership, attachment infant growth in a neonatal intensive care unit: A randomized controlled trial. International Journal of Nursing Studies, 95, 19–27. https://doi.org/10.1016/j.ijnurstu.2019.03.018

Hill, R., & Flanagan, J. (2020), The maternal-infant bond: Clarifying the concept. International Journal of Nursing, 31(1), 14–18. https://doi.org/10.1111/2047-3095.12235

Molmen Lichter, M., Peled, Y., Levy, S., Wiznitzer, A., Krissi, H., & Handelzalts, J. E. (2021). The associations between insecure attachment, rooming-in, and postpartum depression: A 2 months' longitudinal study. Infant Mental Health Journal, 42(1), 74–86. https://doi.org/10.1002/imhj.21895

Olsavsky, A. L., Berrigan, M. N., Schoppe-Sullivan, S. J., Brown, G. L., & Kamp Dush, C. M. (2020). Paternal stimulation and father-infant attachment. Attachment & Human Development, 22(1), 15–26. https://doi.org/10.1080/14616734.2019.1589057

Peñacoba, C., & Catala, P. (2019). Associations between breastfeeding and mother-infant relationships: A systematic review. Breastfeeding Medicine, 14(9), 616–629. https://doi.org/10.1089/bfm.2019.0106

Peralta-Carcelen, M., Schwartz, J., & Carcelen, A. C. (2018). Behavioral and socioemotional development in preterm children. Clinical Perinatology, 45(3), 529–546. https://doi.org/10.1016/j.clp.2018.05.003

+Pinto, T. M., Nunes-Costa, R., & Figueiredo, B. (2022). The Baby Care Scale: A psychometric study with fathers during pregnancy and the postpartum period. Frontiers in Psychology, 12, 751330. https://doi.org/10.3389/fpsyg.2021.751330

P

Parenting Performance   2211

Definition: Parental actions to provide a child a nurturing and constructive physical, emotional, and social environment

OUTCOME TARGET RATING: Maintain at_____ Increase to_____

	Never Demonstrated	Rarely Demonstrated	Sometimes Demonstrated	Often Demonstrated	Consistently Demonstrated	
OUTCOME OVERALL RATING	1	2	3	4	5	
Indicators:						
221132	Provides a clean home environment	1	2	3	4	5	NA
221101	Provides for child's physical needs	1	2	3	4	5	NA
221122	Provides age-appropriate nutrition	1	2	3	4	5	NA
221133	Monitors growth and weight	1	2	3	4	5	NA
221102	Eliminates controllable environmental hazards	1	2	3	4	5	NA

Continued

Parenting Performance—cont'd

		Never Demonstrated	Rarely Demonstrated	Sometimes Demonstrated	Often Demonstrated	Consistently Demonstrated	
221134	Provides age-appropriate toys	1	2	3	4	5	NA
221135	Provides age-appropriate physical activities	1	2	3	4	5	NA
221136	Monitors social contacts	1	2	3	4	5	NA
221137	Supports education	1	2	3	4	5	NA
221130	Provides preventative health care	1	2	3	4	5	NA
221131	Provides episodic health care	1	2	3	4	5	NA
221138	Provides dental care	1	2	3	4	5	NA
221123	Provides structure for child	1	2	3	4	5	NA
221104	Stimulates cognitive development	1	2	3	4	5	NA
221105	Stimulates social development	1	2	3	4	5	NA
221139	Promotes positive self-esteem	1	2	3	4	5	NA
221106	Stimulates emotional growth	1	2	3	4	5	NA
221107	Nurtures spiritual growth	1	2	3	4	5	NA
221124	Stimulates moral growth	1	2	3	4	5	NA
221125	Imparts values that promote functioning in society	1	2	3	4	5	NA
221126	Provides appropriate supervision for child	1	2	3	4	5	NA
221127	Selects appropriate supplemental caregiver	1	2	3	4	5	NA
221128	Monitors supplemental caregiver	1	2	3	4	5	NA
221108	Uses community resources	1	2	3	4	5	NA
221110	Uses interactions appropriate for child's temperament	1	2	3	4	5	NA
221111	Uses behavior management	1	2	3	4	5	NA
221112	Uses age-appropriate discipline	1	2	3	4	5	NA
221113	Provides for child's special needs	1	2	3	4	5	NA
221114	Interacts positively with child	1	2	3	4	5	NA
221115	Empathizes with child	1	2	3	4	5	NA
221129	Maintains open communication	1	2	3	4	5	NA
221116	Verbalizes positive attributes of child	1	2	3	4	5	NA
221117	Exhibits a loving relationship	1	2	3	4	5	NA
221140	Supervises internet activities	1	2	3	4	5	NA
221141	Monitors social media	1	2	3	4	5	NA
221142	Engages with teachers	1	2	3	4	5	NA
221143	Prevents risky behaviors	1	2	3	4	5	NA
221144	Serves as a positive role model	1	2	3	4	5	NA
221118	Expresses realistic expectations of parental role	1	2	3	4	5	NA
221119	Expresses satisfaction with parental role	1	2	3	4	5	NA

Domain-Family Health (VI)   **Class**-Parenting (DD)   *1st edition 1997; revised 2004, 2008, 2013, 2024*

OUTCOME CONTENT REFERENCES:

Hagan, J. F., Shaw, J. S., & Duncan, P. M. (Eds.). (2017). *Bright futures: Guidelines for health supervision of infants, children, and adolescents* (4th ed.). American Academy of Pediatrics.

Hockenberry, M. J., Wilson, D., & Rodgers, C. C. (Eds.). (2019). *Wong's nursing care of infants and children* (11th ed.). Elsevier.

Perry, S. E., Hockenberry, M. J., Lowdermilk, D. J., Wilson, D., Cashion, K., Rodgers, C. C., & Alden, K. R. (2018). *Maternal child nursing care* (6th ed.). Elsevier.

Sebire, S. J., Jago, R., Wood, L., Thompson, J. L., Zahra, J., & Lawlor, D. A. (2016). Examining a conceptual model of parental nurturance, parenting practices and physical activity among 5–6-year-olds. *Social Science & Medicine, 148*, 18–24. https://doi.org/10.1016/j.socscimed.2015.11.022

Parenting Performance: Adolescent   2903

Definition: Parental actions to provide an adolescent with a safe, nurturing, and positive physical, emotional, spiritual, and social environment from 12 years through 17 years

OUTCOME TARGET RATING: Maintain at_____ Increase to_____

		Never Demonstrated	Rarely Demonstrated	Sometimes Demonstrated	Often Demonstrated	Consistently Demonstrated	
OUTCOME OVERALL RATING		1	2	3	4	5	
Indicators:							
290301	Exhibits a loving relationship	1	2	3	4	5	NA
290347	Provides clean home environment	1	2	3	4	5	NA
290302	Maintains open communication with adolescent	1	2	3	4	5	NA
290303	Listens openly, thoughtfully, without interruption	1	2	3	4	5	NA
290304	Promotes appropriate independence	1	2	3	4	5	NA
290305	Serves as role model for personal integrity	1	2	3	4	5	NA
290306	Encourages balance between individual versus group identity	1	2	3	4	5	NA
290348	Discusses strategies to deal with peer pressure	1	2	3	4	5	NA
290307	Assists adolescent to cope constructively with emotions	1	2	3	4	5	NA
290308	Assists adolescent to evaluate consequences of behavior	1	2	3	4	5	NA
290309	Provides clear, consistent rules of behavior	1	2	3	4	5	NA
290310	Enforces family rules of behavior	1	2	3	4	5	NA
290311	Nurtures spiritual growth	1	2	3	4	5	NA
290312	Nurtures moral growth	1	2	3	4	5	NA
290313	Monitors academic performance	1	2	3	4	5	NA
290314	Communicates with teachers about adolescent's academic performance	1	2	3	4	5	NA
290315	Monitors activity involvement to prevent over commitment	1	2	3	4	5	NA
290316	Respects need for emancipation from parental controls	1	2	3	4	5	NA
290317	Respects need for privacy	1	2	3	4	5	NA
290318	Discusses developmental changes with adolescent	1	2	3	4	5	NA
290319	Assists adolescent to develop healthy body image	1	2	3	4	5	NA
290320	Assists adolescent to develop positive self-esteem	1	2	3	4	5	NA
290321	Encourages participation in activities that contribute to lifelong fitness	1	2	3	4	5	NA
290322	Provides appropriate nutrition	1	2	3	4	5	NA
290323	Provides opportunities for family activities	1	2	3	4	5	NA
290324	Monitors for signs of eating disorders	1	2	3	4	5	NA
290325	Discusses age-appropriate sex education	1	2	3	4	5	NA
290326	Teaches to identify predatory, abusive sexual advances	1	2	3	4	5	NA
290327	Teaches to report predatory, abusive sexual advances	1	2	3	4	5	NA

P

Continued

Parenting Performance: Adolescent—cont'd

		Never Demonstrated	Rarely Demonstrated	Sometimes Demonstrated	Often Demonstrated	Consistently Demonstrated	
290349	Monitors internet use	1	2	3	4	5	NA
290350	Monitors social media	1	2	3	4	5	NA
290328	Protects from abuse	1	2	3	4	5	NA
290351	Protects from neglect	1	2	3	4	5	NA
290329	Protects from body mutilation	1	2	3	4	5	NA
290330	Uses strategies to prevent participation in violence	1	2	3	4	5	NA
290331	Assists adolescent to cope with stress	1	2	3	4	5	NA
290332	Discusses problems with substance use	1	2	3	4	5	NA
290333	Establishes clear rules regarding driving	1	2	3	4	5	NA
290334	Establishes clear rules regarding alcohol use	1	2	3	4	5	NA
290335	Establishes clear rules regarding avoidance of drugs	1	2	3	4	5	NA
290336	Reinforces personal hygiene	1	2	3	4	5	NA
290337	Reinforces oral hygiene behaviors	1	2	3	4	5	NA
290338	Maintains recommended dental checkups	1	2	3	4	5	NA
290339	Maintains recommended schedule of health checkups	1	2	3	4	5	NA
290340	Maintains recommended schedule of immunizations	1	2	3	4	5	NA
290341	Promotes adequate sleep	1	2	3	4	5	NA
290342	Teaches danger of hearing damage from portable music devices	1	2	3	4	5	NA
290343	Discusses implications of body piercing and tattoos	1	2	3	4	5	NA
290344	Teaches strategies to prevent injury	1	2	3	4	5	NA
290352	Teaches strategies to prevent infections	1	2	3	4	5	NA
290345	Recognizes symptoms of depression and potential suicide	1	2	3	4	5	NA
290346	Obtains treatment for depressed adolescent	1	2	3	4	5	NA

Domain-Family Health (VI)   **Class**-Parenting (DD)   5th edition 2013; revised 2024

P

OUTCOME CONTENT REFERENCES:

Center for Disease Control and Prevention. (2021, January 22). *CDC's Developmental Milestones.* https://www.cdc.gov/ncbddd/actearly/milestones/index.html

Hagan, J. F., Shaw, J. S., & Duncan, P. M. (Eds.). (2017). *Bright futures: Guidelines for health supervision of infants, children and adolescents* (4th ed.). American Academy of Pediatrics.

Hockenberry, M. J., Wilson, D., & Rodgers, C. C. (Eds.). (2019). *Wong's nursing care of infants and children* (11th ed.). Elsevier.

Hou, Y., Benner, A. D., Kim, S. Y., Chen, S., Spitz, S., Shi, Y., & Beretvas, T. (2020). Discordance in parents' and adolescents' reports of parenting: A meta-analysis and qualitative review. *The American Psychologist, 75*(3), 329–348. https://doi.org/10.1037/amp0000463

Janssen, L., Verkuil, B., van Houtum, L., Wever, M., & Elzinga, B. M. (2021). Perceptions of parenting in daily life: Adolescent-parent differences and associations with adolescent affect. *Journal of Youth and Adolescence, 50*(12), 2427–2443. https://doi.org/10.1007/s10964-021-01489-x

Perry, S. E., Hockenberry, M. J., Lowdermilk, D. J., Wilson, D., Cashion, K., Rodgers, C. C., & Alden, K. R. (2018). *Maternal child nursing care* (6th ed.). Elsevier.

Parenting Performance: Adolescent Physical Safety 2902

Definition: Parental actions to prevent physical injury in an adolescent from 12 years through 17 years of age

OUTCOME TARGET RATING: Maintain at_____ Increase to_____

		Never Demonstrated	Rarely Demonstrated	Sometimes Demonstrated	Often Demonstrated	Consistently Demonstrated	
OUTCOME OVERALL RATING		1	2	3	4	5	
Indicators:							
290201	Uses strategies to protect from sun exposure	1	2	3	4	5	NA
290230	Uses strategies to prevent heat stroke	1	2	3	4	5	NA
290231	Uses strategies to protect from frostbite and hypothermia	1	2	3	4	5	NA
290226	Encourages appropriate clothing for activity	1	2	3	4	5	NA
290203	Maintains home warning devices	1	2	3	4	5	NA
290204	Practices family fire escape plan	1	2	3	4	5	NA
290205	Maintains smoke-free environment	1	2	3	4	5	NA
290206	Monitors use of sport and recreational equipment	1	2	3	4	5	NA
290232	Encourages protective gear use during high-risk activities	1	2	3	4	5	NA
290233	Encourages bicycle safety	1	2	3	4	5	NA
290208	Uses strategies to encourage seat belt use	1	2	3	4	5	NA
290209	Uses strategies to encourage safe driving	1	2	3	4	5	NA
290234	Sets rules against texting while driving	1	2	3	4	5	NA
290235	Uses strategies to prevent impaired driving	1	2	3	4	5	NA
290210	Uses strategies to prevent water accidents	1	2	3	4	5	NA
290236	Uses strategies to prevent concussions	1	2	3	4	5	NA
290237	Uses strategies to prevent diving accidents	1	2	3	4	5	NA
290211	Uses strategies to prevent firearm injuries	1	2	3	4	5	NA
290212	Uses strategies to prevent participation in violence	1	2	3	4	5	NA
290238	Uses strategies to prevent gang participation	1	2	3	4	5	NA
290213	Uses strategies to prevent tobacco use	1	2	3	4	5	NA
290214	Uses strategies to prevent alcohol use	1	2	3	4	5	NA
290239	Uses strategies to prevent vaping	1	2	3	4	5	NA
290215	Uses strategies to prevent recreational drug use	1	2	3	4	5	NA
290216	Uses strategies to prevent medication misuse	1	2	3	4	5	NA
290217	Uses strategies to prevent exposure to toxic chemicals	1	2	3	4	5	NA
290218	Uses strategies to prevent exposure to excessive noise	1	2	3	4	5	NA
290228	Uses strategies to postpone sexual activity	1	2	3	4	5	NA
290220	Uses strategies to prevent high-risk sexual activity	1	2	3	4	5	NA
290229	Uses strategies to prevent communicable disease	1	2	3	4	5	NA
290222	Protects from physical abuse	1	2	3	4	5	NA
290223	Protects from sexual abuse	1	2	3	4	5	NA
290240	Secures firearms to prevent access						
290224	Monitors for warning signs of self-harm	1	2	3	4	5	NA
290227	Obtains training to prepare for emergencies	1	2	3	4	5	NA

Domain-Family Health (VI)   *Class*-Parenting (DD)   *3rd edition 2004; revised 2008, 2013, 2024*

P

OUTCOME CONTENT REFERENCES:

Cox, D. J., Gonder-Frederick, L. A., Shepard, J. A., Campbell, L. K., & Vajda, K. A. (2012). Driving safety: Concerns and experiences of parents of adolescent drivers with type 1 diabetes. *Pediatric Diabetes, 13*(6), 506–509. https://doi.org/10.1111/j.1399-5448.2012.00862.x

Hagan, J. F., Shaw, J. S., & Duncan, P. M. (Eds.). (2017). *Bright futures: Guidelines for health supervision of infants, children and adolescents* (4th ed.). American Academy of Pediatrics.

Hamann, C. J., & Spears, S. (2019). Parent-adolescent bicycling safety communication and bicycling behavior. *Accident: Analysis and Prevention, 131,* 350–356. https://doi.org/10.1016/j.aap.2019.07.017

Hockenberry, M. J., Wilson, D., & Rodgers, C. C. (Eds.). (2019). *Wong's nursing care of infants and children* (11th ed.). Elsevier.

Perry, S. E., Hockenberry, M. J., Lowdermilk, D. J., Wilson, D., Cashion, K., Rodgers, C. C., & Alden, K. R. (2018). *Maternal child nursing care* (6th ed.). Elsevier.

Potter, K., Virtanen, H., Stewart, F., Luca, P., Ho, J., Nettel-Aguirre, A., & Pacaud, D. (2020). Exploring knowledge and safety practices for driving in youth with type 1 diabetes. *Canadian Journal of Diabetes, 44*(2), 169–174.e2. https://doi.org/10.1016/j.jcjd.2019.06.001

Temsah, M. H., Aljamaan, F., Alhaboob, A., Almosned, B., Alsebail, R., Temsah, R., Senjab, A., Alarfaj, A., Aljudi, T., Jamal, A., Habash, A., Alsohime, F., Almazyad, M., Alabdulhafid, M., Hasan, G., Assiri, R. A., Alqahtani, W., Alherbish, A., Alhasan, K., & Al-Eyadhy, A. (2022). Enhancing parental knowledge of childhood and adolescence safety: An interventional educational campaign. *Medicine, 101*(3), e28649. https://doi.org/10.1097/MD.0000000000028649

Parenting Performance: Attention Deficit Hyperactivity Disorder (ADHD) 2908

Definition: Parental actions to provide a child with ADHD a nurturing and supportive environment for optimal functioning

OUTCOME TARGET RATING: Maintain at_____ Increase to_____

		Never Demonstrated	Rarely Demonstrated	Sometimes Demonstrated	Often Demonstrated	Consistently Demonstrated	
OUTCOME OVERALL RATING		1	2	3	4	5	
Indicators:							
290801	Accepts diagnosis based on comprehensive multidisciplinary team evaluation	1	2	3	4	5	NA
290802	Obtains reputable sources of information on ADHD	1	2	3	4	5	NA
290803	Consults experts regarding treatment	1	2	3	4	5	NA
290804	Develops consensus among experts	1	2	3	4	5	NA
290805	Shares diagnosis with family members	1	2	3	4	5	NA
290806	Shares basic ADHD information with family members	1	2	3	4	5	NA
290807	Recognizes importance of supporting child's abilities	1	2	3	4	5	NA
290808	Identifies child's signs and symptoms of ADHD	1	2	3	4	5	NA
290809	Uses tool to record and track symptoms of hyperactivity	1	2	3	4	5	NA
290810	Uses tool to record and track symptoms of inattention	1	2	3	4	5	NA
290811	Uses strategies to reduce environmental stimuli when completing homework	1	2	3	4	5	NA
290812	Uses behavioral approaches recommended by professionals	1	2	3	4	5	NA
290813	Administers prescribed medication	1	2	3	4	5	NA
290814	Monitors therapeutic effects of medication	1	2	3	4	5	NA
290815	Monitors for medication side effects	1	2	3	4	5	NA
290816	Provides positive reinforcement of desired behaviors	1	2	3	4	5	NA

P

Parenting Performance: Attention Deficit Hyperactivity Disorder (ADHD)—cont'd

		Never Demonstrated	Rarely Demonstrated	Sometimes Demonstrated	Often Demonstrated	Consistently Demonstrated	
290817	Models desired problem-solving methods	1	2	3	4	5	NA
290818	Uses appropriate consequences for undesirable behavior	1	2	3	4	5	NA
290819	Provide frequent breaks when sitting for a prolonged time	1	2	3	4	5	NA
290820	Encourages child to make better choices	1	2	3	4	5	NA
290821	Encourages child to take responsibility for behavior	1	2	3	4	5	NA
290822	Communicates treatment plan with teachers	1	2	3	4	5	NA
290823	Seeks periodic evaluation by multidisciplinary team	1	2	3	4	5	NA
290824	Adapts family routines to meet needs of child	1	2	3	4	5	NA
290825	Monitors school performance	1	2	3	4	5	NA
290826	Monitors social interaction skills	1	2	3	4	5	NA
290827	Provides support for learning disabilities	1	2	3	4	5	NA
290828	Obtains therapy for anxiety when needed	1	2	3	4	5	NA
290829	Obtains therapy for depression when needed	1	2	3	4	5	NA
290830	Uses available support groups	1	2	3	4	5	NA
290831	Uses available community resources	1	2	3	4	5	NA

Domain-Family Health (VI)   **Class-** *Parenting (DD)*   *7th edition 2024*

OUTCOME CONTENT REFERENCES:
Aduen, P., Day, A. T., Kofler, M. J., Harmon, S. L., Wells, E. L., & Sarver, D. E. (2018). Social problems in ADHD: Is it a skills acquisition or performance problem? *Journal of Psychopathology and Behavioral Assessment, 40*(3), 440–451. https://doi.org/10.1007/s10862-018-9649-7
Antai-Otong, D., & Zimmerman, M. L. (2016). Treatment approaches to attention deficit hyperactivity disorder. *The Nursing Clinics of North America, 51*(2), 199–211. https://doi.org/10.1016/j.cnur.2016.01.005
Center for Disease Control and Prevention. (2021, September 28.). Attention-Deficit/Hyperactivity Disorder (ADHD). https://www.cdc.gov/ncbddd/adhd/
Hockenberry, M. J., Wilson, D., & Rodgers, C. C. (Eds.). (2019). *Wong's nursing care of infants and children* (11th ed.). Elsevier.
Modesto-Lowe, V., Chaplin, M., Godsay, V., & Soovajian, V. (2014). Parenting teens with attention-deficit/hyperactivity disorder: Challenges and opportunities. *Clinical Pediatrics, 53*(10), 943–948. https://doi.org/10.1177/0009922814540984
Paidipati, C. P., & Deatrick, J. A. (2015). The role of family phenomena in children and adolescents with attention deficit hyperactivity disorder. *Journal of Child and Adolescent Psychiatric Nursing, 28*(1), 3–13. https://doi.org/10.1111/jcap.12097
Ringer, N. (2020). Living with ADHD: A meta-synthesis review of qualitative research on children's experiences and understanding of their ADHD. *International Journal of Disability, Development and Education, 67*(2), 208-224. https://doi.org/10.1080/1034912X.2019.1596226
Spencer, A. E., Oblath, R., Sheldrick, R. C., Ng, L. C., Silverstein, M., & Garg, A. (2022). Social determinants of health and ADHD symptoms in preschool-age children. *Journal of Attention Disorders, 26*(3), 447–455. https://doi.org/10.1177/1087054721996458
Sternhagen, T., Schumacher, H., Ferrell, K., & Willman, A. (2020). Parenting children with ADHD. *South Dakota Medicine: The Journal of the South Dakota State Medical Association, 73*(7), 296–304.
Tandon, M., & Pergjika, A. (2017). Attention deficit hyperactivity disorder in preschool-age children. *Child and Adolescent Psychiatric Clinics of North America, 26*(3), 523–538. https://doi.org/10.1016/j.chc.2017.02.007

P

Parenting Performance: Early Childhood Psychosocial Safety 2909

Definition: Parental actions to protect a child 1 to 5 years old from social contacts that might cause harm or injury

OUTCOME TARGET RATING: Maintain at_____ Increase to_____

		Never Demonstrated	Rarely Demonstrated	Sometimes Demonstrated	Often Demonstrated	Consistently Demonstrated	
OUTCOME OVERALL RATING		1	2	3	4	5	
Indicators:							
290901	Monitors playmates	1	2	3	4	5	NA
290902	Monitors siblings	1	2	3	4	5	NA
290903	Monitors social contacts	1	2	3	4	5	NA
290904	Monitors contacts with family adult friends	1	2	3	4	5	NA
290905	Monitors contacts with extended family	1	2	3	4	5	NA
290906	Fosters open communication	1	2	3	4	5	NA
290907	Selects appropriate supplemental caregiver	1	2	3	4	5	NA
290908	Monitors supplemental caregiver	1	2	3	4	5	NA
290909	Identifies private parts of the body others should not touch	1	2	3	4	5	NA
290910	Teaches to not keep secrets from parents	1	2	3	4	5	NA
290911	Recognizes risk for abuse	1	2	3	4	5	NA
290912	Uses strategies to eliminate risk for abuse	1	2	3	4	5	NA
290913	Protects from neglect	1	2	3	4	5	NA
290914	Protects from physical abuse	1	2	3	4	5	NA
290915	Protects from sexual abuse	1	2	3	4	5	NA
290916	Protects from emotional abuse	1	2	3	4	5	NA
290917	Protects from being bullied	1	2	3	4	5	NA
290918	Provides required level of supervision	1	2	3	4	5	NA
290919	Uses internet to identify sex offenders in neighborhood	1	2	3	4	5	NA
290920	Teaches about bad strangers	1	2	3	4	5	NA
290921	Remains aware of surroundings during outdoor activities	1	2	3	4	5	NA
290922	Teaches to not get in a car without parental permission	1	2	3	4	5	NA
290923	Teaches age-appropriate child lures	1	2	3	4	5	NA
290924	Sets clear rules for behavior	1	2	3	4	5	NA
290925	Maintains structure in child's life	1	2	3	4	5	NA
290926	Maintains daily routine in child's life	1	2	3	4	5	NA

Domain-Family Health (VI)   **Class**-Parenting (DD)   7th edition 2024

OUTCOME CONTENT REFERENCES:

Ahern, N. R., Kemppainen, J., & Thacker, P. (2016). Awareness and knowledge of child and adolescent risky behaviors: A parent's perspective. *Journal of Child and Adolescent Psychiatric Nursing, 29,* 6–14. http//doi.org/10.1111/jcap.12129

Hagan, J. F., Shaw, J. S., & Duncan, P. M. (Eds.). (2017). *Bright futures: Guidelines for health supervision of infants, children, and adolescents* (4th ed.). American Academy of Pediatrics.

Hockenberry, M. J., Wilson, D., & Rodgers, C. C. (Eds.). (2019). *Wong's nursing care of infants and children* (11th ed.). Elsevier.

P

Parenting Performance: Early/Middle Childhood Physical Safety   2901

Definition: Parental actions to avoid physical injury of a child from 3 years through 11 years of age

OUTCOME TARGET RATING: Maintain at_____ Increase to_____

		Never Demonstrated	Rarely Demonstrated	Sometimes Demonstrated	Often Demonstrated	Consistently Demonstrated	
OUTCOME OVERALL RATING		1	2	3	4	5	
Indicators:							
290101	Selects safe, age-appropriate toys	1	2	3	4	5	NA
290102	Provides supervision around pets and animals	1	2	3	4	5	NA
290103	Provides supervision around water	1	2	3	4	5	NA
290104	Avoids leaving child in motor vehicle unsupervised	1	2	3	4	5	NA
290105	Monitors proper use of car seat/seat belt	1	2	3	4	5	NA
290135	Instructs how to safely cross the street	1	2	3	4	5	NA
290106	Supervises selection of weather-appropriate clothing	1	2	3	4	5	NA
290107	Protects from sun exposure	1	2	3	4	5	NA
290136	Protects from frostbite and hypothermia	1	2	3	4	5	NA
290108	Maintains environment to prevent harmful falls	1	2	3	4	5	NA
290137	Maintains environment to prevent burns and electrical shock	1	2	3	4	5	NA
290110	Maintains environment to prevent poisoning	1	2	3	4	5	NA
290111	Practices family fire escape plan	1	2	3	4	5	NA
290112	Keeps medication out of reach	1	2	3	4	5	NA
290113	Maintains home warning devices	1	2	3	4	5	NA
290114	Locks or removes doors from unused appliances	1	2	3	4	5	NA
290115	Maintains smoke-free environment	1	2	3	4	5	NA
290116	Ensures home playground equipment meets safety guidelines	1	2	3	4	5	NA
290117	Provides supervision while on play-ground equipment	1	2	3	4	5	NA
290118	Selects appropriate clothing for activity	1	2	3	4	5	NA
290119	Uses strategies to encourage use of protective helmet	1	2	3	4	5	NA
290120	Uses strategies to encourage use of protective gear during high-risk activities	1	2	3	4	5	NA
290138	Stores matches and lighters to limit access	1	2	3	4	5	NA
290121	Eliminates access to firearms	1	2	3	4	5	NA
290139	Limits access to fireworks and sparklers	1	2	3	4	5	NA
290122	Protects from exposure to violence	1	2	3	4	5	NA
290123	Monitors use of sport and recreational equipment	1	2	3	4	5	NA
290124	Uses strategies to prevent tobacco use	1	2	3	4	5	NA
290125	Uses strategies to prevent alcohol use	1	2	3	4	5	NA
290126	Uses strategies to prevent recreational drug use	1	2	3	4	5	NA
290127	Uses strategies to prevent medication misuse	1	2	3	4	5	NA

P

Continued

Parenting Performance: Early/Middle Childhood Physical Safety—cont'd

		Never Demonstrated	Rarely Demonstrated	Sometimes Demonstrated	Often Demonstrated	Consistently Demonstrated	
290128	Uses strategies to prevent exposure to toxic chemicals	1	2	3	4	5	NA
290129	Uses strategies to prevent exposure to excessive noise	1	2	3	4	5	NA
290130	Uses strategies to prevent precocious sexual behavior	1	2	3	4	5	NA
290140	Uses strategies to prevent communicable disease	1	2	3	4	5	NA
290141	Protects from neglect	1	2	3	4	5	NA
290131	Protects from physical abuse	1	2	3	4	5	NA
290132	Protects from sexual abuse	1	2	3	4	5	NA
290134	Obtains training to prepare for emergencies	1	2	3	4	5	NA

Domain-Family Health (VI)   **Class**-Parenting (DD)   *3rd edition 2004; revised 2008, 2013, 2024*

OUTCOME CONTENT REFERENCES:

Hagan, J. F., Shaw, J. S., & Duncan, P. M. (Eds.). (2017). *Bright futures: Guidelines for health supervision of infants, children and adolescents* (4th ed.). American Academy of Pediatrics.

Hockenberry, M. J., Wilson, D., & Rodgers, C. C. (Eds.). (2019). *Wong's nursing care of infants and children* (11th ed.). Elsevier.

Perry, S. E., Hockenberry, M. J., Lowdermilk, D. J., Wilson, D., Cashion, K., Rodgers, C. C., & Alden, K. R. (2018). *Maternal child nursing care* (6th ed.). Elsevier.

Temsah, M. H., Aljamaan, F., Alhaboob, A., Almosned, B., Alsebail, R., Temsah, R., Senjab, A., Alarfaj, A., Aljudi, T., Jamal, A., Habash, A., Alsohime, F., Almazyad, M., Alabdulhafid, M., Hasan, G., Assiri, R. A., Alqahtani, W., Alherbish, A., Alhasan, K., & Al-Eyadhy, A. (2022). Enhancing parental knowledge of childhood and adolescence safety: An interventional educational campaign. *Medicine, 101*(3), e28649. https://doi.org/10.1097/MD.0000000000028649

Parenting Performance: Infant
2904

Definition: Parental actions to provide an infant a safe, nurturing, and positive physical, emotional, spiritual, and social environment from 28 days to first birthday

OUTCOME TARGET RATING: Maintain at_____ Increase to_____

		Never Demonstrated	Rarely Demonstrated	Sometimes Demonstrated	Often Demonstrated	Consistently Demonstrated	
OUTCOME OVERALL RATING		1	2	3	4	5	
Indicators:							
290401	Exhibits a loving relationship	1	2	3	4	5	NA
290428	Provides a clean home environment	1	2	3	4	5	NA
290402	Provides safe, age-appropriate developmental activities	1	2	3	4	5	NA
290403	Interacts with infant to promote trust	1	2	3	4	5	NA
290404	Interacts with infant to promote language development	1	2	3	4	5	NA
290405	Interacts with infant to promote social development	1	2	3	4	5	NA
290406	Provides transitional objects to reduce anxiety	1	2	3	4	5	NA
290407	Responds appropriately to infant temperament	1	2	3	4	5	NA
290408	Provides appropriate sensory/motor stimulation	1	2	3	4	5	NA
290409	Provides appropriate supervision	1	2	3	4	5	NA

P

Parenting Performance: Infant—cont'd

		Never Demonstrated	Rarely Demonstrated	Sometimes Demonstrated	Often Demonstrated	Consistently Demonstrated	
290410	Uses a social support system to assist with infant	1	2	3	4	5	NA
290411	Selects appropriate supplemental caregiver	1	2	3	4	5	NA
290412	Monitors supplemental caregiver	1	2	3	4	5	NA
290413	Uses strategies to eliminate risk for abuse	1	2	3	4	5	NA
290414	Protects from abuse	1	2	3	4	5	NA
290429	Protects from neglect	1	2	3	4	5	NA
290415	Sets behavioral limits	1	2	3	4	5	NA
290416	Maintains safe sleep environment	1	2	3	4	5	NA
290417	Provides appropriate weaning	1	2	3	4	5	NA
290418	Allows non-nutritive sucking	1	2	3	4	5	NA
290419	Provides age-appropriate nutrition	1	2	3	4	5	NA
290420	Encourages oral hygiene as primary teeth erupt	1	2	3	4	5	NA
290421	Provides a spiritual environment	1	2	3	4	5	NA
290422	Maintains smoke-free environment	1	2	3	4	5	NA
290423	Maintains recommended well-child checkups	1	2	3	4	5	NA
290424	Maintains recommended immunizations	1	2	3	4	5	NA
290425	Uses strategies to prevent injury	1	2	3	4	5	NA
290430	Uses strategies to prevent infections	1	2	3	4	5	NA
290431	Uses strategies to prevent falls	1	2	3	4	5	NA
290432	Monitors other children around infant	1	2	3	4	5	NA
290426	Protects from sun exposure	1	2	3	4	5	NA
290427	Obtains assistance from a health professional when symptoms occur	1	2	3	4	5	NA

Domain-*Family Health (VI)*   **Class**-*Parenting (DD)*   *5th edition 2013; revised 2024*

OUTCOME CONTENT REFERENCES:

Center for Disease Control and Prevention. (2021, January 22). *CDC's Developmental Milestones.* https://www.cdc.gov/ncbddd/actearly/milestones/index.html

Hagan, J. F., Shaw, J. S., & Duncan, P. M. (Eds.). (2017). *Bright futures: Guidelines for health supervision of infants, children and adolescents* (4th ed.). American Academy of Pediatrics.

Hockenberry, M. J., Wilson, D., & Rodgers, C. C. (Eds.). (2019). *Wong's nursing care of infants and children* (11th ed.). Elsevier.

Perry, S. E., Hockenberry, M. J., Lowdermilk, D. J., Wilson, D., Cashion, K., Rodgers, C. C., & Alden, K. R. (2018). *Maternal child nursing care* (6th ed.). Elsevier.

P

Parenting Performance: Infant Physical Safety   2910

Definition: Parental actions to prevent physical injury of a child from birth to first birthday

OUTCOME TARGET RATING: Maintain at_____ Increase to_____

		Never Demonstrated	Rarely Demonstrated	Sometimes Demonstrated	Often Demonstrated	Consistently Demonstrated	
OUTCOME OVERALL RATING		1	2	3	4	5	
Indicators:							
291001	Handles infant properly	1	2	3	4	5	NA
291002	Supports head until neck muscles can provide support	1	2	3	4	5	NA
291003	Uses crib that meets safety regulations	1	2	3	4	5	NA
291004	Positions on back for sleep	1	2	3	4	5	NA
291005	Selects safe, age-appropriate toys	1	2	3	4	5	NA

Continued

Parenting Performance: Infant Physical Safety—cont'd

		Never Demonstrated	Rarely Demonstrated	Sometimes Demonstrated	Often Demonstrated	Consistently Demonstrated	
291006	Keeps sharp objects out of reach	1	2	3	4	5	NA
291007	Feeds infant slowly	1	2	3	4	5	NA
291008	Selects foods that prevent choking	1	2	3	4	5	NA
291009	Stores formula/breastmilk safely	1	2	3	4	5	NA
291010	Prevents falls from furniture	1	2	3	4	5	NA
291011	Provides constant supervision around pets and animals	1	2	3	4	5	NA
291012	Provides constant supervision around water	1	2	3	4	5	NA
291013	Avoids leaving infant in motor vehicle unsupervised	1	2	3	4	5	NA
291014	Uses back facing car seat	1	2	3	4	5	NA
291015	Uses baby monitor	1	2	3	4	5	NA
291016	Selects weather-appropriate clothing	1	2	3	4	5	NA
291017	Protects from sun exposure	1	2	3	4	5	NA
291018	Maintains environment to prevent suffocation	1	2	3	4	5	NA
291019	Maintains environment to prevent harmful falls	1	2	3	4	5	NA
291020	Keeps hot liquids away from infant	1	2	3	4	5	NA
291021	Maintains environment to prevent burns and electrical shock	1	2	3	4	5	NA
291022	Secures household cleaners and poisons	1	2	3	4	5	NA
291023	Keeps medication out of reach	1	2	3	4	5	NA
291024	Secures firearms and ammunition	1	2	3	4	5	NA
291025	Maintains smoke-free environment	1	2	3	4	5	NA
291026	Uses strategies to prevent exposure to excessive noise	1	2	3	4	5	NA
291027	Maintains home warning devices	1	2	3	4	5	NA
291028	Obtains training to prepare for emergencies	1	2	3	4	5	NA
291029	Keeps vaccines up to date	1	2	3	4	5	NA
291030	Protects from neglect	1	2	3	4	5	NA
291031	Protects from physical abuse	1	2	3	4	5	NA
291032	Protects from sexual abuse	1	2	3	4	5	NA

Domain-Family Health (VI)   **Class**-Parenting (DD)   7th edition 2024

OUTCOME CONTENT REFERENCES:

Cashin, M., Wroe, J., & Campbell, L. E. (2021). What parents want to know in the first postnatal year: A Delphi consensus study. *Child Care Health Development, 47*, 47–56. https://doi.org/10.1111/cch.12806

Dao, A., & McMullin, J. (2019). Unintentional injury, supervision, and discourses on childproofing devices. *Medical Anthropology, 38*(1), 15–29. https://doi.org/10.1080/01459740.2018.1482548

Hockenberry, M. J., Wilson, D., & Rodgers, C. C. (Eds.). (2019). *Wong's nursing care of infants and children* (11th ed.). Elsevier.

Perry, S. E., Hockenberry, M. J., Lowdermilk, D. J., Wilson, D., Cashion, K., Rodgers, C. C., & Alden, K. R. (2018). *Maternal child nursing care* (6th ed.). Elsevier.

Staples, A. D., & Bates, J. E. (2018). Parenting of infants and toddlers. In M. R. Sanders, & A. Morawska (Eds.), *Handbook of parenting and child development across the lifespan* (pp. 585–607). Springer International. https://doi.org/10.1007/978-3-319-94598-9_26

Parenting Performance: Infant Psychosocial Safety   2911

Definition: Parental actions to protect an infant from birth to first birthday from social contacts that might cause harm or injury

OUTCOME TARGET RATING: Maintain at_____ Increase to_____

		Never Demonstrated	Rarely Demonstrated	Sometimes Demonstrated	Often Demonstrated	Consistently Demonstrated	
OUTCOME OVERALL RATING		1	2	3	4	5	
Indicators:							
291101	Monitors social contacts	1	2	3	4	5	NA
291102	Monitors contacts with family adult friends	1	2	3	4	5	NA
291103	Monitors contacts with extended family	1	2	3	4	5	NA
291104	Monitors contact with siblings	1	2	3	4	5	NA
291105	Monitors contact with children	1	2	3	4	5	NA
291106	Monitors contact with pets	1	2	3	4	5	NA
291107	Selects appropriate supplemental caregiver	1	2	3	4	5	NA
291108	Monitors supplemental caregiver	1	2	3	4	5	NA
291109	Recognizes risk for abuse	1	2	3	4	5	NA
291110	Uses strategies to eliminate risk for abuse	1	2	3	4	5	NA
291111	Protects from neglect	1	2	3	4	5	NA
291112	Protects from physical abuse	1	2	3	4	5	NA
291113	Protects from sexual abuse	1	2	3	4	5	NA
291114	Protects from emotional abuse	1	2	3	4	5	NA
291115	Provides required level of supervision	1	2	3	4	5	NA
291116	Prevents contact with strangers	1	2	3	4	5	NA

Domain-*Family Health (VI)*   **Class**-*Parenting (DD)*   7th edition 2024

OUTCOME CONTENT REFERENCES:
Hagan, J. F., Shaw, J. S., & Duncan, P. M. (Eds.). (2017). *Bright futures: Guidelines for health supervision of infants, children, and adolescents* (4th ed.). American Academy of Pediatrics.
Hockenberry, M. J., Wilson, D., & Rodgers, C. C. (Eds.). (2019). *Wong's nursing care of infants and children* (11th ed.). Elsevier.

P

Parenting Performance: Middle Childhood   2905

Definition: Parental actions to provide a child with a safe, nurturing, and positive physical, emotional, social, and spiritual environment from 6 years through 11 years

OUTCOME TARGET RATING: Maintain at_____ Increase to_____

		Never Demonstrated	Rarely Demonstrated	Sometimes Demonstrated	Often Demonstrated	Consistently Demonstrated	
OUTCOME OVERALL RATING		1	2	3	4	5	
Indicators:							
290501	Exhibits a loving relationship	1	2	3	4	5	NA
290545	Provides a clean home environment	1	2	3	4	5	NA
290502	Maintains open communication with child	1	2	3	4	5	NA
290503	Promotes appropriate independence	1	2	3	4	5	NA
290504	Encourages safe exploration of environment	1	2	3	4	5	NA

Continued

Parenting Performance: Middle Childhood—cont'd

		Never Demonstrated	Rarely Demonstrated	Sometimes Demonstrated	Often Demonstrated	Consistently Demonstrated	
290505	Provides clear, consistent rules of behavior	1	2	3	4	5	NA
290506	Enforces family rules of behavior	1	2	3	4	5	NA
290507	Uses age-appropriate discipline	1	2	3	4	5	NA
290508	Provides for child's special needs	1	2	3	4	5	NA
290509	Monitors school learning environment	1	2	3	4	5	NA
290510	Monitors academic performance	1	2	3	4	5	NA
290511	Communicates with teachers about child's academic performance	1	2	3	4	5	NA
290512	Provides safe after-school activities	1	2	3	4	5	NA
290513	Encourages peer group involvement	1	2	3	4	5	NA
290514	Encourages completion of activities	1	2	3	4	5	NA
290515	Provides opportunities for learning	1	2	3	4	5	NA
290516	Promotes regular physical exercise	1	2	3	4	5	NA
290517	Assists child to maintain optimum weight	1	2	3	4	5	NA
290518	Encourages participation in team activities	1	2	3	4	5	NA
290519	Monitors activities to prevent over commitment	1	2	3	4	5	NA
290520	Provides opportunities for quiet activities	1	2	3	4	5	NA
290546	Uses strategies to prevent risky behaviors	1	2	3	4	5	NA
290521	Teaches to identify predatory, abusive sexual advances	1	2	3	4	5	NA
290522	Teaches to report predatory, abusive sexual advances	1	2	3	4	5	NA
290523	Protects from abuse	1	2	3	4	5	NA
290547	Protects from neglect	1	2	3	4	5	NA
290548	Protects from bullying	1	2	3	4	5	NA
290524	Prevents exposure to violence	1	2	3	4	5	NA
290525	Maintains sleep routine	1	2	3	4	5	NA
290526	Provides appropriate nutrition	1	2	3	4	5	NA
290527	Discusses prepubescent developmental changes with child	1	2	3	4	5	NA
290528	Discusses age-appropriate sex education	1	2	3	4	5	NA
290529	Accepts child's sexual orientation	1	2	3	4	5	NA
290530	Discusses problems with substance use	1	2	3	4	5	NA
290531	Assists child to cope with stress	1	2	3	4	5	NA
290532	Nurtures spiritual growth	1	2	3	4	5	NA
290533	Nurtures moral growth	1	2	3	4	5	NA
290549	Nurtures self-esteem	1	2	3	4	5	NA
290534	Promotes respect for others	1	2	3	4	5	NA
290535	Reinforces oral hygiene behaviors	1	2	3	4	5	NA
290536	Maintains recommended dental checkups	1	2	3	4	5	NA
290537	Maintains recommended health checkups	1	2	3	4	5	NA
290538	Maintains recommended immunizations	1	2	3	4	5	NA

P

Parenting Performance: Middle Childhood—cont'd

		Never Demonstrated	Rarely Demonstrated	Sometimes Demonstrated	Often Demonstrated	Consistently Demonstrated	
290539	Maintains smoke-free environment	1	2	3	4	5	NA
290540	Teaches personal stranger safety	1	2	3	4	5	NA
290541	Uses strategies to prevent injury	1	2	3	4	5	NA
290550	Uses strategies to prevent infection	1	2	3	4	5	NA
290542	Protects from sun exposure	1	2	3	4	5	NA
290543	Obtains assistance from a health professional for health problems	1	2	3	4	5	NA
290551	Monitors for signs and symptoms of depression	1	2	3	4	5	NA
290544	Obtains treatment for childhood depression	1	2	3	4	5	NA

Domain-Family Health (VI)   **Class**-Parenting (DD)   *5th edition 2013; revised 2024*

OUTCOME CONTENT REFERENCES:

Center for Disease Control and Prevention. (2021, January 22). *CDC's Developmental Milestones*. https://www.cdc.gov/ncbddd/actearly/milestones/index.html
Hagan, J. F., Shaw, J. S., & Duncan, P. M. (Eds.). (2017). *Bright futures: Guidelines for health supervision of infants, children and adolescents* (4th ed.). American Academy of Pediatrics.
Hockenberry, M. J., Wilson, D., & Rodgers, C. C. (Eds.). (2019). *Wong's nursing care of infants and children* (11th ed.). Elsevier.
Perry, S. E., Hockenberry, M. J., Lowdermilk, D. J., Wilson, D., Cashion, K., Rodgers, C. C., & Alden, K. R. (2018). *Maternal child nursing care* (6th ed.). Elsevier.

Parenting Performance: Preschooler   2906

Definition: Parental actions to provide a preschooler with a safe, nurturing, and positive physical, emotional, spiritual, and social environment from 3 through 5 years

OUTCOME TARGET RATING: Maintain at_____ Increase to_____

		Never Demonstrated	Rarely Demonstrated	Sometimes Demonstrated	Often Demonstrated	Consistently Demonstrated	
OUTCOME OVERALL RATING		1	2	3	4	5	
Indicators:							
290601	Exhibits a loving relationship	1	2	3	4	5	NA
290643	Provides a clean home environment	1	2	3	4	5	NA
290602	Provides safe, age-appropriate developmental activities	1	2	3	4	5	NA
290603	Interacts with preschooler to promote trust	1	2	3	4	5	NA
290604	Promotes regular physical exercise	1	2	3	4	5	NA
290605	Assists child to maintain optimum weight	1	2	3	4	5	NA
290606	Encourages activities to promote reading	1	2	3	4	5	NA
290607	Maintains open communication with preschooler	1	2	3	4	5	NA
290608	Verbalizes positive attributes of preschooler	1	2	3	4	5	NA
290609	Assists child to cope with fears	1	2	3	4	5	NA
290610	Provides transitional objects to reduce anxiety	1	2	3	4	5	NA
290611	Responds constructively to negative behavior	1	2	3	4	5	NA
290612	Encourages imagination	1	2	3	4	5	NA
290613	Teaches family rules of behavior	1	2	3	4	5	NA

P

Continued

Parenting Performance: Preschooler—cont'd

		Never Demonstrated	Rarely Demonstrated	Sometimes Demonstrated	Often Demonstrated	Consistently Demonstrated	
290614	Promotes appropriate independence	1	2	3	4	5	NA
290615	Promotes independent dressing	1	2	3	4	5	NA
290616	Promotes independent feeding	1	2	3	4	5	NA
290617	Promotes independent toileting	1	2	3	4	5	NA
290618	Encourages safe exploration of environment	1	2	3	4	5	NA
290619	Nurtures spiritual growth	1	2	3	4	5	NA
290620	Nurtures moral growth	1	2	3	4	5	NA
290644	Nurtures self-esteem	1	2	3	4	5	NA
290621	Encourages interactions with other children	1	2	3	4	5	NA
290622	Monitors preschool learning environment	1	2	3	4	5	NA
290623	Protects from abuse	1	2	3	4	5	NA
290645	Protects from neglect	1	2	3	4	5	NA
290646	Protects from bullying	1	2	3	4	5	NA
290624	Prevents exposure to violence	1	2	3	4	5	NA
290625	Supervises media use	1	2	3	4	5	NA
290626	Monitors supplemental caregiver	1	2	3	4	5	NA
290627	Uses age-appropriate discipline	1	2	3	4	5	NA
290628	Provides for child's special needs	1	2	3	4	5	NA
290629	Maintains safe sleep environment	1	2	3	4	5	NA
290630	Maintains bedtime routine	1	2	3	4	5	NA
290631	Provides age-appropriate nutrition	1	2	3	4	5	NA
290632	Responds constructively to sibling rivalry	1	2	3	4	5	NA
290633	Allows expression of sexual curiosity	1	2	3	4	5	NA
290634	Teaches oral hygiene behaviors	1	2	3	4	5	NA
290635	Maintains recommended dental checkups	1	2	3	4	5	NA
290636	Maintains recommended well-child checkups	1	2	3	4	5	NA
290637	Maintains recommended immunizations	1	2	3	4	5	NA
290638	Maintains smoke-free environment	1	2	3	4	5	NA
290639	Teaches personal stranger safety	1	2	3	4	5	NA
290640	Uses strategies to prevent injury	1	2	3	4	5	NA
290647	Uses strategies to prevent infections	1	2	3	4	5	NA
290641	Protects from sun exposure	1	2	3	4	5	NA
290642	Obtains assistance from a health professional for health problems	1	2	3	4	5	NA

Domain-Family Health (VI)   *Class*-Parenting (DD)   5th edition 2013; revised 2024

OUTCOME CONTENT REFERENCES:

Center for Disease Control and Prevention (2021, January 22). *CDC's Developmental Milestones.* https://www.cdc.gov/ncbddd/actearly/milestones/index.html

Hagan, J. F., Shaw, J. S., & Duncan, P. M. (Eds.). (2017). *Bright futures: Guidelines for health supervision of infants, children and adolescents* (4th ed.). American Academy of Pediatrics.

Hockenberry, M. J., Wilson, D., & Rodgers, C. C. (Eds.). (2019). *Wong's nursing care of infants and children* (11th ed.). Elsevier.

Perry, S. E., Hockenberry, M. J., Lowdermilk, D. J., Wilson, D., Cashion, K., Rodgers, C. C., & Alden, K. R. (2018). *Maternal child nursing care* (6th ed.). Elsevier.

Parenting Performance: School Age Child Psychosocial Safety   2912

Definition: Parental actions to protect a child from 6 to 18 years old from social contacts that might cause harm or injury

OUTCOME TARGET RATING: Maintain at_____ Increase to_____

		Never Demonstrated	Rarely Demonstrated	Sometimes Demonstrated	Often Demonstrated	Consistently Demonstrated	
OUTCOME OVERALL RATING		1	2	3	4	5	
Indicators:							
291201	Monitors playmates	1	2	3	4	5	NA
291202	Monitors school friends	1	2	3	4	5	NA
291203	Monitors social contacts	1	2	3	4	5	NA
291204	Monitors contact with extended family members	1	2	3	4	5	NA
291205	Monitors contact with family adult friends	1	2	3	4	5	NA
291206	Fosters open communication	1	2	3	4	5	NA
291207	Selects appropriate supplemental caregiver	1	2	3	4	5	NA
291208	Monitors supplemental caregiver	1	2	3	4	5	NA
291209	Recognizes risk for abuse	1	2	3	4	5	NA
291210	Uses strategies to eliminate risk for abuse	1	2	3	4	5	NA
291211	Protects from neglect	1	2	3	4	5	NA
291212	Protects from physical abuse	1	2	3	4	5	NA
291213	Protects from sexual abuse	1	2	3	4	5	NA
291214	Protects from emotional abuse	1	2	3	4	5	NA
291215	Protects from being bullied	1	2	3	4	5	NA
291216	Provides required level of supervision	1	2	3	4	5	NA
291217	Uses internet to identify sex offenders in neighborhood	1	2	3	4	5	NA
291218	Teaches to not keep secrets from parents	1	2	3	4	5	NA
291219	Communicates the importance of reporting abuse to an adult	1	2	3	4	5	NA
291220	Uses strategies to prevent high-risk social behavior	1	2	3	4	5	NA
291221	Monitors computer activities and websites	1	2	3	4	5	NA
291222	Monitors phone calls from unknown adults	1	2	3	4	5	NA
291223	Blocks adult programming	1	2	3	4	5	NA
291224	Uses an app to monitor online activity	1	2	3	4	5	NA
291225	Limits daily screen time	1	2	3	4	5	NA
291226	Monitors for problematic internet use	1	2	3	4	5	NA
291227	Teaches about bad strangers	1	2	3	4	5	NA
291228	Discusses examples of fake news	1	2	3	4	5	NA
291229	Teaches to safeguard personal information	1	2	3	4	5	NA
291230	Monitors social media	1	2	3	4	5	NA
291231	Discusses emotional reactions to social media interactions	1	2	3	4	5	NA
291232	Prevents gang participation	1	2	3	4	5	NA
291233	Volunteers to chaperone school activities and trips	1	2	3	4	5	NA
291234	Sets clear rules for behavior	1	2	3	4	5	NA

P

Continued

Parenting Performance: School Age Child Psychosocial Safety—cont'd

		Never Demonstrated	Rarely Demonstrated	Sometimes Demonstrated	Often Demonstrated	Consistently Demonstrated	
291235	Teaches to not get in a car without parental permission	1	2	3	4	5	NA
291236	Teaches age-appropriate child lures	1	2	3	4	5	NA
291237	Encourages to listen to own instincts	1	2	3	4	5	NA
291238	Maintains structure in child's life	1	2	3	4	5	NA
291239	Maintains daily routine in child's life	1	2	3	4	5	NA
291240	Shares ways to cope with emotional issues	1	2	3	4	5	NA

Domain-*Family Health (VI)*   **Class**-*Parenting (DD)*   7th edition 2024

OUTCOME CONTENT REFERENCES:

Ahern, N. R., Kemppainen, J., & Thacker, P. (2016). Awareness and knowledge of child and adolescent risky behaviors: A parent's perspective. *Journal of Child and Adolescent Psychiatric Nursing, 29*, 6–14. https//doi.org/10.1111/jcap.12129

Hagan, J. F., Shaw, J. S., & Duncan, P. M. (Eds.). (2017). *Bright futures: Guidelines for health supervision of infants, children, and adolescents* (4th ed.). American Academy of Pediatrics.

Hockenberry, M. J., Wilson, D., & Rodgers, C. C. (Eds.). (2019). *Wong's nursing care of infants and children* (11th ed.). Elsevier.

Lepkowska, D. (2021). Internet safety: Teaching children to keep themselves safe. *British Journal of Child Health, 1*(6), 265–266. https://doi.org/10.12968/chhe.2020.1.265

Pyrooz, D. C., & Sweeten, G. (2015). Gang membership between ages 5 and 17 years in the United States. *Journal of Adolescent Health, 56*, 414–419. https://doi.org/10.1016/j.jadohealth2014.11.018

Ralph, A. (2018). Parenting of adolescents and emerging adults. In Sanders, M. R., & Morawska, A. (Eds.), *Handbook of parenting and child development across the lifespan* (pp. 651–652). Springer International. https://doi.org/10.1007/978-3-319-94598-9_26

Sebre, S. B., Miltuze1, A., & Limonovs, M. (2020). Integrating adolescent problematic internet use risk factors: Hyperactivity, inconsistent parenting, and maladaptive cognitions. *Journal of Child and Family Studies 29*, 2000–2009. https://doi.org/10.1007/s10826-020-01726-0

Parenting Performance: Toddler   2907

Definition: Parental actions to provide a child with a safe, nurturing, and positive physical, emotional, spiritual, and social environment from 1 year through 2 years

OUTCOME TARGET RATING: Maintain at_____ Increase to_____

		Never Demonstrated	Rarely Demonstrated	Sometimes Demonstrated	Often Demonstrated	Consistently Demonstrated	
OUTCOME OVERALL RATING		1	2	3	4	5	
Indicators:							
290701	Exhibits a loving relationship	1	2	3	4	5	NA
290735	Provides a clean home environment	1	2	3	4	5	NA
290702	Provides safe, age-appropriate developmental activities	1	2	3	4	5	NA
290703	Interacts with toddler to promote trust	1	2	3	4	5	NA
290704	Interacts with toddler to promote language development	1	2	3	4	5	NA
290705	Encourages activities to promote reading	1	2	3	4	5	NA
290706	Encourages interactions with other children	1	2	3	4	5	NA
290735	Limits screen time with electronic devices	1	2	3	4	5	NA
290707	Provides appropriate supervision	1	2	3	4	5	NA
290708	Promotes a sense of autonomy	1	2	3	4	5	NA
290709	Promotes beginning independence	1	2	3	4	5	NA

P

Parenting Performance: Toddler—cont'd

		Never Demonstrated	Rarely Demonstrated	Sometimes Demonstrated	Often Demonstrated	Consistently Demonstrated	
290710	Responds constructively to negative behavior	1	2	3	4	5	NA
290711	Sets realistic expectations for behavior	1	2	3	4	5	NA
290712	Uses a social support system to assist with toddler	1	2	3	4	5	NA
290713	Provides transitional objects to reduce anxiety	1	2	3	4	5	NA
290714	Monitors supplemental caregiver	1	2	3	4	5	NA
290715	Teaches right from wrong	1	2	3	4	5	NA
290716	Nurtures spiritual growth	1	2	3	4	5	NA
290717	Uses strategies to eliminate risk for abuse	1	2	3	4	5	NA
290718	Protects from abuse	1	2	3	4	5	NA
290736	Protects from neglect	1	2	3	4	5	NA
290719	Maintains behavioral limits	1	2	3	4	5	NA
290737	Praises positive behaviors	1	2	3	4	5	NA
290720	Maintains safe sleep environment	1	2	3	4	5	NA
290721	Maintains bedtime routine	1	2	3	4	5	NA
290722	Provides age-appropriate nutrition	1	2	3	4	5	NA
290723	Offers a variety of foods	1	2	3	4	5	NA
290724	Guides toilet training when ready	1	2	3	4	5	NA
290725	Responds constructively to sibling rivalry	1	2	3	4	5	NA
290738	Provides for child's special needs	1	2	3	4	5	NA
290726	Allows expression of sexual curiosity	1	2	3	4	5	NA
290727	Teaches oral hygiene behaviors	1	2	3	4	5	NA
290728	Maintains recommended dental checkups	1	2	3	4	5	NA
290729	Maintains recommended well-child checkups	1	2	3	4	5	NA
290730	Maintains recommended immunizations	1	2	3	4	5	NA
290731	Maintains smoke-free environment	1	2	3	4	5	NA
290732	Uses strategies to prevent injury	1	2	3	4	5	NA
290739	Uses strategies to prevent infections	1	2	3	4	5	NA
290733	Protects from sun exposure	1	2	3	4	5	NA
290734	Obtains assistance from a health professional for health problems	1	2	3	4	5	NA

Domain-Family Health (VI)   *Class*-Parenting (DD)   *5th edition 2013; revised 2024*

OUTCOME CONTENT REFERENCES:

Center for Disease Control and Prevention. (2021, January 22). *CDC's Developmental Milestones.* https://www.cdc.gov/ncbddd/actearly/milestones/index.html

Gubbels, J. S., Gerards, S. M., & Kremers, S. P. (2020). The association of parenting practices with toddlers' dietary intake and BMI, and the moderating role of general parenting and child temperament. *Public Health Nutrition, 23*(14), 2521–2529. https://doi.org/10.1017/S136898002000021X

Hagan, J. F., Shaw, J. S., & Duncan, P. M. (Eds.). (2017). *Bright futures: Guidelines for health supervision of infants, children and adolescents* (4th ed.). American Academy of Pediatrics.

Hockenberry, M. J., Wilson, D., & Rodgers, C. C. (Eds.). (2019). *Wong's nursing care of infants and children* (11th ed.). Elsevier.

Huang, W., Weinert, S., von Maurice, J., & Attig, M. (2022). Specific parenting behaviors link maternal education to toddlers' language and social competence. *Journal of Family Psychology.* Advance online publication. https://doi.org/10.1037/fam0000950

Perry, S. E., Hockenberry, M. J., Lowdermilk, D. J., Wilson, D., Cashion, K., Rodgers, C. C., & Alden, K. R. (2018). *Maternal child nursing care* (6th ed.). Elsevier.

Shin, E., Choi, K., Resor, J., & Smith, C. L. (2021). Why do parents use screen media with toddlers? The role of child temperament and parenting stress in early screen use. *Infant Behavior & Development, 64*, 101595. https://doi.org/10.1016/j.infbeh.2021.101595

Wei, R., Ronfard, S., Leyva, D., & Rowe, M. L. (2019). Teaching a novel word: Parenting styles and toddlers' word learning. *Journal of Experimental Child Psychology, 187*, 104639. https://doi.org/10.1016/j.jecp.2019.05.006

P

Parenting Performance: Toddler Physical Safety   2913

Definition: Parental actions to prevent physical injury of a child from 1 through 2 years of age

OUTCOME TARGET RATING: Maintain at_____ Increase to_____

		Never Demonstrated	Rarely Demonstrated	Sometimes Demonstrated	Often Demonstrated	Consistently Demonstrated	
OUTCOME OVERALL RATING		**1**	**2**	**3**	**4**	**5**	
Indicators:							
291301	Uses crib that meets safety regulations	1	2	3	4	5	NA
291302	Selects safe, age-appropriate toys	1	2	3	4	5	NA
291303	Keeps sharp objects out of reach	1	2	3	4	5	NA
291304	Selects foods that prevent choking	1	2	3	4	5	NA
291305	Provides constant supervision around pets and animals	1	2	3	4	5	NA
291306	Provides constant supervision around water	1	2	3	4	5	NA
291307	Avoids leaving toddler in motor vehicle unsupervised	1	2	3	4	5	NA
291308	Uses correct car seat based on height and weight	1	2	3	4	5	NA
291309	Selects weather-appropriate clothing	1	2	3	4	5	NA
291310	Protects from sun exposure	1	2	3	4	5	NA
291311	Maintains environment to prevent suffocation	1	2	3	4	5	NA
291312	Maintains environment to prevent harmful falls	1	2	3	4	5	NA
291313	Blocks stairs with a small gate or fence	1	2	3	4	5	NA
291314	Maintains environment to prevent burns and electrical shock	1	2	3	4	5	NA
291315	Secures household cleaners and poisons	1	2	3	4	5	NA
291316	Keeps medication out of reach	1	2	3	4	5	NA
291317	Secures firearms and ammunition	1	2	3	4	5	NA
291318	Maintains smoke-free environment	1	2	3	4	5	NA
291319	Uses strategies to prevent exposure to excessive noise	1	2	3	4	5	NA
291320	Maintains home warning devices	1	2	3	4	5	NA
291321	Obtains training to prepare for emergencies	1	2	3	4	5	NA
291322	Ensures home playground equipment meets safety guidelines	1	2	3	4	5	NA
291323	Provides supervision while on playground equipment	1	2	3	4	5	NA
291324	Ensures toddler wears helmet properly	1	2	3	4	5	NA
291325	Protects from neglect	1	2	3	4	5	NA
291326	Protects from physical abuse	1	2	3	4	5	NA
291327	Protects from sexual abuse	1	2	3	4	5	NA

Domain-Family Health (VI)   *Class*-Parenting (DD)   7th edition 2024

OUTCOME CONTENT REFERENCES:

Dao, A., & McMullin, J. (2019). Unintentional injury, supervision, and discourses on childproofing devices. *Medical Anthropology, 38*(1), 15–29. https://doi.org/10.1080/01459740.2018.1482548

Doh, K. F., Morris, C. R., Akbar, T., Chaudhary, S., Lazarus, S. G., Figueroa, J., Agarwal, M., & Simon, H. K. (2021). The relationship between parents' reported storage of firearms and their children's perceived access to firearms: A safety disconnect. *Clinical Pediatrics, 60*(1), 42–49. https://doi.org/10.1177/0009922820944398

Hockenberry, M. J., Wilson, D., & Rodgers, C. C. (Eds.). (2019). *Wong's nursing care of infants and children* (11th ed.). Elsevier.

Perry, S. E., Hockenberry, M. J., Lowdermilk, D. J., Wilson, D., Cashion, K., Rodgers, C. C., & Alden, K. R. (2018). *Maternal child nursing care* (6th ed.). Elsevier.

Staples, A. D., & Bates, J. E. (2018). Parenting of infants and toddlers. In Sanders, M. R., & Morawska, A. (Eds.). *Handbook of parenting and child development across the lifespan.* Springer International. https://doi.org/10.1007/978-3-319-94598-9_26

Participation in Health Care Decisions   1606

Definition: Personal involvement in selecting and evaluating health care options to achieve desired outcomes

OUTCOME TARGET RATING: Maintain at_____ Increase to_____

		Never Demonstrated	Rarely Demonstrated	Sometimes Demonstrated	Often Demonstrated	Consistently Demonstrated	
OUTCOME OVERALL RATING		1	2	3	4	5	
Indicators:							
160601	Claims decision-making responsibility	1	2	3	4	5	NA
160602	Exhibits self-direction in decision-making	1	2	3	4	5	NA
160603	Seeks reputable information	1	2	3	4	5	NA
160604	Defines available options	1	2	3	4	5	NA
160605	Specifies health outcome preferences	1	2	3	4	5	NA
160606	Identifies health outcome priorities	1	2	3	4	5	NA
160607	Identifies barriers to desired outcome achievement	1	2	3	4	5	NA
160608	Uses problem-solving techniques to achieve desired outcomes	1	2	3	4	5	NA
160609	States intent to act on decision	1	2	3	4	5	NA
160610	Identifies available support for achieving desired outcomes	1	2	3	4	5	NA
160611	Seeks health care services to meet desired outcomes	1	2	3	4	5	NA
160617	Uses decision aids provided	1	2	3	4	5	NA
160612	Negotiates for care preferences	1	2	3	4	5	NA
160618	Asks relevant questions to health care providers	1	2	3	4	5	NA
160619	Exhibits emotional ability to participate in decision-making	1	2	3	4	5	NA
160613	Monitors barriers to outcome achievement	1	2	3	4	5	NA
160614	Identifies level of outcome achievement	1	2	3	4	5	NA
160615	Evaluates satisfaction with health care outcomes	1	2	3	4	5	NA

Domain-*Health Knowledge & Behavior (IV)*   **Class**-*Health Behavior (Q)*   *1st edition 1997; revised 2004, 2024*

OUTCOME CONTENT REFERENCES:
Bomhof-Roordink, H., Gärtner, F. R., Stiggelbout, A. M., & Pieterse, A. H. (2019). Key components of shared decision-making models: A systematic review. *British Medical Journal Open, 9*(12), e031763. https://doi.org/10.1136/bmjopen-2019-031763
Clayman, M. L., Bylund, C. L., Chewning, B., & Makoul, G. (2016). The impact of patient participation in health decisions within medical encounters: A systematic review. *Medical Decision Making, 36*(4), 427–452. https://doi.org/10.1177/0272989x15613530
+Ende, J., Kazis, L., Ash, A., & Moskowitz, M. A. (1989). Measuring patient's desire for autonomy: Decision making and information-seeking preferences among medical patients. *Journal of General Internal Medicine, 4*(1), 23–30. https://doi.org/10.1007/BF02596485
Gray, T. F., Nolan, M. T., Clayman, M. L., & Wenzel, J. A. (2019). The decision partner in healthcare decision-making: A concept analysis. *International Journal of Nursing Studies, 92*, 79–89. https://doi.org/10.1016/j.ijnurstu.2019.01.006
Hegyvary, S. T. (1993). Patient care outcomes related to management of symptoms. In J. J. Fitzpatrick & J. J. Stevenson (Eds.), *Annual review of nursing research* (Vol. 11, pp. 145–168). Springer.
Nilsson, M., From, I., & Lindwall, L. (2019). The significance of patient participation in nursing care—A concept analysis. *Scandinavian Journal of Caring Science, 33*(1), 244–251. https://doi.org/10.1111/scs.12609
Scholl, I., LaRussa, A., Hahlweg, P., Kobrin, S., & Elwyn, G. (2018). Organizational- and system-level characteristics that influence implementation of shared decision-making and strategies to address them—A scoping review. *Implementation Science, 13*(1), 40. https://doi.org/10.1186/s13012-018-0731-z

P

Patient Engagement Behavior 1638

Definition: Personal actions to actively participate in one's health care through shared decision-making with health professionals

OUTCOME TARGET RATING: Maintain at_____ Increase to_____

		Never Demonstrated	Rarely Demonstrated	Sometimes Demonstrated	Often Demonstrated	Consistently Demonstrated	
OUTCOME OVERALL RATING		**1**	**2**	**3**	**4**	**5**	
Indicators:							
163801	Obtains reputable health information	1	2	3	4	5	NA
163802	Assesses personal health risk factors	1	2	3	4	5	NA
163803	Identifies causes of illness	1	2	3	4	5	NA
163804	Identifies factors that influence health	1	2	3	4	5	NA
163805	Follows a healthy lifestyle	1	2	3	4	5	NA
163806	Treats minor conditions	1	2	3	4	5	NA
163807	Seeks professional assistance when needed	1	2	3	4	5	NA
163808	Selects appropriate health professional	1	2	3	4	5	NA
163809	Prepares a list of questions to discuss with health professional	1	2	3	4	5	NA
163810	Brings current medication list to discuss with health professional	1	2	3	4	5	NA
163832	Obtains needed prescriptions	1	2	3	4	5	NA
163811	Shares medical information with health professional	1	2	3	4	5	NA
163812	Discusses personal health priorities with health professional	1	2	3	4	5	NA
163813	Shares strategies to meet personal health priorities	1	2	3	4	5	NA
163814	Discusses plan of care with health professional	1	2	3	4	5	NA
163833	Uses communication strategies available in electronic health record	1	2	3	4	5	NA
163815	Seeks second opinion	1	2	3	4	5	NA
163816	Chooses among treatment options	1	2	3	4	5	NA
163817	Monitors treatment effects	1	2	3	4	5	NA
163818	Monitors medication effects	1	2	3	4	5	NA
163819	Shares side effects with health professional	1	2	3	4	5	NA
163820	Follows up with health professional when health status changes	1	2	3	4	5	NA
163834	Obtains required laboratory tests	1	2	3	4	5	NA
163821	Obtains test results	1	2	3	4	5	NA
163822	Obtains appropriate health screenings	1	2	3	4	5	NA
163823	Obtains recommended vaccines	1	2	3	4	5	NA
163824	Maintains personal health record	1	2	3	4	5	NA
163825	Maintains insurance coverage	1	2	3	4	5	NA
163826	Maintains advance directives	1	2	3	4	5	NA
163827	Obtains medical power of attorney	1	2	3	4	5	NA
163828	Shares concerns for personal safety	1	2	3	4	5	NA
163829	Uses strategies to cope with chronic illness	1	2	3	4	5	NA
163830	Manages personal health care	1	2	3	4	5	NA
163831	Uses health care resources consistent with need	1	2	3	4	5	NA

Domain-*Health Knowledge & Behavior (IV)* **Class**-*Health Behavior (Q)* *6th edition 2018; revised 2024*

OUTCOME CONTENT REFERENCES:
+Arvanitis, M., Bailey, S. C., Wismer, G., Griffith, J. W., Freeman, E., Sims, T. J., Paczkowski, R., Klopchin, M., Chung, A. E., Carpenter, D. M., & Wolf, M. S. (2020). Development of the influence, motivation, and patient activation in diabetes (IMPACT-D™) measure. *Diabetes Research and Clinical Practice, 159*, 107965. https://doi.org/10.1016/j.diabres.2019.107965
+Castellon-Lopez, Y., Skrine Jeffers, K., Duru, O. K., Moreno, G., Moin, T., Grotts, J., Mangione, C. M., Norris, K. C., & Hays, R. D. (2020). Psychometric properties of the Altarum Consumer Engagement (ACE) Measure of Activation in patients with prediabetes. *Journal of General Internal Medicine, 35*(11), 3159–3165. https://doi.org/10.1007/s11606-020-05727-z
Coulter, A. (2011). *Engaging patients in healthcare.* McGraw-Hill Education.
Coulter, A. (2012). Patient engagement—What works? *Journal of Ambulatory Care Management, 35*(2), 80–89. https://doi.org/10.1097/JAC.0b013e318249e0fd
+Duke, C., Lynch, W., Smith, B., & Winstanley, J. (2015). Validity of a new patient engagement measure: The Altarum Consumer Engagement (ACE) measure. *Patient, 8*(6), 559–568. https://doi.org/10.1007/s40271-015-0131-2
+Ge, L., Yap, C. W., Kaur, P., Ong, R., & Heng, B. H. (2021). Psychometric evaluation of the 8-item Altarum Consumer Engagement (ACE) Measure™ in community-dwelling adults in Singapore. *BMC Health Services Research, 21*(1), 1347. https://doi.org/10.1186/s12913-021-07369-1
Gruman, J., Holmes-Rovner, M., French, M., Jeffress, D., Sofaer, S., Shaller, D., & Prager, D. (2010). From patient education to patient engagement: Implications for the field of patient education. *Patient Education and Counseling, 78*(3), 350–356. https://doi.org/10.1016/j.pec.2010.02.002
Lauffenburger, J. C., Barlev, R. A., Sears, E. S., Keller, P. A., McDonnell, M. E., Yom-Tov, E., Fontanet, C. P., Hanken, K., Haff, N., & Choudhry, N. K. (2021). Preferences for mHealth technology and text messaging communication in patients with type 2 diabetes: Qualitative interview study. *Journal of Medical Internet Research, 23*(6), e25958. https://doi.org/10.2196/25958
Nelson, L. A., Spieker, A., Greevy, R., LeStourgeon, L. M., Wallston, K. A., & Mayberry, L. S. (2020). User engagement among diverse adults in a 12-month text message-delivered diabetes support intervention: Results from a randomized controlled trial. *JMIR mHealth and uHealth, 8*(7), e17534. https://doi.org/10.2196/17534
+Wolf, M. S., Smith, S. G., Pandit, A. U., Condon, D. M., Curtis, L. M., Griffith, J., O'Conor, R., Rush, S., Bailey, S. C., Kaplan, G., Haufle, V., & Martin, D. (2018). Development and validation of the Consumer Health Activation Index. *Medical Decision Making: An international journal of the Society for Medical Decision Making, 38*(3), 334–343. https://doi.org/10.1177/0272989X17753392

Perimenopause Symptom Severity　　2104

Definition: Severity of reported adverse physical and emotional responses due to declining hormonal levels

OUTCOME TARGET RATING: Maintain at _____ Increase to _____

		Severe	Substantial	Moderate	Mild	None	
OUTCOME OVERALL RATING		1	2	3	4	5	
Indicators:							
210401	Menstrual irregularity	1	2	3	4	5	NA
210402	Abdominal cramps	1	2	3	4	5	NA
210403	Hot flashes	1	2	3	4	5	NA
210404	Night sweats	1	2	3	4	5	NA
210405	Vaginal dryness	1	2	3	4	5	NA
210406	Mood swings	1	2	3	4	5	NA
210407	Menstrual flow	1	2	3	4	5	NA
210408	Insomnia	1	2	3	4	5	NA
210409	Fatigue	1	2	3	4	5	NA
210417	Depression	1	2	3	4	5	NA
210418	Anxiety	1	2	3	4	5	NA
210419	Skin atrophy	1	2	3	4	5	NA
210410	Musculoskeletal pain	1	2	3	4	5	NA
210420	Metabolic changes	1	2	3	4	5	NA
210411	Weight gain	1	2	3	4	5	NA
210412	Decreased libido	1	2	3	4	5	NA
210413	Heart palpitations	1	2	3	4	5	NA
210414	Vertigo	1	2	3	4	5	NA
210415	Memory changes	1	2	3	4	5	NA

Domain-Health & Life Quality (V)　　*Class*-Symptom Status (V)　　2nd edition 2000; revised 2004, 2013, 2024

OUTCOME CONTENT REFERENCES:
Augoulea, A., Moros, M., Lykeridou, A., Kaparos, G., Lyberi, R., & Panoulis, K. (2019). Psychosomatic and vasomotor symptom changes during transition to menopause. *Menopause Review, 18*(2), 110–115. https://doi.org/10.5114/pm.2019.86835
de Kruif, M., Spijker, A. T., & Molendijk, M. L. (2016). Depression during the perimenopause: A meta-analysis. *Journal of Affective Disorders, 206*, 174–180. https://doi.org/10.1016/j.jad.2016.07.040

Delamater, L., & Santoro, N. (2018). Management of the perimenopause. *Clinical Obstetrics and Gynecology, 61*(3), 419–432. https://doi.org/10.1097/GRF.0000000000000389

Gracia, C. R., & Freeman, E. W. (2018). Onset of the menopause transition: The earliest signs and symptoms. *Obstetrics and Gynecology Clinics of North America, 45*(4), 585–597. https://doi.org/10.1016/j.ogc.2018.07.002

Jaeger, M. B., Miná, C. S., Alves, S., Schuh, G. J., Wender, M. C., & Manfro, G. G. (2021). Negative affect symptoms, anxiety sensitivity, and vasomotor symptoms during perimenopause. *Revista Brasileira de Psiquiatria* (Sao Paulo, Brazil), *43*(3), 277–284. https://doi.org/10.1590/1516-4446-2020-0871

Lyndaker, C., & Hulton, L. (2004). The influence of age on symptoms of perimenopause. *Journal of Obstetric, Gynecologic, & Neonatal Nursing, 33*(3), 340–347. https://doi.org/10.1177/0884217504264872

Monteleone, P., Mascagni, G., Giannini, A., Genazzani, A. R., & Simoncini, T. (2018). Symptoms of menopause—Global prevalence, physiology and implications. *Nature Reviews. Endocrinology, 14*(4), 199–215. https://doi.org/10.1038/nrendo.2017.180

Padda, J., Khalid, K., Hitawala, G., Batra, N., Pokhriyal, S., Mohan, A., Zubair, U., Cooper, A. C., & Jean-Charles, G. (2021). Depression and its effect on the menstrual cycle. *Cureus, 13*(7), e16532. https://doi.org/10.7759/cureus.16532

Sander, B., & Gordon, J. L. (2021). Premenstrual mood symptoms in the perimenopause. *Current Psychiatry Reports, 23*(11), 73. https://doi.org/10.1007/s11920-021-01285-1

Peripheral Artery Disease Severity   **2115**

Definition: Severity of signs and symptoms of reduced peripheral blood flow due to atherosclerotic arteries in the extremities

OUTCOME TARGET RATING: Maintain at_____ Increase to_____

		Severe	Substantial	Moderate	Mild	None	
OUTCOME OVERALL RATING		**1**	**2**	**3**	**4**	**5**	
Indicators:							
211501	Intermittent claudication intensity	1	2	3	4	5	NA
211502	Unrelieved muscle pain with rest	1	2	3	4	5	NA
211503	Impaired skin color in extremities	1	2	3	4	5	NA
211504	Impaired skin temperature in extremities	1	2	3	4	5	NA
211505	Impaired skin sensation in extremities	1	2	3	4	5	NA
211506	Tingling in extremities	1	2	3	4	5	NA
211507	Numbness of extremities	1	2	3	4	5	NA
211508	Hair loss on extremities	1	2	3	4	5	NA
211509	Restless leg syndrome	1	2	3	4	5	NA
211510	Impaired physical mobility	1	2	3	4	5	NA
211511	Restricted walking distance	1	2	3	4	5	NA
211512	Muscle pain in upper extremities	1	2	3	4	5	NA
211513	Muscle pain in buttocks	1	2	3	4	5	NA
211514	Muscle pain in thigh	1	2	3	4	5	NA
211515	Erectile dysfunction	1	2	3	4	5	NA
211516	Thrombus formation	1	2	3	4	5	NA
211517	Skin ulceration	1	2	3	4	5	NA

Domain-Health & Life Quality (V)   *Class-Symptom Status (V)*   5th edition 2013; reviewed 2024

OUTCOME CONTENT REFERENCES:

Andrade-Lima, A., da Silva Junior, N., Chehuen, M., Miyasato, R., Souza, R. W. A., Leicht, A. S., Brum, P.C., de Oliveira, E.M., Wolosker, N., & Forjaz, C. L. M. (2021). Local and systemic inflammation and oxidative stress about a single bout of maximal walking in patients with symptomatic peripheral artery disease. *Journal of Cardiovascular Nursing, 36*(5), 498-506. https://doi.org/10.1097/JCN.0000000000000686

Farah, B. Q., Santos, M. F., Cucato, G. G., Kanegusuku, H., Samaio, L. M. M., Monterio, F. A., Wolosker, N., Puech-Leão, P., de Almeida Correia, M., & Ritti-Dias, R. M. (2021). Effect of frailty on physical activity levels and walking capacity in patients with peripheral artery disease: A cross-sectional study. *Journal of Vascular Nursing, 39*, 84–88. https://doi.org/10.1016/j.jvn.2021.07.001

Narcisse, D. L., Ford, C. B., Weissler, E. H., Lippmann, S. J., Smerek, M. M., Greiner, M. A., Hardy, C., O'Brien, B., Sullivan, R. C., Brock, A. J., Long, C., Curtis, L. H., Patel, M. R., & Jones, W. S. (2021). The association of healthcare disparities and patient-specific factors on clinical outcomes in peripheral artery disease. *American Heart Journal, 239*, 135-146. https://doi.org/10.1016/j.ahj.2021.05.014

Peripheral Arterial Disease Coalition. (2007). Gaps in public knowledge of peripheral artery disease: The first national PAD public awareness survey. *Circulation, 116*(18), 2086–2094. https://doi.org/10.1161/circulationaha.107.725101

Peritoneal Dialysis: Disruptive Effects   2307

Definition: Severity of observed or reported disruptive effects of peritoneal dialysis treatments

OUTCOME TARGET RATING: Maintain at _____ Increase to _____

		Severe	Substantial	Moderate	Mild	None	
OUTCOME OVERALL RATING		1	2	3	4	5	
Indicators:							
230701	Catheter-related infection	1	2	3	4	5	NA
230702	Tunnel infections along catheter	1	2	3	4	5	NA
230703	Trauma from unstable catheter	1	2	3	4	5	NA
230704	Dialysate leakage around catheter	1	2	3	4	5	NA
230705	Abdominal pain	1	2	3	4	5	NA
230706	Abdominal tenderness	1	2	3	4	5	NA
230707	Positive dialysate culture	1	2	3	4	5	NA
230708	Peritonitis	1	2	3	4	5	NA
230709	Loss of appetite	1	2	3	4	5	NA
230710	Malnutrition	1	2	3	4	5	NA
230711	Nausea	1	2	3	4	5	NA
230712	Vomiting	1	2	3	4	5	NA
230713	Bloating	1	2	3	4	5	NA
230714	Early satiety	1	2	3	4	5	NA
230715	Weakness	1	2	3	4	5	NA
230716	Fatigue	1	2	3	4	5	NA
230717	Malaise	1	2	3	4	5	NA
230718	Lethargy	1	2	3	4	5	NA
230719	Peritoneal membrane changes	1	2	3	4	5	NA
230720	Development of abdominal hernias	1	2	3	4	5	NA
230721	Bowel perforation	1	2	3	4	5	NA
230722	Genital edema	1	2	3	4	5	NA
230723	Hydrothorax	1	2	3	4	5	NA
230724	Plural effusion	1	2	3	4	5	NA
230725	Gastroesophageal reflux	1	2	3	4	5	NA

Domain-*Physiologic Health (II)*   **Class-***Therapeutic Response (AA)*   *7th edition 2024*

OUTCOME CONTENT REFERENCES:

Ding, X.-R., Huang, H.-E., Liao, Y.-M., Tang, Z. W., Fang, X., & Su, C. (2021). Daily self-care practices influence exit-site condition in patients having peritoneal dialysis: A multicenter cross-sectional survey. *Journal of Advanced Nursing, 77,* 2293–2306. https://doi.org/10.1111/jan.14751

Gilbert, S. J., Weiner, D. E., Bomback, A. S., Perazella, M. A., Tonelli, M., & National Kidney Foundation, issuing body. (2017). *National Kidney Foundation's primer on kidney diseases* (7th ed.). Elsevier and National Kidney Foundation.

Ignatavicius, D. D., Workman, M. L., Rebar, C. R., & Heimgartner, N. M. (2021). *Medical-surgical nursing: Concepts for interprofessional care* (10th ed.). Elsevier.

Khanna, R., & Krediet, R. T. (2020). *Nolph and Gokal's textbook of peritoneal dialysis.* Springer.

Meng, L. F., Yang, L. M., Zhu, X. Y., Zhang, X. X., Li, X. Y., Zhao, J., Liu, S. C., Zhuang, X. H., Luo, P., & Cui, W. P. (2020). Comparison of clinical features and outcomes in peritoneal dialysis-associated peritonitis patients with and without diabetes: A multicenter retrospective cohort study. *World Journal of Diabetes, 11*(10), 435–446. https://doi.org/10.4239/wjd.v11.i10.435

Salamon, K., Woods, J., Paul, E., & Huggins, C. (2013). Peritoneal dialysis patients have higher prevalence of gastrointestinal symptoms than hemodialysis patients. *Journal of Renal Nutrition, 23*(2), 114–118. https://doi.org/10.1053/j.jrn.2012.02.007

Szeto, C.-C., Li, P. K.-T., Johnson, D. W., Bernardini, J., Dong, J., Figueiredo, A. E., Ito, Y., Kazancioglu, R., Moraes, T., Van Esch, S., & Brown, E. A. (2017). ISPD catheter-related infection recommendations: 2017 update. *Peritoneal Dialysis International, 37*(2), 141–154. https://doi.org/10.3747/pdi.2016.00120

Wu, H., Ye, H., Huang, R., Yi, C., Wu, J., Yu, X., & Yang, X. (2020). Incidence and risk factors of peritoneal dialysis-related peritonitis in elderly patients: A retrospective clinical study. *Peritoneal Dialysis International, 40*(1), 26–33. https://doi.org/10.1177/0896860819879868

P

Personal Autonomy

1614

Definition: Personal actions of a competent individual to exercise governance in life decisions

OUTCOME TARGET RATING: Maintain at_____ Increase to_____

		Never Demonstrated	Rarely Demonstrated	Sometimes Demonstrated	Often Demonstrated	Consistently Demonstrated	
OUTCOME OVERALL RATING		1	2	3	4	5	
Indicators:							
161401	Makes informed life decisions	1	2	3	4	5	NA
161402	Considers other opinions when making choices	1	2	3	4	5	NA
161403	Expresses independence with decision-making process	1	2	3	4	5	NA
161404	Makes decisions free from undue pressure by parents	1	2	3	4	5	NA
161405	Makes decisions free from undue pressure by spouse	1	2	3	4	5	NA
161406	Makes decisions free from undue pressure by children	1	2	3	4	5	NA
161407	Makes decisions free from undue pressure by extended family	1	2	3	4	5	NA
161408	Makes decisions free from undue pressure by friends	1	2	3	4	5	NA
161409	Makes decisions free from undue pressure by health provider	1	2	3	4	5	NA
161410	Asserts personal preferences	1	2	3	4	5	NA
161411	Participates in health care decisions	1	2	3	4	5	NA
161412	Expresses satisfaction with life choices	1	2	3	4	5	NA
161413	Expresses ability to cope with present state of health	1	2	3	4	5	NA

Domain-Health Knowledge & Behavior (IV)   *Class*-Health Behavior (Q)   *3rd edition 2004; revised 2018*

OUTCOME CONTENT REFERENCES:

Aveyard, H. (2000). Is there a concept of autonomy that can usefully inform nursing practice? *Journal of Advanced Nursing, 32*(2), 352–358. https://doi.org/10.1046/j.1365-2648.2000.01483.x

Brennan, M. (1997). A concept analysis of consent. *Journal of Advanced Nursing, 25*(3), 477–484. https://doi.org/10.1046/j.1365-2648.2000.01483.x

Dworkin, G. (1988). *The theory and practice of autonomy.* Cambridge University Press.

+Mars, G., van Eijk, J., Post, M., Proot, I., Mesters, I., & Kempen, G. (2014). Development and psychometric properties of the Maastricht Personal Autonomy Questionnaire (MPAQ) in older adults with a chronic physical illness. *Quality of Life Research, 23*(6), 1777–1787. https://doi.org/10.1007/s11136-013-0619-y

Oshana, M. (Ed.). (2015). *Personal autonomy and social oppression: Philosophical perspectives.* Taylor & Francis.

Schüler, J., Sheldon, K., Prentice, M., & Halusic, M. (2014). Do some people need autonomy more than others? Implicit dispositions toward autonomy moderate the effects of felt autonomy on well-being. *Journal of Personality, 84*(1), 5–20. https://doi.org/10.1111/jopy.12133

Wiens, A. G. (1993). Patient autonomy: A theoretical framework for nursing. *Journal of Professional Nursing, 9*(2), 95–103. https://doi.org/10.1016/8755-7223(93)90025-8

P

Personal Health Screening Behavior   1634

Definition: Personal actions to obtain recommended screening for early detection of a communicable or undetected disease

OUTCOME TARGET RATING: Maintain at_____ Increase to_____

		Never Demonstrated	Rarely Demonstrated	Sometimes Demonstrated	Often Demonstrated	Consistently Demonstrated	
OUTCOME OVERALL RATING		1	2	3	4	5	
Indicators:							
163401	Acknowledges disease risk	1	2	3	4	5	NA
163402	Acknowledges need for screening	1	2	3	4	5	NA
163403	Describes timeframes for screening	1	2	3	4	5	NA
163404	Describes benefits of screening	1	2	3	4	5	NA
163405	Describes contraindications to specific screening	1	2	3	4	5	NA
163406	Maintains updated screening record	1	2	3	4	5	NA
163407	Schedules next screening	1	2	3	4	5	NA
163408	Obtains screening at recommended intervals	1	2	3	4	5	NA
163409	Obtains early screening based on family history as recommended by health professional	1	2	3	4	5	NA
163410	Obtains screening based on personal risk factors as recommended by health professional	1	2	3	4	5	NA
163411	Obtains screening for age recommended by experts	1	2	3	4	5	NA
163412	Obtains screening for occupational risk recommended by experts	1	2	3	4	5	NA
163413	Obtains screening for travel recommended by experts	1	2	3	4	5	NA
163414	Obtains genetic screening as recommended by health professional	1	2	3	4	5	NA
163415	Identifies community resources for screening	1	2	3	4	5	NA
163416	Obtains results of screening	1	2	3	4	5	NA
163417	Obtains health care services following abnormal screening results	1	2	3	4	5	NA

Domain-*Health Knowledge & Behavior (IV)*   **Class**-*Health Behavior (Q)*   *5th edition 2013: reviewed 2024*

OUTCOME CONTENT REFERENCES:

American Academy of Pediatrics. (2021). Recommendations for prevention and control of influenza in children, 2021-2022. *Pediatrics, 148*(4), 1–9. https://doi.org/10.1542/peds.2021-053744

American Academy of Pediatrics. (2021). 2021 Recommendations for preventive pediatric health care. *Pediatrics, 147*(3), 1–2. https://doi.org/10.1542/peds.2020-049776

Brenner, D. R., O'Sullivan, D. E., & Hilsden, R. J. (2022). Implications of the United States recommendations for early-age-at-onset colorectal cancer screening in Canada. *Preventive Medicine, 155*, 1–3. https://doi.org/10.1016/j.ypmed.2021.106923

Buterbaugh, J. S. (2021). Pediatric dyslipidemia and screening recommendations. *The Journal for Nurse Practitioners, 17*, 1178-1182. https://doi.org/10.1016/j.nurpra.2021.08.009

Cerqueira, A. G. S., Magno, M. B., Barja-Fidalgo, F., Vicente-Gomila, J., Maia, L. C., & Fonseca-Gonçalves, A. (2020). Recommendations from paediatric dentistry associations of the Americas on breastfeeding and sugar consumption and oral hygiene in infants for the prevention of dental caries: A bibliometric review. *International Journal of Paediatric Dentistry, 31*, 644–675. https://doi.org/10.1111/ipd.12754

Gillespie, G. L., Willis, D. G., & Amar, A. F. (2018). Review and application of the National Academies of Sciences, Engineering, and Medicine bulling or cyber bullying recommendations for screening and lesbian, gay, bisexual, and transgender youth. *Nursing Outlook, 66*, 372–378. https://doi.org/10.1016/j.outlook.2018.03.003

Hill, J. (2021). Screening for colorectal cancer. *Journal of the American Medical Association, 325*, 2026. https://doi.org/10.1001/jama.2021.6238

Jin, J. (2021). Screening for prediabetes and type 2 diabetes. *Journal of the American Medical Association, 326*(8), 778. https://doi.org/10.1001/jama.2021.12531

P

Michaud, P.-A., Visser, A., Vervoort, J. P. M., Kocken, P., Reijneveld, S. A., & Jansen, D. E. M. C. (2020). Availability and accessibility of primary mental health services for adolescents: An overview of national recommendations and services in EU. *The European Journal of Public Health, 30*(6), 1127-1133. https://doi.org/10.1093/eurpub/ckaa102

Smith-Bindman, R., & Bibbins-Domingo, K. (2021). USPSTF recommendations for screening for carotid stenosis to prevent stroke—The need for more data. *JAMA Network Open, 4*(2), 1–4. https://doi.org/10.1001/jamanetworkopen.2020.36218

Ritzwoller, D. P., Meza, R., Carroll, N. M., Blum-Barnett, E., Burnett-Hartman, A. N., Greenlee, R. T., Honda, S. A., Neslund-Dudas, C., Rendle, K. A., & Vachani, A. (2021). Evaluation of population-level changes associated with the 2021 U.S. Preventive Services Task Force lung cancer screening recommendations in community-based health care systems. *JAMA Network Open, 4*(10), 1–10. https://doi.org/10.1001/jamanetworkopen.2021.28176

U.S. Preventive Services Task Force. (2021). Screening for asymptomatic carotid artery stenosis. U.S. Preventive Services Task Force Recommendation Statement. *Journal of the American Medical Association, 325*(5), 1–6. https://doi.org/10.1001/jama.2020.26988

U.S. Preventive Services Task Force. (2021). Screening for hearing loss in older adults. U.S. Preventive Services Task Force Recommendation Statement. *Journal of the American Medical Association, 325*(12), 1–6. https://doi.org/10.1001/jama.2021.2566

U.S. Preventive Services Task Force. (2021). Screening for hepatitis B virus infection in adolescents and adults: Recommendation statement. U.S. Preventive Services Task Force Recommendation Statement. *American Family Physician, 103*(8), 495–501. https://www.aafp.org/afp/2021/0415/p495.html

U.S. Preventive Services Task Force. (2021). Screening for hypertension in adults. U.S. Preventive Services Task Force Reaffirmation Statement. *Journal of the American Medical Association, 325*(16), 1–7. https://doi.org/10.1001/jama.2021.4987

Viswanathan, V., Ramakrishnan, N., Saboo, B., & Agarwal, S. (2021). RSSDI clinical practice recommendations for screening, diagnosis, and treatment in type 2 diabetes mellitus with obstructive sleep apnea. *International Journal of Diabetes in Developing Countries, 41*, 4–21.

Personal Health Status   **2006**

Definition: Overall physical, psychological, social, and spiritual functioning of an adult 18 years or older

OUTCOME TARGET RATING: Maintain at_____ Increase to_____

OUTCOME OVERALL RATING	Severely Compromised	Substantially Compromised	Moderately Compromised	Mildly Compromised	Not Compromised	
	1	**2**	**3**	**4**	**5**	
Indicators:						
200601 Physical fitness level	1	2	3	4	5	NA
200602 Mobility level	1	2	3	4	5	NA
200603 Energy level	1	2	3	4	5	NA
200604 Comfort level	1	2	3	4	5	NA
200605 Performance of activities of daily living	1	2	3	4	5	NA
200606 Performance of instrumental activities of daily living	1	2	3	4	5	NA
200607 Resistance to infection	1	2	3	4	5	NA
200608 Tissue healing	1	2	3	4	5	NA
200609 Sleep-rest pattern	1	2	3	4	5	NA
200610 Gastrointestinal function	1	2	3	4	5	NA
200611 Cardiac function	1	2	3	4	5	NA
200612 Peripheral tissue perfusion	1	2	3	4	5	NA
200613 Neurological function	1	2	3	4	5	NA
200614 Pulmonary function	1	2	3	4	5	NA
200615 Kidney function	1	2	3	4	5	NA
200632 Liver function	1	2	3	4	5	NA
200633 Vision	1	2	3	4	5	NA
200634 Hearing	1	2	3	4	5	NA
200627 Sexual function	1	2	3	4	5	NA
200628 Endocrine function	1	2	3	4	5	NA
200616 Weight	1	2	3	4	5	NA
200635 Oral Health	1	2	3	4	5	NA
200617 Nutritional status	1	2	3	4	5	NA
200618 Cognitive status	1	2	3	4	5	NA
200619 Mental health	1	2	3	4	5	NA
200629 Symptom control	1	2	3	4	5	NA
200630 Pain control	1	2	3	4	5	NA
200620 Mood equilibrium	1	2	3	4	5	NA

P

Personal Health Status—cont'd

		Severely Compromised	Substantially Compromised	Moderately Compromised	Mildly Compromised	Not Compromised	
200621	Spiritual life	1	2	3	4	5	NA
200622	Ability to cope	1	2	3	4	5	NA
200623	Adjustment to chronic conditions	1	2	3	4	5	NA
200636	Adjustment to disability	1	2	3	4	5	NA
200631	Ability to communicate	1	2	3	4	5	NA
200624	Ability to express emotions	1	2	3	4	5	NA
200625	Social relationships	1	2	3	4	5	NA

Domain- *Health & Life Quality (V)*   **Class-***Health Status (JJ)*   *3rd edition 2004; revised 2008, 2024*

OUTCOME CONTENT REFERENCES:

Badhiwala, J. H., Witiw, C. D., Nassiri, F., Akbar, M. A., Jaja, B., Wilson, J. R., & Fehlings, M. G. (2018). FRCSC minimum clinically important difference in SF-36 scores for use in degenerative cervical myelopathy. *SPINE, 43*(21), E1260–E1266. https://doi.org/10.1097/BRS.0000000000002684

+Bergner, M., Bobbit, R. A., Carter, W. B., & Gilson, B. S. (1981). The Sickness Impact Profile: Development and final revision of a health status measure. *Medical Care, 19*(8), 787–805. https://www.jstor.org/stable/3764241

+Hankins, M. (2008). The factor structure of the twelve item General Health Questionnaire (GHQ-12), The result of negative phrasing? *Clinical Practice and Epidemiology in Mental Health, 4*, 10. https://doi.org/10.1186/1745-0179-4-10

LoMartire, R., Äng, B. O., Gerdle, B., & Vixner, L. (2020). Psychometric properties of Short Form-36 Health Survey, EuroQol 5-dimensions, and Hospital Anxiety and Depression Scale in patients with chronic pain. *Pain, 161*(1), 83–95. https://doi.org/10.1097/j.pain.0000000000001700

Mossberg, K., & McFarland, C. (2001). A patient-oriented health status measure in outpatient rehabilitation. *American Journal of Physical Medicine & Rehabilitation, 80*(12), 896–902. https://doi.org/10.1097/00002060-200112000-00005

+Radosevich, D., & Pruit, M. (1995). *Twelve-item Health Status Questionnaire.* Health Outcomes Institute.

+Ware, J. E., & Sherbourne, C. D. (1992). The MOS 36-item Short-Form Health Survey (SF-36): I. Conceptual framework and item selection. *Medical Care, 30*(6), 473–483.

+Ware, J. E., (1999). SF-36 Health Survey. In M. E. Maruish (Ed.), *The use of psychological testing for treatment planning and outcomes assessment* (pp. 1227–1246). Lawrence Erlbaum Associates.

+Ware, J. E. (2000). SF-36 Health Survey Update. *Spine, 25*(24), 3130–3139. https://doi.org/10.1097/00007632-200012150-00008

Personal Identity   1202

Definition: Personal actions that differentiate self and non-self and characterizes one's essence

OUTCOME TARGET RATING: Maintain at_____ Increase to_____

		Never Demonstrated	Rarely Demonstrated	Sometimes Demonstrated	Often Demonstrated	Consistently Demonstrated	
OUTCOME OVERALL RATING		1	2	3	4	5	
Indicators:							
120215	Verbalizes personal feelings	1	2	3	4	5	NA
120216	Verbalizes personal thoughts	1	2	3	4	5	NA
120201	Verbalizes affirmations of personal identity	1	2	3	4	5	NA
120203	Verbalizes clear sense of personal identity	1	2	3	4	5	NA
120217	Verbalizes own uniqueness	1	2	3	4	5	NA
120202	Exhibits congruent verbal and non-verbal behavior about self	1	2	3	4	5	NA
120204	Differentiates self from environment	1	2	3	4	5	NA
120205	Differentiates self from other human beings	1	2	3	4	5	NA
120206	Perceives environment accurately	1	2	3	4	5	NA
120212	Establishes personal boundaries	1	2	3	4	5	NA
120207	Performs social roles	1	2	3	4	5	NA

P

Continued

Personal Identity—cont'd

	Never Demonstrated	Rarely Demonstrated	Sometimes Demonstrated	Often Demonstrated	Consistently Demonstrated	
120208 Verbalizes own value system	1	2	3	4	5	NA
120209 Challenges faulty beliefs about self	1	2	3	4	5	NA
120210 Challenges negative images of self	1	2	3	4	5	NA
120211 Recognizes interpersonal versus intrapersonal conflict	1	2	3	4	5	NA
120213 Verbalizes trust in self	1	2	3	4	5	NA
120218 Verbalizes self-worth	1	2	3	4	5	NA

Domain-Psychosocial Health (III)   **Class**-Psychological Well-Being (M)   *1st edition 1997; revised 2004, 2018*

OUTCOME CONTENT REFERENCES:

+Balistreri, E., Busch-Rossnagel, N. A., & Geisinger, K. F. (1995). Development and preliminary validation of the Ego Identity Process Questionnaire. *Journal of Adolescence, 18*(2), 179–192. https://doi.org/10.1006/jado.1995.1012

Barnard, D. (1990). Healing the damaged self: Identity, intimacy, and meaning in the lives of the chronically ill. *Perspectives in Biology & Medicine, 33*(4), 535–546. https://doi.org/10.1353/pbm.1990.0053

Erickson, E. (1968). *Identity, youth and crisis.* W. W. Norton & Company.

Marcia, J. E. (1966). Development and validations of ego identity status. *Journal of Personality and Social Psychology, 3*(5), 551–558. https://doi.org/10.1037/h0023281

Marcia, J. E. (1967). Ego identity status: Relationships to change in self-esteem, general adjustment, and authoritarianism. *Journal of Personality, 35*(1), 118–133. https://doi.org/10.1111/j.1467-6494.1967.tb01419.x

Pilarska, A. (2014). Self-construal as a mediator between identity structure and subjective well-being. *Current Psychology, 33*(2), 130–154. https://doi.org/10.1007/s12144-013-9202-5

Schwartz, S. J., Luyckx, K., & Vignoles, V. L. (Eds.). (2011). *Handbook of identity theory and research: Vol. 1. Structures and processes.* Springer.

Stuart, G. W. (2013). *Principles and practice of psychiatric nursing* (10th ed.). Elsevier Mosby.

+Tan, A. L., Kendis, R. J., Fine, J. T., & Porac, J. (1977). A short measure of Eriksonian ego identity. *Journal of Personality Assessment, 41*(3), 279–284. https://doi.org/10.1207/s15327752jpa4103_9

Watzlawik, M., & Born, A. (Eds.). (2007). *Capturing identity: Qualitative and quantitative methods.* University Press of America.

Personal Resilience

1309

Definition: Positive psychological adaptation, coping, and function of an individual following significant adversity, crisis, or stress

OUTCOME TARGET RATING: Maintain at_____ Increase to_____

	Never Demonstrated	Rarely Demonstrated	Sometimes Demonstrated	Often Demonstrated	Consistently Demonstrated	
OUTCOME OVERALL RATING	1	2	3	4	5	
Indicators:						
130901 Verbalizes positive outlook	1	2	3	4	5	NA
130902 Uses effective coping strategies	1	2	3	4	5	NA
130903 Expresses emotions	1	2	3	4	5	NA
130904 Clarifies ambiguous communication	1	2	3	4	5	NA
130905 Communicates clearly and appropriately for age	1	2	3	4	5	NA
130906 Exhibits positive mood	1	2	3	4	5	NA
130940 Exhibits self-awareness	1	2	3	4	5	NA
130941 Uses a growth mindset	1	2	3	4	5	NA
130907 Exhibits positive self-esteem	1	2	3	4	5	NA
130908 Expresses comfort with solitude	1	2	3	4	5	NA
130909 Expresses self-efficacy	1	2	3	4	5	NA
130910 Takes responsibility for own actions	1	2	3	4	5	NA
130942 Practices mindfulness	1	2	3	4	5	NA
130911 Verbalizes an enhanced sense of control	1	2	3	4	5	NA

P

Personal Resilience—cont'd

		Never Demonstrated	Rarely Demonstrated	Sometimes Demonstrated	Often Demonstrated	Consistently Demonstrated	
130912	Seeks emotional support	1	2	3	4	5	NA
130943	Expresses feeling supported by friends	1	2	3	4	5	NA
130944	Expresses feeling supported by family	1	2	3	4	5	NA
130945	Identifies appropriate behavior for different social situations	1	2	3	4	5	NA
130946	Learns from past experiences	1	2	3	4	5	NA
130947	Weighs alternatives to resolve problems	1	2	3	4	5	NA
130914	Adapts to adversities as challenges	1	2	3	4	5	NA
130915	Proposes practical, constructive solutions for disputes	1	2	3	4	5	NA
130948	Sets life goals	1	2	3	4	5	NA
130916	Makes progress toward goals	1	2	3	4	5	NA
130917	Uses strategies to promote safety	1	2	3	4	5	NA
130918	Uses strategies to avoid violent situations	1	2	3	4	5	NA
130919	Avoids drug misuse	1	2	3	4	5	NA
130920	Avoids alcohol misuse	1	2	3	4	5	NA
130921	Removes self from abusive relationships	1	2	3	4	5	NA
130922	Practices safe sex	1	2	3	4	5	NA
130923	Refrains from harming others	1	2	3	4	5	NA
130924	Identifies role models	1	2	3	4	5	NA
130925	Identifies available community resources	1	2	3	4	5	NA
130926	Uses available community resources	1	2	3	4	5	NA
130949	Expresses feeling supported by the community	1	2	3	4	5	NA
130927	Uses available support groups	1	2	3	4	5	NA
130928	Participates in employment opportunities	1	2	3	4	5	NA
130950	Expresses importance of obtaining an education	1	2	3	4	5	NA
130934	Verbalizes readiness to learn	1	2	3	4	5	NA
130929	Participates in curricular school activities	1	2	3	4	5	NA
130930	Participates in extracurricular school activities	1	2	3	4	5	NA
130931	Participates in community activities	1	2	3	4	5	NA
130932	Participates in leisure activities	1	2	3	4	5	NA
130933	Uses educational and vocational resources	1	2	3	4	5	NA

Domain-*Psychosocial Health (III)*   **Class**-*Psychosocial Adaptation (N)*   *4th edition 2008; revised 2024*

OUTCOME CONTENT REFERENCES:

Arslan, G. (2019). Mediating role of the self-esteem and resilience in the association between social exclusion and life satisfaction among adolescents. *Personality and Individual Differences, 51*, 109514. https://doi.org/10.1016/j.paid.2019.109514

Babić, R., Babić, M., Rastović, P., Ćurlin, M., Šimić, J., Mandić, K., & Pavlović, K. (2020). Resilience in health and illness. *Psychiatria Danubina, 32*(Suppl. 2), 226–232.

Boullion, A., Withers, M. C., & Lippmann, M. (2021). Mindsets: Investigating resilience. *Personality and Individual Differences, 174*, 110669. https://doi.org/10.1016/j.paid.2021.110669

Burnette, J. L., Knouse, L. E., Vavra, D. T., O'Boyle, E., & Brooks, M. A. (2020). Growth mindsets and psychological distress: A meta-analysis, *Clinical Psychology Review, 77*, 101816. https://doi.org/10.1016/j.cpr.2020.101816

Caldeira, S., & Timmins, F. (2016). Resilience: Synthesis of concept analyses and contribution to nursing classifications. *International Nursing Review, 63*(2), 191–199. https://doi.org/10.1111/inr.12268

Dale, S. K., Reid, R., & Safren, S. A. (2021). Factors associated with resilience among black women living with HIV and histories of trauma. *Journal of Health Psychology, 26*(5), 758–766. https://doi.org/10.1177/1359105319840690

P

Fergus, S., & Zimmerman, M. A. (2005). Adolescent resilience: A framework for understanding healthy development in the face of risk. *Annual Review of Public Health, 26*(1), 399–419.

Liu, J. J. W., Reed, M., & Girard, T. A. (2017). Advancing resilience: An integrative, multi-system model of resilience. *Personality and Individual Differences, 111*, 111–118. https://doi.org/10.1016/j.paid.2017.02.007

+Sinclair, V. G., & Wallston, K. A. (2004). The development and psychometric evaluation of the Brief Resilient Coping Scale. *Assessment, 11*(1), 94–101. https://doi.org/10.1177/1073191103258144

Wesner, A. C., Behenck, A., Finkler, D., Beria, P., Guimarães, L. S. P., Manfro, G. G., Blaya, C., & Heldt, E. (2019). Resilience and coping strategies in cognitive behavioral group therapy for patients with panic disorder. *Archives of Psychiatric Nursing, 33*(4), 428–433. https://doi.org/10.1016/j.apnu.2019.06.003

Yuan, Y. (2021). Mindfulness training on the resilience of adolescents under the COVID-19 epidemic: A latent growth curve analysis. *Personality and Individual Differences, 172*, 110560. https://doi.org/10.1016/j.paid.2020.110560

Personal Safety Behavior 1911

Definition: Personal actions to prevent unintentional physical injury to self

OUTCOME TARGET RATING: Maintain at_____ Increase to_____

		Never Demonstrated	Rarely Demonstrated	Sometimes Demonstrated	Often Demonstrated	Consistently Demonstrated	
OUTCOME OVERALL RATING		**1**	**2**	**3**	**4**	**5**	
Indicators:							
191140	Identifies age-specific safety risks	1	2	3	4	5	NA
191141	Identifies personal high-risk behaviors	1	2	3	4	5	NA
191142	Identifies personal chronic conditions that impact risk	1	2	3	4	5	NA
191119	Avoids high-risk behaviors	1	2	3	4	5	NA
191131	Uses strategies to prevent communicable diseases	1	2	3	4	5	NA
191143	Keeps immunizations current	1	2	3	4	5	NA
191144	Identifies work safety risks	1	2	3	4	5	NA
191110	Uses tools correctly	1	2	3	4	5	NA
191111	Uses machinery correctly	1	2	3	4	5	NA
191145	Identifies community safety risks	1	2	3	4	5	NA
191146	Uses strategies to prevent violence from others	1	2	3	4	5	NA
191147	Practices home safety measures	1	2	3	4	5	NA
191148	Uses home security measures	1	2	3	4	5	NA
191149	Practices safe internet use	1	2	3	4	5	NA
191150	Plans safety measures for weather emergencies	1	2	3	4	5	NA
191151	Practices water safety	1	2	3	4	5	NA
191152	Uses fire safety measures	1	2	3	4	5	NA
191132	Uses strategies to prevent suffocation	1	2	3	4	5	NA
191133	Uses strategies to prevent aspiration	1	2	3	4	5	NA
191102	Stores food to minimize spoilage	1	2	3	4	5	NA
191103	Prepares food to minimize contamination	1	2	3	4	5	NA
191153	Stores poisonous materials safely	1	2	3	4	5	NA
191136	Avoids allergens	1	2	3	4	5	NA
191137	Uses strategies to avoid environmental contaminants	1	2	3	4	5	NA
191154	Uses strategies to prevent falls	1	2	3	4	5	NA
191155	Uses strategies to reduce risk	1	2	3	4	5	NA
191104	Uses protective helmet during high-risk activities	1	2	3	4	5	NA
191134	Uses protective gear during high-risk activities	1	2	3	4	5	NA
191106	Selects appropriate clothing for activity	1	2	3	4	5	NA

P

Personal Safety Behavior—cont'd

		Never Demonstrated	Rarely Demonstrated	Sometimes Demonstrated	Often Demonstrated	Consistently Demonstrated	
191127	Uses strategies to protect from sun exposure	1	2	3	4	5	NA
191128	Uses proper body mechanics	1	2	3	4	5	NA
191107	Uses assistive devices correctly	1	2	3	4	5	NA
191108	Practices safe leisure activities	1	2	3	4	5	NA
191109	Practices safe sexual behaviors	1	2	3	4	5	NA
191156	Uses strategies to prevent intimate partner violence	1	2	3	4	5	NA
191135	Practices firearm safety	1	2	3	4	5	NA
191113	Avoids recreational drug use	1	2	3	4	5	NA
191129	Follows medication precautions	1	2	3	4	5	NA
191117	Avoids tobacco use	1	2	3	4	5	NA
191118	Avoids alcohol misuse	1	2	3	4	5	NA
191125	Avoids operating motor vehicle when using alcohol	1	2	3	4	5	NA
191130	Avoids operating motor vehicle when using substances that impair function	1	2	3	4	5	NA
191105	Uses seat belt	1	2	3	4	5	NA
191156	Avoids using cell phone while driving	1	2	3	4	5	NA
191120	Observes rules of the road	1	2	3	4	5	NA
191138	Uses personal emergency response system	1	2	3	4	5	NA
191139	Seeks safety information related to environment	1	2	3	4	5	NA

Domain-*Health Knowledge & Behavior (IV)*   **Class**-*Safety (HH)*   *1st edition 1997; revised 2004, 2008, 2013, 2024*

OUTCOME CONTENT REFERENCES:
Maxwell, L., Skues, J., Wise, L., Theiler, S., & Pfeifer, J. (2021). Public stranger violence—What makes you vulnerable? A comparison of perspectives from young adults and industry experts. *Journal of Interpersonal Violence*, 36(11/12), 5277–5296. https://doi.org/10.1177/0886260518804836
Potter, P. A., Perry, A. G., Stockert, P. A., & Hall, A. M. (2021). *Fundamentals of nursing* (10th ed.). Elsevier.
Ropaka, M., Nikolaou, D., & Yannis, G. (2020). Investigation of traffic and safety behavior of pedestrians while texting or web-surfing. *Traffic Injury Prevention*, 21(6), 389–394. https://doi.org/10.1080/15389588.2020.1770741
Williams, P. (2020). *Basic geriatric nursing* (7th ed.). Elsevier.

P

Personal Time Management   1635

Definition: Personal actions to complete personal and work commitments within an expected timeframe with minimum stress

OUTCOME TARGET RATING: Maintain at_____ Increase to_____

		Never Demonstrated	Rarely Demonstrated	Sometimes Demonstrated	Often Demonstrated	Consistently Demonstrated	
OUTCOME OVERALL RATING		1	2	3	4	5	
Indicators:							
163501	Prioritizes commitments at home	1	2	3	4	5	NA
163523	Prioritizes work activities	1	2	3	4	5	NA
163524	Sets limits on use of electronic devices	1	2	3	4	5	NA
163502	Sets short-term goals	1	2	3	4	5	NA
163503	Sets long-term goals	1	2	3	4	5	NA
163504	Identifies realistic timeframe for each activity	1	2	3	4	5	NA

Continued

Personal Time Management—cont'd

		Never Demonstrated	Rarely Demonstrated	Sometimes Demonstrated	Often Demonstrated	Consistently Demonstrated	
163505	Sets time for completion of commitments	1	2	3	4	5	NA
163506	Manages commitments within set timeframe	1	2	3	4	5	NA
163507	Balances competing demands	1	2	3	4	5	NA
163508	Monitors progress of multiple commitments	1	2	3	4	5	NA
163509	Plans activities by the week	1	2	3	4	5	NA
163510	Constructs a to-do list	1	2	3	4	5	NA
163511	Keeps reminders in an organized system	1	2	3	4	5	NA
163512	Delegates activities	1	2	3	4	5	NA
163513	Monitors completion of delegated activities	1	2	3	4	5	NA
163514	Defers activities appropriately	1	2	3	4	5	NA
163515	Minimizes interruptions	1	2	3	4	5	NA
163516	Breaks complex activities into manageable activities	1	2	3	4	5	NA
163517	Uses strategies to prevent feeling overwhelmed	1	2	3	4	5	NA
163525	Uses strategies to support changes in work hours or shifts	1	2	3	4	5	NA
163518	Uses strategies to reduce anxiety	1	2	3	4	5	NA
163519	Reassesses commitment priorities	1	2	3	4	5	NA
163520	Maintains organization within personal space	1	2	3	4	5	NA
163521	Uses strategies to manage workload	1	2	3	4	5	NA
163526	Describes impact of work requirements on health behaviors	1	2	3	4	5	NA
163522	Reports low level of stress	1	2	3	4	5	NA

Domain- *Health Knowledge & Behavior (IV)*   **Class-***Health Supporting Life Skills (II)*   *5th edition 2013; revised 2024*

P

OUTCOME CONTENT REFERENCES:

Codina, N., & Pestana, J. V. (2019). Time matters differently in leisure experience for men and women: Leisure dedication and time perspective. *International Journal of Environmental Research and Public Health, 16*(14), 2513. https://doi.org/10.3390/ijerph16142513

Janeslätt, G. K., Holmqvist, K. L., White, S., & Holmefur, M. (2018). Assessment of time management skills: Psychometric properties of the Swedish version. *Scandinavian Journal of Occupational Therapy, 25*(3), 153–161. https://doi.org/10.1080/11038128.2017.1375009

Kelly, J. D., (2019). Your best life: Unlock more time in your day for rest and relaxation—That's an order. *Clinical Orthopaedics and Related Research, 477*(12), 2644–2646. https://doi.org/10.1097/CORR.0000000000001013

+Nakao, T., Takeishi, C., Nunoi, K., Matsuishi, T., Okamura, H., Sato, Y., Uchizono, Y., Mizuno, M., Yokobori, Y., & Shimizu, Y. (2020). Development of the Daily Time Management Scale for use by working people with type 2 diabetes. *Japan Journal of Nursing Science, 17*(2), e12307. https://doi.org/10.1111/jjns.12307

Nakao, T., Takeishi, C., Tsutsumi, C., Sato, Y., Uchizono, Y., & Shimizu, Y. (2021). Employment factors associated with daily time management in working people with type 2 diabetes. *Japan Journal of Nursing Science, 18*(2), 1–8. https://doi.org/10.1111/jjns.12395

Patterson, C. (2021). Keys to success: Motivation combined with time and stress management. *Imprint* (00193062), *68*(4), 30–32.

Wang, W. C. (2019). Exploring the relationship among free-time management, leisure boredom, and internet addiction in undergraduates in Taiwan. *Psychological Reports, 122*(5), 1651–1665. https://doi.org/10.1177/0033294118789034

+White, S. M., Riley, A., & Flom, P. (2013). Assessment of Time Management Skills (ATMS): A practice-based outcome questionnaire. *Occupational Therapy in Mental Health, 29*(3), 215–231, https://doi.org/10.1080/0164212X.2013.819481

Zangerle, C. M. (2021). Two tactics for time management and stress reduction. *Nursing Management, 52*(4), 6–8. https://doi.org/10.1097/01.NUMA.0000737784.64810.4b

Personal Well-Being   2002

Definition: Extent of positive perception of one's current health status

OUTCOME TARGET RATING: Maintain at_____ Increase to_____

		Not at All Satisfied	Somewhat Satisfied	Moderately Satisfied	Very Satisfied	Completely Satisfied	
OUTCOME OVERALL RATING		1	2	3	4	5	
Indicators:							
200201	Performance of activities of daily living	1	2	3	4	5	NA
200212	Performance of usual roles	1	2	3	4	5	NA
200202	Psychological health	1	2	3	4	5	NA
200203	Social relationships	1	2	3	4	5	NA
200204	Spiritual life	1	2	3	4	5	NA
200205	Physical health	1	2	3	4	5	NA
200206	Cognitive status	1	2	3	4	5	NA
200215	Personal achievements	1	2	3	4	5	NA
200207	Ability to cope	1	2	3	4	5	NA
200208	Ability to relax	1	2	3	4	5	NA
200209	Level of happiness	1	2	3	4	5	NA
200210	Ability to express emotions	1	2	3	4	5	NA
200213	Ability to control activities	1	2	3	4	5	NA
200214	Opportunities for health care choices	1	2	3	4	5	NA
200216	Sense of safety	1	2	3	4	5	NA

Domain-Health & Life Quality (V)   *Class-Perceived Health & Life Situation (U)*   *1st edition 1997; revised 2004, 2008, 2013, 2024*

OUTCOME CONTENT REFERENCES:
+Dupuy, H. (1984). The Psychological General Well-Being (PCWB) Index. In N. K. Wenger, M. E. Mattson, C. D. Furberg, & J. Elinson (Eds.), *Assessment of quality of life in clinical trials of cardiovascular therapies* (pp. 170–183, 353–356). Le Jacq.
Grossi, E., Growth, N., Mosconi, P., Cerutti, R., Pace, F., Compare, A., & Apolone, G. (2006). Development and validation of the short version of the Psychological General Well-Being Index (PGWB-S). *Health Quality Life Outcomes, 14*(4), 88. https://doi.org/10.1186/1477-7525-4-88
Mastorci, F., Bastiani, L., Doveri, C., Trivellini, G., Casu, A., Vassalle, C., & Pingitore, A. (2020). Adolescent health: A framework for developing an innovative personalized well-being index. *Frontiers in Pediatrics, 8*, 181. https://doi.org/10.3389/fped.2020.00181
+Misajon, R., Pallant, J., & Bliuc, A. M. (2016). Rasch analysis of the Personal Wellbeing Index. *Quality of Life Research, 25*(10), 2565–2569. https://doi.org/10.1007/s11136-016-1302-x
+Revicki, D. A., Leidy, N. K., & Howland, L. (1996). Evaluating the psychometric characteristics of the Psychological General Well-Being Index with a new response scale. *Quality of Life Research, 5*(4), 419–425. https://doi.org/10.1007/BF00449916
+Tomyn, A. J., Stokes, M. A., Cummins, R. A., & Dias, P. C. (2020). A Rasch analysis of the Personal Well-Being Index in school children. *Evaluation & the Health Professions, 43*(2), 110–119. https://doi.org/10.1177/0163278718819219

P

Physical Aging   0113

Definition: Normal physiologic changes that occur with the natural aging process

OUTCOME TARGET RATING: Maintain at_____ Increase to_____

		Severe Deviation from Normal Range	Substantial Deviation from Normal Range	Moderate Deviation from Normal Range	Mild Deviation from Normal Range	No Deviation from Normal Range	
OUTCOME OVERALL RATING		1	2	3	4	5	
Indicators:							
011318	Memory	1	2	3	4	5	NA
011319	Cognitive status	1	2	3	4	5	NA
011325	Attention span	1	2	3	4	5	NA
011301	Mean body mass	1	2	3	4	5	NA

Continued

Physical Aging—cont'd

		Severe Deviation from Normal Range	Substantial Deviation from Normal Range	Moderate Deviation from Normal Range	Mild Deviation from Normal Range	No Deviation from Normal Range	
011302	Bone density	1	2	3	4	5	NA
011326	Changes in height	1	2	3	4	5	NA
011303	Cardiac output	1	2	3	4	5	NA
011304	Vital capacity	1	2	3	4	5	NA
011305	Blood pressure	1	2	3	4	5	NA
011306	Skin elasticity	1	2	3	4	5	NA
011327	Upper body muscle strength	1	2	3	4	5	NA
011328	Lower body muscle strength	1	2	3	4	5	NA
011320	Joint mobility	1	2	3	4	5	NA
011329	Posture	1	2	3	4	5	NA
011330	Balance	1	2	3	4	5	NA
011331	Gait stability	1	2	3	4	5	NA
011332	Energy level	1	2	3	4	5	NA
011321	Sensory acuity	1	2	3	4	5	NA
011322	Bladder muscle tone	1	2	3	4	5	NA
011333	Swallowing	1	2	3	4	5	NA
011334	Digestion	1	2	3	4	5	NA
011324	Bowel control	1	2	3	4	5	NA
011323	Resistance to infection	1	2	3	4	5	NA
011308	Hearing acuity	1	2	3	4	5	NA
011309	Visual acuity	1	2	3	4	5	NA
011310	Olfactory acuity	1	2	3	4	5	NA
011311	Taste acuity	1	2	3	4	5	NA
011335	Weight	1	2	3	4	5	NA
011312	Basal metabolic rate	1	2	3	4	5	NA
011313	Fat distribution pattern	1	2	3	4	5	NA
011314	Hair distribution pattern	1	2	3	4	5	NA
011315	Menstrual pattern	1	2	3	4	5	NA
011336	Changes in libido	1	2	3	4	5	NA
011316	Sexual functioning	1	2	3	4	5	NA
011337	Sleep pattern changes	1	2	3	4	5	NA

Domain-*Functional Health (I)*   **Class**-*Growth & Development (B)*   *1st edition 1997; revised 2004, 2013, 2024*

OUTCOME CONTENT REFERENCES:

de Carvalho Cordeiro, T. D., Silva, L. M., Monteiro, E. A., de Farias Pontes, M. de L., Golgheto Casemiro, F., & Partezani Rodrigues, R. A. (2021). Physiological changes in vision during aging: Perceptions of older adults and healthcare providers. *Investigacion & Educacion En Enfermeria, 39*(3), 131–147. https://doi.org/10.17533/udea.iee.v39n3e11

Lee, Y.-S., Nichols, J. F., Domingo, A., Kim, Y., Park, S. M., Han, G., Seo, H., & Hovell, M. (2021). Balance performance and related soft tissue components across three age groups. *Health Care for Women International, 42*(1), 67–81. https://doi.org/10.1080/07399332.2019.1678160

Porto, J. M., Spilla, S. B., Cangussu-Oliveira, L. M. R. C. F. Jr., Nakaishi, A. P. M., & de Abreu, D. C. C. (2020). Effect of aging on trunk muscle function and its influence on falls among older adults. *Journal of Aging & Physical Activity, 28*(5), 699–706. https://doi.org/10.1123/japa.2019-0194

Potter, P. A., Perry, A. G., Stockert, P. A., & Hall, A. M. (2021). *Fundamentals of nursing* (10th ed.). Elsevier.

Wang, Z. (2018). *Aging & aging-related disease: Mechanisms and interventions*. Springer.

Williams, P. (2020). *Basic geriatric nursing* (7th ed.). Elsevier.

Wysocki, K. (2021). Genomics of aging: Decreased immune defenses. *Journal of the American Association of Nurse Practitioners, 33*(2), 100–101. https://doi.org/10.1097/JXX.0000000000000579

Physical Fitness   **2004**

Definition: Performance of physical activities with vigor

OUTCOME TARGET RATING: Maintain at_____ Increase to_____

		Severely Compromised	Substantially Compromised	Moderately Compromised	Mildly Compromised	Not Compromised	
OUTCOME OVERALL RATING		1	2	3	4	5	
Indicators:							
200401	Muscle strength	1	2	3	4	5	NA
200402	Muscle endurance	1	2	3	4	5	NA
200403	Joint flexibility	1	2	3	4	5	NA
200415	Range of motion	1	2	3	4	5	NA
200416	Balance	1	2	3	4	5	NA
200417	Speed of movement	1	2	3	4	5	NA
200418	Reaction time	1	2	3	4	5	NA
200404	Performance of physical activities	1	2	3	4	5	NA
200405	Performance of routine exercise	1	2	3	4	5	NA
200406	Cardiovascular function	1	2	3	4	5	NA
200407	Respiratory function	1	2	3	4	5	NA
200408	Aerobic fitness	1	2	3	4	5	NA
200409	Body mass index	1	2	3	4	5	NA
200410	Waist to hip ratio	1	2	3	4	5	NA
200411	Blood pressure	1	2	3	4	5	NA
200412	Target heart rate during exercise	1	2	3	4	5	NA
200414	Resting heart rate	1	2	3	4	5	NA

Domain- *Health & Life Quality (V)*   **Class-** *Health Status (JJ)*   *2nd edition 2000; revised 2004, 2018*

OUTCOME CONTENT REFERENCES:

American College of Sports Medicine. (2013). *Guidelines for exercise testing and prescription* (9th ed.). Williams & Wilkins.

Brown, M., Sinacore, D. R., Ehsani, A. A., Binder, E. F., Holloszy, J. O., & Kohrt, W. M. (2000). Low-intensity exercise as a modifier of physical frailty in older adults. *Archives of Physical Medicine & Rehabilitation, 81*(7), 960–965. https://doi.org/10.1053/apmr.2000.4425

Cauderay, M., Narring, F., & Michaud, P. (2000). A cross-sectional survey assessing physical fitness of 9- to 19-year-old girls and boys in Switzerland. *Pediatric Exercise Science, 12*(4), 398–412. https://doi.org/10.1123/pes.12.4.398

Haskell, W. L., Lee, I., Pate, R. R., Powell, K. E., Blair, S. N., Franklin, B. A., Macera, C. A., Heath, G. W., Thompson, P. D., & Bauman, A. (2007). Physical activity and public health. Updated recommendation for adults from the American College of Sports Medicine and the American Heart Association. *Medicine & Science in Sports & Exercise, 39*(8), 1423–1434. https://doi.org/10.1249/mss.0b013e3180616b27

NIH Consensus Development Panel on Physical Activity and Cardiovascular Health. (1996). Physical activity and cardiovascular health. *Journal of the American Medical Association, 276*(3), 241–246.

U.S. Department of Health and Human Services. (2008). *2008 Physical activity guidelines for Americans.*

U.S. Department of Health and Human Services. (2016). *Healthy people 2020.* https://www.healthypeople.gov/2020/

P

Physical Injury Severity   **1913**

Definition: Severity of signs and symptoms of injuries to the body

OUTCOME TARGET RATING: Maintain at_____ Increase to_____

		Severe	Substantial	Moderate	Mild	None	
OUTCOME OVERALL RATING		1	2	3	4	5	
Indicators:							
191301	Skin abrasions	1	2	3	4	5	NA
191302	Bruises	1	2	3	4	5	NA
191303	Lacerations	1	2	3	4	5	NA
191325	Swelling	1	2	3	4	5	NA

Continued

Physical Injury Severity—cont'd

	Severe	Substantial	Moderate	Mild	None	
191304 Burns	1	2	3	4	5	NA
191305 Extremity sprains	1	2	3	4	5	NA
191306 Back sprains	1	2	3	4	5	NA
191326 Upper extremity fractures	1	2	3	4	5	NA
191327 Lower extremity fractures	1	2	3	4	5	NA
191308 Pelvic fractures	1	2	3	4	5	NA
191309 Hip fractures	1	2	3	4	5	NA
191310 Spinal fractures	1	2	3	4	5	NA
191311 Cranial fractures	1	2	3	4	5	NA
191312 Facial fractures	1	2	3	4	5	NA
191313 Dental injuries	1	2	3	4	5	NA
191314 Open head injuries	1	2	3	4	5	NA
191315 Closed head injuries	1	2	3	4	5	NA
191328 Penetrating neck injuries	1	2	3	4	5	NA
191316 Impaired mobility	1	2	3	4	5	NA
191319 Impaired cognition	1	2	3	4	5	NA
191320 Decreased level of consciousness	1	2	3	4	5	NA
191321 Liver contusion	1	2	3	4	5	NA
191322 Ruptured spleen	1	2	3	4	5	NA
191323 Hemorrhage	1	2	3	4	5	NA
191324 Abdominal trauma	1	2	3	4	5	NA
191329 Eye injuries	1	2	3	4	5	NA

*Domain-*Physiologic Health (II)   *Class-*Tissue Integrity (L)   *1st edition 1997; revised 2004, 2008, 2013, 2018*

OUTCOME CONTENT REFERENCES:

Maas, M. L., Reed, D., Park, M., Specht, J. P., Schutte, D., Kelley, L. S., Swanson, E. A., Tripp-Reimer, T., & Buckwalter, K. C. (2004). Outcomes of family involvement in care intervention for caregivers of individuals with dementia. *Nursing Research, 53*(2):76-86. https://doi.org/10.1097/00006199-200403000-00003

McGrath, A., & Whiting, D. (2015). Recognizing and assessing blunt abdominal trauma. *Emergency Nurse, 22*(10), 1824. https://doi.org/10.7748/en.22.10.18.e1377

McGraw, M. (2014). Getting ahead of penetrating neck injuries. *Nursing, 44*(10), 36–43. https://doi.org/10.1097/01.NURSE.0000453724.85369.e3

Walker, J. (2014). Assessment and management of patients with ankle injuries. *Nursing Standard, 28*(50), 52–59. https://doi.org/10.7748/ns.28.50.52.e9128

P

Physical Maturation: Female   **0114**

Definition: Normal physical changes in the female that occur with the transition from childhood to adulthood

OUTCOME TARGET RATING: Maintain at_____ Increase to_____

	Severe Deviation from Normal Range	Substantial Deviation from Normal Range	Moderate Deviation from Normal Range	Mild Deviation from Normal Range	No Deviation from Normal Range	
OUTCOME OVERALL RATING	1	2	3	4	5	
Indicators:						
011401 Growth spurt between 9.5–14.5 years of age	1	2	3	4	5	NA
011412 Increased growth rate of skeleton	1	2	3	4	5	NA
011413 Increased growth rate of viscera	1	2	3	4	5	NA
011414 Height increase	1	2	3	4	5	NA
011415 Weight increase	1	2	3	4	5	NA
011403 Voice changes	1	2	3	4	5	NA
011404 Adult body hair distribution	1	2	3	4	5	NA

Physical Maturation: Female—cont'd

		Severe Deviation from Normal Range	Substantial Deviation from Normal Range	Moderate Deviation from Normal Range	Mild Deviation from Normal Range	No Deviation from Normal Range	
011405	Breast development	1	2	3	4	5	NA
011416	Hormonal changes	1	2	3	4	5	NA
011406	Menstruation onset	1	2	3	4	5	NA
011407	Increased muscle mass	1	2	3	4	5	NA
011408	Decreased body fat	1	2	3	4	5	NA
011417	Change in body shape of hips	1	2	3	4	5	NA
011409	Increased sebaceous secretions	1	2	3	4	5	NA
011410	Increased perspiration	1	2	3	4	5	NA

Domain-Functional Health (I)   **Class**-Growth & Development (B)   *1st edition 1997; revised 2004, 2024*

OUTCOME CONTENT REFERENCES:
Berk, L. E. (2018). *Development through the lifespan* (7th ed.). Pearson Education.
Hockenberry, M. J., Wilson, D., & Rodgers, C. C. (Eds.). (2019). *Wong's nursing care of infants and children* (11th ed.). Elsevier.
Marcdaute, K. J., & Kliegman, R. M. (2019). *Nelson essentials of pediatrics* (8th ed.). Elsevier.
Potter, P. A., Perry, A. G., Stockert, P. A., & Hall, A. M. (2021). *Fundamentals of nursing* (10th ed.). Elsevier.
Styne, D. M. (2020). Physiology and disorders of puberty. In S. Melmed (Ed.), *Williams textbook of endocrinology*. Elsevier.

Physical Maturation: Male

0115

Definition: Normal physical changes in the male that occur with the transition from childhood to adulthood

OUTCOME TARGET RATING: Maintain at_____ Increase to_____

		Severe Deviation from Normal Range	Substantial Deviation from Normal Range	Moderate Deviation from Normal Range	Mild Deviation from Normal Range	No Deviation from Normal Range	
OUTCOME OVERALL RATING		1	2	3	4	5	
Indicators:							
011501	Growth spurt between 10.5 and 16 years of age	1	2	3	4	5	NA
011513	Increased growth rate of skeleton	1	2	3	4	5	NA
011514	Increased growth rate of viscera	1	2	3	4	5	NA
011515	Height increase	1	2	3	4	5	NA
011516	Weight increase	1	2	3	4	5	NA
011517	Hormonal changes	1	2	3	4	5	NA
011503	Voice changes	1	2	3	4	5	NA
011504	Adult body hair distribution	1	2	3	4	5	NA
011505	Testicular descent	1	2	3	4	5	NA
011506	Penis enlargement	1	2	3	4	5	NA
011507	First ejaculation of sperm (wet dream)	1	2	3	4	5	NA
011508	Increased muscle mass	1	2	3	4	5	NA
011509	Decreased body fat	1	2	3	4	5	NA
011510	Increased sebaceous secretions	1	2	3	4	5	NA
011511	Increased perspiration	1	2	3	4	5	NA

Domain-Functional Health (I)   **Class**-Growth & Development (B)   *1st edition 1997; revised 2004, 2024*

OUTCOME CONTENT REFERENCES:
Berk, L. E. (2018). *Development through the lifespan* (7th ed.). Pearson Education.
Hockenberry, M. J., Wilson, D., & Rodgers, C. C. (Eds.). (2019). *Wong's nursing care of infants and children* (11th ed.). Elsevier.
Marcdaute, K. J., & Kliegman, R. M. (2019). *Nelson essentials of pediatrics* (8th ed.). Elsevier.
Potter, P. A., Perry, A. G., Stockert, P. A., & Hall, A. M. (2021). *Fundamentals of nursing* (10th ed.). Elsevier.
Styne, D. M. (2020). Physiology and disorders of puberty. In S. Melmed (Ed.), *Williams textbook of endocrinology* (Ch. 26). Elsevier.

P

Play Participation

0116

Definition: Use of activities by a child to foster age-appropriate social and physical skills that are enjoyable and entertaining

OUTCOME TARGET RATING: Maintain at_____ Increase to_____

		Never Demonstrated	Rarely Demonstrated	Sometimes Demonstrated	Often Demonstrated	Consistently Demonstrated	
OUTCOME OVERALL RATING		1	2	3	4	5	
Indicators:							
011601	Participates in play activities	1	2	3	4	5	NA
011610	Expresses satisfaction with play activities	1	2	3	4	5	NA
011603	Enjoys play activities	1	2	3	4	5	NA
011604	Uses social skills during play activities	1	2	3	4	5	NA
011605	Uses physical skills during play activities	1	2	3	4	5	NA
011606	Uses imagination during play activities	1	2	3	4	5	NA
011607	Expresses emotions during play activities	1	2	3	4	5	NA
011608	Uses role-playing	1	2	3	4	5	NA
011611	Plays with pets	1	2	3	4	5	NA
011612	Dances as part of play activities	1	2	3	4	5	NA
011613	Participates in organized sports	1	2	3	4	5	NA
011614	Participates in gymnastics	1	2	3	4	5	NA
011615	Participates in water activities	1	2	3	4	5	NA
011616	Participates in outdoor activities	1	2	3	4	5	NA
011617	Plays computer games	1	2	3	4	5	NA

Domain-Functional Health (I) **Class-***Growth & Development (B)* *1st edition 1997; revised 2004, 2018*

OUTCOME CONTENT REFERENCES:

Goltz, H., & Brown, T. (2014). Are children's psychological self-concepts predictive of their self-reported activity preferences and leisure participation? *Australian Occupational Therapy Journal, 61*(3), 177–186. https://doi.org/10.1111/1440-1630.12101

Kolehmainen, N., Francis, J. J., Ramsay, C. R., Owen, C., McKee, L., Ketelaar, M., & Rosenbaum, P. (2011). Participation in physical play and leisure: Developing a theory- and evidence-based intervention for children with motor impairments. *BMC Pediatrics, 11*(100). https://doi.org/10.1186/1471-2431-11-100

Kolehmainen, N., Ramsay, C., McKee, L., Missiuna, C., Owen, C., & Francis, J. (2015). Participation in physical play and leisure in children with motor impairments: Mixed-methods study to generate evidence for developing an intervention. *Physical Therapy, 95*(10), 1374–1386. https://doi.org/10.2522/ptj.20140404

Powrie, B., Kolehmainen, N., Turpin, M., Ziviani, J., & Copley, J. (2015). The meaning of leisure for children and young people with physical disabilities: A systematic evidence synthesis. *Developmental Medicine & Child Neurology, 57*(11), 993–1010. https://doi.org/10.1111/dmcn.12788

Silva, P., & Santos, M. P. (2017). Playing outdoor and practicing sport: A study of physical activity levels in Portuguese children. *European Journal of Sport Science, 17*(2), 208–214. https://doi.org/10.1080/17461391.2016.1226389

P

Postpartum Maternal Health Behavior

1624

Definition: Personal actions to promote health of a mother in the period following birth of infant

OUTCOME TARGET RATING: Maintain at_____ Increase to_____

		Never Demonstrated	Rarely Demonstrated	Sometimes Demonstrated	Often Demonstrated	Consistently Demonstrated	
OUTCOME OVERALL RATING		1	2	3	4	5	
Indicators:							
162401	Adapts to maternal role	1	2	3	4	5	NA
162402	Bonds with infant	1	2	3	4	5	NA
162403	Checks uterine fundus	1	2	3	4	5	NA
162404	Monitors lochia changes	1	2	3	4	5	NA
162405	Maintains perineum care	1	2	3	4	5	NA

Postpartum Maternal Health Behavior—cont'd

		Never Demonstrated	Rarely Demonstrated	Sometimes Demonstrated	Often Demonstrated	Consistently Demonstrated	
162406	Maintains care of surgical incision	1	2	3	4	5	NA
162407	Maintains care of episiotomy	1	2	3	4	5	NA
162408	Monitors discomfort from episiotomy	1	2	3	4	5	NA
162409	Monitors for signs and symptoms of infection	1	2	3	4	5	NA
162410	Monitors for signs of postpartum depression	1	2	3	4	5	NA
162411	Monitors for nipple tenderness	1	2	3	4	5	NA
162412	Monitors breasts for engorgement	1	2	3	4	5	NA
162413	Monitors for stress incontinence	1	2	3	4	5	NA
162414	Monitors for development of new health problems	1	2	3	4	5	NA
162415	Uses water-based vaginal lubricant	1	2	3	4	5	NA
162416	Obtains health care when warning signs occur	1	2	3	4	5	NA
162417	Uses effective pain management strategies	1	2	3	4	5	NA
162418	Uses stress management techniques	1	2	3	4	5	NA
162419	Monitors anxiety level	1	2	3	4	5	NA
162420	Monitors comfort status	1	2	3	4	5	NA
162421	Maintains adequate nutrient intake	1	2	3	4	5	NA
162422	Maintains adequate fluid intake	1	2	3	4	5	NA
162423	Performs regular physical activity	1	2	3	4	5	NA
162424	Performs pelvic floor exercises	1	2	3	4	5	NA
162425	Balances activity and rest	1	2	3	4	5	NA
162426	Monitors sleep patterns	1	2	3	4	5	NA
162427	Uses strategies to obtain needed sleep	1	2	3	4	5	NA
162428	Obtains assistance from health professional for depression as needed	1	2	3	4	5	NA
162429	Discusses options for birth control with health professional	1	2	3	4	5	NA
162430	Follows recommendations for sexual activity restrictions	1	2	3	4	5	NA
162431	Obtains assistance from health professional as needed	1	2	3	4	5	NA
162432	Uses family support	1	2	3	4	5	NA
162433	Uses available support groups	1	2	3	4	5	NA
162434	Participates in postpartum checkups	1	2	3	4	5	NA
162435	Maintains bowel elimination	1	2	3	4	5	NA

Domain-*Health Knowledge & Behavior (IV)*   **Class**-*Health Behavior (Q)*   *4th edition 2008; revised 2024*

OUTCOME CONTENT REFERENCES:

Almalik, M. M. (2017). Understanding maternal postpartum needs: A descriptive survey of current maternal health services. *Journal of Clinical Nursing, 26*(23-24), 4654–4663. https://doi.org/10.1111/jocn.13812

Baratieri, T., & Natal, S. (2019). Postpartum program actions in primary health care: An integrative review. *Ciência & Saúde Coletiva, 24*(11), 4227–4238. https://doi.org/10.1590/1413-812320182411.28112017

Dipietro, L., Evenson, K. R., Bloodgood, B., Sprow, K., Troiano, R. P., Piercy, K. L., Vaux-Bjerke, A., & Powell, K. E. (2019). Benefits of physical activity during pregnancy and postpartum: An umbrella review. *Medicine & Science in Sports & Exercise, 51*(6), 1292–1302. https://doi.org/10.1249/MSS.0000000000001941

Esmkhani, M., Ahmadi, L., & Maleki, A. (2020). The effect of client needs counseling on the postpartum quality of life of women. *Journal of Perinatal Education, 29*(2), 95–102. https://doi.org/10.1891/J-PE-D-18-00044

Fallon. V., Groves, R., Halford, J. C., Bennett, K. M., & Harrold, J. A. (2016). Postpartum anxiety and infant-feeding outcomes. *Journal of Human Lactation, 32*(4), 740–758. https://doi.org/10.1177/0890334416662241

Kristoschek, J. H., Moreira de Sá, R. A., & Silva, F. C. D., & Vellarde, G. C. (2017). Ultrasonographic evaluation of uterine involution in the early puerperium. *Revista Brasileira de Ginecologia e Obstetrícia, 39*(4), 149–154. English. https://doi.org/10.1055/s-0037-1601418

Mattson, S. (Ed.). (2015). *Core curriculum for maternal-newborn nursing* (5th ed.). W.B. Saunders.

Murray, S. S., & McKinney, E. S. (2018). *Foundations of maternal-newborn and women's health nursing* (7th ed.). Elsevier.

Oyetunji. A., & Chandra, P. (2020). Postpartum stress and infant outcome: A review of current literature. *Psychiatry Research, 284*, 112769. https://doi.org/10.1016/j.psychres.2020.112769

Ricci, S. (2017). *Essentials of maternity, newborn, and women's health nursing* (4th ed.). Wolters Kluwer.

P

Post-Procedure Recovery 2303

Definition: Extent to which an individual returns to baseline function following a procedure or minor surgery requiring anesthesia or sedation

OUTCOME TARGET RATING: Maintain at_____ Increase to_____

OUTCOME OVERALL RATING	Severe Deviation from Normal Range	Substantial Deviation from Normal Range	Moderate Deviation from Normal Range	Mild Deviation from Normal Range	No Deviation from Normal Range	
	1	2	3	4	5	
Indicators:						
230301 Patent airway	1	2	3	4	5	NA
230328 Apical heart rate	1	2	3	4	5	NA
230302 Spontaneous respirations	1	2	3	4	5	NA
230303 Respiratory rate	1	2	3	4	5	NA
230304 Depth of inspiration	1	2	3	4	5	NA
230305 Forceful cough	1	2	3	4	5	NA
230306 Oxygen saturation	1	2	3	4	5	NA
230307 Systolic blood pressure	1	2	3	4	5	NA
230329 Diastolic blood pressure	1	2	3	4	5	NA
230308 Aldrete score	1	2	3	4	5	NA
230334 Passing gas	1	2	3	4	5	NA
230309 Gag reflex	1	2	3	4	5	NA
230310 Swallowing ability	1	2	3	4	5	NA
230311 Retains oral fluids	1	2	3	4	5	NA
230312 Answers questions	1	2	3	4	5	NA
230313 Fully awake	1	2	3	4	5	NA
230314 Moves extremities on command	1	2	3	4	5	NA
230315 Ambulation tolerance	1	2	3	4	5	NA
230330 Body temperature	1	2	3	4	5	NA
230318 Voiding	1	2	3	4	5	NA
230317 Urine output	1	2	3	4	5	NA
230325 Fluid balance	1	2	3	4	5	NA
230326 Electrolyte and acid/base balance	1	2	3	4	5	NA
230327 Wound tissue perfusion	1	2	3	4	5	NA
230331 Amount of drainage from wound drains/tubes	1	2	3	4	5	NA
230332 Amount of drainage on dressing	1	2	3	4	5	NA

	Severe	Substantial	Moderate	Mild	None	
230333 Bleeding	1	2	3	4	5	NA
230335 Orthostatic hypotension	1	2	3	4	5	NA
230336 Atelectasis	1	2	3	4	5	NA
230321 Nausea	1	2	3	4	5	NA
230322 Vomiting	1	2	3	4	5	NA
230323 Shivering	1	2	3	4	5	NA
230324 Pain	1	2	3	4	5	NA

Domain-Physiologic Health (II)   **Class**-Therapeutic Response (AA)   *3rd edition 2004; revised 2008, 2013, 2024*

OUTCOME CONTENT REFERENCES:

Cansino, C., Denny, C., Carlisle, A. S., & Stubblefield, P. (2021). Society of family planning clinical recommendations: Pain control in surgical abortion part 2—Moderate sedation, deep sedation, and general anesthesia. *Contraception, 104*, 583–592. https://doi.org/10.1015/j.contraception.2021.08.007

Cen, L., & Cao, Y. (2021). Therapeutic effects of auricular point acupressure on the recovery of patients after pterygium surgery: A pilot study: *Complementary Therapies in Clinical Practice, 43*, https://doi.org/10.1016/j.ctcp.2021.101339

Hagstrom, S., Hall, J., Sakhitab-Kerestes, A., & Tracy, M. F. (2021). Pediatric critical care nurses' practices related to sedation and analgesia. *Dimensions of Critical Care Nursing, 40*(5), 280–287. https://doi.org/10.1097/DCC.0000000000000491

Hogan, A. M., Luck, C., Woods, S., Ortu, A., & Petkov, S. (2021). The effect of orthostatic hypotension detected pre-operatively on post-operative outcome. *Journal of the American Geriatrics Society, 69*, 767–772. https://doi.org/10.1111/jgs.16966

Jeong, H., Tanatpom, P., Ahn, H. J., Yang, M., Kim, J. A., Yeo, H., & Kim, W. (2021). Pressure support versus spontaneous ventilation during anesthetic emergence—Effects on postoperative atelectasis: a randomized controlled trial. *Anesthesiology, 135*(6), 1004–1014. https://doi.org/10.1097/ALN.0000000000003997

Laporta, M. L., O'Brien, E. K., Stokken, J. K., Choby, G., Spring, J., & Weingarten, T. N. (2021). *The Laryngoscope, 131*, E815–E820. https://doi.org/10.1002/lary.28862

Premenstrual Syndrome (PMS) Severity   2105

Definition: Severity of reported and adverse physical and emotional responses due to cyclic hormonal fluctuations

OUTCOME TARGET RATING: Maintain at _____ Increase to _____

		Severe	Substantial	Moderate	Mild	None	
OUTCOME OVERALL RATING		1	2	3	4	5	
Indicators:							
210521	Pain	1	2	3	4	5	NA
210501	Abdominal bloating	1	2	3	4	5	NA
210502	Abdominal cramps	1	2	3	4	5	NA
210522	Menstrual blood loss	1	2	3	4	5	NA
210503	Disrupted bowel patterns	1	2	3	4	5	NA
210504	Decreased urine output	1	2	3	4	5	NA
210505	Acne	1	2	3	4	5	NA
210506	Anxiety	1	2	3	4	5	NA
210507	Backache	1	2	3	4	5	NA
210508	Breast tenderness	1	2	3	4	5	NA
210509	Decreased energy	1	2	3	4	5	NA
210510	Depression	1	2	3	4	5	NA
210511	Fluid retention	1	2	3	4	5	NA
210512	Food cravings	1	2	3	4	5	NA
210513	Headaches	1	2	3	4	5	NA
210514	Insomnia	1	2	3	4	5	NA
210523	Disturbed sleep	1	2	3	4	5	NA
210515	Irritability	1	2	3	4	5	NA
210516	Mood swings	1	2	3	4	5	NA
210517	Nausea	1	2	3	4	5	NA
210518	Vertigo	1	2	3	4	5	NA
210519	Vomiting	1	2	3	4	5	NA

Domain-*Health & Life Quality (V)*   **Class**-*Symptom Status (V)*   *2nd edition 2000; revised 2004, 2013, 2024*

OUTCOME CONTENT REFERENCES:

Abdi, F., Ozgoli, G., & Rahnemaie, F. S. (2019). A systematic review of the role of vitamin D and calcium in premenstrual syndrome. *Obstetrics & Gynecology Science, 62*(2), 73–86. https://doi.org/10.5468/ogs.2019.62.2.73

Baker, F. C., & Lee, K. A. (2018). Menstrual cycle effects on sleep. *Sleep Medicine Clinics, 13*(3), 283–294. https://doi.org/10.1016/j.jsmc.2018.04.002

Czajkowska, M., Drosdzol-Cop, A., Naworska, B., Galazka, I., Gogola, C., Rutkowska, M., & Skrzypulec-Plinta, V. (2020). The impact of competitive sports on menstrual cycle and menstrual disorders, including premenstrual syndrome, premenstrual dysphoric disorder and hormonal imbalances. *Ginekologia Polska, 91*(9), 503–512. https://doi.org/10.5603/GP.2020.0097

Le, J., Thomas, N., & Gurvich, C. (2020). Cognition, the menstrual cycle, and premenstrual disorders: A review. *Brain Sciences, 10*(4), 198. https://doi.org/10.3390/brainsci10040198

Magnay, J. L., O'Brien, S., Gerlinger, C., & Seitz, C. (2018). A systematic review of methods to measure menstrual blood loss. *BMC Women's Health, 18*(1), 142. https://doi.org/10.1186/s12905-018-0627-8

Richards, M., Rubinow, D. R., Daly, R. C., & Schmidt, P. J. (2006). Premenstrual symptoms and perimenopausal depression. *American Journal of Psychiatry, 163*(1), 133–137. https://doi.org/10.1176/appi.ajp.163.1.133

Santer, M., Wyke, S., & Warner, P. (2007). What aspects of periods are most bothersome for women reporting heavy menstrual bleeding? Community survey and qualitative study. *BMC Women's Health, 7*, 8. https://doi.org/10.1186/1472-6874-7-8

Schoep, M. E., Nieboer, T. E., van der Zanden, M., Braat, D., & Nap, A. W. (2019). The impact of menstrual symptoms on everyday life: A survey among 42,879 women. *American Journal of Obstetrics and Gynecology, 220*(6), 569.e1–569.e7. https://doi.org/10.1016/j.ajog.2019.02.048

+Steiner, M., Macdougall, M., & Brown, E. (2003). The Premenstrual Symptoms Screening Tool (PSST) for clinicians. *Archives of Women's Mental Health, 6*, 203–209. https://doi.org/10.1007/s00737-003-0018-4

P

Prenatal Health Behavior

1607

Definition: Personal actions to promote a healthy pregnancy and a healthy newborn

OUTCOME TARGET RATING: Maintain at_____ Increase to_____

		Never Demonstrated	Rarely Demonstrated	Sometimes Demonstrated	Often Demonstrated	Consistently Demonstrated	
OUTCOME OVERALL RATING		**1**	**2**	**3**	**4**	**5**	
Indicators:							
160701	Maintains healthy preconceptual state	1	2	3	4	5	NA
160702	Uses proper body mechanics	1	2	3	4	5	NA
160703	Keeps appointments for prenatal care	1	2	3	4	5	NA
160704	Maintains healthy weight gain pattern	1	2	3	4	5	NA
160705	Receives proper dental care	1	2	3	4	5	NA
160722	Participates in genetic testing	1	2	3	4	5	NA
160706	Uses motor vehicle safety devices correctly	1	2	3	4	5	NA
160707	Attends childbirth education classes	1	2	3	4	5	NA
160709	Participates in regular exercise	1	2	3	4	5	NA
160710	Maintains adequate nutrient intake for pregnancy	1	2	3	4	5	NA
160711	Practices safe sex	1	2	3	4	5	NA
160721	Uses medication as prescribed	1	2	3	4	5	NA
160712	Consults health professional about non-prescription medication use	1	2	3	4	5	NA
160723	Uses iron supplements	1	2	3	4	5	NA
160724	Uses daily multivitamin	1	2	3	4	5	NA
160713	Avoids environmental hazards	1	2	3	4	5	NA
160714	Avoids exposure to infectious diseases	1	2	3	4	5	NA
160715	Avoids recreational drug use	1	2	3	4	5	NA
160716	Avoids alcohol use	1	2	3	4	5	NA
160717	Avoids tobacco use	1	2	3	4	5	NA
160718	Avoids teratogenic agents	1	2	3	4	5	NA
160719	Avoids abusive situations	1	2	3	4	5	NA

Domain-Health Knowledge & Behavior (IV) **Class**-Health Behavior (Q) *2nd edition 2000; revised 2004, 2018*

P

OUTCOME CONTENT REFERENCES:

Bollini, P., & Quack-Lötscher, K. (2013). Guidelines-based indicators to measure quality of antenatal care. *Journal of Evaluation in Clinical Practice, 19*(6), 1060–1066. https://doi.org/10.1111/jep.12027

Centers for Disease Control and Prevention. (2012). Preconception health indicators among women—Texas, 2002–2010. *MMWR: Morbidity & Mortality Weekly Report, 61*(29), 550–555.

Cohen, T., Plourde, H., & Koski, K. (2010). Are Canadian women achieving a fit pregnancy? A pilot study. *Canadian Journal of Public Health, 101*(1), 87–91. https://doi.org/10.1007/BF03405570

Gollenberg, A., Pekow, P., Markenson, G., Tucker, K., & Taber, L. (2008). Dietary behaviors, physical activity, and cigarette smoking among pregnant Puerto Rican women. *American Journal of Clinical Nutrition, 87*(6), 1844–1851. https://doi.org/10.1093/ajcn/87.6.1844

Henn, B., Coull, B., & Wright, R. (2014). Chemical mixtures and children's health. *Current Opinion in Pediatrics, 26*(2), 223–229. https://doi.org/10.1097/MOP.0000000000000067

Pre-Procedure Readiness   1921

Definition: Personal actions of a patient to safely prepare for a procedure requiring anesthesia or sedation

OUTCOME TARGET RATING: Maintain at_____ Increase to_____

		Never Demonstrated	Rarely Demonstrated	Sometimes Demonstrated	Often Demonstrated	Consistently Demonstrated	
OUTCOME OVERALL RATING		1	2	3	4	5	
Indicators:							
192121	Completes required physical exam	1	2	3	4	5	NA
192122	Participates in pre-procedure checklist	1	2	3	4	5	NA
192123	Identifies procedural site	1	2	3	4	5	NA
192124	Participates in marking procedural site	1	2	3	4	5	NA
192125	Identifies known allergies	1	2	3	4	5	NA
192126	Signs consent for procedure	1	2	3	4	5	NA
192127	Reports basic knowledge of procedure	1	2	3	4	5	NA
192128	Identifies potential risks and complications of procedure	1	2	3	4	5	NA
192129	Participates in pre-procedure routines	1	2	3	4	5	NA
192130	Reports knowledge of post-procedure routines	1	2	3	4	5	NA
192131	Identifies recent changes in health status	1	2	3	4	5	NA
192132	Reports past adverse reaction to anesthetics	1	2	3	4	5	NA
192133	Reports completion of bowel preparation	1	2	3	4	5	NA
192134	Confirms adherence to intake restrictions	1	2	3	4	5	NA
192135	Completes skin preparation	1	2	3	4	5	NA
192136	Acknowledges patient identification procedures	1	2	3	4	5	NA
192137	Completes required laboratory tests	1	2	3	4	5	NA
192138	Completes personal preparation for procedure	1	2	3	4	5	NA
192139	Reports modification of regimen	1	2	3	4	5	NA
192140	Reports changes in medication required for procedure	1	2	3	4	5	NA
192141	Reports concerns about procedure	1	2	3	4	5	NA
192142	Asks questions prior to procedure	1	2	3	4	5	NA

Domain-*Health Knowledge & Behavior (IV)*   **Class**-*Safety (HH)*   *4th edition 2008; revised 2024*

P

OUTCOME CONTENT REFERENCES:

AL-Sagarat, A. Y., Al-Oran, H. M., Obeidat, H., Hamlan, A. M., & Moxham, L. (2017). Preparing the family and children for surgery. *Critical Care Nursing Quarterly, 40*(2), 99–107. https://doi.org/10.1097/CNQ.0000000000000146

American Organization of Perioperative Nurses. (2020). *Guidelines for perioperative practice.*

Goodman, T., & Spry, C. (2017). *Essentials of perioperative nursing* (6th ed.). Jones & Bartlett Learning.

Haynes, A. B., Weiser, T. G., Berry, W. R., Lipsitz, S. R., Breizat, A.-H. S., Dellinger, E. P., Herbosa, T., Joseph, S., Kibatala, P. L., Lapitan, M. C. M., Merry, A. F., Moorthy, K., Reznick, R. K., Taylor, B., & Gawande, A. A. (2009). A surgical safety checklist to reduce morbidity and mortality in a global population. *New England Journal of Medicine, 360*(5), 491–499. https://doi.org/10.1056/NEJMsa0810119

Hinkle, J. L., Cheever, K. H., & Overbaugh, K. (2021). *Brunner & Suddarth's textbook of medical-surgical nursing* (15th ed.). Wolters Kluwer.

Ignatavicius, D. D., Workman, M. L., Rebar, C. R., & Heimgartner, N. M. (2021). *Medical-surgical nursing: Concepts for interprofessional care* (10th ed.). Elsevier.

Pugel, A. E., Simianu, V. V., Flum, D. R., & Patchen Dellinger, E. (2015). Use of the surgical safety checklist to improve communication and reduce complications. *Journal of Infection and Public Health, 8*(3), 219–225. https://doi.org/10.1016/j.jiph.2015.01.001

Preterm Infant Organization   0117

Definition: Extrauterine integration of physiological and behavioral function by the infant born 24 to 37 (term) weeks gestation

OUTCOME TARGET RATING: Maintain at_____ Increase to_____

		Severely Compromised	Substantially Compromised	Moderately Compromised	Mildly Compromised	Not Compromised	
OUTCOME OVERALL RATING		1	2	3	4	5	
Indicators:							
011701	Apical heart rate (120–160 bpm)	1	2	3	4	5	NA
011702	Gestational age index	1	2	3	4	5	NA
011703	Respiratory rate (30–60)	1	2	3	4	5	NA
011704	Oxygen saturation > 85%	1	2	3	4	5	NA
011705	Thermoregulation	1	2	3	4	5	NA
011706	Skin color	1	2	3	4	5	NA
011707	Feeding tolerance	1	2	3	4	5	NA
011722	Coordination of breathing, sucking, and swallowing	1	2	3	4	5	NA
011708	Relaxed muscle tone	1	2	3	4	5	NA
011709	Smooth synchronous movement	1	2	3	4	5	NA
011710	Flexed posture	1	2	3	4	5	NA
011711	Hands brought to mouth	1	2	3	4	5	NA
011712	Deep sleep	1	2	3	4	5	NA
011713	Light sleep	1	2	3	4	5	NA
011714	Quiet-alert	1	2	3	4	5	NA
011715	Active-alert	1	2	3	4	5	NA
011716	Attentiveness to stimuli	1	2	3	4	5	NA
011717	Response to stimuli	1	2	3	4	5	NA
011718	Appropriate time-out signals	1	2	3	4	5	NA
011719	Sustained alertness during interaction	1	2	3	4	5	NA
011720	Interaction with caregiver	1	2	3	4	5	NA
011721	Self-consolability	1	2	3	4	5	NA
011723	Growth	1	2	3	4	5	NA

Domain-*Functional Health (I)*   **Class**-*Growth & Development (B)*   *2nd edition 2000; revised 2004, 2018*

P

OUTCOME CONTENT REFERENCES:

Jackson, B., Kelly, B., McCann, C., & Purdy, S. (2016). Predictors of the time to attain full oral feeding in late preterm infants. *Acta Paediatrica, 105*(1), e1–e6. https://doi.org/10.1111/apa.13227

Medoff-Cooper, B., Rankin, K., Li, Z., Liu, L., & White-Traut, R. (2015). Multisensory intervention for preterm infants improves sucking organization. *Advances in Neonatal Care, 15*(2), 142–149. https://doi.org/10.1097/ANC.0000000000000166

Neubauer, V., Fuchs, T., Griesmaier, E., Pupp-Peglow, U., & Kiechl-Kohlendorder, U. (2016). Comparing growth charts demonstrated significant deviations between the interpretation of postnatal growth patterns in very preterm infants. *Acta Paediatrica, 105*(3), 268–273. https://doi.org/10.1111/apa.13175

Ravn, I., Smith, L., Lindemann, R., Smeby, N., Kyno, N., Bunch, E., & Sandvik, L. (2011). Effect of early intervention on social interaction between mothers and preterm infants at 12 months of age: A randomized controlled trial. *Infant Behavior & Development, 34*(2), 215–225. https://doi.org/10.1016/j.infbeh.2010.11.004

Vinall, J., & Grunau, R. (2014). Impact of repeated procedural pain-related stress in infants born very preterm. *Pediatric Research, 75*(5), 584–587. https://doi.org/10.1038/pr.2014.16

White-Traut, R., Norr, K., Fabiyi, C., Rankin, K., & Li, Z. (2013). Mother-infant interaction improves with a developmental intervention for mother-preterm infant dyads. *Infant Behavior & Development, 36*(4), 694–706. https://doi.org/10.1016/j.infbeh.2013.07.004

White-Traut, R., Wink, T., Minehart, T., & Holditch-Davis, D. (2012). Frequency of premature infant engagement and disengagement behaviors during two maternally administered interventions. *Newborn & Infant Nursing Reviews, 12*(3), 124–131. https://doi.org/10.1053/j.nainr.2012.06.005

Psychomotor Energy 0006

Definition: Personal drive and energy to maintain activities of daily living, nutrition, and personal safety

OUTCOME TARGET RATING: Maintain at_____ Increase to_____

		Never Demonstrated	Rarely Demonstrated	Sometimes Demonstrated	Often Demonstrated	Consistently Demonstrated	
OUTCOME OVERALL RATING		1	2	3	4	5	
Indicators:							
000601	Exhibits affect that fits situation	1	2	3	4	5	NA
000602	Exhibits concentration	1	2	3	4	5	NA
000603	Maintains personal grooming and hygiene	1	2	3	4	5	NA
000604	Exhibits normal appetite	1	2	3	4	5	NA
000613	Complies with medication regimen	1	2	3	4	5	NA
000614	Complies with therapeutic regimen	1	2	3	4	5	NA
000606	Shows interest in surroundings	1	2	3	4	5	NA
000608	Exhibits stable energy level	1	2	3	4	5	NA
000615	Completes daily tasks	1	2	3	4	5	NA
000616	Sets goals for the future	1	2	3	4	5	NA
		Consistently Demonstrated	Often Demonstrated	Sometimes Demonstrated	Rarely Demonstrated	Never Demonstrated	
000607	Suicide ideation	1	2	3	4	5	NA
000611	Lethargy	1	2	3	4	5	NA
000612	Depression	1	2	3	4	5	NA

Domain-*Functional Health (I)* **Class**-*Energy Maintenance (A)* 2nd edition 2000; revised 2004, 2008, 2024

OUTCOME CONTENT REFERENCES:

American Psychiatric Association. (2022). *Diagnostic and statistical manual of mental disorders* (5th ed., text rev.). https://doi.org/10.1176/appi. books.9780890425787

Faurholt-Jepsen, M., Brage, S., Vinberg, M., Christensen, E. M., Knorr, U., Jensen, H. M., & Kessing, L. V. (2012). Differences in psychomotor activity in patients suffering from unipolar and bipolar affective disorder in the remitted or mild/moderate depressive state. *Journal of Affective Disorders, 141*(2–3), 457–463. https://doi.org/10.1016/j.jad.2012.02.020

Freyberg, J., Brage, S., Kessing, L. K., & Faurholt-Jepsen, M. (2020). Differences in psychomotor activity and heart rate variability in patients with newly diagnosed bipolar disorder, unaffected relatives, and healthy individuals. *Journal of Affective Disorders, 266*, 30–36. https://doi.org/10.1016/j.jad.2020.01.110

Gorby, H. E., Brownawell, A. M., & Falk, M. C. (2010). Do specific dietary constituents and supplements affect mental energy? Review of the evidence. *Nutrition Reviews, 68*(12), 697–718. https://doi.org/10.1111/j.1753-4887.2010.00340.x

Lieberman, H. R. (2006). Mental energy: Assessing the cognition dimension. *Nutrition Reviews*, 64(3), S10–S13. https://doi.org/10.1111/j.1753-4887.2006.tb00252.x

Lieberman, H. R. (2007). Cognitive methods for assessing mental energy. *Nutritional Neuroscience*, 10(5-6), 229–42. https://doi.org/10.1080/10284150701722273

O'Connor, P. J. (2006). Mental energy: Assessing the mood dimension. *Nutrition Reviews*, 64(3), S7–S9. https://doi.org/10.1111/j.1753-4887.2006.tb00256.x

P

Psychosocial Adjustment: Life Change 1305

Definition: Adaptive psychosocial response of an individual to a significant life circumstance

OUTCOME TARGET RATING: Maintain at_____ Increase to_____

OUTCOME OVERALL RATING	Never Demonstrated	Rarely Demonstrated	Sometimes Demonstrated	Often Demonstrated	Consistently Demonstrated	
	1	2	3	4	5	
Indicators:						
130516 Shares feelings with others	1	2	3	4	5	NA
130517 Monitors psychosocial impact of change	1	2	3	4	5	NA
130518 Monitors changes in mood	1	2	3	4	5	NA
130502 Maintains self-esteem	1	2	3	4	5	NA
130519 Expresses confidence in managing change	1	2	3	4	5	NA
130520 Maintains positive self-image	1	2	3	4	5	NA
130521 Maintains positive thinking	1	2	3	4	5	NA
130501 Sets realistic goals	1	2	3	4	5	NA
130505 Verbalizes optimism about present	1	2	3	4	5	NA
130506 Verbalizes optimism about future	1	2	3	4	5	NA
130507 Reports feeling empowered	1	2	3	4	5	NA
130503 Maintains productivity	1	2	3	4	5	NA
130504 Reports feeling useful	1	2	3	4	5	NA
130522 Expresses acceptance of new role	1	2	3	4	5	NA
130523 Expresses satisfaction with personal role performance	1	2	3	4	5	NA
130508 Identifies multiple coping strategies	1	2	3	4	5	NA
130509 Uses effective coping strategies	1	2	3	4	5	NA
130524 Uses effective stress reduction techniques	1	2	3	4	5	NA
130510 Uses effective financial management strategies	1	2	3	4	5	NA
130513 Uses available social support	1	2	3	4	5	NA
130511 Expresses satisfaction with living arrangements	1	2	3	4	5	NA
130525 Expresses feeling comfortable with physical environment	1	2	3	4	5	NA
130526 Expresses feeling comfortable with social environment	1	2	3	4	5	NA
130514 Participates in leisure activities	1	2	3	4	5	NA
130512 Reports feeling socially engaged	1	2	3	4	5	NA

Domain-*Psychosocial Health (III)* **Class**-*Psychosocial Adaptation (N)* *1st edition 1997; revised 2004, 2018*

OUTCOME CONTENT REFERENCES:

Conley, C. S., Travers, L. V., & Bryant, F. B. (2013). Promoting psychosocial adjustment and stress management in first-year college students: The benefits of engagement in a psychosocial wellness seminar. *Journal of American College Health, 61*(2), 75–86. https://doi.org/10.1080/07448481.2012.754757

Hertz, J. E., Koren, M. E., Rossetti, J., & Tibbits, K. (2016). Management of relocation in cognitively intact older adults. *Journal of Gerontological Nursing, 42*(11), 14–23. https://doi.org/10.3928/00989134-20071101-05

+Liang, J. (1984). Dimensions of the Life Satisfaction Index A: A structural formulation. *Journal of Gerontology, 39*(5), 613–622. https://doi.org/10.1093/geronj/39.5.613

+Neugarten, B. L., Havighurst, R. J., & Tobin, S. (1961). The measurement of life satisfaction. *Journal of Gerontology, 16*(2), 134–143. https://doi.org/10.1093/geronj/16.2.134

Rodrigue, J. R., Kanasky, W. F. Jr., Jackson, S. I., & Perri, M. G. (2000). The Psychosocial Adjustment to Illness Scale--Self-Report: Factor structure and item stability. *Psychological Assessment, 12*(4), 409–413.

Rosenkoetter, M. M., McKethan, T., Chernecky, C., & Looney, S. (2016). Assessment of the psychosocial adjustment of well elderly residing in retirement communities. *Issues in Mental Health Nursing, 37*(11), 858–867. https://doi.org/10.1080/01612840.2016.1226998

P

Quality of Life   2000

Definition: Extent of positive perception of current life circumstances

OUTCOME TARGET RATING: Maintain at_____ Increase to_____

		Not at All Satisfied	Somewhat Satisfied	Moderately Satisfied	Very Satisfied	Completely Satisfied	
OUTCOME OVERALL RATING		1	2	3	4	5	
Indicators:							
200001	Health status	1	2	3	4	5	NA
200002	Social circumstances	1	2	3	4	5	NA
200003	Environmental circumstances	1	2	3	4	5	NA
200013	Privacy	1	2	3	4	5	NA
200014	Dignity	1	2	3	4	5	NA
200015	Autonomy	1	2	3	4	5	NA
200004	Economic status	1	2	3	4	5	NA
200005	Education level	1	2	3	4	5	NA
200006	Occupational achievements	1	2	3	4	5	NA
200017	Interpersonal relationships	1	2	3	4	5	NA
200008	Achievement of life goals	1	2	3	4	5	NA
200009	Ability to cope	1	2	3	4	5	NA
200018	Ability to adapt	1	2	3	4	5	NA
200010	Self-concept	1	2	3	4	5	NA
200011	Pervasive mood	1	2	3	4	5	NA
200019	Independence in self-care	1	2	3	4	5	NA
200020	Spiritual well-being	1	2	3	4	5	NA

Domain-Health & Life Quality (V)   **Class**-Perceived Health & Life Situation (U)   1st edition 1997; revised 2004, 2008, 2024

OUTCOME CONTENT REFERENCES:

Cheng, C., Yang, C., Inder, K., & Chan, S. W. (2020). Illness perceptions, coping strategies, and quality of life in people with multiple chronic conditions. *Journal of Nursing Scholarship, 52*(2), 145–154. https://doi.org/10.1111/jnu.12540

+Diener, E., Emmons, R. A., Larsen, R. J., & Griffin, S. (1985). The Satisfaction with Life Scale. *Journal of Personality Assessment, 49*(1), 71–75. https://doi.org/10.1207/s15327752jpa4901_13

Manson, A., Ciro, C., Williams, K. C., & Maliski, S. L. (2020). Identity and perceptions of quality of life in Alzheimer's disease. *Applied Nursing Research, 52*, 151225. https://doi.org/10.1016/j.apnr.2019.151225

+Mezzich, J., Cohen, N., Ruiperez, M., Banzato, C., & Zapata-Vega, M. (2011). The Multicultural Quality of Life Index: Presentation and validation. *Journal of Evaluation in Clinical Practice, 17*(2), 357–364. https://doi.org/10.1111/j.1365-2753.2010.01609.x

Nguyen, H., Lee, J., Sorkin, D. H., & Gibbs, L. (2019). Living happily despite having an illness: Perceptions of healthy aging among Korean American, Vietnamese American, and Latino older adults. *Applied Nursing Research, 48*, 30–36. https://doi.org/10.1016/j.apnr.2019.04.002

Paterniani, A., Sperati, F., Esposito, G., Cognetti, G., Pulimeno, A. M. L., Rocco, G., Diamanti, P., Bertini, L., Baldeschi, G. C., Varrassi, G., Giannarelli, D., De Marinis, M. G., Ricci, S., & Latina, R. (2020). Quality of life and disability of chronic non-cancer pain in adult patients attending pain clinics: A prospective, multicenter, observational study. *Applied Nursing Research, 56*, 151332. https://doi.org/10.1016/j.apnr.2020.151332

Timonet-Andreu, E., Morales-Asencio, J. M., Alcalá Gutierrez, P., Cruzado Alvarez, C., López-Moyano, G., Mora Banderas, A., López-Leiva, I., & Canca-Sanchez, J. C. (2020). Health-related quality of life and use of hospital services by patients with heart failure and their family caregivers: A multicenter case-control study. *Journal of Nursing Scholarship, 52*(2), 217–228. https://doi.org/10.1111/jnu.12545

Yilmaz, M., & Cengiz, H. Ö. (2020). The relationship between spiritual well-being and quality of life in cancer survivors. *Palliative and Supportive Care 18*, 55–62. https://doi.org/10.1017/S1478951519000464

Q

Relocation Adaptation 1311

Definition: Adaptive emotional and behavioral response of a cognitively intact individual to a required change in living environment

OUTCOME TARGET RATING: Maintain at_____ Increase to_____

		Never Demonstrated	Rarely Demonstrated	Sometimes Demonstrated	Often Demonstrated	Consistently Demonstrated	
OUTCOME OVERALL RATING		1	2	3	4	5	
Indicators:							
131101	Recognizes reason for change in living environment	1	2	3	4	5	NA
131102	Participates in decision-making in new environment	1	2	3	4	5	NA
131103	Expresses satisfaction with daily routine	1	2	3	4	5	NA
131104	Expresses satisfaction with level of independence	1	2	3	4	5	NA
131105	Compares care needs with available resources	1	2	3	4	5	NA
131106	Expresses satisfaction with social relationships	1	2	3	4	5	NA
131107	Expresses satisfaction with variety of food	1	2	3	4	5	NA
131108	Expresses satisfaction with food preparation	1	2	3	4	5	NA
131109	Expresses satisfaction with retained personal belongings	1	2	3	4	5	NA
131110	Expresses satisfaction with living arrangements	1	2	3	4	5	NA
131111	Exhibits positive mood	1	2	3	4	5	NA
131112	Appears content	1	2	3	4	5	NA
131113	Respects others' rights	1	2	3	4	5	NA
131114	Maintains positive relationship with family	1	2	3	4	5	NA
131115	Maintains positive relationships with friends	1	2	3	4	5	NA
131116	Maintains positive relationships with others in new environment	1	2	3	4	5	NA
131117	Participates in social activities	1	2	3	4	5	NA

		Never Demonstrated	Rarely Demonstrated	Sometimes Demonstrated	Often Demonstrated	Consistently Demonstrated	
131118	Agitation	1	2	3	4	5	NA
131119	Anxiety	1	2	3	4	5	NA
131120	Fear	1	2	3	4	5	NA
131121	Worry	1	2	3	4	5	NA
131122	Frustration	1	2	3	4	5	NA
131123	Anger	1	2	3	4	5	NA
131124	Depression	1	2	3	4	5	NA
131130	Loss	1	2	3	4	5	NA
131125	Withdrawal	1	2	3	4	5	NA
131126	Loneliness	1	2	3	4	5	NA
131127	Boredom	1	2	3	4	5	NA
131128	Apathy	1	2	3	4	5	NA
131129	Suspicion	1	2	3	4	5	NA

Domain-*Psychosocial Health (III)*   **Class**-*Psychosocial Adaptation (N)*   5th edition 2013; revised 2024

OUTCOME CONTENT REFERENCES:

Bekhet, A., Fouad, R., & Zauszniewski, A. (2010). The role of positive cognitions in Egyptian elders' relocation adjustment. *Western Journal of Nursing Research,* 33(1), 121–135. https://doi.org/10.1177/0193945910381763

Chen, F. (2010). Assisting adults with severe mental illness in transitioning from parental homes to independent living. *Community Mental Health Journal,* 46(4), 372–380. https://doi.org/10.1007/s10597-009-9263-y

Hertz, J. E., Koren, M. E., Rossetti. J., & Robertson, J. F. (2008). Early identification of relocation risk in older adults with critical illness. *Critical Care Nursing Quarterly,* 31(1), 59–64. https://doi.org/10.1097/01.CNQ.0000306398.32648.26

Lee, G. E. (2010). Predictors of adjustment to nursing home life of elderly residents: A cross-sectional survey. *International Journal of Nursing Studies,* 47(8), 957–964. https://doi.org/10.1016/j.ijnurstu.2009.12.020

R

Regier, N. G., & Parmelee, P. A. (2021). Selective optimization with compensation strategies utilized by older adults newly-transitioned to assisted living. *Aging & Mental Health, 25*(10), 1877-1886. https://doi.org/10.1080/13607863.2020.1856776

Yong, B., Lin, R., & Xiao, H. (2021). Factors associated with nursing home adjustment in older adults: A systematic review. *International Journal of Nursing Studies, 113*, 1–10. https://doi.org/10.1016/j.ijnurstu.2020.103790

Respiratory Function   0415

Definition: Movement of air in and out of the lungs and exchange of carbon dioxide and oxygen at the alveolar level

OUTCOME TARGET RATING: Maintain at_____ Increase to_____

		Severe Deviation from Normal Range	Substantial Deviation from Normal Range	Moderate Deviation from Normal Range	Mild Deviation from Normal Range	No Deviation from Normal Range	
OUTCOME OVERALL RATING		1	2	3	4	5	
Indicators:							
041501	Respiratory rate	1	2	3	4	5	NA
041502	Respiratory rhythm	1	2	3	4	5	NA
041503	Depth of inspiration	1	2	3	4	5	NA
041504	Auscultated breath sounds	1	2	3	4	5	NA
041532	Airway patency	1	2	3	4	5	NA
041505	Tidal volume	1	2	3	4	5	NA
041506	Achievement of expected incentive spirometer	1	2	3	4	5	NA
041507	Vital capacity	1	2	3	4	5	NA
041533	Diffusion capacity	1	2	3	4	5	NA
041508	Oxygen saturation	1	2	3	4	5	NA
041509	Pulmonary function tests	1	2	3	4	5	NA
041534	Pulmonary ultrasound	1	2	3	4	5	NA
		Severe	Substantial	Moderate	Mild	None	
041535	Arrythmias	1	2	3	4	5	NA
041510	Accessory muscle use	1	2	3	4	5	NA
041511	Chest retraction	1	2	3	4	5	NA
041512	Pursed lips breathing	1	2	3	4	5	NA
041513	Cyanosis	1	2	3	4	5	NA
041536	Dyspnea	1	2	3	4	5	NA
041516	Restlessness	1	2	3	4	5	NA
041517	Somnolence	1	2	3	4	5	NA
041518	Diaphoresis	1	2	3	4	5	NA
041519	Impaired cognition	1	2	3	4	5	NA
041520	Accumulation of sputum	1	2	3	4	5	NA
041521	Atelectasis	1	2	3	4	5	NA
041522	Adventitious breath sounds	1	2	3	4	5	NA
041523	Impaired expiration	1	2	3	4	5	NA
041524	Gasping	1	2	3	4	5	NA
041525	Agonal respirations	1	2	3	4	5	NA
041526	Grunting	1	2	3	4	5	NA
041527	Clubbing of fingers	1	2	3	4	5	NA
041528	Nasal flaring	1	2	3	4	5	NA
041530	Fever	1	2	3	4	5	NA
041531	Coughing	1	2	3	4	5	NA

R

Domain-*Physiologic Health (II)*   **Class**-*Cardiopulmonary (E)*   *4th edition 2008; revised 2013, 2024*

OUTCOME CONTENT REFERENCES:

Boutou, A. K., Georgopoulou, A., Pitsiou, G., Stanopoulos, I., Kontakiotis, T., & Kioumis, I. (2021). Changes in the respiratory function of COVID-19 survivors during follow-up: A novel respiratory disorder on the rise? *International Journal of Clinical Practice, 75*, e14301. https://doi.org/10.1111/ijcp.14301

Chatterjee, N. A., Jensen, P. N., Harris, A. W., Nguyen, D. D., Huang, H. D., Cheng, R. K., Savla, J. J., Larsen, T. R., Gomez, J. M. D., Du-Fay-de-Lavallaz, J. M., Lemaitre, R. N., McKnight, B., Gharib, S. A., & Sotoodehnia, N. (2021). Admission respiratory status predicts mortality in COVID-19. *Influenza and Other Respiratory Viruses, 15*(5), 569–572. https://doi.org/10.1111/irv.12869

Cloutier, M. M. (2019). *Respiratory physiology* (2nd ed.). Elsevier.

da Silva, V. M., de Oliveira Lopes, M. V., de Araujo, T. L., Beltrao, B. A., Monteiro, F. P. M., Cavalcante, T. F., Moreira, R. P., & Santos, F. A. A. S. (2011). Operational definitions of outcome indicators related to ineffective breathing patterns in children with congenital heart disease. *Heart & Lung, 40*(3), e70–e77. https://doi.org/10.1016/j.hrtlng.2010.12.002

Duncan, D. (2017). *Respiratory care: Assessment and management.* M&K Publishing.

Fumagalli, A., Misuraca, C., Bianchi, A., Borsa, N., Limonta, S., Maggiolini, S., Bonardi, D. R., Corsonello, A., Di Rosa, M., Soraci, L., Lattanzio, F., & Colombo, D. (2021). Pulmonary function in patients surviving to COVID-19 pneumonia. *Infection, 49*(1), 153–157. https://doi.org/10.1007/s15010-020-01474-9

Huether, S. E., McCance, K. L., & Brashers, V. L. (2020). *Understanding pathophysiology* (7th ed.). Elsevier.

Ignatavicius, D. D., Workman, M. L., Rebar, C. R., & Heimgartner, N. M. (2021). *Medical-surgical nursing: Concepts for interprofessional care* (10th ed.). Elsevier.

Raimondi, F., Migliaro, F., Verdoliva, L., Gragnaniello, D., Poggi, G., Kosova, R., Sansone, C., Vallone, G., & Capasso, L. (2018). Visual assessment versus computer-assisted gray scale analysis in the ultrasound evaluation of neonatal respiratory status. *PLOS One, 13*(10), e0202397. https://doi.org/10.1371/journal.pone.0202397

Torres-Castro, R., Vasconcello-Castillo, L., Alsina-Restoy, X., Solis-Navarro, L., Burgos, F., Puppo, H., & Vilaró, J. (2021). Respiratory function in patients post-infection by COVID-19: A systematic review and meta-analysis. *Pulmonology, 27*(4), 328–337. https://doi.org/10.1016/j.pulmoe.2020.10.013

Valenzuela, A., Sibuet, N., Hornero, G., & Casas, O. (2021). Non-contact video-based assessment of the respiratory function using a RGB-D camera. *Sensors* (Basel, Switzerland), *21*(16), 5605. https://doi.org/10.3390/s21165605

Respiratory Function: Airway Patency   0410

Definition: Open, clear tracheobronchial passages for air exchange

OUTCOME TARGET RATING: Maintain at_____ Increase to_____

	Severe Deviation from Normal Range	Substantial Deviation from Normal Range	Moderate Deviation from Normal Range	Mild Deviation from Normal Range	No Deviation from Normal Range	
OUTCOME OVERALL RATING	1	2	3	4	5	
Indicators:						
041004 Respiratory rate	1	2	3	4	5	NA
041005 Respiratory rhythm	1	2	3	4	5	NA
041017 Depth of inspiration	1	2	3	4	5	NA
041012 Ability to clear secretions	1	2	3	4	5	NA
041022 Body mass index (BMI)	1	2	3	4	5	NA
041023 Heart rate	1	2	3	4	5	NA
041024 Mallampati score	1	2	3	4	5	NA
041025 Effective cough	1	2	3	4	5	NA
	Severe	Substantial	Moderate	Mild	None	
041002 Anxiety	1	2	3	4	5	NA
041003 Choking	1	2	3	4	5	NA
041013 Nasal flaring	1	2	3	4	5	NA
041026 Dyspnea	1	2	3	4	5	NA
041014 Gasping	1	2	3	4	5	NA
041018 Accessory muscle use	1	2	3	4	5	NA
041019 Coughing	1	2	3	4	5	NA
041027 Snoring	1	2	3	4	5	NA
041028 Secretions in airway	1	2	3	4	5	NA
041029 Stridor	1	2	3	4	5	NA
041030 Swelling of tissues in airway	1	2	3	4	5	NA
041021 Agonal respirations	1	2	3	4	5	NA

R

Domain-Physiologic Health (II)   *Class*-Cardiopulmonary (E)   *2nd edition 2000; revised 2004, 2008, 2024*

OUTCOME CONTENT REFERENCES:
Abrons, R. O., Ten Eyck, P., & Sheffield, I. D. (2021). The articulated oral airway as an aid to mask ventilation: A prospective, randomized, interventional, non-inferiority study. *BMC Anesthesiology, 21*(1), 1–8. https://doi.org/10.1186/s12871-021-01315-8
Cloutier, M. M. (2019). *Respiratory physiology* (2nd ed.). Elsevier.
Huether, S. E., McCance, K. L., & Brashers, V. L. (2020). *Understanding pathophysiology* (7th ed.). Elsevier.
Ignatavicius, D. D., Workman, M. L., Rebar, C. R., & Heimgartner, N. M. (2021). *Medical-surgical nursing: Concepts for interprofessional care* (10th ed.). Elsevier.
Li, J., Perez, A., Schehl, J., Albers, A., & Husain, I. A. (2021). The association between upper airway patency and speaking valve trial tolerance for patients with tracheostomy: A clinical retrospective study and an in vitro study. *American Journal of Speech-Language Pathology, 30*, 1728–1736. https://doi.org/10.1044/2021_AJSLP-20-00331
McMurray, R., & Becker, L. (2020). Airway management for deep sedation: Current practice, limitations, and needs as identified by clinical observation and survey results. *AANA Journal, 88*(2), 123–129.
Primov-Fever, A., Zaretsky, U., Elad, D., & Wolf, M. (2016). Evaluation of nasal airway patency by analysis of breathing sounds. *Acta Oto-Laryngologica, 136*(2), 219–224. https://doi.org/10.3109/00016489.2015.1100325

Respiratory Function: Gas Exchange   0402

Definition: Alveolar exchange of carbon dioxide and oxygen to maintain arterial blood gas concentrations

OUTCOME TARGET RATING: Maintain at_____ Increase to_____

		Severe Deviation from Normal Range	Substantial Deviation from Normal Range	Moderate Deviation from Normal Range	Mild Deviation from Normal Range	No Deviation from Normal Range	
OUTCOME OVERALL RATING		1	2	3	4	5	
Indicators:							
040208	Partial pressure of oxygen in arterial blood (PaO$_2$)	1	2	3	4	5	NA
040209	Partial pressure of carbon dioxide in arterial blood (PaCO$_2$)	1	2	3	4	5	NA
040210	Arterial pH	1	2	3	4	5	NA
040211	Oxygen saturation	1	2	3	4	5	NA
040212	End-tidal carbon dioxide	1	2	3	4	5	NA
040213	Chest x-ray results	1	2	3	4	5	NA
040214	Ventilation perfusion balance	1	2	3	4	5	NA
		Severe	Substantial	Moderate	Mild	None	
040217	Dyspnea	1	2	3	4	5	NA
040205	Restlessness	1	2	3	4	5	NA
040218	Irritability	1	2	3	4	5	NA
040206	Cyanosis	1	2	3	4	5	NA
040207	Somnolence	1	2	3	4	5	NA
040219	Headache	1	2	3	4	5	NA
040220	Diaphoresis	1	2	3	4	5	NA
040221	Agitation	1	2	3	4	5	NA
040216	Impaired cognition	1	2	3	4	5	NA

Domain-Physiologic Health (II) *Class*-Cardiopulmonary (E) 1st edition 1997; revised 2000, 2004, 2008, 2024

R

OUTCOME CONTENT REFERENCES:
Fernandes, C. J., Luppino Assad, A. P., Alves, J. L. Jr., Jardim, C., & de Souza, R. (2019). Pulmonary embolism and gas exchange. *Respiration: International Review of Thoracic Diseases, 98*(3), 253–262. https://doi.org/10.1159/000501342
Gochicoa-Rangel, L., Hernández-Morales, A. P., Salles-Rojas, A., Madrid-Mejía, W., Guzmán-Valderrábano, C., González-Molina, A., Salas-Escamilla, I., Durán-Cuellar, A., Silva-Cerón, M., Hernández-Morales, V., Reyes-García, A., Alvarado-Amador, I., Lozano-Martínez, L., Enright, P., Pensado-Piedra, L. E., & Torre-Bouscoulet, L. (2021). Gas exchange impairment during COVID-19 recovery. *Respiratory Care, 66*(10), 1610–1617. https://doi.org/10.4187/respcare.09114
Hassan, A., Lai, W., Alison, J., Huang, S., & Milross, M. (2021). Effect of intrapulmonary percussive ventilation on intensive care unit length of stay, the incidence of pneumonia and gas exchange in critically ill patients: A systematic review. *PLOS One, 16*(7), e0255005. https://doi.org/10.1371/journal.pone.0255005

Huether, S. E., McCance, K. L., & Brashers, V. L. (2020). *Understanding pathophysiology* (7th ed.). Elsevier.

Ignatavicius, D. D., Workman, M. L., Rebar, C. R., & Heimgartner, N. M. (2021). *Medical-surgical nursing: Concepts for interprofessional care* (10th ed.). Elsevier.

Pascoal, L. M., de Oliveira Lopes, M. V., da Silva, V. M., Diniz, C. M., Nunes, M. M., Carvalho de Sousa Freire, V. E., & Amorim, B. B. (2021). Content analysis of clinical indicators for impaired gas exchange. *Revista Gaucha de Enfermagem, 42,* 1–9. https://doi.org/10.1590/1983-1447.2021.20200099

Schenck, E. J., Hoffman, K., Goyal, P., Choi, J., Torres, L., Rajwani, K., Tam, C. W., Ivascu, N., Martinez, F. J., & Berlin, D. A. (2020). Respiratory mechanics and gas exchange in COVID-19-associated respiratory failure. *Annals of the American Thoracic Society, 17*(9), 1158–1161. https://doi.org/10.1513/AnnalsATS.202005-427RL

Tsareva, N. A., Avdeev, S. N., Kosanovic, D., Schermuly, R. T., Trushenko, N. V., & Nekludova, G. V. (2021). Inhaled iloprost improves gas exchange in patients with COVID-19 and acute respiratory distress syndrome. *Critical Care* (London, England), *25*(1), 258. https://doi.org/10.1186/s13054-021-03690-7

Respiratory Function: Ventilation   0403

Definition: Movement of air in and out of the lungs

OUTCOME TARGET RATING: Maintain at_____ Increase to_____

		Severe Deviation from Normal Range	Substantial Deviation from Normal Range	Moderate Deviation from Normal Range	Mild Deviation from Normal Range	No Deviation from Normal Range	
OUTCOME OVERALL RATING		**1**	**2**	**3**	**4**	**5**	
Indicators:							
040301	Respiratory rate	1	2	3	4	5	NA
040302	Respiratory rhythm	1	2	3	4	5	NA
040303	Depth of inspiration	1	2	3	4	5	NA
040318	Percussed sounds	1	2	3	4	5	NA
040324	Tidal volume	1	2	3	4	5	NA
040325	Vital capacity	1	2	3	4	5	NA
040326	Chest x-ray results	1	2	3	4	5	NA
040327	Pulmonary function tests	1	2	3	4	5	NA
		Severe	**Substantial**	**Moderate**	**Mild**	**None**	
040309	Accessory muscle use	1	2	3	4	5	NA
040310	Adventitious breath sounds	1	2	3	4	5	NA
040311	Chest retraction	1	2	3	4	5	NA
040312	Pursed lips breathing	1	2	3	4	5	NA
040329	Dyspnea	1	2	3	4	5	NA
040315	Orthopnea	1	2	3	4	5	NA
040317	Tactile fremitus	1	2	3	4	5	NA
040329	Asymmetrical chest expansion	1	2	3	4	5	NA
040330	Impaired vocalization	1	2	3	4	5	NA
040331	Accumulation of sputum	1	2	3	4	5	NA
040332	Impaired expiration	1	2	3	4	5	NA
040333	Distorted voice sounds on auscultation	1	2	3	4	5	NA
040334	Atelectasis	1	2	3	4	5	NA

Domain-*Physiologic Health (II)*   **Class**-*Cardiopulmonary (E)*   *1st edition 1997; revised 2004, 2008, 2024*

OUTCOME CONTENT REFERENCES:
Cloutier, M. M. (2019). *Respiratory physiology* (2nd ed.). Elsevier.

Duncan, D. (2017). *Respiratory care: Assessment and management.* M&K Publishing.

Huether, S. E., McCance, K. L., & Brashers, V. L. (2020). *Understanding pathophysiology* (7th ed.). Elsevier.

Ignatavicius, D. D., Workman, M. L., Rebar, C. R., & Heimgartner, N. M. (2021). *Medical-surgical nursing: Concepts for interprofessional care* (10th ed.). Elsevier.

Jünger, C., Reimann, M., Krabbe, L., Gaede, K. I., Lange, C., Herzmann, C., & Rüller, S. (2020). Non-invasive ventilation with pursed lips breathing mode for patients with COPD and hypercapnic respiratory failure: A retrospective analysis. *PLOS One, 15*(9), e0238619. https://doi.org/10.1371/journal.pone.0238619

Rest   0003

Definition: Quantity and pattern of diminished activity for mental, physical, and spiritual rejuvenation

OUTCOME TARGET RATING: Maintain at_____ Increase to_____

		Severely Compromised	Substantially Compromised	Moderately Compromised	Mildly Compromised	Not Compromised	
OUTCOME OVERALL RATING		**1**	**2**	**3**	**4**	**5**	
Indicators:							
000301	Amount of rest	1	2	3	4	5	NA
000302	Rest pattern	1	2	3	4	5	NA
000311	Napping pattern	1	2	3	4	5	NA
000303	Rest quality	1	2	3	4	5	NA
000304	Physically rested	1	2	3	4	5	NA
000305	Mentally rested	1	2	3	4	5	NA
000308	Emotionally rested	1	2	3	4	5	NA
000312	Spiritually rested	1	2	3	4	5	NA
000309	Energy restored after rest	1	2	3	4	5	NA
000310	Rested appearance	1	2	3	4	5	NA
000313	Environment supportive of rest	1	2	3	4	5	NA

Domain-*Functional Health (I)*   **Class**-*Energy Maintenance (A)*   *1st edition 1997; revised 2004, 2008, 2024*

OUTCOME CONTENT REFERENCES:

Horváth, K., & Plunkett, K. (2018). Spotlight on daytime napping during early childhood. *Nature and Science of Sleep, 10,* 97–104. https://doi.org/10.2147/NSS.S126252

Inazumi, C. K., Andrechuk, C. R. S., Lima, M. G., Zancanella, E., de Azevedo Barros, M. B., de Oliveira Cardoso, T. A. M., & Ceolim, M. F. (2020). Is napping related with health-related behaviors and sleep habits among adolescents? A population-based study. *Applied Nursing Research, 56,* 151373. https://doi.org/10.1016/j.apnr.2020.151373

Nassery, W., & Landgren, K. (2019). Parents' experience of their sleep and rest when admitted to hospital with their ill child: A qualitative study. *Comprehensive Child and Adolescent Nursing, 42*(4), 265–279. https//doi.org/10.1080/24694193.2018.1528310

Owusu, J. T., Wennberg, A. M. V., Holingue, C. B., Tzuang, M., Abeson, K. D., & Spira, A. P. (2019). Napping characteristics and cognitive performance in older adults. *International Journal of Geriatric Psychiatry, 34*(1), 87–96. https://doi.org/10.1002/gps.4991

Potter, P. A., Perry, A. G., Stockert, P., & Hall, A. (2021). *Fundamentals of nursing* (10th ed.). Elsevier.

Williams, P. (2020). *Basic geriatric nursing* (7th ed.). Elsevier.

Risk Control   1902

Definition: Personal actions to understand, prevent, eliminate, or reduce modifiable health threats

OUTCOME TARGET RATING: Maintain at_____ Increase to_____

		Never Demonstrated	Rarely Demonstrated	Sometimes Demonstrated	Often Demonstrated	Consistently Demonstrated	
OUTCOME OVERALL RATING		**1**	**2**	**3**	**4**	**5**	
Indicators:							
190219	Seeks current information about health risks	1	2	3	4	5	NA
190220	Identifies risk factors	1	2	3	4	5	NA
190201	Acknowledges personal risk factors	1	2	3	4	5	NA
190221	Acknowledges ability to change behavior	1	2	3	4	5	NA
190202	Monitors environmental risk factors	1	2	3	4	5	NA
190203	Monitors personal risk factors	1	2	3	4	5	NA
190204	Develops effective risk control strategies	1	2	3	4	5	NA

Continued

Risk Control—cont'd

		Never Demonstrated	Rarely Demonstrated	Sometimes Demonstrated	Often Demonstrated	Consistently Demonstrated	
190205	Adjusts risk control strategies	1	2	3	4	5	NA
190206	Commits to risk control strategies	1	2	3	4	5	NA
190207	Follows selected risk control strategies	1	2	3	4	5	NA
190208	Modifies lifestyle to reduce risk	1	2	3	4	5	NA
190209	Avoids exposure to health threats	1	2	3	4	5	NA
190210	Participates in screening for health problems	1	2	3	4	5	NA
190211	Participates in screening for identified risks	1	2	3	4	5	NA
190212	Obtains recommended immunizations	1	2	3	4	5	NA
190213	Uses health care services congruent with needs	1	2	3	4	5	NA
190214	Uses personal support systems to reduce risk	1	2	3	4	5	NA
190215	Uses community resources to reduce risk	1	2	3	4	5	NA
190216	Recognizes changes in health status	1	2	3	4	5	NA
190217	Monitors changes in general health status	1	2	3	4	5	NA

Domain-Health Knowledge & Behavior (IV) *Class*-Risk Control (T) 1st edition 1997; revised 2004, 2013; reviewed 2024

OUTCOME CONTENT REFERENCES:

+Hettler, B. (1982). Wellness promotion and risk reduction on a university campus. In M. Faber & A. Reinhardt (Eds.), *Promoting health through risk reduction.* Macmillan.

Hughes, E., Kilmer, G., Li, Y., Valluru, B., Brown, J., Colclough, G., Gethers, S., Roberts, H., Elam-Evans, L., & Balluz, L. (2010). Surveillance for certain health behaviors among states and selected local areas-United States, 2008. *Morbidity and Mortality Weekly Report Surveillance Summaries, 59*(SS-10), 1–221.

Kliche, T., Plaumann, M., Nocker, G., Dubben, S., & Walter, U. (2011). Disease prevention and health promotion programs: Benefits, implementation, quality assurance and open questions—a summary of the evidence. *Journal of Public Health, 19*(4), 283–292. https://doi.org/10.1007/s10389-011-0413-7

Peters, R. M. (2000). Using NOC outcome of risk control in prevention, early detection, and control of hypertension: Nursing Outcomes Classification system. *Outcomes Management for Nursing Practice, 4*(1), 39–45.

Pincus, H., Pechura, C., Keyser, D., Bachman, J., & Houtsinger, J. (2006). Depression in primary care: Learning lessons in a national quality improvement program. *Administration and Policy in Mental Health and Mental Health Services Research, 33*(1), 2–15. https://doi.org/10.1007/s10488-005-4227-1

Ruffin, M., IV., Nease, D. Jr., Sen, A., Pace, W., Wang, C., Acheson, L., Rubinstein, W., & Gramling, R. (2011). Effect of preventive messages tailored to family history on health behaviors: The family healthcare impact trials. *Annuals of Family Medicine, 9*(1), 3–11. https://doi.org/10.1370/afm.1197

Zortea, T. C., Cleare, S., Melson, A. J., Wetherall, K., & O'Connor, R. C. (2020). Understanding and managing suicide risk. *British Medical Bulletin, 134*(1), 73–84. https://doi.org/10.1093/bmb/ldaa013

Risk Control: Alcohol Use — 1903

Definition: Personal actions to understand, prevent, eliminate, or reduce the threats to health associated with alcohol use

OUTCOME TARGET RATING: Maintain at_____ Increase to_____

		Never Demonstrated	Rarely Demonstrated	Sometimes Demonstrated	Often Demonstrated	Consistently Demonstrated	
OUTCOME OVERALL RATING		1	2	3	4	5	
Indicators:							
190318	Seeks current information about alcohol use	1	2	3	4	5	NA
190319	Identifies risk factors for alcohol misuse	1	2	3	4	5	NA
190301	Acknowledges personal risk for alcohol misuse	1	2	3	4	5	NA
190321	Acknowledges impact of early exposure to alcohol	1	2	3	4	5	NA
190302	Acknowledges consequences associated with alcohol misuse	1	2	3	4	5	NA

Risk Control: Alcohol Use—cont'd

		Never Demonstrated	Rarely Demonstrated	Sometimes Demonstrated	Often Demonstrated	Consistently Demonstrated	
190320	Acknowledges ability to change behavior	1	2	3	4	5	NA
190303	Monitors environment for factors encouraging alcohol misuse	1	2	3	4	5	NA
190304	Monitors personal alcohol use patterns	1	2	3	4	5	NA
190305	Develops effective alcohol use control strategies	1	2	3	4	5	NA
190306	Adjusts alcohol use control strategies	1	2	3	4	5	NA
190307	Commits to alcohol use control strategies	1	2	3	4	5	NA
190308	Follows selected alcohol use control strategies	1	2	3	4	5	NA
190309	Participates in screening for health problems	1	2	3	4	5	NA
190310	Uses health care services congruent with needs	1	2	3	4	5	NA
190322	Uses strategies to control stress	1	2	3	4	5	NA
190311	Uses personal support systems to control alcohol misuse	1	2	3	4	5	NA
190312	Uses support group to control alcohol misuse	1	2	3	4	5	NA
190313	Uses community resources to control alcohol misuse	1	2	3	4	5	NA
190314	Recognizes changes in general health status	1	2	3	4	5	NA
190315	Monitors changes in general health status	1	2	3	4	5	NA
190316	Controls alcohol intake	1	2	3	4	5	NA

Domain-Health Knowledge & Behavior (IV)   **Class**-Risk Control (T)   *1st edition 1997; revised 2004, 2013; revised 2024*

OUTCOME CONTENT REFERENCES:
Deutsch, A. R., Lustfield, R., & Hanson, J. D. (2021). Where there's a will, there's a way? Strategies to reduce or abstain from alcohol use developed by Northern Plains American Indian women participating in a brief, alcohol-exposed pregnancy preconceptual intervention. *Alcoholism: Clinical and Experimental Research, 45,* 2383–2395. https://doi.org/10.1111/acer.14721
Haeny, A. M., Gueorguieva, R., Jackson, A., Morean, M .E., Krishnan-Sarin, S., DeMartini, K. S., Pearlson, G. D., Anticevic, A., Krystal, J. H., & O'Malley, S. S. (2021). Individual differences in the associations between risk factors for alcohol use disorder and alcohol use-related outcomes. *Psychology of Addictive Behaviors, 35*(5), 501–513. https://doi.org/10.1037/adb0000733
Kendler, K. S., Ohlsson, H., Sundquist, J., & Sundquist, K. (2021). The rearing environment and the risk for alcohol use disorder: A Swedish national high-risk home-reared, adopted co-sibling control study. *Psychological Medicine, 51,* 2370–2377. https://doi.org/10.1017/S0033291720000963
+MacNeil, G. (1991). A short-form scale to measure alcohol abuse. *Research on Social Work Practice, 1*(1), 68–75. https://doi.org/10.1177/104973159100100104
McGill, E., Petticrew, M., Marks, D., McGrath, M., Rinaldi, C., & Egan, M. (2021). Applying a complex systems perspective to alcohol consumption and the prevention of alcohol-related harms in the 21st century: A scoping review. *Addiction, 116*(9), 2260–2288. https://doi.org/10.1111/add.15341
McMullin, S. D., Shields, G. S., Slavich, G. M., & Buchanan, T. W. (2021). Cumulative lifetime stress exposure predicts greater impulsivity and addictive behaviors. *Journal of Health Psychology, 26*(14), 2921–2936. https://doi.org/10.1177/1359105320937055
Palmer, R., Corbin, W., & Cronce, J. (2010). Protective strategies: A mediator of risk associated with age of drinking onset. *Addictive Behaviors, 35*(5), 486–491. https://doi.org/10.1016/j.addbeh.2009.12.028
Rodriguez, L. M., Litt, D. M., & Stewart, S. H. (2021). COVID-19 psychological and financial stress and their links to drinking: A dyadic analysis in romantic couples. *Psychology of Addictive Behaviors, 35*(4), 377-390. https://doi.org/10.1037/adb0000724
Talashek, M. L., Gerace, L. M., & Starr, K. L. (1994). The substance abuse pandemic: Determinants to guide interventions. *Public Health Nursing, 11*(2), 131–139. https://doi.org/10.1111/j.1525-1446.1994.tb00780.x
Weyerer, S., Schäufele, M., Eifflaender-Gorfer, S., Köhler, L., Maier, W., Haller, F., Cvetanocska-Pllashiniku, G., Pentzek, M., Fuchs, A., van den Bussche, H., Zimmermann, T., Eisele, M., Bickel, H., Mösch, E., Wiese, B., Angermeyer, M. C., Riedel-Heller, S. G., & German AgeCoDe Study group (German Study on Ageing, Cognition, Dementia in Primary Care Patients). (2009). At-risk alcohol drinking in primary care patients aged 75 years and older. *International Journal of Geriatric Psychiatry, 24*(12), 1376–1385. https://doi.org/10.1002/gps.2274

R

Risk Control: Aspiration

Definition: Personal actions to understand and prevent the passage of fluid and solid particles into the lung

OUTCOME TARGET RATING: Maintain at_____ Increase to_____

		Never Demonstrated	Rarely Demonstrated	Sometimes Demonstrated	Often Demonstrated	Consistently Demonstrated	
OUTCOME OVERALL RATING		**1**	**2**	**3**	**4**	**5**	
Indicators:							
193501	Seeks current information about aspiration prevention	1	2	3	4	5	NA
193502	Identifies risk factors for aspiration	1	2	3	4	5	NA
193503	Acknowledges personal risk factors for aspiration	1	2	3	4	5	NA
193504	Notifies others of swallowing difficulties	1	2	3	4	5	NA
193505	Selects foods based on swallowing ability	1	2	3	4	5	NA
193506	Selects food of proper consistency	1	2	3	4	5	NA
193507	Selects fluid of proper consistency	1	2	3	4	5	NA
193508	Uses liquid thickeners as needed	1	2	3	4	5	NA
193509	Positions self upright for eating and drinking	1	2	3	4	5	NA
193510	Remains upright for 30 minutes after eating	1	2	3	4	5	NA
193511	Uses caution when swallowing pills	1	2	3	4	5	NA
193512	Brushes teeth after eating	1	2	3	4	5	NA
193513	Cleans dentures daily	1	2	3	4	5	NA
193514	Obtains assistance when choking	1	2	3	4	5	NA
193515	Maintains recommended nutritional requirements	1	2	3	4	5	NA
193516	Uses strategies to reduce stress when eating	1	2	3	4	5	NA
193517	Uses strategies to reduce coughing when eating	1	2	3	4	5	NA
193518	Obtains recommended pneumonia vaccine	1	2	3	4	5	NA

Domain-Health Knowledge & Behavior (IV)   **Class**-Risk Control (T)   6th edition 2018

R

OUTCOME CONTENT REFERENCES:

Cabrera, G., & Schub, T. (2016). *Pneumonia, aspiration (anaerobic)*. Cinahl Information Systems.

DiBardino, D., & Wunderink, R. (2015). Aspiration pneumonia: A review of modern trends. *Journal of Critical Care, 30*(1), 40–48. https://doi.org/10.1016/j.jcrc.2014.07.011

Echevarría, I. M., & Schwoebel, A. (2012). Development of an intervention model for the prevention of aspiration pneumonia in high-risk patients on a medical-surgical unit. *MEDSURG Nursing, 21*(5), 303–308.

Liantonio, J., Salzman, B., & Snyderman, D. (2014). Preventing aspiration pneumonia by addressing three key risk factors: Dysphagia, poor oral hygiene, and medication use. *Annals of Long-Term Care, 22*(10), 42–48.

Maarel-Wierink, C., Vanobbergen, J., Bronkhorst, E., Schols, J., & Baat, C. (2012). Oral health care and aspiration pneumonia in frail older people: A systematic literature review. *Gerodontology, 30*(1), 3–9. https://doi.org/10.1111/j.1741-2358.2012.00637.x

Richards, M., Bice, E., & Hobbs, A. (2015). Reducing aspiration pneumonia risk. *Annals of Long Term Care, 23*(10), 21–26.

Risk Control: Cancer   1917

Definition: Personal actions to understand, prevent, or reduce the threat of cancer

OUTCOME TARGET RATING: Maintain at_____   Increase to_____

		Never Demonstrated	Rarely Demonstrated	Sometimes Demonstrated	Often Demonstrated	Consistently Demonstrated	
OUTCOME OVERALL RATING		**1**	**2**	**3**	**4**	**5**	
Indicators:							
191701	Seeks current information about cancer prevention	1	2	3	4	5	NA
191713	Identifies risk factors for cancer	1	2	3	4	5	NA
191714	Acknowledges personal risk factors for cancer	1	2	3	4	5	NA
191718	Monitors for warning signs of cancer	1	2	3	4	5	NA
191724	Identifies recommended screenings based on age and gender	1	2	3	4	5	NA
191707	Obtains recommended cancer screening	1	2	3	4	5	NA
191719	Obtains genetic screening as recommended by health professional	1	2	3	4	5	NA
191720	Obtains oral screening	1	2	3	4	5	NA
191712	Obtains health care services following abnormal screening results	1	2	3	4	5	NA
191706	Performs recommended self-screening for cancer detection	1	2	3	4	5	NA
191721	Participates in regular exercise	1	2	3	4	5	NA
191722	Uses strategies to maintain adequate sleep	1	2	3	4	5	NA
191725	Eats a healthy diet	1	2	3	4	5	NA
191705	Follows dietary recommendations	1	2	3	4	5	NA
191723	Protects from sun exposure	1	2	3	4	5	NA
191702	Avoids exposure to carcinogens	1	2	3	4	5	NA
191704	Modifies environment to eliminate exposure to carcinogens	1	2	3	4	5	NA
191710	Eliminates tobacco use	1	2	3	4	5	NA
191716	Uses personal support systems to follow risk strategies	1	2	3	4	5	NA
191717	Uses community resources to reduce cancer risk	1	2	3	4	5	NA
191715	Monitors changes in general health status	1	2	3	4	5	NA
191711	Obtains recommended vaccinations	1	2	3	4	5	NA

Domain-*Health Knowledge & Behavior (IV)*   *Class*-*Risk Control (T)*   *2nd edition 2000; revised 2004, 2008, 2013, 2018, 2024*

OUTCOME CONTENT REFERENCES:

Caple, C., & Schub, T. (2015). *Prostate cancer: Risk factors and prevention.* Cinahl Information Systems.

Chang, V. C., Cotterchio, M., De, P., & Tinmouth, J. (2021). Risk factors for early-onset colorectal cancer: A population-based case-control study in Ontario, Canada. *Cancer Causes Control, 32,* 1063–1083. https://doi.org/10.1007/s10552-021-01456-8

Cooley, J., & Quale, L. (2013). Skin cancer preventive behavior and sun protection recommendations. *Seminars in Oncology Nursing, 29*(3), 223–226. https://doi.org/10.1016/j.soncn.2013.06.008

Forstner, R. (2020). Early detection of ovarian cancer. *European Radiology, 30*(10), 5370–5373. https://doi.org/10.1007/s00330-020-06937-z

Gray, T. F., Cudjoe, J., Murphy, J., Thorpe, R. J. Jr., Wenzel, J., & Han, H. R. (2017). Disparities in cancer screening practices among minority and underrepresented populations. *Seminars in Oncology Nursing, 33*(2), 184–198. https://doi.org/10.1016/j.soncn.2017.02.008

Klemp, J. (2015). Breast cancer prevention across the cancer care continuum. *Seminars in Oncology Nursing, 31*(2), 89–99. https://doi.org/10.1016/j.soncn.2015.03.002

Ladabaum, U., Dominitz, J. A., Kahi, C., & Schoen, R. E. (2020). Strategies for colorectal cancer screening. *Gastroenterology, 158*(2), 418–432. https://doi.org/10.1053/j.gastro.2019.06.043

Lehto, R. (2014). Lung cancer screening guidelines: The nurse's role in patient education and advocacy. *Clinical Journal of Oncology Nursing, 18*(3), 338–342. https://doi.org/10.1188/14.CJON.338-342

R

Nagao, T., & Warnakulasuriya, S. (2020). Screening for oral cancer: Future prospects, research and policy development for Asia. *Oral Oncology*, *105*, 104632. https://doi.org/10.1016/j.oraloncology.2020.104632

Patel, S. G., May, F. P., Anderson, J. C., Burke, C. A., Dominitz, J. A., Gross, S. A., Jacobson, B. C., Shaukat, A., & Robertson, D. J. (2022). Updates on age to start and stop colorectal cancer screening: Recommendations from the U.S. Multi-Society Task Force on Colorectal Cancer. *Gastrointestinal Endoscopy*, *95*(1), 1–15. https://doi.org/10.1016/j.gie.2021.06.012

Saunders, C. L., Massou, E., Waller, J., Meads, C., Marlow, L. A. V., & Usher-Smith, J. A. (2021). Cervical screening attendance and cervical cancer risk among women who have sex with women. *Journal of Medical Screening*, *28*(3), 349–356. https://doi.org/10.1177/0969141320987271

Stuckey, A., & Onstad, M. (2015). Hereditary breast cancer: An update on risk assessment and genetic testing in 2015. *American Journal of Obstetrics & Gynecology, 213*(2), 161–165. https://doi.org/10.1016/j.ajog.2015.03.003

Tumwebaze, J., Carter, V. L., & Dawkins, N. L. (2021). Enhancing the awareness of modifiable risk factors for cancer prevention in the Alabama black belt region: A follow-up study. *Journal of Health Care for the Poor and Underserved, 32*(4), 1995–2011. https://doi.org/10.1353/hpu.2021.0178

Vidrine, J., Stewart, D., Stuyck, S., Ward, J., Brown, A., Smith, C., & Wetter, D. (2013). Lifestyle and cancer prevention in women: Knowledge, perceptions, and compliance with recommended guidelines. *Journal of Women's Health, 22*(6), 487–492. https://doi.org/10.1089/jwh.2012.4015

Risk Control: Cardiovascular Disease   1914

Definition: Personal actions to understand, prevent, eliminate, or reduce the threat of cardiovascular disease

OUTCOME TARGET RATING: Maintain at_____ Increase to_____

		Never Demonstrated	Rarely Demonstrated	Sometimes Demonstrated	Often Demonstrated	Consistently Demonstrated	
OUTCOME OVERALL RATING		1	2	3	4	5	
Indicators:							
191418	Seeks current information about cardio-vascular disease	1	2	3	4	5	NA
191419	Identifies risk factors for cardiovascular disease	1	2	3	4	5	NA
191401	Acknowledges personal risk for cardio-vascular disease	1	2	3	4	5	NA
191402	Acknowledges ability to change behavior	1	2	3	4	5	NA
191403	Eliminates tobacco use	1	2	3	4	5	NA
191420	Eliminates recreational drug use	1	2	3	4	5	NA
191404	Monitors blood pressure	1	2	3	4	5	NA
191405	Monitors radial pulse rate	1	2	3	4	5	NA
191421	Monitors changes in general health status	1	2	3	4	5	NA
191406	Uses strategies to reduce stress	1	2	3	4	5	NA
191407	Uses effective weight control strategies	1	2	3	4	5	NA
191408	Follows heart healthy diet	1	2	3	4	5	NA
191409	Uses health care services congruent with needs	1	2	3	4	5	NA
191410	Follows non-prescription medication precautions	1	2	3	4	5	NA
191411	Seeks information about strategies to maintain cardiovascular health	1	2	3	4	5	NA
191412	Monitors effects of stimulants	1	2	3	4	5	NA
191413	Participates in cholesterol screening	1	2	3	4	5	NA
191422	Maintains glycemic control	1	2	3	4	5	NA
191414	Uses medication as prescribed	1	2	3	4	5	NA
191415	Participates in regular exercise	1	2	3	4	5	NA
191416	Participates in aerobic exercise	1	2	3	4	5	NA
191425	Participates in resistance training exercise	1	2	3	4	5	NA
191423	Uses personal support systems to reduce cardiovascular risk	1	2	3	4	5	NA
191424	Uses community resources to reduce cardiovascular risk	1	2	3	4	5	NA

***Domain**-Health Knowledge & Behavior (IV)*   ***Class**-Risk Control (T)*   *2nd edition 2000; revised 2004, 2013, 2024*

OUTCOME CONTENT REFERENCES:

Andersen, E., van der Ploeg, H. P., van Mechelen, W., Gray, C. M., Mutrie, N., van Nassau, F., Jelsma, J. G. M., Anderson, A. S., Silva, M. N., Pereira, H. V., McConnachie, A., Sattar, N., Sørensen, M., Røynesdal, Ø. B., Hunt, K., Roberts, G. C., Wyke, S., & Gill, J. M. R. (2021). Contributions of changes in physical activity, sedentary time, diet and body weight to changes in cardiometabolic risk. *International Journal of Behavioral Nutrition and Physical Activity, 18,* 1–13. https://doi.org/10.1186/s12966-021-01237-1

Andersen, L., Riddoch, C., Kriemler, S., & Hills, A. (2011). Physical activity and cardiovascular risk factors in children. *British Journal of Sports Medicine, 45*(11), 871–876. https://doi.org/10.1136/bjsports-2011-090333

Chen, X., Zhao, S., Hsue, C., Dai, X., Liu, L., Miller, J. D., Fang, Z., Feng, J., Huang, Y., Wang, X., & Lou, Q. (2021). Effects of aerobic training and resistance training in reducing cardiovascular disease risk for patients with prediabetes: A multi-center randomized controlled trial. *Primary Care Diabetes, 15,* 1063–1070. https://doi.org/10.1016/j.pcd.2021.08.013

Cooney, M., Cooney, H., Dudina, A., & Graham, I. (2011). Total cardiovascular disease risk assessment: A review. *Current Opinion in Cardiology, 26*(5), 429–437. https://doi.org/10.1097/HCO.0b013e3283499f06

Jemigan, V., Duran, B., Ahn, D., & Winkleby, M. (2010). Changing patterns in health behaviors and risk factors related to cardiovascular disease among American indians and Alaska natives. *American Journal of Public Health, 100*(4), 677–683. https://doi.org/10.2105/AJPH.2009.164285

King, K., Thomlinson, E., Sanguins, J., & LeBlanc, P. (2006). Men and women managing coronary artery disease risk: Urban-rural contrasts. *Social Science & Medicine, 62*(5), 1091–1102. https://doi.org/10.1016/j.socscimed.2005.07.012

Mochari-Greenberger, H., Mills, T., Simpson, S., & Mosca, L. (2010). Knowledge, preventive action, and barriers to cardiovascular disease prevention by race and ethnicity in women: An American Heart Association national survey. *Journal of Women's Health, 19*(7), 1243–1249. https://doi.org/10.1089/jwh.2009.1749

Ramos, S. R., O'Hare, O. M., Colon, A. H., Jacobs, S. K., Campbell, B., Kershaw, T., Vorderstrasse, A., & Reynolds, H. R. (2021). Purely behavioral: A scoping review of nonpharmacological behavioral and lifestyle interventions to prevent cardiovascular disease in persons living with HIV. *Journal of the Association of Nurses in AIDS Care, 32*(5), 536–547. https://doi.org/10.1097/JNC.0000000000000230

Soltani, S., Saraf-Bank, S., Basirat, R., Salehi-Abargouei, A., Mohammadifard, N., Sadeghi, M., Khosravi, A., Fadhil, I., Puska, P., & Sarrafzadegan, N. (2021). Community-based cardiovascular disease prevention programmes and cardiovascular risk factors: A systematic review and meta-analysis. *Public Health, 200,* 59–70. https://doi.org/10.1016/j.puhe.2021.09.006

Risk Control: Child Bullying   1936

Definition: Personal actions to understand, prevent, eliminate, or reduce the threat of becoming a victim of childhood bullying

OUTCOME TARGET RATING: Maintain at_____ Increase to_____

OUTCOME OVERALL RATING	Never Demonstrated	Rarely Demonstrated	Sometimes Demonstrated	Often Demonstrated	Consistently Demonstrated	
	1	2	3	4	5	
Indicators:						
193601 Obtains information about bullying	1	2	3	4	5	NA
193602 Identifies risk factors	1	2	3	4	5	NA
193603 Identifies personal risk factors	1	2	3	4	5	NA
193604 Identifies parental relationship risk factors	1	2	3	4	5	NA
193605 Identifies supportive family relationships	1	2	3	4	5	NA
193606 Identifies the power balance between persons	1	2	3	4	5	NA
193607 Develops positive peer relationships	1	2	3	4	5	NA
193608 Develops social competence	1	2	3	4	5	NA
193609 Develops supportive family network	1	2	3	4	5	NA
193610 Participates in peer group activities	1	2	3	4	5	NA
193611 Uses effective problem-solving strategies	1	2	3	4	5	NA
193612 Exhibits positive self-esteem	1	2	3	4	5	NA
193613 Develops resilience	1	2	3	4	5	NA
193614 Uses effective task-oriented coping strategies	1	2	3	4	5	NA
193615 Uses strategies to avoid bullying situations	1	2	3	4	5	NA
193616 Talks with a trusted adult	1	2	3	4	5	NA
193617 Notifies an adult of physical bullying	1	2	3	4	5	NA
193618 Notifies an adult of cyber-bullying	1	2	3	4	5	NA
193619 Notifies an adult of verbal bullying	1	2	3	4	5	NA
193620 Notifies an adult of social bullying	1	2	3	4	5	NA
193621 Notifies an adult of sibling bullying	1	2	3	4	5	NA
193622 Notifies school official of bullying event	1	2	3	4	5	NA

R

Domain*-Health Knowledge & Behavior (IV)   **Class**-Risk Control (T)   6th edition 2018*

OUTCOME CONTENT REFERENCES:
Lemstra, M., Nielsen, G., Rogers, M., Thompson, A., & Moraros, J. (2012). Risk indicators and outcomes associated with bullying in youth aged 9–15 years. *Canadian Public Health Association 103*(1), 9–13. https://doi.org/10.1007/BF03404061
Marvicsin, D., Boucher, N., & Eagle, M. J. (2013). Youth bullying: Implications for primary care providers. *The Journal for Nurse Practitioners, 9*(1), 523–527. https://doi.org/10.1016/j.nurpra.2013.05.006
Vivolo, A. M., Holt, M. K., & Massetti, G. M. (2011). Individual and contextual factors for bullying and peer victimization: Implications for prevention. *Journal of School Violence, 10*(2), 201–211.https://doi.org/10.1080/15388220.2010.539169
Waasdorp, T., Pas, E., O'Brennan, L., & Bradshaw, C. (2011). A multilevel perspective on the climate of bullying: Discrepancies among students, school staff and parents. *Journal of School Violence, 10*(2), 115–132. https://doi.org/10.1080/15388220.2010.539164

Risk Control: Dehydration 1937

Definition: Personal actions to understand, prevent, eliminate, or reduce the threat of inadequate water in the intracellular and extracellular compartments of the body

OUTCOME TARGET RATING: Maintain at_____ Increase to_____

		Never Demonstrated	Rarely Demonstrated	Sometimes Demonstrated	Often Demonstrated	Consistently Demonstrated	
OUTCOME OVERALL RATING		1	2	3	4	5	
Indicators:							
193701	Identifies risk factors for dehydration	1	2	3	4	5	NA
193702	Acknowledges personal risk factors for dehydration	1	2	3	4	5	NA
193703	Drinks 64 to 80 ounces of water daily	1	2	3	4	5	NA
193704	Eliminates caffeine use	1	2	3	4	5	NA
193705	Identifies environmental factors for increased fluid intake	1	2	3	4	5	NA
193706	Maintains fluid intake based on activity	1	2	3	4	5	NA
193707	Monitors weight	1	2	3	4	5	NA
193708	Monitors changes in pulse	1	2	3	4	5	NA
193709	Monitors blood pressure	1	2	3	4	5	NA
193710	Monitors for generalized weakness	1	2	3	4	5	NA
193711	Monitors thirst	1	2	3	4	5	NA
193712	Monitors skin turgor	1	2	3	4	5	NA
193713	Monitors for muscle cramps	1	2	3	4	5	NA
193714	Monitors urinary pattern	1	2	3	4	5	NA
193715	Monitors urine color	1	2	3	4	5	NA
193716	Monitors loss of fluid through stool	1	2	3	4	5	NA
193717	Monitors loss of fluid through vomiting	1	2	3	4	5	NA
193718	Identifies potential fluid loss from medication side effects	1	2	3	4	5	NA

Domain-Health Knowledge & Behavior (IV)   **Class**-Risk Control (T)   6th edition 2018

OUTCOME CONTENT REFERENCES:
Hodgkinson, B., Evans, D., & Wood, J. (2003). Maintaining oral hydration in older adults: A systematic review. *International Journal of Nursing Practice, 9*(3), S19–S28. https://doi.org/10.1046/j.1440-172x.2003.00425.x
Wakefield, B. J., Mentes, J., Holman, J. E., & Culp, K. (2008). Risk factors and outcomes associated with hospital admission for dehydration. *Rehabilitation Nursing, 33*(6), 233–241. https://doi.org/10.1002/j.2048-7940.2008.tb00234.x
Wakefield, B. J., Mentes, J., Holman, J. E., & Culp, K. (2009). Postadmission dehydration: Risk factors, indicators, and outcomes. *Rehabilitation Nursing, 34*(5), 209–216. https://doi.org/10.1002/j.2048-7940.2009.tb00281.x

Risk Control: Drug Use   1904

Definition: Personal actions to understand, prevent, eliminate, or reduce the threats to health associated with drug use

OUTCOME TARGET RATING: Maintain at_____ Increase to_____

		Never Demonstrated	Rarely Demonstrated	Sometimes Demonstrated	Often Demonstrated	Consistently Demonstrated	
OUTCOME OVERALL RATING		1	2	3	4	5	
Indicators:							
190418	Seeks current information about drug misuse	1	2	3	4	5	NA
190419	Identifies risk factors for drug misuse	1	2	3	4	5	NA
190401	Acknowledges personal risk for drug misuse	1	2	3	4	5	NA
190402	Acknowledges consequences associated with drug misuse	1	2	3	4	5	NA
190420	Acknowledges ability to change behavior	1	2	3	4	5	NA
190403	Monitors environment for factors encouraging drug misuse	1	2	3	4	5	NA
190404	Monitors personal drug use pattern	1	2	3	4	5	NA
190405	Develops effective drug misuse control strategies	1	2	3	4	5	NA
190406	Adjusts drug misuse control strategies	1	2	3	4	5	NA
190407	Commits to drug misuse control strategies	1	2	3	4	5	NA
190408	Follows selected drug misuse control strategies	1	2	3	4	5	NA
190409	Participates in screening for health problems	1	2	3	4	5	NA
190410	Uses health care services congruent with needs	1	2	3	4	5	NA
190421	Uses strategies to control anxiety	1	2	3	4	5	NA
190421	Uses strategies to control depression	1	2	3	4	5	NA
190422	Uses strategies to control stress	1	2	3	4	5	NA
190411	Uses personal support systems to control drug misuse	1	2	3	4	5	NA
190412	Uses support group to control drug misuse	1	2	3	4	5	NA
190413	Uses community resources to control drug misuse	1	2	3	4	5	NA
190414	Recognizes changes in general health status	1	2	3	4	5	NA
190415	Monitors changes in general health status	1	2	3	4	5	NA
190416	Eliminates adverse drug use	1	2	3	4	5	NA

Domain-*Health Knowledge & Behavior (IV)*   **Class**-*Risk Control (T)*   *1st edition 1997; revised 2004, 2013, 2024*

R

OUTCOME CONTENT REFERENCES:
Afuseh, E., Pike, C. A., & Oruche, U. M. (2020). Individualized approach to primary prevention of substance use disorder: Age-related risks. *Substance Abuse Treatment, Prevention, and Policy, 15*(1), 58. https://doi.org/10.1186/s13011-020-00300-7

Cho, J., Kelley-Quon, L. I., Barrington-Trimis, J. L., Kechter, A., Axeen, S., & Leventhal, A. M. (2021). Behavioral health risk factors for nonmedical prescription opioid use in adolescence. *Pediatrics, 148*(3), 1–11. https://doi.org/10.1542/peds.2021-051451

de Barros, G. M., de Moraes Horta, A. L., Diehl, A., da Rocha Miranda, R. O., de Moura, A. A. M., Seleghim, M. R., da Silva, C. J., dos Santos, M. A., Wagstaff, C., & Pillon, S. C. (2021). Prevalence, consequences and factors associated with drug use among individuals over 50 years of age in the family perspective. *Aging & Mental Health, 25*(11), 2140–2148. https://doi.org/10.1080/13607863.2020.1808879

El Hayek, S., Geagea, L., El Bourji, H., Kadi, T., & Talih, F. (2022). Prevention strategies of alcohol and substance use disorders in older adults. *Clinics in Geriatric Medicine, 38*(1), 169–179. https://doi.org/10.1016/j.cger.2021.07.011

Kumar, N., Janmohamed, K., Nyhan, K., Martins, S. S., Cerda, M., Hasin, D., Scott, J., Sarpong Frimpong, A., Pates, R., Ghandour, L. A., Wazaify, M., & Khoshnood, K. (2022). Substance, use in relation to COVID-19: A scoping review. *Addictive Behaviors, 127*, 107213. https://doi.org/10.1016/j.addbeh.2021.107213

Nelson, L. F., Weitzman, E. R., & Levy, S. (2022). Prevention of substance use disorders. *The Medical Clinics of North America, 106*(1), 153–168. https://doi.org/10.1016/j.mcna.2021.08.005

Ornell, F., Moura, H. F., Scherer, J. N., Pechansky, F., Kessler, F., & von Diemen, L. (2020). The COVID-19 pandemic and its impact on substance use: Implications for prevention and treatment. *Psychiatry Research, 289*, 113096. https://doi.org/10.1016/j.psychres.2020.113096

Perrenoud, L. O., Oikawa, K. F., Williams, A. V., Laranjeira, R., Fischer, B., Strang, J., & Ribeiro, M. (2021). Factors associated with crack-cocaine early initiation: A Brazilian multicenter study. *BMC Public Health, 21*, 1–14. https://doi.org/10.1186/s12889-021-10769-x

Risk Control: Dry Eye 1927

Definition: Personal actions to understand, prevent, eliminate, or reduce the threat of dry eye

OUTCOME TARGET RATING: Maintain at_____ Increase to_____

OUTCOME OVERALL RATING	Never Demonstrated	Rarely Demonstrated	Sometimes Demonstrated	Often Demonstrated	Consistently Demonstrated	
	1	2	3	4	5	
Indicators:						
192701 Seeks current information about dry eye	1	2	3	4	5	NA
192702 Identifies risk factors for dry eye	1	2	3	4	5	NA
192703 Identifies incomplete eyelid closure	1	2	3	4	5	NA
192704 Acknowledges personal risk factors for dry eye	1	2	3	4	5	NA
192705 Produces adequate tears	1	2	3	4	5	NA
192706 Acknowledges relationship of age and dry eye	1	2	3	4	5	NA
192707 Acknowledges relationship of gender and dry eye	1	2	3	4	5	NA
192708 Acknowledges relationship of hormones and dry eye	1	2	3	4	5	NA
192709 Acknowledges relationship of autoimmune diseases and dry eye	1	2	3	4	5	NA
192710 Identifies signs and symptoms of dry eye	1	2	3	4	5	NA
192711 Reduces contact lenses wearing time	1	2	3	4	5	NA
192712 Uses eye drops when wearing contact lenses	1	2	3	4	5	NA
192713 Avoids injury to the eye	1	2	3	4	5	NA
192714 Protects ocular surface integrity	1	2	3	4	5	NA
192715 Limits exposure to prolonged air conditioning	1	2	3	4	5	NA
192716 Limits exposure to strong wind	1	2	3	4	5	NA
192717 Limits exposure to direct sunlight	1	2	3	4	5	NA
192718 Limits exposure to air pollution	1	2	3	4	5	NA
192719 Limits exposure to low humidity	1	2	3	4	5	NA
192720 Limits prolonged reading	1	2	3	4	5	NA
192721 Limits prolonged use of computer	1	2	3	4	5	NA
192722 Avoids tobacco use	1	2	3	4	5	NA
192723 Blinks at frequent intervals	1	2	3	4	5	NA
192724 Closes eyelids completely	1	2	3	4	5	NA
192725 Obtains periodic eye exam	1	2	3	4	5	NA
192726 Uses ointments and lubricants as prescribed	1	2	3	4	5	NA
192727 Identifies medication that contribute to dry eye	1	2	3	4	5	NA
192728 Uses devices to protect eyes	1	2	3	4	5	NA
192729 Uses moisture chamber to prevent tear evaporation	1	2	3	4	5	NA

Domain-*Health Knowledge & Behavior (IV)*   **Class**-*Risk Control (T)*   *5th edition 2013; reviewed 2024*

OUTCOME CONTENT REFERENCES:

Alanazi, M.A., El-Hiti, G.A., Al-Madani, A., & Fagehi, R. (2021). Analysis of tear ferning patterns in young female subjects with refractive errors. *Journal of Ophthalmology,* https://doi.org/10.1155/2021/9524143

Kanski, J. J., & Bowling, B. (2011). *Clinical ophthalmology: A systematic approach* (7th ed., pp. 121–130). Elsevier.

O'Neil, E. C., Henderson, M., Massaro-Giordano, M., & Bunya, V. Y. (2019). Advances in dry eye disease treatment. *Current Opinion in Ophthalmology, 30*(3), 166–178. https://doi.org/10.1097/ICU.0000000000000569

Sahai, A., & Malik, P. (2005). Dry eye: Prevalence and attributable risk factors in a hospital-based population. *Indian Journal of Ophthalmology, 53*(2), 87–91. https://doi.org/10.4103/0301-4738.16170

Sendecka, M., Baryluk, A., Polz-Dacewicz, M. (2004). Prevalence and risk factors of dry eye syndrome. *Przeglad Epidemiologiczny, 58*(1), 227–233. https://doi.org/10.1001/archopht.118.9.1264

Risk Control: Environmental Hazards   1938

Definition: Personal actions to understand, prevent, eliminate, or reduce the threat of exposure to biological, chemical, physical, biomechanical, or psychosocial hazards in personal environment

OUTCOME TARGET RATING: Maintain at_____ Increase to_____

		Never Demonstrated	Rarely Demonstrated	Sometimes Demonstrated	Often Demonstrated	Consistently Demonstrated	
OUTCOME OVERALL RATING		1	2	3	4	5	
Indicators:							
193801	Monitors indoor pollutants	1	2	3	4	5	NA
193802	Monitors indoor allergens	1	2	3	4	5	NA
193803	Uses air purifier	1	2	3	4	5	NA
193804	Conforms to safety guidelines for appliances	1	2	3	4	5	NA
193805	Maintains carbon monoxide alarms	1	2	3	4	5	NA
193806	Maintains smoke detector alarms	1	2	3	4	5	NA
193807	Monitors the level of indoor radon	1	2	3	4	5	NA
193808	Removes lead-based paint	1	2	3	4	5	NA
193809	Eliminates tobacco use	1	2	3	4	5	NA
193810	Eliminates mold	1	2	3	4	5	NA
193811	Monitors hand-washing with soaps	1	2	3	4	5	NA
193812	Uses water filter device	1	2	3	4	5	NA
193813	Conforms to safety guidelines for aerosols	1	2	3	4	5	NA
193814	Conforms to safety guidelines for insecticides	1	2	3	4	5	NA
193815	Conforms to safety guidelines for herbicides	1	2	3	4	5	NA
193816	Conforms to safety guidelines for fungicides	1	2	3	4	5	NA
193817	Conforms to safety guidelines for rodenticides	1	2	3	4	5	NA
193818	Checks for weather warnings	1	2	3	4	5	NA
193819	Complies with safety instructions during inclement weather	1	2	3	4	5	NA

Domain-*Health Knowledge & Behavior (IV)*   **Class**-*Risk Control (T)*   *6th edition 2018*

OUTCOME CONTENT REFERENCES:
Diette, G. B., Hansel, N. N., Buckley, T. J., Curtin-Brosnan, J., Eggleston, P. A., Matsui, E. C., McCormack, C., Williams, D. L., & Breysse, P. N. (2007). Home indoor pollutant exposures among inner-city children with and without asthma. *Environmental Health Perspectives, 115*(11), 1665–1669. https://doi.org/10.1289/ehp.10088
Fabian, M. P., Stout, N. K., Adamkiewicz, G., Geggel, A., Ren, C., Sandel, M., & Levy, J. I. (2012). The effects of indoor environmental exposures on pediatric asthma: A discrete event simulation model. *Environmental Health, 11*, 1–16. https://doi.org/10.1186/1476-069X-11-66
Logue, J. M., Klepeis, N. E., Lobscheid, A. B., & Singer, B. C. (2014). Pollutant exposures from natural gas cooking burners: A simulation-based assessment for Southern California. *Environmental Health Perspectives, 122*(1), 43–50. https://doi.org/10.1289/ehp.1306673

R

Risk Control: Falls

Definition: Personal actions to understand, prevent, eliminate, or reduce falls

OUTCOME TARGET RATING: Maintain at_____ Increase to_____

		Never Demonstrated	Rarely Demonstrated	Sometimes Demonstrated	Often Demonstrated	Consistently Demonstrated	
OUTCOME OVERALL RATING		1	2	3	4	5	
Indicators:							
193901	Seeks information about fall risks	1	2	3	4	5	NA
193902	Identifies risk factors for falls	1	2	3	4	5	NA
193903	Acknowledges personal risks for falls	1	2	3	4	5	NA
193904	Acknowledges potential consequences of falls	1	2	3	4	5	NA
193905	Acknowledges ability to change behavior	1	2	3	4	5	NA
193906	Participates in screening for risk for falls	1	2	3	4	5	NA
193907	Uses strategies to compensate visual limitations	1	2	3	4	5	NA
193908	Monitors environment for risk factors	1	2	3	4	5	NA
193909	Uses assistive devices to reduce risk for falls	1	2	3	4	5	NA
193910	Commits to performing strategies to reduce risk for falls	1	2	3	4	5	NA
193911	Maintains pathways free of objects	1	2	3	4	5	NA
193912	Maintains adequate lighting	1	2	3	4	5	NA
193913	Wears good fitting shoes or slippers with soles that grip walking surfaces	1	2	3	4	5	NA
193914	Performs regular exercises to maintain strength and balance	1	2	3	4	5	NA
193915	Maintains nutrition and hydration to maintain strength and balance	1	2	3	4	5	NA
193916	Modifies lifestyle to reduce risk for falls	1	2	3	4	5	NA
193917	Uses assistive devices if needed to reduce risk for falls	1	2	3	4	5	NA
193918	Schedules routine wheelchair maintenance	1	2	3	4	5	NA
193919	Uses strategies to reduce risk when transferring from one surface to another	1	2	3	4	5	NA
193920	Operates wheelchair safely	1	2	3	4	5	NA
193921	Follows wheelchair safety guidelines	1	2	3	4	5	NA
193922	Uses strategies to compensate for standing balance issues	1	2	3	4	5	NA
193923	Uses strategies to compensate for sitting balance issues	1	2	3	4	5	NA
193924	Obtains financial resources for adding safety devices to home	1	2	3	4	5	NA
193925	Uses strategies to compensate for mobility limitations	1	2	3	4	5	NA
193926	Adjusts strategies to compensate for disabilities	1	2	3	4	5	NA
193927	Requests needed assistance for ambulation to reduce risk for falls	1	2	3	4	5	NA
193928	Uses precautions when taking medication that increase risk for falls	1	2	3	4	5	NA

Domain-*Health Knowledge & Behavior (IV)*   **Class**-*Risk Control (T)*   *6th edition 2018; reviewed 2024*

OUTCOME CONTENT REFERENCES:

Costa, A. G., de Araujo, T. L., Cavalcante, T. F., Lopes, M. V., Oliveira-Kumakura, A. R., & Costa, F. B. (2017). Clinical validation of the nursing outcomes Fall Prevention Behavior in people with stroke. *Applied Nursing Research, 33*, 67–71. https://doi.org/10.1016/j.apnr.2016.10.003

Jehu, D. A., Davis, J. C., & Liu-Ambrose, T. (2020). Risk factors for recurrent falls in older adults: A study protocol for a systematic review with meta-analysis. *BMJ Open, 10*(5), e033602. https://doi.org/10.1136/bmjopen-2019-033602

Mikos, M., Kucharska, E., Lulek, A. M., Kłosiński, M., & Batko, B. (2020). Evaluation of risk factors for falls in patients with rheumatoid arthritis. *Medical Science Monitor: International Medical Journal of Experimental and Clinical Research, 26*, e921862. https://doi.org/10.12659/MSM.921862

Park, S. H. (2018). Tools for assessing fall risk in the elderly: A systematic review and meta-analysis. *Aging Clinical and Experimental Research, 30*(1), 1–16. https://doi.org/10.1007/s40520-017-0749-0

Pereira, C., Veiga, G., Almeida, G., Matias, A. R., Cruz-Ferreira, A., Mendes, F., & Bravo, J. (2021). Key factor cutoffs and interval reference values for stratified fall risk assessment in community-dwelling older adults: The role of physical fitness, body composition, physical activity, health condition, and environmental hazards. *BMC Public Health, 21*, 1–10. https://doi.org/10.1186/s12889-021-10947-x

Rosenblatt, N. J., & Madigan, M. L. (2021). Exploring the association between measures of obesity and measures of trip-induced fall risk among older adults. *Archives of Physical Medicine and Rehabilitation, 102*, 2362–2368. https://doi.org/10.1016/j.apmr.2021.06.013

Risk Control: Food Insecurity   1943

Definition: Personal actions to understand, prevent, eliminate, or reduce the threat of inadequate access to quality, affordable, nutritious food due to financial restrictions

OUTCOME TARGET RATING: Maintain at_____ Increase to_____

		Never Demonstrated	Rarely Demonstrated	Sometimes Demonstrated	Often Demonstrated	Consistently Demonstrated	
OUTCOME OVERALL RATING		1	2	3	4	5	
Indicators:							
194301	Acknowledges personal risk of food insecurity	1	2	3	4	5	NA
194302	Acknowledges potential consequences of food insecurity	1	2	3	4	5	NA
194303	Acknowledges impact of food insecurity on health	1	2	3	4	5	NA
194304	Seeks current information on healthy food choices	1	2	3	4	5	NA
194305	Seeks current information on how to reduce food costs	1	2	3	4	5	NA
194306	Attends nutrition education classes	1	2	3	4	5	NA
194307	Identifies neighborhood food stores	1	2	3	4	5	NA
194308	Shares food needs with support network	1	2	3	4	5	NA
194309	Seeks assistance from supplemental nutrition assistance programs (SNAP)	1	2	3	4	5	NA
194310	Attends congregate meal sites	1	2	3	4	5	NA
194311	Uses local food pantries	1	2	3	4	5	NA
194312	Participates in senior meal delivery programs	1	2	3	4	5	NA
194313	Monitors body weight	1	2	3	4	5	NA
194314	Monitors changes in general health status	1	2	3	4	5	NA
194315	Uses available community resources	1	2	3	4	5	NA
194316	Acquires food for current short-term needs	1	2	3	4	5	NA
194317	Stabilizes access to food	1	2	3	4	5	NA

Domain-Health Knowledge & Behavior (IV)   *Class*-Risk Control (T)   7th edition 2024

OUTCOME CONTENT REFERENCES:

Ashby, S., Kleve, S., McKechnie, R., & Palermo, C. (2016). Measurement of the dimensions of food insecurity in developed countries: A systematic literature review. *Public Health Nutrition, 19*(16), 2887–2896. https://doi.org/10.1017/S1368980016001166

Banerjee, S., Radak, T., Khubchandani, J., & Dunn, P. (2021). Food insecurity and mortality in American adults: Results from the NHANES-linked mortality study. *Health Promotion Practice, 22*(2), 204–214. https://doi.org/10.1177/1524839920945927

Cockerham, M., Camel, S., James, L., & Neill, D. (2021). Food insecurity in baccalaureate nursing students: A cross-sectional survey. *Journal of Professional Nursing, 37*(2), 249–254. https://doi.org/10.1016/j.profnurs.2020.12.015

Coleman-Jensen, A., Rabbitt, C. A., & Singh, G. A. (2019). *Household food security in the United States in 2018.* U.S. Department of Agriculture Economic Research Service. https://www.ers.usda.gov/webdocs/publications/94849/err-270.pdf?v=963.1

Diallo, A. F., Falls, K., Hicks, K., Gibson, E. M., Obaid, R., Slattum, P., Zanjani, F., Price, E., & Parsons, P. (2020). The Healthy Meal Program: A food insecurity screening and referral program for urban dwelling older adults. *Public Health Nursing, 37,* 671–676. https://doi.org/10.1111/phn.12778

Dush, J. L. (2020). Adolescent food insecurity: A review of contextual and behavioral factors. *Public Health Nursing, 37,* 327–338. https://doi.org/10.1111/phn.12708

Hawkins, M., & Panzera, A. (2021). Food insecurity: A key determinant of health. *Archives of Psychiatric Nursing, 35,* 113–117. https://doi.org/10.1016/j.apnu.2020.10.01

+Johnson, C. M., Ammerman, A. S., Adair, L. S., Aiello, A. E., Flax, V. L., Elliott, S., Hardison-Moody, A., & Bowen, S. K. (2020). The Four Domain Food Insecurity Scale (4D-FIS): Development and evaluation of a complementary food insecurity measure. *Translational Behavioral Medicine, 10*(6), 1255–1265. https://doi.org/10.1093/tbm/ibaa125

Pinstrup-Andersen, P. (2009). Food security: Definition and measurement. *Food Security, 1,* 5–7. https://doi.org/10.1007/s12571-008-0002-y

Potter, P. A., & Perry, A. G. (2021). *Fundamentals of nursing* (10th ed.). Elsevier.

U.S. Department of Agriculture. (2019). *Definitions of food security.* https://www.ers.usda.gov/topics/food-nutrition-assistance/food-security-in-the-us/definitions-of-food-security.aspx

Risk Control: Hearing Impairment   1915

Definition: Personal actions to understand, prevent, eliminate, or reduce threats to hearing function

OUTCOME TARGET RATING: Maintain at_____ Increase to_____

		Never Demonstrated	Rarely Demonstrated	Sometimes Demonstrated	Often Demonstrated	Consistently Demonstrated	
OUTCOME OVERALL RATING		1	2	3	4	5	
Indicators:							
191513	Seeks current information about hearing impairment	1	2	3	4	5	NA
191514	Identifies risk factors for hearing impairment	1	2	3	4	5	NA
191515	Acknowledges personal risk factors for hearing impairment	1	2	3	4	5	NA
191501	Monitors symptoms of hearing deterioration	1	2	3	4	5	NA
191502	Protects eardrum integrity	1	2	3	4	5	NA
191503	Avoids trauma to the ear	1	2	3	4	5	NA
191504	Reduces noise exposure	1	2	3	4	5	NA
191517	Limits use of personal listening devices	1	2	3	4	5	NA
191516	Seeks assistance in removing excessive cerumen	1	2	3	4	5	NA
191506	Manages ear infections	1	2	3	4	5	NA
191507	Uses hearing protective devices	1	2	3	4	5	NA
191508	Obtains periodic ear examinations	1	2	3	4	5	NA
191509	Obtains periodic hearing tests	1	2	3	4	5	NA
191510	Uses ear medication as prescribed	1	2	3	4	5	NA
191511	Avoids placing objects in ear	1	2	3	4	5	NA

Domain-Health Knowledge & Behavior (IV)   **Class**-Risk Control (T)   2nd edition 2000; revised 2004, 2013, 2024

OUTCOME CONTENT REFERENCES:

Asghari, M. (2021). Tinnitus characteristics at high-and low-risk occupations from occupational noise expose standpoint. *The International Tinnitus Journal, 25*(1), 87–93. https://doi.org/10.5935/0946-5448.20210016

Butcher, E., Dezateux, C., & Knowles, R. L. (2020). Risk factors for permanent childhood hearing impairment. *Archives of Disease in Childhood, 105*(2), 187–189. https://doi.org/10.1136/archdischild-2018-315866

Crawford, K., Fethke, N. B., Peters, T. M., & Anthony, R. (2021). Assessment of occupational personal sound exposures for music instructors. *Journal of Occupational and Environmental Hygiene, 18*(3), 139–148. https://doi.org/10.1080/15459624.2020.1867729

Lee, H.-J., & Jeong, I. S. (2021). Personal listening device use habits, listening beliefs, and perceived change in hearing among adolescents. *Asian Nursing Research, 15,* 113–120. https://doi.org/10.1016/j.anr.2021.01.001

U.S. Preventive Services Task Force. (2021). Screening for hearing loss in older adults. U.S. Preventive Services Task Force Recommendation Statement. *Journal of the American Medical Association, 325* (12), 1–6. https://doi.org/10.1001/jama.2021.2566

Vos, B., Noll, D., Pigeon, M., Bagatto, M., & Fitzpatrick, E. M. (2019). Risk factors for hearing loss in children: A systematic literature review and meta-analysis protocol. *Systematic Reviews, 8*(1), 172. https://doi.org/10.1186/s13643-019-1073-x

Risk Control: Housing Insecurity   1944

Definition: Personal actions to understand, prevent, or reduce the threat of homelessness or inadequate living arrangements

OUTCOME TARGET RATING: Maintain at_____ Increase to_____

OUTCOME OVERALL RATING		Never Demonstrated	Rarely Demonstrated	Sometimes Demonstrated	Often Demonstrated	Consistently Demonstrated	
		1	2	3	4	5	
Indicators:							
194401	Acknowledges financial challenges	1	2	3	4	5	NA
194402	Ability to save money for housing expenses	1	2	3	4	5	NA
194403	Ability to pay rent or mortgage each month	1	2	3	4	5	NA
194404	Acknowledges personal risk of housing insecurity	1	2	3	4	5	NA
194405	Acknowledges potential consequences of housing insecurity	1	2	3	4	5	NA
194406	Acknowledges impact of housing insecurity on mental health	1	2	3	4	5	NA
194407	Acknowledges impact of housing insecurity on physical health	1	2	3	4	5	NA
194408	Acknowledges impact of housing insecurity on social support network	1	2	3	4	5	NA
194409	Seeks current information on safe housing options	1	2	3	4	5	NA
194410	Seeks current information on how to reduce housing costs	1	2	3	4	5	NA
194411	Seeks current information on housing subsidies available	1	2	3	4	5	NA
194412	Shares housing needs with support network	1	2	3	4	5	NA
194413	Solves problems with landlord of rental property	1	2	3	4	5	NA
194414	Recognizes difficulty of renting property as a pet owner	1	2	3	4	5	NA
194415	Recognizes difficulty of renting property without personal vehicle	1	2	3	4	5	NA
194416	Recognizes difficulty of renting property as a smoker	1	2	3	4	5	NA
194417	Uses community shelter facilities	1	2	3	4	5	NA
194418	Seeks housing with family members	1	2	3	4	5	NA
194419	Seeks housing with friends	1	2	3	4	5	NA
194420	Applies for government housing assistance	1	2	3	4	5	NA
194421	Uses available community resources	1	2	3	4	5	NA
194422	Uses temporary housing for short-term needs	1	2	3	4	5	NA
194423	Stabilizes housing arrangements	1	2	3	4	5	NA

Domain-Health Knowledge & Behavior (IV)   *Class*-Risk Control (T)   7th edition 2024

OUTCOME CONTENT REFERENCES:

Aurand, A., Emmanuel, D., Yentel, D., Errico, E., & Pang, M. (2018). *The gap: A shortage of affordable homes*. National Low Income Housing Coalition. https://nlihc.org/sites/default/files/gap/Gap-Report_2018.pdf

Carnemolla, P., & Skinner, V. (2021). Outcomes associated with providing secure, stable, and permanent housing for people who have been homeless: An international scoping review. *Journal of Planning Literature, 36*(4), 508–525. https://doi.org/10.1177/08854122211012911

Daoud, N., Matheson, F. I., Pedersen, C., Hamilton-Wright, S., Minh, A., Zhang, J., & O'Campo, P. (2016). Pathways and trajectories linking housing instability and poor health among low-income women experiencing intimate partner violence (IPV): Toward a conceptual framework. *Women & Health, 56*(2), 208–225. https://doi.org/10.1080/03630242.2015.1086465

Darab, S., Hartman, Y., & Holdsworth, L. (2017). What women want: Single older women and their housing preferences. *Housing Studies, 33*(4), 525–543. https://doi.org/10.1080/02673037.2017.1359501

Grenier, A., Barken, R., Sussman, T., Rothwell, D., Bourgeois-Guerin, V., & Lavoie, J. P. (2016). Homelessness among older people: Assessing strategies and frameworks across Canada. *Canadian Review of Social Policy, 74*, 1–39.

Hoke, M. K., & Boen, C. E. (2021). The health impacts of eviction: Evidence from the national longitudinal study of adolescent to adult health. *Social Science & Medicine, 273*, 113742. https://doi.org/10.1016/j.socscimed.2021.113742

Kang, S. (2021). Beyond households: Regional determinants of housing instability among low-income renters in the United States. *Housing Studies, 36*(1), 80–109. https://doi.org/10.1080/02673037.2019.1676402

Martin, P., Liaw, W., Bazemore, A., Jetty, A., Petterson, S., & Kushel, M. (2019). Adults with housing insecurity have worse access to primary and preventive care. *Journal of the American Board of Family Medicine: JABFM, 32*(4), 521–530. https://doi.org/10.3122/jabfm.2019.04.180374

O'Campo, P., Daoud, N., Hamilton-Wright, S., & Dunn, J. (2016). Conceptualizing housing instability: Experiences with material and psychological instability among women living with partner violence. *Housing Studies, 31*(1), 1–19. https://doi.org/10.1080/02673037. 2015

O'Neil, K., Aubrecht, K., & Keefe, J. (2021). Dimensions of housing insecurity for older women living with a low income. *Journal of Aging and Environment, 35*(1), 1–27. https://doi.org/10.1080/26892618.2020.1744498

Power, E. R. (2017). Renting with pets: A pathway to housing insecurity? *Housing Studies, 32*(3), 336–360. https://doi.org/10.1080/02673037.2016.1210095

Stanhope, M., & Lancaster, J. (2020). *Public health nursing: Population-centered health care in the community* (10th ed.). Elsevier.

Risk Control: Hypertension

1928

Definition: Personal actions to understand, prevent, eliminate, or reduce the threat of high blood pressure

OUTCOME TARGET RATING: Maintain at_____ Increase to_____

		Never Demonstrated	Rarely Demonstrated	Sometimes Demonstrated	Often Demonstrated	Consistently Demonstrated	
OUTCOME OVERALL RATING		1	2	3	4	5	
Indicators:							
192801	Seeks current information about hypertension	1	2	3	4	5	NA
192802	Identifies risk factors for hypertension	1	2	3	4	5	NA
192803	Acknowledges personal risk factors for hypertension	1	2	3	4	5	NA
192804	Acknowledges ability to change behavior	1	2	3	4	5	NA
192805	Identifies signs and symptoms of hypertension	1	2	3	4	5	NA
192806	Checks blood pressure at recommended intervals	1	2	3	4	5	NA
192807	Monitors health status changes	1	2	3	4	5	NA
192808	Follows dietary recommendations	1	2	3	4	5	NA
192809	Adheres to sodium intake recommendations	1	2	3	4	5	NA
192810	Maintains recommended body weight	1	2	3	4	5	NA
192811	Participates in regular exercise	1	2	3	4	5	NA
192812	Uses relaxation techniques	1	2	3	4	5	NA
192813	Uses strategies to facilitate sleep	1	2	3	4	5	NA
192814	Uses strategies to reduce stress	1	2	3	4	5	NA
192815	Monitors medication effects that influence blood pressure	1	2	3	4	5	NA
192816	Eliminates tobacco use	1	2	3	4	5	NA
192817	Consumes alcohol in moderation	1	2	3	4	5	NA
192818	Consumes caffeine in moderation	1	2	3	4	5	NA
192819	Monitors changes in general health status	1	2	3	4	5	NA
192820	Uses health care services to screen for hypertension	1	2	3	4	5	NA
192821	Uses personal support systems to modify lifestyle	1	2	3	4	5	NA
192822	Uses community resources to reduce hypertension risk	1	2	3	4	5	NA

Domain-Health Knowledge & Behavior (IV)   **Class**-Risk Control (T)   5th edition 2013: reviewed 2024

OUTCOME CONTENT REFERENCES:

Mancia, G., Masi, S., Palatini, P., Tsioufis, C., & Grassi, G. (2021). Elevated heart rate and cardiovascular risk in hypertension. *Journal of Hypertension*, *39*(6), 1060–1069. https://doi.org/10.1097/HJH.0000000000002760

Moroi, M. K., Ruzieh, M., Ahmed, A., Kanjwal, S., & Kanjwal, K. (2021). Preventions and management of supine hypertension in patients with orthostatic hypotension. *American Journal of Therapeutics, 28*, e228-e231. https://doi.org/10.1097/MJT.0000000000001054

Putra, M., Balasooriya, M. M., Boscia, A. L., Dalkiran, E., & Sokol, R. (2021). The impact of the new hypertension guidelines to low-dose aspirin prophylaxis eligibility for the prevention of preeclampsia: A cost-benefit analysis. *American Journal of Perinatology, 38*, 363–369. https://doi.org/10.1055/s-0039-1697588

U.S. Preventive Services Task Force. (2021). Screening for hypertension in adults. U.S. Preventive Services Task Force Reaffirmation Statement. *Journal of the American Medical Association, 325*(16), 1–7. https://doi.org/10.1001/jama.2021.4987

Risk Control: Hyperthermia   1922

Definition: Personal actions to understand, prevent, eliminate, or reduce the threat of high body temperature

OUTCOME TARGET RATING: Maintain at_____ Increase to_____

		Never Demonstrated	Rarely Demonstrated	Sometimes Demonstrated	Often Demonstrated	Consistently Demonstrated	
OUTCOME OVERALL RATING		1	2	3	4	5	
Indicators:							
192220	Seeks current information about hyperthermia	1	2	3	4	5	NA
192221	Identifies risk factors for hyperthermia	1	2	3	4	5	NA
192201	Acknowledges personal risk factors for hyperthermia	1	2	3	4	5	NA
192202	Identifies signs and symptoms of hyperthermia	1	2	3	4	5	NA
192203	Identifies health conditions that accelerate heat production	1	2	3	4	5	NA
192222	Monitors environment for factors that increase body temperature	1	2	3	4	5	NA
192206	Identifies relationship of age to body temperature	1	2	3	4	5	NA
192207	Modifies living environment to control body temperature	1	2	3	4	5	NA
192223	Monitors changes in general health status	1	2	3	4	5	NA
192208	Modifies fluid intake as appropriate	1	2	3	4	5	NA
192209	Modifies physical activity to control body temperature	1	2	3	4	5	NA
192210	Wears appropriate clothing to protect skin	1	2	3	4	5	NA
192211	Maintains intact skin integument	1	2	3	4	5	NA
192212	Participates in screening for health problems that increase risk	1	2	3	4	5	NA
192213	Performs self-protective actions to control body temperature	1	2	3	4	5	NA
192214	Identifies prescribed medication effects on body temperature	1	2	3	4	5	NA
192215	Avoids strenuous activities to reduce risk	1	2	3	4	5	NA
192216	Avoids alcohol consumption	1	2	3	4	5	NA
192217	Uses community shelters to reduce risk	1	2	3	4	5	NA
192218	Performs outdoor activities at coolest part of day	1	2	3	4	5	NA
192219	Allows for acclimatization to warmer temperatures	1	2	3	4	5	NA

Domain-*Health Knowledge & Behavior (IV)*   **Class**-*Risk Control (T)*   *4th edition 2008; revised 2013; reviewed 2024*

R

OUTCOME CONTENT REFERENCES:

Bouchama, A., Abuyassin, B., Lehe, C., Laitano, O., Jay, O., O'Connor, F. G., & Leon, L. R. (2022). Classic and exertional heatstroke. *Nature Reviews. Disease Primers, 8*(1), 8. https://doi.org/10.1038/s41572-021-00334-6

Douma, M. J., Aves, T., Allan, K. S., Bendall, J. C., Berry, D. C., Chang, W. T., Epstein, J., Hood, N., Singletary, E. M., Zideman, D., Lin, S., & First Aid Task Force of the International Liaison Committee on Resuscitation. (2020). First aid cooling techniques for heat stroke and exertional hyperthermia: A systematic review and meta-analysis. *Resuscitation, 148*, 173–190. https://doi.org/10.1016/j.resuscitation.2020.01.007

Foster, J., Hodder, S. G., Lloyd, A. B., & Havenith, G. (2020). Individual responses to heat stress: Implications for hyperthermia and physical work capacity. *Frontiers in Physiology, 11*, 541483. https://doi.org/10.3389/fphys.2020.541483

Gleich, S. J., Strupp, K., Wilder, R. T., Kor, D. J., & Flick, R. (2016). An automated real-time method for the detection of patients at risk for malignant hyperthermia. *Paediatric Anaesthesia, 26*(9), 876–882. https://doi.org/10.1111/pan.12954

Hall, C., Ha, S., Yen, I. H., & Goldman-Mellor, S. (2021). Risk factors for hyperthermia mortality among emergency department patients. *Annals of Epidemiology, 64*, 90–95. https://doi.org/10.1016/j.annepidem.2021.09.009

Kare, J., & Shneiderman, A. (2001). Hyperthermia and hypothermia in the older population. *Topics in Emergency Medicine, 23*(3), 39–52.

McLafferty, E. (2010). Prevention and management of hyperthermia during a heat wave. *Nursing Older People, 22*(7), 23–27.

McLaren, C., Null, J., & Quinn, J. (2005). Heat stress from enclosed vehicles: Moderate ambient temperatures cause significant temperature rise in enclosed vehicles. *Pediatrics, 116*(1), 109–112. https://doi.org/10.1542/peds.2004-2368

Nixdorf-Miller, A., Hunsaker, D. M., & Hunsaker, J. C., III. (2006). Hypothermia and hyperthermia medicolegal investigation of morbidity and mortality from exposure to environmental temperature extremes. *Archives of Pathologic Laboratory Medicine, 130*(9), 1297–1304. https://doi.org/10.5858/2006-130-1297-HAHMIO

Wood, L. (2004). Heat resistant: How to identify the rationale with which to support the frequency and type of health monitoring of employees, in relation to heat exposure in their working roles. *Occupational Health, 56*(7), 25–30.

Risk Control: Hypotension   1933

Definition: Personal actions to understand, prevent, eliminate, or reduce the threat of low blood pressure

OUTCOME TARGET RATING: Maintain at_____ Increase to_____

	Never Demonstrated	Rarely Demonstrated	Sometimes Demonstrated	Often Demonstrated	Consistently Demonstrated	
OUTCOME OVERALL RATING	1	2	3	4	5	
Indicators:						
193301 Seeks current information about hypotension	1	2	3	4	5	NA
193302 Identifies risk factors for hypotension	1	2	3	4	5	NA
193303 Identifies signs and symptoms of hypotension	1	2	3	4	5	NA
193304 Identifies signs and symptoms of shock	1	2	3	4	5	NA
193305 Monitors blood pressure at recommended intervals	1	2	3	4	5	NA
193306 Identifies tolerance for low blood pressure	1	2	3	4	5	NA
193307 Develops effective strategies to take medication as prescribed	1	2	3	4	5	NA
193308 Report episodes of lightheadedness or dizziness to health provider	1	2	3	4	5	NA
193309 Monitors frequency of hypotensive episodes	1	2	3	4	5	NA
193310 Monitors for orthostatic hypotension when changing positions	1	2	3	4	5	NA
193311 Avoids standing for long periods of time	1	2	3	4	5	NA
193312 Wears compression stockings	1	2	3	4	5	NA
193313 Maintains hydration	1	2	3	4	5	NA
193314 Eats frequent low-carbohydrate meals	1	2	3	4	5	NA
193315 Includes more sodium in diet	1	2	3	4	5	NA
193316 Includes caffeinated drinks with meals	1	2	3	4	5	NA
193317 Acknowledges risk for hypotension when taking pain medication	1	2	3	4	5	NA
193318 Acknowledges risk for hypotension when taking antidepressants	1	2	3	4	5	NA
193319 Commits to alcohol use control strategies	1	2	3	4	5	NA
193320 Acknowledges higher risk for falls with hypertension medication	1	2	3	4	5	NA

Domain-Health Knowledge & Behavior (IV)   *Class*-Risk Control (T)   5th edition 2013; reviewed 2024

OUTCOME CONTENT REFERENCES:

Biaggioni I. (2018). Orthostatic hypotension in the hypertensive patient. *American Journal of Hypertension*, *31*(12), 1255–1259. https://doi.org/10.1093/ajh/hpy089

Fanciulli, A., Leys, F., Falup-Pecurariu, C., Thijs, R., & Wenning, G. K. (2020). Management of orthostatic hypotension in Parkinson's disease. *Journal of Parkinson's Disease*, *10*(Suppl. 1), S57–S64. https://doi.org/10.3233/JPD-202036

Koudelka, M., & Sovová, E. (2021). COVID-19 causing hypotension in frail geriatric hypertensive patients? *Medicina* (Kaunas, Lithuania), *57*(6), 633. https://doi.org/10.3390/medicina57060633

Potter, P. A., Perry, A. G., Stockert, P. A., & Hall, A. (2021). *Fundamentals of Nursing* (10th ed.). Elsevier.

Rivasi, G., Rafanelli, M., Mossello, E., Brignole, M., & Ungar, A. (2020). Drug-related orthostatic hypotension: Beyond anti-hypertensive medications. *Drugs & Aging*, *37*(10), 725–738. https://doi.org/10.1007/s40266-020-00796-5

Rivasi, G., & Ungar, A. (2020). Orthostatic hypotension in older adults: The role of medications. *Monaldi Archives for Chest Disease*, *90*(4), 1254. https://doi.org/10.4081/monaldi.2020.1254

Risk Control: Hypothermia   1923

Definition: Personal actions to understand, prevent, eliminate, or reduce the threat of low body temperature

OUTCOME TARGET RATING: Maintain at_____ Increase to_____

		Never Demonstrated	Rarely Demonstrated	Sometimes Demonstrated	Often Demonstrated	Consistently Demonstrated	
OUTCOME OVERALL RATING		1	2	3	4	5	
Indicators:							
192319	Seeks current information about hypothermia	1	2	3	4	5	NA
192320	Identifies risk factors for hypothermia	1	2	3	4	5	NA
192301	Acknowledges personal risk factors for hypothermia	1	2	3	4	5	NA
192302	Identifies signs and symptoms of hypothermia	1	2	3	4	5	NA
192303	Identifies health conditions that decrease heat production	1	2	3	4	5	NA
192304	Identifies conditions that jeopardize ability to conserve heat	1	2	3	4	5	NA
192305	Identifies health conditions that accelerate heat loss	1	2	3	4	5	NA
192321	Monitors environment for factors that decrease body temperature	1	2	3	4	5	NA
192307	Identifies relationship of age to body temperature	1	2	3	4	5	NA
192319	Identifies relationship of body mass to body temperature	1	2	3	4	5	NA
192322	Monitors changes in general health status	1	2	3	4	5	NA
192308	Modifies living environment to promote heat conservation	1	2	3	4	5	NA
192309	Modifies physical activity to maintain body temperature	1	2	3	4	5	NA
192310	Maintains emergency cold weather supplies in vehicle	1	2	3	4	5	NA
192311	Maintains intact skin integument	1	2	3	4	5	NA
192312	Participates in screening for health problems that increase risk	1	2	3	4	5	NA
192319	Limits time in cold environment	1	2	3	4	5	NA
192313	Performs self-protective actions to control body temperature	1	2	3	4	5	NA
192314	Modifies fluid intake as appropriate	1	2	3	4	5	NA
192315	Wears appropriate clothing to protect skin	1	2	3	4	5	NA

R

Continued

Risk Control: Hypothermia—cont'd

		Never Demonstrated	Rarely Demonstrated	Sometimes Demonstrated	Often Demonstrated	Consistently Demonstrated	
192316	Performs outdoor activities at warmest part of day	1	2	3	4	5	NA
192317	Identifies prescribed medication effects on body temperature	1	2	3	4	5	NA
192318	Allows for acclimatization to colder temperatures	1	2	3	4	5	NA

Domain-*Health Knowledge & Behavior (IV)* **Class**-*Risk Control (T)* 4th edition 2008; revised 2013, 2024

OUTCOME CONTENT REFERENCES:

Drigny, J., Rolland, M., Pla, R., Chesneau, C., Lebreton, T., Marais, B., Outin, P., Moussay, S., Racinais, S., & Mauvieux, B. (2021). Risk factors and predictors of hypothermia and dropouts during open-water swimming competitions. *International Journal of Sports Physiology and Performance, 16,* 1692–1699. https://doi.org/10.1123/ijspp.2020-0875

Fudge, J. (2016). Preventing and managing hypothermia and frostbite injury. *Sports Health, 8*(2), 133–139. https://doi.org/10.1177/1941738116630542

Min, J. Y., Choi, Y. S., Lee, H. S., Lee, S., & Min, K. B. (2021). Increased cold injuries and the effect of body mass index in patients with peripheral vascular disease. *BMC Public Health, 21*(1), 294. https://doi.org/10.1186/s12889-020-09789-w

Oshiro, K., Tanioka, Y., Schweizer, J., Zafren, K., Brugger, H., & Paal, P. (2022). Prevention of hypothermia in the aftermath of natural disasters in areas at risk of avalanches, earthquakes, tsunamis and floods. *International Journal of Environmental Research and Public Health, 19*(3), 1098. https://doi.org/10.3390/ijerph19031098

Rathjen, N. A., Shahbodaghi, S. D., & Brown, J. A. (2019). Hypothermia and cold weather injuries. *American Family Physician, 100*(11), 680–686.

Risk Control: Infant Allergies   **1940**

Definition: Parental actions to prevent the onset of eczema and food allergies in an infant

OUTCOME TARGET RATING: Maintain at_____ Increase to_____

		Never Demonstrated	Rarely Demonstrated	Sometimes Demonstrated	Often Demonstrated	Consistently Demonstrated	
OUTCOME OVERALL RATING		1	2	3	4	5	
Indicators:							
194001	Shares family history of allergy with health providers	1	2	3	4	5	NA
19402	Explains the relationship between eczema and allergy development	1	2	3	4	5	NA
194003	Prevents skin barrier interruption	1	2	3	4	5	NA
194004	Applies moisturizer daily to prevent eczema in high-risk infants	1	2	3	4	5	NA
194005	Identifies the common food allergens	1	2	3	4	5	NA
194006	Introduces new foods one at a time from 4 to 6 months of age	1	2	3	4	5	NA
194007	Introduces new foods in home environment	1	2	3	4	5	NA
194008	Introduces peanut, egg, and cow's milk in diet progression	1	2	3	4	5	NA
194009	Exposes tolerated allergic foods regularly once introduced	1	2	3	4	5	NA
194010	Rotates foods in diet using a 4-day cycle	1	2	3	4	5	NA
194011	Avoids genetically modified foods	1	2	3	4	5	NA
194012	Avoids foods in the same food family as a known allergen	1	2	3	4	5	NA
194013	Avoids processed foods with a long list of ingredients	1	2	3	4	5	NA
194014	Seeks assistance from an allergist for high-risk infants	1	2	3	4	5	NA

Domain-*Health Knowledge & Behavior (IV)* **Class**-*Risk Control (T)* 6th edition 2018; reviewed 2024

OUTCOME CONTENT REFERENCES:

Abrams, E., & Becker, A. (2015). Food introduction and allergy prevention in infants. *CMAJ: Canadian Medical Association Journal, 187*(17), 1297–1301. https://doi.org/10.1503/cmaj.150364

Güngör, D., Nadaud, P., LaPergola, C. C., Dreibelbis, C., Wong, Y. P., Terry, N., Abrams, S. A., Beker, L., Jacobovits, T., Järvinen, K. M., Nommsen-Rivers, L. A., O'Brien, K. O., Oken, E., Pérez-Escamilla, R., Ziegler, E. E., & Spahn, J. M. (2019). Infant milk-feeding practices and food allergies, allergic rhinitis, atopic dermatitis, and asthma throughout the life span: A systematic review. *The American Journal of Clinical Nutrition, 109*(Suppl. 7), 772S–799S. https://doi.org/10.1093/ajcn/nqy283

Gupta, R. S., Warren, C. M., Smith, B. M., Blumenstock, J. A., Jiang, J., Davis, M. M., & Nadeau, K. C. (2018). The public health impact of parent-reported childhood food allergies in the United States. *Pediatrics, 142*(6), e20181235. https://doi.org/10.1542/peds.2018-1235

Koksal, B. T., Barıs, Z., Ozcay, F., & Yilmaz Ozbek, O. (2018). Single and multiple food allergies in infants with proctocolitis. *Allergologia et Immunopathologia, 46*(1), 3–8. https://doi.org/10.1016/j.aller.2017.02.006

Sicherer, S. H., Warren, C. M., Dant, C., Gupta, R. S., & Nadeau, K. C. (2020). Food allergy from infancy through adulthood. *The Journal of Allergy and Clinical Immunology. In Practice, 8*(6), 1854–1864. https://doi.org/10.1016/j.jaip.2020.02.010

Skypala, I., & Vlieg-Boerstra, B. (2014). Food intolerance and allergy: Increased incidence or contemporary inadequate diets? *Current Opinion in Clinical Nutrition & Metabolic Care, 17*(5), 442–447. https://doi.org/10.1097/MCO.0000000000000086

Smith, M. (2015). The facts about food allergies. *Better Nutrition, 77*(8), 50–52.

Waserman, S. (2016). Doctor, can we prevent food allergy and eczema in our baby? *Current Opinion in Allergy & Clinical Immunology, 16*(3), 265–271. https://doi.org/10.1097/ACI.0000000000000267

Risk Control: Infectious Process   1924

Definition: Personal actions to understand, prevent, eliminate, or reduce the threat of acquiring an infection

OUTCOME TARGET RATING: Maintain at_____ Increase to_____

		Never Demonstrated	Rarely Demonstrated	Sometimes Demonstrated	Often Demonstrated	Consistently Demonstrated	
OUTCOME OVERALL RATING		1	2	3	4	5	
Indicators:							
192425	Seeks current information about infection control	1	2	3	4	5	NA
192426	Identifies risk factors for infection	1	2	3	4	5	NA
192401	Acknowledges personal risk factors for infection	1	2	3	4	5	NA
192402	Acknowledges consequences associated with infection	1	2	3	4	5	NA
192403	Acknowledges behaviors associated with risk for infection	1	2	3	4	5	NA
192404	Identifies infection risk in daily activities	1	2	3	4	5	NA
192427	Identifies risk from contact with animals	1	2	3	4	5	NA
192405	Identifies signs and symptoms of infection	1	2	3	4	5	NA
192406	Seeks validation of perceived infection risk	1	2	3	4	5	NA
192407	Identifies strategies to protect self from others with infection	1	2	3	4	5	NA
192408	Monitors personal behaviors for factors associated with infection risk	1	2	3	4	5	NA
192409	Monitors environment for factors associated with infection risk	1	2	3	4	5	NA
192410	Monitors time of infectious disease incubation period	1	2	3	4	5	NA
192428	Restricts contact with family members who are infected	1	2	3	4	5	NA
192411	Maintains a clean environment	1	2	3	4	5	NA
192412	Uses strategies to disinfect supplies	1	2	3	4	5	NA
192413	Develops effective infection control strategies	1	2	3	4	5	NA
192414	Uses universal precautions	1	2	3	4	5	NA

R

Continued

Risk Control: Infectious Process—cont'd

		Never Demonstrated	Rarely Demonstrated	Sometimes Demonstrated	Often Demonstrated	Consistently Demonstrated	
192429	Follows guidance from public health experts	1	2	3	4	5	NA
192415	Practices hand sanitization	1	2	3	4	5	NA
192416	Practices infection control strategies	1	2	3	4	5	NA
192417	Adjusts infection control strategies	1	2	3	4	5	NA
192420	Monitors changes in general health status	1	2	3	4	5	NA
192421	Takes immediate actions to reduce risk	1	2	3	4	5	NA
192422	Obtains recommended immunizations	1	2	3	4	5	NA
192423	Uses reputable sources of information	1	2	3	4	5	NA
192424	Uses health care services congruent with needs	1	2	3	4	5	NA
192427	Seeks information on health risks prior to travel	1	2	3	4	5	NA

Domain-Health Knowledge & Behavior (IV)   *Class*-Risk Control (T)   4th edition 2008; revised 2013, 2024

OUTCOME CONTENT REFERENCES:

Aleksejeva, V., Dovbenko, A., Kroiča, J., & Skadiņš, I. (2021). Toys in the playrooms of children's hospitals: A potential source of nosocomial bacterial infections? *Children* (Basel, Switzerland), 8(10), 914. https://doi.org/10.3390/children8100914

Chaabna, K., Doraiswamy, S., Mamtani, R., & Cheema, S. (2021). Facemask use in community settings to prevent respiratory infection transmission: A rapid review and meta-analysis. *International Journal of Infectious Diseases, 104,* 198–206. https://doi.org/10.1016/j.ijid.2020.09.1434

Krein, S. L., Olmsted, R. N., Hofer, T. P., Kowalski, C., Forman, J., Banaszak, J., & Saint, S. (2006). Translating infection prevention evidence into practice using quantitative and qualitative research. *American Journal of Infection Control, 34,* 507–512. https://doi.org/10.1016/j.ajic.2005.05.017

Li, H., Yuan, K., Sun, Y. K., Zheng, Y. B., Xu, Y. Y., Su, S. Z., Zhang, Y. X., Zhong, Y., Wang, Y. J., Tian, S. S., Gong, Y. M., Fan, T. T., Lin, X., Gobat, N., Wong, S., Chan, E., Yan, W., Sun, S. W., Ran, M. S., Bao, Y. P., & Lu, L. (2022). Efficacy and practice of facemask use in general population: A systematic review and meta-analysis. *Translational Psychiatry, 12*(1), 49. https://doi.org/10.1038/s41398-022-01814-3

McGuckin, M., Storr, J. A., & Govednik, J. (2021). Patient awareness of healthcare-associated infection risk and prevention: Has there been a change in 3 decades (1989-2019)? *American Journal of Infection Control, 49*(11), 1448–1449. https://doi.org/10.1016/j.ajic.2021.05.009

Mahon, M. M., Sheehan, M. C., Kelleher, P. F., Johnson, A. J., & Doyle, S. M. (2017). An assessment of Irish farmers' knowledge of the risk of spread of infection from animals to humans and their transmission prevention practices. *Epidemiology and Infection, 145*(12), 2424–2435. https://doi.org/10.1017/S0950268817001418

Querido, M. M., Aguiar, L., Neves, P., Pereira, C. C., & Teixeira, J. P. (2019). Self-disinfecting surfaces and infection control. *Colloids and Surfaces. Biointerfaces, 178,* 8–21. https://doi.org/10.1016/j.colsurfb.2019.02.009

Risk Control: Lipid Disorder

1929

Definition: Personal actions to understand, prevent, eliminate, or reduce the threat of hyperlipidemia

OUTCOME TARGET RATING: Maintain at_____ Increase to_____

		Never Demonstrated	Rarely Demonstrated	Sometimes Demonstrated	Often Demonstrated	Consistently Demonstrated	
OUTCOME OVERALL RATING		**1**	**2**	**3**	**4**	**5**	
Indicators:							
192901	Seeks current information about lipid disorders	1	2	3	4	5	NA
192902	Identifies risk factors for lipid disorders	1	2	3	4	5	NA
192903	Acknowledges personal risk factors for lipid disorder	1	2	3	4	5	NA
192904	Modifies lifestyle to reduce risk	1	2	3	4	5	NA
192905	Develops effective risk control strategies	1	2	3	4	5	NA
192906	Commits to risk control strategies	1	2	3	4	5	NA
192907	Monitors changes in general health status	1	2	3	4	5	NA

R

Risk Control: Lipid Disorder—cont'd

		Never Demonstrated	Rarely Demonstrated	Sometimes Demonstrated	Often Demonstrated	Consistently Demonstrated	
192908	Participates in aerobic exercise	1	2	3	4	5	NA
192909	Follows dietary recommendations	1	2	3	4	5	NA
192910	Maintains recommended body weight	1	2	3	4	5	NA
192911	Avoids tobacco use	1	2	3	4	5	NA
192912	Obtains prescribed laboratory tests	1	2	3	4	5	NA
192913	Uses medication as prescribed	1	2	3	4	5	NA
192914	Uses significant others to support behavior changes	1	2	3	4	5	NA
192915	Uses reputable sources of information	1	2	3	4	5	NA
192916	Uses community resources to identify lipid disorder risk	1	2	3	4	5	NA

Domain-Health Knowledge & Behavior (IV)   *Class*-Risk Control (T)   5th edition 2013; reviewed 2024

OUTCOME CONTENT REFERENCES:

Bertolotti, M., Lancellotti, G., & Mussi, C. (2019). Management of high cholesterol levels in older people. *Geriatrics & Gerontology International*, *19*(5), 375–383. https://doi.org/10.1111/ggi.13647

Gatti, A., Maranghi, M., Bacci, S., Carallo, C., Gnasso, A., Mandosi, E., Fallarino, M., Morano, S., Trischitta, V., & Filetti, S. (2009). Poor glycemic control is an independent risk factor for low HDL cholesterol in patients with type 2 diabetes. *Diabetes Care, 32*(8), 1550–1552. https://doi.org/10.2337/dc09-0256

Hemmer, A., Mareschal, J., Dibner, C., Pralong, J. A., Dorribo, V., Perrig, S., Genton, L., Pichard, C., & Collet, T.-H. (2021). The effects of shift work on cardio-metabolic diseases and eating patterns. *Nutrients, 13*, 1–15. https://doi.org/10.3390/nu131141780/nu13114178

Michos, E. D., McEvoy, J. W., & Blumenthal, R. S. (2019). Lipid management for the prevention of atherosclerotic cardiovascular disease. *The New England Journal of Medicine, 381*(16), 1557–1567. https://doi.org/10.1056/NEJMra1806939

Sarraju, A., Ward, A., Li, J., Valencia, A., Palaniappan, L., Scheinker, D., & Rodriguez, F. (2022). Personalizing cholesterol treatment recommendations for primary cardiovascular disease prevention. *Scientific Reports, 12*(1), 23. https://doi.org/10.1038/s41598-021-03796-6

Sobhani, S. R., Mortazavi, M., Kazemifar, M., & Azadbakht, L. (2021). The association between fast-food consumption with cardiovascular diseases risk factors and kidney function in patients with diabetic nephropathy. *Journal of Cardiovascular and Thoracic Research, 13*(3), 241–249. https//doi.org/10.34172/jcvtr.2021.42

Risk Control: Obesity   1941

Definition: Personal actions to understand, prevent, or reduce the threat of obesity

OUTCOME TARGET RATING: Maintain at_____ Increase to_____

		Never Demonstrated	Rarely Demonstrated	Sometimes Demonstrated	Often Demonstrated	Consistently Demonstrated	
OUTCOME OVERALL RATING		1	2	3	4	5	
Indicators:							
194101	Acknowledges personal risk factors	1	2	3	4	5	NA
194102	Acknowledges consequences of obesity	1	2	3	4	5	NA
194103	Obtains reputable information about obesity	1	2	3	4	5	NA
194104	Commits to healthy eating plan	1	2	3	4	5	NA
194105	Monitors body weight regularly	1	2	3	4	5	NA
194106	Monitors factors that encourage overeating	1	2	3	4	5	NA
194107	Monitors personal eating pattern	1	2	3	4	5	NA
194108	Monitors family eating pattern	1	2	3	4	5	NA
194109	Monitors food portions to maintain healthy weight	1	2	3	4	5	NA
194110	Chooses healthy food	1	2	3	4	5	NA
194111	Prepares healthy meals	1	2	3	4	5	NA

R

Continued

Risk Control: Obesity—cont'd

	Never Demonstrated	Rarely Demonstrated	Sometimes Demonstrated	Often Demonstrated	Consistently Demonstrated	
194112 Eats breakfast every day	1	2	3	4	5	NA
194113 Chooses healthy snacks	1	2	3	4	5	NA
194114 Drinks water for adequate hydration	1	2	3	4	5	NA
194115 Adjusts recipes to decrease calories	1	2	3	4	5	NA
194116 Reads food labels for nutritional content	1	2	3	4	5	NA
194117 Introduces healthy new items into diet	1	2	3	4	5	NA
194118 Makes healthy choices when eating out	1	2	3	4	5	NA
194119 Avoids high-caloric food	1	2	3	4	5	NA
194120 Limits consumption of high-caloric fluid	1	2	3	4	5	NA
194121 Limits saturated fat intake	1	2	3	4	5	NA
194122 Avoids use of weight loss medication	1	2	3	4	5	NA
194123 Participates in regular exercise	1	2	3	4	5	NA
194124 Maintains healthy sleep routine	1	2	3	4	5	NA
194125 Obtains advice from a health professional for weight loss strategies	1	2	3	4	5	NA
194126 Uses available community resources to increase activity	1	2	3	4	5	NA

Domain-Health Knowledge & Behavior (IV)   **Class**-Risk Control (T)   6th edition 2018; reviewed 2024

OUTCOME CONTENT REFERENCES:

Dabas, A., & Seth, A. (2018). Prevention and management of childhood obesity. *Indian Journal of Pediatrics, 85*(7), 546–553. https://doi.org/10.1007/s12098-018-2636-x

Demir, D., & Bektas, M. (2021). The effect of an obesity prevention program on children's eating behaviors, food addiction, physical activity, and obesity status. *Journal of Pediatric Nursing, 61*, 355–363. https://doi.org/10.1016/j.pedn.2021.09.001

Elagizi, A., Kachur, S., Carbone, S., Lavie, C. J., & Blair, S. N. (2020). A review of obesity, physical activity, and cardiovascular disease. *Current Obesity Reports, 9*(4), 571–581. https://doi.org/10.1007/s13679-020-00403-z

Franco, L., Morais, C., & Cominetti, C. (2016). Normal-weight obesity syndrome: Diagnosis, prevalence, and clinical implications. *Nutrition Reviews, 74*(9), 558–570. https://doi.org/10.1093/nutrit/nuw019

Golden, N., Schneider, M., & Wood, C. (2016). Preventing obesity and eating disorders in adolescents. *Pediatrics, 138*(3), e1–e10. https://doi.org/10.1542/peds.2016-1649

Lanigan, J. (2018). Prevention of overweight and obesity in early life. *The Proceedings of the Nutrition Society, 77*(3), 247–256. https://doi.org/10.1017/S0029665118000411

Sal, S., & Bektas, M. (2022). Effectiveness of obesity prevention program developed for secondary school students. *American Journal of Health Education, 53*(1), 45–55. https://doi.org/10.1080/19325037.2021.2001774

Smith, J. D., Fu, E., & Kobayashi, M. A. (2020). Prevention and management of childhood obesity and its psychological and health comorbidities. *Annual Review of Clinical Psychology, 16*, 351–378. https://doi.org/10.1146/annurev-clinpsy-100219-060201

Tamayo, M. C., Dobbs, P. D., & Pincu, Y. (2021). Family-centered interventions for treatment and prevention of childhood obesity in Hispanic families: A systematic review. *Journal of Community Health, 46*(3), 635–643. https://doi.org/10.1007/s10900-020-00897-7

Thomas, A., & Janusek, L. (2018). Obesity prevention behaviors in Asian Indian adolescent girls: A pilot study. *Journal of Pediatric Nursing, 42*, 9–15. https://doi.org/10.1016/j.pedn.2018.05.007

Weihrauch-Blüher, S., Kromeyer-Hauschild, K., Graf, C., Widhalm, K., Korsten-Reck, U., Jödicke, B., Markert, J., Müller, M. J., Moss, A., Wabitsch, M., & Wiegand, S. (2018). Current guidelines for obesity prevention in childhood and adolescence. *Obesity Facts, 11*(3), 263–276. https://doi.org/10.1159/000486512

R

Risk Control: Osteoporosis 1930

Definition: Personal actions to understand, prevent, eliminate, or reduce the threat of osteoporosis

OUTCOME TARGET RATING: Maintain at_____ Increase to_____

		Never Demonstrated	Rarely Demonstrated	Sometimes Demonstrated	Often Demonstrated	Consistently Demonstrated	
OUTCOME OVERALL RATING		1	2	3	4	5	
Indicators:							
193001	Seeks current information about osteoporosis	1	2	3	4	5	NA
193002	Identifies risk factors for osteoporosis	1	2	3	4	5	NA
193003	Acknowledges personal risk factors for osteoporosis	1	2	3	4	5	NA
193004	Monitors personal risk factors	1	2	3	4	5	NA
193005	Selects foods that provide calcium to meet requirement	1	2	3	4	5	NA
193006	Uses calcium supplements within recommended guidelines	1	2	3	4	5	NA
193007	Uses vitamin D supplements within recommended guidelines	1	2	3	4	5	NA
193008	Avoids alcohol misuse	1	2	3	4	5	NA
193009	Avoids tobacco use	1	2	3	4	5	NA
193010	Maintains recommended body weight	1	2	3	4	5	NA
193011	Participates in weight-bearing activities appropriate for age	1	2	3	4	5	NA
193012	Obtains periodic prescribed physical examination	1	2	3	4	5	NA
193013	Reports family history of osteoporosis	1	2	3	4	5	NA
193014	Reports history of fractures	1	2	3	4	5	NA
193015	Identifies medication that may reduce bone density	1	2	3	4	5	NA
193016	Reports use of medication that may reduce bone density	1	2	3	4	5	NA
193017	Obtains standardized bone mineral density evaluation	1	2	3	4	5	NA
193018	Follows recommendations based on bone mineral density evaluation	1	2	3	4	5	NA
193019	Takes anti-resorptive medication as prescribed	1	2	3	4	5	NA
193020	Reports side effects of prescribed anti-resorptive medication	1	2	3	4	5	NA
193021	Follows proper procedure for oral bisphosphonate therapy	1	2	3	4	5	NA
193022	Monitors changes in general health status	1	2	3	4	5	NA
193023	Uses personal support systems to reduce osteoporosis risk	1	2	3	4	5	NA
193024	Uses community resources to reduce osteoporosis risk	1	2	3	4	5	NA

Domain-Health Knowledge & Behavior (IV)   *Class*-Risk Control (T)   5th edition 2013; reviewed 2024

R

OUTCOME CONTENT REFERENCES:

Chen, L., & Yu, Y. (2020). Exercise and osteoarthritis. *Advances in Experimental Medicine and Biology, 1228*, 219–231. https://doi.org/10.1007/978-981-15-1792-1-15

Cherukuri, L., Kinninger, A., Birudaraju, D., Lakshmanan, S., Li, D., Flores, F., Mao, S. S., & Budoff, M. J. (2021). Effect of body mass index on bone mineral density is age-specific. *Nutrition, Metabolism, & Cardiovascular Diseases, 31*, 1767–1773. https://doi.org/10.1016/j.numecd.2021.02.027

Clark, P., & Lavielle, P. (2021). Are women ready to prevent osteoporosis? Change stages for preventive behaviors. *Health Education & Behavior, 48*(6), 892–898.

Cox, S. I., & Hopper, G. (2020). Improving bone health and detection of osteoporosis. *The Journal for Nurse Practitioners, 17*(2), 233–235. https://doi.org/10.1016/j.nurpra.2020.05.008

Kim, B., Cho, Y. J., & Lim, W. (2021). Osteoporosis therapies and their mechanisms of action (Review). *Experimental and Therapeutic Medicine, 22*(6), 1379. https://doi.org/10.3892/etm.2021.10815

NAMS Position Statement. (2021). Management of osteoporosis in postmenopausal women: The 2021 position statement of The North American Menopause Society. *Menopause, 28*(9), 973–997. https://doi.org/10.1007/GME.0000000000001831

Roos, E. M., & Arden, N. K. (2016). Strategies for the prevention of knee osteoarthritis. *Nature Reviews. Rheumatology, 12*(2), 92–101. https://doi.org/10.1038/nrrheum.2015.135

Rosen, H. (2010). *Drugs that affect bone metabolism.* https://www.uptodate.com/contents/drugs-that-affect-bone-metabolism

Wu, L.-C., Chen, H.-J., Lin, W., Kao, H.-H., Huang, P.-F. (2021). Using a simple preliminary screening tool to explore related factors of osteoporosis in the elderly of southern Taiwan. *Medicine, 100*(9), 1–8. https://doi.org/10.1097/MD.0000000000024950

Risk Control: Prediabetes   1945

Definition: Personal actions to understand, prevent, delay, or reduce the threat of type 2 diabetes

OUTCOME TARGET RATING: Maintain at_____ Increase to_____

		Never Demonstrated	Rarely Demonstrated	Sometimes Demonstrated	Often Demonstrated	Consistently Demonstrated	
OUTCOME OVERALL RATING		1	2	3	4	5	
Indicators:							
194501	Acknowledges personal risk of developing type 2 diabetes	1	2	3	4	5	NA
197502	Acknowledges family history of type 2 diabetes	1	2	3	4	5	NA
197503	Identifies risk factors of developing type 2 diabetes	1	2	3	4	5	NA
197504	Seeks current information on preventing type 2 diabetes	1	2	3	4	5	NA
197505	Identifies role of diet in prevention of type 2 diabetes	1	2	3	4	5	NA
197506	Acknowledges ability to change behavior	1	2	3	4	5	NA
197507	Monitors changes in general health status	1	2	3	4	5	NA
197508	Uses effective weight control strategies	1	2	3	4	5	NA
197509	Uses strategies to reduce body weight	1	2	3	4	5	NA
197510	Eats a healthy diet	1	2	3	4	5	NA
197511	Participates in regular exercise	1	2	3	4	5	NA
197512	Participates in aerobic exercise	1	2	3	4	5	NA
197513	Seeks support from fitness coach	1	2	3	4	5	NA
197514	Monitors blood pressure	1	2	3	4	5	NA
197515	Monitors heart rate	1	2	3	4	5	NA
197516	Uses medication as prescribed	1	2	3	4	5	NA
197517	Obtains fasting glucose screening as recommended	1	2	3	4	5	NA
197518	Obtains A1C blood screening as recommended	1	2	3	4	5	NA
197519	Participates in cholesterol screening	1	2	3	4	5	NA
197520	Eliminates tobacco use	1	2	3	4	5	NA
197521	Shares personal dietary goals with health professional	1	2	3	4	5	NA
197522	Shares personal physical activity goals with health providers	1	2	3	4	5	NA

R

Risk Control: Prediabetes—cont'd

		Never Demonstrated	Rarely Demonstrated	Sometimes Demonstrated	Often Demonstrated	Consistently Demonstrated	
197523	Follows recommendations from health professional	1	2	3	4	5	NA
197524	Keeps appointments with health professional	1	2	3	4	5	NA
197525	Seeks nutritional consultation	1	2	3	4	5	NA
197526	Uses personal social support	1	2	3	4	5	NA
197527	Modifies lifestyle to reduce risk	1	2	3	4	5	NA
197528	Uses community resources to reduce risk for developing type 2 diabetes	1	2	3	4	5	NA

Domain-Health Knowledge & Behavior (IV)   *Class*-Risk Control (T)   7th edition 2024

OUTCOME CONTENT REFERENCES:

Braga, T., Kraemer-Aguiar, L. G., Docherty, N. G., & Le Roux, C. W. (2019). Treating prediabetes: Why and how should we do it? *Minerva Medica*, *110*(1), 52–61. https://doi.org/10.23736/S0026-4806.18.05897-4

Daftarian, Z., & Bowen, P. G. (2020). Improving outcomes in patients with prediabetes through a lifestyle modification program. *Journal of the American Association of Nurse Practitioners*, *32*(3), 244–251. https://doi.org/10.1097/JXX.0000000000000213

Dorman, J. S., Valdez, R., Liu, T., Wang, C., Rubinstein, W. S., O'Neill, S. M., Acheson, L. S., Ruffin, M. T., & Khoury, M. J., (2012). Health beliefs among individuals at increased familial risk for type 2 diabetes: Implications for prevention. *Diabetes Research & Clinical Practice*, *96*(2), 156–162. https://doi.org/10.1016/j.diabres.2011.12.017

Epstein, L. H., Paluch, R. A., Stein, J. S., Quattrin, T., Mastrandrea, L. D., Bree, K. A., Sze, Y. Y., Greenawald, M. H., Biondolillo, M. J., & Bickel, W. K. (2021). Delay discounting, glycemic regulation and health behaviors in adults with prediabetes. *Behavioral Medicine*, *47*(3), 194–204. https://doi.org/10.1080/08964289.2020.1712581

Glechner, A., Harreiter, J., Gartlehner, G., Rohleder, S., Kautzky, A., Tuomilehto, J., Van Noord, M., Kaminski-Hartenthaler, A., & Kautzky-Willer, A. (2015). Sex-specific differences in diabetes prevention: A systematic review and meta-analysis. *Diabetologia*, *58*(2), 242–254. https://doi.org/10.1007/s00125-014-3439-x

Glechner, A., Keuchel, L., Affengruber, L., Titscher, V., Sommer, I., Matyas, N., Wagner, G., Kien, C., Klerings, I., & Gartlehner, G. (2018). Effects of lifestyle changes on adults with prediabetes: A systematic review and meta-analysis. *Primary Care Diabetes*, *12*(5), 393–408. https://doi.org/10.1016/j.pcd.2018.07.003

Ledford, C. J. W., Seehusen, D. A., & Crawford, P. F. (2019). The relationship between patient perceptions of diabetes and glycemic control: A study of patients living with prediabetes or type 2 diabetes. *Patient Education & Counseling*, *102*(11), 2097–2101. https://doi.org/10.1016/j.pec.2019.05.023

Owei, I., Umekwe, N., Ceesay, F., & Dagogo-Jack, S. (2019). Awareness of prediabetes status and subsequent health behavior, body weight, and blood glucose levels. *Journal of the American Board of Family Medicine*, *32*(1), 20–27. https://doi.org/10.3122/jabfm.2019.01.180242

Pestoni, G., Riedl, A., Breuninger, T. A., Wawro, N., Krieger, J.-P., Meisinger, C., Rathmann, W., Thorand, B., Harris, C., Peters, A., Rohrmann, S., & Linseisen, J. (2021). Association between dietary patterns and prediabetes, undetected diabetes or clinically diagnosed diabetes: Results from the KORA FF4 study. *European Journal of Nutrition*, *60*(5), 2331–2341. https://doi.org/10.1007/s00394-020-02416-9

Risk Control: Pressure Injury   1942

Definition: Personal actions to understand, prevent, eliminate, or reduce the threat of developing pressure induced tissue damage

R

OUTCOME TARGET RATING: Maintain at_____ Increase to_____

		Never Demonstrated	Rarely Demonstrated	Sometimes Demonstrated	Often Demonstrated	Consistently Demonstrated	
OUTCOME OVERALL RATING		1	2	3	4	5	
Indicators:							
194201	Identifies risk factors for pressure ulcer development	1	2	3	4	5	NA
194202	Acknowledges personal risk factors for pressure ulcer development	1	2	3	4	5	NA
194203	Identifies signs and symptoms of pressure ulcer	1	2	3	4	5	NA
194204	Checks for redness on bony prominences	1	2	3	4	5	NA
194205	Monitors changes in sensory perception	1	2	3	4	5	NA
194206	Uses tight-fitting bed linen	1	2	3	4	5	NA

Continued

Risk Control: Pressure Injury—cont'd

		Never Demonstrated	Rarely Demonstrated	Sometimes Demonstrated	Often Demonstrated	Consistently Demonstrated	
194207	Uses effective strategies to control skin moisture	1	2	3	4	5	NA
194208	Identifies skin irritants	1	2	3	4	5	NA
194209	Reduces skin exposure to urine	1	2	3	4	5	NA
194210	Reduces skin exposure to stool	1	2	3	4	5	NA
194211	Monitors body edema	1	2	3	4	5	NA
194212	Identifies mobility limitations	1	2	3	4	5	NA
194213	Shifts position at least every 2 hours	1	2	3	4	5	NA
194214	Monitors medication effects that influence tissue perfusion	1	2	3	4	5	NA
194215	Maintains a healthy diet	1	2	3	4	5	NA
194216	Uses reputable sources of information	1	2	3	4	5	NA

Domain-Health Knowledge & Behavior (IV)   **Class**-Risk Control (T)   6th edition 2018

OUTCOME CONTENT REFERENCES:
Campbell, J. L., Coyer, F. M., & Osborne, S. R. (2016). The skin safety model: Reconceptualizing skin vulnerability in older patients. *Journal of Nursing Scholarship, 48*(1), 14–22. https://doi.org/10.1111/jnu.12176
Edsberg, L. E., Langemo, D., Baharestani, M. M., Posthauer, M. E., & Goldberg, M. (2014). Unavoidable pressure injury: State of the science and consensus outcomes. *Journal of Wound Ostomy & Continence Nursing, 41*(4), 313–334. https://doi.org/10.1097/WON.0000000000000050
Gefen, A., Farid, K. J., & Shaywitz, I. (2013). A review of deep tissue injury development, detection, and prevention: Shear savvy. *Ostomy Wound Management, 59*(2), 26–35.
National Pressure Ulcer Advisory Panel, European Pressure Ulcer Advisory Panel, & Pan Pacific Pressure Injury Alliance. (2014). *Prevention and treatment of pressure ulcers: Clinical practice guideline.* Cambridge Media.

Risk Control: Problematic Internet Use   1946

Definition: Personal actions to understand, prevent, eliminate, or reduce the threat of compulsive use of the internet and internet gaming

OUTCOME TARGET RATING: Maintain at_____ Increase to_____

		Never Demonstrated	Rarely Demonstrated	Sometimes Demonstrated	Often Demonstrated	Consistently Demonstrated	
OUTCOME OVERALL RATING		1	2	3	4	5	
Indicators:							
194601	Acknowledges personal preoccupation with the internet	1	2	3	4	5	NA
194602	Seeks current information on negative consequences of excessive internet use	1	2	3	4	5	NA
194603	Recognizes a strong personal desire to engage in internet gaming activities	1	2	3	4	5	NA
194604	Recognizes a strong personal desire to engage in social media	1	2	3	4	5	NA
194605	Identifies impact of gaming on sleep quality and duration	1	2	3	4	5	NA
194606	Identifies impact on general health	1	2	3	4	5	NA
194607	Identifies impact on social relationships	1	2	3	4	5	NA
194608	Monitors feelings of depression	1	2	3	4	5	NA
194609	Monitors feelings of restlessness	1	2	3	4	5	NA
194610	Monitors impact on sleep quality	1	2	3	4	5	NA
194611	Identifies time spent on social media	1	2	3	4	5	NA

R

Risk Control: Problematic Internet Use—cont'd

		Never Demonstrated	Rarely Demonstrated	Sometimes Demonstrated	Often Demonstrated	Consistently Demonstrated	
194612	Sets time limits on personal gaming interactions	1	2	3	4	5	NA
194613	Maintains a diary of time spent on internet activities	1	2	3	4	5	NA
194614	Evaluates impact on educational performance	1	2	3	4	5	NA
194615	Evaluates impact on work performance	1	2	3	4	5	NA
194616	Evaluates impact on financial status	1	2	3	4	5	NA
194617	Validates threat to health with others	1	2	3	4	5	NA

Domain-Health Knowledge & Behavior (IV)   **Class**-Risk Control (T)   7th edition 2024

OUTCOME CONTENT REFERENCES:

Başdaş, Ö., & Özbey, H. (2020). Digital game addiction, obesity, and social anxiety among adolescents. *Archives of Psychiatric Nursing, 34*(2), 17–20. https://doi.org/10.1016/j.apnu.2019.12.010

Dienlin, T., & Johannes, N. (2020). The impact of digital technology use on adolescent well-being. *Dialogues in Clinical Neuroscience, 22*(2), 135–142. https://doi.org/10.31887/DCNS.2020.22.2

Knell, G., Durand, C. P., Kohl, H. W., III, Wu, I. H. C., & Pettee, G. K. (2019). Prevalence and likelihood of meeting sleep, physical activity, and screen-time guidelines among U.S. youth. *Journal of American Medical Association Pediatrics,173*(4), 387–389. https://doi.org/10.1001/jamapediatrics.2018.4847

Männikkö, N., Ruotsalainen, H., Miettunen, J., Pontes, H. M., & Kääriäinen, M. (2020). Problematic gaming behavior and health-related outcomes: A systematic review and meta-analysis. *Journal of Health Psychology, 25*(1), 67–81. https://doi.org/10.1177/1359105317740414

Mills, K. L. (2016). Possible effects of internet use on cognitive development in adolescence. *Media and Communication, 4*(3), 4–12. https://doi.org/10.17645/mac.v4i3.516

Sebre, S. B., Miltuze1, A., & Limonovs, M. (2020). Integrating adolescent problematic internet use risk factors: Hyperactivity, inconsistent parenting, and maladaptive cognitions. *Journal of Child and Family Studies, 29,* 2000–2009. https://doi.org/10.1007/s10826-020-01726-0

Stevens, C., Zhang, E., Cherkerzian, S., Chen, J. A., & Liu, C. H. (2020). Problematic internet use/computer gaming among U.S. college students: Prevalence and correlates with mental health symptoms. *Depression & Anxiety, 37,* 1127–1136. https://doi.org/10.1002/da.23094

Risk Control: Sexually Transmitted Diseases (STD)   1905

Definition: Personal actions to understand, prevent, eliminate, or reduce the threat of acquiring a sexually transmitted disease

OUTCOME TARGET RATING: Maintain at_____ Increase to_____

		Never Demonstrated	Rarely Demonstrated	Sometimes Demonstrated	Often Demonstrated	Consistently Demonstrated	
OUTCOME OVERALL RATING		1	2	3	4	5	
Indicators:							
190519	Seeks current information about sexually transmitted diseases	1	2	3	4	5	NA
190520	Identifies risk factors for sexually transmitted diseases	1	2	3	4	5	NA
190501	Acknowledges personal risk factors for sexually transmitted disease	1	2	3	4	5	NA
190502	Acknowledges consequences associated with sexually transmitted disease	1	2	3	4	5	NA
190521	Acknowledges ability to change behavior	1	2	3	4	5	NA
190505	Develops effective strategies to reduce sexually transmitted disease exposure	1	2	3	4	5	NA
190522	Limits number of partners	1	2	3	4	5	NA

R

Continued

Risk Control: Sexually Transmitted Diseases (STD)—cont'd

		Never Demonstrated	Rarely Demonstrated	Sometimes Demonstrated	Often Demonstrated	Consistently Demonstrated	
190509	Inquires of partner's sexually transmitted disease status before sexual activity	1	2	3	4	5	NA
190523	Negotiates safe sexual practices with partner	1	2	3	4	5	NA
190524	Uses a condom	1	2	3	4	5	NA
190525	Practices safe anal sex	1	2	3	4	5	NA
190529	Abstains from drug use	1	2	3	4	5	NA
190510	Uses strategies to prevent sexually transmitted disease transmission	1	2	3	4	5	NA
190511	Recognizes signs and symptoms of sexually transmitted disease	1	2	3	4	5	NA
190526	Monitors for signs and symptoms of sexually transmitted disease	1	2	3	4	5	NA
190512	Participates in screening for sexually transmitted disease	1	2	3	4	5	NA
190527	Obtains health care services when necessary	1	2	3	4	5	NA
190528	Uses community resources to reduce sexually transmitted disease risk	1	2	3	4	5	NA
190517	Maintains absence of sexually transmitted disease	1	2	3	4	5	NA

Domain-Health Knowledge & Behavior (IV)   **Class**-Risk Control (T)   *1st edition 1997; revised 2004, 2013, 2024*

OUTCOME CONTENT REFERENCES:

Du, X., Zhang, L., Luo, H., Rong, W., Meng, X., Yu, H., & Tan, X. (2021). Factors associated with risk sexual behaviours of HIV/STDs infection among university students in Henan, China: A cross-sectional study. *Reproductive Health, 18,* 172–183. https://doi.org/10.1186/s12978-021-012193

Jenkins, W. D., Williams, L. D., & Pearson, W. S. (2021). Sexually transmitted infection epidemiology and care in rural areas: A narrative review. *Sexually Transmitted Diseases, 48*(12), e236-e240. https://doi.org/10.1097/OLQ.0000000000001512

Jones, K., Williams, J., Sipsma, H., & Patil, C. (2019). Adolescent and emerging adults' evaluation of a Facebook site providing sexual health education. *Public Health Nursing* (Boston, Mass.), *36*(1), 11–17. https://doi.org/10.1111/phn.12555

Kalichman, S., Banas, E., Kalichman, M., Dewing, S., Jennings, K., Daniels, J., Berteler, M., & Mathews, C. (2021). Brief enhanced partner notification and risk reduction counseling to prevent sexually transmitted infections, Cape Town, South Africa. *Sexually Transmitted Diseases, 48*(3), 174–182. https://doi.org/10.1097/OLQ.0000000000001295

Kumar, S., Haderxhanaj, L. T., & Spicknall, I. H. (2021). Reviewing PrEP's effect on STI incidence among men who have sex with men: Balancing increased STI screening and potential behavioral sexual risk compensation. *AIDS and Behavior, 25,* 1810–1818. https://doi.org/10.1007/s10461-020-03110-x

Reynolds, C., Sutherland, M. A., & Palacios, I. (2019). Exploring the use of technology for sexual health risk-reduction among Ecuadorean adolescents. *Annals of Global Health, 85*(1), 57. https://doi.org/10.5334/aogh.35

R

Risk Control: Stroke   1931

Definition: Personal actions to understand, prevent, eliminate, or reduce the threat of a cerebral vascular accident

OUTCOME TARGET RATING: Maintain at_____ Increase to_____

		Never Demonstrated	Rarely Demonstrated	Sometimes Demonstrated	Often Demonstrated	Consistently Demonstrated	
OUTCOME OVERALL RATING		1	2	3	4	5	
Indicators:							
193101	Seeks current information about stroke prevention	1	2	3	4	5	NA
193102	Identifies risk factors for stroke	1	2	3	4	5	NA
193103	Acknowledges personal risk factors for stroke	1	2	3	4	5	NA

Risk Control: Stroke—cont'd

		Never Demonstrated	Rarely Demonstrated	Sometimes Demonstrated	Often Demonstrated	Consistently Demonstrated	
193125	Monitors for warning signs and symptoms of stroke	1	2	3	4	5	NA
193115	Participates in vascular screening	1	2	3	4	5	NA
193126	Uses risk control strategies	1	2	3	4	5	NA
193105	Acknowledges ability to change modifiable risk factors	1	2	3	4	5	NA
193119	Eliminates tobacco use	1	2	3	4	5	NA
193127	Uses strategies to manage hypertension	1	2	3	4	5	NA
193120	Follows recommended alcohol restrictions	1	2	3	4	5	NA
193110	Uses effective weight control strategies	1	2	3	4	5	NA
193116	Maintains glycemic control	1	2	3	4	5	NA
193118	Complies with treatment regimen for comorbid conditions	1	2	3	4	5	NA
193114	Participates in screening for dyslipidemia	1	2	3	4	5	NA
193128	Participates in screening for atrial fibrillation	1	2	3	4	5	NA
193129	Follows recommendations for physical activity	1	2	3	4	5	NA
193121	Uses strategies to reduce stress	1	2	3	4	5	NA
193130	Uses strategies to manage chronic bacterial infections	1	2	3	4	5	NA
193111	Follows dietary recommendations	1	2	3	4	5	NA
193113	Reduces sodium intake	1	2	3	4	5	NA
193131	Maintains hydration	1	2	3	4	5	NA
193132	Follows anticoagulant therapy	1	2	3	4	5	NA
193117	Uses medication as prescribed	1	2	3	4	5	NA
193124	Monitors for changes in general health status	1	2	3	4	5	NA

Domain-Health Knowledge & Behavior (IV)   **Class**-Risk Control (T)   5th edition 2013; revised 2018; reviewed 2024

OUTCOME CONTENT REFERENCES:

Caprio, F. Z., & Sorond, F. A. (2019). Cerebrovascular disease: Primary and secondary stroke prevention. *The Medical Clinics of North America, 103*(2), 295–308. https://doi.org/10.1016/j.mcna.2018.10.001

Hill, V. A., & Towfighi, A. (2017). Modifiable risk factors for stroke and strategies for stroke prevention. *Seminars in Neurology, 37*(3), 237–258. https://doi.org/10.1055/s-0037-1603685

Jame, S., & Barnes, G. (2020). Stroke and thromboembolism prevention in atrial fibrillation. *Heart, 106*(1), 10–17. https://doi.org/10.1136/heartjnl-2019-314898

Kernan, W., Ovbiagele, B., Black, H., Bravata, D., Chimowitz, M., Ezekowitz, M., Fang, M. C., Fisher, M., Furie, K. L., Heck, D. V., Jonston, C., Kasner, S. E., Kittner, S. J., Michell, P. H., Rich, M. W., Richardson, D., Schwamm, L. H., & Wilson, J. A. (2014). Guidelines for the prevention of stroke in patients with stroke and transient ischemic attack: A guideline for healthcare professionals from the American Heart Association/American Stroke Association. *Stroke, 45*(7), 2160–2236. https://doi.org/10.1161/STR.0000000000000024

Spence, J. D. (2018). Diet for stroke prevention. *Stroke and Vascular Neurology, 3*(2), 44–50. https://doi.org/10.1136/svn-2017-000130

Spence, J. D., Azarpazhooh, M. R., Larsson, S. C., Bogiatzi, C., & Hankey, G. J. (2020). Stroke prevention in older adults: Recent advances. *Stroke, 51*(12), 3770–3777. https://doi.org/10.1161/STROKEAHA.120.031707

Milionis, H., Ntaios, G., Korompoki, E., Vemmos, K., & Michel, P. (2020). Statin-based therapy for primary and secondary prevention of ischemic stroke: A meta-analysis and critical overview. *International Journal of Stroke, 15*(4), 377–384. https://doi.org/10.1177/1747493019873594

Yeh, C. H., Chang, W. L., Chan, P. C., Mou, C. H., Chang, K. S., Hsu, C. Y., Tsay, S. L., Tsai, M. T., Hsu, M. H., & Sung, F. C. (2021). Women with osteoarthritis are at increased risk of ischemic stroke: A population-based cohort study. *Journal of Epidemiology, 31*(12), 628–634. https://doi.org/10.2188/jea.JE20200042

R

Risk Control: Sun Exposure 1925

Definition: Personal actions to understand, prevent, or reduce threats to skin and eyes from sun exposure

OUTCOME TARGET RATING: Maintain at_____ Increase to_____

		Never Demonstrated	Rarely Demonstrated	Sometimes Demonstrated	Often Demonstrated	Consistently Demonstrated	
OUTCOME OVERALL RATING		1	2	3	4	5	
Indicators:							
192516	Seeks current information about control of sun exposure	1	2	3	4	5	NA
192517	Identifies risk of sun exposure	1	2	3	4	5	NA
192501	Acknowledges personal risk factors of sun exposure	1	2	3	4	5	NA
192518	Modifies lifestyle to reduce risk	1	2	3	4	5	NA
192519	Participates in sun protection counseling	1	2	3	4	5	NA
192502	Selects sunscreen with recommended sun protection factor or greater	1	2	3	4	5	NA
192503	Applies appropriate amount of sunscreen	1	2	3	4	5	NA
192504	Reapplies sunscreen as needed	1	2	3	4	5	NA
192505	Avoids sun exposure between 10 a.m. and 3 p.m.	1	2	3	4	5	NA
192506	Monitors length of sun exposure	1	2	3	4	5	NA
192507	Seeks outdoor activities in the shade	1	2	3	4	5	NA
192508	Wears appropriate clothing to protect skin	1	2	3	4	5	NA
192509	Wears hat with 4-inch brim to protect head and face	1	2	3	4	5	NA
192510	Uses ointment to protect lips	1	2	3	4	5	NA
192511	Wears ultraviolet (UV) protection glasses when outdoors	1	2	3	4	5	NA
192512	Avoids use of ultraviolet (UV) devices	1	2	3	4	5	NA
192513	Follows recommendations for regular skin inspection	1	2	3	4	5	NA
192514	Checks medication side effects for photosensitivity	1	2	3	4	5	NA
192515	Uses reputable sources of information	1	2	3	4	5	NA

Domain-*Health Knowledge & Behavior (IV)* **Class**-*Risk Control (T)* *4th edition 2008; revised 2013, 2024*

OUTCOME CONTENT REFERENCES:

Buller, D. B., Heckman, C. J., & Manne, S. L. (2018). The potential of behavioral counseling to prevent skin cancer. *Journal of the American Medical Association Dermatology, 154*(5), 519-521. https://doi.org/10.1001/jamadermatol.2018.0325

Hedges, T., & Scriven, A. (2010). Young park users' attitudes and behavior to sun protection. *Global Health Promotion, 17*(4), 24–31. https://doi.org/10.1177/1757975910383928

Nickasch, B. L., Sauer, T., & Lehr, M. (2020). The impact of increasing sun protection counseling and skin cancer screening. *Journal of Doctoral Nursing Practice, 13*(03), 249-253. https://doi.org/10.1891/JDNP-D-20-00012

Siegel, J. A., Yudkin, J. S., Craker, K., Hwang, A., & Libby, T. J. (2021). Uncapping the bottle: A proposal to allow full-sized sunscreens in carry-on luggage to promote sun protection and prevent skin cancer. *Journal of the American Academy of Dermatology, 84*(4), 1206-1207. https://doi.org/10.1016/j.jaad.2020.10.066

U.S. Preventive Services Task Force Recommendation Statement. (2018). Behavioral counseling to prevent skin cancer. *Journal of the American Medical Association, 319*(11), 1134. https://doi.org/10.1001/jama.2018.1623

R

Risk Control: Thrombus   1932

Definition: Personal actions to understand, prevent, eliminate, or reduce the threat of thrombus formation or embolus

OUTCOME TARGET RATING: Maintain at_____ Increase to_____

		Never Demonstrated	Rarely Demonstrated	Sometimes Demonstrated	Often Demonstrated	Consistently Demonstrated	
OUTCOME OVERALL RATING		1	2	3	4	5	
Indicators:							
193201	Seeks current information about embolus prevention	1	2	3	4	5	NA
193202	Identifies risk factors for thrombus formation	1	2	3	4	5	NA
193203	Acknowledges personal risk factors for thrombus formation	1	2	3	4	5	NA
193205	Monitors for warning signs and symptoms of thrombus formation or embolus	1	2	3	4	5	NA
193212	Uses effective weight control strategies	1	2	3	4	5	NA
193222	Uses strategies to reduce vascular intimal injury	1	2	3	4	5	NA
193223	Uses strategies to reduce venous stasis	1	2	3	4	5	NA
193224	Uses strategies to manage hypertension	1	2	3	4	5	NA
193211	Follows recommendations for physical activity	1	2	3	4	5	NA
193214	Follows recommended alcohol restrictions	1	2	3	4	5	NA
193213	Eliminates tobacco use	1	2	3	4	5	NA
193209	Monitors medication side effects	1	2	3	4	5	NA
193219	Follows non-prescription medication precautions	1	2	3	4	5	NA
193220	Obtains periodic laboratory tests	1	2	3	4	5	NA
193208	Uses medication as prescribed	1	2	3	4	5	NA
193207	Complies with treatment regimen for comorbid conditions	1	2	3	4	5	NA
193210	Uses therapeutic stockings as recommended	1	2	3	4	5	NA
193215	Follows fluid intake recommendations	1	2	3	4	5	NA
193216	Avoids sitting for long time periods	1	2	3	4	5	NA
193218	Shifts position while sitting	1	2	3	4	5	NA
193217	Follows activity recommendations for travel	1	2	3	4	5	NA
193221	Monitors changes in general health status	1	2	3	4	5	NA
193225	Obtains immediate treatment if signs and symptoms of thrombus occur	1	2	3	4	5	NA

Domain-*Health Knowledge & Behavior (IV)*   *Class*-*Risk Control (T)*   *5th edition 2013; revised 2018*

OUTCOME CONTENT REFERENCES:
Agnelli, G., & Becattini, C. (2008). Treatment of DVT: How long is enough and how do you predict recurrence. *Journal of Thrombosis and Thrombolysis, 25*(1), 37–44. https://doi.org/10.1007/s11239-007-0103-z

Andrews, P. L., & Habashi, N. M. (2010). Detecting, managing, and preventing pulmonary embolism. *American Nurse Today, 5*(9), 21–26.

Farley, A. H., McLafferty, E., & Hendry, C. (2009). Pulmonary embolism: Identification, clinical features and management. *Nursing Standard, 23*(28), 49–56. https://doi.org/10.7748/ns2009.03.23.28.49.c6924

Findlay, J., Keogh, M., & Cooper, L. (2010). Venous thromboembolism prophylaxis: The role of the nurse. *British Journal of Nursing, 19*(16), 1028–1032. https://doi.org/10.12968/bjon.2010.19.16.78190

Fitzgerald, J. (2010). Venous thromboembolism: Have we made headway? *Orthopaedic Nursing, 29*(4), 226–234. https://doi.org/10.1097/NOR. 0b013e3181e517af

Headley, C. M., & Melander, S. (2011). When it may be a pulmonary embolism. *Nephrology Nursing Journal, 38*(2), 127–137, 152.

Houman Fekrazad, M., Lopes, R. D., Stashenko, G. J., Alexander, J. H., & Garcia, D. (2009). Treatment of venous thromboembolism: Guidelines translated for the clinician. *Journal of Thrombosis and Thrombolysis, 28*(3), 270–275. https://doi.org/10.1007/s11239-009-0374-7

R

Kearon, C., Kahn, S. R., Agnelli, G., Goldhaber, S., Raskob, G. E., & Comerota, A. J., American College of Chest Physicians. (2008). Antithrombotic therapy for venous thromboembolic disease: American College of Chest Physicians evidence-based clinical practice guidelines (8th ed.). *Chest, 133*(Suppl. 6), 454S–545S. https://doi.org/10.1378/chest.08-0658suppl

Lancaster, S. L., Owens, A., Bryant, A. S., Ramey, L. S., Nicholson, J., Gossett, K., Forni, J. T., & Padgett, T. M. (2010). Emergency: Upper-extremity deep vein thrombosis. *AJN, American Journal of Nursing, 110*(5), 48–52. https://doi.org/10.1097/01.NAJ.0000372072.24134.a5

Meetoo, D. (2010). In too deep: Understanding, detecting and managing DVT. *British Journal of Nursing, 19*(16), 1021–1027. https://doi.org/10.12968/bjon.2010.19.16.78188

Perry, M. (2008). Knowing the early signs of pulmonary embolism. *Practice Nursing, 19*(12), 620–623.

Yee, C. A. (2010). Conquering pulmonary embolism. *OR Nurse, 4*(5), 18–24.

Risk Control: Tobacco Use   1906

Definition: Personal actions to understand, prevent, eliminate, or reduce the threats to health associated with tobacco use

OUTCOME TARGET RATING: Maintain at_____ Increase to_____

		Never Demonstrated	Rarely Demonstrated	Sometimes Demonstrated	Often Demonstrated	Consistently Demonstrated	
OUTCOME OVERALL RATING		**1**	**2**	**3**	**4**	**5**	
Indicators:							
190627	Seeks current information about hazards of tobacco use	1	2	3	4	5	NA
190632	Identifies products containing tobacco	1	2	3	4	5	NA
190628	Acknowledges addictive property of tobacco	1	2	3	4	5	NA
190629	Identifies risk factors for tobacco use	1	2	3	4	5	NA
190601	Acknowledges personal risk factors for tobacco use	1	2	3	4	5	NA
190619	Acknowledges personal satisfaction associated with tobacco use	1	2	3	4	5	NA
190630	Acknowledges personal disadvantages associated with tobacco use	1	2	3	4	5	NA
190602	Acknowledges consequences associated with tobacco use	1	2	3	4	5	NA
190633	Acknowledges risk of cancer and heart disease linked to tobacco use	1	2	3	4	5	NA
190631	Acknowledges ability to change behavior	1	2	3	4	5	NA
190603	Monitors environment for factors encouraging tobacco use	1	2	3	4	5	NA
190620	Acknowledges influence of peer pressure	1	2	3	4	5	NA
190621	Uses strategies to prevent tobacco use around peers	1	2	3	4	5	NA
190622	Recognizes social influences to engage in tobacco use	1	2	3	4	5	NA
190623	Recognizes cultural influences to engage in tobacco use	1	2	3	4	5	NA
190610	Uses health care services congruent with needs	1	2	3	4	5	NA
190612	Uses personal support systems to prevent tobacco use	1	2	3	4	5	NA
190613	Uses support group to prevent tobacco use	1	2	3	4	5	NA
190625	Avoids situations that encourage tobacco use	1	2	3	4	5	NA

R

Risk Control: Tobacco Use—cont'd

		Never Demonstrated	Rarely Demonstrated	Sometimes Demonstrated	Often Demonstrated	Consistently Demonstrated	
190626	Uses reputable sources of information	1	2	3	4	5	NA
190614	Uses community resources to prevent tobacco use	1	2	3	4	5	NA
190634	Identifies financial cost of tobacco use	1	2	3	4	5	NA

Domain-Health Knowledge & Behavior (IV)   *Class*-Risk Control (T)   *1st edition 1997; revised 2004, 2008, 2013, 2024*

OUTCOME CONTENT REFERENCES:

Fried, N. D., & Gardner, J. D. (2020). Heat-not-burn tobacco products: An emerging threat to cardiovascular health. *American Journal of Physiology. Heart and Circulatory Physiology*, *319*(6), H1234–H1239. https://doi.org/10.1152/ajpheart.00708.2020

Gupta, A. K., & Mehrotra, R. (2021). Increasing use of flavored tobacco products amongst youth. *The Indian Journal of Tuberculosis*, *68S*, S105–S107. https://doi.org/10.1016/j.ijtb.2021.07.020

Hu, M., Griesler, P., Schaffran, C., & Kandel, D. (2011). Risk and protective factors for nicotine dependence in adolescence. *Journal of Child Psychology & Psychiatry*, *52*(10), 1063–1072.

Johnson, A. C., Simmens, S. J., Turner, M. M., Evans, W. D., Strasser, A. A., & Mays, D. (2022). Longitudinal effects of cigarette pictorial warning labels among young adults. *Journal of Behavioral Medicine*, *45*(1), 124–132. https://doi.org/10.1007/s10865-021-00258-2

Kaufman, A. R., Twesten, J. E., Suls, J., McCaul, K. D., Ostroff, J. S., Ferrer, R. A., Brewer, N. T., Cameron, L. D., Halpern-Felsher, B., Hay, J. L., Park, E. R., Peters, E., Strong, D. R., Waters, E. A., Weinstein, N. D., Windschitl, P. D., & Klein, W. (2020). Measuring cigarette smoking risk perceptions. *Nicotine & Tobacco Research*, *22*(11), 1937–1945. https://doi.org/10.1093/ntr/ntz213

Kim-Mozeleski, J. E., & Pandey, R. (2020). The intersection of food insecurity and tobacco use: A scoping review. *Health Promotion Practice*, *21*(Suppl. 1), 124S–138S. https://doi.org/10.1177/1524839919874054

Klesges, R., Sherrill-Mittleman, D., Ebbert, J., Talcott, W., & DeBon, M. (2010). Tobacco use harm reduction, elimination, and escalation in a large military cohort. *American Journal of Public Health, 100*(12), 2487–2492.

Kondo, T., Nakano, Y., Adachi, S., & Murohara, T. (2019). Effects of tobacco smoking on cardiovascular disease. *Circulation Journal, 83*(10), 1980–1985. https://doi.org/10.1253/circj.CJ-19-0323

Middlekauff, H. R. (2020). Cardiovascular impact of electronic-cigarette use. *Trends in Cardiovascular Medicine, 30*(3), 133–140. https://doi.org/10.1016/j.tcm.2019.04.006

Puleo, G. E., Borger, T., Bowling, W. R., & Burris, J. L. (2022). The state of the science on cancer diagnosis as a "teachable moment" for smoking cessation: A scoping review. *Nicotine & Tobacco Research, 24*(2), 160–168. https://doi.org/10.1093/ntr/ntab139

Risk Control: Unintended Pregnancy   1907

Definition: Personal actions to understand, prevent, or reduce the possibility of unintended pregnancy

OUTCOME TARGET RATING: Maintain at_____ Increase to_____

		Never Demonstrated	Rarely Demonstrated	Sometimes Demonstrated	Often Demonstrated	Consistently Demonstrated	
OUTCOME OVERALL RATING		1	2	3	4	5	
Indicators:							
190717	Seeks current information about family planning strategies	1	2	3	4	5	NA
190718	Identifies risk factors for unintended pregnancy	1	2	3	4	5	NA
190701	Acknowledges personal risk factors for unintended pregnancy	1	2	3	4	5	NA
190703	Acknowledges consequences associated with unintended pregnancy	1	2	3	4	5	NA
190705	Understands physiological processes of conception	1	2	3	4	5	NA
190719	Monitors changes in general health status	1	2	3	4	5	NA
190706	Develops effective pregnancy prevention strategies	1	2	3	4	5	NA

R

Continued

Risk Control: Unintended Pregnancy—cont'd

		Never Demonstrated	Rarely Demonstrated	Sometimes Demonstrated	Often Demonstrated	Consistently Demonstrated	
190707	Adjusts pregnancy prevention strategies	1	2	3	4	5	NA
190708	Commits to pregnancy prevention strategies	1	2	3	4	5	NA
190709	Follows selected pregnancy prevention strategies	1	2	3	4	5	NA
190710	Uses personal support systems to enhance prevention strategies	1	2	3	4	5	NA
190711	Uses available community resources	1	2	3	4	5	NA
190712	Identifies personal contraceptive method	1	2	3	4	5	NA
190713	Obtains contraceptive supplies and devices	1	2	3	4	5	NA
190714	Uses contraceptive methods correctly	1	2	3	4	5	NA
190715	Uses health care services congruent with needs	1	2	3	4	5	NA

Domain-Health Knowledge & Behavior (IV)   **Class**-Risk Control (T)   1st edition 1997; revised 2004, 2013; reviewed 2024

OUTCOME CONTENT REFERENCES:

Lin, T. K., Law, R., Beaman, J., & Foster, D. G. (2021). The impact of the COVID-19 pandemic on economic security and pregnancy intentions among people at risk of pregnancy. *Contraception, 103,* 380–385. https://doi.org/10.1016/j.contraception.2021.02.001

Luca, D. L., Stevens, J., Rotz, D., Goesling, B., & Lutz, R. (2021). Evaluating teen options for preventing pregnancy: Impacts and mechanisms. *Journal of Health Economics, 77,* https://doi.org/10.1016/j.jhealeco.2021.102459

Roy, N., Adhikary, P., Kiarie, J., Mburu, G., Dhabhai, N., Chowdhury, R., & Mazumder, S. (2021). *BMC Pregnancy and Childbirth, 21,* 1–8. https://doi.org/10.1186/s12884-021-04294-3

Sherwood, J., Lankiewicz, E., Roose-Snyder, B., Cooper, B., Jones, A., & Honermann, B. (2021). The role of contraception in preventing HIV-positive births: Global estimates and projections. *BMC Public Health, 21,* 1–11. https://doi.org/10.1186/s12889-021-10570-w

---

Risk Control: Visual Impairment   1916

Definition: Personal actions to understand, prevent, eliminate, or reduce threats to visual function

OUTCOME TARGET RATING: Maintain at_____ Increase to_____

		Never Demonstrated	Rarely Demonstrated	Sometimes Demonstrated	Often Demonstrated	Consistently Demonstrated	
OUTCOME OVERALL RATING		1	2	3	4	5	
Indicators:							
191613	Seeks current information about visual impairment	1	2	3	4	5	NA
191614	Identifies risk factors for visual impairment	1	2	3	4	5	NA
191615	Acknowledges personal risk factors for visual impairment	1	2	3	4	5	NA
191601	Monitors symptoms of vision deterioration	1	2	3	4	5	NA
191602	Monitors environment for eye hazards	1	2	3	4	5	NA
191616	Monitors changes in general health status	1	2	3	4	5	NA
191603	Avoids trauma to the eye	1	2	3	4	5	NA
191604	Uses adequate lighting for activity	1	2	3	4	5	NA
191618	Limits screen time on electronic devices	1	2	3	4	5	NA

R

Risk Control: Visual Impairment—cont'd

		Never Demonstrated	Rarely Demonstrated	Sometimes Demonstrated	Often Demonstrated	Consistently Demonstrated	
191605	Takes breaks from activity causing eye strain	1	2	3	4	5	NA
191606	Monitors for symptoms of eye disease	1	2	3	4	5	NA
191619	Properly cleans and maintains contact lenses	1	2	3	4	5	NA
191607	Uses eye medication as prescribed	1	2	3	4	5	NA
191608	Uses devices to protect eyes	1	2	3	4	5	NA
191617	Wears ultraviolet (UV) protection glasses when outdoors	1	2	3	4	5	NA
191609	Obtains routine eye exams	1	2	3	4	5	NA
191611	Obtains glaucoma screening	1	2	3	4	5	NA
191612	Obtains macular degeneration screening	1	2	3	4	5	NA

Domain-*Health Knowledge & Behavior (IV)*   **Class**-*Risk Control (T)*   *2nd edition 2000; revised 2004, 2013, 2024*

OUTCOME CONTENT REFERENCES:

Alabdulkader, B. (2021). Effect of digital device use during COVID-19 on digital eye strain. *Clinical & Experimental Optometry*, *104*(6), 698–704. https://doi.org/10.1080/08164622.2021.1878843

Dhoot, A. S., Popovic, M. M., Lee, S., El-Defrawy, S., & Schlenker, M. B. (2021). Eye protection following cataract surgery: A systematic review. *Canadian Journal of Ophthalmology*. S0008-4182(21)00396-3. Advance online publication. https://doi.org/10.1016/j.jcjo.2021.11.001

Lundälv, J., & Thodelius, C. (2021). Risk of injury events in patients with visual impairments: A Swedish survey study among hospital social workers. *Journal of Visual Impairment & Blindness*, *115*(5), 426–435. https://doi.org/10.1177/0145482X211046666

McGoldrick, M. (2019). Personal protective equipment: Protecting the eyes. *Home Healthcare Now*, *37*(4), 234–235. https://doi.org/10.1097/NHH.0000000000000804

Monaco, W. A., Crews, J. E., Nguyen, A. T. H., & Arif, A. (2021). Prevalence of vision loss and associations with age-related eye diseases among nursing home residents aged ≥65 years. *Journal of the American Medical Directors Association*, *22*(6), 1156–1161. https://doi.org/10.1016/j.jamda.2020.08.036

Sert, Z. E., Özsoy, S. A., & Kalkım, A. (2021). Eye health screening for students in an elementary school within the scope of school health nursing roles. *Journal of Education & Research in Nursing*, *18*(2), 227–233. https://doi.org/10.5152/jern.2021.68889

Woodward, M. A., Hughes, K., Ballouz, D., Hirth, R. A., Errickson, J., & Newman-Casey, P. A. (2022). Assessing eye health and eye care needs among North American native individuals. *JAMA Ophthalmology*, *140*(2), 134–142. https://doi.org/10.1001/jamaophthalmol.2021.5507

Risk Control: Voice Disorder   1948

Definition: Personal actions to understand, prevent, delay, or reduce the threat of voice dysphonia

OUTCOME TARGET RATING: Maintain at_____ Increase to_____

		Never Demonstrated	Rarely Demonstrated	Sometimes Demonstrated	Often Demonstrated	Consistently Demonstrated	
OUTCOME OVERALL RATING		1	2	3	4	5	
Indicators:							
194801	Seeks current information about vocal function	1	2	3	4	5	NA
194802	Seeks information on ways to avoid extremes of vocal range	1	2	3	4	5	NA
194803	Seeks education about voice use	1	2	3	4	5	NA
194804	Seeks information about acid reflux	1	2	3	4	5	NA
194805	Identifies risk factors for vocal impairment	1	2	3	4	5	NA
194806	Acknowledges impact on daily living	1	2	3	4	5	NA
194807	Acknowledges personal risk factors of vocal impairment	1	2	3	4	5	NA
194808	Acknowledges ability to change behavior	1	2	3	4	5	NA

R

Continued

Risk Control: Voice Disorder—cont'd

		Never Demonstrated	Rarely Demonstrated	Sometimes Demonstrated	Often Demonstrated	Consistently Demonstrated	
194809	Acknowledges importance of exercise	1	2	3	4	5	NA
194810	Monitors changes in general health status	1	2	3	4	5	NA
194811	Participates in vocal health screenings	1	2	3	4	5	NA
194812	Participates in vocal training	1	2	3	4	5	NA
194813	Participates in speech therapy	1	2	3	4	5	NA
194814	Seeks respiratory training therapy	1	2	3	4	5	NA
194815	Seeks information about appropriate medication therapy	1	2	3	4	5	NA
194816	Seeks treatment for acid reflux	1	2	3	4	5	NA
194817	Monitors symptoms of vocal impairment	1	2	3	4	5	NA
194818	Avoids vocal trauma	1	2	3	4	5	NA
194819	Reduces voice strain	1	2	3	4	5	NA
194820	Avoids smoking	1	2	3	4	5	NA
194821	Limits exposure to second-hand smoke	1	2	3	4	5	NA
194822	Avoids spicy foods	1	2	3	4	5	NA
194823	Uses voice rest	1	2	3	4	5	NA
194824	Manages throat irritation	1	2	3	4	5	NA
194825	Uses hydration therapy	1	2	3	4	5	NA
194826	Uses laryngeal hydration therapy	1	2	3	4	5	NA
194827	Uses nasal hygiene techniques	1	2	3	4	5	NA
194828	Avoids mouthwash with alcohol	1	2	3	4	5	NA
194829	Uses humidifier in living space	1	2	3	4	5	NA
194830	Seeks information on medication causing dryness of mouth	1	2	3	4	5	NA
194831	Drinks plenty of fluids	1	2	3	4	5	NA
194832	Avoids talking loudly	1	2	3	4	5	NA
194833	Consults with health professionals if signs and symptoms persistent	1	2	3	4	5	NA

Domain-*Health Knowledge & Behavior (IV)* **Class**-*Risk Control (T)* 7th edition 2024

OUTCOME CONTENT REFERENCES:

Enclade, H. X., Chow, M. S., Sund, L. T., O'Dell, K., Hapner, E. R., & Johns, M. M., III. (2021). Pilot evaluation of community-based vocal health screenings. *Journal of Voice, 35*(4), 666.e1–666.e5. https://doi.org/10.1016/j.jvoice.2019.12.018

Grillo, E. U. (2021). Functional voice assessment and therapy methods supported by telepractice, VoiceEvalU8, and Estill voice training. *Seminars in Speech and Language, 42*(1), 41–53. https://doi.org/10.1055/s-0040-1722753

Huttunen, K., & Rantala, L. (2021). Effects of humidification on the vocal tract and respiratory muscle training in women with voice symptoms—A pilot study. *Journal of Voice, 35*(1), 158.e21–158.e33. https://doi.org/10.1016/j.jvoice.2019.07.019

Lee, J. M., Roy, N., Park, A., Muntz, H., Meier, J., Skirko, J., & Smith, M. (2021). Personality in children with vocal fold nodules: A multitrait analysis. *Journal of Speech, Language, and Hearing Research, 64*, 3742–3758. https://doi.org/10.1044/2021_JSLHR-21-00144

Nusseck, M., Spahn, C., Echternach, M., Immerz, A., & Richter, B. (2020). Vocal health, voice self-concept and quality of life in German school teachers. *Journal of Voice, 34*(3), 488.e29–488.e39. https://doi.org/10.1016/j.jvoice.2018.11.008

Porcaro, C. K., Howery, S., Suhandron, A., & Gollery, T. (2021). Impact of vocal hygiene training on teachers' willingness to change vocal behaviors. *Journal of Voice, 35*(3), 499.e1–499.e11. https://doi.org/10.1016/j.jvoice.2019.11.011

Slavych, B. K., Zraick, R. I., Bursac, Z., Tulunay-Ugur, O., & Hadden, K. (2021). An investigation of the relationship between adherence to voice therapy for muscle tension dysphonia and employment, social support, and life satisfaction. *Journal of Voice, 35*(3), 386–393. https://doi.org/10.1016/j.jvoice.2019.10.015

Titze, I. (2020). Long hours of vocalization over electronic media. *Journal of Singing, 77*(1), 71–72.

National Institute on Deafness and Other Communication Disorders. (2021, April 15). *Taking care of your voice* (NIH Publication No. 14-5160, pp. 1–4), U.S. Department of Health and Human Service, National Institutes of Health. https://www.nidcd.nih.gov/health/taking-care-your-voice

Vermeulen, R., van der Linde, J., Abdoola, S., van Lierde, K., & Graham, M. A. (2021). The effect of superficial hydration, with or without systematic hydration, on voice quality in future female professional singers. *Journal of Voice, 35*(5), 728–738. https://doi.org/10.1016/j.jvoice.2020.01.008

Zalvan, C., Yuen, E., Geliebter, J., & Tiwari, R. (2021). A trigger reduction approach to treatment of paradoxical vocal fold motion disorder in the pediatric population. *Journal of Voice, 35*(2), 323.e9–323.e15. https://doi.org/10.1016/j.jvoice.2019.08.013

R

Risk Detection   1908

Definition: Personal actions to identify personal health threats

OUTCOME TARGET RATING: Maintain at_____   Increase to_____

		Never Demonstrated	Rarely Demonstrated	Sometimes Demonstrated	Often Demonstrated	Consistently Demonstrated	
OUTCOME OVERALL RATING		1	2	3	4	5	
Indicators:							
190801	Recognizes signs and symptoms that indicate risks	1	2	3	4	5	NA
190802	Identifies potential health risks	1	2	3	4	5	NA
190803	Seeks validation of perceived risks	1	2	3	4	5	NA
190804	Performs self-examinations at recommended intervals	1	2	3	4	5	NA
190805	Participates in screening at recommended intervals	1	2	3	4	5	NA
190806	Acquires knowledge of family history	1	2	3	4	5	NA
190814	Shares identified risks with family members also at risk	1	2	3	4	5	NA
190807	Maintains updated knowledge of family health history	1	2	3	4	5	NA
190808	Maintains updated knowledge of personal health history	1	2	3	4	5	NA
190809	Uses resources to stay informed about personal risks	1	2	3	4	5	NA
190815	Seeks information about available screening options	1	2	3	4	5	NA
190816	Discusses frequency of screening based on risk and age	1	2	3	4	5	NA
190813	Monitors changes in general health status	1	2	3	4	5	NA
190810	Uses health care services congruent with needs	1	2	3	4	5	NA
190812	Obtains information about changes in health recommendations	1	2	3	4	5	NA

Domain-Health Knowledge & Behavior (IV)   ***Class*-Risk Control (T)**   *1st edition 1997; revised 2004, 2013, 2024*

OUTCOME CONTENT REFERENCES:

Bibbins-Domingo, K., Grossman, D. C., Curry, S. J., Davidson, K. W., Ebell, M., Epling, J. W., Jr, García, F. A. R., Gillman, M. W., Kemper, A. R., Krist, A. H., Kurth, A. E., Landefeld, C. S., Mangione, C. M., Phillips, W. R., Phipps, M. G., Pignone, M. P., & Siu, A. L. (2016). Screening for skin cancer: U.S. Preventive Services Task Force Recommendation Statement. *Journal of the American Medical Association, 316*(4), 429–435. https://doi.org/10.1001/jama.2016.8465

Gaddam, S., Heller, S. L., Babb, J. S., & Gao, Y. (2021). Male breast cancer risk assessment and screening recommendations in high-risk men who undergo genetic counseling and multigene panel testing. *Clinical Breast Cancer, 21*(1), e74–e79. https://doi.org/10.1016/j.clbc.2020.07.014

Gilbert, F. J., Hickman, S. E., Baxter, G. C., Allajbeu, I., James, J., Caraco, C., Vinnicombe, S., & Carraco, C. (2021). Opportunities in cancer imaging: Risk-adapted breast imaging in screening. *Clinical Radiology, 76*(10), 763–773. https://doi.org/10.1016/j.crad.2021.02.013

Gilfoyle, M., Chaurasia, A., Garcia, J., & Oremus, M. (2021). Perceived susceptibility to developing cancer and screening for colorectal and prostate cancer: A longitudinal analysis of Alberta's Tomorrow Project. *Journal of Medical Screening, 28*(2), 148–157. https://doi.org/10.1177/0969141320941900

Kates, F. R., Romero, R., Jones, D., Egelfeld, J., & Datta, S. (2021). A comparison of web-based cancer risk calculators that inform shared decision-making for lung cancer screening. *JGIM: Journal of General Internal Medicine, 36*(6), 1543–1552. https://doi.org/10.1007/s11606-021-06754-0

Li, J., Hart, T., Aronson, M., Crangle, C., & Govindarajan, A. (2016). Cancer worry, perceived risk and cancer screening in first-degree relatives of patients with familial gastric cancer. *Journal of Genetic Counseling, 25*(3), 520–528. https://doi.org/10.1007/s10897-015-9903-z

Obermair, H. M., McCaffery, K. J., & Dodd, R. H. (2020). "A Pap smear saved my life": Personal experiences of cervical abnormalities shape attitudes to cervical screening renewal. *Journal of Medical Screening, 27*(4), 223–226. https://doi.org/10.1177/0969141319889648

Özkan, İ., & Taylan, S. (2021). Barriers to women's breast cancer screening behaviors in several countries: A meta-synthesis study. *Health Care for Women International, 42*(7–9), 1013–1043. https://doi.org/10.1080/07399332.2020.1814777

Patel, S. G., May, F. P., Anderson, J. C., Burke, C. A., Dominitz, J. A., Gross, S. A., Jacobson, B. C., Shaukat, A., & Robertson, D. J. (2022). Updates on age to start and stop colorectal cancer screening: Recommendations from the U.S. Multi-Society Task Force on Colorectal Cancer. *Gastrointestinal Endoscopy, 95*(1), 1–15. https://doi.org/10.1016/j.gie.2021.06.012

Phelan, D. L., Oliveria, S. A., Christos, P. J., Dusza, S. W., & Halpern, A. C. (2003). Skin self-examination in patients at high risk for melanoma: A pilot study. *Oncology Nursing Forum, 30*(6), 1029–1036. https://doi.org/10.1188/03.ONF.1029-1036

R

Rainey, L., van der Waal, D., Donnelly, L. S., Southworth, J., French, D. P., Evans, D. G., & Broeders, M. J. M. (2022). Women's health behaviour change after receiving breast cancer risk estimates with tailored screening and prevention recommendations. *BMC Cancer, 22*(1), 1–13. https://doi.org/10.1186/s12885-022-09174-3

Schifferdecker, K. E., Tosteson, A. N. A., Kaplan, C., Kerlikowske, K., Buist, D. S. M., Henderson, L. M., Johnson, D., Jaworski, J., Jackson-Nefertiti, G., Ehrlich, K., Marsh, M. W., Vu, L., Onega, T., & Wernli, K. J. (2020). Knowledge and perception of breast density, screening mammography, and supplemental screening: In search of "informed." *JGIM: Journal of General Internal Medicine, 35*(6), 1654–1660. https://doi.org/10.1007/s11606-019-05560-z

Role Performance 1501

Definition: Personal actions to convey congruence of an individual's role behavior with role expectations

OUTCOME TARGET RATING: Maintain at_____ Increase to_____

	Never Demonstrated	Rarely Demonstrated	Sometimes Demonstrated	Often Demonstrated	Consistently Demonstrated	
OUTCOME OVERALL RATING	1	2	3	4	5	
Indicators:						
150118 Reports role changes with illness or disability	1	2	3	4	5	NA
150119 Reports role changes with death of family member	1	2	3	4	5	NA
150120 Reports role changes with elderly dependents	1	2	3	4	5	NA
150121 Reports role changes with new family member	1	2	3	4	5	NA
150122 Reports role changes when family member leaves home	1	2	3	4	5	NA
150123 Reports strategies for role change(s)	1	2	3	4	5	NA
150124 Performs strategies to aid with role change(s)	1	2	3	4	5	NA
150125 Performs role expectations	1	2	3	4	5	NA
150126 Reports knowledge of role transition periods	1	2	3	4	5	NA
150127 Performs family role behaviors	1	2	3	4	5	NA
150128 Performs parental role behaviors	1	2	3	4	5	NA
150129 Performs intimate role behaviors	1	2	3	4	5	NA
150130 Performs community role behaviors	1	2	3	4	5	NA
150131 Performs work role behaviors	1	2	3	4	5	NA
150132 Performs friendship role behaviors	1	2	3	4	5	NA
150133 Reports comfort with role expectations	1	2	3	4	5	NA
150134 Reports comfort with role change(s)	1	2	3	4	5	NA
150135 Reports satisfaction with role changes	1	2	3	4	5	NA
150136 Reports satisfaction with non-traditional role choices	1	2	3	4	5	NA

Domain-Psychosocial Health (III)   **Class**-Social Interaction (P)   *1st edition 1997; revised 2004, 2013, 2024*

OUTCOME CONTENT REFERENCES:

Brass, N. R., & Ryan, A. M. (2021). Changes in behavioral correlates of social status during early adolescence: Does school contact matter? *Developmental Psychology, 57*(7), 1136–1148. https://doi.org/10.1037/dev0000957

Chesley, N., & Flood, S. (2017). Signs of change? At-home and breadwinner parents' housework and child-care time. *Journal of Marriage and Family, 79*, 511–534. https://doi.org/10.1111/jomf.12376

Hodkinson, P., & Brooks, R. (2018). Interchangeable parents? The roles and identities of primary and equal carer fathers of young children. *Current Sociology, 68*(6), 780–797. https://doi.org/10.1177/0011392118807530

Kim, C. Y. (2021). Perceived social loafing congruence between leaders and members: Effect on performance. *Social Behavior and* Personality: *An International Journal, 49*(6), e10266, 1–13. https://doi.org/10.2224/sbp.10266

Pinho, M., & Gaunt, R. (2021). Doing and undoing gender in male carer/female breadwinner families. *Community, Work & Family, 24*(3), 315–330. https://doi.org/10.1080/13668803.2019.1681940

Richter, N., Bondü, R., & Trommsdorff, G. (2021). Linking transition to motherhood to parenting, children's emotion regulation, and life satisfaction: A longitudinal study. *Journal of Family Psychology, 27*(5), 773–783. https://doi.org/10.1037/fam0000868

Stanford, N., Carlock, S., & Jia, F. (2021). The role of community in black identity development and occupational choice. *Societies, 11*, 1–11. https://doi.org/10.3390/soc11030111

Willroth, E. C., Atherton, O. E., & Robins, R. W. (2021). Life satisfaction trajectories during adolescence and the transition to young adulthood: Findings from a longitudinal study of Mexican-origin youth. *Journal of Personality and Social Psychology: Personality Processes and Individual Differences, 120*(1), 192–205. https://doi.org/10.1037/pspp0000294

Xing, M., Xia, Y., Zhao, M., & Lan, Y. (2021). Perceived negative gossip of coworkers: Effect on newcomers' work outcomes during social adjustment. *Social Behavior and Personality, 49*(4), e9817. https://doi.org/10.2224/sbp.9817

Safe Health Care Environment   1934

Definition: Physical and system arrangements to minimize factors that might cause physical harm or injury in the health care facility

OUTCOME TARGET RATING: Maintain at_____ Increase to_____

	Poor	Fair	Good	Very Good	Excellent	
OUTCOME OVERALL RATING	1	2	3	4	5	
Indicators:						
193429 Provision of lighting	1	2	3	4	5	NA
193430 Placement of handrails	1	2	3	4	5	NA
193431 Use of personal alarm system	1	2	3	4	5	NA
193432 Nurse call system within reach	1	2	3	4	5	NA
193433 Bed in low position	1	2	3	4	5	NA
193434 Arrangement of furniture to reduce risks based on patient needs	1	2	3	4	5	NA
193435 Room temperature regulation	1	2	3	4	5	NA
193436 Elimination of harmful noise levels	1	2	3	4	5	NA
193437 Provision of assistive devices in accessible locations	1	2	3	4	5	NA
193438 Equipment safety alarms on and working	1	2	3	4	5	NA
193439 Provision of equipment that meets safety standards	1	2	3	4	5	NA
193440 Security systems in place in nursery	1	2	3	4	5	NA
193441 Provision of safe play area	1	2	3	4	5	NA
193442 Provision of age-appropriate toys	1	2	3	4	5	NA
193443 Use of electrical outlet covers	1	2	3	4	5	NA
193444 Safe storage of hazardous materials	1	2	3	4	5	NA
193445 Falls prevention policy	1	2	3	4	5	NA
193446 Patient identification system	1	2	3	4	5	NA
193447 Computerized physician order entry	1	2	3	4	5	NA
193448 High alert medication policy	1	2	3	4	5	NA
193449 Point of care bedside medication charting	1	2	3	4	5	NA
193450 Barcoding system for patients and medication	1	2	3	4	5	NA
193451 Medication reconciliation activity	1	2	3	4	5	NA
193452 Allergy alert system	1	2	3	4	5	NA
193453 Safe storage of medication	1	2	3	4	5	NA
193454 Error reporting system including near miss	1	2	3	4	5	NA
193455 Patient safety program	1	2	3	4	5	NA
193456 Use of evidence-based practice protocols	1	2	3	4	5	NA
193457 Care management systems in place	1	2	3	4	5	NA
193458 Evaluation of physical restraints use and reassessment policy	1	2	3	4	5	NA
193459 Evaluation of chemical restraints use and reassessment policy	1	2	3	4	5	NA

S

Continued

Safe Health Care Environment—cont'd

		Poor	Fair	Good	Very Good	Excellent	
193460	Visitation policy in place	1	2	3	4	5	NA
193461	Fire evacuation policy	1	2	3	4	5	NA
193462	Adverse weather policy	1	2	3	4	5	NA
193463	Leadership support for patient safety	1	2	3	4	5	NA
193464	Teamwork across units	1	2	3	4	5	NA
193465	Surveillance systems for hospital acquired infections	1	2	3	4	5	NA
193466	Computerized clinical decision support	1	2	3	4	5	NA
193467	Surgical checklist to prevent adverse events in surgery	1	2	3	4	5	NA
193468	Security procedures in mental health units	1	2	3	4	5	NA
193469	Security procedures in emergency rooms	1	2	3	4	5	NA
193470	Open communication about safety with patients and families	1	2	3	4	5	NA
193471	Communication between nurses and other health care professionals	1	2	3	4	5	NA

Domain-Health Knowledge & Behavior (IV) **Class**-Safety (HH) 5th edition 2013; revised 2024

OUTCOME CONTENT REFERENCES:

Bates, D. W., & Singh, H. (2018). Two decades since *To Err is Human*: An assessment of progress and emerging priorities in patient safety. *Health Affairs, 37*(11), 1736–1743. https://doi.org/10.1377/hlthaff.2018.0738

Burrus, S., Hall, M., & Tooley, E. (2021). Factors related to serious safety events in a Children's Hospital Patient Safety Collaborative. *Pediatrics, 148*(3), 1–7. https://doi.org/10.1542/peds.2020-030346

Desmedt, M., Bergs, J., Willaert, B., Schrooten, W., Vlayen, A., Hellings, J., Claes, N., & Vandijck, D. (2021). Exploring and evaluating patient safety culture in a community-based primary care setting. *Journal of Patient Safety, 17*(8), e1216–e1222. https://doi.org/10.1097/PTS.0000000000000458

Groves, P. S., Bunch, J. L., Sabadosa, K. A., Cannava, K. E., & Williams, J. K. (2021). A grounded theory of creating space for open safety communication between hospitalized patients and nurses. *Nursing Outlook, 69*(4), 632–640. https://doi.org/10.1016/j.outlook.2021.01.005

Merner, B., Hill, S., & Taylor, M. (2019). "I'm trying to stop things before they happen": Carers' contributions to patient safety in hospitals. *Qualitative Health Research, 29*(10), 1508–1518. https://doi.org/10.1177/1049732319841021

+Monaca, C., Bestmann, B., Kattein, M., Langner, D., Müller, H., & Manser, T. (2020). Assessing patients' perceptions of safety culture in the hospital setting: Development and initial evaluation of the Patients' Perceptions of Safety Culture Scale. *Journal of Patient Safety, 16*(1), 90–97. https://doi.org/10.1097/PTS.0000000000000436

Sauro, K., Machan, M., Whalen-Browne, L., Owen, V., Wu, G., & Stelfox, H. (2021). Evolving factors in hospital safety. A systematic review and meta-analysis of hospital adverse events. *Journal of Patient Safety, 17*(8), e1285–e1295. https://doi.org/10.1097/PTS.0000000000000889

Shah, R. K., & Godambe, S. A. (2021). *Patient safety and quality improvement in healthcare*. Springer.

Tlili, M. A., Aouicha, W., Sahli, J., Zedini, C., Ben Dhiab, M., Chelbi, S., Mtiraoui, A., Said Latiri, H., Ajmi, T., Ben Rejeb, M., & Mallouli, M. (2021). A baseline assessment of patient safety culture and its associated factors from the perspective of critical care nurses: Results from 10 hospitals. *Australian Critical Care, 34*(4), 363–369. https://doi.org/10.1016/j.aucc.2020.09.004

Torrente, G., & de Fátima Faria Barbosa, S. (2021). Questionnaire for assessing patient safety culture in emergency services: An integrative review. *Brazilian Journal of Nursing, 74*(2), 1–8. https://doi.org/10.1590/0034-7167-2019-0693

Wachter, R., & Gupta, K. (2018). *Understanding patient safety* (3rd ed.). McGraw-Hill.

Safe Home Environment 1910

Definition: Physical arrangements and protective actions to minimize environmental factors that can cause physical injury in the home

OUTCOME TARGET RATING: Maintain at _____ Increase to _____

		Poor	Fair	Good	Very Good	Excellent	
OUTCOME OVERALL RATING		1	2	3	4	5	
Indicators:							
191044	Exterior building maintenance	1	2	3	4	5	NA
191045	Exterior lighting	1	2	3	4	5	NA
191046	Interior home maintenance	1	2	3	4	5	NA
191047	Interior lighting	1	2	3	4	5	NA

Safe Home Environment—cont'd

		Poor	Fair	Good	Very Good	Excellent	
191048	Availability of clean water	1	2	3	4	5	NA
191049	Safe food storage	1	2	3	4	5	NA
191050	Safe food preparation	1	2	3	4	5	NA
191051	Knives stored to prevent access by children	1	2	3	4	5	NA
191052	Cleanliness of dwelling	1	2	3	4	5	NA
191053	Elimination of pests	1	2	3	4	5	NA
191054	Space to move safely in dwelling	1	2	3	4	5	NA
191055	Locks on windows	1	2	3	4	5	NA
191056	Locks on doors	1	2	3	4	5	NA
191057	Use of home security system	1	2	3	4	5	NA
191058	Placement of handrails on stairs	1	2	3	4	5	NA
191059	Stairs free of clutter	1	2	3	4	5	NA
191060	Removal of throw rugs	1	2	3	4	5	NA
191061	Carbon monoxide detector maintenance	1	2	3	4	5	NA
191062	Smoke detector maintenance	1	2	3	4	5	NA
191063	Availability of emergency response system	1	2	3	4	5	NA
191064	Accessibility of telephone or cell phone	1	2	3	4	5	NA
191065	Accessibility of bathroom	1	2	3	4	5	NA
191066	Safety bars in bathroom	1	2	3	4	5	NA
191067	Toilet at correct height	1	2	3	4	5	NA
191068	Safe storage of medication	1	2	3	4	5	NA
191069	Proper disposal of medication	1	2	3	4	5	NA
191070	Accessibility of assistive devices	1	2	3	4	5	NA
191071	Equipment maintained to meet safety standards	1	2	3	4	5	NA
191072	Safe storage of firearms	1	2	3	4	5	NA
191073	Safe storage of hazardous materials	1	2	3	4	5	NA
191074	Safe disposal of hazardous materials	1	2	3	4	5	NA
191075	Safe storage of matches/lighters	1	2	3	4	5	NA
191076	Safe use of ladders and step stools	1	2	3	4	5	NA
191077	Elimination of mold	1	2	3	4	5	NA
191078	Elimination of radon	1	2	3	4	5	NA
191079	Elimination of toxic fumes	1	2	3	4	5	NA
191080	Elimination of tobacco smoke	1	2	3	4	5	NA
191081	Arrangement of furniture to reduce risks	1	2	3	4	5	NA
191082	Safety of outdoor play area	1	2	3	4	5	NA
191083	Removal of doors from unused appliances	1	2	3	4	5	NA
191084	Correction of lead hazard risks	1	2	3	4	5	NA
191085	Safety of age-appropriate toys	1	2	3	4	5	NA
191086	Use of electrical outlet covers	1	2	3	4	5	NA
191087	Inspection of electrical cords for damage	1	2	3	4	5	NA
191088	Avoidance of extension cord use	1	2	3	4	5	NA
191089	Room temperature regulation	1	2	3	4	5	NA
191090	Use of motion activated lights	1	2	3	4	5	NA
191091	Elimination of harmful noise levels	1	2	3	4	5	NA
191092	Placement of window guards	1	2	3	4	5	NA
191093	Safe use of space heaters	1	2	3	4	5	NA

S

Continued

Safe Home Environment—cont'd

		Poor	Fair	Good	Very Good	Excellent	
191094	Development of an emergency escape plan	1	2	3	4	5	NA
191095	Maintenance of fire extinguishers	1	2	3	4	5	NA
191096	Maintenance of emergency contact list	1	2	3	4	5	NA
191097	Keep garage and door locked	1	2	3	4	5	NA
191098	Supervision of children around pets	1	2	3	4	5	NA

Domain-Health Knowledge & Behavior (IV)   **Class**-Safety (HH)   1st edition 1997; revised 2004, 2008, 2013, 2024

OUTCOME CONTENT REFERENCES:

Byrne, A., Hagen, M. G., & Thompson, L. (2021). Gun safety for children. *Journal of the American Medical Association Pediatrics*, *175*(3), 332. https://doi.org/10.1001/jamapediatrics.2020.5989

Casteel, C., Bruening, R., Carson, M., Berard-Reed, K., & Ashida, S. (2020). Evaluation of a falls and fire safety program for community-dwelling older adults. *Journal of Community Health*, *45*(4), 717–727. https://doi.org/10.1007/s10900-019-00786-8

Jennissen, C. A., Wetjen, K. M., Wymore, C. C., Stange, N. R., Denning, G. M., Liao, J., & Wood, K. E. (2021). Firearm exposure and storage practices in the homes of rural adolescents. *Western Journal of Emergency Medicine: Integrating Emergency Care with Population Health*, *22*, 74–85. https://doi.org/10.5811/westjem.2021.3.50263

Keglovits, M., Clemson, L., Hu, Y., Nguyen, A., Neff, A. J., Mandelbaum, C., Hudson, M., Williams, R., Silianoff, T., & Stark, S. (2020). A scoping review of fall hazards in the homes of older adults and development of a framework for assessment and intervention. *Australian Occupational Therapy Journal*, *67*(5), 470–478. https://doi.org/10.1111/1440-1630.12682

Kivimäki, T., Stolt, M., Charalambous, A., & Suhonen, R. (2020). Safety of older people at home: An integrative literature review. *International Journal of Older People Nursing*, *15*(1), e12285. https://doi.org/10.1111/opn.12285

Powell-Cope, G., Thomason, S., Bulat, T., Pippins, K. M., & Young, H. M. (2018). Preventing falls and fall-related injuries at home: Teaching family caregivers about home modification and what to do if a fall occurs. *AJN, American Journal of Nursing*, *118*(1), 58–61. https://doi.org/10.1097/01.NAJ.0000529720.67793.60

Smith, G. A., Chounthirath, T., & Splaingard, M. (2020). Do sleeping children respond better to a smoke alarm that uses their mother's voice? *Academic Pediatrics*, *20*(3), 319–326. https://doi.org/10.1016/j.acap.2019.06.016

Vane, J., Fullerton, L., & Sapién, R. (2021). Identification of household dangers by parents from adult versus child visual perspective. *Journal of Injury & Violence Research*, *13*(2), 121–126. https://doi.org/10.5249/jivr.v13i2.1654

Safe Home Environment: Nursery

1947

Definition: Physical arrangements and protective actions to minimize environmental factors that can cause physical injury to an infant or toddler

OUTCOME TARGET RATING: Maintain at _____ Increase to _____

		Poor	Fair	Good	Very Good	Excellent	
OUTCOME OVERALL RATING		1	2	3	4	5	

Indicators:

194701	Furniture secured to wall to prevent tip-overs	1	2	3	4	5	NA
194702	Avoidance of glass doors in furniture	1	2	3	4	5	NA
194703	Dresser drawers secured with child proof locks	1	2	3	4	5	NA
194704	Crib positioned away from window	1	2	3	4	5	NA
194705	Crib meets current safety standards	1	2	3	4	5	NA
194706	Use of a firm mattress that properly fits the crib	1	2	3	4	5	NA
194707	Lowering of mattress level over time as infant grows	1	2	3	4	5	NA
194708	Use of a fitted sheet in crib	1	2	3	4	5	NA
194709	Use of cordless window treatments	1	2	3	4	5	NA
194710	Use of overhead lighting rather than freestanding lamps	1	2	3	4	5	NA
194711	Use of sleep sacks or sleepers rather than blankets	1	2	3	4	5	NA
194712	Use of window guards or window stops	1	2	3	4	5	NA
194713	Avoidance of chairs or furniture near window	1	2	3	4	5	NA
194714	Infant monitor placed at least 3 feet from crib with cords secured	1	2	3	4	5	NA
194715	Pillows and bumper guards not used in crib	1	2	3	4	5	NA

S

Safe Home Environment: Nursery—cont'd

	Poor	Fair	Good	Very Good	Excellent	
194716 Storage of toys outside of crib	1	2	3	4	5	NA
194717 Avoids hanging pictures or heavy objects over crib	1	2	3	4	5	NA
194718 Mobiles hung at safe height over crib (out of reach) with less than 7 inches of cord	1	2	3	4	5	NA
194719 Smoke detector used in nursery	1	2	3	4	5	NA
194720 Electrical outlet protectors in place	1	2	3	4	5	NA
194721 Use of a toy chest without a lid	1	2	3	4	5	NA

Domain-Health Knowledge & Behavior (IV)   **Class**-Safety (HH)   7th edition 2024

OUTCOME CONTENT REFERENCES:

American Academy of Pediatrics, Task Force on Sudden Infant Death Syndrome. (2016). SIDS and other sleep-related infant deaths: Updated 2016 recommendations for a safe infant sleeping environment. *Pediatrics, 138*(5), e20162938. https://doi.org/10.1542/peds.2016-2938

Carrow, J. N., Vladescu, J. C., Reeve, S. A., & Kisamore, A. N. (2020). Back to sleep: Teaching adults to arrange safe infant sleep environments. *Journal of Applied Behavior Analysis, 53*(3), 1321–1336. https://doi.org/10.1002/jaba.681

Cole, R., Young, J., Kearney, L., & Thompson, J. M. D. (2021). Challenges parents encounter when implementing infant safe sleep advice. *Acta Paediatrics, 110*(11), 1–11. https://doi.org/10.1111/apa.16040

Hockenberry, M. J., Wilson, D., & Rodgers, C. C. (Eds.). (2019). *Wong's nursing care of infants and children* (11th ed.). Elsevier.

Vladescu, J. C., Schnell, L. K., & Day-Watkins, J. (2020). Infant positioning: A brief review. *Journal of Applied Behavioral Analysis, 53*(3), 1237–1241. https://doi.org/10.1002/jaba.746

Safe Wandering   1926

Definition: Safe, socially acceptable moving about without apparent purpose in an individual with cognitive impairment

OUTCOME TARGET RATING: Maintain at_____ Increase to_____

	Never Demonstrated	Rarely Demonstrated	Sometimes Demonstrated	Often Demonstrated	Consistently Demonstrated	
OUTCOME OVERALL RATING	1	2	3	4	5	
Indicators:						
192601 Moves about without harming self	1	2	3	4	5	NA
192602 Moves about without harming others	1	2	3	4	5	NA
192623 Moves about without bumping into obstacles	1	2	3	4	5	NA
192624 Moves about without upsetting others	1	2	3	4	5	NA
192625 Engages respectfully with others	1	2	3	4	5	NA
192626 Engages in relevant conversation	1	2	3	4	5	NA
192627 Maintains consistent emotional expression	1	2	3	4	5	NA
192603 Sits for more than 5 minutes at a time	1	2	3	4	5	NA
192604 Paces a given route	1	2	3	4	5	NA
192605 Appears content in calm environment	1	2	3	4	5	NA
192606 Remains in secure area when unaccompanied	1	2	3	4	5	NA
192628 Moves about own space	1	2	3	4	5	NA
192629 Moves about in public space	1	2	3	4	5	NA
192608 Uses own toileting facilities	1	2	3	4	5	NA
192609 Performs purposeful activities	1	2	3	4	5	NA
192630 Performs diversional activities	1	2	3	4	5	NA

Continued

S

Safe Wandering—cont'd

		Never Demonstrated	Rarely Demonstrated	Sometimes Demonstrated	Often Demonstrated	Consistently Demonstrated	
192610	Locates landmarks in familiar setting	1	2	3	4	5	NA
192611	Can be redirected from unsafe activities	1	2	3	4	5	NA
192612	Distracts easily	1	2	3	4	5	NA
192613	Dresses appropriately	1	2	3	4	5	NA

Domain-Health Knowledge & Behavior (IV) **Class**-Safety (HH) 4th edition 2008; revised 2024

OUTCOME CONTENT REFERENCES:

Aud, M. A. (2004). Dangerous wandering: Elopements of older adults with dementia from long-term care facilities. *American Journal of Alzheimer's Disorders and Other Dementias, 19*(6), 361–368. https://doi.org/10.1177/153331750401900602

Barnard-Brak, L., & Parmelee, P. (2021). Measuring risk of wandering and symptoms of dementia via caregiver report. *Journal of Applied Gerontology, 40*(10), 1372–1376. https://doi.org/10.1177/0733464820947287

Barrett, B., Bulat, T., Schultz, S. K., & Luther, S. L. (2018). Factors associated with wandering behaviors in veterans with mild dementia: A prospective longitudinal community-based study. *American Journal of Alzheimer's Disease & Other Dementias, 33*(2), 100–111. https://doi.org/10.1177/1533317517735168

Brak-Barnard, L., Richman, D. M., & Owen, D. C. (2018). Assessing wandering risk among individuals with Alzheimer's disease and dementia: A pilot study. *Psychogeriatrics, 18*(5), 388–392. https://doi.org/10.1111/psyg.12336

Ko-Xin, C. H. E. N., Miao-Hsin, K. O., Mei-Yin, L. I. U., & Jing-Jy, W. A. N. G. (2022). Getting lost in people with dementia: A scoping review. *Journal of Nursing, 69*(1), 100–113. https://doi.org/10.6224/JN.202202_69(1).12

Lee, K. H., Algase, D. L., & McConnell, E. S. (2014). Relationship between observable emotional expression and wandering behavior of people with dementia. *International Journal of Geriatric Psychiatry, 29*(1), 85–92. https://doi.org/10.1002/gps.3977

MacAndrew, M., Beattie, E., O'Reilly, M., Kolanowski, A., & Windsor, C. (2017). The trajectory of tolerance for wandering-related boundary transgression: An exploration of care staff and family perceptions. *The Gerontologist, 57*(3), 451–460. https://doi.org/10.1093/geront/gnv136

MacAndrew, M., Brooks, D., & Beattie, E. (2017). Nonpharmacological interventions for managing wandering in the community: A narrative review of the evidence base. *Health and Social Care, 27*(2), 306–319. https://doi.org/10.1111/hsc.12590

Neubauer, N., & Liu, L. (2020). Evaluation of antecedent behaviors of dementia-related wandering in community and facility settings. *Neurodegenerative Disease Management, 10*(3), 125–135. https://doi.org/10.2217/nmt-2019-0030

Seizure Self-Control

1620

Definition: Personal actions to reduce or minimize the occurrence of seizure episodes and impact on life quality

OUTCOME TARGET RATING: Maintain at _____ Increase to _____

		Never Demonstrated	Rarely Demonstrated	Sometimes Demonstrated	Often Demonstrated	Consistently Demonstrated	
OUTCOME OVERALL RATING		1	2	3	4	5	
Indicators:							
162018	Participates in educational programs to learn about seizure prevention	1	2	3	4	5	NA
162001	Describes precipitating seizure factors	1	2	3	4	5	NA
162019	Adheres to medication regimen	1	2	3	4	5	NA
162002	Uses medication as prescribed	1	2	3	4	5	NA
162016	Obtains needed medication	1	2	3	4	5	NA
162004	Contacts health professional when medication side effects occur	1	2	3	4	5	NA
162006	Avoids seizure triggers/risk factors	1	2	3	4	5	NA
162017	Obtains medical attention immediately if seizure frequency increases	1	2	3	4	5	NA
162008	Uses effective stress reduction techniques	1	2	3	4	5	NA
162009	Maintains positive attitude toward seizure disorder	1	2	3	4	5	NA

S

Seizure Self-Control—cont'd

		Never Demonstrated	Rarely Demonstrated	Sometimes Demonstrated	Often Demonstrated	Consistently Demonstrated	
162010	Maintains role performance	1	2	3	4	5	NA
162011	Maintains social relationships	1	2	3	4	5	NA
162012	Maintains sleep-wake pattern	1	2	3	4	5	NA
162013	Follows prescribed exercise program	1	2	3	4	5	NA
162015	Implements safety practices in environment	1	2	3	4	5	NA
162020	Lowers self to floor if experiencing impending seizure	1	2	3	4	5	NA
162021	Monitors seizure frequency	1	2	3	4	5	NA
162022	Monitors impact of fatigue	1	2	3	4	5	NA
162023	Monitors for signs of depression	1	2	3	4	5	NA
162024	Monitors quality of life	1	2	3	4	5	NA

Domain-*Health Knowledge & Behavior (IV)*   **Class**-*Health Behavior (Q)*   *3rd edition 2004; revised 2008, 2013, 2024*

OUTCOME CONTENT REFERENCES:

Edward, K., Cook, M., Stephenson, J., & Giandinoto, J. A. (2019). The impact of brief lifestyle self-management education for the control of seizures. *British Journal of Nursing, 28*(6), 348–354. https://doi.org/10.12968/bjon.2019.28.6.348

Freedman, D. A., & Albert, D. V. F. (2021). Seizure safety education should be provided to pediatric patients with suspected seizures. *Pediatric Neurology, 114*, 53–54. https://doi.org/10.1016/j.pediatrneurol.2020.08.018

Hu, M., Zhang, C., Xiao, X., Guo, J., & Sun, H. (2020). Effect of intensive self-management education on seizure frequency and quality of life in epilepsy patients with prodromes or precipitating factors. *Seizure, 78*, 38–42. https://doi.org/10.1016/j.seizure.2020.03.003

Luedke, M. W., Blalock, D. V., Goldstein, K. M., Kosinski, A. S., Sinha, S. R., Drake, C., Lewis, J. D., Husain, A. M., Lewinski, A. A., Shapiro, A., Gierisch, J. M., Tran, T. T., Gordon, A. M., Van Noord, M. G., Bosworth, H. B., & Williams, J. W. (2019). Self-management of epilepsy: A systematic review. *Annals of Internal Medicine, 171*(2), 117–126. https://doi.org/10.7326/M19-0458

Mahmoud, S. H., Zhou, X. Y., & Ahmed, S. N. (2020). Managing the patient with epilepsy and renal impairment. *Seizure, 76*, 143–152. https://doi.org/j.seizure.2020.02.006

Seizure Severity   **2118**

Definition: Severity of signs and symptoms of an observed convulsion

OUTCOME TARGET RATING: Maintain at_____ Increase to_____

		Severe	Substantial	Moderate	Mild	None	
OUTCOME OVERALL RATING		1	2	3	4	5	
Indicators:							
211801	Jaw clenching	1	2	3	4	5	NA
211802	Fidgeting	1	2	3	4	5	NA
211803	Lip smacking	1	2	3	4	5	NA
211804	Nystagmus	1	2	3	4	5	NA
211805	Dilated pupils	1	2	3	4	5	NA
211806	Involuntary head movement	1	2	3	4	5	NA
211807	Involuntary neck movement	1	2	3	4	5	NA
211808	Involuntary body movement	1	2	3	4	5	NA
211809	Flailing lower extremities	1	2	3	4	5	NA
211810	Flailing upper extremities	1	2	3	4	5	NA
211811	Dystonic posturing	1	2	3	4	5	NA
211812	Asynchronous movement	1	2	3	4	5	NA
211813	Cyanosis	1	2	3	4	5	NA

S

Continued

Seizure Severity—cont'd

		Severe	Substantial	Moderate	Mild	None	
211814	Drooling	1	2	3	4	5	NA
211815	Tongue biting	1	2	3	4	5	NA
211816	Urinary incontinence	1	2	3	4	5	NA
211817	Bowel incontinence	1	2	3	4	5	NA
211818	Rhythmic contractions	1	2	3	4	5	NA
211819	Bizarre behaviors	1	2	3	4	5	NA
211820	Confusion	1	2	3	4	5	NA
	Length of seizure (minutes)_____						

Domain-Health & Life Quality (V)   *Class*-Symptom Status (V)   6th edition 2018

OUTCOME CONTENT REFERENCES:

+Baker, G., Smith, D., Jacoby, A., Hayes, J., & Chadwick, D. (1998). Liverpool Seizure Severity Scale revisited. *Seizure, 7*(3), 201–205. https://doi.org/10.1016/s1059-1311(98)80036-8

Core, E. T. (2010). Seizure precautions for pediatric bedside nurses. *Pediatric Nursing, 36*(4), 190–194.

Cramer J. A. (2001). Assessing the severity of seizures and epilepsy: Which scales are valid? *Current Opinion Neurology, 14*(2), 225–229. https://doi.org/10.1097/00019052-200104000-00015

Hinkel, J. L., & Cheever, K. H. (2014). *Brunner and Suddarth's textbook of medical–surgical* (13th ed.). Wolters Kluwer Health/Lippincott, Williams & Wilkins.

Kue, S. (2009). The 'fit chart', fit for purpose? A review of seizure chart documentation. *British Journal of Neuroscience Nursing, 5*(3), 106–112. https://doi.org/10.12968/bjnn.2009.5.3.40608

O'Dell, C., O'Hara, K., Kiel, S., & McCullough, K. (2007). Emergency management of seizures in the school setting. *The Journal of School Nursing, 23*(3), 158–165. https://doi.org/10.1177/10598405070230030601

Self-Awareness

1215

Definition: Acknowledges one's strengths, limitations, values, feelings, attitudes, thoughts, and behaviors in relationship to the environment and others

OUTCOME TARGET RATING: Maintain at_____ Increase to_____

		Never Demonstrated	Rarely Demonstrated	Sometimes Demonstrated	Often Demonstrated	Consistently Demonstrated	
OUTCOMES OVERALL RATING		1	2	3	4	5	

Indicators:

121501	Differentiates self from environment	1	2	3	4	5	NA
121502	Differentiates self from others	1	2	3	4	5	NA
121503	Recognizes personal physical abilities	1	2	3	4	5	NA
121504	Recognizes personal mental abilities	1	2	3	4	5	NA
121505	Recognizes personal emotional abilities	1	2	3	4	5	NA
121506	Recognizes personal physical limitations	1	2	3	4	5	NA
121507	Recognizes personal mental limitations	1	2	3	4	5	NA
121508	Recognizes personal emotional limitations	1	2	3	4	5	NA
121509	Recognizes personal behavioral patterns	1	2	3	4	5	NA
121510	Recognizes personal values	1	2	3	4	5	NA
121511	Recognizes subjective response to others	1	2	3	4	5	NA
121512	Recognizes subjective response to situations	1	2	3	4	5	NA
121513	Maintains awareness of internal signals to situations	1	2	3	4	5	NA
121514	Maintains awareness of external signals to situations	1	2	3	4	5	NA
121515	Maintains awareness of thoughts	1	2	3	4	5	NA

Self-Awareness—cont'd

		Never Demonstrated	Rarely Demonstrated	Sometimes Demonstrated	Often Demonstrated	Consistently Demonstrated	
121516	Maintains awareness of feelings	1	2	3	4	5	NA
121517	Reflects on thoughts for self-discovery	1	2	3	4	5	NA
121518	Reflects on feelings for self-discovery	1	2	3	4	5	NA
121519	Reflects on intentions for self-discovery	1	2	3	4	5	NA
121520	Expresses feelings to others	1	2	3	4	5	NA
121521	Reflects on interactions with others	1	2	3	4	5	NA
121528	Reflects on self-knowledge	1	2	3	4	5	NA
121522	Expresses needs to others	1	2	3	4	5	NA
121523	Accepts ownership of thoughts	1	2	3	4	5	NA
121524	Accepts ownership of feelings	1	2	3	4	5	NA
121525	Accepts ownership of behaviors	1	2	3	4	5	NA
121526	Remembers oneself in the past	1	2	3	4	5	NA
121527	Imagines oneself in the future	1	2	3	4	5	NA

Domain-Psychosocial Health (III)   Class-Psychological Well-Being (M)   5th edition 2013; revised 2024

OUTCOME CONTENT REFERENCES:

Amanzio, M., Bartoli, M., Cipriani, G. E., & Palermo, S. (2020). Executive dysfunction and reduced self-awareness in patients with neurological disorders. A mini-review. *Frontiers in Psychology, 11*, 1697. https://doi.org/10.3389/fpsyg.2020.01697

Eckroth-Bucher, M. (2010). Self-awareness: A review and analysis of a basic nursing concept. *ANS. Advances in Nursing Science, 33*(4), 297–309. https://doi.org/10.1097/ANS.0b013e3181fb2e4c

Herwig, U., Kaffenberger, T., Jäncke, L., & Brühl, A. B. (2010). Self-related awareness and emotion regulation. *Neuro Image, 50*(2), 734–741. https://doi.org/10.1016/j.neuroimage.2009.12.089

Leary, M. R., & Buttermore, N. R. (2003). The evolution of the human self: Tracing the natural history of self-awareness. *Journal for the Theory of Social Behaviour, 33*(4), 365–404. https://doi.org/10.10461/j1468-5914.2003.00223.x

Rasheed, S. P., Sundus, A., Younas, A., Fakhar, J., & Inayat, S. (2020). Development and testing of a measure of self-awareness among nurses. *Western Journal of Nursing Research, 43*(1), 36–44. https://doi.org/10.1177/0193945920923079

Rasheed, S. P., Younas, A., & Sundus, A. (2019). Self-awareness in nursing: A scoping review. *Journal of Clinical Nursing, 28*(5-6), 762–774. https://doi.org/10.1111/jocn.14708

Rochat, P. (2003). Five levels of self-awareness as they unfold early in life. *Consciousness and Cognition, 12*(4), 717–731. https://doi.org/10.1016/s1053-8100(03)00081-3

Rochat, P. (2021). Clinical pointers from developing self-awareness. *Developmental Medicine and Child Neurology, 63*(4), 382–386. https://doi.org/10.1111/dmcn.14767

Williamson, C., Alcantar, O., Rothlind, J., Cahn-Weiner, D., Miller, B. L., & Rosen, H. J. (2010). Standardised measurement of self-awareness deficits in FTD and AD. *Journal of Neurology, Neurosurgery, and Psychiatry, 81*(2), 140–145. https://doi.org/10.1136/jnnp.2008.166041

Younas, A., Rasheed, S. P., Sundus, A., & Inayat, S. (2020). Nurses' perspectives of self-awareness in nursing practice: A descriptive qualitative study. *Nursing & Health Sciences, 22*(2), 398–405. https://doi.org/10.1111/nhs.12671

Self-Care Behavior   0313

S

Definition: Personal actions to perform basic personal care activities and instrumental activities of daily living

OUTCOME TARGET RATING: Maintain at _____ Increase to _____

		Never Demonstrated	Rarely Demonstrated	Sometimes Demonstrated	Often Demonstrated	Consistently Demonstrated	
OUTCOME OVERALL RATING		1	2	3	4	5	
Indicators:							
031316	Bathes self	1	2	3	4	5	NA
031317	Dresses self	1	2	3	4	5	NA
031318	Prepares food and fluid for eating	1	2	3	4	5	NA
031319	Feeds self	1	2	3	4	5	NA
031320	Maintains personal cleanliness	1	2	3	4	5	NA

Continued

Self-Care Behavior—cont'd

		Never Demonstrated	Rarely Demonstrated	Sometimes Demonstrated	Often Demonstrated	Consistently Demonstrated	
031321	Maintains oral hygiene	1	2	3	4	5	NA
031322	Toilets self independently	1	2	3	4	5	NA
031323	Manages own non-parenteral medication	1	2	3	4	5	NA
031324	Manages own parenteral medication	1	2	3	4	5	NA
031325	Performs household tasks	1	2	3	4	5	NA
031326	Manages household finances	1	2	3	4	5	NA
031327	Arranges for own transportation	1	2	3	4	5	NA
031328	Obtains required household items	1	2	3	4	5	NA
031329	Recognizes safety needs in the home	1	2	3	4	5	NA

Domain-Functional Health (I)   **Class**-Self-Care (D)   *3rd edition 2004; revised 2008, 2013, 2024*

OUTCOME CONTENT REFERENCES:

Dahlgren, A., Sand, Å., Larsson, Å., Karlsson, A. K., & Claesson, L. (2013). Linking the Klein–Bell Activities of Daily Living Scale to the International Classification of Functioning, Disability, and Health. *Journal of Rehabilitation Medicine, 45*(4), 351–357. https://doi.org/10.2340/16501977-1111

Ferreira, P. L., Simões, A. L., Dourado, M., Holm, M. B., & Rogers, J. C. (2021). The Portuguese Performance Assessment of Self-Care Skills Measure: Validity and reliability. *OTJR: Occupation, Participation and Health, 41*(4), 299–308. https://doi.org/10.1177/15394492211021309

Graham, J. E., Granger, C. V., Karmarkar, A. M., Deutsch, A., Niewczyk, P., DiVita, M., & Ottenbacher, K. J. (2014). The uniform data system for medical rehabilitation: Report of follow-up information on patients discharged from rehabilitation programs in 2002–2010. *American Journal of Physical Medicine & Rehabilitation/Association of Academic Physiatrists, 93*(3), 231. https://doi.org/10.1097/PHM.0b013e3182a92c58

+Klein, R. M., & Bell, B. (1982). Self-care skills: Behavioral measurement with Klein-Bell ADL Scale. *Archives of Physical Medicine and Rehabilitation, 63*(7), 335–338.

Luciana, M., Montali, L., Nicolò, G., Fabrizi, D., Di Mauro, S., & Ausili, D. (2021). Self-care is renouncement, routine, and control: The experience of adults with type 2 diabetes mellitus. *Clinical Nursing Research, 30*(6), 892–900. https://doi.org/10.1177/1054773820969540

Morgan, J. C., Kemp, C. L., Barmon, C., Fitzroy, A., & Bell, M. M. (2021). Limiting and promoting resident self-care in assisted living. *The Journals of Gerontology: Series B, 76*(8), 1664–1672. https://doi.org/10.1093/geronb/gbab016

Oliveira–Kumakura, A. R. D. S., Sousa, C. M. F. M., Biscaro, J. A., Silva, K. C. R. D., Silva, J. L. G., Morais, S. C. R. V., & Lopes, M. V. D. O. (2021). Clinical validation of nursing diagnoses related to self-care deficits in patients with stroke. *Clinical Nursing Research, 30*(4), 494–501. https://doi.org/10.1177/1054773819883352

Queirós, C., Silva, M. A. T. C. P., Cruz, I., Cardoso, A., & Morais, E. J. (2021). Nursing diagnoses focused on universal self-care requisites. *International Nursing Review, 68*(3), 328–340. https://doi.org/10.1111/inr.12654

Singh, J. A., Tornberg, H., & Goodman, S. M. (2021). Pop a pill or give myself a shot? Patient perspectives of disease-modifying anti-rheumatic drug choice for rheumatoid arthritis. *Joint Bone Spine, 88*(1), 1–7. https://doi.org/10.1016/j.jbspin.2020.07.002

Tulu, S. N., Cook, P., Oman, K. S., Meek, P., & Gudina, E. K. (2020). Chronic disease self-care: A concept analysis. *Nursing Forum, 56*(3), 734–741. https://doi.org/10.1111/nuf.12577

Yang, C., Hui, Z., Wang, X., Tang, G., & Lee, D. T. F. (2021). A medication self-management intervention to improve adherence for older people with multimorbidity: A pilot study. *Age and Ageing, 50*(1), i12–i42. https://doi.org/10.1093/ageing/afab030.44

Self-Care Behavior: Activities of Daily Living (ADL)   **0300**

Definition: Personal actions to perform the most basic physical tasks and personal care activities independently with or without assistive device

OUTCOME TARGET RATING: Maintain at _____ Increase to _____

		Never Demonstrated	Rarely Demonstrated	Sometimes Demonstrated	Often Demonstrated	Consistently Demonstrated	
OUTCOME OVERALL RATING		1	2	3	4	5	
Indicators:							
030013	Eating	1	2	3	4	5	NA
030014	Dressing	1	2	3	4	5	NA
030015	Toileting	1	2	3	4	5	NA
030016	Bathing	1	2	3	4	5	NA

S

Self-Care Behavior: Activities of Daily Living (ADL)—cont'd

		Never Demonstrated	Rarely Demonstrated	Sometimes Demonstrated	Often Demonstrated	Consistently Demonstrated	
030017	Grooming	1	2	3	4	5	NA
030018	Hygiene performance	1	2	3	4	5	NA
030019	Oral hygiene performance	1	2	3	4	5	NA
030020	Walking	1	2	3	4	5	NA
030021	Wheelchair mobility	1	2	3	4	5	NA
030022	Transfer performance	1	2	3	4	5	NA
030023	Positioning self	1	2	3	4	5	NA

Domain-Functional Health (I)   **Class**-Self-Care (D)   1st edition 1997; revised 2004, 2013, 2024

OUTCOME CONTENT REFERENCES:

Ćwirlej-Sozańska, A., Wiśniowska-Szurlej, A., Wilmowska-Pietrusyńska, A., & Sozański, B. (2019). Determinants of ADL and IADL disability in older adults in southeastern Poland. *BMC Geriatrics, 19*(1), 1–13. https://doi.org/10.1186/s12877-019-1319-4

+Dahlgren, A., Sand, Å., Larsson, Å., Karlsson, A. K., & Claesson, L. (2013). Linking the Klein–Bell Activities of Daily Living Scale to the International Classification of Functioning, Disability, and Health. *Journal of Rehabilitation Medicine, 45*(4), 351–357. https://doi.org/10.2340/16501977-1111

Head, B. J., Maas, M., & Johnson, M. (2003). Validity and community health nursing sensitivity of six outcomes for community health nursing with older clients. *Public Health Nursing, 20*(5), 385–398. https://doi.org/10.1046/j.1525-1446.2003.20507.x

Hopman-Rock, M., van Hirtum, H., de Vreede, P., & Freiberger, E. (2019). Activities of daily living in older community-dwelling persons: A systematic review of psychometric properties of instruments. *Aging Clinical and Experimental Research, 31*(7), 917–925. https://doi.org/10.1007/s40520-018-1034-6

+Katz, S., Ford, A. B., Moskowitz, R. W., Jackson, B. A., & Jaffe, M. W. (1963). Studies of illness in the aged. The Index of ADL: A standardized measure of biological and psychosocial function. *Journal of the American Medical Association, 185*(12), 914–919. https://doi.org/10.1001/jama.1963.03060120024016

+Klein, R. M., & Bell, B. (1982). Self-care skills: Behavioral measurement with Klein-Bell ADL Scale. *Archives of Physical Medicine and Rehabilitation, 63*(7), 335–338.

Tok Yildiz, F., & Kaşikçi, M. (2020). Impact of training based on Orem's theory on self-care agency and quality of life in patients with coronary artery disease. *The Journal of Nursing Research, 28*(6), 1–10. https://doi.org/10.1097/jnr.0000000000000406

Self-Care Behavior: Bathing   0301

Definition: Personal actions to cleanse own body independently with or without assistive device

OUTCOME TARGET RATING: Maintain at _____   Increase to _____

		Never Demonstrated	Rarely Demonstrated	Sometimes Demonstrated	Often Demonstrated	Consistently Demonstrated	
OUTCOME OVERALL RATING		1	2	3	4	5	
Indicators:							
030117	Gets in and out of bathroom	1	2	3	4	5	NA
030118	Gets bath supplies	1	2	3	4	5	NA
030119	Turns on water	1	2	3	4	5	NA
030120	Regulates water temperature	1	2	3	4	5	NA
030121	Regulates water flow	1	2	3	4	5	NA
030122	Bathes at sink	1	2	3	4	5	NA
030123	Uses bath wipes	1	2	3	4	5	NA
030124	Bathes in tub	1	2	3	4	5	NA
030125	Bathes in shower	1	2	3	4	5	NA
030126	Washes face	1	2	3	4	5	NA
030127	Washes upper body	1	2	3	4	5	NA
030128	Washes lower body	1	2	3	4	5	NA
030129	Cleans perineal area	1	2	3	4	5	NA
030130	Dries body	1	2	3	4	5	NA

Domain-Functional Health (I)   **Class**-Self-Care (D)   1st edition 1997; revised 2004, 2013, 2024

S

OUTCOME CONTENT REFERENCES:

Archer, V., Smyth, W., & Nagle, C. (2021). Bathing wipes, a valuable hygiene option for frail older persons at home: A proof-of-concept study. *Australian Journal of Advanced Nursing, 38*(3), 43–46. https://doi.org/10.37464/2020.383.458

+Dahlgren, A., Sand, Å., Larsson, Å., Karlsson, A. K., & Claesson, L. (2013). Linking the Klein-Bell Activities of Daily Living Scale to the International Classification of Functioning, Disability, and Health. *Journal of Rehabilitation Medicine, 45*(4), 351–357. https://doi.org/10.2340/16501977-1111

Graham, J. E., Granger, C. V., Karmarkar, A. M., Deutsch, A., Niewczyk, P., DiVita, M., & Ottenbacher, K. J. (2014). The Uniform Data System for Medical Rehabilitation: Report of follow-up information on patients discharged from rehabilitation programs in 2002–2010. *American Journal of Physical Medicine & Rehabilitation, 93*(3), 231–244. https://doi.org/10.1097/PHM.0613e3182a92058

Hopman–Rock, M., van Hirtum, H., de Vreede, P., & Freiberger, E. (2019). Activities of daily living in older community-dwelling persons: A systematic review of psychometric properties of instruments. *Aging Clinical and Experimental Research, 31*(7), 917–925. https://doi.org/10.1007/s40520-018-1034-6

+Katz, S., Ford, A. B., Moskowitz, R. W., Jackson, B. A., & Jaffe, M. W. (1963). Studies of illness in the aged. The Index of ADL: A standardized measure of biological and psychosocial function. *Journal of the American Medical Association, 185*(12), 914–919. https://doi.org/10.1001/jama.1963.03060120024016

+Klein, R. M., & Bell, B. (1982). Self-care skills: Behavioral measurement with Klein–Bell ADL Scale. *Archives of Physical Medicine and Rehabilitation, 63*(7), 335–338.

Oliveira–Kumakura, A. R. D. S., Sousa, C. M. F. M., Biscaro, J. A., Silva, K. C. R. D., Silva, J. L. G., Morais, S. C. R. V., & Lopes, M. V. D. O. (2021). Clinical validation of nursing diagnoses related to self-care deficits in patients with stroke. *Clinical Nursing Research, 30*(4), 494–501. https://doi.org/10.1177/1054773819883352

Sagari, A., Tabira, T., Maruta, M., Miyata, H., Han, G., & Kawagoe, M. (2020). Causes of changes in basic activities of daily living in older adults with long-term care needs. *Australasian Journal on Ageing, 40*(1), e54–e61. https://doi.org/10.1111/ajag.12848

Self-Care Behavior: Dressing

0302

Definition: Personal actions to dress self independently with or without assistive device

OUTCOME TARGET RATING: Maintain at _____ Increase to _____

		Never Demonstrated	Rarely Demonstrated	Sometimes Demonstrated	Often Demonstrated	Consistently Demonstrated	
OUTCOME OVERALL RATING		1	2	3	4	5	
Indicators:							
030217	Selects clothing	1	2	3	4	5	NA
030218	Gets clothing from drawer	1	2	3	4	5	NA
030219	Gets clothing from closet	1	2	3	4	5	NA
030220	Picks up clothing	1	2	3	4	5	NA
030221	Puts clothing on upper body	1	2	3	4	5	NA
030222	Puts clothing on lower body	1	2	3	4	5	NA
030223	Buttons clothing	1	2	3	4	5	NA
030224	Uses fasteners	1	2	3	4	5	NA
030225	Uses zippers	1	2	3	4	5	NA
030226	Puts on socks	1	2	3	4	5	NA
030227	Puts on shoes	1	2	3	4	5	NA
030228	Ties shoes	1	2	3	4	5	NA
030229	Removes clothes from upper body	1	2	3	4	5	NA
030230	Removes clothes from lower body	1	2	3	4	5	NA
030231	Uses assistive devices	1	2	3	4	5	NA

Domain-Functional Health (I)   **Class**-Self-Care (D)   *1st edition 1997; revised 2004, 2008, 2013, 2024*

OUTCOME CONTENT REFERENCES:

+Dahlgren, A., Sand, Å., Larsson, Å., Karlsson, A. K., & Claesson, L. (2013). Linking the Klein-Bell Activities of Daily Living Scale to the International Classification of Functioning, Disability, and Health. *Journal of Rehabilitation Medicine, 45*(4), 351–357. https://doi.org/10.2340/16501977-1111

El Kass, S. A., Ragheb, M. M., Hamed, S. M., Turkman, A. M., & Zaki, A. T. (2021). Needs and self-care efficacy for cancer patients suffering from side effects of chemotherapy. *Journal of Oncology, 2021*, 1–9. https://doi.org/10.1155/2021/8880366

+ Graham, J. E., Granger, C. V., Karmarkar, A. M., Deutsch, A., Niewczyk, P., DiVita, M., & Ottenbacher, K. J. (2014). The uniform data system for medical rehabilitation: Report of follow-up information on patients discharged from rehabilitation programs in 2002–2010. *American Journal of Physical Medicine & Rehabilitation, 93*(3), 231–244. https://doi.org/10.1097/PHM.0613e3182a92058

S

Oliveira-Kumakura, A. R. D. E. S., Sousa, C. M. F. M., Biscaro, J. A., da Silva, K. C. R., Silva, J. L. G., Morais, S. C. R. V., & Lopes, M. V. O. (2021). Clinical validation of nursing diagnoses related to self-care deficits in patients with stroke. *Clinical Nursing Research, 30*(4), 494–501. https://doi.org/10.1177/1054773819883352

Queirós, C., Silva, M. A. T. C. P., Cruz, I., Cardoso, A., & Morais, E. J. (2021). Nursing diagnoses focused on universal self-care requisites. *International Nursing Review, 68*(3), 328–340. https://doi.org/10.1111/inr.12654

Self-Care Behavior: Eating   0303

Definition: Personal actions to prepare and ingest food and fluid independently with or without assistive device

OUTCOME TARGET RATING: Maintain at _____ Increase to _____

OUTCOME OVERALL RATING	Never Demonstrated	Rarely Demonstrated	Sometimes Demonstrated	Often Demonstrated	Consistently Demonstrated	
	1	2	3	4	5	
Indicators:						
030318 Prepares food for ingestion	1	2	3	4	5	NA
030319 Opens containers	1	2	3	4	5	NA
030320 Cuts up food	1	2	3	4	5	NA
030321 Uses utensils	1	2	3	4	5	NA
030322 Gets food onto the utensil	1	2	3	4	5	NA
030323 Picks up cup or glass	1	2	3	4	5	NA
030324 Brings food to mouth with fingers	1	2	3	4	5	NA
030325 Brings food to mouth with container	1	2	3	4	5	NA
030326 Brings food to mouth with utensil	1	2	3	4	5	NA
030327 Drinks from a cup or glass	1	2	3	4	5	NA
030328 Places food in mouth	1	2	3	4	5	NA
030329 Manipulates food in mouth	1	2	3	4	5	NA
030330 Chews food	1	2	3	4	5	NA
030331 Safely swallows food	1	2	3	4	5	NA
030332 Safely swallows fluid	1	2	3	4	5	NA
030333 Completes a meal	1	2	3	4	5	NA
030334 Eats in an acceptable manner	1	2	3	4	5	NA

Domain-*Functional Health (I)*   **Class**-*Self-Care (D)*   *1st edition 1997; revised 2004, 2013, 2024*

OUTCOME CONTENT REFERENCES:

Dahlgren, A., Sand, Å., Larsson, Å., Karlsson, A. K., & Claesson, L. (2013). Linking the Klein-Bell Activities of Daily Living Scale to the International Classification of Functioning, Disability, and Health. *Journal of Rehabilitation Medicine, 45*(4), 351–357. https://doi.org/10.2340/16501977-1111

El-Kvass, S. A., Ragheb, M. M., Hamed, S. M., Turkman, A. M., & Zaki, A. T. (2021). Needs and self-care efficacy for cancer patients suffering from side effects of chemotherapy. *Journal of Oncology, 2021*, 1–9. https://doi.org/10.1155/2021/8880366

+ Graham, J. E., Granger, C. V., Karmarkar, A. M., Deutsch, A., Niewczyk, P., DiVita, M., & Ottenbacher, K. J. (2014). The Uniform Data System for Medical Rehabilitation: Report of follow-up information on patients discharged from rehabilitation programs in 2002–2010. *American Journal of Physical Medicine & Rehabilitation, 93*(3), 231–244. https://doi.org/10.1097/PHM.0613e3182a92058

Hopman-Rock, M., van Hirtum, H., de Vreede, P., & Freiberger, E. (2019). Activities of daily living in older community-dwelling persons: A systematic review of psychometric properties of instruments. *Aging Clinical and Experimental Research, 31*(7), 917–925. https://doi.org/10.1007/s40520-018-1034-6

Queirós, C., Silva, M. A. T. C. P., Cruz, I., Cardoso, A., & Morais, E. J. (2021). Nursing diagnoses focused on universal self-care requisites. *International Nursing Review, 68*(3), 328–340. https://doi.org/10.1111/inr.12654

Sagari, A., Tabira, T., Maruta, M., Miyata, H., Han, G., & Kawagoe, M. (2020). Causes of changes in basic activities of daily living in older adults with long-term care needs. *Australasian Journal on Ageing, 40*(1), e54–e61. https://doi.org/10.1111/ajag.12848

S

Self-Care Behavior: Feet 0314

Definition: Personal actions to inspect, protect, and care for feet independently or with assistance

OUTCOME TARGET RATING: Maintain at_____ Increase to_____

OUTCOME OVERALL RATING	Never Demonstrated 1	Rarely Demonstrated 2	Sometimes Demonstrated 3	Often Demonstrated 4	Consistently Demonstrated 5	
Indicators:						
031401 Tests bath water temperature	1	2	3	4	5	NA
031402 Washes feet daily	1	2	3	4	5	NA
031403 Dries feet after bathing	1	2	3	4	5	NA
031404 Uses exfoliates or files to remove dead skin	1	2	3	4	5	NA
031405 Monitors for foot odor	1	2	3	4	5	NA
031406 Monitors for nail fungus	1	2	3	4	5	NA
031407 Trims nails correctly	1	2	3	4	5	NA
031408 Wears clean socks	1	2	3	4	5	NA
031409 Ensures proper fit of shoes and slippers	1	2	3	4	5	NA
031410 Protects feet from injury by avoiding walking barefoot	1	2	3	4	5	NA
031411 Inspects bottom of feet using mirror	1	2	3	4	5	NA
031412 Inspects for marks on feet when removing shoes and socks	1	2	3	4	5	NA
031413 Inspects feet for injury	1	2	3	4	5	NA
031414 Inspects feet for signs and symptoms of infection	1	2	3	4	5	NA
031415 Inspects toes for ingrown nails	1	2	3	4	5	NA
031416 Inspects feet for blisters	1	2	3	4	5	NA
031417 Inspects skin between toes for athletes foot	1	2	3	4	5	NA
031418 Inspects feet for signs and symptoms of edema	1	2	3	4	5	NA
031419 Inspects feet for signs and symptoms of poor circulation	1	2	3	4	5	NA
031420 Inspects feet for signs of skin breakdown	1	2	3	4	5	NA
031421 Inspects feet for signs of necrosis	1	2	3	4	5	NA
031422 Removes corns or calluses	1	2	3	4	5	NA
031423 Applies moisturizer to dry areas of legs and feet	1	2	3	4	5	NA
031424 Exercises feet	1	2	3	4	5	NA
031425 Reports signs of infection to health professional	1	2	3	4	5	NA
031426 Reports signs of skin breakdown to health professional	1	2	3	4	5	NA
031427 Reports foot pain to health professional	1	2	3	4	5	NA
031428 Reports numbness or tingling to health professional	1	2	3	4	5	NA
031429 Seeks professional evaluation of changes in boney structures	1	2	3	4	5	NA
031430 Seeks help for care of feet as needed	1	2	3	4	5	NA

Domain-Functional Health (I)   *Class*-Self-Care (D)   *7th edition 2024*

S

OUTCOME CONTENT REFERENCES:

Ataseven, M., Namoglu, S. S., & Akin, S. (2020). Assessment of knowledge level and training needs about diabetic foot care practices of diabetic patients undergoing hemodialysis. *International Journal of Caring Sciences, 13*(3), 1878–1889.

Hanley, G., Chiou, P., Liu, C., Chen, H., & Pfeiffer, S. (2020). Foot care knowledge, attitudes and practices among patients with diabetic foot and amputation in St. Kitts and Nevis. *International Wound Journal, 17*(5), 1142–1152. https://doi.org/10.1111/iwj.13446

Hodgson, L., Growcott, C., Williams, A., Nester, C., & Morrison, S. (2020). First steps: Parent health behaviours related to children's foot health. *Journal of Child Health Care, 24*(2), 221–232. https://doi.org/10.1177/1367493519864752

Miikkola, M., Lantta, T., Suhonen, R., & Stolt, M. (2019). Challenges of foot self-care in older people: A qualitative focus-group study. *Journal of Foot and Ankle Research, 12*(5), 5. https://doi.org/10.1186/s13047-019-0315-4

Morrison, S. C., Barrett, L., & Haines, D. (2020). Foot care needs for children and young people with intellectual and developmental disabilities. *British Journal of Learning Disabilities, 48*(1), 4–9. https://doi.org/10.1111/bld.12291

O'Connor, J. J., Deroche, C. B., & Wipke-Tevis, D. D. (2021). Foot care self-management in non–diabetic older adults: A pilot controlled trial. *Western Journal of Nursing Research, 43*(8), 751–761. https://doi.org/10.1177/0193945920962712

Omote, S., Watanabe, A., Hiramatsu, T., Saito, E., Yokogawa, M., Okamoto, R., Sakakibara, C., Ichimori, A., Kyota, K., & Tsukasaki, K. (2017). A foot-care program to facilitate self-care by the elderly: A non-randomized intervention study. *BMC Research Notes, 10*(1), 586. https://doi.org/10.1186/s13104-017-2898-9

Paton, J., Abey, S., Hendy, P., Williams, J., Collings, R., & Callaghan, L. (2021). Behaviour change approaches for individuals with diabetes to improve foot self-management: A scoping review. *Journal of Foot and Ankle Research, 14*(1). https://doi.org/10.1186/s13047-020-00440-w

Ramirez-Perdomo, C., Perdomo-Romero. A., & Rodríguez-Vélez. M. (2019). Knowledge and practices for diabetic foot prevention. *Revista Gaúcha de Enfermagem, 40*, e20180161. https://doi.org/10.1590/19831447.2019.20180161

Yılmaz Karadağ, F., Saltoğlu, N., Ak, Ö., Çınar Aydın, G., Şenbayrak, S., Erol, S., Mıstanoğlu Özatağ, D., Kadanalı, A., Küçükardalı, Y., Çomoğlu, Ş., Yörük, G., Akkoyunlu, Y., Meriç Koç, M., & Altunçekiç Yıldırım, A. (2019). Foot self-care in diabetes mellitus: Evaluation of patient awareness. *Primary Care Diabetes, 13*(6), 515–520. https://doi.org/10.1016/j.pcd.2019.06.003

Self-Care Behavior: Hygiene   0305

Definition: Personal actions to maintain own personal cleanliness and neat appearance independently with or without assistive device

OUTCOME TARGET RATING: Maintain at _____ Increase to _____

		Never Demonstrated	Rarely Demonstrated	Sometimes Demonstrated	Often Demonstrated	Consistently Demonstrated	
OUTCOME OVERALL RATING		1	2	3	4	5	
Indicators:							
031518	Washes hands	1	2	3	4	5	NA
031519	Uses body wipes	1	2	3	4	5	NA
031520	Cleans ears	1	2	3	4	5	NA
031521	Keeps nose blown and clean	1	2	3	4	5	NA
031522	Maintains oral hygiene	1	2	3	4	5	NA
031523	Shampoos hair	1	2	3	4	5	NA
031524	Combs or brushes hair	1	2	3	4	5	NA
031525	Safely shaves	1	2	3	4	5	NA
031526	Applies makeup	1	2	3	4	5	NA
031527	Cares for fingernails	1	2	3	4	5	NA
031528	Cares for toenails	1	2	3	4	5	NA
031529	Cleans perineal area	1	2	3	4	5	NA
031530	Wears protective pads	1	2	3	4	5	NA
031531	Uses a mirror	1	2	3	4	5	NA
031532	Maintains neat appearance	1	2	3	4	5	NA
031533	Maintains body hygiene	1	2	3	4	5	NA

Domain-Functional Health (I)   Class-Self-Care (D)   1st edition 1997; revised 2004, 2008, 2013, 2024

S

OUTCOME CONTENT REFERENCES:

Archer, V., Smyth, W., & Nagle, C. (2021). Bathing wipes, a valuable hygiene option for frail older persons at home: A proof-of-concept study. *Australian Journal of Advanced Nursing, 38*(3). 43–46. https://dpoi.org/10.37464/2020.383458

+Dahlgren, A., Sand, Å., Larsson. Å., Karlsson, A. K., & Claesson, L. (2013). Linking the Klein-Bell Activities of Daily Living Scale to the International Classification of Functioning, Disability, and Health. *Journal of Rehabilitation Medicine, 45*(4), 351–357. https://doi.org/10.2340/16501977-1111

+Graham, J. E., Granger, C. V., Karmarkar, A. M., Deutsch, A., Niewczyk, P., DiVita, M., & Ottenbacher, K. J. (2014). The Uniform Data System for Medical Rehabilitation: Report of follow-up information on patients discharged from rehabilitation programs in 2002–2010. *American Journal of Physical Medicine & Rehabilitation, 93*(3), 231–244. https://doi.org/10.1097/PHM.0613e3182a92058

Hopman–Rock, M., van Hirtum, H., de Vreede, P., & Freiberger, E. (2019). Activities of daily living in older community–dwelling persons: A systematic review of psychometric properties of instruments. *Aging Clinical and Experimental Research, 31*(7), 917–925. https://doi.org/10.1007/s40520-018-1034-6

Queirós, C., Silva, M. A. T. C. P., Cruz, I., Cardoso, A., & Morais, E. J. (2021). Nursing diagnoses focused on universal self-care requisites. *International Nursing Review, 68*(3), 328–340. https://doi.org/10.1111/inr.12654

Sagari, A., Tabira, T., Maruta, M., Miyata, H., Han, G., & Kawagoe, M. (2020). Causes of changes in basic activities of daily living in older adults with long-term care needs. *Australasian Journal on Ageing, 40*(1), e54–e61. https://doi.org/10.1111/ajag.12848

Self-Care Behavior: Instrumental Activities of Daily Living (IADL)   0306

Definition: Personal actions to perform activities needed to function in the home or community independently with or without assistive device

OUTCOME TARGET RATING: Maintain at _____ Increase to _____

		Never Demonstrated	Rarely Demonstrated	Sometimes Demonstrated	Often Demonstrated	Consistently Demonstrated	
OUTCOME OVERALL RATING		1	2	3	4	5	
Indicators:							
030620	Shops for groceries	1	2	3	4	5	NA
030621	Shops for clothing	1	2	3	4	5	NA
030622	Shops for household supplies	1	2	3	4	5	NA
030623	Prepares meals	1	2	3	4	5	NA
030624	Serves meals	1	2	3	4	5	NA
030625	Uses landline or cell phone	1	2	3	4	5	NA
030626	Uses computer or electronic device	1	2	3	4	5	NA
030627	Handles written communication	1	2	3	4	5	NA
030628	Manages social relationships	1	2	3	4	5	NA
030629	Opens containers	1	2	3	4	5	NA
030630	Performs housework	1	2	3	4	5	NA
030631	Performs household repairs	1	2	3	4	5	NA
030632	Performs yard work	1	2	3	4	5	NA
030633	Manages money	1	2	3	4	5	NA
030634	Manages business affairs	1	2	3	4	5	NA
030635	Manages job responsibilities	1	2	3	4	5	NA
030636	Travels on public transportation	1	2	3	4	5	NA
030637	Drives own car	1	2	3	4	5	NA
030638	Does own laundry	1	2	3	4	5	NA
030639	Manages own non-parenteral medication	1	2	3	4	5	NA
030640	Manages own parenteral medication	1	2	3	4	5	NA

Domain-*Functional Health (I)*   **Class**-*Self-Care (D)*   *1st edition 1997; revised 2004, 2008, 2013, 2024*

OUTCOME CONTENT REFERENCES:

+Ferreira, P. L., Simões, A. L., Dourado, M., Holm, M. B., & Rogers, J. C. (2021). The Portuguese Performance Assessment of Self-Care Skills Measure: Validity and reliability. *OTRJ: Occupation, Participation & Health, 41*(4), 299–308. https://doi.org/10.1177/15394492211021309

Gentizon, J., Hirt, J., Jaques, C, Lang, P. O., & Mabire, C. (2021). Instruments assessing medication literacy in adult recipients of care: A systematic review of measurement. *International Journal of Nursing Studies, 113*, 1–17. https://doi.org/10.1016/j.ijnurstu.2020.103785

Head, B. J., Maas, M., & Johnson, M. (2003). Validity and community health nursing sensitivity of six outcomes for community health nursing with older clients. *Public Health Nursing, 20*(5), 385–398. https://doi.org/10.1046/j.1525-1446.2003.20507.x

+Katz, S., Ford, A. B., Moskowitz, R. W., Jackson, B. A., & Jaffe, M. W. (1963). Studies of illness in the aged. The Index of ADL: A standardized measure of biological and psychosocial function. *Journal of the American Medical Association, 185*(12), 914–919. https://doi.org/10.1001/jama.1963.03060120024016

Koolen, E. H., Spruit, M. A., deMan, M., Antons, J. C., Nijhuis, E., Nakken, N., Janssen, D. J. A., & Vant, A. J. (2021). Effectiveness of home-based occupational therapy on COPM performance and satisfaction scores in patients with COPD. *Canadian Journal of Occupational Therapy, 88*(1), 26–37. https://doi.org/10.1177/0008417420971124

Linn, M. W., & Linn, B. S. (1982). The Rapid Disability Rating Scale-2. *Journal of the American Geriatric Society, 30*(6), 378–382. https://doi.org/10.1111/j.1532-5415.1982.tb02835.x

Makhinova, T., Barner, J. C., Brown, C. M., Richards, K. M., Rascati, K. L., Rush, S., & Nag, A. (2021). Examination of barriers to medications adherence, asthma management, and control among community pharmacy patients with asthma. *Journal of Pharmacy Practice, 34*(4), 515–522. https://doi.org/10.1177/0897190019840117

Nastasi, J. A., & Harris, L. (2021). Evidence of occupational therapy interventions supporting work and social participation for adults with multiple sclerosis: A systemic review. *American Journal of Occupational Therapy, 75*(4), 1–13. https://doi.org/10.5014/ajot.2021.048058

Self-Care Behavior: Non-Parenteral Medication 0307

Definition: Personal actions to administer oral, topical, and inhaler medications to meet therapeutic goals independently with or without assistive device

OUTCOME TARGET RATING: Maintain at _____ Increase to _____

		Never Demonstrated	Rarely Demonstrated	Sometimes Demonstrated	Often Demonstrated	Consistently Demonstrated	
OUTCOME OVERALL RATING		1	2	3	4	5	
Indicators:							
030720	Identifies medication	1	2	3	4	5	NA
030721	Reports importance of taking medication	1	2	3	4	5	NA
030722	Identifies preferred medication route	1	2	3	4	5	NA
030723	Maintains up-to-date medication list	1	2	3	4	5	NA
030724	Administers correct dose	1	2	3	4	5	NA
030725	Follows medication plan	1	2	3	4	5	NA
030726	Monitors therapeutic effects	1	2	3	4	5	NA
030727	Adjusts medication to achieve therapeutic effects	1	2	3	4	5	NA
030728	Follows medication precautions	1	2	3	4	5	NA
030729	Monitors medication side effects	1	2	3	4	5	NA
030730	Uses memory aids	1	2	3	4	5	NA
030731	Uses mobile health technology to support medication adherence	1	2	3	4	5	NA
030732	Performs self-monitoring activities	1	2	3	4	5	NA
030733	Uses monitoring equipment accurately	1	2	3	4	5	NA
030734	Maintains required supplies	1	2	3	4	5	NA
030745	Uses medication as prescribed	1	2	3	4	5	NA
030736	Stores medication properly	1	2	3	4	5	NA
030737	Disposes of medication properly	1	2	3	4	5	NA
030738	Obtains required laboratory tests	1	2	3	4	5	NA
030739	Understands implications of test results	1	2	3	4	5	NA

Domain-Functional Health (I) **Class-***Self-Care (D)* *1st edition 1997; revised 2004, 2008, 2013, 2024*

OUTCOME CONTENT REFERENCES:

Adama, S., Wallace, L. J., Arthur, J., Kwakye, S., & Adongo, P. B. (2021). Self-medication practice of pregnant women attending antenatal clinic in Northern Ghana: An analytical cross-sectional study. *African Journal of Reproductive Health, 25*(4), 89–98. https://doi.org/10.29063/ajrh2021/v25i4.10

Chlebowy, D. O. (2021). The complexity of diabetes self-care. *Western Journal of Nursing Research, 43*(4), 287. https://doi.org/10.1177/0193945920976602

Gentizon, J., Hirt, J., Jaques, C., Lang, P. O., & Mabire ,C. (2021). Instruments assessing medication literacy in adult recipients of care: A systemic review of measurement properties. *International Journal of Nursing Studies, 113*, 1–17. https://doi.org/10.1016/j.ijnurstu.2020.103785

Karaaslan–Eşer, A., & Ayaz–Alkaya, S. (2021). The effect of a mobile application on treatment adherence and symptom management in patients using oral anticancer agents: A randomized controlled trial. *European Journal of Oncology Nursing, 52*, 101969. https://doi.org/10.1016/j.ejon.2021.101969

Makhinova, T., Barner, J. C., Brown, C. M., Richards, K. M., Rascati, K. L., Rush, S., & Nag, A. (2021). Examination of barriers to medication adherence, asthma management, and control among community pharmacy patients with asthma. *Journal of Pharmacy Practice, 34*(4), 515–522. https://doi.org/10.1177/0897190019840117

Marseille, B. R., Commodore-Mensah, Y., Davidson, P. M., Baker, D., D'Aoust, R., & Baptiste, D. L. (2021). Improving hypertension knowledge, medication adherence, and blood pressure control: A feasibility study. *Journal of Clinical Nursing, 30*(19/20), 2960–2967. https://doi.org/10.1111/jocn.15803

Singh, J. A., Tornberg, H., & Goodman, S. M. (2021). Pop a pill or give myself a shot? Patient perspectives of disease-modifying anti-rheumatic drug choice for rheumatoid arthritis. *Joint Bone Spine, 88*(1), 1–7. https://doi.org/10.1016/j.jbspin.2020.07.002

Yang, C., Hui, Z., Wang, X., Tang, G., & Lee, D. T. F. (2021). A medication intervention to improve adherence for older people with multimorbidity: A pilot study. *Age and Ageing, 50*(1), i12–i42. https://doi.org/10.1093/ageing/afab030.44

Self-Care Behavior: Oral Hygiene   0308

Definition: Personal actions to care for own mouth and teeth independently with or without assistive device

OUTCOME TARGET RATING: Maintain at _____ Increase to _____

	Never Demonstrated	Rarely Demonstrated	Sometimes Demonstrated	Often Demonstrated	Consistently Demonstrated	
OUTCOME OVERALL RATING	1	2	3	4	5	
Indicators:						
030711 Brushes teeth	1	2	3	4	5	NA
030712 Flosses teeth	1	2	3	4	5	NA
030713 Uses mouthwash	1	2	3	4	5	NA
030714 Cleans mouth, gums, and tongue	1	2	3	4	5	NA
030715 Cleans dentures or dental appliances	1	2	3	4	5	NA
030716 Uses a special toothbrush to clean teeth while wearing braces	1	2	3	4	5	NA
030717 Uses fluoridation	1	2	3	4	5	NA
030718 Uses plaque-disclosing methods	1	2	3	4	5	NA
030719 Obtains regular dental care	1	2	3	4	5	NA

Domain-Functional Health (I)   *Class*-Self-Care (D)   *1st edition 1997; revised 2004, 2013, 2024*

OUTCOME CONTENT REFERENCES:

Bomfim, R. A., Schneider, I. J. C., de Andrade, F. B., Lima-Costa, M. F., Corrêa, V. P., Frazão, P., Watt, R. G., Bastos, J. L., & de Oliveira, C. (2020). Racial inequities in tooth loss among older Brazilian adults: A decomposition analysis. *Community Dentistry and Oral Epidemiology, 49*, 119–127. https://doi.org/10.1111/cdoe.12583

Curtis, S. A., Scambler, S., Manthorpe, J., Samsi, K., Rooney, Y. M., & Gallaher, J. E. (2021). Everyday experiences of people living with dementia and their carers relating to oral health and dental care. *Dementia, 20*(6), 1925–1939. https://doi.org/10.1177/1471301220975942

McKelvey, V., Darlow, B. A., Horwood, L. J., & Martin, J. (2020). Dental status of young adults born with very low birthweight: A national cohort study. *Community Dentistry Oral Epidemiology, 49*(3), 240–248. https://doi.org/10.1111/cdoe.12595

+Niederman, R., & Sullivan, T. M. (1981). Oral Hygiene Skill Achievement Index I. *Journal of Periodontology, 52*(3), 143–149. https://doi.org/10.1902/jop.1981.52.3.143

+Niederman, R., Sullivan, T. M., Weiss, D., Morhart, R., Robbins, W., & Maier, D. (1981). Oral Hygiene Skill Achievement Index II. *Journal of Periodontology. 52*(3), 150–154. https://doi.org/10.1902/jop.1981.52.3.150

Oliveira, L. M., Pazinatto, J., & Zanatta, F. B. (2020). Are oral hygiene instructions with aid of plaque-disclosing methods effective in improving self-performed dental plaque control? A systematic review of randomized controlled trials. *International Journal of Dental Hygiene, 19*(3), 239–254. https://doi.org/10.1111/idh.12491

Timmesfeld, N., Kunst, M., Fondel, F., & Güldner, C. (2020). Mechanical tongue cleaning is a worthwhile procedure to improve the taste sensation. *Journal of Oral Rehabilitation, 48*(1), 45–54. https://doi.org/10.1111/joor.13099

S

Self-Care Behavior: Parenteral Medication   0309

Definition: Personal actions to administer medications by injection or infusion to meet therapeutic goals independently with or without assistive device

OUTCOME TARGET RATING: Maintain at _____ Increase to _____

OUTCOME OVERALL RATING		Never Demonstrated	Rarely Demonstrated	Sometimes Demonstrated	Often Demonstrated	Consistently Demonstrated	
		1	2	3	4	5	
Indicators:							
030922	Identifies medication	1	2	3	4	5	NA
030923	Reports importance of taking medication	1	2	3	4	5	NA
030924	Administers correct dose	1	2	3	4	5	NA
030925	Follows tailored medication plan	1	2	3	4	5	NA
030926	Monitors therapeutic effects	1	2	3	4	5	NA
030927	Adjusts medication to achieve therapeutic effects	1	2	3	4	5	NA
030928	Provides a list of medication to health professional	1	2	3	4	5	NA
030929	Participates in medication reconciliation with health professional	1	2	3	4	5	NA
030930	Follows medication precautions	1	2	3	4	5	NA
030931	Monitors medication side effects	1	2	3	4	5	NA
030932	Uses memory aids	1	2	3	4	5	NA
030933	Performs self-monitoring activities	1	2	3	4	5	NA
030934	Uses monitoring equipment accurately	1	2	3	4	5	NA
030935	Maintains required supplies	1	2	3	4	5	NA
030936	Uses medication as prescribed	1	2	3	4	5	NA
030937	Stores medication properly	1	2	3	4	5	NA
030938	Disposes of medication properly	1	2	3	4	5	NA
030939	Disposes of syringes and needles properly	1	2	3	4	5	NA
030940	Maintains asepsis	1	2	3	4	5	NA
030941	Monitors injection sites	1	2	3	4	5	NA
030942	Obtains required laboratory tests	1	2	3	4	5	NA

Domain-Functional Health (I)   *Class*-Self-Care (D)   *1st edition 1997; revised 2004, 2008, 2024*

OUTCOME CONTENT REFERENCES:

Adama, S., Wallace, L. J., Arthur, J., Kwakye, S., & Adongo, P. B. (2021). Self-medication practice of pregnant women attending antenatal clinic in Northern Ghana: An analytical cross-sectional study. *African Journal of Reproductive Health, 25*(4), 89–98. https://doi.org/10.29063/ajrh2021/v25i4.10

Chlebowy, D. O. (2021). The complexity of diabetes self-care. *Western Journal of Nursing Research, 43*(4), 287. https://doi.org/10.1177/0193945920976602

Gentizon, J., Hirt, J., Jaques, C., Lang, P. O., & Mabire, C. (2021). Instruments assessing medication literacy in adult recipients of care: A systemic review of measurement properties. *International Journal of Nursing Studies, 113*, 1–17. https://doi.org/10.1016/j.ijnurstu.2020.103785

Makhinova, T., Barner, J. C., Brown, C. M., Richards, K. M., Rascati, K. L., Rush, S., & Nag, A. (2021). Examination of barriers to medication adherence, asthma management, and control among community pharmacy patients with asthma. *Journal of Pharmacy Practice, 34*(4), 515–522. https://doi.org/10.1177/0897190019840117

Marseille, B. R., Commodore-Mensah, Y., Davidson, P. M., Baker, D., D'Aoust, R., & Baptiste, D. L. (2021). Improving hypertension knowledge, medication adherence, and blood pressure control: A feasibility study. *Journal of Clinical Nursing, 30*(19/20), 2960–2967. https://doi.org/10.1111/jocn.15803

Pierik, A., Martins, D. S., Casey, L., & Piper, H. G. (2021). Use of instructional videos to reduce central venous catheter complications in children with intestinal failure receiving home parental nutrition. *Nutrition in Clinical Practice, 36*(4), 872–876. https://doi.org/10.1002/ncp.10638

S

Self-Care Behavior: Toileting   0310

Definition: Personal actions to toilet self independently with or without assistive device

OUTCOME TARGET RATING: Maintain at _____ Increase to _____

OUTCOME OVERALL RATING		Never Demonstrated	Rarely Demonstrated	Sometimes Demonstrated	Often Demonstrated	Consistently Demonstrated	
		1	2	3	4	5	
Indicators:							
031016	Responds to full bladder in timely manner	1	2	3	4	5	NA
031017	Responds to urge to have a bowel movement in timely manner	1	2	3	4	5	NA
031018	Uses safety handrails	1	2	3	4	5	NA
031019	Uses elevated toilet seat	1	2	3	4	5	NA
031020	Positions self on toilet or commode	1	2	3	4	5	NA
031021	Gets to toilet between urge and passage of urine	1	2	3	4	5	NA
031022	Gets to toilet between urge and evacuation of stool	1	2	3	4	5	NA
031023	Removes clothing	1	2	3	4	5	NA
031024	Empties bladder	1	2	3	4	5	NA
031025	Empties bowel	1	2	3	4	5	NA
031026	Wipes self after urinating	1	2	3	4	5	NA
031027	Wipes self after bowel movement	1	2	3	4	5	NA
031028	Gets up from toilet or commode	1	2	3	4	5	NA
031029	Adjusts clothing after toileting	1	2	3	4	5	NA
031030	Washes hands after toileting	1	2	3	4	5	NA

Domain-Functional Health (I)   *Class*-Self-Care (D)   *1st edition 1997; revised 2004, 2008, 2013, 2024*

OUTCOME CONTENT REFERENCES:

Duong, T., Braid, J., Staunton, H., Barriere, A., Petridis, F., Reithinger, J., Cruz, R., Jarecki, J., De Lemus, M., Gusser, N., Broekgaarden, R., Randhawa, S., Flynn, J., Arbuckle, R., Reif, S., Yang, L., De Martini, A., & Vuillerot, C. (2021). Understanding the relationship between the 32-item motor function measure and daily activities from an individual with spinal muscular atrophy and their caregivers' perspective: A two-part study. *BMC Neurology, 21*(1), 143–158. https://doi.org/10.1186/s12883-021-02166-z

+Graham, J. E., Granger, C. V., Karmarkar, A. M., Deutsch, A., Niewczyk, P., DiVita, M., & Ottenbacher, K. J. (2014). The Uniform Data System for Medical Rehabilitation: Report of follow-up information on patients discharged from rehabilitation programs in 2002–2010. *American Journal of Physical Medicine & Rehabilitation, 93*(3), 231–244. https://doi.org/10.1097/PHM.0613e3182a92058

+Katz, S., Ford, A. B., Moskowitz, R. W., Jackson, B. A., & Jaffe, M. W. (1963). Studies of illness in the aged. The Index of ADL: A standardized measure of biological and psychosocial function. *Journal of the American Medical Association, 185*(12), 914–919. https://doi.org/10.1001/jama.1963.03060120024016

Oliveira-Kumakura, A. R. D. E. S., Sousa, C. M. F. M., Biscaro, J. A., da Silva, K. C. R., Silva, J. L. G., Morais, S. C. R. V., & Lopes, M. V. O. (2021). Clinical validation of nursing diagnoses related to self-care deficits in patients with stroke. *Clinical Nursing Research, 30*(4), 494–501. https://doi.org/10.1177/1054773819883352

Queirós, C., Silva, M. A. T. C. P., Cruz, I., Cardoso, A., & Morais, E. J. (2021). Nursing diagnoses focused on universal self-care requisites. *International Nursing Review, 68*(3), 328–340. https://doi.org/10.1111/inr.12654

S

Self-Direction of Care   1613

Definition: Care recipient actions taken to direct others who assist with or perform physical tasks and personal health care

OUTCOME TARGET RATING: Maintain at _____ Increase to _____

		Never Demonstrated	Rarely Demonstrated	Sometimes Demonstrated	Often Demonstrated	Consistently Demonstrated	
OUTCOME OVERALL RATING		1	2	3	4	5	
Indicators:							
161312	Describes impact of condition to others	1	2	3	4	5	NA
161313	Sets personal health care goals	1	2	3	4	5	NA
161314	Determines personal care needs	1	2	3	4	5	NA
161315	Writes action care plan	1	2	3	4	5	NA
161316	Expresses need for control	1	2	3	4	5	NA
161302	Describes appropriate care	1	2	3	4	5	NA
161317	Chooses services to be used	1	2	3	4	5	NA
161318	Acknowledges consequences of choices	1	2	3	4	5	NA
161311	Obtains needed resources	1	2	3	4	5	NA
161304	Instructs others in appropriate care behaviors	1	2	3	4	5	NA
161305	Evaluates the care given by others	1	2	3	4	5	NA
161319	Evaluates performance of paid care provider	1	2	3	4	5	NA
161306	Determines that care is completed appropriately	1	2	3	4	5	NA
161320	Evaluates progress on personal health care goals	1	2	3	4	5	NA
161307	Expresses confidence in problem-solving	1	2	3	4	5	NA
161308	Takes corrective action when care is not appropriate	1	2	3	4	5	NA
161321	Self-reliant in tasks able to perform	1	2	3	4	5	NA
161322	Develops partnership with care provider	1	2	3	4	5	NA
161309	Instructs others in appropriate health maintenance activities	1	2	3	4	5	NA
161323	Instructs others in organizing social interactions	1	2	3	4	5	NA
161324	Takes appropriate action when condition changes	1	2	3	4	5	NA
161325	Conveys to others emergency plans	1	2	3	4	5	NA
161326	Instructs others when health professional to be consulted	1	2	3	4	5	NA
161327	Writes a backup plan for continuity of care	1	2	3	4	5	NA

Domain-*Health Knowledge & Behavior (IV)*   **Class**-*Health Behavior (Q)*   *2nd edition 2000; revised 2004, 2008, 2024*

OUTCOME CONTENT REFERENCES:

Arman, M., & HöK, J. (2016). Self-care follows from compassionate care: Chronic pain patients' experience of integrative rehabilitation. *Scandinavian Journal of Caring Sciences, 30*(2), 374–381. https://doi.org/10.1111/scs.12258

Bogenschutz, M. D., DeCarlo, M., Hall-Lande, J., & Hewitt, A. (2019). Fiscal stewardship, choice, and control: The context of self-directed services for people with intellectual and developmental disabilities in the United States. *Intellectual and Development Disabilities, 57*(2), 158–171. https://doi.org/10.1352/1934-9556-57.2.158

Bolscher–Niehuis, M. J. T., Uitdehaag, M. J., & Francke, A. L. (2019). Community nurses' self-management support in older adults: A qualitative study on view, dilemmas and strategies. *Health and Social Care in Community, 28*(1), 195–203. https://doi.org/10.1111/hsc.12853

Goetti. T., Buren, T., Graham, S., Streich, B., Waterman, E., Ho, S., Self, H., Bulatao, M., & Yoshida, K. (2020). Getting on with life: A qualitative evaluation of an independent living skills education program for people with physical disabilities. *Disability and Rehabilitation, 42*(25), 3621–3627. https://doi.org/10.1080/09638288.2019.1604820

S

Kulnik, S. T., Hollinshead, L., & Jones, F. (2019). "I'm still me – I'm still here!" Understanding the person's sense of self in the provision of self-management support for people with progressive neurological long-term conditions. *Disability and Rehabilitation, 41*(11), 1296–1306. https://doi.org/10.1080/09638288.2018.1424953

McClure, J., & Leah, C. (2021). Is independence enough? Rehabilitation should include autonomy and social engagement to achieve quality of life. *Clinical Rehabilitation, 35*(1), 3–12. https://doi.org/10.1177/0269215520954344

McIntyre, A., Marrocco, S. L., McRae, S. A., Sleeth, L., Hitzig, S., Jaglal, S., Linassi, G., Munce, S., & Wolfe, D. L. (2020. A scoping review of self-management interventions following spinal cord injury. *Topics in Spinal Cord Injury Rehabilitation, 26*(1), 36–63. https://doi.org/10.1310/sci12601-36

Meng, K., Reusch, A., Musekamp, G., Seekatz, B., Zietz, B., Steimann, G., Altstidl, R., Haug, G., Worringen, U., & Faller, H. (2018). Self-management education for rehabilitation inpatients: A cluster-randomized controlled trail. *Patient Education and Counseling, 101*(9), 1630–1638. https://doi.org/10.1016/j.pec.2018.03.027

Self-Direction of Instrumental Activities of Daily Living   1639

Definition: Personal actions to direct others who assist with or perform duties needed to live independently

OUTCOME TARGET RATING: Maintain at_____ Increase to_____

OUTCOME OVERALL RATING	Never Demonstrated 1	Rarely Demonstrated 2	Sometimes Demonstrated 3	Often Demonstrated 4	Consistently Demonstrated 5	
Indicators:						
163901 Identifies assistance needed to maintain home	1	2	3	4	5	NA
163902 Instructs others in assistance needed for shopping	1	2	3	4	5	NA
163903 Instructs others in assistance with meal preparation	1	2	3	4	5	NA
163904 Obtains assistance with house maintenance	1	2	3	4	5	NA
163905 Obtains assistance with house safety equipment	1	2	3	4	5	NA
163906 Obtains assistance with housework	1	2	3	4	5	NA
163907 Obtains assistance with laundry	1	2	3	4	5	NA
163908 Obtains assistance arranging transportation	1	2	3	4	5	NA
163909 Asks for assistance with financial affairs	1	2	3	4	5	NA
163910 Obtains assistance with yard work	1	2	3	4	5	NA
163911 Obtains assistance with communication needs	1	2	3	4	5	NA
163912 Asks for assistance with medication management	1	2	3	4	5	NA
163913 Supervises delegated tasks to others	1	2	3	4	5	NA

Domain-Health Knowledge & Behavior (IV)   *Class*-Health Behavior (Q)   6th edition 2018

OUTCOME CONTENT REFERENCES:
Mahoney, K., Sciegaj, M., & Mahoney, E. (2014). The future of participant direction in aging services. *Generations, 38*(2), 85–93. https://www.jstor.org/stable/26556054

Ruggiano, N. (2012). Consumer direction in long-term care policy: Overcoming barriers to promoting older adults' opportunity for self-direction. *Journal of Gerontological Social Work, 55*(2), 146–159. https://doi.org/10.1080/01634372.2011.638701

Yen, L., McRae, I., Jeon, Y., Essue, B., & Herath, P. (2011). The impact of chronic illness on workforce participation and the need for assistance with household tasks and personal care by older Australians. *Health & Social Care in the Community, 19*(5), 485–494. https://doi.org/10.1111/j.1365-2524.2011.00994.x

Self-Esteem   1205

Definition: Personal judgment of self-worth

OUTCOME TARGET RATING: Maintain at _____ Increase to _____

		Never Positive	Rarely Positive	Sometimes Positive	Often Positive	Consistently Positive	
OUTCOME OVERALL RATING		1	2	3	4	5	
Indicators:							
120501	Verbalizations of self-acceptance	1	2	3	4	5	NA
120502	Acceptance of self-limitations	1	2	3	4	5	NA
120523	Verbalizations of self-compassion	1	2	3	4	5	NA
120503	Maintenance of erect posture	1	2	3	4	5	NA
120504	Maintenance of eye contact	1	2	3	4	5	NA
120505	Description of self	1	2	3	4	5	NA
120524	Verbalization of personal opinions	1	2	3	4	5	NA
120525	Shares personal needs with others	1	2	3	4	5	NA
120526	Self-images on social media	1	2	3	4	5	NA
120506	Regard for others	1	2	3	4	5	NA
120507	Open communication	1	2	3	4	5	NA
120508	Fulfillment of personally significant roles	1	2	3	4	5	NA
120509	Maintenance of grooming and hygiene	1	2	3	4	5	NA
120510	Balance of speaking and listening in groups	1	2	3	4	5	NA
120511	Confidence level	1	2	3	4	5	NA
120512	Acceptance of compliments from others	1	2	3	4	5	NA
120513	Expected response from others	1	2	3	4	5	NA
120514	Acceptance of constructive criticism	1	2	3	4	5	NA
120515	Willingness to confront others	1	2	3	4	5	NA
120521	Description of success in work	1	2	3	4	5	NA
120522	Description of success in school	1	2	3	4	5	NA
120517	Description of success in social groups	1	2	3	4	5	NA
120518	Description of pride in self	1	2	3	4	5	NA
120519	Feelings of self-worth	1	2	3	4	5	NA
120527	Satisfaction with lifestyle	1	2	3	4	5	NA

Domain-Psychosocial Health (III)   *Class*-Psychological Well-Being (M)   *1st edition 1997; revised 2008, 2024*

OUTCOME CONTENT REFERENCES:

Arsandaux, J., Galéra, C., & Salamon, R. (2021), The association of self-esteem and psychosocial outcomes in young adults: A 10-year prospective study. *Child and Adolescent Mental Health, 26*(2), 106–113. https://doi.org/10.1111/camh.12392

Blascovich, J., & Tomaka, J. (2013). Measures of self-esteem. In J. P. Robinson, P. R. Shaver & L. S. Wrightsman (Eds.), *Measures of personality and social psychological attitudes: Measures of social psychological attitudes* (pp. 115–23). Academic Press.

De Ruiter, N. M. P., van Geert, P. L. C., & Kunnen, E. S. (2017). Explaining the "how" of self-esteem development: The Self-Organizing Self-Esteem Model. *Review of General Psychology, 21*(1), 49–68. https://doi.org/10.1037/gpr0000099

Fox, J., Vendemia, M. A., Smith, M. A., & Brehm, N. R. (2021). Effects of taking selfies on women's self-objectification, mood, self-esteem, and social aggression toward female peers. *Body Image, 36*, 193–200. https://doi.org/10.1016/j.bodyim.2020.11.011

Opheim, R., Moum, B., Grimstad, B., Jahnsen, J., Berset, I. P., Hovde, Ø., Huppertz-Hauss, G., Bernklev, T., & Jelsness-Jørgensen, L.-P. (2020). Self-esteem in patients with inflammatory bowel disease. *Quality of Life Research, 29*(7), 1839–1846. https://doi.org/10.1007/s11136-020-02467-9

Orth, U., Maes, J., & Schmitt, M. (2015). Self-esteem development across the life span: A longitudinal study with a large sample from Germany. *Developmental Psychology, 51*(2), 248–59. https://doi.org/10.1037/a0038481

Pandey, R., Tiwari, G. K., Parihar, P., & Rai, P. K. (2021). Positive, not negative, self-compassion mediates the relationship between self-esteem and well-being. *Psychology Psychotherapy—Theory Research and Practice, 94*, 1–15. https://doi.org/10.1111/papt.12259

+Rosenberg M. (1965). *Society and the adolescent self-image.* Princeton University Press.

von Soest, T., Wagner, J., Hansen, T., & Gerstorf, D. (2018). Self-esteem across the second half of life: The role of socioeconomic status, physical health, social relationships, and personality factors. *Journal of Personality and Social Psychology, 114*(6), 945–958. https://doi.org/10.1037/pspp0000123

Wang, S., Xu, H., Zhang, S., Yang, R., Li, D., Sun, Y., Wan, Y., & Tao, F. (2022). Linking childhood maltreatment and psychological symptoms: The role of social support, coping styles, and self-esteem in adolescents. *Journal of Interpersonal Violence, 37*(1/2), NP620–NP650. https://doi.org/10.1177/0886260520918571

Wang, Y., Wang, X., Liu, H., Xie, X., Wang, P., & Lei, L. (2020). Selfie posting and self-esteem among young adult women: A mediation model of positive feedback and body satisfaction. *Journal of Health Psychology, 25*(2), 161–172. https://doi.org/10.1177/1359105318787624

S

Self-Harm Restraint

1414

Definition: Personal actions to refrain from intentional non-lethal self-inflicted injury

OUTCOME TARGET RATING: Maintain at_____ Increase to_____

OUTCOME OVERALL RATING		Never Demonstrated 1	Rarely Demonstrated 2	Sometimes Demonstrated 3	Often Demonstrated 4	Consistently Demonstrated 5	
Indicators:							
141401	Refrains from gathering means for self-injury	1	2	3	4	5	NA
141402	Upholds contract to not harm self	1	2	3	4	5	NA
141403	Refrains from breaking skin	1	2	3	4	5	NA
141404	Refrains from cutting self	1	2	3	4	5	NA
141405	Refrains from ingesting harmful substances	1	2	3	4	5	NA
141406	Refrains from injuring self	1	2	3	4	5	NA
141407	Maintains self-control without supervision	1	2	3	4	5	NA
141408	Follows a well-balanced diet	1	2	3	4	5	NA
141409	Follows treatment regimen	1	2	3	4	5	NA
141410	Uses medication as prescribed	1	2	3	4	5	NA
141411	Obtains treatment for depression	1	2	3	4	5	NA
141412	Obtains treatment for substance abuse	1	2	3	4	5	NA
141413	Reports adequate chronic pain control	1	2	3	4	5	NA
141414	Uses effective coping strategies	1	2	3	4	5	NA
141415	Uses available support groups	1	2	3	4	5	NA
141416	Obtains assistance as needed	1	2	3	4	5	NA
141417	Participates in mental health promotion activities	1	2	3	4	5	NA

Domain *Psychosocial Health (III)*   **Class**-*Psychosocial Adaptation (N)*   7th edition, 2024

OUTCOME CONTENT REFERENCES:

Allen, D., Mistler, L., Ray, R., Batscha, C., Delaney, K., Loucks, J., Nadler-Moodie, M., & Sharp, D. (2019). A call to action from the APNA Council for safe environments: Defining violence and aggression for research and practice improvement purposes. *Journal of the American Psychiatric Nurses Association, 25*(1), 7–10. https://doi.org/10.1177/1078390318809159

de Sousa, G. S., Perrelli, J. G. A., de Oliveira Mangueira, S., de Oliveira Lopes, M. V., & Sougey, E. B. (2020). Clinical validation of the nursing diagnosis risk for suicide in the older adults. *Archives of Psychiatric Nursing, 34*(2), 21–28. https://doi.org/10.1016/j.apnu.2020.01.003

Ji, Y. D., Robertson, F. C., Patel, N. A., Peacock, Z .S., & Resnick, C. M. (2020). Assessment of risk factors for suicide among U.S. health care professionals. *JAMA Surgery, 155*(8), 713–721. https://doi.org/10.1001/jamasurg.20201338

Kang, M., Bushell, H., Lee, S., Berry, C., Hollander, Y., Rauchberger, I., & Whitecross, F. (2020). Exploring behaviours of concern including aggression, self-harm, sexual harm and absconding within an Australian inpatient mental health service. *Australasian Psychiatry, 28*(4), 394–400. https://doi.org/10.1177/1039856220926940

Kellerman, Q. D., Hartoonian, N., Beier, M. L., Leipertz, S. L., Maynard, C., Hostetter, T. A., Haselkorn, J. K., & Turner, A. P. (2020). Risk factors for suicide in a national sample of veterans with multiple sclerosis. *Archives of Physical Medicine and Rehabilitation, 101*(7), 1138–43. https://doi.org/10.1016/j.apmr.2020.03.0

Liberatore, K. (2019). Preventing self-harm in the nonpsychiatric health care setting. *AJN, American Journal of Nursing, 119*(11). 67–69. https://doi.org/10.1097/01.NAJ.0000605396.83183.d2

Moore, C., Damari, N., Liles, E. A., & Bramson, B. (2019). Who you gonna call? Outcomes of a team-based approach to respond to disruptive behavioral issues in hospitalized patients. *The Joint Commission Journal on Quality and Patient Safety, 45*(11), 781–785. https://doi.org/10.1016/j.jcjq.2019.08.006

Nelson, P. A., & Adams, S. M. (2020). Role of primary care in suicide prevention during the COVID-19 pandemic. *The Journal of Nurse Practitioners, 16*(9), 654–659, https://doi.org/10.1016/j.nursra.2020.07.015

Nyberg, J., Gustavsson, S., Åberg, M. A., Kuhn, H. G., & Waern, M. (2020). Late-adolescent risk factors for suicide and self-harm in middle-aged men: Explorative prospective population-based study. *The British Journal of Psychiatry, 217*(1), 370–376. https://doi.org/10.1192/bjp.2019.243

Schmutte, T., Olfson, M., Xie, M., & Marcus, S. C. (2020). Self-harm, suicidal ideation, and attempted suicide in older adults: A national study of emergency department visits and follow-up care. The *American Journal of Geriatric Psychiatry, 28*(6), 646–658. https://doi.org/10.1016/j.jagp.2019.12.003

S

Self-Management: Acute Illness   3100

Definition: Personal actions to manage a reversible illness, its treatment, and to prevent complications

OUTCOME TARGET RATING: Maintain at _____ Increase to _____

		Never Demonstrated	Rarely Demonstrated	Sometimes Demonstrated	Often Demonstrated	Consistently Demonstrated	
OUTCOME OVERALL RATING		1	2	3	4	5	
Indicators:							
310001	Monitors signs and symptoms of illness	1	2	3	4	5	NA
310002	Follows recommended precautions	1	2	3	4	5	NA
310003	Monitors for signs and symptoms of complications	1	2	3	4	5	NA
310030	Monitors temperature	1	2	3	4	5	NA
310004	Obtains required laboratory test	1	2	3	4	5	NA
310005	Identifies cultural beliefs that impact treatment	1	2	3	4	5	NA
310006	Discusses cultural beliefs that impact treatment with health provider	1	2	3	4	5	NA
310007	Follows recommended treatment	1	2	3	4	5	NA
310008	Performs prescribed procedure	1	2	3	4	5	NA
310009	Uses treatment devices correctly	1	2	3	4	5	NA
310010	Monitors treatment therapeutic effects	1	2	3	4	5	NA
310011	Monitors treatment side effects	1	2	3	4	5	NA
310012	Uses strategies to reduce transmission of illness to others	1	2	3	4	5	NA
310013	Follows medication regimen	1	2	3	4	5	NA
310014	Monitors medication therapeutic effects	1	2	3	4	5	NA
310015	Monitors medication side effects	1	2	3	4	5	NA
310016	Monitors medication adverse effects	1	2	3	4	5	NA
310017	Seeks assistance for self-care	1	2	3	4	5	NA
310018	Adjusts activity level during illness	1	2	3	4	5	NA
310019	Adjusts diet during illness	1	2	3	4	5	NA
310031	Monitors fluid intake	1	2	3	4	5	NA
310020	Avoids behaviors that potentiate illness	1	2	3	4	5	NA
310021	Uses strategies to cope with illness	1	2	3	4	5	NA
310022	Uses strategies to enhance comfort	1	2	3	4	5	NA
310023	Uses strategies to maintain adequate sleep	1	2	3	4	5	NA
310024	Balances activity and rest	1	2	3	4	5	NA
310025	Monitors changes in illness	1	2	3	4	5	NA
310026	Uses reputable sources of information	1	2	3	4	5	NA
310027	Obtains advice from health provider as needed	1	2	3	4	5	NA
310028	Uses health care services congruent with needs	1	2	3	4	5	NA
310029	Schedules appointments with health professional as needed	1	2	3	4	5	NA

Domain-*Health Knowledge & Behavior (IV)*   **Class**-*Health Management (FF)*   *5th edition 2013; revised 2024*

S

OUTCOME CONTENT REFERENCES:

Jones, R., White, P., Armstrong, D., Ashworth, M., & Peters, M. (2010). *Managing acute illness.* The King's Fund.

Lange, P. W., Gazzard, M., Walker, S., Hilton, J. J., Haycock, S., Wagstaff, J. F. R., & Ward, G. A. (2020). Where are our patients? Retrospective cohort study of acute medical unit admissions during and prior to the COVID-19 pandemic. *Internal Medicine Journal, 50,* 1132–1134. https://doi.org/10.1111/imj.14983

Long S. S. (2016). Diagnosis and management of undifferentiated fever in children. *The Journal of Infection,* (Suppl. 72), S68–S76. https://doi.org/10.1016/j.jinf.2016.04.025

Potter, P., Perry, A., Stockert, P., & Hall, A. (2021). *Fundamentals of nursing* (10th ed.). Elsevier.

Self-Management: Anticoagulation Therapy   3101

Definition: Personal actions to manage therapy to maintain blood clotting time within a prescribed range and prevent complications

OUTCOME TARGET RATING: Maintain at_____ Increase to_____

		Never Demonstrated	Rarely Demonstrated	Sometimes Demonstrated	Often Demonstrated	Consistently Demonstrated	
OUTCOME OVERALL RATING		**1**	**2**	**3**	**4**	**5**	
Indicators:							
310101	Seeks information about anticoagulation therapy	1	2	3	4	5	NA
310102	Seeks information about actions of anti-coagulation agent	1	2	3	4	5	NA
310103	Participates in health care decisions	1	2	3	4	5	NA
310104	Uses medication as prescribed	1	2	3	4	5	NA
310105	Seeks information about potential complications	1	2	3	4	5	NA
310106	Seeks information about laboratory test for clotting time	1	2	3	4	5	NA
310107	Obtains laboratory tests	1	2	3	4	5	NA
310108	Monitors for signs and symptoms of thromboembolism	1	2	3	4	5	NA
310109	Monitors for signs and symptoms of bleeding	1	2	3	4	5	NA
310110	Monitors for signs and symptoms of atrial fibrillation	1	2	3	4	5	NA
310111	Monitors for signs and symptoms of stroke	1	2	3	4	5	NA
310112	Monitors for signs and symptoms of transient ischemic attack	1	2	3	4	5	NA
310113	Reports symptoms of complications	1	2	3	4	5	NA
310114	Notifies health professionals of anticoagulation therapy	1	2	3	4	5	NA
310115	Uses strategies to reduce venous stasis	1	2	3	4	5	NA
310116	Uses strategies to prevent internal bleeding	1	2	3	4	5	NA
310117	Uses strategies to prevent physical injuries	1	2	3	4	5	NA
310118	Monitors vital signs	1	2	3	4	5	NA
310119	Follows dietary restrictions	1	2	3	4	5	NA
310120	Avoids substances that interact with anticoagulant agent	1	2	3	4	5	NA
310121	Eliminates alcohol use	1	2	3	4	5	NA
310122	Eliminates tobacco use	1	2	3	4	5	NA
310123	Discusses use of non-prescription medication with health provider	1	2	3	4	5	NA

S

Self-Management: Anticoagulation Therapy—cont'd

	Never Demonstrated	Rarely Demonstrated	Sometimes Demonstrated	Often Demonstrated	Consistently Demonstrated	
310127 Uses smart phone or app to support self-management	1	2	3	4	5	NA
310128 Uses monitor to check blood clotting time	1	2	3	4	5	NA
310124 Develops plan for medical emergencies	1	2	3	4	5	NA
310125 Informs caregiver about management of anticoagulation therapy	1	2	3	4	5	NA
310126 Shares plan for immediate treatment with family caregiver	1	2	3	4	5	NA

Domain-Health Knowledge & Behavior (IV)   **Class-**Health Management (FF)   5th edition 2013; revised 2024

OUTCOME CONTENT REFERENCES:

Cabellos-García, A. C., Martínez-Sabater, A., Castro-Sánchez, E., Kangasniemi, M., Juárez-Vela, R., & Gea-Caballero, V. (2018). Relation between health literacy, self-care and adherence to treatment with oral anticoagulants in adults: A narrative systematic review. BMC Public Health, 18(1), 1157. https://doi.org/10.1186/s12889-018-6070-9

Corrochano, M., Jiménez, B., Millón, J., Gich, I., Rambla, M., Gil, E., Caparrós, P., Macho, R., & Souto, J. C. (2020). Patient self-management of oral anticoagulation with vitamin K antagonists in everyday practice: Clinical outcomes in a single centre cohort after long-term follow-up. BMC Cardiovascular Disorders, 20(1), 166. https://doi.org/10.1186/s12872-020-01448-7

Ritchie, L. A., Penson, P. E., & Lane, D. A. (2019). Warfarin therapy and improved anticoagulation control by patient self-management. Thrombosis and Haemostasis, 119(10), 1550–1552. https://doi.org/10.1055/s-0039-1696982

Sølvik, U. Ø., Løkkebø, E., Kristoffersen, A. H., Brodin, E., Averina, M., & Sandberg, S. (2019). Quality of warfarin therapy and quality of life are improved by self-management for two years. Thrombosis and Haemostasis, 119(10), 1632–1641. https://doi.org/10.1055/s-0039-1693703

Vegt, J., & Guest, P. C. (2018). A user-friendly app for blood coagulation disorders. Methods in Molecular Biology, 1735, 499–504. https://doi.org/10.1007/978-1-4939-7614-0_37

Vogeler, E., Dieterlen, M. T., Garbade, J., Lehmann, S., Jawad, K., Borger, M. A., & Meyer, A. L. (2021). Benefit of self-managed anticoagulation in patients with left ventricular assist device. The Thoracic and Cardiovascular Surgeon, 69(6), 518–525. https://doi.org/10.1055/s-0040-1719153

Witt, D. M., Nieuwlaat, R., Clark, N. P., Ansell, J., Holbrook, A., Skov, J., Shehab, N., Mock, J., Myers, T., Dentali, F., Crowther, M. A., Agarwal, A., Bhatt, M., Khatib, R., Riva, J. J., Zhang, Y., & Guyatt, G. (2018). American Society of Hematology 2018 guidelines for management of venous thromboembolism: Optimal management of anticoagulation therapy. Blood Advances, 2(22), 3257–3291. https://doi.org/10.1182/bloodadvances.2018024893

Self-Management: Arthritis   3112

Definition: Personal actions to manage arthritis, its treatment, and to prevent or limit disease progression and complications

OUTCOME TARGET RATING: Maintain at_____ Increase to_____

	Never Demonstrated	Rarely Demonstrated	Sometimes Demonstrated	Often Demonstrated	Consistently Demonstrated	
OUTCOME OVERALL RATING	1	2	3	4	5	
Indicators:						
311201 Participates in health care decisions	1	2	3	4	5	NA
311202 Uses complementary therapies as approved by health professional	1	2	3	4	5	NA
311203 Uses strategies to control pain	1	2	3	4	5	NA
311204 Monitors for signs and symptoms of depression	1	2	3	4	5	NA
311205 Monitors for signs and symptoms of anxiety	1	2	3	4	5	NA
311206 Uses strategies to control flare up of arthritis	1	2	3	4	5	NA
311207 Seeks information about methods to maintain joint mobility	1	2	3	4	5	NA

S

Continued

Self-Management: Arthritis—cont'd

		Never Demonstrated	Rarely Demonstrated	Sometimes Demonstrated	Often Demonstrated	Consistently Demonstrated	
311208	Identifies ways to cope with functional changes	1	2	3	4	5	NA
311209	Uses effective weight control strategies	1	2	3	4	5	NA
311210	Uses medication as prescribed	1	2	3	4	5	NA
311211	Monitors prescribed medication therapeutic effects	1	2	3	4	5	NA
311212	Monitors medication adverse effects	1	2	3	4	5	NA
311213	Uses only non-prescription medication approved by health professional	1	2	3	4	5	NA
311214	Seeks assistance for self-care	1	2	3	4	5	NA
311215	Follows recommended activity level	1	2	3	4	5	NA
311216	Participates in stretching exercises	1	2	3	4	5	NA
311217	Participates in aerobic exercises	1	2	3	4	5	NA
311218	Participates in periarticular muscle strengthening exercises	1	2	3	4	5	NA
311219	Participates in flexibility exercises	1	2	3	4	5	NA
311220	Participates in joint range of motion exercises	1	2	3	4	5	NA
311221	Participates in weight-bearing exercises	1	2	3	4	5	NA
311222	Participates in muscle-strengthening exercises	1	2	3	4	5	NA
311223	Practices joint protective strategies	1	2	3	4	5	NA
311224	Uses assistive devices correctly						
311225	Uses fall prevention strategies	1	2	3	4	5	NA
311226	Uses energy conservation techniques	1	2	3	4	5	NA
311227	Uses strategies to maintain adequate sleep	1	2	3	4	5	NA
311228	Balances activity and rest	1	2	3	4	5	NA
311229	Paces daily activities	1	2	3	4	5	NA
311230	Keeps appointments with health professional	1	2	3	4	5	NA
311231	Uses available community resources	1	2	3	4	5	NA
311232	Uses support group	1	2	3	4	5	NA

Domain-*Health Knowledge & Behavior* **Class**-*Health Management (FF)* 6th edition 2018

OUTCOME CONTENT REFERENCES:

Bernatsky, S., Rusu, C., O'Donnell, S., Mackay, C., Hawker, G., Canizares, M., & Badley, E. (2012). Self-management strategies in overweight and obese Canadians with arthritis. *Arthritis Care & Research, 64*(2), 280–286. https://doi.org/10.1002/acr.20654

Breedland, I., van Scheppingen, C., Leijsma, M., Verheij-Jansen, N. P., & van Weert, E. (2011). Effects of a group-based exercise and educational program on physical performance and disease self-management in rheumatoid arthritis: A randomized controlled study. *Physical Therapy, 91*(6), 879–893. https://doi.org/10.2522/ptj.20090010

Fitzcharles, M., Lussier, D., & Shir, Y. (2010). Management of chronic arthritis pain in the elderly. *Drugs & Aging, 27*(6), 471–490. https://doi.org/10.2165/11536530-000000000-00000

Home, D., & Carr, M. (2009). Rheumatoid arthritis: The role of early intervention and self-management. *British Journal of Community Nursing, 14*(10), 432–436. https://doi.org/10.12968/bjcn.2009.14.10.44495

Manning, V., Hurley, M., Scott, D., Coker, B., Choy, E., & Bearne, L. (2014). Education, self-management, and upper extremity exercise training in people with rheumatoid arthritis: A randomized controlled trial. *Arthritis Care & Research, 66*(2), 217–227. https://doi.org/10.1002/acr.22102

Trudeau, K., Pujol, L., DasMahapatra, P., Wall, R., Black, R., & Zacharoff, K. (2015). A randomized controlled trial of an online self-management program for adults with arthritis pain. *Journal of Behavioral Medicine, 38*(3), 483–496. https://doi.org/10.1007/s10865-015-9622-9

S

Self-Management: Asthma   0704

Definition: Personal actions to manage asthma, its treatment, and to prevent complications

OUTCOME TARGET RATING: Maintain at_____ Increase to_____

		Never Demonstrated	Rarely Demonstrated	Sometimes Demonstrated	Often Demonstrated	Consistently Demonstrated	
OUTCOME OVERALL RATING		1	2	3	4	5	
Indicators:							
070436	Accepts diagnosis	1	2	3	4	5	NA
070437	Obtains reputable information about asthma	1	2	3	4	5	NA
070438	Identifies health beliefs that impact treatment	1	2	3	4	5	NA
070418	Describes causal factors	1	2	3	4	5	NA
070439	Identifies personal asthma triggers	1	2	3	4	5	NA
070401	Initiates action to avoid personal triggers	1	2	3	4	5	NA
070440	Identifies triggers in work, school, or other community environments	1	2	3	4	5	NA
070419	Recognizes onset of asthma symptoms	1	2	3	4	5	NA
070402	Initiates action to manage personal triggers	1	2	3	4	5	NA
070426	Shares acute asthma management with relevant individual(s)	1	2	3	4	5	NA
070427	Shares emergency plan with relevant individual(s)	1	2	3	4	5	NA
070428	Follows emergency plan for acute attacks	1	2	3	4	5	NA
070441	Identifies emergency medical services in community	1	2	3	4	5	NA
070429	Adjusts life routine for optimal health	1	2	3	4	5	NA
070442	Considers impact of lifestyle changes on asthma management	1	2	3	4	5	NA
070403	Makes appropriate environmental modifications	1	2	3	4	5	NA
070420	Uses diary or app to monitor symptoms over time	1	2	3	4	5	NA
070430	Obtains early treatment for infections	1	2	3	4	5	NA
070443	Obtains recommended immunizations	1	2	3	4	5	NA
070405	Participates in age-appropriate activities	1	2	3	4	5	NA
070444	Follows prescribed activity recommendations	1	2	3	4	5	NA
070406	Sleeps through the night with no cough or wheeze	1	2	3	4	5	NA
070431	Reports energy restored after rest	1	2	3	4	5	NA
070432	Maintains access to medication	1	2	3	4	5	NA
070445	Adheres to medication regimen	1	2	3	4	5	NA
070433	Monitors medication side effects	1	2	3	4	5	NA
070446	Monitors medication adverse effects	1	2	3	4	5	NA
070447	Monitors impact of stress on symptoms	1	2	3	4	5	NA
070410	Monitors peak flow routinely	1	2	3	4	5	NA

S

Continued

Self-Management: Asthma—cont'd

		Never Demonstrated	Rarely Demonstrated	Sometimes Demonstrated	Often Demonstrated	Consistently Demonstrated	
070411	Monitors peak flow when symptoms occur	1	2	3	4	5	NA
070412	Makes appropriate medication choices	1	2	3	4	5	NA
070434	Uses inhalers, spacers, and nebulizers correctly	1	2	3	4	5	NA
070414	Self-manages exacerbations	1	2	3	4	5	NA
070415	Reports uncontrolled symptoms	1	2	3	4	5	NA
070448	Participates smoking cessation regimen	1	2	3	4	5	NA
070449	Monitors changes in general health	1	2	3	4	5	NA
070450	Keeps appointments with health professional	1	2	3	4	5	NA
070451	Discusses treatment goals with health professional	1	2	3	4	5	NA
070452	Reviews written action plan with health professional	1	2	3	4	5	NA
070453	Shares treatment plan with school nurse	1	2	3	4	5	NA
070454	Obtains family support for treatment	1	2	3	4	5	NA
070435	Uses support group	1	2	3	4	5	NA
070455	Uses available community resources	1	2	3	4	5	NA
070421	Reports asthma controlled	1	2	3	4	5	NA

Domain-*Health Knowledge & Behavior (IV)*   **Class**-*Health Management (FF)*   *2nd edition 2000; revised 2004, 2008, 2013, 2024*

OUTCOME CONTENT REFERENCES:

Cloutier, M. M., Dixon, A. E., Krishnan, J. A., Lemanske, R. F., Pace, W., & Schatz, M. (2020). Managing asthma in adolescents and adults: 2020 asthma guideline update from the National Asthma Education and Prevention Program. *Journal of American Medical Association, 324*(22), 2301–2317. https://doi.org/10.1001/jama.2020.21974

Curto, E., Crespo-Lessmann, A., González-Gutiérrez, M. V., Bardagí, S., Pellicer, C., Bazús, T., del Carmen Vennera, M., Martínez, C., & Plaza, V. (2019). Is asthma in the elderly different? Functional and clinical characteristics of asthma in individuals aged 65 years and older. *Asthma Research and Practice, 5*(2), 2. https://doi.org/10.1186/s40733-019-0049-x

Dilber, O. M. F., & Kurtuluş, A. A. D. S. (2021). Obstructive sleep apnea is a determinant of asthma control independent of smoking, reflux, and rhinitis. *Allergy and Asthma Proceedings, 42*(1), e25–e29. https://doi.org/10.2500/aap.2021.42.200098

Expert Panel Working Group of the National Heart, Lung, and Blood Institute (NHLBI) administered and coordinated National Asthma Education and Prevention Program Coordinating Committee (NAEPPCC), Cloutier, M. M., Baptist, A. P., Blake, K. V., Brooks, E. G., Bryant-Stephens, T., DiMango, E., Dixon, A. E., Elward, K. S., Hartert, T., Krishnan, J. A., Lemanske, R. F. Jr., Ouellette, D. R., Pace, W. D., Schatz, M., Skolnik, N. S., Stout, J. W., Teach, S. J., & Walsh, C. G. (2020). 2020 focused updates to the asthma management guidelines: A report from the National Asthma Education and Prevention Program Coordinating Committee Expert Panel Working Group. *Journal of Allergy and Clinical Immunology, 146*(6), 1217–1270. https://doi.org/10.1016/j.jaci.2020.10.003

Gruffydd-Jones, K., & Hansen, K. (2019). Working for better asthma control: How can we improve the dialogue between patients and healthcare professionals? *Advanced Therapy, 37*(1), 1–9. https://doi.org/10.6084/m9.figshare.9994856.v2

Lovinsky-Desir, S., & O'Connor, G. T. (2020). Evolving strategies for long-term asthma management. *Journal of American Medical Association, 324*(22), 2265–2267. https://doi.org/10.1001/jama.2020.16895

Marcano Belisario, J. S., Huckvale, K., Greenfield, G., Car, J., & Gunn, L. H. (2013). Smartphone and tablet self-management apps for asthma. *The Cochrane Database of Systematic Reviews, 2013*(11), CD010013. https://doi.org/10.1002/14651858.CD010013.pub2

Nanda, A., & Wasan, A. N. (2020). Asthma in adults. *Medical Clinics of North America, 104*(1), 95–108. https://doi.org/10.1016/j.mcna.2019.08.013

Rhee, H., Love, T., Harrington, D., & Walters, L. (2020). Comparing three measures of self-efficacy of asthma self-management in adolescents. *Academic Pediatrics, 20*(7), 983–990. https://doi.org/10.1016/j.acap.2020.03.001

S

Self-Management: Autism Spectrum Disorder   3113

Definition: Personal actions to manage autism, use positive behavior practices, its treatment, and to prevent complications

OUTCOME TARGET RATING: Maintain at_____ Increase to_____

		Never Demonstrated	Rarely Demonstrated	Sometimes Demonstrated	Often Demonstrated	Consistently Demonstrated	
OUTCOME OVERALL RATING		1	2	3	4	5	
Indicators:							
311301	Accepts diagnosis	1	2	3	4	5	NA
311302	Obtains reputable information about autism	1	2	3	4	5	NA
311303	Identifies learning style	1	2	3	4	5	NA
311304	Monitors for signs and symptoms of complications	1	2	3	4	5	NA
311305	Uses strategies to prevent complications	1	2	3	4	5	NA
311306	Performs treatment regimen as prescribed	1	2	3	4	5	NA
311307	Monitors treatment therapeutic effects	1	2	3	4	5	NA
311308	Alters behavior to meet treatment requirements	1	2	3	4	5	NA
311309	Uses medication as prescribed	1	2	3	4	5	NA
311310	Monitors medication therapeutic effects	1	2	3	4	5	NA
311311	Monitors medication side effects	1	2	3	4	5	NA
311312	Obtains assistance for activities of daily living	1	2	3	4	5	NA
311313	Obtains assistance for instrumental activities of daily living	1	2	3	4	5	NA
311314	Uses strategies to cope with effects of autism	1	2	3	4	5	NA
311315	Uses strategies to reduce anxiety	1	2	3	4	5	NA
311316	Maintains socially accepted behavior during stress	1	2	3	4	5	NA
311317	Monitors intensity of anxiety	1	2	3	4	5	NA
311318	Develops transition plan with others	1	2	3	4	5	NA
311319	Uses time management skills	1	2	3	4	5	NA
311320	Uses strategies to minimize the impact of change	1	2	3	4	5	NA
311321	Uses strategies to balance environmental stimuli	1	2	3	4	5	NA
311322	Uses effective relaxation techniques	1	2	3	4	5	NA
311323	Maintains role performance	1	2	3	4	5	NA
311324	Uses strategies to communicate effectively	1	2	3	4	5	NA
311325	Exchanges messages accurately with others	1	2	3	4	5	NA
311326	Communicates awareness of interpersonal environment	1	2	3	4	5	NA
311327	Uses strategies to adapt to social situations	1	2	3	4	5	NA
311328	Participates in health care decisions	1	2	3	4	5	NA

S

Continued

Self-Management: Autism Spectrum Disorder—cont'd

		Never Demonstrated	Rarely Demonstrated	Sometimes Demonstrated	Often Demonstrated	Consistently Demonstrated	
311329	Uses case manager to coordinate care	1	2	3	4	5	NA
311330	Uses health care services congruent with needs	1	2	3	4	5	NA
311331	Uses strategies to maintain routine	1	2	3	4	5	NA
311332	Uses available family support system	1	2	3	4	5	NA
311333	Participates in peer group activities	1	2	3	4	5	NA
311334	Uses appropriate social interaction skills	1	2	3	4	5	NA
311335	Uses support group	1	2	3	4	5	NA
311336	Uses available community resources	1	2	3	4	5	NA

Domain-*Health Knowledge & Behavior* **Class**-*Health Management (FF)* *6th edition 2018*

OUTCOME CONTENT REFERENCES:

American Psychiatric Association. (2013). *Diagnostic and statistical manual of mental disorders* (5th ed.). https://doi.org/10.1176/appi.books.9780890425596
Carr, M. (2016). Self-management of challenging behaviors associated with autism spectrum disorder: A meta-analysis. *Australian Psychologist, 51*(4), 316–333. https://doi.org/10.1111/ap.12227
Hume, K., Loftin, R., & Lantz, J. (2009). Increasing independence in autism spectrum disorders: A review of three focused interventions. *Journal of Autism and Developmental Disorders, 39*(9), 1329–1338. https://doi.org/10.1007/s10803-009-0751-2
Johnson, T., & Joshi, A. (2016). Dark clouds or silver linings? A stigma threat perspective on the implications of an autism diagnosis for workplace well-being. *Journal of Applied Psychology, 101*(3), 430–449. https://doi.org/10.1037/apl0000058
Roberts, K. (2010). Topic areas to consider when planning transition from high school to postsecondary education for students with autism spectrum disorders. *Focus on Autism and Other Developmental Disabilities, 25*(3), 158–162. https://doi.org/10.1177/1088357610371476

Self-Management: Cancer

3114

Definition: Personal actions to manage cancer, its treatment, and the prevention of disease progression and complications

OUTCOME TARGET RATING: Maintain at_____ Increase to_____

	Never Demonstrated	Rarely Demonstrated	Sometimes Demonstrated	Often Demonstrated	Consistently Demonstrated	
OUTCOME OVERALL RATING	1	2	3	4	5	

Indicators:

		Never Demonstrated	Rarely Demonstrated	Sometimes Demonstrated	Often Demonstrated	Consistently Demonstrated	
311401	Accepts diagnosis	1	2	3	4	5	NA
311402	Obtains information about cancer	1	2	3	4	5	NA
311403	Identifies cultural beliefs that impact treatment	1	2	3	4	5	NA
311404	Collaborates with health professional to create an individualized plan of care	1	2	3	4	5	NA
311405	Sets realistic short-term goals	1	2	3	4	5	NA
311406	Sets realistic long-term goals	1	2	3	4	5	NA
311407	Monitors signs and symptoms of disease	1	2	3	4	5	NA
311408	Follows treatment schedule	1	2	3	4	5	NA
311409	Monitors chemotherapy effects	1	2	3	4	5	NA
311410	Monitors radiation effects	1	2	3	4	5	NA
311411	Discusses benefits of medication with health professional	1	2	3	4	5	NA

S

Self-Management: Cancer—cont'd

		Never Demonstrated	Rarely Demonstrated	Sometimes Demonstrated	Often Demonstrated	Consistently Demonstrated	
311412	Discusses non-prescription medication use with health professional	1	2	3	4	5	NA
311413	Maintains positive attitude	1	2	3	4	5	NA
311414	Monitors for signs and symptoms of depression	1	2	3	4	5	NA
311415	Obtains assistance for depression	1	2	3	4	5	NA
311416	Uses strategies to cope with adverse effects of disease	1	2	3	4	5	NA
311417	Uses strategies to control fatigue	1	2	3	4	5	NA
311418	Balances activity and rest	1	2	3	4	5	NA
311419	Uses strategies to cope with changes in body image	1	2	3	4	5	NA
311420	Uses strategies to control pain	1	2	3	4	5	NA
311421	Maintains healthy lifestyle	1	2	3	4	5	NA
311422	Obtains assistance with activities of daily living	1	2	3	4	5	NA
311423	Obtains assistance with instrumental activities of daily living	1	2	3	4	5	NA
311424	Modifies work schedule	1	2	3	4	5	NA
311425	Obtains financial resources for assistance	1	2	3	4	5	NA
311426	Maintains positive relationships with family	1	2	3	4	5	NA
311427	Maintains positive relationships with friends	1	2	3	4	5	NA
311428	Keeps appointments with health professional	1	2	3	4	5	NA
311429	Informs family members of genetic risk for cancer	1	2	3	4	5	NA
311430	Reports signs and symptoms of disease reoccurrence	1	2	3	4	5	NA
311431	Uses support group	1	2	3	4	5	NA
311432	Uses available community resources	1	2	3	4	5	NA

Specify cancer_____

Domain-*Health Knowledge & Behavior (IV)*   **Class**-*Health Management (FF)*   6th edition 2018

OUTCOME CONTENT REFERENCES:
Graves, S., Young, L., & Cousin, C. (2014). Current knowledge and perceptions of cancer held by African American seniors in the District of Columbia. *American Journal of Health Education, 45*(3), 166–173. https://doi.org/10.1080/19325037.2014.901111

Jansen, F., van Uden–Kraan, C., van Zwieten, V., Witte, B., & Leeuw, I. (2015). Cancer survivors' perceived need for supportive care and their attitude towards self-management and ehealth. *Support Care Cancer, 23*(6), 1679–1688. https://doi.org/10.1007/s00520-014-2514-7

McCorkle, R., Ercolano, E., Lazenby, M., Schulman–Green, D., Schilling, L., Lorig, K., & Wagner, E. (2011). Self-management: Enabling and empowering patients living with cancer as a chronic illness. *CA: A Cancer Journal for Clinicians, 61*(1), 50–62. https://doi.org/10.3322/caac.20093

Rosenberg, C., Flanagan, C., Brockstein, B., Obel, J., Dragon, L., Merkel, D., Wade, E. L., Law, T. M., Khandekar, J. D., & Hensing, T. A. (2016). Promotion of self-management for post treatment cancer survivors: Evaluation of a risk-adapted visit. *Journal of Cancer Survivorship, 10*(1), 206–219. https://doi.org/10.1007/s11764-015-0467-6

S

Self-Management: Cardiac Disease 1617

Definition: Personal actions to manage heart disease, its treatment, and to prevent disease progression and complications

OUTCOME TARGET RATING: Maintain at_____ Increase to_____

		Never Demonstrated	Rarely Demonstrated	Sometimes Demonstrated	Often Demonstrated	Consistently Demonstrated	
OUTCOME OVERALL RATING		1	2	3	4	5	
Indicators:							
161701	Accepts the diagnosis	1	2	3	4	5	NA
161702	Seeks information about methods to maintain cardiovascular health	1	2	3	4	5	NA
161703	Participates in health care decisions	1	2	3	4	5	NA
161704	Participates in prescribed cardiac rehabilitation	1	2	3	4	5	NA
161705	Performs treatment regimen as prescribed	1	2	3	4	5	NA
161706	Monitors symptom onset	1	2	3	4	5	NA
161707	Monitors symptom persistence	1	2	3	4	5	NA
161708	Monitors symptom severity	1	2	3	4	5	NA
161709	Monitors symptom frequency	1	2	3	4	5	NA
161710	Reports symptoms of worsening disease	1	2	3	4	5	NA
161748	Reports signs and symptoms of anxiety	1	2	3	4	5	NA
161711	Reports signs and symptoms of depression	1	2	3	4	5	NA
161712	Uses diary to monitor symptoms over time	1	2	3	4	5	NA
161713	Uses preventive measures to reduce risk of complications	1	2	3	4	5	NA
161714	Uses symptom relief methods	1	2	3	4	5	NA
161744	Obtains health care when warning signs occur	1	2	3	4	5	NA
161716	Monitors pulse rate and rhythm	1	2	3	4	5	NA
161717	Monitors blood pressure	1	2	3	4	5	NA
161718	Limits sodium intake	1	2	3	4	5	NA
161719	Limits fat and cholesterol intake	1	2	3	4	5	NA
161720	Follows recommended diet	1	2	3	4	5	NA
161721	Follows fluid restrictions	1	2	3	4	5	NA
161749	Monitors caffeine intake	1	2	3	4	5	NA
161723	Monitors body weight	1	2	3	4	5	NA
161724	Uses effective weight control strategies	1	2	3	4	5	NA
161725	Maintains optimum weight	1	2	3	4	5	NA
161726	Follows recommendations for alcohol use	1	2	3	4	5	NA
161727	Participates in smoking cessation regimen	1	2	3	4	5	NA
161728	Participates in recommended exercise	1	2	3	4	5	NA
161729	Uses energy conservation techniques	1	2	3	4	5	NA
161730	Balances activity and rest	1	2	3	4	5	NA
161731	Performs usual life routine	1	2	3	4	5	NA
161750	Obtains information about impact on sexual activity	1	2	3	4	5	NA

S

Self-Management: Cardiac Disease—cont'd

		Never Demonstrated	Rarely Demonstrated	Sometimes Demonstrated	Often Demonstrated	Consistently Demonstrated	
161732	Follows recommendations for sexual activity	1	2	3	4	5	NA
161733	Obtains required medication	1	2	3	4	5	NA
161734	Uses medication as prescribed	1	2	3	4	5	NA
161735	Monitors prescribed medication therapeutic effects	1	2	3	4	5	NA
161751	Monitors side effects of medication	1	2	3	4	5	NA
161736	Uses only non-prescription medication approved by health professional	1	2	3	4	5	NA
161752	Participates in medication reconciliation with health professional	1	2	3	4	5	NA
161737	Uses stress management strategies	1	2	3	4	5	NA
161753	Obtains recommended vaccines	1	2	3	4	5	NA
161739	Uses health care services congruent with needs	1	2	3	4	5	NA
161740	Participates in screening for cholesterol	1	2	3	4	5	NA
161754	Participates in cardiac rehabilitation	1	2	3	4	5	NA
161741	Reports need for financial assistance	1	2	3	4	5	NA
161742	Keeps appointments with health professional	1	2	3	4	5	NA
161755	Maintains plan for symptom occurrence	1	2	3	4	5	NA
161743	Maintains plan for medical emergencies	1	2	3	4	5	NA
161745	Adjusts life routine for optimal health	1	2	3	4	5	NA

Domain-Health Knowledge & Behavior (IV)   **Class**-Health Management (FF)   3rd edition 2004; revised 2008, 2013, 2024

OUTCOME CONTENT REFERENCES:
Cavalcante, A., Lopes, C. T., Brunori, E., Swanson, E., Moorhead, S. A., Bachion, M. M., & de Barros, A. (2018). Self-care behaviors in heart failure. *International Journal of Nursing Knowledge, 29*(3), 146–155. https://doi.org/10.1111/2047-3095.12170

Cavalcante, A. M, Lopes, C. T., Swanson, E., Moorhead, S. A., Bachion, M. M., Barros, A. L. (2020). Validation of definitions of the indicators for Nursing Outcomes Classification outcomes: Self-management: Cardiac Disease. *Acta Paulista de Enfermagem, 33*(1), 1–9. https://doi.org/10.37689/acta-ape/2020AO0265

Guo, P., & Harris, R. (2016). The effectiveness and experience of self-management following acute coronary syndrome: A review of the literature. *International Journal of Nursing Studies, 61*, 29–51. https://doi.org/10.1016/j.iinurstu.2016.05.008S

Hendriks, J., Andreae, C., Ågren, S., Eriksson, H., Hjelm, C., Walfridsson, U., Ski, C. F., Thylén, I., & Jaarsma, T. (2020). Cardiac disease and stroke: Practical implications for personalized care in cardiac-stroke patients. A state-of-the-art review supported by the Association of Cardiovascular Nursing and Allied Professions. *European Journal of Cardiovascular Nursing: Journal of the Working Group on Cardiovascular Nursing of the European Society of Cardiology, 19*(6), 495–504. https://doi.org/10.1177/1474515119895734

Riegel, B., Moser, D. K., Buck, H. G., Dickson, V. V., Dunbar, S. B., Lee, C. S., Lennie, T. A., Lindenfeld, J., Mitchell, J. E., Treat-Jacobson, D. J., Webber, D. E., & American Heart Association Council on Cardiovascular and Stroke Nursing: Council on Peripheral Vascular Disease; and Council on Quality of Care and Outcomes Research. (2017). Self-care for the prevention and management of cardiovascular disease and stroke: A scientific statement for healthcare professionals from the American Heart Association. *Journal of the American Heart Association, 6*(9), e006997. https://doi.org/10.1161.JAHA.117006997

Zhang, L., Gallagher, R., Ding, D., & Neubeck, L. (2018). Self-management following a cardiac event in people of Chinese ethnicity living in western countries: A scoping review. *Journal of Immigrant and Minority Health, 20*(3), 744–754. https://doi.org/10.1007/s1090-017-0584-6

S

Self-Management: Celiac Disease   3115

Definition: Personal actions to manage celiac disease, its treatment, and to prevent or limit disease progression and complications

OUTCOME TARGET RATING: Maintain at_____ Increase to_____

OUTCOME OVERALL RATING	Never Demonstrated 1	Rarely Demonstrated 2	Sometimes Demonstrated 3	Often Demonstrated 4	Consistently Demonstrated 5	
Indicators:						
311501 Monitors for signs and symptoms of gluten intolerance	1	2	3	4	5	NA
311502 Reports potential long-term consequences of untreated celiac disease	1	2	3	4	5	NA
311503 Participates in educational program	1	2	3	4	5	NA
311504 Identifies gluten in food sources	1	2	3	4	5	NA
311505 Identifies gluten in non-food sources	1	2	3	4	5	NA
311506 Adheres to a gluten-free diet	1	2	3	4	5	NA
311507 Chooses gluten-free foods consistent with cultural beliefs	1	2	3	4	5	NA
311508 Identifies retailers of gluten-free food	1	2	3	4	5	NA
311509 Interprets information on food labels correctly	1	2	3	4	5	NA
311510 Monitors for possible cross contamination	1	2	3	4	5	NA
311511 Uses supplemental vitamins as recommended	1	2	3	4	5	NA
311512 Plans for eating out	1	2	3	4	5	NA
311513 Plans for social situations	1	2	3	4	5	NA
311514 Adjusts life routine for optimal health	1	2	3	4	5	NA
311515 Obtains reputable information about celiac disease	1	2	3	4	5	NA
311516 Obtains financial resources for assistance	1	2	3	4	5	NA
311517 Uses support group	1	2	3	4	5	NA
311518 Keeps appointments with health professional for celiac	1	2	3	4	5	NA
311519 Keeps appointments with health professional for comorbid conditions	1	2	3	4	5	NA
311520 Uses available community resources	1	2	3	4	5	NA

Domain-*Health Knowledge & Behavior (IV)*   **Class**-*Health Management (FF)*   *6th edition 2018*

S

OUTCOME CONTENT REFERENCES:

Dowd, A., Jung, M., Chen, M., & Beauchamp, M. (2016). Prediction of adherence to a gluten-free diet using protection motivation theory among adults with celiac disease. *Journal of Human Nutrition & Dietetics, 29*(3), 391–398. https://doi.org/10.1111/jhn.1232

Ogden, J. (2016). Improving recognition and management of coeliac disease. *Prescriber, 27*(3), 44–47. https://doi.org/10.1002/psb.1446

Paul, S., Krikham, E., & Pidgeon, S. (2015). Coeliac disease in children. *Nursing Standard, 29*(49), 36–41. https://doi.org/10.7748/ns.29.49.36.e10022

Silvester, J., Weiten, D., Graff, L., Walker, J., & Duerksen, D. (2016). Living gluten-free: Adherence, knowledge, lifestyle adaptations and feelings towards a gluten-free diet. *Journal of Human Nutrition & Dietetics, 29*(3), 374–382. https://doi.org/10.1111/jhn.12316

Self-Management: Chronic Anemia   3116

Definition: Personal actions to manage persistent anemia, its treatment, and to prevent complications

OUTCOME TARGET RATING: Maintain at_____ Increase to_____

		Never Demonstrated	Rarely Demonstrated	Sometimes Demonstrated	Often Demonstrated	Consistently Demonstrated	
OUTCOME OVERALL RATING		1	2	3	4	5	
Indicators:							
311601	Monitors signs and symptoms of anemia	1	2	3	4	5	NA
311602	Obtains information about anemia	1	2	3	4	5	NA
311603	Obtains information about methods to prevent cardiac complications	1	2	3	4	5	NA
311604	Monitors for signs and symptoms of cardiac complications	1	2	3	4	5	NA
311605	Reports signs and symptoms of cardiac complications	1	2	3	4	5	NA
311606	Monitors fatigue level	1	2	3	4	5	NA
311607	Uses energy conservation techniques	1	2	3	4	5	NA
311608	Uses symptom relief measures	1	2	3	4	5	NA
311609	Monitors factors that decrease the ability to perform activity	1	2	3	4	5	NA
311610	Monitors factors that impact ability to perform activity	1	2	3	4	5	NA
311611	Uses strategies to ambulate safely	1	2	3	4	5	NA
311612	Participates in health care decisions	1	2	3	4	5	NA
311613	Monitors medication therapeutic effects	1	2	3	4	5	NA
311614	Monitors medication side effects	1	2	3	4	5	NA
311615	Monitors medication adverse effects	1	2	3	4	5	NA
311616	Follows recommended diet	1	2	3	4	5	NA
311629	Monitors hydration intake	1	2	3	4	5	NA
311617	Follows recommended dietary restrictions	1	2	3	4	5	NA
311618	Uses nutritional supplements as recommended	1	2	3	4	5	NA
311619	Uses iron supplements as prescribed	1	2	3	4	5	NA
311620	Obtains assistance from a health professional	1	2	3	4	5	NA
311621	Obtains needed tests	1	2	3	4	5	NA
311622	Follows instructions for test procedures	1	2	3	4	5	NA
311623	Keeps appointments with health professional	1	2	3	4	5	NA
311624	Adjusts life routine for optimal health	1	2	3	4	5	NA
311625	Obtains recommended vaccines	1	2	3	4	5	NA
311627	Uses reputable resources of anemia-specific information	1	2	3	4	5	NA
311628	Reports need for financial assistance	1	2	3	4	5	NA

Domain-Health Knowledge & Behavior (IV)   *Class*-Health Management (FF)   6th edition 2018; revised 2024

OUTCOME CONTENT REFERENCES:
de Miranda, F. R., Ivo, M. L., Teston, E. F., Lino, I. G. T., Mandetto, M. A., & Marcheti, M. A. (2020). Families' experiences in managing children with sickle cell anemia: Implications for care. *Revista Enfermagem UERJ,* (Rio de Janeiro, Brazil), *28*, e51594. https://doi.org/10.12957/reuerj.2020.S1594

Hockenberry, M. J., Rodgers, C. C., & Wilson, D. (2022). *Wong's essential of pediatric nursing* (11th ed.). Elsevier.

Marchi, G., Busti, F., Vianello, A., & Girelli, D. (2021). Anemia and iron deficiency in heart failure: Extending evidence from chronic to acute setting. *Internal and Emergency Medicine, 16*(1), 167–170. https://doi.org/10.1007/s11739-020-02434-9

Pasini, E., Corsetti, G., Romano, C., Aquilani, R., Scarabelli, T., Chen-Scarabelli, C., & Dioguardi, F. S. (2021). Management of anemia of chronic disease: Beyond iron-only supplementation. *Nutrients, 13*(1), 237. https://doi.org/10.3390/nu13010237

S

Stabell, N., Averina, M., & Flægstad, T. (2021). Chronic iron deficiency and anaemia were highly prevalent in a population-based longitudinal study among adolescent girls. *Acta Paediatrica, 110*(10), 2842–2849. https://doi.org/10.1111/apa.1601

Wiciński, M., Liczner, G., Cadelski, K., Kolnierzk, T., Nowaczewska, M., & Malinowski, B. (2020). Anemia of chronic diseases: Wider diagnostics—Better treatment? *Nutrients, 12*(6), 1784. https://doi.org/10.3390/nu12061784

Self-Management: Chronic Disease   3102

Definition: Personal actions to manage a chronic disease, its treatment, and to prevent disease progression and complications

OUTCOME TARGET RATING: Maintain at _____ Increase to _____

		Never Demonstrated	Rarely Demonstrated	Sometimes Demonstrated	Often Demonstrated	Consistently Demonstrated	
OUTCOME OVERALL RATING		1	2	3	4	5	
Indicators:							
310201	Accepts diagnosis	1	2	3	4	5	NA
310202	Seeks information about disease	1	2	3	4	5	NA
310203	Monitors signs and symptoms of disease	1	2	3	4	5	NA
310252	Monitors pattern of signs and symptoms	1	2	3	4	5	NA
310204	Follows recommended precautions	1	2	3	4	5	NA
310205	Seeks information about methods to prevent complications	1	2	3	4	5	NA
310206	Monitors for signs and symptoms of complications	1	2	3	4	5	NA
310207	Reports signs and symptoms of complications	1	2	3	4	5	NA
310208	Uses symptom relief strategies	1	2	3	4	5	NA
310209	Identifies cultural beliefs that impact treatment	1	2	3	4	5	NA
310210	Discusses cultural beliefs that impact treatment with health provider	1	2	3	4	5	NA
310211	Follows recommended treatment	1	2	3	4	5	NA
310212	Performs prescribed procedure	1	2	3	4	5	NA
310213	Uses treatment devices correctly	1	2	3	4	5	NA
310214	Monitors treatment therapeutic effects	1	2	3	4	5	NA
310215	Monitors treatment side effects	1	2	3	4	5	NA
310216	Alters roles to meet treatment requirements	1	2	3	4	5	NA
310217	Obtains required laboratory tests	1	2	3	4	5	NA
310218	Follows medication regimen	1	2	3	4	5	NA
310219	Monitors medication therapeutic effects	1	2	3	4	5	NA
310220	Monitors medication side effects	1	2	3	4	5	NA
310221	Monitors medication adverse effects	1	2	3	4	5	NA
310253	Participates in medication reconciliation with health professional	1	2	3	4	5	NA
310222	Uses only non-prescription medication approved by health professional	1	2	3	4	5	NA
310223	Seeks assistance for self-care	1	2	3	4	5	NA
310224	Follows recommended diet	1	2	3	4	5	NA
310225	Follows recommended activity level	1	2	3	4	5	NA
310226	Participates in recommended exercises	1	2	3	4	5	NA

S

Self-Management: Chronic Disease—cont'd

		Never Demonstrated	Rarely Demonstrated	Sometimes Demonstrated	Often Demonstrated	Consistently Demonstrated	
310227	Eliminates tobacco use	1	2	3	4	5	NA
310228	Uses stress management strategies	1	2	3	4	5	NA
310229	Maintains optimum weight	1	2	3	4	5	NA
310230	Monitors vital signs	1	2	3	4	5	NA
310231	Avoids behaviors that potentiate disease progression	1	2	3	4	5	NA
310232	Uses strategies to prevent complications	1	2	3	4	5	NA
310254	Uses strategies to manage continuous care	1	2	3	4	5	NA
310233	Adjusts life routine for optimal health	1	2	3	4	5	NA
310234	Uses strategies to cope with effects of disease	1	2	3	4	5	NA
310235	Uses strategies to enhance comfort	1	2	3	4	5	NA
310236	Uses strategies to control pain	1	2	3	4	5	NA
310237	Uses strategies to maintain adequate sleep	1	2	3	4	5	NA
310238	Balances activity and rest	1	2	3	4	5	NA
310255	Obtains recommended vaccines	1	2	3	4	5	NA
310241	Participates in prescribed educational program	1	2	3	4	5	NA
310242	Monitors changes in disease	1	2	3	4	5	NA
310256	Obtains advice from health professional for follow-up treatment	1	2	3	4	5	NA
310243	Uses reputable sources of information	1	2	3	4	5	NA
310244	Participates in health care decisions	1	2	3	4	5	NA
310245	Uses case manager to coordinate care	1	2	3	4	5	NA
310246	Uses health care services congruent with needs	1	2	3	4	5	NA
310247	Develops plan for medical emergencies	1	2	3	4	5	NA
310248	Obtains advice from health professional as needed	1	2	3	4	5	NA
310249	Keeps appointments with health professional	1	2	3	4	5	NA
310250	Uses support group	1	2	3	4	5	NA
310251	Uses available community resources	1	2	3	4	5	NA

Domain-Health Knowledge & Behavior (IV)   **Class**-Health Management (FF)   5th edition 2013; revised 2024

OUTCOME CONTENT REFERENCES:

Bauer, M. S., Weaver, K., Kim, B., Lew, R., Stolzmann, K., Sullivan, J. L., Riendeau, R., Connolly, S., Pitcock, J., Ludvigsen, S. M., & Elwy, A. R. (2019). The Collaborative Chronic Care Model for mental health conditions. *Medical Care, 67*, S221–S227. https://doi.org/10.1097/MLR.0000000000001145

Cody, S. L. (2021). Managing sleep disorders with chronic illness across the lifespan. *Nursing Clinics of North America, 56*(2), xiii–xiv. https://doi.org/10.1016/j.cnur.2021.03.003

Crespo, R., Christiansen, M., Tieman, K., & Wittberg, R. (2020). An emerging model for community health worker-based chronic care management for patients with high health care costs in rural Appalachia. *Preventing Chronic Disease, 17*, 190316. https://doi.org/10.58888/pcd17.190316

Favarato, M. H., Germani, A. C. C. G., & Martins, M. de A. (2021). Glimpsing the raging seas that stop swans: A qualitative look at living with multimorbidity and pain in patients from a tertiary care service. *Journal of Multimorbidity and Comorbidity, 11*. https://doi.org/10.1177/2633556521999509

Francesconi, P., Ballo, P., Profili, F., Policardo, L., Roti, L., & Zuppiroli, A. (2019). Chronic care model for the management of patients with heart failure in primary care. *Health Services Insights, 12*, 1–2. https://doi.org/10.1177/1178632919866200

Kong, L. N., Zhu, W. F., Li, L., Lei, Q. S., Wang, T., & Li, Y. L. (2021). Self-management behaviors in adults with chronic hepatitis B: A structural equation model. *International Journal of Nursing Studies, 116*, 1–7. https://doi.org/10.1016/j.inurstu.2019.06.013

Pany, M. J., Chen, L., Sheridan, B., & Huckman, R. S. (2021). Provider teams outperform solo providers in managing chronic diseases and could improve the value of care. *Health Affairs, 40*(3), 435–444. https://doi.org/10.1377/hlthaff.2020.01580

+Robinson, L., Newton, J. L., Jones, D., & Dawson, P. (2014). Promoting self-management and adherence with strength and balance training for older people with long-term conditions: A mixed methods study. *Journal of Evaluation in Clinical Practice, 20*(4), 318–326. https://doi.org/10.1111/jep.12128

Sand, C. D., Rahbek, K., Willadsen, T. G., & Jønsson, A. R. (2021). Prioritizing social identities: Patients' perspective on living with multimorbidity. *Journal of Comorbidity, 11*. https://doi.org/10.1177/26335565211009375

S

Self-Management: Chronic Obstructive Pulmonary Disease   3103

Definition: Personal actions to manage chronic obstructive pulmonary disease, its treatment, and to prevent disease progression and complications

OUTCOME TARGET RATING: Maintain at_____ Increase to_____

OUTCOME OVERALL RATING	Never Demonstrated	Rarely Demonstrated	Sometimes Demonstrated	Often Demonstrated	Consistently Demonstrated	
	1	2	3	4	5	
Indicators:						
310301 Accepts diagnosis	1	2	3	4	5	NA
310302 Seeks information about methods to prevent progression of disease	1	2	3	4	5	NA
310303 Seeks information about methods to prevent complications	1	2	3	4	5	NA
310304 Participates in health care decisions	1	2	3	4	5	NA
310305 Performs treatment regimen as prescribed	1	2	3	4	5	NA
310306 Avoids environmental risk factors	1	2	3	4	5	NA
310307 Participates in pulmonary rehabilitation	1	2	3	4	5	NA
310308 Monitors pulse rate and rhythm	1	2	3	4	5	NA
310309 Monitors respiratory rate and rhythm	1	2	3	4	5	NA
310310 Monitors body temperature	1	2	3	4	5	NA
310311 Monitors oxygen saturation	1	2	3	4	5	NA
310342 Maintains optimum weight	1	2	3	4	5	NA
310312 Monitors food intake effects on breathing	1	2	3	4	5	NA
310313 Monitors fluid intake effects on breathing	1	2	3	4	5	NA
310314 Monitors symptom onset	1	2	3	4	5	NA
310315 Monitors symptom persistence	1	2	3	4	5	NA
310316 Monitors symptom severity	1	2	3	4	5	NA
310317 Monitors symptom frequency	1	2	3	4	5	NA
310318 Monitors disease progression	1	2	3	4	5	NA
310319 Reports symptoms of worsening disease	1	2	3	4	5	NA
310343 Uses strategies to manage exacerbations	1	2	3	4	5	NA
310320 Obtains health care when warning signs occur	1	2	3	4	5	NA
310321 Uses symptom relief methods	1	2	3	4	5	NA
310322 Obtains required medication	1	2	3	4	5	NA
310323 Uses medication as prescribed	1	2	3	4	5	NA
310324 Monitors prescribed medication therapeutic effects	1	2	3	4	5	NA
310325 Monitors medication side effects	1	2	3	4	5	NA
310344 Participates in medication reconciliation with health professional	1	2	3	4	5	NA
310326 Uses oxygen correctly	1	2	3	4	5	NA
310327 Participates in smoking cessation regimen	1	2	3	4	5	NA
310328 Participates in recommended exercise	1	2	3	4	5	NA
310345 Participates in pulmonary rehabilitation	1	2	3	4	5	NA
310329 Uses energy conservation techniques	1	2	3	4	5	NA
310330 Balances activity and rest	1	2	3	4	5	NA
310331 Uses strategies to cope with functional changes	1	2	3	4	5	NA

S

Self-Management: Chronic Obstructive Pulmonary Disease—cont'd

		Never Demonstrated	Rarely Demonstrated	Sometimes Demonstrated	Often Demonstrated	Consistently Demonstrated	
310332	Monitors for signs and symptoms of depression	1	2	3	4	5	NA
310333	Uses relaxation techniques	1	2	3	4	5	NA
310334	Adjusts life routine for optimal health	1	2	3	4	5	NA
310346	Obtains recommended vaccines	1	2	3	4	5	NA
310337	Uses health care services congruent with needs	1	2	3	4	5	NA
310338	Reports need for financial assistance	1	2	3	4	5	NA
310339	Keeps appointments with health professional	1	2	3	4	5	NA
310340	Maintains plan for medical emergencies	1	2	3	4	5	NA
310347	Uses available educational opportunities	1	2	3	4	5	NA
310341	Uses available community resources	1	2	3	4	5	NA

Domain-*Health Knowledge & Behavior (IV)*   **Class**-*Health Management (FF)*   *5th edition 2013; revised 2024*

OUTCOME CONTENT REFERENCES:

Criner, G., & Duffy, S. (2021). Reducing and managing chronic obstructive pulmonary disease exacerbations with tiotropium + olodaterol. *Current Medical Research and Opinion. 37*(2), 275–284. https://doi.org/10.1080/03007995.2020.1841615

Janssen, S. M., Vlieland, T. P. V., Volker, G., Spruit, M. A., & Abbink, J. J. (2021). Pulmonary rehabilitation improves self-management ability in subjects with obstructive lung disease. *Respiratory Care, 66*(8), 1271–1281. https://doi.org/10.4187/respcare.07852

Luckett, T., San Martin, A., Currow, D. C., Johnson, M. J., Barnes-Harris, M. M., & Phillips, J. L. (2020). A systematic review and meta-analysis of studies comparing burden from lung cancer and chronic obstructive pulmonary disease. *Palliative Medicine, 34*(10), 1291–1304. https://doi.org/10.1177/0269216320940153

O'Connell, S., McCarthy, V. J. C., Queally, M., & Savage, E. (2021). The preferences of people with asthma or chronic obstructive pulmonary disease for self-management support: A qualitative descriptive study. *Journal of Clinical Nursing, 30*(19/20), 2832–2841. https://doi.org/10.1111/jocn.15790

Politis, J., Eastman, P., Le, B., Furler, J., Irving, L., & Smallwood, N. (2021). Managing severe chronic breathlessness in chronic obstructive pulmonary disease is challenging for general practitioners. *American Journal of Hospice & Palliative Medicine, 38*(5), 472–479. https://doi.org/10.1177/1049909120959061

Ratarasarn, K., & Kundu, A. (2020). Yoga and tai chi: A mind-body approach in managing respiratory symptoms in obstructive lung diseases. *Current Opinion in Pulmonary Medicine, 26*(2), 186–192. https://doi.org/10.1097/MCP.0000000000000654

Tumilty, E., Doolan-Noble, F., Latu, A. T. F., McAuley, K., Dummer, J., Baxter, J., Hannah, D., Donlevy, S., & Stokes, T. (2020). 'A balancing act'. Living with severe chronic obstructive pulmonary disease in Southern New Zealand: A qualitative study. *Journal of Primary Health Care, 12*(2), 166–172. https://doi.org/10.1071/HC20007

Self-Management: Coronary Artery Disease   3104

Definition: Personal actions to manage coronary artery disease, its treatment, and to prevent disease progression and complications

OUTCOME TARGET RATING: Maintain at_____ Increase to_____

		Never Demonstrated	Rarely Demonstrated	Sometimes Demonstrated	Often Demonstrated	Consistently Demonstrated	
OUTCOME OVERALL RATING		1	2	3	4	5	
Indicators:							
310401	Accepts diagnosis	1	2	3	4	5	NA
310402	Seeks information about methods to manage disease	1	2	3	4	5	NA
310444	Obtains information on treatment options	1	2	3	4	5	NA
310403	Participates in health care decisions	1	2	3	4	5	NA
310404	Participates in prescribed cardiac rehabilitation	1	2	3	4	5	NA

S

Continued

Self-Management: Coronary Artery Disease—cont'd

		Never Demonstrated	Rarely Demonstrated	Sometimes Demonstrated	Often Demonstrated	Consistently Demonstrated	
310405	Performs treatment regimen as prescribed	1	2	3	4	5	NA
310406	Monitors heart rate and rhythm	1	2	3	4	5	NA
310407	Monitors blood pressure	1	2	3	4	5	NA
310408	Monitors for pain	1	2	3	4	5	NA
310409	Monitors for shortness of breath	1	2	3	4	5	NA
310445	Monitors fatigue level	1	2	3	4	5	NA
310410	Monitors symptom onset	1	2	3	4	5	NA
310411	Monitors symptom persistence	1	2	3	4	5	NA
310412	Monitors symptom severity	1	2	3	4	5	NA
310413	Monitors symptom frequency	1	2	3	4	5	NA
310414	Reports symptoms of worsening disease	1	2	3	4	5	NA
310415	Uses diary or app to monitor symptoms over time	1	2	3	4	5	NA
310416	Uses symptom relief methods	1	2	3	4	5	NA
310417	Uses preventive strategies to reduce risk of complications	1	2	3	4	5	NA
310418	Obtains health care for change in symptoms	1	2	3	4	5	NA
310419	Uses medication as prescribed	1	2	3	4	5	NA
310420	Monitors medication therapeutic effects	1	2	3	4	5	NA
310446	Participates in medication reconciliation with health professional	1	2	3	4	5	NA
310421	Monitors medication side effects	1	2	3	4	5	NA
310422	Avoids stopping medication suddenly	1	2	3	4	5	NA
310423	Uses only non-prescription medication approved by health professional	1	2	3	4	5	NA
310447	Obtains information on treatment plan relationship to comorbid conditions	1	2	3	4	5	NA
310424	Follows prescribed diet	1	2	3	4	5	NA
310425	Monitors effects of stimulants	1	2	3	4	5	NA
310426	Uses effective weight control strategies	1	2	3	4	5	NA
310427	Maintains optimum weight	1	2	3	4	5	NA
310428	Follows recommendations for alcohol use	1	2	3	4	5	NA
310429	Eliminates tobacco use	1	2	3	4	5	NA
310430	Avoids second-hand smoke	1	2	3	4	5	NA
310431	Participates in recommended exercise	1	2	3	4	5	NA
310432	Follows recommendations for sexual activity	1	2	3	4	5	NA
310433	Uses stress management strategies	1	2	3	4	5	NA
310434	Uses anger management techniques	1	2	3	4	5	NA
310435	Obtains influenza seasonal vaccine	1	2	3	4	5	NA
310436	Obtains pneumonia vaccine	1	2	3	4	5	NA
310437	Uses health care services congruent with needs	1	2	3	4	5	NA
310438	Participates in screening for cholesterol	1	2	3	4	5	NA
310439	Participates in screening for blood glucose level	1	2	3	4	5	NA

S

Self-Management: Coronary Artery Disease—cont'd

		Never Demonstrated	Rarely Demonstrated	Sometimes Demonstrated	Often Demonstrated	Consistently Demonstrated	
310440	Uses social support	1	2	3	4	5	NA
310441	Keeps appointments with health professional	1	2	3	4	5	NA
310442	Maintains plan for medical emergencies	1	2	3	4	5	NA
310443	Adapts life routine for optimal health	1	2	3	4	5	NA

Domain-Health Knowledge & Behavior (IV)   **Class**-Health Management (FF)   5th edition 2013; revised 2024

OUTCOME CONTENT REFERENCES:

Dale, L. P., Whittaker, R., Jiang, Y., Stewart, R., Rolleston, A., & Maddison, R. (2014). Improving coronary heart disease self-management using mobile technologies (Text4Heart): A randomised controlled trial protocol. *Trials, 15*, 71. https://doi.org/10.1186/1745-6215-15-71

Ignatavicius, D. D., Workman, M. L., Rebar, C. R., & Heimgartner, N. M. (2021). *Medical-surgical nursing: Concepts for interprofessional collaborative care,* (10th ed.). Elsevier.

Jung, H. G., & Yang, Y. K. (2021). Factors influencing health behavior practice in patients with coronary artery diseases. *Health and Quality of Life Outcomes, 19*(3), 1–9. https://doi.org/10.1186/s12955-020-01635-2

Lu, M., Xia, H., Ma, J., Lin, Y., Zhang, X., Shen, Y., & Hravnak, M. (2020). Relationship between adherence to secondary prevention and health literacy, self-efficacy and disease knowledge among patients with coronary artery disease in China. *European Journal of Cardiovascular Nursing, 19*(3), 230–237. https://doi.org/10.1177/1474515119880059

Mares, M., Salamonson, Y., Maneze, D., Elmir, R., & Everett, B. (2022). Development and validation of a scale to measure self-efficacy and self-management in people with coronary heart disease. *The Journal of Cardiovascular Nursing, 37*(4), E81–E88. https://doi.org/10.1097/JCN.0000000000000777

Palacios, J., Lee, G. A., Duaso, M., Clifton, A., Norman, I. J., Richards, D., & Barley, E. A. (2017). Internet-delivered self-management support for improving coronary heart disease and self-management-related outcomes: A systematic review. *The Journal of Cardiovascular Nursing, 32*(4), E9–E23. https://doi.org/10.1097/JCN.0000000000000392

Pfaeffli Dale, L. P., Whittaker, R., Jiang, Y., Stewart, R., Rolleston, A., & Maddison, R. (2015). Text message and internet support for coronary heart disease self-management: Results from the Text4Heart Randomized Controlled Trial. *Journal of Medical Internet Research, 17*(10), e237. https://doi.org/10.2196/jmir.4944

Williams, P. (2020). *Basic geriatric nursing* (6th ed.). Elsevier.

Self-Management: Diabetes   1619

Definition: Personal actions to manage diabetes, its treatment, and to prevent complications

OUTCOME TARGET RATING: Maintain at_____ Increase to_____

		Never Demonstrated	Rarely Demonstrated	Sometimes Demonstrated	Often Demonstrated	Consistently Demonstrated	
OUTCOME OVERALL RATING		1	2	3	4	5	
Indicators:							
161901	Accepts diagnosis	1	2	3	4	5	NA
161902	Seeks information about methods to prevent complications	1	2	3	4	5	NA
161903	Performs preventive foot care practices	1	2	3	4	5	NA
161904	Obtains dilated vision examination as recommended	1	2	3	4	5	NA
161905	Adjusts medication when acutely ill	1	2	3	4	5	NA
161906	Reports non-healing breaks in skin to primary care provider	1	2	3	4	5	NA
161907	Participates in health care decisions	1	2	3	4	5	NA
161908	Participates in prescribed educational program	1	2	3	4	5	NA
161909	Performs treatment regimen as prescribed	1	2	3	4	5	NA
161910	Performs correct procedure for blood glucose testing	1	2	3	4	5	NA

Continued

Self-Management: Diabetes—cont'd

		Never Demonstrated	Rarely Demonstrated	Sometimes Demonstrated	Often Demonstrated	Consistently Demonstrated	
161911	Monitors blood glucose	1	2	3	4	5	NA
161912	Treats symptoms of hyperglycemia	1	2	3	4	5	NA
161913	Treats symptoms of hypoglycemia	1	2	3	4	5	NA
161914	Monitors frequency of hypoglycemia episodes	1	2	3	4	5	NA
161915	Reports symptoms of complications	1	2	3	4	5	NA
161916	Uses diary or app to monitor blood glucose level over time	1	2	3	4	5	NA
161917	Uses preventive measures to reduce risk for complications	1	2	3	4	5	NA
161941	Obtains health care if blood glucose levels fluctuate outside of recommendations	1	2	3	4	5	NA
161919	Monitors urinary glucose and ketones	1	2	3	4	5	NA
161920	Follows recommended diet	1	2	3	4	5	NA
161921	Follows recommended activity level	1	2	3	4	5	NA
161922	Monitors body weight	1	2	3	4	5	NA
161923	Uses effective weight control strategies	1	2	3	4	5	NA
161924	Maintains optimum weight	1	2	3	4	5	NA
161925	Follows recommendations for alcohol use	1	2	3	4	5	NA
161926	Participates in smoking cessation regimen	1	2	3	4	5	NA
161927	Participates in recommended exercise	1	2	3	4	5	NA
161928	Performs usual life routine	1	2	3	4	5	NA
161929	Uses correct procedure for insulin administration	1	2	3	4	5	NA
161930	Stores insulin correctly	1	2	3	4	5	NA
161931	Obtains required medication	1	2	3	4	5	NA
161932	Uses medication as prescribed	1	2	3	4	5	NA
161933	Monitors medication therapeutic effects	1	2	3	4	5	NA
161934	Rotates injection sites	1	2	3	4	5	NA
161935	Uses only non-prescription medication approved by health professional	1	2	3	4	5	NA
161947	Obtains recommended vaccines	1	2	3	4	5	NA
161937	Uses health care services congruent with needs	1	2	3	4	5	NA
161938	Reports need for financial assistance	1	2	3	4	5	NA
161939	Keeps appointments with health professional	1	2	3	4	5	NA
161940	Maintains plan for medical emergencies	1	2	3	4	5	NA
161948	Completes medication reconciliation with health professional	1	2	3	4	5	NA
161949	Commits to partnering with health professional to control diabetes	1	2	3	4	5	NA
161943	Obtains preconception counseling	1	2	3	4	5	NA
161944	Monitors for signs and symptoms of depression	1	2	3	4	5	NA
161942	Adjusts life routine for optimal health	1	2	3	4	5	NA
161050	Seeks social support	1	2	3	4	5	NA

Domain-Health Knowledge & Behavior (IV)   **Class**-Health Management (FF)   *3rd edition 2004; revised 2008, 2013, 2024*

OUTCOME CONTENT REFERENCES:

American Diabetes Association, ADA. (2019). Lifestyle management: Standards of medical care in diabetes. *Diabetes Care, 42*(Suppl. 1), S46–S60. https://doi.org/10.2337/dc19-S005

Beck, J., Greenwood, D. A., Blanton, L., Bollinger, S. T., Butcher, M. K., Condon, J. E., Cypress, M., Faulkner, P., Fischl, A. H., Francis, T., Kolb, L. K., Lavin–Tompkins, J. M., MaLeod, J., Maryniuk, M., Mensing, C., Orzeck, E. A., Pope, D. D., Pulizzi, J. L., Reed, A. A., Rhinehart, A. S., Siminerio, L., & Wang, J. (2017). National standards for diabetes self-management education and support. *The Diabetes Educator, 43*(5), 449–464. https://doi.org/10.1177/0145721717722968

Can, S., Cicek, S. C., & Ankarali, H. (2020). The effect of illness acceptance on diabetes self-care activities in diabetic individuals. *International Journal of Caring Sciences, 13*(3), 2191–2200.

Chasens, A. R., Imes, C. C., Kariuki, J. K., Luyster, F. S., Morris, J. L., DiNardo, M. M., Godzik, C. M., Jeon, B., & Yang, K. (2021). Sleep and metabolic syndrome. *Nursing Clinics of North America, 56*(2), 203–217. https://doi.org/10.1016/j.cnur.2020.10.012

Cradock, K. A., ÓLaighin, G., Finucane, F. M., McKay, R., Quinlan, L. R., Martin Ginis, K. A., & Gainforth, H. L. (2017). Diet behavior change techniques in type 2 diabetes: A systematic review and meta-analysis. *Diabetes Care, 40*(12), 1800–1810. https://doi.org/10.2337/dc17-0462

García, A. A., Bose, E., Zuñiga, J. A., & Wenhui Zhang, W. (2019). Mexican Americans' diabetes symptom prevalence, burden, and clusters. *Applied Nursing Research, 46,* 37–42. https://doi.org/10.1016/j.apnr.2019.02.002

Hernandez, L., Leutwyler, H., Cataldo, J., Kanaya, A., Swislocki, A., & Chesla, C. (2019). Symptom experience of older adults with type 2 diabetes and diabetes-related distress. *Nursing Research, 68*(5), 374–382. https://doi.org/10.1097/NNR.0000000000000370

Ji, M., Ren, D., Dunbar-Jacob, J., Gary-Webb, T. L., & Erlen, J. A. (2020). Self-management behaviors, glycemic control, and metabolic syndrome in type 2 diabetes. *Nursing Research, 69*(2), E9–E17. https://doi.org/10.1097/NNR.0000000000000401

Kim, S. H., & Utz, S. (2019). Effectiveness of a social media-based, health literacy-sensitive diabetes self-management intervention: A randomized controlled trial. *Journal of Nursing Scholarship, 51*(6), 661–669. https://doi.org/10.1111/jnu.12521

Lavdaniti, M. (2020). The impact of smoking on individuals with diabetes type 2. *International Journal of Caring Sciences, 13*(3), e2304.

Levesque, C. (2017). Therapeutic lifestyle changes for diabetes mellitus. *Nursing Clinics of North America, 52*(4), 679–692. https://doi.org/10.1016/j.cnur.2017.07.012

Oh, H., & Moorhead, S. (2019). Validation of the knowledge and self-management Nursing Outcomes Classification for adults with diabetes. *CIN: Computers, Informatics, Nursing, 37*(4), 222–228. https://doi.org/10.1097/CIN.0000000000000495

Self-Management: Dysrhythmia   3105

Definition: Personal actions to manage abnormal heart rhythms, its treatment, and to prevent disease progression and complications

OUTCOME TARGET RATING: Maintain at_____ Increase to_____

		Never Demonstrated	Rarely Demonstrated	Sometimes Demonstrated	Often Demonstrated	Consistently Demonstrated	
OUTCOME OVERALL RATING		1	2	3	4	5	
Indicators:							
310501	Accepts diagnosis	1	2	3	4	5	NA
310502	Seeks information about methods to manage dysrhythmia	1	2	3	4	5	NA
310543	Obtains information on treatment options	1	2	3	4	5	NA
310503	Participates in health care decisions	1	2	3	4	5	NA
310504	Performs treatment regimen as prescribed	1	2	3	4	5	NA
310505	Monitors radial pulse rate and rhythm	1	2	3	4	5	NA
310506	Monitors for heart palpitations	1	2	3	4	5	NA
310507	Monitors blood pressure	1	2	3	4	5	NA
310508	Monitors factors that precede dysrhythmia onset	1	2	3	4	5	NA
310509	Monitors symptom persistence	1	2	3	4	5	NA
310510	Monitors symptom severity	1	2	3	4	5	NA
310511	Monitors symptom frequency	1	2	3	4	5	NA
310512	Reports significant change in radial pulse immediately	1	2	3	4	5	NA
310513	Reports redness or pain at site	1	2	3	4	5	NA
310514	Reports painful shocks	1	2	3	4	5	NA
310515	Reports increase in severity or frequency of dysrhythmia	1	2	3	4	5	NA
310516	Monitors effects of stimulants	1	2	3	4	5	NA
310544	Monitors effects of fatigue	1	2	3	4	5	NA
310517	Uses diary to monitor symptoms over time	1	2	3	4	5	NA

S

Continued

Self-Management: Dysrhythmia—cont'd

		Never Demonstrated	Rarely Demonstrated	Sometimes Demonstrated	Often Demonstrated	Consistently Demonstrated	
310518	Uses preventive measures to reduce episodes of dysrhythmia	1	2	3	4	5	NA
310519	Obtains health care when warning signs occur	1	2	3	4	5	NA
310520	Obtains required medication	1	2	3	4	5	NA
310521	Uses medication as prescribed	1	2	3	4	5	NA
310522	Follows schedule for taking medication	1	2	3	4	5	NA
310523	Monitors prescribed medication therapeutic effects	1	2	3	4	5	NA
310545	Participates in medication reconciliation with health professional	1	2	3	4	5	NA
310524	Monitors medication side effects	1	2	3	4	5	NA
310525	Uses only non-prescription medication approved by health professional	1	2	3	4	5	NA
310546	Obtains information on treatment plan relationship to comorbid conditions	1	2	3	4	5	NA
310526	Uses anxiety-reducing techniques	1	2	3	4	5	NA
310527	Performs usual life routine	1	2	3	4	5	NA
310528	Follows recommendations for alcohol use	1	2	3	4	5	NA
310529	Participates in smoking cessation regimen	1	2	3	4	5	NA
310530	Participates in physical activities that do not cause dysrhythmia	1	2	3	4	5	NA
310531	Follows recommendations for sexual activity	1	2	3	4	5	NA
310532	Reports need for financial assistance	1	2	3	4	5	NA
310533	Keeps appointments with health professional	1	2	3	4	5	NA
310534	Maintains plan for medical emergencies	1	2	3	4	5	NA
310535	Follows recommendations for site care immediately post-surgery	1	2	3	4	5	NA
310536	Wears loose fitting clothes over implant site	1	2	3	4	5	NA
310547	Wears medical identification bracelet	1	2	3	4	5	NA
310538	Avoids contact activities that could cause trauma to site	1	2	3	4	5	NA
310539	Avoids devices that can disrupt pacemaker or defibrillator function	1	2	3	4	5	NA
310540	Follows manufacturer's instructions for device	1	2	3	4	5	NA
310541	Follows maintenance schedule for device	1	2	3	4	5	NA
310542	Notifies health professional of pacemaker or defibrillator prior to procedures	1	2	3	4	5	NA

Domain-Health Knowledge & Behavior (IV)   **Class**-Health Management (FF)   5th edition 2013; revised 2024

OUTCOME CONTENT REFERENCES:

Bond, C., Morgenstern, J., Heitz, C., & Milne, W. K. (2020). Hot off the press: Chemical versus electrical cardioversion for atrial fibrillation. *Academic Emergency Medicine, 27*(4), 333–335. https://doi.org/10.1111/acem13874

Gammone, M. A., & D'Orazio, N. (2021). Cocoa overconsumption and cardiac rhythm: Potential arrhythmogenic trigger or beneficial pleasure? *Current Research in Nutrition and Food Science, 9*(1), 40–51. https://doi.org/10.12944/CRNFSJ.9.1.05 ISSN:2347-467X

National Heart and Lung Blood Institute. (2011). *Arrhythmia.* https://www.nhlbi.nih.gov/health–topics/arrhythmia

Normand, C., Kaye, D. M., Povsic, T. J., & Dickstein, K. (2019). Beyond pharmacological treatment: An insight into therapies that target specific aspects of heart failure pathophysiology. *Lancet, 393*(10175), 1045–1055. https://doi.org/10.1016/S0140-6736(18)32216-5

Potter, P. A., Perry, A. G., Stockert, P. A., & Hall, A. M. (2021). *Fundamentals of nursing* (10th ed.). Elsevier.

Ravid, J. D., Kamel, M. H., & Chitalia, V. C. (2021). Uraemic solutes as therapeutic targets in CKD-associated cardiovascular disease. *Nature, 17*(6), 402–416. https://doi.org/10.1038/s41581-021-00408-4

Xu, W., Sun, G., Lin, Z., Chen, M., Yang, B., Chen, H., & Cao, K. (2010). Knowledge, attitude, and behavior in patients with atrial fibrillation undergoing radio frequency catheter ablation. *Journal of Interventional Cardiac Electrophysiology, 28*(3), 199–207. https://doi.org/10.1007/s10840-010-9496-2

Self-Management: Heart Failure   3106

Definition: Personal actions to manage heart failure, its treatment, and to prevent disease progression and complications

OUTCOME TARGET RATING: Maintain at_____ Increase to_____

		Never Demonstrated	Rarely Demonstrated	Sometimes Demonstrated	Often Demonstrated	Consistently Demonstrated	
OUTCOME OVERALL RATING		1	2	3	4	5	
Indicators:							
310601	Accepts diagnosis	1	2	3	4	5	NA
310644	Understands diagnosis	1	2	3	4	5	NA
310602	Seeks information about heart failure management	1	2	3	4	5	NA
310603	Participates in health care decisions	1	2	3	4	5	NA
310645	Uses strategies to prevent infections	1	2	3	4	5	NA
310604	Obtains required laboratory tests	1	2	3	4	5	NA
310605	Monitors heart rate and rhythm	1	2	3	4	5	NA
310606	Monitors respiratory rate	1	2	3	4	5	NA
310607	Monitors for shortness of breath	1	2	3	4	5	NA
310608	Monitors blood pressure	1	2	3	4	5	NA
310609	Monitors for edema	1	2	3	4	5	NA
310610	Monitors for complications of edema	1	2	3	4	5	NA
310646	Monitors for sleep problems	1	2	3	4	5	NA
310611	Obtains assistance for a symptom exacerbation	1	2	3	4	5	NA
310612	Performs treatment regimen as prescribed	1	2	3	4	5	NA
310613	Follows prescribed diet	1	2	3	4	5	NA
310614	Follows sodium intake recommendations	1	2	3	4	5	NA
310615	Follows fluid restrictions	1	2	3	4	5	NA
310616	Limits alcohol use	1	2	3	4	5	NA
310617	Eliminates tobacco, e-cigarette, and water-pipe use	1	2	3	4	5	NA
310618	Avoids second-hand smoke	1	2	3	4	5	NA
310619	Monitors body weight daily	1	2	3	4	5	NA
310620	Uses effective weight control strategies	1	2	3	4	5	NA
310621	Maintains optimum weight	1	2	3	4	5	NA
310622	Elevates legs when sitting	1	2	3	4	5	NA
310623	Applies elastic stockings correctly	1	2	3	4	5	NA
310624	Follows recommendations for physical activity	1	2	3	4	5	NA
310625	Uses energy conservation techniques	1	2	3	4	5	NA
310626	Balances activity and rest	1	2	3	4	5	NA
310627	Manages basic activities of daily living	1	2	3	4	5	NA
310628	Manages instrumental activities of daily living	1	2	3	4	5	NA
310646	Obtains recommended immunizations	1	2	3	4	5	NA
310631	Uses pulse oximetry monitor correctly	1	2	3	4	5	NA
310632	Uses oxygen correctly	1	2	3	4	5	NA
310633	Uses medication as prescribed	1	2	3	4	5	NA
310647	Adjusts diuretics when necessary	1	2	3	4	5	NA
310634	Monitors prescribed medication therapeutic effects	1	2	3	4	5	NA

S

Continued

Self-Management: Heart Failure—cont'd

		Never Demonstrated	Rarely Demonstrated	Sometimes Demonstrated	Often Demonstrated	Consistently Demonstrated	
310635	Monitors side effects of medication	1	2	3	4	5	NA
310636	Uses only non-prescription medication approved by health professional	1	2	3	4	5	NA
310637	Uses stress management strategies	1	2	3	4	5	NA
310648	Reports signs and symptoms of anxiety	1	2	3	4	5	NA
310638	Reports signs and symptoms of depression	1	2	3	4	5	NA
310649	Obtains assistance for anxiety	1	2	3	4	5	NA
310639	Obtains assistance for depression	1	2	3	4	5	NA
310650	Obtains sexual counseling	1	2	3	4	5	NA
310640	Obtains support from family	1	2	3	4	5	NA
310641	Uses support group	1	2	3	4	5	NA
310642	Keeps appointments with health professional	1	2	3	4	5	NA
310643	Adjusts life routine for optimal health	1	2	3	4	5	NA

Domain-Health Knowledge & Behavior (IV)   **Class**-Health Management (FF)   5th edition 2013; revised 2024

OUTCOME CONTENT REFERENCES:

Clays, E., Puddu, P. E., Luštrek, M., Pioggia, G., Derboven, J., Vrana, M., De Sutter, J., Donne, R. L., Baert, A., Bohanec, M., Ciancarelli, M. C., Dawodu, A. A., Pauw, M. D., Smedt, D. D., Marino, F., Pardaens, S., Schiariti, M. S., Valič, J., Vanderheyden, M., Vodopija, A., & Tartarisco, G. (2021). Proof-of-concept trial results of the HeartMan mobile personal health system for self-management in congestive heart failure. *Science Reports, 11*(1), 5663. https://doi.org/10.1038/s41598-021-84920-4

Ignatavicius, D. D., Workman, M. L., Rebar, C. R., & Heimgartner, N. M. (2021). *Medical-surgical nursing: Concepts for interprofessional care* (10th ed.). Elsevier.

Jaarsma, T., Hill, L., Bayes-Genis, A., La Rocca, H.-P. B., Castiello, T., Čelutkienė, J., Marques-Sule, E., Plymen, C. M., Piper, S. E., Riegel, B., Rutten, F. H., Ben Gal, T., Bauersachs, J., Coats, A. J., Chioncel, O., Lopatin, Y., Lund, L. H., Lainscak, M., Moura, B., Mullens, W., Piepoli, M. F., Rosano, G., Seferovic, P., & Strömberg, A. (2021). Self-care of heart failure patients: Practical management recommendations from the Heart Failure Association of the European Society of Cardiology. *European Journal of Heart Failure, 23*(1), 157–174. https://doi.org/10.1002/ejhf.2008

Kabbani, S., Al Habeeb, W., Liew, H. B., Mohan, J. C., Ogola, E., Sim, D., & Tsabedze, N. (2019). Supporting the management of patients with heart failure within Asia-Pacific, Middle East, and African Countries: A toolbox for healthcare providers. *Cardiology, 142*(Suppl. 1), 1–10. https://doi.org/10.1159/000496663

Mizukawa, M., Moriyama, M., Yamamoto, H., Rahman, M. M., Naka, M., Kitagawa, T., Kobayashi, S., Oda, N., Yasunobu, Y., Tomiyama, M., Morishima, N., Matsuda, K., & Kihara, Y. (2019). Nurse-led collaborative management using telemonitoring improves quality of life and prevention of rehospitalization in patients with heart failure. *International Heart Journal, 60*(6), 1293–1302. https://doi.org/10.1536/ihj.19-313

Zhao, Q., Chen, C., Zhang, J., Ye, Y., & Fan, X. (2020). Effects of self-management interventions on heart failure: Systematic review and meta-analysis of randomized controlled trials. *International Journal of Nursing Studies, 110*, 103689. https://doi.org/10.1016/j.ijnurstu.2020.103689

Self-Management: Human Immunodeficiency Virus   3117

Definition: Personal actions to manage human immunodeficiency virus (HIV), its treatment, and to prevent disease progression and complications

OUTCOME TARGET RATING: Maintain at_____ Increase to_____

		Never Demonstrated	Rarely Demonstrated	Sometimes Demonstrated	Often Demonstrated	Consistently Demonstrated	
OUTCOME OVERALL RATING		1	2	3	4	5	
Indicators:							
311701	Accepts diagnosis	1	2	3	4	5	NA
311702	Obtains information about human immunodeficiency virus	1	2	3	4	5	NA
311703	Collaborates with health professional to create an individualized plan of care	1	2	3	4	5	NA
311704	Monitors signs and symptoms of disease	1	2	3	4	5	NA

S

Self-Management: Human Immunodeficiency Virus—cont'd

		Never Demonstrated	Rarely Demonstrated	Sometimes Demonstrated	Often Demonstrated	Consistently Demonstrated	
311705	Follows recommended precautions	1	2	3	4	5	NA
311706	Discloses human immunodeficiency virus positive status to intimate partners	1	2	3	4	5	NA
311707	Adheres to prescribed antiretroviral medication	1	2	3	4	5	NA
311708	Monitors medication side effects	1	2	3	4	5	NA
311709	Monitors medication adverse effects	1	2	3	4	5	NA
311710	Obtains required laboratory tests	1	2	3	4	5	NA
311711	Monitors CD4 T lymphocyte count	1	2	3	4	5	NA
311712	Monitors viral load	1	2	3	4	5	NA
311713	Disposes contaminated materials safely	1	2	3	4	5	NA
311714	Modifies unhealthy behaviors	1	2	3	4	5	NA
311715	Participates in exercise	1	2	3	4	5	NA
311716	Follows healthy diet	1	2	3	4	5	NA
311739	Refrains from smoking	1	2	3	4	5	NA
311717	Refrains from intravenous drug use	1	2	3	4	5	NA
311718	Practices safe sex	1	2	3	4	5	NA
311740	Uses strategies to manage depression	1	2	3	4	5	NA
311741	Uses strategies to manage fatigue	1	2	3	4	5	NA
311719	Uses strategies to prevent infection	1	2	3	4	5	NA
311742	Uses strategies to manage treatment burden	1	2	3	4	5	NA
311720	Verbalizes awareness of social inequities	1	2	3	4	5	NA
311721	Discusses the stigma associated with human immunodeficiency virus	1	2	3	4	5	NA
311722	Engages in spiritual practices to cope	1	2	3	4	5	NA
311723	Engages in religious practices to cope	1	2	3	4	5	NA
311724	Verbalizes a clear trajectory of change in self-image	1	2	3	4	5	NA
311725	Sets realistic goals	1	2	3	4	5	NA
311726	Uses strategies to meet goals	1	2	3	4	5	NA
311727	Forgives self for life circumstances	1	2	3	4	5	NA
311728	Forgives others for life circumstances	1	2	3	4	5	NA
311729	Uses strategies to manage stress	1	2	3	4	5	NA
311730	Reports depressive symptoms to health professional	1	2	3	4	5	NA
311743	Obtains recommended vaccines	1	2	3	4	5	NA
311733	Attends peer support groups	1	2	3	4	5	NA
311734	Shares information about human immunodeficiency virus with others	1	2	3	4	5	NA
311744	Obtains assistance to complete activities of daily living	1	2	3	4	5	NA
311735	Obtains support from friends	1	2	3	4	5	NA
311736	Obtains support from family	1	2	3	4	5	NA
311745	Obtains financial assistance as needed	1	2	3	4	5	NA
311737	Keeps appointments with health professional	1	2	3	4	5	NA
311738	Uses available community resources	1	2	3	4	5	NA

Domain-*Health Knowledge & Behavior (IV)*   **Class**-*Health Management (FF)*   *6th edition 2018; revised 2024*

S

OUTCOME CONTENT REFERENCES:

Bernard, C., Seydi, M., Tanon, A., Messou, E., Minga, A., Font, H., Dabis, F., & the International Epidemiological Database to evaluate Aids (IeDEA) West Africa Collaboration. (2021). Barriers influencing task-shifting for the management of depression in people living with HIV: A study from West Africa IeDEA cohort collaboration, *AIDS Care, 33*(3), 352–356. https://doi.org/10.1080/09540121.2020.1739202

Boucher, L. M., O'Brien, K. K., Baxter, L. N., Fitzgerald, M. L., Liddy, C. E., & Kendall, C. E. (2019). Healthy aging with HIV: The role of self-management support. *Patient Education and Counseling, 102*(8), 1565–1569. https://doi.org/10.1016/j.pec.2019.02.019

Ignatavicius, D. D., Workman, M. L., Rebar, C. R., & Heimgartner, N. M. (2021). *Medical-surgical nursing: Concepts for interprofessional collaborative care.* Elsevier.

Schreiner, N., Perazzo, J., Digennaro, S., Currie, J., Daly, B., & Webel, A. (2019). A descriptive, cross-sectional study examining treatment burden in people living with HIV. *Applied Nursing Research, 46*, 31–36. https://doi.org/10.1016/j.apnr.2019.02.009

Schreiner, N., Perazzo, J., Digennaro, S., Currie, J., Daly, B., & Webel, A. (2020). Associations between symptom severity and treatment burden in people living with HIV. *Journal of Advanced Nursing, 76*, 2348–2358. https://doi.org/10.1111/jan.14461

Schreiner, N., Perazzo, J., Digennaro, S., Currie, J., Daly, B., & Webel, A. (2020). Examining the association between item specific treatment burden and adherence in people living with HIV. *Western Journal of Nursing Research, 42*(7), 495–502. https://doi.org/10.1177/01939-45919880317

Self-Management: Hypertension 3107

Definition: Personal actions to manage high blood pressure, its treatment, and to prevent complications

OUTCOME TARGET RATING: Maintain at_____ Increase to_____

		Never Demonstrated	Rarely Demonstrated	Sometimes Demonstrated	Often Demonstrated	Consistently Demonstrated	
OUTCOME OVERALL RATING		1	2	3	4	5	
Indicators:							
310701	Monitors blood pressure	1	2	3	4	5	NA
310702	Performs correct procedure for blood pressure measurement	1	2	3	4	5	NA
310703	Checks calibration of home blood pressure device	1	2	3	4	5	NA
310704	Maintains target blood pressure	1	2	3	4	5	NA
310705	Uses medication as prescribed	1	2	3	4	5	NA
310706	Monitors medication therapeutic effects	1	2	3	4	5	NA
310707	Monitors medication adverse effects	1	2	3	4	5	NA
310708	Monitors medication side effects	1	2	3	4	5	NA
310709	Uses only non-prescription medication approved by health professional	1	2	3	4	5	NA
310710	Participates in recommended exercises	1	2	3	4	5	NA
310711	Uses strategies for weight reduction	1	2	3	4	5	NA
310712	Maintains optimum body weight	1	2	3	4	5	NA
310713	Follows recommended diet	1	2	3	4	5	NA
310714	Limits sodium intake	1	2	3	4	5	NA
310715	Limits high calorie fluids	1	2	3	4	5	NA
310716	Limits high calorie snacks	1	2	3	4	5	NA
310717	Decreases food portions	1	2	3	4	5	NA
310718	Limits caffeine consumption	1	2	3	4	5	NA
310719	Uses stress management strategies	1	2	3	4	5	NA
310720	Uses relaxation techniques	1	2	3	4	5	NA
310721	Participates in smoking cessation regimen	1	2	3	4	5	NA
310722	Eliminates tobacco use	1	2	3	4	5	NA
310723	Follows recommendations for alcohol use	1	2	3	4	5	NA

S

Self-Management: Hypertension—cont'd

		Never Demonstrated	Rarely Demonstrated	Sometimes Demonstrated	Often Demonstrated	Consistently Demonstrated	
310724	Uses strategies to maintain adequate sleep	1	2	3	4	5	NA
310725	Uses diary or app to monitor blood pressure over time	1	2	3	4	5	NA
310726	Monitors for complications of hypertension	1	2	3	4	5	NA
310727	Contacts health provider when not in target range	1	2	3	4	5	NA
310728	Keeps appointments with health professional	1	2	3	4	5	NA
310734	Completes medication reconciliation with health professional	1	2	3	4	5	NA
310735	Commits to partnering with health professional to control hypertension	1	2	3	4	5	NA
310729	Uses support group	1	2	3	4	5	NA
310730	Uses reputable sources of information	1	2	3	4	5	NA
310731	Uses available community resources	1	2	3	4	5	NA
310732	Seeks financial resources	1	2	3	4	5	NA
310733	Uses social support	1	2	3	4	5	NA

Domain-*Health Knowledge & Behavior (IV)*   **Class**-*Health Management (FF)*   *5th edition 2013; revised 2024*

OUTCOME CONTENT REFERENCES:
Abegaz, T. M., Shehab, A., Gebreyohannes, E. A., Bhagavathula, A. S., & Elnour, A. A. (2017). Nonadherence to antihypertensive drugs: A systematic review and meta-analysis. *Medicine, 96*(4), e5641. https://doi.org/10.1097/MD.0000000000005641
Kario, K. (2020). Management of hypertension in the digital era. *Hypertension, 76*(3), 640–650. https://doi.org/10.1161/HYPERTENSIONAHA.120.14742
Li, R., Liang, N., Bu, F., & Hesketh, T. (2020). The effectiveness of self-management of hypertension in adults using mobile health: Systematic review and meta-analysis. *JMIR mHealth and uHealth, 8*(3), e17776. https://doi.org/10.2196/17776
Moss, K. O., Still, C. H., Jones, L. M., Blackshire, G., & Wright, K. D. (2019). Hypertension self-management perspectives from African American older adults. *Western Journal of Nursing Research, 41*(5), 667–684. https://doi.org/10.1177/0193945918780331
Oh, H., & Moorhead, S. (2020). Validation of the knowledge and self-management Nursing Outcomes Classification outcomes for adults with hypertension and lipid disorder. *Online Journal of Nursing Informatics, 24*(2), 1.
Peacock, E., & Krousel-Wood, M. (2017). Adherence to antihypertensive therapy. *The Medical Clinics of North America, 101*(1), 229–245. https://doi.org/10.1016/j.mcna.2016.08.005
Shahaj, O., Denneny, D., Schwappach, A., Pearce, G., Epiphaniou, E., Parke, H., Taylor, S., & Pinnock, H. (2019). Supporting self-management for people with hypertension. *Journal of Hypertension, 37*(2), 264–279. https://doi.org/10.1097/HJH.0000000000001867
Swaminathan, R., Cohen, E., Philley, M., Hokanson, J., & Young, K. (2020). Impact of self-measured blood pressure monitoring on hypertension management. *Blood Pressure Monitoring, 25*(5), 259–262. https://doi.org/10.1097/MBP.0000000000000455
Warren-Findlow, J., Krinner, L. M., Vinoski, T. E., Coffman, M. J., Gordon, B., & Howden, R. (2020). Relative and cumulative effects of hypertension self-care behaviors on blood pressure. *Western Journal of Nursing Research, 42*(3), 157–164. https://doi.org/10.1177/0193945919851111
Whelton, P. K., Carey, R. M., Aronow, W. S., Casey, D. E., Collins, K. J., Dennison Himmelfarb, C., & Wright, J. T. (2018). 2017 ACC/AHA/AAPA/ABC/ACPM/AGS/APhA/ASH/ASPC/NMA/PCNA guideline for the prevention, detection, evaluation, and management of high blood pressure in adults: A report of the American College of Cardiology/American Heart Association Task Force on Clinical Practice Guidelines. *Journal of the American College of Cardiology, 71*(19), e127–e248. https://doi.org/10.1016/j.jacc.2017.11.006
Wright, K., Harmon Still, C., Jones, L. M., & Moss, K. O. (2018). Design of a co-created intervention to self-manage stress and blood pressure in African American older adults with hypertension. *International Journal of Hypertension, 7591289.* https://doi.org/10.1155/2018/7591289

S

Self-Management: Infection 3118

Definition: Personal actions to manage infection, its treatment, and to prevent complications

OUTCOME TARGET RATING: Maintain at_____ Increase to_____

OUTCOME OVERALL RATING		Never Demonstrated 1	Rarely Demonstrated 2	Sometimes Demonstrated 3	Often Demonstrated 4	Consistently Demonstrated 5	
Indicators:							
311801	Obtains screening for early detection	1	2	3	4	5	NA
311802	Obtains treatment for diagnosed infection	1	2	3	4	5	NA
311803	Obtains information about infection	1	2	3	4	5	NA
311804	Performs treatment regimen as prescribed	1	2	3	4	5	NA
311824	Self-isolates as recommended by health professional	1	2	3	4	5	NA
311825	Wears mask to prevent spread of virus	1	2	3	4	5	NA
311805	Monitors signs and symptoms of infection	1	2	3	4	5	NA
311806	Monitors body temperature	1	2	3	4	5	NA
311807	Uses symptom relief methods	1	2	3	4	5	NA
311808	Uses strategies to prevent complications	1	2	3	4	5	NA
311809	Uses strategies to avoid infection transmission to others	1	2	3	4	5	NA
311810	Monitors health status for exacerbation	1	2	3	4	5	NA
311811	Practices hand hygiene	1	2	3	4	5	NA
311812	Practices body hygiene	1	2	3	4	5	NA
311813	Uses medication as prescribed	1	2	3	4	5	NA
311814	Monitors medication therapeutic effects	1	2	3	4	5	NA
311815	Monitors medication side effects	1	2	3	4	5	NA
311816	Monitors medication adverse effects	1	2	3	4	5	NA
311817	Monitors for potential medication interactions	1	2	3	4	5	NA
311818	Monitors for potential medication resistance	1	2	3	4	5	NA
311819	Uses probiotics	1	2	3	4	5	NA
311820	Follows healthy diet	1	2	3	4	5	NA
311821	Increases fluid intake	1	2	3	4	5	NA
311822	Promotes restful sleep	1	2	3	4	5	NA
311826	Disposes of infectious waste material	1	2	3	4	5	NA
311823	Keeps appointments with health professional	1	2	3	4	5	NA

Domain-Health Knowledge & Behavior (IV)   **Class**-Health Management (FF)   6th edition 2018; revised 2024

OUTCOME CONTENT REFERENCES:

Aleksejeva, V., Dovbenko, A., Kroiča, J., & Skadiņš, I. (2021). Toys in the playrooms of children's hospitals: A potential source of nosocomial bacterial infections? *Children* (Basel, Switzerland), 8(10), 914. https://doi.org/10.3390/children8100914

Chaabna, K., Doraiswamy, S., Mamtani, R., & Cheema, S. (2021). Facemask use in community settings to prevent respiratory infection transmission: A rapid review and meta-analysis. *International Journal of Infectious Diseases*, 104, 198–206. https://doi.org/10.1016/j.ijid.2020.09.1434

Grundmann, H., Aires-de-Sousa, M., Boyce, J., & Tiemersma, E. (2006). Emergence and resurgence of methicillin-resistant staphylococcus aureus as a public-health threat. *Lancet, 368*, 874-885. https://doi.org/10.1016/S0140-6736(06)68853-3

Krein, S. L., Olmsted, R. N., Hofer, T. P., Kowalski, C., Forman, J., Banaszak, J., & Saint, S. (2006). Translating infection prevention evidence into practice using quantitative and qualitative research. *American Journal of Infection Control, 34*, 507–512. https://doi.org/10.1016/j.ajic.2005.05.017

Lelie-van der Zande, R., Koster, E. S., Teichert, M., & Bouvy, M. L. (2021). Womens' self-management skills for prevention and treatment of recurring urinary tract infection. *International Journal of Clinical Practice, 75*(8), e14289. https://doi.org/10.1111/ijcp.14289

Li, H., Yuan, K., Sun, Y. K., Zheng, Y. B., Xu, Y. Y., Su, S. Z., Zhang, Y. X., Zhong, Y., Wang, Y. J., Tian, S. S., Gong, Y. M., Fan, T. T., Lin, X., Gobat, N., Wong, S., Chan, E., Yan, W., Sun, S. W., Ran, M. S., Bao, Y. P., & Lu, L. (2022). Efficacy and practice of facemask use in general population: A systematic review and meta-analysis. *Translational Psychiatry, 12*(1), 49. https://doi.org/10.1038/s41398-022-01814-3

McGuckin, M., Storr, J. A., & Govednik, J. (2021). Patient awareness of healthcare-associated infection risk and prevention: Has there been a change in 3 decades (1989-2019)? *American Journal of Infection Control, 49*(11), 1448–1449. https://doi.org/10.1016/j.ajic.2021.05.009

Querido, M. M., Aguiar, L., Neves, P., Pereira, C. C., & Teixeira, J. P. (2019). Self-disinfecting surfaces and infection control. *Colloids and Surfaces. Biointerfaces, 178*, 8–21. https://doi.org/10.1016/j.colsurfb.2019.02.009

S

Self-Management: Inflammatory Bowel Disease   3119

Definition: Personal actions to manage inflammatory bowel disease, its treatment, and to prevent disease progression and complications

OUTCOME TARGET RATING: Maintain at_____ Increase to_____

		Never Demonstrated	Rarely Demonstrated	Sometimes Demonstrated	Often Demonstrated	Consistently Demonstrated	
OUTCOME OVERALL RATING		1	2	3	4	5	
Indicators:							
311901	Accepts diagnosis	1	2	3	4	5	NA
311902	Monitors for signs and symptoms	1	2	3	4	5	NA
311903	Obtains treatment for the disease	1	2	3	4	5	NA
311904	Monitors risk factors of progression	1	2	3	4	5	NA
311905	Obtains reputable information about inflammatory bowel disease	1	2	3	4	5	NA
311906	Obtains information about treatment options	1	2	3	4	5	NA
311937	Obtains laboratory testing regularly	1	2	3	4	5	NA
311907	Obtains information on diagnostic tests	1	2	3	4	5	NA
311908	Follows treatment regimen	1	2	3	4	5	NA
311909	Monitors health status for exacerbation	1	2	3	4	5	NA
311938	Monitors comorbidities for worsening signs and symptoms	1	2	3	4	5	NA
311910	Obtains health care with worsening signs and symptoms	1	2	3	4	5	NA
311911	Uses strategies to adapt lifestyle	1	2	3	4	5	NA
311912	Monitors medication therapeutic effects	1	2	3	4	5	NA
311913	Monitors medication side effects	1	2	3	4	5	NA
311914	Monitors medication adverse effects	1	2	3	4	5	NA
311915	Monitors for potential medication interactions	1	2	3	4	5	NA
311939	Monitors bone density	1	2	3	4	5	NA
311940	Monitors weight	1	2	3	4	5	NA
311916	Uses energy conservation techniques	1	2	3	4	5	NA
311917	Uses strategies to regulate bowel function	1	2	3	4	5	NA
311918	Uses strategies to control stress	1	2	3	4	5	NA
311919	Uses strategies to control pain	1	2	3	4	5	NA
311920	Uses strategies to promote regular exercise	1	2	3	4	5	NA
311941	Uses strategies to promote well-being	1	2	3	4	5	NA
311942	Identifies sources of social support	1	2	3	4	5	NA
311921	Avoids tobacco use	1	2	3	4	5	NA
311922	Avoids alcohol use	1	2	3	4	5	NA
311923	Avoids caffeine	1	2	3	4	5	NA
311924	Avoids dairy products	1	2	3	4	5	NA
311925	Avoids trigger foods	1	2	3	4	5	NA
311926	Follows prescribed diet	1	2	3	4	5	NA
311927	Increases fluid intake as recommended	1	2	3	4	5	NA
311928	Uses strategies to promote restful sleep	1	2	3	4	5	NA
311929	Balances activity and rest	1	2	3	4	5	NA

S

Continued

Self-Management: Inflammatory Bowel Disease—cont'd

	Never Demonstrated	Rarely Demonstrated	Sometimes Demonstrated	Often Demonstrated	Consistently Demonstrated	
311930 Uses strategies to avoid reoccurrence	1	2	3	4	5	NA
311931 Identifies disease impact on lifestyle	1	2	3	4	5	NA
311932 Identifies disease impact on pregnancy	1	2	3	4	5	NA
311933 Identifies disease impact on growth and development	1	2	3	4	5	NA
311934 Uses support groups	1	2	3	4	5	NA
311935 Uses available community resources	1	2	3	4	5	NA
311936 Keeps appointments with health professional	1	2	3	4	5	NA

Domain-Health Knowledge & Behavior (IV)   *Class*-Health Management (FF)   6th edition 2018; revised 2024

OUTCOME CONTENT REFERENCES:
Conley, S., & Redeker, N. (2016). A systematic review of self-management interventions for inflammatory bowel disease. *Journal of Nursing Scholarship, 48*(2), 118127. https://doi.org/10.1111/jnu.12189
Crosby, S., Schuh, M. J., Cladera, F., & Farraye, F. A. (2021). Vaccination of patients with inflammatory bowel disease during the COVID-19 pandemic. *Gastroenterology & Hepatology, 17*(1), 18–30.
Grover, Z., & Alex, A. (2019). Management of inflammatory bowel disease in children: It is time for an individualized approach. *Journal of Paediatrics and Child Health, 56*, 1677–1684. https://doi.org/10.1111/jpc.14652
Kamp. K. J., West, P., Holmstrom, A., Luo, Z., Wyatt, G., & Given, B. (2019). Systematic review of social support on psychological symptoms and self-management behaviors among adults with inflammatory bowel disease. *Journal of Nursing Scholarship, 51*(4), 380–389. https://doi.org/10.1111/jnu.12487
Tran, L., & Mulligan, K. (2019). A systematic review of self-management interventions for children and adolescents with inflammatory bowel disease. *Inflammatory Bowel Diseases, 25*(4). https://doi.org/10.1093/ibd/izy299
Tun, G. S. Z., Cripps, S., & Lobo, A. J. (2018). Crohn's disease: Management in adults, children and young people—Concise guidance. *Clinical Medicine, 18*(3), 1–8. https://doi.org/10.7861/clinmedicine.18-3-231

Self-Management: Kidney Disease   3108

Definition: Personal actions to manage kidney disease, its treatment, and to prevent disease progression and complications

OUTCOME TARGET RATING: Maintain at_____ Increase to_____

	Never Demonstrated	Rarely Demonstrated	Sometimes Demonstrated	Often Demonstrated	Consistently Demonstrated	
OUTCOME OVERALL RATING	1	2	3	4	5	
Indicators:						
310801 Accepts diagnosis	1	2	3	4	5	NA
310802 Seeks information about methods to maintain kidney function	1	2	3	4	5	NA
310803 Participates in health care decisions	1	2	3	4	5	NA
310804 Performs treatment regimen as prescribed	1	2	3	4	5	NA
310805 Monitors symptom persistence	1	2	3	4	5	NA
310806 Monitors symptom severity	1	2	3	4	5	NA
310807 Monitors symptom frequency	1	2	3	4	5	NA
310808 Reports symptoms of worsening disease	1	2	3	4	5	NA
310809 Monitors weight	1	2	3	4	5	NA
310810 Monitors intake and output	1	2	3	4	5	NA
310811 Monitors blood pressure	1	2	3	4	5	NA
310812 Monitors for signs and symptoms of fluid excess	1	2	3	4	5	NA

S

Self-Management: Kidney Disease—cont'd

		Never Demonstrated	Rarely Demonstrated	Sometimes Demonstrated	Often Demonstrated	Consistently Demonstrated	
310842	Monitors for signs and symptoms of kidney infection	1	2	3	4	5	NA
310843	Monitors for signs and symptoms of kidney stones	1	2	3	4	5	NA
310813	Monitors for edema	1	2	3	4	5	NA
310814	Monitors for disequilibrium syndrome	1	2	3	4	5	NA
310815	Reports shortness of breath	1	2	3	4	5	NA
310844	Obtains information on treatment options	1	2	3	4	5	NA
310816	Obtains needed medication	1	2	3	4	5	NA
310817	Uses medication as prescribed	1	2	3	4	5	NA
310818	Uses only non-prescription medication approved by health professional	1	2	3	4	5	NA
310819	Reports side effects of medication	1	2	3	4	5	NA
310820	Monitors prescribed medication therapeutic effects	1	2	3	4	5	NA
310845	Participates in medication reconciliation with health professional	1	2	3	4	5	NA
310821	Follows recommended diet	1	2	3	4	5	NA
310822	Follows fluid restrictions	1	2	3	4	5	NA
310846	Uses strategies to support sleep	1	2	3	4	5	NA
310823	Uses strategies to control nausea	1	2	3	4	5	NA
310824	Uses strategies to prevent infection	1	2	3	4	5	NA
310825	Obtains influenza seasonal vaccine	1	2	3	4	5	NA
310826	Obtains pneumonia vaccine	1	2	3	4	5	NA
310827	Obtains adequate sleep	1	2	3	4	5	NA
310828	Balances activity and rest	1	2	3	4	5	NA
310829	Monitors for activity tolerance	1	2	3	4	5	NA
310847	Uses strategies to cope with lifestyle changes	1	2	3	4	5	NA
310830	Uses strategies to conserve energy	1	2	3	4	5	NA
310831	Uses strategies to relieve dry skin	1	2	3	4	5	NA
310848	Obtains information on catheter care	1	2	3	4	5	NA
310832	Assesses fistula bruit daily	1	2	3	4	5	NA
310833	Performs correct procedure for care of dialysis access site	1	2	3	4	5	NA
310834	Monitors blood clotting time	1	2	3	4	5	NA
310835	Uses strategies to prevent bleeding	1	2	3	4	5	NA
310836	Uses precautions with shunt arm	1	2	3	4	5	NA
310837	Keeps appointments with health professional	1	2	3	4	5	NA
310838	Maintains plans for medical emergencies	1	2	3	4	5	NA
310839	Uses support group	1	2	3	4	5	NA
310840	Uses available community resources	1	2	3	4	5	NA
310841	Uses federal health care resources	1	2	3	4	5	NA

Domain-Health Knowledge & Behavior (IV)   **Class**-Health Management (FF)   5th edition 2013; revised 2024

S

OUTCOME CONTENT REFERENCES:

Chan, W. (2021). Chronic kidney disease and nutrition support. *Nutrition in Clinical Practice, 36*(2), 312–330. https://doi.org/10.1002/ncp.10658

Cheng, E., Evangelidis, N., Guha, C., Hanson, C., Unruh, M., Wilkie, M., Schell, J., Hecking, M., Gonzalez, A. M., Ju, A., Eckert, D. J., Craig, J. C., & Tong, A. (2021). Patient experiences of sleep in dialysis: Systematic review of qualitative studies. *Sleep Medicine, 80*, 66–76. https://doi.org/10.1016/j.sleep.2021.01.019

Diaz-González de Ferris, M. E., Pierce, C. B., Gipson, D. S., Furth, S. L., Warady, B. A., Hooper, S. R., & authoring group for the CKID study. Health-related quality of life in children with chronic kidney disease is affected by the number of medications. *Pediatric Nephrology, 36*(5), 1307–1310. https://doi.org/10.1007/s00467-021-04919-x-

Levi, A., Simard, T., & Glover, C. (2020). Coronary artery disease in patients with end-stage kidney disease: Current perspective and gaps in knowledge. *Seminars in Dialysis, 33*(3), 187–197. https://doi.org/10.1111/sdi.12886

Premachandra, K. H., Day, R. O., & Roberts, D. M. (2021). Managing hyperuricemia and gout in chronic kidney disease: A clinical conundrum. *Current Opinion in Nephrology and Hypertension, 30*(2), 245–251. https://doi.org/10.1097/MNH.0000000000000691

Smith Brown, J., & Elliott, R. W. (2021). Social determinants of health: Understanding the basics and their impact on chronic kidney disease. *Nephrology Nursing Journal, 48*(2), 131–135. https://doi.org/10.37526/1526-744X

Stømer, U. E., Wahl, A. K., Gøransson, L. G., & Urstad, K. H. (2020). Health literacy in kidney disease: Associations with quality of life and adherence. *Journal of Renal Care, 46*(2), 85–94. https://doi.org/10.1111/jorc.12328

Wembenyui, C., Douglas, C., & Bonner, A. (2021). Validation of the Australian version of the Chronic Kidney Disease Self-Management Instrument. *International Journal of Nursing Practice, 27*(2), 1–9. https://doi.org/10.1111/ijn.12857

Self-Management: Kidney Failure   3125

Definition: Personal actions to manage kidney failure, its treatment, and to prevent disease progression and complications

OUTCOME TARGET RATING: Maintain at_____ Increase to_____

		Never Demonstrated	Rarely Demonstrated	Sometimes Demonstrated	Often Demonstrated	Consistently Demonstrated	
OUTCOME OVERALL RATING		**1**	**2**	**3**	**4**	**5**	
Indicators:							
312501	Accepts diagnosis	1	2	3	4	5	NA
312502	Seeks information about kidney failure management	1	2	3	4	5	NA
312503	Uses reputable sources of kidney failure information	1	2	3	4	5	NA
312504	Identifies personal systemic effects of kidney failure	1	2	3	4	5	NA
312505	Participates in health care decisions as kidney function declines	1	2	3	4	5	NA
312506	Discusses replacement treatment options with health provider	1	2	3	4	5	NA
312507	Shares cultural influences on compliance to treatment regimen with health professional	1	2	3	4	5	NA
312508	Discusses eligibility for kidney transplant with health provider	1	2	3	4	5	NA
312509	Obtains required laboratory tests	1	2	3	4	5	NA
312510	Monitors heart rate and rhythm	1	2	3	4	5	NA
312511	Monitors respiratory rate	1	2	3	4	5	NA
312512	Monitors blood pressure	1	2	3	4	5	NA
312513	Monitors for edema	1	2	3	4	5	NA
312514	Monitors for complications of edema	1	2	3	4	5	NA
312515	Monitors urinary output	1	2	3	4	5	NA
312516	Obtains assistance for symptom exacerbations	1	2	3	4	5	NA
312517	Adheres to hemodialysis or peritoneal treatment schedule	1	2	3	4	5	NA
312518	Uses strategies to limit treatment side effects	1	2	3	4	5	NA
312519	Uses strategies for managing symptom burden	1	2	3	4	5	NA

S

Self-Management: Kidney Failure—cont'd

		Never Demonstrated	Rarely Demonstrated	Sometimes Demonstrated	Often Demonstrated	Consistently Demonstrated	
312520	Provides routine care of dialysis vascular access site	1	2	3	4	5	NA
312521	Protects vascular access site	1	2	3	4	5	NA
312522	Seeks emergency care for access site problems	1	2	3	4	5	NA
312523	Follows prescribed diet	1	2	3	4	5	NA
312524	Uses strategies to increase diet compliance	1	2	3	4	5	NA
312525	Adheres to recommended fluid intake per day	1	2	3	4	5	NA
312526	Uses strategies to limit fluid intake	1	2	3	4	5	NA
312527	Spread fluid intake over 24-hour day	1	2	3	4	5	NA
312528	Follows dietary sodium restrictions	1	2	3	4	5	NA
312529	Follows dietary protein restrictions	1	2	3	4	5	NA
312530	Follows dietary phosphorus restrictions	1	2	3	4	5	NA
312531	Limits alcohol use	1	2	3	4	5	NA
312532	Eliminates tobacco, e-cigarette, and waterpipe use	1	2	3	4	5	NA
312533	Avoids second-hand smoke	1	2	3	4	5	NA
312534	Monitors body weight daily	1	2	3	4	5	NA
312535	Identifies dry body weight	1	2	3	4	5	NA
312536	Uses effective weight control strategies	1	2	3	4	5	NA
312537	Follows recommendations for physical activity	1	2	3	4	5	NA
312538	Monitors fatigue level	1	2	3	4	5	NA
312539	Uses energy conservation techniques	1	2	3	4	5	NA
312540	Manages basic activities of daily living	1	2	3	4	5	NA
312541	Manages instrumental activities of daily living	1	2	3	4	5	NA
312542	Obtains recommended immunizations	1	2	3	4	5	NA
312543	Uses medication as prescribed	1	2	3	4	5	NA
312544	Monitors prescribed medication therapeutic effects	1	2	3	4	5	NA
312545	Monitors side effects of medication	1	2	3	4	5	NA
312546	Monitors adverse effects of medications	1	2	3	4	5	NA
312547	Uses only non-prescription medication approved by health professional	1	2	3	4	5	NA
312548	Prevents infections	1	2	3	4	5	NA
312549	Uses stress management strategies	1	2	3	4	5	NA
312550	Reports signs and symptoms of anxiety	1	2	3	4	5	NA
312551	Reports signs and symptoms of depression	1	2	3	4	5	NA
312552	Obtains assistance psychological symptoms	1	2	3	4	5	NA
312553	Obtains support from family	1	2	3	4	5	NA
312554	Obtains support from friends	1	2	3	4	5	NA
312555	Uses support group	1	2	3	4	5	NA
312556	Keeps appointments with health professional	1	2	3	4	5	NA
312557	Reframes life goals	1	2	3	4	5	NA
312558	Uses available support groups	1	2	3	4	5	NA

S

Continued

Self-Management: Kidney Failure—cont'd

		Never Demonstrated	Rarely Demonstrated	Sometimes Demonstrated	Often Demonstrated	Consistently Demonstrated	
312559	Reputable sources of kidney disease information	1	2	3	4	5	NA
312560	Adjusts life routine for optimal health	1	2	3	4	5	NA
312561	Uses community resources	1	2	3	4	5	NA

Domain-*Health Knowledge & Behavior (IV)*   **Class**-*Health Management (FF)*   *7th edition 2024*

OUTCOME CONTENT REFERENCES:

Bertschi, L. A. (2020). Abnormal basic metabolic panel findings: Implications for nursing. *AJN, American Journal of Nursing, 120*(6), 58–66. https://doi.org/10.1097/01.naj.0000668764.99872.89

Chen, J., Fowler, K. J., & Grams, M. E. (2020). Knowledge is power: Patient education as a tool for patient activation. *American Journal of Kidney Diseases, 76*(2), 163–165. https://doi.org/10.1053/j.ajkd.2020.03.012

Chen, T. K., Knicely, D. H., & Grams, M. E. (2020). Chronic kidney disease diagnosis and management: A review. *Journal of American Medical Association, 322*(3), 1294–1304. https://doi.org/10.1001/jama.2019.14745

Correia, B. R., Brandão, M. A. G., Lopes, R. O. P., Silva, P. C. G., Zaccaro, K. R. L., Benevides, A. B., Duarte, S. C. M., & Silva, R. C. (2021). Arteriovenous fistula maturation clinical assessment for hemodialysis: A scoping review. *Acta Paulista de Enfermagen, 34*, eAPE00232. https://doi.org/10.37689/acta-ape/2021AR00232

El Monem, M. M. A., & Salim, H. M. (2020). Nursing guidelines to improve sexual function and quality of life among women undergoing hemodialysis. *Central European Journal of Nursing & Midwifery, 11*(4), 171–179. https://doi.org/10.15452/CEJNM.2020.11.0029

Frament, J., Hall, R. K., & Manley, H. J. (2020). Medication reconciliation: The foundation of medication safety for patients requiring dialysis. *American Journal of Kidney Diseases, 76*(6), 868–876.

González, A. M., Gutman, T., Lopez-Vargas, P., Anumudu, S., Arce, C. M., Craig, J. C., Eckardt, K. U., Harris, T., Levey, A. S., Lightstone, L., Scholes–Robertson, N., Shen, J. I., Teixeira-Pinto, A., Wheeler, D. C., White, D., Wilkie, M., Jadoul, M., Winkelmayer, W. C., & Tong, A. (2020). Patient and caregiver priorities for outcomes in CKD: A multinational nominal group technique study. *American Journal of Kidney Diseases, 76*(5), 679–689.

Guerra-Guerrero, V., Camargo Plazas, P., Cameron, B. L., Santos Salas, A. V., & Cofre González, C. G. (2020). Understanding the life experience of people on hemodialysis: Adherence to treatment and quality of life. *CANNT Journal, 30*(4), 24–32.

Huether, S. E., McCance, K. L., & Brashers, V. L. (2020). *Understanding pathophysiology* (7th ed.). Elsevier.

Ignatavicius, D. D., Workman, M. L., Rebar, C. R., & Heimgartner, N. M. (2021). *Medical-surgical nursing: Concepts for interprofessional care* (10th ed.). Elsevier.

Ikizler, T. A., Burrowes, J. D., Byham-Gray, L. D., Campbell, K. L., Carrero, J., Chan, W., Fouque, D., Friedman, A. N., Ghaddar, S., D., Goldstein-Fuchs, J., Kaysen, G. A., Kopple, J. D., Teta, D., Wang, A. Y.-M., & Cuppari, L. (2020). KDOQI Clinical practice guideline for nutrition in CKD: 2020 update. *American Journal of Kidney Diseases, 76*(3), S1–S107. https://doi.org/10.1053/j.ajkd.2020.05.006

Murali, K. M., Mullan, J., Roodenrys, S., Hassan, H. C., Lambert, K., & Lonergan, M. (2019). Strategies to improve dietary, fluid, dialysis or medication adherence in patients with end stage kidney disease on dialysis: A systematic review and meta-analysis of randomized intervention trials. *PLOS One, 14*(1), e0211479. https://doi.org/10.1371/journal.pone.0211479

Ng, M. S. N., Wong, C. L., Ho, E. H. S., Hui, Y. H., Miaskowski, C., & So, W. K. W. (2020). Burden of living with multiple concurrent symptoms in patients with end-stage renal disease. *Journal of Clinical Nursing, 29*(13/14), 2589–2601. https://doi.org/10.1111/jocn.15282

Perl, J., Fuller, D. S., Bieber, B. A., Boudville, N., Kanjanabuch, T., Ito, Y., Nessim, S. J., Piraino, B. M., Pisoni, R. L., Robinson, B. M., Schaubel, D. E., Schreiber, M. J., Teitelbaum, I., Woodrow, G., Zhao, J., & Johnson, D. W. (2020). Peritoneal dialysis-related infection rates and outcomes: Results from the Peritoneal Dialysis Outcomes and Practice Patterns Study (PDOPPS). *American Journal of Kidney Diseases, 76*(1), 42–53. https://doi.org/10.1053/j.ajkd.2019.09.016

Sousa, H., Ribeiro, O., Paúl, C., Costa, E., Miranda, V., Ribeiro, F., & Figueiredo, D. (2019). Social support and treatment adherence in patients with end-stage renal disease: A systematic review. *Seminars in Dialysis, 32*(6), 562–574. https://doi.org/10.1111/sdi.12831

Self-Management: Known Allergy   **3120**

Definition: Personal actions to manage a known allergy and to prevent episodes of a hypersensitivity response to a specific antigen

OUTCOME TARGET RATING: Maintain at_____ Increase to_____

		Never Demonstrated	Rarely Demonstrated	Sometimes Demonstrated	Often Demonstrated	Consistently Demonstrated	
OUTCOME OVERALL RATING		1	2	3	4	5	
Indicators:							
312001	Monitors environment for triggering allergens	1	2	3	4	5	NA
312002	Reduces triggering elements in home environment	1	2	3	4	5	NA

S

Self-Management: Known Allergy—cont'd

		Never Demonstrated	Rarely Demonstrated	Sometimes Demonstrated	Often Demonstrated	Consistently Demonstrated	
312003	Avoids use of products with triggering allergens	1	2	3	4	5	NA
312004	Interprets information on food labels correctly	1	2	3	4	5	NA
312005	Monitors for possible cross contamination	1	2	3	4	5	NA
312006	Educates self about risk of allergic response	1	2	3	4	5	NA
312007	Shares signs and symptoms of allergic response with others	1	2	3	4	5	NA
312008	Informs childcare provider about severity risk of allergic response	1	2	3	4	5	NA
312009	Informs friends about risk of allergic response	1	2	3	4	5	NA
312010	Informs work colleagues about risk of allergic response	1	2	3	4	5	NA
312011	Uses reputable sources of information about allergy	1	2	3	4	5	NA
312012	Monitors for signs and symptoms of allergic response	1	2	3	4	5	NA
312013	Uses medication as prescribed	1	2	3	4	5	NA
312014	Uses reputable alternative therapies as indicated	1	2	3	4	5	NA
312015	Undergoes desensitization if indicated	1	2	3	4	5	NA
312016	Informs all health professionals of allergens	1	2	3	4	5	NA
312017	Wears medical alert bracelet	1	2	3	4	5	NA
312018	Uses proper technique for self-administration of rescue inhaler	1	2	3	4	5	NA
312019	Uses proper technique for self-administration of epinephrine auto-injection	1	2	3	4	5	NA
312020	Carries emergency anaphylaxis kit at all times	1	2	3	4	5	NA
312021	Replaces epinephrine auto-injection as prescribed	1	2	3	4	5	NA
312022	Takes immediate action to prevent allergic response	1	2	3	4	5	NA
312023	Maintains plan for medical emergencies	1	2	3	4	5	NA
312024	Seeks medical attention immediately for systemic allergic response	1	2	3	4	5	NA

Domain-Health Knowledge & Behavior (IV)   *Class*-Health Management (FF)   6th edition 2018

OUTCOME CONTENT REFERENCES:
Gupta, R., Lau, C., Dyer, A., Sohn, M.–W., Altshuler, B., Kaye, B., & Necheles, J. (2014). Food allergy diagnosis and management practices among pediatricians. *Clinical Pediatrics, 53*(6), 524–230. https://doi.org/10.1177/0009922813518425
Herbert, L., Lin, A., Matsui, E., Wood, R., & Sharma, H. (2016). Development of a tool to measure youths' food allergy management facilitators and barriers. *Journal of Pediatric Psychology, 41*(3), 363–372. https://doi.org/10.1093/jpepsy/jsv099
Jones, C., Smith, H., Frew, A., Toit, G., Mukhopadhyay, S., & Llewellyn, C. (2014). Explaining adherence to self-care behaviors amongst adolescents with food allergy: A comparison of the Health Belief Model and the Common Sense Self-Regulation Model. *British Journal of Health Psychology, 19*(1), 65–82. https://doi.org/10.1111/bjhp.12033
Pistiner, M., & Devore, C. (2013). The role of pediatricians in school food allergy management. *Pediatric Annals, 42*(8), 334–340. https://doi.org/10.3928/00904481-20130723-14

S

Self-Management: Lipid Disorder 3109

Definition: Personal actions to manage hyperlipidemia, its treatment, and to prevent complications

OUTCOME TARGET RATING: Maintain at_____ Increase to_____

		Never Demonstrated	Rarely Demonstrated	Sometimes Demonstrated	Often Demonstrated	Consistently Demonstrated	
OUTCOME OVERALL RATING		**1**	**2**	**3**	**4**	**5**	
Indicators:							
310901	Seeks information about methods to manage disorder	1	2	3	4	5	NA
310902	Participates in health care decisions	1	2	3	4	5	NA
310903	Discusses benefits of medication with health professional	1	2	3	4	5	NA
310904	Obtains required laboratory tests	1	2	3	4	5	NA
310905	Monitors lipid levels	1	2	3	4	5	NA
310906	Adapts life routine for optimal health	1	2	3	4	5	NA
310907	Uses effective weight control strategies	1	2	3	4	5	NA
310908	Maintains optimum weight	1	2	3	4	5	NA
310909	Follows recommended diet	1	2	3	4	5	NA
310910	Limits fat and cholesterol intake	1	2	3	4	5	NA
310926	Monitors vitamin D intake	1	2	3	4	5	NA
310911	Participates in recommended aerobic exercise	1	2	3	4	5	NA
310912	Follows recommendations for alcohol use	1	2	3	4	5	NA
310913	Eliminates tobacco use	1	2	3	4	5	NA
310914	Avoids second-hand smoke	1	2	3	4	5	NA
310915	Uses medication as prescribed	1	2	3	4	5	NA
310916	Monitors medication therapeutic effects	1	2	3	4	5	NA
310917	Monitors medication adverse effects	1	2	3	4	5	NA
310918	Monitors medication side effects	1	2	3	4	5	NA
310919	Avoids stopping medication suddenly	1	2	3	4	5	NA
310920	Uses only non-prescription medication approved by health professional	1	2	3	4	5	NA
310927	Completes medication reconciliation with health professional	1	2	3	4	5	NA
310921	Monitors changes in general health	1	2	3	4	5	NA
310922	Uses health care services congruent with needs	1	2	3	4	5	NA
310923	Keeps appointments with health professional	1	2	3	4	5	NA
310924	Uses significant others to support behavior changes	1	2	3	4	5	NA
310925	Uses available community resources	1	2	3	4	5	NA

Domain-Health Knowledge & Behavior (IV)   *Class*-Health Management (FF)   5th edition 2013; revised 2024

OUTCOME CONTENT REFERENCES:

Berman, A. N., & Blankstein, R. (2019). Optimizing dyslipidemia management for the prevention of cardiovascular disease: A focus on risk assessment and therapeutic options. *Current Cardiology Reports*, 21(9), 110. https://doi.org/10.1007/s11886-019-1175-z

Dombalis, S., & Nash, A. (2021). The effect of statins in children and adolescents with familial hypercholesterolemia: A systematic review. *Journal of Pediatric Healthcare*, 35(3), 292–303. https://doi.org/10.1016/j.pedhc.2020.11.007

Ko, S. H., & Kim, H. S. (2020). Menopause-associated lipid metabolic disorders and foods beneficial for postmenopausal women. *Nutrients*, 12(1), 202. https://doi.org/10.3390/nu12010202

S

Liang, T., Wu, L., Xi, Y., Li, Y., Xie, X., Fan, C., Yang, L., Yang, S., Chen, X., Zhang, J., & Wu, Q. (2021). Probiotics supplementation improves hyperglycemia, hypercholesterolemia, and hypertension in type 2 diabetes mellitus: An update of meta-analysis. *Critical Reviews in Food Science & Nutrition, 61*(10), 1670–1688. https://doi.org/10.1080/10408398.2020.1764488

Newman, C. B., Blaha, M. J., Boord, J. B., Cariou, B., Chait, A., Fein, H. G., Ginsberg, H. N., Goldberg, I. J., Murad, M. H., Subramanian, S., & Tannock, L. R. (2020). Lipid management in patients with endocrine disorders: An Endocrine Society Clinical Practice Guideline. *The Journal of Clinical Endocrinology and Metabolism, 105*(12), 3613–3682. https://doi.org/10.1210/clinem/dgaa674

Oh, H., & Moorhead, S. (2020). Validation of the knowledge and self-management Nursing Outcomes Classification outcomes for adults with hypertension and lipid disorder. *Online Journal of Nursing Informatics, 24*(2), 1.

Silverman, M. G., Ference, B. A., Im, K., Wiviott, S. D., Giugliano, R. P., Grundy, S. M., Baunwald, E., & Sabatine, M. S. (2016). Association between lowering LDL-C and cardiovascular risk reduction among different therapeutic interventions: A systematic review and meta-analysis. *Journal of the American Medical Association, 316*(12), 1289–1297. https://doi.org/10.1001/jama.2016.13985

Vázquez-Manjarrez, N., Guevara-Cruz, M., Flores-López, A., Pichardo-Ontiveros, E., Tovar, A. R., & Torres, N. (2021). Effect of a dietary intervention with functional foods on LDL-C concentrations and lipoprotein subclasses in overweight subjects with hypercholesterolemia: Results of a controlled trial. *Clinical Nutrition, 40*(5), 2527–2534. https://doi.org/10.1016/j.clnu.2021.02.048

Self-Management: Liver Disease   3126

Definition: Personal actions to manage liver disease, its treatment, and to prevent disease progression and complications

OUTCOME TARGET RATING: Maintain at_____ Increase to_____

		Never Demonstrated	Rarely Demonstrated	Sometimes Demonstrated	Often Demonstrated	Consistently Demonstrated	
OUTCOME OVERALL RATING		1	2	3	4	5	
Indicators:							
312601	Accepts diagnosis	1	2	3	4	5	NA
312602	Seeks information about disease and symptoms	1	2	3	4	5	NA
312603	Monitors signs and symptoms	1	2	3	4	5	NA
312604	Reports unusual or new signs and symptoms	1	2	3	4	5	NA
312605	Manages signs and symptoms	1	2	3	4	5	NA
312606	Seeks information about managing symptoms	1	2	3	4	5	NA
312607	Seeks information about treatment	1	2	3	4	5	NA
312608	Uses strategies to comply with treatment regimen	1	2	3	4	5	NA
312609	Seeks information on preventing complications	1	2	3	4	5	NA
312610	Obtains information on managing complications	1	2	3	4	5	NA
312611	Obtains information on relapse prevention	1	2	3	4	5	NA
312612	Implements actions to manage complications	1	2	3	4	5	NA
312613	Follows recommended treatment	1	2	3	4	5	NA
312614	Performs prescribed procedure	1	2	3	4	5	NA
312615	Uses treatment devices correctly	1	2	3	4	5	NA
312616	Monitors treatment therapeutic effects	1	2	3	4	5	NA
312617	Monitors treatment side effects	1	2	3	4	5	NA
312618	Commits to lifestyle improvement	1	2	3	4	5	NA
312619	Adapts lifestyle to restrictions	1	2	3	4	5	NA
312620	Uses strategies to cope	1	2	3	4	5	NA
312621	Uses reputable sources of information	1	2	3	4	5	NA
312622	Identifies reputable e-health sources of information	1	2	3	4	5	NA

Continued

Self-Management: Liver Disease—cont'd

		Never Demonstrated	Rarely Demonstrated	Sometimes Demonstrated	Often Demonstrated	Consistently Demonstrated	
312623	Educates self about alcohol consumption and consequences	1	2	3	4	5	NA
312624	Monitors alcohol consumption	1	2	3	4	5	NA
312625	Uses strategies to address fatigue	1	2	3	4	5	NA
312626	Uses strategies to address pain	1	2	3	4	5	NA
312627	Uses strategies to address depression	1	2	3	4	5	NA
312628	Uses strategies to address anxiety	1	2	3	4	5	NA
312629	Uses strategies to promote sleep	1	2	3	4	5	NA
312630	Uses strategies to promote exercise	1	2	3	4	5	NA
312631	Participates in health screening	1	2	3	4	5	NA
312632	Obtains recommended vaccinations	1	2	3	4	5	NA
312633	Avoids hepatotoxic medication	1	2	3	4	5	NA
312634	Monitors changes in disease	1	2	3	4	5	NA
312635	Monitors changes in comorbid conditions	1	2	3	4	5	NA
312636	Records weight as recommended	1	2	3	4	5	NA
312637	Records blood pressure as recommended	1	2	3	4	5	NA
312638	Participates in laboratory tests and scans as ordered	1	2	3	4	5	NA
312639	Develops plan for medical emergencies	1	2	3	4	5	NA
312640	Collaborates with health professionals	1	2	3	4	5	NA
312641	Obtains advice from health professional as needed	1	2	3	4	5	NA
312642	Keeps appointments with health professional	1	2	3	4	5	NA
312643	Participates in health care decisions	1	2	3	4	5	NA
312644	Seeks information about risks prior to travelling outside of the country	1	2	3	4	5	NA

Domain-Health Knowledge & Behavior (IV)   **Class**-Health Management (FF)   7th edition 2024

OUTCOME CONTENT REFERENCES:

+Beg, S., Curtis, S., & Shariff, M. (2016). Patient education and its effect on self-management in cirrhosis: A pilot study. *European Journal of Gastroenterology & Hepatology, 28*(5), 582–587. https://doi.org/10.1097/MEG.0000000000000579

Brewer, C. (2019). Hepatitis A and B: Updates for general practice nurses. *Practice Nursing, 30*(4), 120–125. https://doi.org/10.12968/pnur.2019.30.4.120

+Boundreault, S., Chen, J., Wu, K. Y., Plüddemann, A., & Heneghan, C. (2020). Self-management programmes for cirrhosis: A systematic review. *Journal of Clinical Nursing, 29*(19/20), 3625–3637, https://doi.org/10.1111/jocn.15416

+Hansen, L., Leo, M. C., Chang, M. F., Zucker, B. L., & Sasaki, A. (2014). Pain and self-care behaviours in adult patients with end-stage liver disease. *Journal of Palliative Care, 30*(1), 32–40.

+Hayward, K. L., Horsfall, L. U., Ruffin, B. J., Cottrell, W. N., Chachay, V. S., Irvine, K. M., Martin, J. H., Powell, E. E., & Valery, P.C. (2017). Optimizing care of patients with chronic disease: Patient-oriented education may improve disease knowledge and self-management. *Internal Medicine Journal, 47*(8), 952–955. https://doi.org/10.1111/imj.13505

+Lau-Walker, M., Presky, J., Webzell, I., Murrells, T., & Heaton, N. (2015). Patients with alcohol-related liver disease—Beliefs about their illness and factors that influence their self-management. *Journal of Advanced Nursing, 72*(1), 173–185.

+Lin, W.-S., Lee, T.-T., Yang, Y.-H., & Mills, M. E. (2019). Environmental factors affecting self-management of chronic hepatis B from the patients' perspective. *Journal of Clinical Nursing, 28*(21-22), 4128–4138. https://doi.org/10.1111/jocn.14973

Moore, M. P., Cunninham, R. P., Dashek, R. J., Mucinski, J. M., & Rector, R. S. (2020). A fad too far? Dietary strategies for the prevention and treatment of NAFLD. *Obesity, 28*(10), 1843–1852. https://doi.org/10.1002/oby.22964

O'Gorman, P., Monaghan, A., McGrath, M., Naimimohasses, S., Gormley, J., & Norris, S. (2021). Determinants of physical activity engagement in patients with nonalcoholic fatty liver disease: The need for an individualized approach to lifestyle interventions. *PTJ: Physical Therapy & Rehabilitation Journal, 101*(2), 1–11. https://doi.org/10.1093/ptj/pzaa195

+Robinson, L., Newton, J. L., Jones, D., & Dawson, P. (2014). Promoting self-management and adherence with strength and balance training for older people with long-term conditions: A mixed methods study. *Journal of Evaluation in Clinical Practice, 20*(4), 318–326. https://doi.org/10.1111/jep.12128

Stelmach, M., Medeiros, K. A. A., Carvalho, B. J., Pipek, L. Z., Mesquita, G. H. A., Nii, F., Martines, D. R., Iuamoto, L. R., D'Albuquerque, L. A. C., Meyer, A., & Andraus, W. (2021). Instrument to evaluate the knowledge of patient with cirrhosis on his disease: Construction and validity. *BMC Gastroenterology, 21*, 83. https://doi.org/10.1186/s12876-021-01665-0

S

Self-Management: Lymphedema   3121

Definition: Personal actions to manage lymphedema, its treatment, and to prevent disease progression and complications

OUTCOME TARGET RATING: Maintain at_____ Increase to_____

		Never Demonstrated	Rarely Demonstrated	Sometimes Demonstrated	Often Demonstrated	Consistently Demonstrated	
OUTCOME OVERALL RATING		1	2	3	4	5	
Indicators:							
312101	Accepts diagnosis	1	2	3	4	5	NA
312102	Obtains reputable information about lymphedema	1	2	3	4	5	NA
312103	Monitors signs and symptoms of lymphedema	1	2	3	4	5	NA
312104	Monitors for signs and symptoms of complications	1	2	3	4	5	NA
312105	Follows intensive treatment plan with combined decongestive therapy	1	2	3	4	5	NA
312106	Applies bandages correctly	1	2	3	4	5	NA
312107	Performs manual lymphatic therapy	1	2	3	4	5	NA
312108	Uses intermittent pneumatic compression pump	1	2	3	4	5	NA
312109	Reports medication adverse effects	1	2	3	4	5	NA
312110	Reports medication side effects	1	2	3	4	5	NA
312124	Obtains information about surgical options	1	2	3	4	5	NA
312111	Uses strategies to cope with physiological impact	1	2	3	4	5	NA
312112	Uses strategies to cope with psychosocial impact	1	2	3	4	5	NA
312113	Uses strategies to cope with functional changes	1	2	3	4	5	NA
312114	Uses strategies to cope with changes in body image	1	2	3	4	5	NA
312115	Uses strategies to cope with perceived diminished sexuality	1	2	3	4	5	NA
312116	Uses strategies to promote self-esteem	1	2	3	4	5	NA
312117	Obtains modifications for physical limitations at work	1	2	3	4	5	NA
312118	Identifies health beliefs that impact treatment	1	2	3	4	5	NA
312119	Obtains family support for treatment	1	2	3	4	5	NA
312120	Obtains financial resources for assistance	1	2	3	4	5	NA
312121	Uses available support groups	1	2	3	4	5	NA
312122	Uses available community resources	1	2	3	4	5	NA
312123	Keeps appointments with health professional	1	2	3	4	5	NA

Domain-Health Knowledge & Behavior (IV)   ***Class***-Health Management (FF)   *6th edition 2018; revised 2024*

OUTCOME CONTENT REFERENCES:
Brown, J. C., Kumar, A., Cheville, A. L., Tchou, J. C., Troxel, A. B., Harris, S. R., & Schmitz, K. H. (2015). Association between lymphedema self-care adherence and lymphedema outcomes among women with breast cancer-related lymphedema. *American Journal of Physical Medicine & Rehabilitation*, 94(4), 288–296. https://doi.org/10.1097/PHM.0000000000000178

Fu, M. R., Ridner, S. H., Hu, S. H., Stewart, B. R., Cormier, J. N., & Armer, J. M. (2013). Psychosocial impact of lymphedema: A systematic review of literature from 2004 to 2011. *Psychooncology*, 22(7), 1466–1484. https://doi.org/10.1002/pon.3201

Johansson, K., Ochalek, K., & Hayes, S. (2020). Prevention of arm lymphedema through the use of compression sleeves following breast cancer: Results from a targeted literature review. *Physical Therapy Reviews*, 25(4), 213–218. https://doi.org/10.1080/10833196.2020.1822140

Kristiansen, M., Halle, M., Pignatti, M., & Skogh, A.-C. D. (2021). Evaluation and selection of lower limb lymphedema patients for lymphaticovenular anastomosis: A prospective study. *Injury, 9*, S108–S113. https://doi.org/10.1016/j.injury.2020.02.110

McDuff, S. G. R., Mina, A. I., Brunelle, C. L., Salama, L., Warren, L. E. G., Abouegylah, M., Swaroop, M., Skolny, M. N., Asdourian, M., Gillespie, T., Daniell, K., Sayegh, H. E., Naoum, G. E., Zheng, H., & Taghian, A. G. (2019). Timing of lymphedema after treatment for breast cancer: When are patients most at risk? *International Journal of Radiation Oncology, Biology, Physics, 103*(1), 62–70. https://doi.org/10.1016/j.ijrobp.2018.08.036

McLaughlin, S. A., Brunelle, C. L., & Taghian, A. (2020). Breast cancer-related lymphedema: Risk factors, screening, management, and the impact of locoregional treatment. *Journal of Clinical Oncology: Official Journal of the American Society of Clinical Oncology, 38*(20), 2341–2350. https://doi.org/10.1200/JCO.19.02896

Ostby, P. L., & Armer, J. M. (2015). Complexities of adherence and post-cancer lymphedema management. *Journal of Personalized Medicine, 5*(4), 370–388. https://doi.org/10.3390/jpm5040370

Self-Management: Multiple Sclerosis 1631

Definition: Personal actions to manage multiple sclerosis and to prevent relapses and complications

OUTCOME TARGET RATING: Maintain at_____ Increase to_____

	Never Demonstrated	Rarely Demonstrated	Sometimes Demonstrated	Often Demonstrated	Consistently Demonstrated	
OUTCOME OVERALL RATING	1	2	3	4	5	
Indicators:						
163101 Accepts diagnosis	1	2	3	4	5	NA
163102 Seeks information about methods to maintain muscular skeletal health	1	2	3	4	5	NA
163103 Participates in health care decisions	1	2	3	4	5	NA
163104 Performs treatment regimen as prescribed	1	2	3	4	5	NA
163105 Identifies symptoms of disease progression	1	2	3	4	5	NA
163106 Identifies ways to cope with functional changes	1	2	3	4	5	NA
163107 Monitors symptom onset	1	2	3	4	5	NA
163108 Monitors symptom persistence	1	2	3	4	5	NA
163109 Monitors symptom severity	1	2	3	4	5	NA
163110 Monitors symptom frequency	1	2	3	4	5	NA
163111 Reports symptoms of worsening disease	1	2	3	4	5	NA
163112 Reports signs and symptoms of mood changes	1	2	3	4	5	NA
163141 Uses strategies to manage depression	1	2	3	4	5	NA
163142 Uses strategies to manage anxiety	1	2	3	4	5	NA
163113 Obtains health care when warning signs occur	1	2	3	4	5	NA
163114 Uses symptom relief methods	1	2	3	4	5	NA
163115 Obtains required medication	1	2	3	4	5	NA
163116 Uses medication as prescribed	1	2	3	4	5	NA
163117 Monitors prescribed medication therapeutic effects	1	2	3	4	5	NA
163118 Monitors medication side effects	1	2	3	4	5	NA
163119 Uses correct procedure for injection administration	1	2	3	4	5	NA
163120 Rotates injection sites	1	2	3	4	5	NA
163121 Stores medication correctly	1	2	3	4	5	NA
163122 Uses preventive measures to reduce medication side effects	1	2	3	4	5	NA

S

Self-Management: Multiple Sclerosis—cont'd

		Never Demonstrated	Rarely Demonstrated	Sometimes Demonstrated	Often Demonstrated	Consistently Demonstrated	
163123	Follows recommended diet	1	2	3	4	5	NA
163143	Evaluate needs for sleep disorder assessment	1	2	3	4	5	NA
163124	Uses strategies to control fatigue	1	2	3	4	5	NA
163125	Balances activity and rest	1	2	3	4	5	NA
163144	Uses strategies to decrease falls	1	2	3	4	5	NA
163145	Obtains assistance as needed	1	2	3	4	5	NA
163146	Structures physical environment to support physical limitations	1	2	3	4	5	NA
163147	Uses strategies to enhance cognitive function	1	2	3	4	5	NA
163148	Uses weight control strategies	1	2	3	4	5	NA
163126	Participates in recommended exercise	1	2	3	4	5	NA
163127	Uses energy conservation techniques	1	2	3	4	5	NA
163128	Adjusts life routine for optimal health	1	2	3	4	5	NA
163149	Uses problem-focused coping strategies	1	2	3	4	5	NA
163129	Uses stress management strategies	1	2	3	4	5	NA
163150	Uses strategies to promote well-being	1	2	3	4	5	NA
163130	Uses alterative treatment techniques	1	2	3	4	5	NA
163151	Obtains required vaccines	1	2	3	4	5	NA
163132	Obtains required liver function tests	1	2	3	4	5	NA
163133	Uses strategies to enhance bladder function	1	2	3	4	5	NA
163134	Uses strategies to enhance bowel function	1	2	3	4	5	NA
163135	Avoids extremes of temperatures	1	2	3	4	5	NA
163136	Keeps appointments with health professional	1	2	3	4	5	NA
163137	Maintains plan for medical emergencies	1	2	3	4	5	NA
163152	Identifies person to act as legal representative	1	2	3	4	5	NA
163153	Uses reputable e-health resources	1	2	3	4	5	NA
163154	Uses mental health resources	1	2	3	4	5	NA
163155	Uses rehabilitation resources	1	2	3	4	5	NA
163156	Uses support groups	1	2	3	4	5	NA
163157	Uses reputable sources of information	1	2	3	4	5	NA

Domain *Health Knowledge & Behavior (IV)*   **Class**-*Health Management (FF)*   *4th edition 2008; reviewed 2013; revised 2024*

S

OUTCOME CONTENT REFERENCES:

Bromley, L., Horvath, P. J., Bennett, S. E., Weinstock-Guttman, B., & Ray, A. D. (2019). Impact of nutritional intake on function in people with mild-to-moderate multiple sclerosis. *International Journal of MS Care, 21*(1), 1–9. https://doi.org/10.7224/1537-2073.2017-039

Carletto, S., Cavalera, C., Sadowski, I., Rovaris, M., Borghi, M., Khoury, B., Ostacoli, L., & Pagnini, F. (2020). Mindfulness-based intervention for the improvement of well-being in people with multiple sclerosis: A systematic review and meta–analysis. *Psychosomatic Medicine, 82*(6), 600–613. https://doi.org/10.1097/PSY.0000000000000819

Coote, S., Comber, L., Quinn, G., Santoyo–Medina, C., Kalron, A., & Gunn, H. (2020). Falls in people with multiple sclerosis. *International Journal of MS Care. 22*, 247–255. https://doi.org/10.7224/1537-2073.2020-014

Eldridge-Smith, E. D., Loew, M., & Stepleman, L. M. (2019). The adaptation and validation of a stigma measure for individuals with multiple sclerosis. *Disability and Rehabilitation, 43*(2), 262–269. https://doi.org/10.1080/096338288.2019.1617793

Matthews, P. M., Block, V. J., & Leocani, L. (2020). E-health and multiple sclerosis. *Current Opinion in Neurology, 33*(3), 271–276. https://doi.org/10.1097/WCO.0000000000000823

Nelson, L. M., & Bourdette, D. (2020). Two decades of research. Time to incorporate comorbidity management into the care of MS? *Neurology, 95*(5), 193–194. https://doi.org/10.1212/WNL.0000000000010036

Rahn, A. C., Solari, A., Beckerman, H., Nicholas, R., Wilkie, D., Heesen, C., & Giordano, A. (2020). "I will respect the autonomy of my patient:" A scoping review of shared decision making in multiple sclerosis. *International Journal of MS Care, 22*(6), 285–293. https://doi.org/10.7224/1537-2073.2020-027

Salter, A., Kowalec, K., Fitzgerald, K. C., Cutter, G., & Marrie, R. A. (2020). Comorbidity is associated with disease activity in MS: Findings from the CombiRx trial. *Neurology, 95*(5), e446–e456. https://doi.org/10.1212/WNL.0000000000010024

Schirda, B., Duraney, E., Lee, H. K., Manglani, H. R., Andridge, R. R., Plate, A., Nicholas, J., & Prakash, R. S. (2020). Mindfulness training for emotion dysregulations in multiple sclerosis: A pilot randomized controlled trial. *Rehabilitation Psychology, 65*(3), 206–218. https://doi.org/10.1037/rep0000324

White, E. K., Sullivan, A. B., & Drerup, M. (2019). Impact of sleep disorders on depression and patient-perceived health-related quality of life in multiple sclerosis. *International Journal of MS Care, 21*(1), 10–14. https://doi.org/10.7224/1537-2073.2017-068

Self-Management: Osteoporosis 3110

Definition: Personal actions to manage osteoporosis, its treatment, and to prevent disease progression and complications

OUTCOME TARGET RATING: Maintain at_____ Increase to_____

		Never Demonstrated	Rarely Demonstrated	Sometimes Demonstrated	Often Demonstrated	Consistently Demonstrated	
OUTCOME OVERALL RATING		1	2	3	4	5	
Indicators:							
311001	Uses medication as prescribed	1	2	3	4	5	NA
311002	Monitors medication side effects	1	2	3	4	5	NA
311003	Follows treatment regimen	1	2	3	4	5	NA
311004	Discusses non-prescription medication use with health provider	1	2	3	4	5	NA
311005	Follows recommendations for calcium supplements	1	2	3	4	5	NA
311006	Follows recommendations for vitamin D supplements	1	2	3	4	5	NA
311007	Follows recommended diet	1	2	3	4	5	NA
311008	Eliminates tobacco use	1	2	3	4	5	NA
311009	Follows recommendations for alcohol use	1	2	3	4	5	NA
311010	Participates in weight-bearing exercises	1	2	3	4	5	NA
311011	Participates in muscle-strengthening exercises	1	2	3	4	5	NA
311012	Uses fall prevention strategies	1	2	3	4	5	NA
311013	Reports a fall to health professional	1	2	3	4	5	NA
311014	Reports a fracture to health professional	1	2	3	4	5	NA
311015	Keeps appointment with health professional	1	2	3	4	5	NA
311016	Uses available community resources	1	2	3	4	5	NA

Domain-*Health Knowledge & Behavior (IV)* **Class**-*Health Management (FF)* 5th edition 2013

OUTCOME CONTENT REFERENCES:

Alexander, L., LaRosa, J. H., Bader, H., Garfield, S., & Alexander, W. J. (2010). *New dimensions in women's health* (5th ed.). Jones & Bartlett.

Bhalla, A. (2010). Management of osteoporosis in a pre-menopausal woman. *Best Practice & Research Clinical Rheumatology, 24*(3), 313–327. https://doi.org/10.1016/j.berh.2010.01.006

Daly, R., Ahlborg, H., Ringsberg, K., Gardsell, P., Sembo, I., & Karlsson, M. (2008). Association between changes in habitual physical activity and changes in bone density, muscle strength, and functional performance in elderly men and women. *Journal of the American Geriatrics Society, 56*(12), 2252–2260. https://doi.org/10.1111/j.1532-5415.2008.02039.x

Gates, B., & Das, S. (2011). Management of osteoporosis in elderly men. *Maturitas, 69*(2), 113–119. https://doi.org/10.1016/j.maturitas.2011.03.009

International Society for Clinical Densitometry (ISCD). (2004). *Pocket guide to bone mineral density testing.* https://www.iscd.org/visitors/pdfs/ISCD–CANADIANPanelOfficialPositions-BMDcard.pdf

Matheson, E., Mainous, A., & Carnemolla, M. (2009). The association between onion consumption and bone density in perimenopausal and postmenopausal non-Hispanic white women 50 years and older. *Menopause, 16*(4), 756–759. https://doi.org/10.1097/gme.0b013e31819581a5

Papaioannou, A., Morin, S., Cheung, A. M., Atkinson, S., Brown, J. P., Feldman, S., Hanley, D. A., Hodsman, A., Jamal, S. A., Kaiser, S. M., Kvern, B., Siminoski, K., & Leslie, W. D. (2010). 2010 clinical practice guidelines for the diagnosis and management of osteoporosis in Canada: Summary. *Canadian Medical Association Journal, 182*(17), 1864–1873. https://doi.org/10.1097/gme.0b013e31819581a5

Self-Management: Ostomy   1615

Definition: Personal actions to maintain ostomy for elimination

OUTCOME TARGET RATING: Maintain at_____ Increase to_____

OUTCOME OVERALL RATING	Never Demonstrated	Rarely Demonstrated	Sometimes Demonstrated	Often Demonstrated	Consistently Demonstrated	
	1	2	3	4	5	
Indicators:						
161524 Accepts diagnosis	1	2	3	4	5	NA
161525 Expresses acceptance of colostomy	1	2	3	4	5	NA
161526 Reports acceptance of body image change	1	2	3	4	5	NA
161527 Washes hands before procedure	1	2	3	4	5	NA
161528 Views stoma during care	1	2	3	4	5	NA
161529 Inspects the stoma	1	2	3	4	5	NA
161530 Cleanses skin around stoma	1	2	3	4	5	NA
161531 Monitors skin condition around stoma	1	2	3	4	5	NA
161504 Measures stoma for proper appliance fit	1	2	3	4	5	NA
161532 Follow regular daily schedule for irrigation	1	2	3	4	5	NA
161521 Uses correct irrigation technique	1	2	3	4	5	NA
161507 Empties ostomy bag	1	2	3	4	5	NA
161508 Changes ostomy bag	1	2	3	4	5	NA
161509 Monitors for complications related to stoma	1	2	3	4	5	NA
161510 Monitors amount, character, and consistency of stool	1	2	3	4	5	NA
161533 Monitors for intestinal complications	1	2	3	4	5	NA
161511 Follows schedule for changing ostomy bag	1	2	3	4	5	NA
161512 Obtains ostomy supplies	1	2	3	4	5	NA
161534 Avoids extreme temperatures for storage of supplies	1	2	3	4	5	NA
161513 Avoids flatus producing food and drink	1	2	3	4	5	NA
161514 Maintains adequate fluid intake	1	2	3	4	5	NA
161515 Follows recommended diet	1	2	3	4	5	NA
161516 Avoids odor producing foods	1	2	3	4	5	NA
161535 Monitors medication therapeutic effects	1	2	3	4	5	NA
161536 Monitors medication side effects	1	2	3	4	5	NA
161522 Modifies daily activities to optimize self-care	1	2	3	4	5	NA
161537 Asks for assistance as needed	1	2	3	4	5	NA
161538 Seeks family support	1	2	3	4	5	NA
161539 Uses support group	1	2	3	4	5	NA
161523 Obtains assistance from a health professional	1	2	3	4	5	NA
161540 Engages in activities of daily living as directed	1	2	3	4	5	NA

Domain-Health Knowledge & Behavior (IV)   *Class*-Health Behavior (Q)   *3rd edition 2004; revised 2008, 2024*

OUTCOME CONTENT REFERENCES:

Chabal, L. O., Prentice, J. L., & Ayello, E. A. (2021). Practice implications from the WCET* international ostomy guideline 2020. *Advances in Skin & Wound Care, 34*(6), 293–300. https://doi.org/10.1097/01.ASW.0000742888.02025.d6

Ignatavicius, D. D., Workman, M. L., Rebar, C. R., & Heimgartner, N. M. (2021). *Medical-surgical nursing, Concepts for interprofessional collaborative care* (10th ed.). Elsevier.

Lataillade, L., & Chabal, L. (2021). Therapeutic patient education: A multifaceted approach to ostomy care. *Advances in Skin & Wound Care, 34*(1), 36–42. https://doi.org/10.1097/01.ASW.0000722756.35017.02

Potter, P. A., Perry, A. G., Stockert, P. A., & Hall, A. M. (2021). *Fundamentals of nursing* (10th ed.). Elsevier.

Stetzer, M. N. (2021). Essential ostomy knowledge for nurses: Promoting adaptation in children with new ostomy and their caregivers. *Pediatric Nursing, 47*(2), 71–78.

Wang, W., Ding, Y., Lu, Q., Qi, J., & Zhang, S. (2021). The development of a behavior questionnaire for stoma self-management for persons with bladder cancer and an ileal conduit. *Journal of Advanced Nursing, 77*(2), 1085–1095. https://doi.org/10.1111/jan.14662

Self-Management: Parkinson Disease   3127

Definition: Personal actions to manage Parkinson disease, its treatment, and to prevent or limit disease progression and complications

OUTCOME TARGET RATING: Maintain at_____ Increase to_____

		Never Demonstrated	Rarely Demonstrated	Sometimes Demonstrated	Often Demonstrated	Consistently Demonstrated	
OUTCOME OVERALL RATING		1	2	3	4	5	
Indicators:							
312701	Accepts diagnosis	1	2	3	4	5	NA
312702	Obtains reputable information	1	2	3	4	5	NA
310703	Participates in health care decisions considering stage of disease	1	2	3	4	5	NA
310704	Involves family in health care decisions	1	2	3	4	5	NA
310705	Identifies health beliefs that impact treatment	1	2	3	4	5	NA
310706	Monitors motor symptoms of disease	1	2	3	4	5	NA
310707	Monitors non-motor symptoms of disease	1	2	3	4	5	NA
310708	Uses symptom relief measures	1	2	3	4	5	NA
310709	Monitors for signs and symptoms of disease progression	1	2	3	4	5	NA
310710	Follows medication regimen to control motor symptoms	1	2	3	4	5	NA
310711	Adapts life routine for optimal health	1	2	3	4	5	NA
310712	Balances activity and rest	1	2	3	4	5	NA
310713	Uses strategies to cope with functional changes	1	2	3	4	5	NA
310714	Uses strategies to prevent falls	1	2	3	4	5	NA
310715	Uses assistive devices for mobility	1	2	3	4	5	NA
310716	Modifies home environment for safety issues	1	2	3	4	5	NA
310717	Participates in recommended physical exercise	1	2	3	4	5	NA
310718	Practices yoga to improve body awareness	1	2	3	4	5	NA
310719	Monitors nutritional intake	1	2	3	4	5	NA
310720	Includes nutritious snacks in daily routine	1	2	3	4	5	NA
310721	Monitors medication therapeutic effects	1	2	3	4	5	NA
310722	Reports medication adverse effects	1	2	3	4	5	NA
310723	Reports medication side effects	1	2	3	4	5	NA
310724	Reports medication and food interactions	1	2	3	4	5	NA

S

Self-Management: Parkinson Disease—cont'd

		Never Demonstrated	Rarely Demonstrated	Sometimes Demonstrated	Often Demonstrated	Consistently Demonstrated	
310725	Uses strategies to prevent pressure injuries	1	2	3	4	5	NA
310726	Uses strategies to improve sleep	1	2	3	4	5	NA
310727	Monitors for daytime drowsiness	1	2	3	4	5	NA
310728	Uses strategies to cope with changes in body image	1	2	3	4	5	NA
310729	Monitors for signs of depression	1	2	3	4	5	NA
310730	Uses strategies to cope with cognitive changes	1	2	3	4	5	NA
310731	Monitors for changes in elimination patterns	1	2	3	4	5	NA
310732	Uses strategies to facilitate elimination	1	2	3	4	5	NA
310733	Uses strategies to cope with changes in communication ability	1	2	3	4	5	NA
310734	Identifies family care provider when needed	1	2	3	4	5	NA
310735	Obtains assistance for self-care needs	1	2	3	4	5	NA
310736	Uses available support groups	1	2	3	4	5	NA
310737	Uses available community resources	1	2	3	4	5	NA
310738	Keeps appointments with health professional	1	2	3	4	5	NA
310739	Uses home health care services as needed	1	2	3	4	5	NA
310740	Uses health care services congruent with need	1	2	3	4	5	NA
310741	Revises care support needs as disease progresses	1	2	3	4	5	NA
310742	Clarifies personal wishes for support-ive care when dependent	1	2	3	4	5	NA

***Domain**-Health Knowledge & Behavior (IV)*   ***Class**-Health Condition (GG)*   *7th edition 2024*

OUTCOME CONTENT REFERENCES:

Hellqvist, C., Berterö, C., Dizdar, N., Sund-Levander, M., & Hagell, P. (2020). Self-management education for persons with Parkinson's disease and their care partners: A quasi-experimental case-control study in clinical practice. *Parkinson's Disease, 2020*, Article 6920943. https://doi.org/10.1155/2020/6920943

Ignatavicius, D. D., Workman, M. L., Rebar, C. R., & Heimgartner, N. M. (2021). *Medical-surgical nursing: Concepts for interprofessional care* (10th ed.). Elsevier.

Iwasa, Y., Saito, I., & Suzuki, M. (2021). Differences in home health nursing care for patients with Parkinson's disease by stage of progress: Patients in Hoehn and Yahr stages III, IV, and V. *Parkinson's Disease, 2021*, Article 8834998. https://doi.org/10.1155/2021/8834998

Kessler, D., Hatch, S., Alexander, L., Grimes, D., Côté, D., Liddy, C., & Mestre, T. (2021). The integrated Parkinson's Disease Care Network (IPCN), Qualitative evaluation of a new approach to care for Parkinson's disease. *Patient Education and Counseling, 104*(1), 136–142. https://doi.org/10.1016/j.pec.2020.07.002

Lim, K. E., Kim, S. R., Sung, Y. H., Oh, S., Kim, M. S., & Chung, S. J. (2020). Factors influencing self-management in Parkinson's disease: A cross-sectional study. *Geriatric Nursing, 41*(3), 254–260. https://doi.org/10.1016/j.gerinurse.2019.10.005

Martignon, C., Pedrinolla, A., Ruzzante, F., Giuriato, G., Laginestra, F. G., Bouça–Machado, R., Ferreira, J. J., Tinazzi, M., Schena, F., & Venturelli, M. (2021). Guidelines on exercise testing and prescription for patients at different stages of Parkinson's disease. *Aging Clinical & Experimental Research, 33*(2), 221–246. https://doi.org/10.1007/s40520-020-01612-1

Rosqvist, K., Kylberg, M., Löfqvist, C., Schrag, A., Odin, P., & Iwarsson, S. (2021). Perspectives on care for late-stage Parkinson's disease. *Parkinson's Disease 2021*, Article 9475026. https://doi.org/10.1155/2021/9475026

Tuijt, R., Tan, A., Armstrong, M., Pigott, J., Read, J., Davies, N., Walters, K., & Schrag, A. (2020). Self-management components as experienced by people with Parkinson's disease and their carers: A systematic review and synthesis of the qualitative literature. *Parkinson's Disease, 2020*, Article 8857385. https://doi.org/10.1155/2020/8857385

S

Self-Management: Peripheral Artery Disease

3111

Definition: Personal actions to manage peripheral artery disease, its treatment, and prevent disease progression

OUTCOME TARGET RATING: Maintain at_____ Increase to_____

OUTCOME OVERALL RATING		Never Demonstrated	Rarely Demonstrated	Sometimes Demonstrated	Often Demonstrated	Consistently Demonstrated	
		1	2	3	4	5	
Indicators:							
311101	Monitors signs and symptoms of peripheral artery disease	1	2	3	4	5	NA
311102	Monitors signs and symptoms of claudication	1	2	3	4	5	NA
311103	Seeks information about peripheral artery disease	1	2	3	4	5	NA
311104	Seeks information about claudication	1	2	3	4	5	NA
311105	Uses medication as prescribed	1	2	3	4	5	NA
311106	Participates in prescribed exercise	1	2	3	4	5	NA
311107	Uses effective weight control strategies	1	2	3	4	5	NA
311108	Maintains optimum weight	1	2	3	4	5	NA
311109	Eliminates tobacco use	1	2	3	4	5	NA
311110	Monitors blood cholesterol	1	2	3	4	5	NA
311111	Limits fat and cholesterol intake	1	2	3	4	5	NA
311112	Monitors blood pressure	1	2	3	4	5	NA
311113	Monitors for symptoms of thromboembolism	1	2	3	4	5	NA
311114	Controls blood glucose level	1	2	3	4	5	NA
311115	Monitors for signs and symptoms of worsening peripheral artery disease	1	2	3	4	5	NA
311116	Monitors sensation in lower extremities	1	2	3	4	5	NA
311117	Monitors temperature in lower extremities	1	2	3	4	5	NA
311118	Monitors color in lower extremities	1	2	3	4	5	NA
311119	Monitors muscle strength in lower extremities	1	2	3	4	5	NA
311120	Monitors changes in general health	1	2	3	4	5	NA
311121	Discusses treatment options with health provider	1	2	3	4	5	NA
311122	Schedules appointments at regular intervals	1	2	3	4	5	NA
311123	Keeps appointments with health professional	1	2	3	4	5	NA
311124	Develops plan for medical emergencies	1	2	3	4	5	NA

Domain-*Health Knowledge & Behavior (IV)*   **Class**-*Health Management (FF)*   *5th edition 2013*

OUTCOME CONTENT REFERENCES:

Hirsch, A., Haskal, Z., Hertzer, N., Bakal, C., Creager, M., Halperin, J., Hiratzka, L. F., Murphy, W. R. C., Olin, J. W., Puschett, J. B., Rosenfield, K. A., Sacks, D., Stanley, J. C., Tayler, L. M. Jr., White, C. J., White, J., & White, R. A. (2006). ACC/AHA 2005 practice guidelines for the management of patients with peripheral arterial disease (lower extremity, renal, mesenteric, and abdominal aortic. *Circulation, 113*(11), e463–e654. https://doi.org/10.1161/CIRCULATIONAHA.106.174526

Hirsch, A. T., Murphy, T. P., Lovell, M. B., Twillman, G., Treat-Jacobson, D., Harwood, E. M., Mohler, E. R., III, Creager, M. A. Hobson, R. W., II, Robertson, R. M., Howard, W. J., Criqui, M. H., & Peripheral Arterial Disease Coalition. (2007). Gaps in public knowledge of peripheral artery disease: The first national PAD public awareness survey. *Circulation, 116*(18), 2086–2094. https://doi.org/10.1161/CIRCULATIONAHA.107.725101

Lewis, S., Dirksen, S., Heitkemper, M., Bucher, L., & Camera, I. (2011). *Medical–surgical nursing: Assessment and management of clinical problems* (8th ed., pp. 874–880). Elsevier Mosby.

Self-Management: Pneumonia   3122

Definition: Personal actions to manage pneumonia, its treatment, and to prevent complications

OUTCOME TARGET RATING: Maintain at_____ Increase to_____

		Never Demonstrated	Rarely Demonstrated	Sometimes Demonstrated	Often Demonstrated	Consistently Demonstrated	
OUTCOME OVERALL RATING		1	2	3	4	5	
Indicators:							
312201	Accepts diagnosis	1	2	3	4	5	NA
312202	Seeks treatment for pneumonia	1	2	3	4	5	NA
312203	Monitors for signs and symptoms	1	2	3	4	5	NA
312204	Obtains reputable information about methods to prevent complications	1	2	3	4	5	NA
312205	Follows treatment regimen	1	2	3	4	5	NA
312206	Monitors body temperature	1	2	3	4	5	NA
312207	Monitors respiratory rate	1	2	3	4	5	NA
312208	Monitors for shortness of breath	1	2	3	4	5	NA
312209	Monitors health status for exacerbation	1	2	3	4	5	NA
312210	Obtains health care with worsening signs and symptoms	1	2	3	4	5	NA
312211	Completes prescribed antibiotics	1	2	3	4	5	NA
312212	Monitors medication therapeutic effects	1	2	3	4	5	NA
312213	Monitors medication side effects	1	2	3	4	5	NA
312214	Monitors medication adverse effects	1	2	3	4	5	NA
312215	Monitors for potential medication interactions	1	2	3	4	5	NA
312216	Conducts deep breathing exercises	1	2	3	4	5	NA
312217	Uses bulb syringe to clear nasal airways	1	2	3	4	5	NA
312218	Uses nebulizer treatments as prescribed	1	2	3	4	5	NA
312219	Uses postural drainage procedure	1	2	3	4	5	NA
312220	Avoids smoking	1	2	3	4	5	NA
312221	Avoids alcohol use	1	2	3	4	5	NA
312222	Uses strategies to increase humidification	1	2	3	4	5	NA
312223	Obtains diagnostic tests	1	2	3	4	5	NA
312231	Obtains vaccine as recommended	1	2	3	4	5	NA
312224	Follows healthy diet	1	2	3	4	5	NA
312225	Increases fluid intake as recommended	1	2	3	4	5	NA
312226	Uses strategies to promote sleep	1	2	3	4	5	NA
312227	Balances activity and rest	1	2	3	4	5	NA
312228	Uses energy conservation techniques	1	2	3	4	5	NA
312229	Uses strategies to avoid reoccurrence	1	2	3	4	5	NA
312230	Keeps appointments with health professional	1	2	3	4	5	NA

Domain-Health Knowledge & Behavior (IV)   *Class*-Health Management (FF)   6th edition 2018; revised 2024

S

OUTCOME CONTENT REFERENCES:

Burman, M. E., & Wright, W. L. (2007). Diagnosis and management of community-acquired pneumonia: Evidence-based practice. *The Journal for Nurse Practitioners, 3*(9), 633–640. https://doi.org/10.1016/j.nurpra.2007.07.019

Kaysin, A., & Viera, A. (2016). Community-acquired pneumonia in adults: Diagnosis and management. *American Family Physician, 94*(9), 698–706.

Lanks, C. W., Musani, A. I., & Hsia, D. W. (2019). Community-acquired pneumonia and hospital-acquired pneumonia. *The Medical Clinics of North America*, *103*(3), 487–501. https://doi.org/10.1016/j.mcna.2018.12.008

Scelfo, C., Menzella, F., Fontana, M., Ghidoni, G., Galeone, C., & Facciolongo, N. C. (2021). Pneumonia and invasive pneumococcal diseases: The role of pneumococcal conjugate vaccine in the era of multi-drug resistance. *Vaccines*, *9*(5), 420. https://doi.org/10.3390/vaccines9050420

van Werkhoven, C. H., & Huijts, S. M. (2018). Vaccines to prevent pneumococcal community-acquired pneumonia. *Clinics in Chest Medicine*, *39*(4), 733–752. https://doi.org/10.1016/j.ccm.2018.07.007

Self-Management: Stroke 3123

Definition: Personal actions to manage the consequences of a stroke, its treatment, rehabilitation, and to prevent reoccurrences

OUTCOME TARGET RATING: Maintain at_____ Increase to_____

	Never Demonstrated	Rarely Demonstrated	Sometimes Demonstrated	Often Demonstrated	Consistently Demonstrated	
OUTCOME OVERALL RATING	1	2	3	4	5	
Indicators:						
312301 Obtains information about stroke	1	2	3	4	5	NA
312302 Reports signs and symptoms of stroke	1	2	3	4	5	NA
312303 Follows treatment regimen	1	2	3	4	5	NA
312304 Uses medication as prescribed	1	2	3	4	5	NA
312305 Monitors medication therapeutic effects	1	2	3	4	5	NA
312306 Monitors medication adverse effects	1	2	3	4	5	NA
312307 Monitors medication side effects	1	2	3	4	5	NA
312308 Monitors anticoagulant therapy	1	2	3	4	5	NA
312309 Monitors blood pressure	1	2	3	4	5	NA
312310 Monitors low-density lipoprotein cholesterol	1	2	3	4	5	NA
312311 Monitors glucose levels	1	2	3	4	5	NA
312312 Monitors body weight	1	2	3	4	5	NA
312313 Follows recommended diet	1	2	3	4	5	NA
312314 Avoids substances that interact with medication	1	2	3	4	5	NA
312315 Expresses self-confidence to do daily tasks	1	2	3	4	5	NA
312316 Adapts to sensory loss	1	2	3	4	5	NA
312317 Adapts to cognitive changes	1	2	3	4	5	NA
312331 Uses strategies to manage changes in communication ability	1	2	3	4	5	NA
312318 Uses assistive devices correctly	1	2	3	4	5	NA
312319 Participates in physical activity	1	2	3	4	5	NA
312320 Participates in rehabilitation	1	2	3	4	5	NA
312321 Monitors sleep apnea	1	2	3	4	5	NA
312322 Participates in smoking cessation	1	2	3	4	5	NA
312323 Follows recommended alcohol use	1	2	3	4	5	NA
312324 Adjusts life routine for optimal health	1	2	3	4	5	NA
312332 Modifies leisure activities	1	2	3	4	5	NA
312325 Uses strategies to cope with effects of stroke	1	2	3	4	5	NA
312326 Uses others to support behavior changes	1	2	3	4	5	NA
312327 Participates in health care decisions	1	2	3	4	5	NA

S

Self-Management: Stroke—cont'd

		Never Demonstrated	Rarely Demonstrated	Sometimes Demonstrated	Often Demonstrated	Consistently Demonstrated	
312328	Maintains plan for medical emergencies	1	2	3	4	5	NA
312329	Uses social support	1	2	3	4	5	NA
312330	Uses community resources	1	2	3	4	5	NA
312331	Keeps appointments with health professional	1	2	3	4	5	NA

Domain-Health Knowledge & Behavior (IV)   **Class**-Health Management (FF)   6th edition 2018; revised 2024

OUTCOME CONTENT REFERENCES:

Boger, E. J., Demain, S., & Latter, S. (2013). Self-management: A systematic review of outcome measures adopted in self-management interventions for stroke. *Disability and Rehabilitation, 35*(17), 1415–1428. https://doi.org/10.3109/09638288.2012.737080

Boger, E. J., Demain, S. H., & Latter, S. M. (2015). Stroke self-management: A focus group study to identify the factors influencing self-management following stroke. *International Journal of Nursing Studies, 52*(1), 175–187. https://doi.org/10.1016/j.ijnurstu.2014.05.006

Church, G., Ali, A., Smith, C. L., Broom, D., & Sage, K. (2022). Examining clinical practice guidelines for exercise and physical activity as part of rehabilitation for people with stroke: A systematic review. *International Journal of Environmental Research and Public Health, 19*(3), 1707. https://doi.org/10.3390/ijerph19031707

Fugazzaro, S., Denti, M., Accogli, M. A., Costi, S., Pagliacci, D., Calugi, S., Cavalli, E., Taricco, M., Bardelli, R., & On Behalf of Look After Yourself Project (2021). Self-management in stroke survivors: Development and implementation of the Look after Yourself (LAY) intervention. *International Journal of Environmental Research and Public Health, 18*(11), 5925. https://doi.org/10.3390/ijerph18115925

Lo, S., Chau, J., & Chang, A. M. (2021). Strategies adopted to manage physical and psychosocial challenges after returning home among people with stroke: A qualitative study. *Medicine, 100*(10), e25026. https://doi.org/10.1097/MD.0000000000025026

Nott, M., Wiseman, L., Seymour, T., Pike, S., Cuming, T., & Wall, G. (2021). Stroke self-management and the role of self-efficacy. *Disability and Rehabilitation, 43*(10), 1410–1419. https://doi.org/10.1080/09638288.2019.1666431

Winstein, C. J., Stein, J., Arena, R., Bates, B., Cherney, L. R., Cramer, S. C., Deruyter, F., Eng, J. J., Fisher, B., Harvey, R. L., Lang, C. E., MacKay-Lyons, M., Ottenbacher, K. J., Pugh, S., Reeves, M. J., Richards, L. G., Stiers, W., Zorowitz, R. D., & American Heart Association Stroke Council, Council on Cardiovascular and Stroke Nursing, Council on Clinical Cardiology, and Council on Quality of Care and Outcomes Research (2016). Guidelines for adult stroke rehabilitation and recovery: A guideline for healthcare professionals from the American Heart Association/American Stroke Association. *Stroke, 47*(6), e98–e169. https://doi.org/10.1161/STR.0000000000000098

Wray, F., Clarke, D., & Forster, A. (2019). How do stroke survivors with communication difficulties manage life after stroke in the first year? A qualitative study. *International Journal of Language & Communication Disorders, 54*(5), 814–827. https://doi.org/10.1111/1460-6984.12487

Self-Management: Treatment Procedure   **3128**

Definition: Personal actions to manage a procedure(s) required as a part of a treatment plan for an on-going condition

OUTCOME TARGET RATING: Maintain at_____ Increase to_____

		Never Demonstrated	Rarely Demonstrated	Sometimes Demonstrated	Often Demonstrated	Consistently Demonstrated	
OUTCOME OVERALL RATING		1	2	3	4	5	
Indicators:							
312801	Verbalizes purpose of procedure	1	2	3	4	5	NA
312802	Verbalizes steps of procedure	1	2	3	4	5	NA
312803	Verbalizes benefits of procedure	1	2	3	4	5	NA
312804	Secures financial resource	1	2	3	4	5	NA
312805	Practices steps of procedure with health professional	1	2	3	4	5	NA
312806	Washes hands before procedure	1	2	3	4	5	NA
312807	Carries out steps of procedure correctly	1	2	3	4	5	NA
312808	Develops schedule for the procedure	1	2	3	4	5	NA
312809	Takes precautions during procedure	1	2	3	4	5	NA
312810	Follows restrictions related to procedure	1	2	3	4	5	NA

S

Continued

Self-Management: Treatment Procedure—cont'd

		Never Demonstrated	Rarely Demonstrated	Sometimes Demonstrated	Often Demonstrated	Consistently Demonstrated	
312811	Uses equipment correctly	1	2	3	4	5	NA
312812	Verbalizes complications that could occur	1	2	3	4	5	NA
312813	Maintains equipment correctly	1	2	3	4	5	NA
312814	Disposes of equipment correctly	1	2	3	4	5	NA
312815	Maintains needed supplies	1	2	3	4	5	NA
312816	Identifies impact of procedure on lifestyle	1	2	3	4	5	NA
312817	Adapts procedure to lifestyle	1	2	3	4	5	NA
312818	Verbalizes complications that could occur	1	2	3	4	5	NA
312819	Takes action when complications occur	1	2	3	4	5	NA
312820	Monitors treatment effects	1	2	3	4	5	NA
312821	Involves others in procedure as needed	1	2	3	4	5	NA
312822	Keeps appointments with health professional	1	2	3	4	5	NA
312823	Obtains advice from health professional as needed	1	2	3	4	5	NA
312824	Consults with health professional on when to stop procedure	1	2	3	4	5	NA

***Domain**-Health Knowledge & Behavior (IV)*   ***Class**-Health Management (FF)*   *7th edition 2024*

OUTCOME CONTENT REFERENCES:

McConville, H., Harvey, M., Callahan, C., Motley, L., Difilippo, H., & White, C. (2017). CAR T-cell therapy effects. Review of procedures and patient education. *Clinical Journal of Oncology Nursing, 21*(3), E79–E86.

Van Halsema, E. E., Hoen, C. A., de Koning, P. S., Rosmolen, W. D., van Hooft, J. E., & Bergman, J. J. (2018). Self-dilation for therapy-resistant benign esophageal strictures. *Surgical Endoscopy, 32*, 3200–3207. https://doi10.1007//s00464-018-6037-z

Walter, E., Avgush, S., Daly, C., & Crump, C. (2020). The impact of the great recession on diabetes management in a high-risk population. *Journal of Health Care for the Poor and Underserved, 31*(2), 1007–1017. https://doi.org/10.1353/hpu.2020.0074

Self-Management: Treatment Regimen   3129

Definition: Personal actions to manage a therapeutic plan of care

OUTCOME TARGET RATING: Maintain at_____ Increase to_____

		Never Demonstrated	Rarely Demonstrated	Sometimes Demonstrated	Often Demonstrated	Consistently Demonstrated	
OUTCOME OVERALL RATING		1	2	3	4	5	
Indicators:							
312901	Verbalizes relationship between regimen and disease	1	2	3	4	5	NA
312902	Identifies impact of regimen on lifestyle	1	2	3	4	5	NA
312903	Adapts regimen to lifestyle	1	2	3	4	5	NA
312904	Verbalizes purpose of regimen	1	2	3	4	5	NA
312905	Verbalizes parts of regimen	1	2	3	4	5	NA
312906	Verbalizes benefits of regimen	1	2	3	4	5	NA
312907	Reviews regimen with health professional	1	2	3	4	5	NA
312908	Secures financial resource	1	2	3	4	5	NA

Self-Management: Treatment Regimen—cont'd

		Never Demonstrated	Rarely Demonstrated	Sometimes Demonstrated	Often Demonstrated	Consistently Demonstrated	
312909	Follows diet correctly	1	2	3	4	5	NA
312910	Follows physical activity plan	1	2	3	4	5	NA
312911	Takes medication as prescribed	1	2	3	4	5	NA
312912	Follows treatment procedure(s) correctly	1	2	3	4	5	NA
312913	Follows restrictions related to regimen	1	2	3	4	5	NA
312914	Uses equipment correctly	1	2	3	4	5	NA
312915	Maintains equipment correctly	1	2	3	4	5	NA
312916	Disposes of equipment correctly	1	2	3	4	5	NA
312917	Maintains needed supplies	1	2	3	4	5	NA
312918	Verbalizes complications that could occur	1	2	3	4	5	NA
312919	Take actions when complications occur	1	2	3	4	5	NA
312920	Monitors treatment effects	1	2	3	4	5	NA
312921	Involves others in treatment regimen as needed	1	2	3	4	5	NA

Domain-Health Knowledge & Behavior (IV)   **Class**-Health Management (FF)   7th edition 2024

OUTCOME CONTENT REFERENCES:

Despins, L. A., & Wakefield, B. J. (2020). Making sense of blood glucose data and self-management in individuals with type 2 diabetes mellitus: A qualitative study. *Journal of Clinical Nursing, 29*, 2572–2588. https://doi.org/10.1111/jocn.15280

McConville, H., Harvey, M., Callahan, C., Motley, L., Difilippo, H., & White, C. (2017). CAR T-cell therapy effects. Review of procedures and patient education. *Clinical Journal of Oncology Nursing, 21*(3), E79–E86. https://doi.org/10.1007/s11912-018-0662-5

Peltola, M., & Isotalus, P. (2020). Competing discourses of professional-patient relationships in type 2 diabetes management. *Health Communication, 35*(14), 1811–1820. https://doi.org/10.1080/10410236.2019.1663586

Racine, M., Sánchez-Rodríguez, E., de la Veg, R., Galán, S., Solé, E., Jensen, M. P., Miró, J., Moulin, D. E., & Nielson, W. R. (2020). Pain-related activity management patterns as predictors of treatment outcomes in patients with fibromyalgia syndrome. *Pain Medicine, 21*(2), e191–e200. https://doi.org/10.1093/pm/pnz259

Walter, E., Avgush, S., Daly, C., & Crump, C. (2020). The impact of the great recession on diabetes management in a high-risk population. *Journal of Health Care for the Poor and Underserved, 31*(2), 1007–1017. https://doi.org/10.1353/hpu.2020.0074

Self-Management: Wound   **3124**

Definition: Personal actions to manage a surgical incision, puncture, ulcer, or open wound following tissue injury

OUTCOME TARGET RATING: Maintain at_____   Increase to_____

		Never Demonstrated	Rarely Demonstrated	Sometimes Demonstrated	Often Demonstrated	Consistently Demonstrated	
OUTCOME OVERALL RATING		1	2	3	4	5	
Indicators:							
312401	Identifies type of wound and associated risks	1	2	3	4	5	NA
312402	Identifies type of wound closure	1	2	3	4	5	NA
312403	Obtains information about wound care	1	2	3	4	5	NA
312404	Identifies wound care products needed	1	2	3	4	5	NA
312405	Uses pain control strategies	1	2	3	4	5	NA
312406	Obtains needed supplies	1	2	3	4	5	NA
312407	Washes hands prior to wound care	1	2	3	4	5	NA
312408	Uses mirror if needed to view affected area	1	2	3	4	5	NA

Continued

S

Self-Management: Wound—cont'd

		Never Demonstrated	Rarely Demonstrated	Sometimes Demonstrated	Often Demonstrated	Consistently Demonstrated	
312409	Monitors for signs and symptoms of infection	1	2	3	4	5	NA
312410	Monitors affected area with each dressing change	1	2	3	4	5	NA
312411	Cleans wound as instructed	1	2	3	4	5	NA
312412	Follows wound irrigation regimen	1	2	3	4	5	NA
312413	Manages wound drainage system	1	2	3	4	5	NA
312414	Debrides wound as instructed	1	2	3	4	5	NA
312415	Packs wound as instructed	1	2	3	4	5	NA
312416	Uses ointments as prescribed	1	2	3	4	5	NA
312417	Applies dressing to cover wound	1	2	3	4	5	NA
312418	Monitors wound drainage	1	2	3	4	5	NA
312419	Reinforces dressing as needed	1	2	3	4	5	NA
312420	Follows bathing instructions	1	2	3	4	5	NA
312421	Monitors body temperature as instructed	1	2	3	4	5	NA
312422	Reports elevated temperature to health provider	1	2	3	4	5	NA
312423	Reports wound dehiscence to health provider	1	2	3	4	5	NA
312424	Reports increased bleeding to health provider	1	2	3	4	5	NA
312425	Reports increased drainage to health provider	1	2	3	4	5	NA
312426	Washes hands after wound care	1	2	3	4	5	NA
312427	Disposes of contaminated material safely	1	2	3	4	5	NA
312428	Obtains assistance from family member as needed	1	2	3	4	5	NA
312429	Completes antibiotic therapy as prescribed	1	2	3	4	5	NA
312430	Shares history of tape sensitivity with health provider	1	2	3	4	5	NA
312431	Reviews tetanus immunization status with health provider	1	2	3	4	5	NA
312432	Uses sunscreen on skin after healing	1	2	3	4	5	NA
312433	Keeps appointments with health professional	1	2	3	4	5	NA

Domain-Health Knowledge & Behavior (IV)   **Class**-Health Management (FF)   6th edition 2018; reviewed 2024

OUTCOME CONTENT REFERENCES:

Black, K., Cico, S., & Caglar, D. (2015). Wound management. *Pediatrics in Review, 36*(5), 207–216.

Chen, Y.-C., Wang, Y.-C., Chen, W.-K., Smith, M., Huang, H.-M., & Huang, L.-C. (2013). The effectiveness of a health education intervention on self-care of traumatic wounds. *Journal of Clinical Nursing, 22*(17/18), 2499–2508. https://doi.org/10.1111/j.1365-2702.2012.04295.x

Cousins, Y. (2014). Wound care considerations in neonates. *Nursing Standards, 28*(46), 61–70. https://doi.org/10.7748/ns.28.46.61.e8402

Hunt, D. S. (2016). Self-care and postoperative dressing management. *British Journal of Nursing, 25*(Suppl. 15), S34–S41. https://doi.org/10.12968/bjon.2016.25.15.S34

Kapp, S., Miller, C., & Santamaria, N. (2018). The quality of life of people who have chronic wounds and who self-treat. *Journal of Clinical Nursing, 27*(1-2), 182–192. https://doi.org/10.1111/jocn.13870

Kapp, S., & Santamaria, N. (2017). How and why patients self-treat chronic wounds. *International Wound Journal, 14*(6), 1269–1275. https://doi.org/10.1111/iwj.12796

Sensory Function   2405

Definition: Ability to correctly sense skin stimulation, sounds, proprioception, taste and smell, and visual images

OUTCOME TARGET RATING: Maintain at _____ Increase to _____

		Severely Compromised	Substantially Compromised	Moderately Compromised	Mildly Compromised	Not Compromised	
OUTCOME OVERALL RATING		1	2	3	4	5	
Indicators:							
240501	Skin stimulation perception	1	2	3	4	5	NA
240502	Hearing acuity	1	2	3	4	5	NA
240507	Head position perception	1	2	3	4	5	NA
240508	Body position perception	1	2	3	4	5	NA
240504	Odor discrimination	1	2	3	4	5	NA
240505	Taste discrimination	1	2	3	4	5	NA
240506	Visual acuity	1	2	3	4	5	NA

Domain-*Physiologic Health (II)*   **Class**-*Sensory (Y)*   *3rd edition 2004; revised 2008, 2013*

OUTCOME CONTENT REFERENCES:

Chung, J. (2006). Measuring sensory processing patterns of older Chinese people: Psychometric validation of the adult sensory profile. *Aging & Mental Health, 10*(6), 648–655. https://doi.org/10.1080/13607860600648080
LeMone, P., Burke, K., & Bauldoff, G. (2011). *Medical-surgical nursing: Critical thinking in patient care* (5th ed., pp. 258). Pearson Education.
Smeltzer, S., Bare, B., Hinkle, J., & Cheever, K. (2010). *Brunner and Suddarth's textbook of medical-surgical nursing* (12th ed., pp. 325–326). Wolters Kluwer Health.
Swanson, E. A., & Drury, J. (2001). Sensory/perceptual alterations. In M. Maas, K. Buckwalter, M. Hardy, T. Tripp–Reimer, M. Titler, & J. Specht (Eds.), *Nursing care of older adults: Diagnoses, outcomes & interventions* (pp. 476–491). Mosby.

Sensory Function: Hearing   2401

Definition: Ability to correctly sense sounds

OUTCOME TARGET RATING: Maintain at _____ Increase to _____

		Severely Compromised	Substantially Compromised	Moderately Compromised	Mildly Compromised	Not Compromised	
OUTCOME OVERALL RATING		1	2	3	4	5	
Indicators:							
240101	Auditory acuity (left)	1	2	3	4	5	NA
240102	Auditory acuity (right)	1	2	3	4	5	NA
240103	Air conduction of sound (left)	1	2	3	4	5	NA
240112	Air conduction of sound (right)	1	2	3	4	5	NA
240104	Bone conduction of sound (left)	1	2	3	4	5	NA
240113	Bone conduction of sound (right)	1	2	3	4	5	NA
240105	Ratio of air and bone conduction	1	2	3	4	5	NA
240107	Auditory discrimination of discrete sounds	1	2	3	4	5	NA
240108	Hears a whisper 6 inches from left ear (voice test)	1	2	3	4	5	NA
240114	Hears a whisper 6 inches from right ear (voice test)	1	2	3	4	5	NA
240109	Turns to sound	1	2	3	4	5	NA
240110	Responds to auditory stimuli	1	2	3	4	5	NA

S

Continued

Sensory Function: Hearing—cont'd

	Severe	Substantial	Moderate	Mild	None	
240106 Tinnitus (left)	1	2	3	4	5	NA
240115 Tinnitus (right)	1	2	3	4	5	NA
240116 Loss of high-pitched tones	1	2	3	4	5	NA
240117 Loss of ability to distinguish conversation from background environmental noise	1	2	3	4	5	NA

Assistive device YES / NO

Domain-*Physiologic Health (II)*   **Class**-*Sensory (Y)*   *2nd edition 2000; revised 2004, 2008, 2013*

OUTCOME CONTENT REFERENCES:

LeMone, P., Burke, K., & Bauldoff, G. (2011). *Medical-surgical nursing: Critical thinking in patient care* (5th ed., pp. 258). Pearson Education.
Lieu, J., Kenna, M., Anne, S., & Davidson, L. (2020). Hearing loss in children: A review. *Journal of the American Medical Association, 324*(21), 2195–2205. https://doi.org/10.1001/jama.2020.17647
May, J. J. (2000). Occupational hearing loss. *American Journal of Industrial Medicine, 37*(1), 112–120.
Sataloff, J., & Roberts, B. (1999). Differential diagnosis in occupation hearing loss compensation claims. *Journal of Occupation Hearing Loss, 2*(4), 183–189.
Smeltzer, S., Bare, B., Hinkle, J., & Cheever, K. (2010). *Brunner and Suddarth's textbook of medical-surgical nursing* (12th ed., pp. 325–326). Wolters Kluwer Health.
Swanson, E. A., & Drury, J. (2001). Sensory/perceptual alterations. In M. Maas, K. Buckwalter, M. Hardy, T. Tripp–Reimer, M. Titler, & J. Specht (Eds.), *Nursing care of older adults: Diagnoses, outcomes & interventions* (pp. 476–491). Mosby.

Sensory Function: Proprioception   2402

Definition: Ability to correctly sense position and movement of the head and body

OUTCOME TARGET RATING: Maintain at _____ Increase to _____

	Severely Compromised	Substantially Compromised	Moderately Compromised	Mildly Compromised	Not Compromised	
OUTCOME OVERALL RATING	**1**	**2**	**3**	**4**	**5**	
Indicators:						
240201 Head position discrimination	1	2	3	4	5	NA
240202 Head movement discrimination	1	2	3	4	5	NA
240214 Upper limb movement discrimination (right)	1	2	3	4	5	NA
240215 Upper limb movement discrimination (left)	1	2	3	4	5	NA
240216 Lower limb movement discrimination (right)	1	2	3	4	5	NA
240217 Lower limb movement discrimination (left)	1	2	3	4	5	NA
240218 Upper limb position discrimination (right)	1	2	3	4	5	NA
240219 Upper limb position discrimination (left)	1	2	3	4	5	NA
240220 Lower limb position discrimination (right)	1	2	3	4	5	NA
240221 Lower limb position discrimination (left)	1	2	3	4	5	NA
240212 Trunk movement discrimination	1	2	3	4	5	NA
240213 Trunk position discrimination	1	2	3	4	5	NA
240205 Sense of balance	1	2	3	4	5	NA

S

Sensory Function: Proprioception—cont'd

		Severe	Substantial	Moderate	Mild	None	
240206	Vertigo	1	2	3	4	5	NA
240207	Lightheadedness	1	2	3	4	5	NA
240208	Nystagmus	1	2	3	4	5	NA

Domain-Physiologic Health (II)   *Class*-Sensory (Y)   *2nd edition 2000; revised 2004, 2013*

OUTCOME CONTENT REFERENCES:
Boerboom, A., Huizinga, M., Kaan, W., Stewart, R., Hof, A., Bulstra, S., & Diercks, R. (2008). Validation of a method to measure the proprioception of the knee. *Gait & Posture, 28*(4), 610–614. https://doi.org/10.1016/j.gaitpost.2008.04.007
LeMone, P., Burke, K., & Bauldoff, G. (2011). *Medical-surgical nursing: Critical thinking in patient care* (5th ed., pp. 258). Pearson Education.
Smeltzer, S., Bare, B., Hinkle, J., & Cheever, K. (2010). *Brunner and Suddarth's textbook of medical-surgical nursing* (12th ed., pp. 325–326). Wolter Kluwer Health.
Swanson, E. A., & Drury, J. (2001). Sensory/perceptual alterations. In M. Maas, K. Buckwalter, M. Hardy, T. Tripp-Reimer, M. Titler, & J. Specht (Eds.), *Nursing care of older adults: Diagnoses, outcomes & interventions* (pp. 476–491). Mosby.

Sensory Function: Smell 2406

Definition: Ability to correctly sense chemicals or particles that are inhaled

OUTCOME TARGET RATING: Maintain at _____ Increase to _____

		Severely Compromised	Substantially Compromised	Moderately Compromised	Mildly Compromised	Not Compromised	
OUTCOME OVERALL RATING		1	2	3	4	5	
Indicators:							
240601	Odor discrimination	1	2	3	4	5	NA
240602	Fragrance recognition (flowers or perfume)	1	2	3	4	5	NA
240603	Fruity recognition (non-citrus fruits)	1	2	3	4	5	NA
240604	Citrus fruit recognition	1	2	3	4	5	NA
240605	Woody recognition (pine or fresh cut grass)	1	2	3	4	5	NA
240606	Chemical recognition (bleach or ammonia)	1	2	3	4	5	NA
240607	Sweet recognition (chocolate, vanilla, caramel)	1	2	3	4	5	NA
240608	Mint recognition (peppermint)	1	2	3	4	5	NA
240609	Toasted or nut recognition (popcorn or peanut butter)	1	2	3	4	5	NA
240610	Pungent recognition (blue cheese or cigar smoke)	1	2	3	4	5	NA
240611	Decay recognition (sour milk or rotting meat)	1	2	3	4	5	NA

		Severe	Substantial	Moderate	Mild	None	
240612	Odor distortion	1	2	3	4	5	NA
240613	Hemianosmia	1	2	3	4	5	NA
240614	Hyposmia	1	2	3	4	5	NA
240615	Smoking	1	2	3	4	5	NA
240616	Nasal mucous	1	2	3	4	5	NA

Domain-Physiologic Health (II)   *Class*-Sensory (Y)   *7th edition 2024*

S

OUTCOME CONTENT REFERENCES:

Aziz, M., Goyal, H., Haghbin, H., Lee-Smith, W. M., Gajendran, M., & Perisetti, A. (2021). The association of "loss of smell" to COVID-19: A systematic review and meta-analysis. *The American Journal of the Medical Sciences, 361*(2), 216–225. https://doi.org/10.1016/j.amjms.2020.09.017

Fluitman, K. S., Hesp, A. C., Kaihatu, R. F., Nieuwdorp, M., Keijser, B. J. F., Ijzerman, R. G., & Visser, M. (2021). Poor taste and smell are associated with poor appetite, macronutrient intake, and dietary quality but not with undernutrition in older adults. *Journal of Nutrition, 151*(3), 605–614. https://doi.org/10.1093/jn/nxaa400

Huether, S. E., McCance, K. L., & Brashers, V .L. (2020). *Understanding pathophysiology* (7th ed.). Elsevier.

Ignatavicius, D. D., Workman, M. L., Rebar, C. R., & Heimgartner, N. M. (2021). *Medical-surgical nursing: Concepts for interprofessional care* (10th ed.). Elsevier.

McGettigan, N., Dhuibhir, P. U., Barrett, M., Sui, J., Balding, L., Higgins, S., O'Leary, N., Kennedy, A., & Walsh, D. (2019). Subjective and objective assessment of taste and smell sensation in advanced cancer. *American Journal of Hospice & Palliative Medicine, 36*(8), 688–696. https://doi.org/10.1177/1049909119832836

Sensory Function: Tactile 2400

Definition: Ability to correctly sense stimulation of the skin

OUTCOME TARGET RATING: Maintain at _____ Increase to _____

OUTCOME OVERALL RATING	Severely Compromised 1	Substantially Compromised 2	Moderately Compromised 3	Mildly Compromised 4	Not Compromised 5	
Indicators:						
240013 Sharp discrimination	1	2	3	4	5	NA
240014 Dull discrimination	1	2	3	4	5	NA
240002 2-point discrimination	1	2	3	4	5	NA
240003 Vibration discrimination	1	2	3	4	5	NA
240015 Temperature discrimination	1	2	3	4	5	NA
240016 Light touch	1	2	3	4	5	NA
240007 Noxious stimulus discrimination	1	2	3	4	5	NA
240017 Pressure discrimination	1	2	3	4	5	NA
	Severe	**Substantial**	**Moderate**	**Mild**	**None**	
240008 Paresthesia	1	2	3	4	5	NA
240009 Hyperparesthesia	1	2	3	4	5	NA
240011 Tingling	1	2	3	4	5	NA
240012 Loss of sensation	1	2	3	4	5	NA

Domain-*Physiologic Health (II)* **Class**-*Sensory (Y)* 2nd edition 2000; revised 2004, 2013

OUTCOME CONTENT REFERENCES:

LeMone, P., Burke, K., & Bauldoff, G. (2011). *Medical-surgical nursing: Critical thinking in patient care* (5th ed., pp. 258). Pearson Education.

McPoil, T., & Cornwall, M. (2006). Plantar tactile sensory thresholds in healthy men and women. *Foot, 16*(4), 192–397. https://doi.org/10.1111/ajag.12558

Smeltzer, S., Bare, B., Hinkle, J., & Cheever, K. (2010). *Brunner and Suddarth's textbook of medical-surgical nursing* (12th ed., pp. 325–326). Wolters Kluwer Health.

Swanson, E. A., & Drury, J. (2001). Sensory/perceptual alterations. In M. Maas, K. Buckwalter, M. Hardy, T. Tripp-Reimer, M. Titler, & J. Specht (Eds.), *Nursing care of older adults: Diagnoses, outcomes & interventions* (pp. 476–491). Mosby.

S

Sensory Function: Taste

2407

Definition: Ability to correctly sense chemicals or substances dissolved in saliva

OUTCOME TARGET RATING: Maintain at _____ Increase to _____

		Severely Compromised	Substantially Compromised	Moderately Compromised	Mildly Compromised	Not Compromised	
OUTCOME OVERALL RATING		1	2	3	4	5	
Indicators:							
240701	Sweet flavor recognition	1	2	3	4	5	NA
240702	Salty flavor recognition	1	2	3	4	5	NA
240703	Bitter flavor recognition	1	2	3	4	5	NA
240704	Sour flavor recognition	1	2	3	4	5	NA
		Severe	**Substantial**	**Moderate**	**Mild**	**None**	
240705	Taste distortion	1	2	3	4	5	NA
240706	Metallic taste	1	2	3	4	5	NA

Domain-Physiologic Health (II)   *Class*-Sensory (Y)   7th edition 2024

OUTCOME CONTENT REFERENCES:
Aziz, M., Goyal, H., Haghbin, H., Lee-Smith, W. M., Gajendran, M., & Perisetti, A. (2021). The association of "loss of smell" to COVID-19: A systematic review and meta-analysis. *The American Journal of the Medical Sciences, 361*(2), 216–225. https://doi.org/10.1016/j.amjms.2020.09.017
Fluitman, K. S., Hesp, A. C., Kaihatu, R. F., Nieuwdorp, M., Keijser, B. J. F., IJzerman, R. G., & Visser, M. (2021). Poor taste and smell are associated with poor appetite, macronutrient intake, and dietary quality but not with undernutrition in older adults. *Journal of Nutrition, 151*(3), 605–614. https://doi.org/10.1093/jn/nxaa400
Huether, S. E., McCance, K. L., & Brashers, V. L. (2020). *Understanding pathophysiology* (7th ed.). Elsevier.
Ignatavicius, D. D., Workman, M. L., Rebar, C. R., & Heimgartner, N. M. (2021). *Medical-surgical nursing: Concepts for interprofessional care* (10th ed.). Elsevier.
McGettigan, N., Dhuibhir, P. U., Barrett, M., Sui, J., Balding, L., Higgins, S., O'Leary, N., Kennedy, A., & Walsh, D. (2019). Subjective and objective assessment of taste and smell sensation in advanced cancer. *American Journal of Hospice & Palliative Medicine, 36*(8), 688–696. https://doi.org/10.1177/1049909119832836
Sakai, M., Ikeda, M., Kazui, H., Shigenobu, K., & Nishikawa, T. (2016). Decline of gustatory sensitivity with the progression of Alzheimer's disease. *International Psychogeriatrics, 28*(3), 511–517. https://doi.org/10.1017/S1041610215001337
Timmesfeld, N., Kunst, M., Fondel, F., Güldner, C., & Steinbach, S. (2021). Mechanical tongue cleaning is a worthwhile procedure to improve the taste sensation. *Journal of Oral Rehabilitation, 48*(1), 45–54. https://doi.org/10.1111/joor.13099

Sensory Function: Vision

2404

Definition: Ability to correctly sense visual images

OUTCOME TARGET RATING: Maintain at _____ Increase to _____

		Severely Compromised	Substantially Compromised	Moderately Compromised	Mildly Compromised	Not Compromised	
OUTCOME OVERALL RATING		1	2	3	4	5	
Indicators:							
240401	Central visual acuity (left)	1	2	3	4	5	NA
240421	Central visual acuity (right)	1	2	3	4	5	NA
240402	Peripheral visual acuity (left)	1	2	3	4	5	NA
240422	Peripheral visual acuity (right)	1	2	3	4	5	NA
240403	Central visual fields (left)	1	2	3	4	5	NA
240423	Central visual fields (right)	1	2	3	4	5	NA
240404	Peripheral visual fields (left)	1	2	3	4	5	NA
240424	Peripheral visual fields (right)	1	2	3	4	5	NA
240416	Response to visual stimuli	1	2	3	4	5	NA

S

Continued

Sensory Function: Vision—cont'd

		Severe	Substantial	Moderate	Mild	None	
240405	Hemianopia	1	2	3	4	5	NA
240406	Floaters	1	2	3	4	5	NA
240407	Flashes of light	1	2	3	4	5	NA
240408	Halos around lights	1	2	3	4	5	NA
240409	Spiderwebs	1	2	3	4	5	NA
240410	Double vision	1	2	3	4	5	NA
240411	Blurred vision	1	2	3	4	5	NA
240412	Distorted vision	1	2	3	4	5	NA
240413	Color vision distortions	1	2	3	4	5	NA
240414	Night blindness	1	2	3	4	5	NA
240415	Day blindness	1	2	3	4	5	NA
240417	Headaches	1	2	3	4	5	NA
240418	Dizziness	1	2	3	4	5	NA
240419	Eye strain	1	2	3	4	5	NA

Assistive device YES / NO

Domain-*Physiologic Health (II)*   **Class**-*Sensory (Y)*   *2nd edition 2000; revised 2004, 2013*

OUTCOME CONTENT REFERENCES:

LeMone, P., Burke, K., & Bauldoff, G. (2011). *Medical-surgical nursing: Critical thinking in patient care* (5th ed., pp. 258). Pearson Education.

Smeltzer, S., Bare, B., Hinkle, J., & Cheever, K. (2010). *Brunner and Suddarth's textbook of medical-surgical nursing* (12th ed., pp. 325–326). Wolters Kluwer Health.

Swanson, E. A., & Drury, J. (2001). Sensory/perceptual alterations. In M. Maas, K. Buckwalter, M. Hardy, T. Tripp-Reimer, M. Titler, & J. Specht (Eds.), *Nursing care of older adults: Diagnoses, outcomes & interventions* (pp. 476–491). Mosby.

Sexual Functioning   **0119**

Definition: Integration of physical, socioemotional, and intellectual aspects of sexual expression and performance through the stages of sexual desire, arousal, and orgasm, as well as subjective satisfaction

OUTCOME TARGET RATING: Maintain at _____ Increase to _____

		Never Demonstrated	Rarely Demonstrated	Sometimes Demonstrated	Often Demonstrated	Consistently Demonstrated	
OUTCOME OVERALL RATING		1	2	3	4	5	
Indicators:							
011901	Attains sexual arousal	1	2	3	4	5	NA
011902	Sustains penile/clitoral erection through orgasm	1	2	3	4	5	NA
011903	Sustains arousal through orgasm	1	2	3	4	5	NA
011927	Expresses experiencing no pain with intercourse	1	2	3	4	5	NA
011904	Uses assistive device as needed	1	2	3	4	5	NA
011905	Adapts sexual techniques as needed	1	2	3	4	5	NA
011906	Refrains from substance use that adversely affects sexual function	1	2	3	4	5	NA
011928	Uses hormone replacement therapy as needed	1	2	3	4	5	NA

S

Sexual Functioning—cont'd

		Never Demonstrated	Rarely Demonstrated	Sometimes Demonstrated	Often Demonstrated	Consistently Demonstrated	
011929	Expresses ability to perform sexually despite physical disabilities	1	2	3	4	5	NA
011908	Expresses comfort with sexual expression	1	2	3	4	5	NA
011909	Expresses self-esteem	1	2	3	4	5	NA
011910	Expresses comfort with body	1	2	3	4	5	NA
011911	Expresses sexual interest	1	2	3	4	5	NA
011930	Expresses desire to be intimate	1	2	3	4	5	NA
011913	Expresses willingness to be sexual	1	2	3	4	5	NA
011914	Reports available consenting partner	1	2	3	4	5	NA
011915	Expresses respect for partner	1	2	3	4	5	NA
011916	Expresses acceptance of partner	1	2	3	4	5	NA
011917	Expresses knowledge of partner's sexual capabilities	1	2	3	4	5	NA
011918	Expresses knowledge of personal sexual capabilities	1	2	3	4	5	NA
011919	Expresses knowledge of partner's sexual needs	1	2	3	4	5	NA
011920	Expresses knowledge of personal sexual needs	1	2	3	4	5	NA
011921	Communicates comfortably with partner	1	2	3	4	5	NA
011922	Communicates sexual needs with partner	1	2	3	4	5	NA
011923	Communicates sexual preferences with partner	1	2	3	4	5	NA
011924	Performs sexually if environment conducive	1	2	3	4	5	NA
011931	Discusses level of commitment with partner	1	2	3	4	5	NA
011925	Performs sexually without coercion of partner	1	2	3	4	5	NA
011932	Expresses satisfaction with sexual experiences	1	2	3	4	5	NA

Domain-Functional Health (I)   **Class**-Growth & Development (B)   2nd edition 2000; revised 2004, 2008, 2024

OUTCOME CONTENT REFERENCES:

Aepfelbacher, J. A., Chaudhury, C. S., Mee, T., Purdy, J. B., Hawkins, K., Curl, K. A., Dee, N., & Hadigan, C. (2020). Reproductive and sexual health knowledge, experiences, and milestones in young adults with life-long HIV. *AIDS Care, 32*(3), 354–361. https://doi.org/10.1080/09540121.2019.1679711

Byers, E. S., O'Sullivan, L. F., & Hughes, K. (2021). Sexual functioning of late adolescents and young adults in relationships: Association with individual characteristics and relationship factors. *Sexual & Relationship Therapy, 36*(2/3), 178–197. https://doi.org/10.1080/14681994.2019.1626982

Den Ouden, M. E. M., Pelgrum-Keurhorst, M. N., Uitdehaag, M. J., & De Vocht, H. M. (2019). Intimacy and sexuality in women with breast cancer: Professional guidance needed. *Breast Cancer, 26*(3), 326–332. https://doi.org/10.1007/s12282018-0927-8

Ejegi-Memeh, S., Hinchliff, S., & Johnson, M. (2021). Sexual health discussions between healthcare professionals and midlife-older women living with type 2 diabetes: An interpretative phenomenological study. *Journal of Advanced Nursing, 77*(3), 1411–1421. https://doi.org/10.1111/jan.14688

Heath, H. (2019). Sexuality and sexual intimacy in later life. *Nursing Older People, 31*(1), 40–48. https://doi.org/10.7748/nop.2019.e1102

Nimbi, F. M., Rossi, V., Tripodi, F., Luria, M., Flinchum, M., Tambelli, R., & Simonelli, C. (2020). Genital pain and sexual functioning: Effects on sexual experience, psychological health, and quality of life. *The Journal of Sexual Medicine, 17*(4), 771–783. https://doi.org/10.1016/j.jsxm.2020.01.014

Tarkowska, M., Głowacka-Mrotek, I., Nowikiewicz, T., Monastyrska-Waszak, E., Gastecka, A., Goch, A., & Zegarski, W. (2020). Sexual functioning and self-esteem in women after mastectomy—A single-centre, non-randomised, cross-sectional study. *Contemporary Oncology* (Poznan, Poland), *24*(2), 106–111. https://doi.org/10.5114/wo.2020.95876

Wang, P., Ai, J., Davidson, P. M., Slater, T., Du, R., & Chen, C. (2019). Nurses' attitudes, beliefs and practices on sexuality for cardiovascular care: A cross-sectional study. *Journal of Clinical Nursing, 28*(5–6), 980–986. https://doi.org/10.1111/jocn.14692

S

Sexual Identity

Definition: Acknowledgment and acceptance of one's personal sexual orientation, desires, romantic or sexual attractions, and behaviors

OUTCOME TARGET RATING: Maintain at _____ Increase to _____

	Never Demonstrated	Rarely Demonstrated	Sometimes Demonstrated	Often Demonstrated	Consistently Demonstrated	
OUTCOME OVERALL RATING	**1**	**2**	**3**	**4**	**5**	
Indicators:						
120701	Affirms self as a sexual being	1	2	3	4	5	NA
120702	Exhibits clear sense of sexual orientation	1	2	3	4	5	NA
120703	Exhibits comfort with sexual orientation	1	2	3	4	5	NA
120716	Shares sexual orientation with others	1	2	3	4	5	NA
120704	Integrates sexual orientation into life roles	1	2	3	4	5	NA
120706	Uses healthy coping behaviors to resolve sexual identity issues	1	2	3	4	5	NA
120717	Shares stressful or negative feelings about sexual identity	1	2	3	4	5	NA
120707	Challenges negative images of sexual self	1	2	3	4	5	NA
120708	Seeks social support	1	2	3	4	5	NA
120709	Reports healthy intimate relationships	1	2	3	4	5	NA
120710	Reports healthy sexual functioning	1	2	3	4	5	NA
120711	Describes risks associated with sexual activity	1	2	3	4	5	NA
120712	Uses precautions to minimize risks associated with sexual activity	1	2	3	4	5	NA
120713	Describes personal sexual value system	1	2	3	4	5	NA
120714	Sets personal sexual boundaries	1	2	3	4	5	NA

Domain-*Psychosocial Health (III)*   **Class**-*Psychological Well-Being (M)*   *2nd edition 2000; revised 2004, 2008, 2024*

OUTCOME CONTENT REFERENCES:

Bjarnadottir, R. I., Bockting, W., Trifilio, M., & Dowding, D. W. (2019). Assessing sexual orientation and gender identity in home health care: Perceptions and attitudes of nurses. *LGBT Health*, 6(8), 409–416. https://doi.org/10.1089/lgbt.2019.0030

Evans-Polce, R. J., Veliz, P. T., Boyd, C. J., Hughes, T. L., & McCabe, S. E. (2020). Associations between sexual orientation discrimination and substance use disorders: Differences by age in U.S. adults. *Social Psychiatry and Psychiatric Epidemiology*, 55(1), 101–110. https://doi.org/10.1007/s00127-019-01694-x

Hockenberry, M. J., Wilson, D., & Rodgers, C. C. (Eds.). (2019). *Wong's nursing care of infants and children* (11th ed.). Elsevier.

Luctkar-Flude, M., Tyerman, J., Ziegler, E., Carroll, B., Shortall, C., Chumbley, L., & Tregunno, D. (2020). Developing a sexual orientation and gender identity nursing education toolkit. *Journal of Continuing Education in Nursing*, 51(9), 412–419. https://doi.org/10.3928/00220124-20200812-06

Stewart, J. L., Spivey, L. A., Widman, L., Choukas-Bradley, S., & Prinstein, M. J. (2019). Developmental patterns of sexual identity, romantic attraction, and sexual behavior among adolescents over three years. *Journal of Adolescence*, 77, 90–97. https://doi.org/10.1016/j.adolescence.2019.10.006

Suen, L. W., Lunn, M. R., Katuzny, K., Finn, S., Duncan, L., Sevelius, J., Flentje, A., Capriotti, M. R., Lubensky, M. E., Hunt, C., Weber, S., Bibbins-Domingo, K., & Obedin-Maliver, J. (2020). What sexual and gender minority people want researchers to know about sexual orientation and gender identity questions: A qualitative study. *Archives of Sexual Behavior*, 49(7), 2301–2318. https://doi.org/10.1007/s10508-020-01810-y

Veliz, P. T., McCabe, S. E., Hughes, T. L., Everett, B. G., Caceres, B. A., & Arslanian-Engoren, C. (2020). Sexual orientation and hypertension risk reduction behaviors among adults with high blood pressure. *Annals of LGBTQ Public and Population Health, 1*(2), 115–127. https://doi.org/10.1891/lgbtq-2019-0011

S

Shock Severity: Anaphylactic   0417

Definition: Severity of signs and symptoms of blood flow inadequate to perfuse tissues due to vasodilation and capillary permeability with a rapid-onset systemic hypersensitivity reaction

OUTCOME TARGET RATING: Maintain at_____ Increase to_____

		Severe	Substantial	Moderate	Mild	None	
OUTCOME OVERALL RATING		1	2	3	4	5	
Indicators:							
041701	Decreased systolic blood pressure	1	2	3	4	5	NA
041702	Decreased diastolic blood pressure	1	2	3	4	5	NA
041703	Increased heart rate	1	2	3	4	5	NA
041704	Arrhythmias	1	2	3	4	5	NA
041705	Rhinitis	1	2	3	4	5	NA
041706	Respiratory wheezes	1	2	3	4	5	NA
041707	Respiratory stridor	1	2	3	4	5	NA
041708	Laryngospasm	1	2	3	4	5	NA
041709	Bronchospasm	1	2	3	4	5	NA
041710	Dyspnea	1	2	3	4	5	NA
041711	Decrease in arterial oxygen	1	2	3	4	5	NA
041712	Warm, flushed skin	1	2	3	4	5	NA
041713	Edema of the lips, eyelids, tongue	1	2	3	4	5	NA
041714	Angioedema	1	2	3	4	5	NA
041715	Edema of hands and feet	1	2	3	4	5	NA
041716	Edema of genitalia	1	2	3	4	5	NA
041717	Parathesias	1	2	3	4	5	NA
041718	Pruritus	1	2	3	4	5	NA
041719	Abdominal cramps	1	2	3	4	5	NA
041720	Vomiting	1	2	3	4	5	NA
041721	Diarrhea	1	2	3	4	5	NA
041722	Decreased urine output	1	2	3	4	5	NA
041723	Panic	1	2	3	4	5	NA
041724	Decreased level of consciousness	1	2	3	4	5	NA

Domain-*Physiologic Health (II)*   **Class**-*Cardiopulmonary (E)*   *5th edition 2013*

OUTCOME CONTENT REFERENCES:

LeMone, P., Burke, K., & Bauldoff, G. (2011). *Medical-surgical nursing: Critical thinking in patient care* (5th ed., pp. 260–261). Pearson Education.

Limsuwan, T., & Demoly, P. (2010). Acute symptoms of drug hypersensitivity (urticaria, angioedema, anaphylaxis, anaphylactic shock). *Medical Clinics of North America, 94*(4), 691–710. https://doi.org/10.1016/j.mcna.2010.03.007

Smeltzer, S., Bare, B., Hinkle, J., & Cheever, K. (2010). *Brunner and Suddarth's textbook of medical-surgical nursing* (12th ed., pp. 327–332). Wolters Kluwer Health.

Wilmot, L. (2010). Shock: Early recognition and management. *Journal of Emergency Nursing, 36*(2), 134–139. https://doi.org/10.1016/j.jen.2009.05.021

Younker, J., & Soar, J. (2010). Recognition and treatment of anaphylaxis. *Nursing in Critical Care, 15*(2), 94–98. https://doi.org/10.1111/j.1478-5153.2010.00366.x

S

Shock Severity: Cardiogenic   0418

Definition: Severity of signs and symptoms of blood flow inadequate to perfuse tissues due to the heart's inability to contract and pump blood

OUTCOME TARGET RATING: Maintain at_____ Increase to_____

OUTCOME OVERALL RATING		Severe	Substantial	Moderate	Mild	None	
		1	2	3	4	5	
Indicators:							
041801	Decreased pulse pressure	1	2	3	4	5	NA
041802	Decreased mean arterial pressure	1	2	3	4	5	NA
041803	Decreased systolic blood pressure	1	2	3	4	5	NA
041804	Decreased diastolic blood pressure	1	2	3	4	5	NA
041805	Prolonged capillary refill time	1	2	3	4	5	NA
041806	Increased central venous pressure	1	2	3	4	5	NA
041807	Increased heart rate	1	2	3	4	5	NA
041808	Weak, thready pulse	1	2	3	4	5	NA
041809	Arrhythmias	1	2	3	4	5	NA
041810	Chest pain	1	2	3	4	5	NA
041811	Increased respiratory rate	1	2	3	4	5	NA
041812	Crackles in lungs	1	2	3	4	5	NA
041813	Pulmonary edema	1	2	3	4	5	NA
041814	Decreased arterial oxygen	1	2	3	4	5	NA
041815	Increased arterial carbon dioxide	1	2	3	4	5	NA
041816	Cyanosis	1	2	3	4	5	NA
041817	Cold moist skin	1	2	3	4	5	NA
041818	Pallor	1	2	3	4	5	NA
041819	Distention of veins in neck	1	2	3	4	5	NA
041820	Dependent edema	1	2	3	4	5	NA
041821	Decreased urine output	1	2	3	4	5	NA
041822	Restlessness	1	2	3	4	5	NA
041823	Anxiety	1	2	3	4	5	NA
041824	Feelings of doom	1	2	3	4	5	NA
041825	Decreased level of consciousness	1	2	3	4	5	NA
041826	Metabolic acidosis	1	2	3	4	5	NA

Domain-*Physiologic Health (II)*   **Class**-*Cardiopulmonary (E)*   *5th edition 2013*

OUTCOME CONTENT REFERENCES:
Garrestson, G., & Malberti, S. (2007). Understanding hypovolaemic, cardiogenic, and septic shock. *Nursing Standard, 21*(50), 46–55. https://doi.org/10.7748/ns2007.08.21.50.46.c4608

Josephson, L. (2008). Cardiogenic shock. *Dimensions of Critical Care Nursing, 27*(4), 160–170.

Kelley, D. (2005). Hypovolemic shock: An overview. *Critical Care Nursing Quarterly, 28*(1), 2–19. https://doi.org/10.1097/00002727-200501000-00002

LeMone, P., Burke, K., & Bauldoff, G. (2011). *Medical-surgical nursing: Critical thinking in patient care* (5th ed., pp. 258). Pearson Education.

Scottish Intercollegiate Guidelines Network (SIGN). (2007). *Acute coronary syndromes. A national clinical guideline.*

Smeltzer, S., Bare, B., Hinkle, J., & Cheever, K. (2010). *Brunner and Suddarth's textbook of medical-surgical nursing* (12th ed., pp. 325–326). Wolters Kluwer Health.

Wilmot, L. (2010). Shock: Early recognition and management. *Journal of Emergency Nursing, 36*(2), 134–139. https://doi.org/10.1111/j.1478-5153.2010.00366.x

S

Shock Severity: Hypovolemic   0419

Definition: Severity of signs and symptoms of blood flow inadequate to perfuse tissues due to a severe decrease in intravascular fluid volume

OUTCOME TARGET RATING: Maintain at_____ Increase to_____

		Severe	Substantial	Moderate	Mild	None	
OUTCOME OVERALL RATING		1	2	3	4	5	
Indicators:							
041901	Decreased pulse pressure	1	2	3	4	5	NA
041902	Decreased mean arterial pressure	1	2	3	4	5	NA
041903	Decreased systolic blood pressure	1	2	3	4	5	NA
041904	Decreased diastolic blood pressure	1	2	3	4	5	NA
041905	Delayed capillary refill	1	2	3	4	5	NA
041906	Increased heart rate	1	2	3	4	5	NA
041907	Weak, thready pulse	1	2	3	4	5	NA
041908	Arrhythmias	1	2	3	4	5	NA
041909	Chest pain	1	2	3	4	5	NA
041910	Increased respiratory rate	1	2	3	4	5	NA
041911	Shallow respirations	1	2	3	4	5	NA
041912	Crackles in lungs	1	2	3	4	5	NA
041913	Decreased arterial oxygen	1	2	3	4	5	NA
041914	Increased arterial carbon dioxide	1	2	3	4	5	NA
041915	Cold clammy skin	1	2	3	4	5	NA
041916	Pallor	1	2	3	4	5	NA
041917	Prolonged coagulation times	1	2	3	4	5	NA
041918	Hypoactive bowel sounds	1	2	3	4	5	NA
041919	Thirst	1	2	3	4	5	NA
041920	Decreased urine output	1	2	3	4	5	NA
041921	Confusion	1	2	3	4	5	NA
041922	Lethargy	1	2	3	4	5	NA
041923	Decreased level of consciousness	1	2	3	4	5	NA
041924	Sluggish pupil response	1	2	3	4	5	NA
041925	Metabolic acidosis	1	2	3	4	5	NA
041926	Hyperkalemia	1	2	3	4	5	NA

Domain-*Physiologic Health (II)*   *Class*-*Cardiopulmonary (E)*   *5th edition 2013*

OUTCOME CONTENT REFERENCES:

Garrestson, G., & Malberti, S. (2007). Understanding hypovolaemic, cardiogenic, and septic shock. *Nursing Standard, 21*(50), 46–55. https://doi.org/10.7748/ns2007.08.21.50.46.c4608

LeMone, P., Burke, K., & Bauldoff, G. (2011). *Medical-surgical nursing: Critical thinking in patient care* (5th ed., pp. 253–267). Pearson Education.

Smeltzer, S., Bare, B., Hinkle, J., & Cheever, K. (2010). *Brunner and Suddarth's textbook of medical-surgical nursing* (12th ed., pp. 322–324). Wolters Kluwer Health.

Wilmot, L. (2010). Shock: Early recognition and management. *Journal of Emergency Nursing, 36*(2), 134–139. https://doi.org/10.1111/j.1478-5153.2010.00366.x

S

Shock Severity: Neurogenic

0420

Definition: Severity of signs and symptoms of blood flow inadequate to perfuse tissues due to sustained vasodilation resulting from a parasympathetic-sympathetic system imbalance

OUTCOME TARGET RATING: Maintain at_____ Increase to_____

	Severe	Substantial	Moderate	Mild	None	
OUTCOME OVERALL RATING	1	2	3	4	5	
Indicators:						
042001 Bounding pulse	1	2	3	4	5	NA
042002 Decreased heart rate	1	2	3	4	5	NA
042003 Decreased systolic blood pressure	1	2	3	4	5	NA
042004 Decreased diastolic blood pressure	1	2	3	4	5	NA
042005 Increased heart rate	1	2	3	4	5	NA
042006 Arrhythmias	1	2	3	4	5	NA
042007 Respiratory changes	1	2	3	4	5	NA
042008 Decreased arterial oxygen	1	2	3	4	5	NA
042009 Warm, dry skin	1	2	3	4	5	NA
042010 Cold, clammy skin	1	2	3	4	5	NA
042011 Decreased body temperature	1	2	3	4	5	NA
042012 Decreased urine output	1	2	3	4	5	NA
042013 Hypoactive bowel sounds	1	2	3	4	5	NA
042014 Restlessness	1	2	3	4	5	NA
042015 Anxiety	1	2	3	4	5	NA
042016 Lethargy	1	2	3	4	5	NA
042017 Decreased level of consciousness	1	2	3	4	5	NA
042018 Dilated pupils	1	2	3	4	5	NA
042019 Sluggish pupil response	1	2	3	4	5	NA

Domain-*Physiologic Health (II)*   **Class**-*Cardiopulmonary (E)*   *5th edition 2013*

OUTCOME CONTENT REFERENCES:

Guly, H., Bouamra, O., & Lecky, F. (2007). The incidence of neurogenic shock in patients with isolated spinal cord injury in the emergency department. *Resuscitation, 76*(1), 57–62.

King, K., & Olson, D. (2007). What you should know about neurogenic shock. *American Nurse Today, 2*(2), 36, 38.

LeMone, P., Burke, K., & Bauldoff, G. (2011). *Critical thinking in patient care* (5th ed., pp. 259–260). Pearson Education.

Smeltzer, S., Bare, B., Hinkle, J., & Cheever, K. (2010). *Brunner and Suddarth's textbook of medical-surgical nursing* (12th ed., pp. 328). Wolters Kluwer Health.

Wilmot, L. (2010). Shock: Early recognition and management. *Journal of Emergency Nursing, 36*(2), 134–139. https://doi.org/10.1111/j.1478-5153.2010.00366.x

S

Shock Severity: Septic

0421

Definition: Severity of signs and symptoms of blood flow inadequate to perfuse tissues due to vasodilation resulting from the release of endotoxins with widespread infection

OUTCOME TARGET RATING: Maintain at_____ Increase to_____

	Severe	Substantial	Moderate	Mild	None	
OUTCOME OVERALL RATING	1	2	3	4	5	
Indicators:						
042101 Decreased systolic blood pressure	1	2	3	4	5	NA
042102 Decreased diastolic blood pressure	1	2	3	4	5	NA
042103 Increased heart rate	1	2	3	4	5	NA
042104 Weak, thready pulse	1	2	3	4	5	NA

Shock Severity: Septic—cont'd

		Severe	Substantial	Moderate	Mild	None	
042105	Arrhythmias	1	2	3	4	5	NA
042106	Increased respiratory rate	1	2	3	4	5	NA
042107	Increased depth of respirations	1	2	3	4	5	NA
042108	Shallow respirations	1	2	3	4	5	NA
042109	Dyspnea	1	2	3	4	5	NA
042110	Decreased arterial oxygen	1	2	3	4	5	NA
042111	Increased body temperature	1	2	3	4	5	NA
042112	Chills	1	2	3	4	5	NA
042113	Warm, flushed skin	1	2	3	4	5	NA
042114	Decreased body temperature	1	2	3	4	5	NA
042115	Cold, clammy skin	1	2	3	4	5	NA
042116	Pallor	1	2	3	4	5	NA
042117	Intravascular clotting	1	2	3	4	5	NA
042118	Decreased urine output	1	2	3	4	5	NA
042119	Hypoactive bowel sounds	1	2	3	4	5	NA
042120	Nausea	1	2	3	4	5	NA
042121	Vomiting	1	2	3	4	5	NA
042122	Diarrhea	1	2	3	4	5	NA
042123	Confusion	1	2	3	4	5	NA
042124	Lethargy	1	2	3	4	5	NA
042125	Decreased level of consciousness	1	2	3	4	5	NA
042126	Metabolic acidosis	1	2	3	4	5	NA

Domain-Physiologic Health (II)   **Class**-Cardiopulmonary (E)   5th edition 2013

OUTCOME CONTENT REFERENCES:

Chen, W., & Kuo, C. (2007). Characteristics of heart rate variability can predict impending septic shock in emergency department patients with sepsis. *Academic Emergency Medicine, 14*(5), 392–397. https://doi.org/10.1197/j.aem.2006.12.015

Garrestson, G., & Malberti, S. (2007). Understanding hypovolaemic, cardiogenic, and septic shock. *Nursing Standard, 21*(50), 46–55.

LeMone, P., Burke, K., & Bauldoff, G. (2011). *Medical-surgical nursing: Critical thinking in patient care* (5th ed., pp. 259). Pearson Education.

Smeltzer, S., Bare, B., Hinkle, J., & Cheever, K. (2010). *Brunner and Suddarth's textbook of medical-surgical nursing* (12th ed., pp. 328–331). Wolters Kluwer Health.

Wilmot, L. (2010). Shock: Early recognition and management. *Journal of Emergency Nursing, 36*(2), 134–139. https://doi.org/10.1111/j.1478-5153.2010.00366.x

Skeletal Function

0211

Definition: Ability of the bones to support the body and facilitate movement

OUTCOME TARGET RATING: Maintain at _____ Increase to _____

		Severely Compromised	Substantially Compromised	Moderately Compromised	Mildly Compromised	Not Compromised	
OUTCOME OVERALL RATING		1	2	3	4	5	
Indicators:							
021101	Bone integrity	1	2	3	4	5	NA
021102	Bone density	1	2	3	4	5	NA
021103	Joint movement	1	2	3	4	5	NA
021104	Weight bearing	1	2	3	4	5	NA
021105	Skeletal alignment	1	2	3	4	5	NA
021106	Joint stability	1	2	3	4	5	NA

Domain-Functional Health (I)   **Class**-Mobility (C)   2nd edition 2000; revised 2004; reviewed 2018

S

OUTCOME CONTENT REFERENCES:

Kindler, J. M., Lewis, R. D., & Hamrick, M. W. (2015). Skeletal muscle and pediatric bone development. *Current Opinion in Endocrinology, Diabetes & Obesity, 22*(6), 467–474. https://doi.org/10.1097/MED.000000000000201

Maier, G. S., Seeger, J. B., Horas, K., Roth, K. E., Kurth, A. A., & Maus, U. (2015). The prevalence of vitamin D deficiency in patients with vertebral fragility fractures. *Bone & Joint Journal, 97-B*(1), 89–93. https://doi.org/10.1302/0301-620X.97B1.34558

Specker, B., Thiex, N. W., & Sudhagoni, R. G. (2015). Does exercise influence pediatric bone? A systematic review. *Clinical Orthopaedics & Related Research, 473*(11), 3658–3672. https://doi.org/10.1007/s11999-015-4467-7

Turner, B., Ali, S., Drudge-Coates, L., Pati, J., Nargund, V., & Wells, P. (2016). Skeletal health part 1: Overview of bone health and management in the cancer setting. *Urologic Nursing, 36*(1), 17–21, 26.

Turner, B., Ali, S., Drudge-Coates, L., Pati, J., Nargund, V., & Wells, P. (2016). Skeletal health part 2: Development of a nurse practitioner bone support clinic for urologic patients. *Urologic Nursing, 36*(1), 22–26.

Sleep 0004

Definition: Natural periodic suspension of consciousness and decreased physical activity every 24 hours during which the body is restored

OUTCOME TARGET RATING: Maintain at _____ Increase to _____

	Severely Compromised	Substantially Compromised	Moderately Compromised	Mildly Compromised	Not Compromised	
OUTCOME OVERALL RATING	1	2	3	4	5	
Indicators:						
000401 Hours of sleep per night	1	2	3	4	5	NA
000402 Observed hours of sleep	1	2	3	4	5	NA
000403 Sleep pattern	1	2	3	4	5	NA
000404 Sleep quality	1	2	3	4	5	NA
000405 Sleep efficiency	1	2	3	4	5	NA
000407 Sleep routine	1	2	3	4	5	NA
000418 Sleeps through the night	1	2	3	4	5	NA
000408 Feelings of rejuvenation after sleep	1	2	3	4	5	NA
000410 Wakeful at appropriate times	1	2	3	4	5	NA

Domain-*Functional Health (I)* **Class**-*Energy Maintenance (A)* *1st edition 1997; revised 2000, 2004, 2008, 2024*

OUTCOME CONTENT REFERENCES:

+Buysse, D. J., Reynolds, C. F., III, Monk, T. H., Berman, S. R., & Kupfer, D. J. (1989). The Pittsburgh Sleep Quality Index: A new instrument for psychiatric practice and research. *Psychiatry Research, 28*(2), 193–213. https://doi.org/10.1016/0165-1781(89)90047-4

Chaiard, J., & Weaver, T. E. (2019). Update on research and practices in major sleep disorders: Part I. Obstructive sleep apnea syndrome. *Journal of Nursing Scholarship, 51*(5), 500–508. https://doi.org/10.1111/jnu.12489

Chaiard, J., & Weaver, T. E. (2019). Update on research and practices in major sleep disorders: Part II-Insomnia, Willis Ekbom disease (restless leg syndrome), and narcolepsy. *Journal of Nursing Scholarship, 51*(6), 624–633. https://doi.org/10.1111/jnu.12515

Chasens, E. R., Imes, C. C., Kariuki, J. K., Luyster, F. S., Morris, J. L., DiNardo, C. M., Jeon, G. B., & Yang, K. (2021). Sleep and metabolic syndrome. *Nursing Clinics of North America, 56*(2), 203–217. https://doi.org/10.1016/j.cnur.2020.10.012

Khubchandani, J., & Price, J. H. (2020). Short sleep duration in working American adults, 2010–2018. *Journal of Community Health, 45*(2), 219–227. https://doi.org/10.1007/s10900-019-00731-9

Knell, G., Durand, C. P., Kohl, H. W., III., Wu, I. H. C., & Pettee Gabriel, K. (2019). Prevalence and likelihood of meeting sleep, physical activity, and screen-time guidelines among U.S. youth. *Journal of American Medical Association Pediatrics, 173*(4), 387–389. https://doi.org/10.1001/jamapediatrics.2018.4847

Paruthi, S., Brooks, L. J., D'Ambrosio, C., Hall, W. A., Kotagal, S., Lloyd, R. M., Malow, B. A., Maski, K., Nichols, C., Quan, S. F., Rosen, C. L., Troester, M. M., & Wise, M. S. (2016). Consensus statement of the American Academy of Sleep Medicine on the recommended amount of sleep for healthy children: Methodology and discussion. *Journal of Clinical Sleep Medicine (JCSM), 12*(11), 1549–1561. https://doi.org/10.5664/jcsm.6288

Potter, P. A., Perry, A. G., Stockert, P., & Hall, A. (2021). *Fundamentals of nursing* (10th ed.). Elsevier.

Williams, P. (2020). *Basic geriatric nursing* (7th ed.). Elsevier.

Sleep Disruption Severity   **2119**

Definition: Severity of sleep pattern interferences in adults

OUTCOME TARGET RATING: Maintain at_____ Increase to_____

		Severe	Substantial	Moderate	Mild	None	
OUTCOME OVERALL RATING		1	2	3	4	5	
Indicators:							
211901	Difficulty getting to sleep	1	2	3	4	5	NA
211902	Difficulty staying asleep	1	2	3	4	5	NA
211903	Early morning awakening	1	2	3	4	5	NA
211904	Non-restorative sleep	1	2	3	4	5	NA
211905	Insomnia	1	2	3	4	5	NA
211906	Interrupted sleep	1	2	3	4	5	NA
211907	Daytime sleepiness	1	2	3	4	5	NA
211908	Pain	1	2	3	4	5	NA
211909	Discomfort	1	2	3	4	5	NA
211910	Disruptive leg cramps	1	2	3	4	5	NA
211911	Disruptive muscle aches	1	2	3	4	5	NA
211912	Night-time coughing	1	2	3	4	5	NA
211913	Sleep apnea	1	2	3	4	5	NA
211914	Snoring	1	2	3	4	5	NA
211915	Dependence on sleep aids	1	2	3	4	5	NA
211916	Nightmares	1	2	3	4	5	NA
211917	Racing thoughts	1	2	3	4	5	NA
211918	Nocturia	1	2	3	4	5	NA
211919	Noisy sleep environment	1	2	3	4	5	NA
211920	Lighted sleep environment	1	2	3	4	5	NA
211921	Emotional distress	1	2	3	4	5	NA
211922	Sleep walking	1	2	3	4	5	NA
211923	Disruptions from sleep partner	1	2	3	4	5	NA
211924	Disruptions from family members	1	2	3	4	5	NA

Domain-*Health & Life Quality (V)*   **Class**-*Symptom Status (V)*   *7th edition 2024*

OUTCOME CONTENT REFERENCES:

Aydın Sayılan, A., Kulakaç, N., & Sayılan S. (2021). The effects of noise levels on pain, anxiety, and sleep in patients. *Nursing in Critical Care, 26*, 79–85. https://doi.org/10.1111/nicc.12525

Bani Younis, M., Hayajneh, F., & Alshraideh, J. A. (2021). Effect of noise and light levels on sleep of intensive care unit patients. *Nursing in Critical Care, 26*(2), 73–78. https://doi.org/10.1111/nicc.12490

Chaiard, J., & Weaver, T.E. (2019), Update on research and practices in major sleep disorders: Part II-Insomnia, Willis Ekbom disease (restless leg syndrome), and narcolepsy. *Journal of Nursing Scholarship, 5*(6), 624–633. https://doi.org/10.1111/jnu.12515

Chasens, E. R., Imes, C. C., Kariuki, J. K., Luyster, F. S., Morris, J. L., DiNardo, C. M., Jeon, G. B., & Yang, K. (2021). Sleep and metabolic syndrome. *Nursing Clinics of North America, 56*(2), 203–217. https://doi.org/10.1016/j.cnur.2020.10.012

Ignatavicius, D. D., Workman, M. L., Rebar, C. R., & Heimgartner, N. M. (2021). *Medical-surgical nursing: Concepts for interprofessional care* (10th ed.). Elsevier.

Lichuan Ye, R. L., & Owens, P. D. (2019). Individualized sleep promotion in acute care hospitals: Identifying factors that affect patient sleep. *Applied Nursing Research, 48*, 63–67. https://doi.org/10.1016/j.apnr.2019.05.006

Potter, P. A., Perry, A. G., Stockert, P., & Hall, A. (2021). *Fundamentals of nursing* (10th ed.). Elsevier.

Reuter-Rice, K., McMurray, M. G., Christoferson, E., Yeager, H., & Wiggins, B. (2020). Sleep in the intensive care unit: Biological, environmental, and pharmacologic implications for nurses. *Critical Care Nursing Clinics of North America, 32*(2), 191–201. https://doi.org/10.1016/j.cnc.2020.02.002

Williams, P. (2020). *Basic geriatric nursing* (7th ed.). Elsevier.

S

Sleep Enhancement Behavior   1642

Definition: Personal actions to enhance sleep quality, pattern, efficiency, and routine to improve health and illness recovery

OUTCOME TARGET RATING: Maintain at_____ Increase to_____

		Never Demonstrated	Rarely Demonstrated	Sometimes Demonstrated	Often Demonstrated	Consistently Demonstrated	
OUTCOME OVERALL RATING		1	2	3	4	5	
Indicators:							
164201	Recognizes the important role of sleep in staying healthy	1	2	3	4	5	NA
164202	Sets a bedtime early enough for at least 7 to 8 hours of sleep	1	2	3	4	5	NA
164203	Adjusts work-life balance to improve sleep	1	2	3	4	5	NA
164204	Keeps a specific sleep schedule	1	2	3	4	5	NA
164205	Adjusts sleep schedule gradually for time change	1	2	3	4	5	NA
164206	Evaluates the impact of work schedule on sleep pattern	1	2	3	4	5	NA
164207	Exercises daily	1	2	3	4	5	NA
164208	Uses bed for only sleep and sex	1	2	3	4	5	NA
164209	Maintains a healthy diet with plenty of fiber	1	2	3	4	5	NA
164210	Limits daytime napping to 20 minutes early in the afternoon	1	2	3	4	5	NA
164211	Limits exposure to bright lights in the evening	1	2	3	4	5	NA
164212	Develops a relaxing bedtime routine	1	2	3	4	5	NA
164213	Uses relaxation techniques as part of bedtime routine when needed	1	2	3	4	5	NA
164214	Takes a warm bath or shower at bedtime	1	2	3	4	5	NA
164215	Goes to bed only when sleepy	1	2	3	4	5	NA
164216	Uses light-blocking curtains in bedroom	1	2	3	4	5	NA
164217	Maintains a cool temperature in bedroom	1	2	3	4	5	NA
164218	Uses aroma therapy in bedroom	1	2	3	4	5	NA
164219	Uses a fan to provide air circulation and low-level noise	1	2	3	4	5	NA
164220	Creates a personalized sleep sanctuary	1	2	3	4	5	NA
164221	Listens to white and pink noise using a sound machine	1	2	3	4	5	NA
164222	Avoids large meals before bedtime	1	2	3	4	5	NA
164223	Eats a small snack at bedtime if hungry	1	2	3	4	5	NA
164224	Reduces fluid intake before bedtime	1	2	3	4	5	NA
164225	Avoids caffeine products at least 4 hours before bedtime	1	2	3	4	5	NA
164226	Avoids alcohol before bedtime	1	2	3	4	5	NA
164227	Avoids nicotine products before bedtime	1	2	3	4	5	NA
164228	Avoids exciting activities before bedtime	1	2	3	4	5	NA
164229	Uses an eye mask to block light	1	2	3	4	5	NA
164230	Avoids caffeine 7 hours before bedtime	1	2	3	4	5	NA
164231	Avoids gaming, tweeting, and posting to social media in bed	1	2	3	4	5	NA

S

Sleep Enhancement Behavior—cont'd

		Never Demonstrated	Rarely Demonstrated	Sometimes Demonstrated	Often Demonstrated	Consistently Demonstrated	
164232	Stops using electronic devices at least an hour before bedtime	1	2	3	4	5	NA
164233	Recognizes the impact of blue light on melatonin production	1	2	3	4	5	NA
164234	Keeps hands and feet warm	1	2	3	4	5	NA
164235	Avoids arguments close to bedtime	1	2	3	4	5	NA
164236	Resolves worries or concerns before bedtime when possible	1	2	3	4	5	NA
164237	Gets out of bed after 20 minutes if not asleep	1	2	3	4	5	NA
164238	Maintains a sleep journal	1	2	3	4	5	NA
164239	Seeks help from a health professional for persistent sleep problems	1	2	3	4	5	NA

Domain-*Functional Health (IV)*   **Class**-*Health Behavior (Q)*   *7th edition 2024*

OUTCOME CONTENT REFERENCES:

Chaiard, J., & Weaver, T. E. (2019). Update on research and practices in major sleep disorders: Part I. Obstructive sleep apnea syndrome. *Journal of Nursing Scholarship, 51*(5), 500–508. https://doi.org/10.1111/jnu.12489

Gupta, R., Grover, S., Basu, A., Krishnan, V., Tripathi, A., Subramanyam, A., Nischal, A., Hussain, A., Mehra, A., Ambekar, A., Saha, G., Mishra, K. K., Bathla, M., Jagiwala, M., Manjunatha, N., Nebhinani, N., Gaur, N., Kumar, N., Dalal, P. K., & Kumar, P. (2020). Changes in sleep pattern and sleep quality during COVID-19 lockdown. *Indian Journal of Psychiatry, 62*(4), 370–378. https://doi.org/10.4103/psychiatry.IndianJPsychiatry_523_20

Khubchandani, J., & Price, J. H. (2020). Short sleep duration in working American adults, 2010–2018. *Journal of Community Health* 45, 219–227. https://doi.org/10.1007/s10900-019-00731-9

Knell, G., Durand, C. P., Kohl, H. W., III., Wu, I. H. C., & Pettee Gabriel, K. (2019). Prevalence and likelihood of meeting sleep, physical activity, and screen-time guidelines among U.S. youth. *Journal of American Medical Association Pediatrics,173*(4), 387–389. https://doi.org/10.1001/jamapediatrics.2018.4847

Paruthi, S., Brooks, L. J., D'Ambrosio, C., Hall, W. A., Kotagal, S., Lloyd, R. M., Malow, B. A., Maski, K., Nichols, C., Quan, S. F., Rosen, C. L., Troester, M. M., & Wise, M. S. (2016). Consensus statement of the American Academy of Sleep Medicine on the recommended amount of sleep for healthy children: Methodology and discussion. *Journal of Clinical Sleep Medicine (JCSM), 12*(11), 1549–1561. https://doi.org/10.5664/jcsm.6288

Pérez-Carbonell, L., Meurling, I. J., Wassermann, D., Gnoni, V., Leschziner, G., Weighall, A., Ellis, J., Durrant, S., Hare, A., & Steier, J. (2020). Impact of the novel coronavirus (COVID-19) pandemic on sleep. *Journal of Thoracic Disease, 12*(2), S163–S175. https://doi.org/10.21037/jtd-cus-2020-015

Potter, P. A., Perry, A. G., Stockert, P., & Hall, A. (2021). *Fundamentals of nursing* (10th ed.). Elsevier.

Shriane, A. E., Ferguson, S. A., Jay, S. M., & Vincent, G. E. (2020). Sleep hygiene in shift workers: A systematic literature review. *Sleep Medicine Reviews*, 53, 101336. https://doi.org/10.1016/j.smrv.2020.101336

Smith, K. N. (2021). Need better sleep? Consider changing up your food choices. *Environmental Nutrition, 44*(3), 7.

Williams, P. (2020). *Basic geriatric nursing* (7th ed.). Elsevier.

Smoking Cessation Behavior 1625

Definition: Personal actions to eliminate tobacco use

OUTCOME TARGET RATING: Maintain at_____ Increase to_____

		Never Demonstrated	Rarely Demonstrated	Sometimes Demonstrated	Often Demonstrated	Consistently Demonstrated	
OUTCOME OVERALL RATING		**1**	**2**	**3**	**4**	**5**	
Indicators:							
162501	Expresses willingness to stop smoking	1	2	3	4	5	NA
162502	Expresses belief in the ability to stop smoking	1	2	3	4	5	NA
162530	Identifies co-existence of smoking and alcohol abuse	1	2	3	4	5	NA
162503	Identifies benefits of smoking cessation	1	2	3	4	5	NA

Continued

Smoking Cessation Behavior—cont'd

		Never Demonstrated	Rarely Demonstrated	Sometimes Demonstrated	Often Demonstrated	Consistently Demonstrated	
162504	Identifies negative consequences of tobacco use	1	2	3	4	5	NA
162505	Develops effective strategies to eliminate tobacco use	1	2	3	4	5	NA
162506	Identifies barriers to tobacco elimination	1	2	3	4	5	NA
162507	Adjusts tobacco elimination strategies as needed	1	2	3	4	5	NA
162508	Commits to tobacco elimination strategies	1	2	3	4	5	NA
162529	Commits to tobacco abstinence	1	2	3	4	5	NA
162509	Follows selected tobacco elimination strategies	1	2	3	4	5	NA
162510	Participates in screening for associated health problems	1	2	3	4	5	NA
162531	Recognizes the presence of smoking related illness	1	2	3	4	5	NA
162511	Uses strategies to cope with withdrawal symptoms	1	2	3	4	5	NA
162532	Uses strategies to control cravings for alcohol	1	2	3	4	5	NA
162512	Uses behavior modification strategies	1	2	3	4	5	NA
162513	Uses effective coping strategies	1	2	3	4	5	NA
162533	Uses strategies to address mental health issues	1	2	3	4	5	NA
162514	Obtains assistance from health professional	1	2	3	4	5	NA
162515	Uses personal support system	1	2	3	4	5	NA
162534	Uses psychosocial support system	1	2	3	4	5	NA
162516	Uses reputable sources of information	1	2	3	4	5	NA
162535	Uses reputable e-Health resources	1	2	3	4	5	NA
162517	Uses nicotine replacement therapy	1	2	3	4	5	NA
162536	Uses nicotine replacement therapy with additional strategies	1	2	3	4	5	NA
162537	Monitors side effects of nicotine replacement therapy	1	2	3	4	5	NA
162538	Uses strategies to control weight	1	2	3	4	5	NA
162519	Identifies emotional states that affect tobacco use	1	2	3	4	5	NA
162539	Monitors emotions that affect tobacco use	1	2	3	4	5	NA
162520	Adjusts lifestyle to promote tobacco elimination	1	2	3	4	5	NA
162540	Adopts smoke-free home environment	1	2	3	4	5	NA
162541	Adopts smoke-free car policy	1	2	3	4	5	NA
162521	Uses prescribed medication as recommended	1	2	3	4	5	NA
162522	Uses non-prescription medication as recommended	1	2	3	4	5	NA
162542	Understands the mechanisms of action of prescribed medication	1	2	3	4	5	NA
162543	Understands the mechanisms of the side effects of medication	1	2	3	4	5	NA
162544	Uses strategies to control stress	1	2	3	4	5	NA

S

Smoking Cessation Behavior—cont'd

	Never Demonstrated	Rarely Demonstrated	Sometimes Demonstrated	Often Demonstrated	Consistently Demonstrated	
162523 Uses available support groups	1	2	3	4	5	NA
162524 Uses available community resources	1	2	3	4	5	NA
162525 Participates in counseling	1	2	3	4	5	NA
162526 Participates in telephone counseling	1	2	3	4	5	NA
162527 Monitors for signs of depression	1	2	3	4	5	NA
162545 Recognizes possible challenges to remain abstinent	1	2	3	4	5	NA
162546 Uses strategies to eliminate binge drinking	1	2	3	4	5	NA
162547 Adjusts lifestyle to limit alcohol consumption	1	2	3	4	5	NA
162528 Eliminates tobacco use	1	2	3	4	5	NA

Domain-Health Knowledge & Behavior (IV)   **Class**-Health Behavior (Q)   4th edition 2008; revised 2024

OUTCOME CONTENT REFERENCES:

American Cancer Society. (2022). How to quit using tobacco. https://cancer.org/healthy/stay-away-from-tobacco/guide-quitting-smoking/deciding-to-quit-smoking-and-making-a-plan.html

Blackwell, C. W., & Castillo, H. L. (2020). Use of electronic nicotine delivery systems (ENDS) in lesbian, gay, bisexual, transgender and queer persons: Implications for public health nursing. *Public Health Nursing, 37*(4), 569–580. https://doi.org/10.1111/phn.12746

Bold, K. W., Rosen, R. L., Steinberg, M. L., Epstein, E. E., McCrady, B. S., & Williams, J. M. (2020). Smoking characteristics and alcohol use among women in treatment for alcohol use disorder. *Addictive Behaviors, 101*, 1–8. https://doi.org/10.1016/j.addbeh.2019.106137

Case, K. R., Hinds, J. T., Creamer, M. R., Loukas, A., & Perry, C. L. (2020). Who is JUULing and why? An examination of young adult electronic nicotine delivery systems users. *Journal of Adolescent Health, 66*(1), 48–55. https://doi.org/10.1016/j.jadohealth.2019.05.030

DiSilvio, B., Baqdunes, M., Alhajbusain, A., & Cheema, T. (2021). Smoking addiction and strategies for cessation. *Critical Care Nursing Quarterly, 44*(1), 33–48. https://doi.org/10.1097/CNQ.0000000000000338

Haass-Koffler, C. L., Souza, R. D., Wilmott, J. P., Aston, E. R., & Song, J. H. (2021). A combined alcohol and smoking cue-reactivity paradigm in people who drink heavily and smoke cigarettes: Preliminary findings. *Alcohol and Alcoholism, 56*(1), 47–56. https://doi.org/10.1093/alcalc/agaa089

Hughes, J. R. (2020). An update on hardening: A qualitative review. *Nicotine & Tobacco Research, 22*(6), 867–871. https://doi.org/10.1093/ntr/ntz042

Kurti, A. N. (2020). Reducing tobacco use among women of childbearing age: Contributions of tobacco regulatory science and tobacco control. *Experimental and Clinical Psychopharmacology, 28*(5), 501–516. https://doi.org/10.1037/pha0000342

Sharifpour, A., Taghizadeh, F., Zarghami, M., & Alipour, A. (2021). The effectiveness of individual interventions on smoking cessation of chronic obstructive pulmonary disease patients. *Journal of Nursing Midwifery Science, 7*(1), 13–21. https://doi.org/10.4103/JNMS.JMNS_38_19

The Royal Australian College of General Practitioners. (2019). *Supporting smoking cessation: A guide for health professionals* (2nd ed.). RACGP.

U.S. Preventive Services Task Force. (2021). Interventions for tobacco smoking cessation in adults, including pregnant persons: U.S. Preventive Services Task Force recommendation statement. *JAMA, 325*(3), 265–279. https://doi.org/10.1001/jama.2020.25019

Wootton, R. E., Greenstone, H. S. R., Abdellaoui, A., Denys, D., Verweij, K. J. H., Munafò, M. R., & Treur, J. L. (2020). Bidirectional effects between loneliness, smoking, and alcohol use: Evidence from a Mendelian randomization study. *Addiction, 116*(2), 400–406. https://doi.org/10.1111/add.15142

Social Anxiety Level   **1216**

Definition: Severity of irrational avoidance, apprehension, and distress in anticipation of or during social situations

OUTCOME TARGET RATING: Maintain at_____ Increase to_____

	Severe	Substantial	Moderate	Mild	None	
OUTCOME OVERALL RATING	1	2	3	4	5	
Indicators:						
121601 Avoidance of social situations	1	2	3	4	5	NA
121602 Avoidance of unfamiliar people	1	2	3	4	5	NA
121603 Avoidance of leaving home	1	2	3	4	5	NA
121604 Anxious anticipation of social situations	1	2	3	4	5	NA
121605 Anxious anticipation of encountering unfamiliar people	1	2	3	4	5	NA

Continued

S

Social Anxiety Level—cont'd

		Severe	Substantial	Moderate	Mild	None	
121606	Activation of sympathetic nervous system responses	1	2	3	4	5	NA
121607	Negative self-perceptions of social skills	1	2	3	4	5	NA
121608	Negative self-perceptions of acceptance by others	1	2	3	4	5	NA
121618	Parental criticism	1	2	3	4	5	NA
121619	Parental rejection	1	2	3	4	5	NA
121609	Fear of scrutiny by others	1	2	3	4	5	NA
121610	Fear of interacting with members of the opposite sex	1	2	3	4	5	NA
121611	Fear of interacting with superiors	1	2	3	4	5	NA
121612	Discomfort during social encounters	1	2	3	4	5	NA
121613	Discomfort with changing routine	1	2	3	4	5	NA
121614	Concern about judgment of others after social encounters	1	2	3	4	5	NA
121615	Panic symptoms in social situations	1	2	3	4	5	NA
121616	Interference with role functioning	1	2	3	4	5	NA
121617	Interference with relationships	1	2	3	4	5	NA

Domain-Psychosocial Health (III)   **Class**-Psychological Well-Being (M)   5th edition 2013; revised 2018

OUTCOME CONTENT REFERENCES:

Alfano, C. A., Pina, A. A., Villanlta, I. K., Beidel, D. C., Ammerman, R. T., & Crosby, L. E. (2009). Mediators and moderators of outcome in the behavioral treatment of childhood social phobia. *Journal of the American Academy of Child and Adolescent Psychiatry, 48*(9), 945–953. https://doi.org/10.1097/CHI.0b013e3181af8216

American Psychiatric Association. (2013). *Diagnostic and statistical manual of mental disorders* (5th ed.). https://doi.org/10.1176/appi.books.9780890425596

Borge, F., Hoffart, A., & Sexton, H. (2010). Predictors of outcome in residential cognitive and interpersonal treatment for social phobia: Do cognitive and social dysfunction moderate treatment outcome? *Journal of Behavior Therapy and Experimental Psychiatry, 41*(3), 212–219. https://doi.org/10.1016/j.jbtep.2010.01.005

Kneisl, C. R., Wilson, H. S., & Trigoboff, E. (2004). *Contemporary psychiatric-mental health nursing.* Prentice Hall.

Mohr, W. K. (2006). *Psychiatric-mental health nursing* (6th ed.). Lippincott, Williams, & Wilkins.

Nanda, M., Reichert, E., Jones, U., & Flannery-Schroeder, E. (2016). Childhood maltreatment and symptoms of social anxiety: Exploring the role of emotional abuse, neglect, and cumulative trauma. *Journal of Child & Adolescent Trauma, 9*(3), 201–207. https://doi.org/10.1007/s40653-0150-0070-z

Stuart, G. W. (2009). *Principles and practice of psychiatric nursing* (9th ed.). Mosby Elsevier.

Social Identity

1223

Definition: An overall sense of self based on social group memberships that strongly impact feelings about self and self-esteem

S

OUTCOME TARGET RATING: Maintain at_____ Increase to_____

		Never Demonstrated	Rarely Demonstrated	Sometimes Demonstrated	Often Demonstrated	Consistently Demonstrated	
OUTCOME OVERALL RATING		1	2	3	4	5	
Indicators:							
122301	Acknowledges how group memberships impact personal views	1	2	3	4	5	NA
122302	Acknowledges how group memberships impact personal choices	1	2	3	4	5	NA
122303	Verbalizes impact of race as a social group	1	2	3	4	5	NA
122304	Verbalizes impact of ethnic origin as a social group	1	2	3	4	5	NA

Social Identity—cont'd

		Never Demonstrated	Rarely Demonstrated	Sometimes Demonstrated	Often Demonstrated	Consistently Demonstrated	
122305	Verbalizes impact of gender as a social group	1	2	3	4	5	NA
122306	Verbalizes impact of sexual orientation as a social group	1	2	3	4	5	NA
122307	Verbalizes impact of social class as a social group	1	2	3	4	5	NA
122308	Verbalizes impact of world views such as religion as a social group	1	2	3	4	5	NA
122309	Verbalizes impact of functional ability status as a social group	1	2	3	4	5	NA
122310	Verbalizes impact of first language as a social group	1	2	3	4	5	NA
122311	Verbalizes impact of country-of-origin as a social group	1	2	3	4	5	NA
122312	Verbalizes impact of generational group (age) as a social group	1	2	3	4	5	NA
122313	Identifies other important group memberships impacting social identity	1	2	3	4	5	NA
122314	Evaluates how group memberships impact "us vs. them" thinking	1	2	3	4	5	NA

Domain-Psychosocial Health (III)   *Class*-Psychological Well-Being (M)   *7th edition 2024*

OUTCOME CONTENT REFERENCES:
Bagci, S. C., Verkuyten, M., Koc, Y., Turnuklu, A., Piyale, Z. F., & Bekmezci, E. (2020). Being tolerated and being discriminated against: Links to psychological well-being through threatened social identity needs. *European Journal of Social Psychology, 50*(7), 1463–1477. https://doi.org/10.1002/ejsp.2699

Haslam, S. A., Jetten, J., Postmes, T., & Haslam, C. (2009). Social identity, health and well-being: An emerging agenda for applied psychology. *Applied Psychology-An International Review–Psychologie Appliquee-Revue Internationale, 58*(1), 1–23. https://doi.org/10.1111/j.1464-0597.2008.00379.x

Jenkins R. (2014). *Social identity* (4th ed.). Routledge.

McLeod, S. A. (2019, October 24). Social identity theory. *Simply Psychology*. https://www.simplypsychology.org/social-identity-theory.html

Sand, C. D., Rahbek, K., Willadsen, T. G., & Jønsson, A. R. (2021). Prioritizing social identities: Patients' perspective on living with multimorbidity. *Journal of Comorbidity, 11*, 1–10. https://doi.org/10.1177/26335565211009375

Tajfel, H., Billig, M. G., Bundy, R. P., & Flament, C. (1971). Social categorization and intergroup behaviour. *European Journal of Social Psychology, 1*(2), 149–178. https://doi.org/10.1002/ejsp.2420010202

Tajfel, H. (1982). Social psychology of intergroup relations. *Annual Review of Psychology, 33*(1), 1–39. https://doi.org/10.1146/annurev.ps.33.020182.000245

Tajfel, H., & Turner, J. C. (1986). The social identity theory of inter-group behavior. In S. Worchel & L. W. Austin (Eds.), *Psychology of intergroup relations* (pp. 7–24). Nelson-Hall.

Veelen, R., Veldman, J., Van Laar, C., & Derks, B. (2020). Distancing from a stigmatized social identity: State of the art and future research agenda on self-group distancing. *European Journal of Social Psychology, 50*(6), 1089–1107. https://doi.org/10.1002/ejsp.2714

Social Interaction Skills   1502

S

Definition: Personal behaviors that promote effective relationships

OUTCOME TARGET RATING: Maintain at _____ Increase to _____

	Never Demonstrated	Rarely Demonstrated	Sometimes Demonstrated	Often Demonstrated	Consistently Demonstrated	
OUTCOME OVERALL RATING	1	2	3	4	5	
Indicators:						
150201 Uses disclosure as appropriate	1	2	3	4	5	NA
150202 Exhibits receptiveness	1	2	3	4	5	NA
150203 Cooperates with others	1	2	3	4	5	NA
150204 Exhibits sensitivity to others	1	2	3	4	5	NA

Continued

Social Interaction Skills—cont'd

		Never Demonstrated	Rarely Demonstrated	Sometimes Demonstrated	Often Demonstrated	Consistently Demonstrated	
150205	Uses assertive behaviors as appropriate	1	2	3	4	5	NA
150217	Uses strategies to address communication limitations	1	2	3	4	5	NA
150218	Exhibits non-verbal behavior congruent with verbal communication	1	2	3	4	5	NA
150206	Uses confrontation as appropriate	1	2	3	4	5	NA
150207	Exhibits consideration	1	2	3	4	5	NA
150208	Exhibits genuineness	1	2	3	4	5	NA
150209	Exhibits warmth	1	2	3	4	5	NA
150210	Exhibits poise	1	2	3	4	5	NA
150211	Appears relaxed	1	2	3	4	5	NA
150212	Engages others	1	2	3	4	5	NA
150213	Exhibits trust	1	2	3	4	5	NA
150214	Uses compromise as appropriate	1	2	3	4	5	NA
150216	Uses conflict resolution strategies	1	2	3	4	5	NA

Domain-Psychosocial Health (III)   **Class**-Social Interaction (P)   1st edition 1997; revised 2004, 2018

OUTCOME CONTENT REFERENCES:

Erickson, D. H., Beiser, M., Iacono, W. G., Fleming, J. A., & Lin, T. (1989). The role of social relationships in the course of first-episode schizophrenia and affective psychosis. *American Journal of Psychiatry, 146*(11), 1456–1461. https://doi.org/10.1176/ajp.146.11.1456

Gotcher, J. M. (1992). Interpersonal communication and psychosocial adjustment. *Journal of Psychosocial Oncology, 10*(3), 21–39. https://doi.org/10.1300/j077v10N05_02

Heltsley, M. E., & Powers, R. C. (1975). Social interaction and perceived adequacy of interaction of the rural aged. *The Gerontologist, 15*(6), 533–536. https://doi.org/10.1093/geront/15.6.533

Levin, J., & Levin, W. C. (1981). Willingness to interact with an old person. *Research on Aging, 3*(2), 211–217. https://doi.org/10.1177/016402758132006

Nussbaum, J. F. (1983). Relational closeness of elderly interaction: Implications for life satisfaction. *Western Journal of Speech Communication, 47*(3), 229–243. https://doi.org/10.1080/1057318309374120

Palmer, A. D., Newsom, J. T., & Rook, K. S. (2016). How does difficulty communicating affect the social relationship of older adults? An exploration using data from a national survey. *Journal of Communication Disorders, 62*, 131–143. https://doi.org/10.1016/j.jcomdis.2016.06.002

+Ruehlman, L. S., & Karoly, P. (1991). With a little flak from my friends: Development and preliminary validation of the Test of Negative Social Exchange (TENSE). *Psychological Assessment: A Journal of Consulting and Clinical Psychology, 3*(1), 97–104. https://doi.org/10.1037/1040-3590.3.1.97

Social Involvement

1503

Definition: Social interactions with persons, groups, or organizations

OUTCOME TARGET RATING: Maintain at _____ Increase to _____

		Never Demonstrated	Rarely Demonstrated	Sometimes Demonstrated	Often Demonstrated	Consistently Demonstrated	
OUTCOME OVERALL RATING		1	2	3	4	5	
Indicators:							
150314	Connects daily with others	1	2	3	4	5	NA
150301	Interacts with close friends	1	2	3	4	5	NA
150302	Interacts with neighbors	1	2	3	4	5	NA
150303	Interacts with family members	1	2	3	4	5	NA
150304	Interacts with members of work group(s)	1	2	3	4	5	NA
150315	Evaluates personal social network	1	2	3	4	5	NA
150316	Establishes intergenerational connections	1	2	3	4	5	NA
150317	Establishes new relationships	1	2	3	4	5	NA
150318	Attends group activities	1	2	3	4	5	NA

S

Social Involvement—cont'd

		Never Demonstrated	Rarely Demonstrated	Sometimes Demonstrated	Often Demonstrated	Consistently Demonstrated	
150319	Attends educational offerings	1	2	3	4	5	NA
150320	Participates in school activities	1	2	3	4	5	NA
150321	Participates in mentoring opportunities	1	2	3	4	5	NA
150305	Participates as member of church	1	2	3	4	5	NA
150306	Participates in active church work	1	2	3	4	5	NA
150307	Participates in organized activity	1	2	3	4	5	NA
150308	Participates as officer in organization	1	2	3	4	5	NA
150309	Participates as a volunteer	1	2	3	4	5	NA
150311	Participates in leisure activities with others	1	2	3	4	5	NA
150313	Participates in team sports	1	2	3	4	5	NA

Domain-*Psychosocial Health (III)*   **Class**-*Social Interaction (P)*   *1st edition 1997; revised 2004, 2018*

OUTCOME CONTENT REFERENCES:

Cutting, A. L., & Dunn, J. (2006). Conversations with siblings and with friends: Links between relationship quality and social understanding. *British Journal of Developmental Psychology, 24*(1), 73–87. https://doi.org/10/1348/1026151005X70337
Isherwood, L. M., King, D. S., & Luszcz, M. A. (2017). Widowhood in the fourth age: Support exchange, relationships and social participation. *Ageing & Society, 37*(1), 188–212. https://doi.org/10.1017/s0144686X15001166
Pettigrew, S., Donovan, R., Boldy, D., & Newton, R. (2014). Older people's perceived causes of and strategies for dealing with social isolation. *Aging & Mental Health, 18*(7), 914–920. https://doi.org/10.1080/13607863.2014.89997
Ristau, S. (2011). People do need people: Social interaction boosts brain health in older age. *Generations, 35*(2), 70–76.
Yu, R. P., McCammon, R. J., Ellison, N. B., & Langa, K. M. (2016). The relationships that matter: Social network site use and social well-being among older adults in the United States of America. *Ageing & Society, 36*(9), 1826–1852. https://doi.org/10.1017/S014468X15000677

Social Support   1504

Definition: Reliable support from others

OUTCOME TARGET RATING: Maintain at _____ Increase to _____

		None	Limited	Moderate	Substantial	Extensive	
OUTCOME OVERALL RATING		1	2	3	4	5	
Indicators:							
150414	Willingness to call on others for assistance	1	2	3	4	5	NA
150415	Money available from others when needed	1	2	3	4	5	NA
150416	Assistance offered from others	1	2	3	4	5	NA
150417	Time provided by others	1	2	3	4	5	NA
150418	Labor provided by others	1	2	3	4	5	NA
150419	Communication about assistance needs	1	2	3	4	5	NA
150420	Individuals available to assist	1	2	3	4	5	NA
150421	Individuals physically able to assist	1	2	3	4	5	NA
150422	Information provided by others	1	2	3	4	5	NA
150423	Emotional support from others	1	2	3	4	5	NA
150424	Confidant relationship(s)	1	2	3	4	5	NA
150425	Persons who can help as needed	1	2	3	4	5	NA
150426	Assistive social network	1	2	3	4	5	NA
150427	Supportive social contacts	1	2	3	4	5	NA
150428	Stable social network	1	2	3	4	5	NA

Domain-*Psychosocial Health (III)*   **Class**-*Social Interaction (P)*   *1st edition 1997; revised 2004, 2008, 2024*

S

OUTCOME CONTENT REFERENCES:

Alananzeh, I., Lord, H., & Fernandez, R. (2021). Social support for Arab people with chronic conditions: A scoping review. *Clinical Nursing Research, 30*(4), 380–391. https://doi.org/10.1177/1054773820932262

Bumble, J. L., Sanderson, K. A., Zemke, K. E., & Hodapp, R. M. (2021). Marrying into it: Siblings-in-law in the social support networks of adults with intellectual and developmental disabilities. *Journal of Intellectual Disability Research, 65*(9), 849–862. https://doi.org/10.1111/jir.12864

Canavan, M., Gallo, W. T., & Marshall, G. L. (2021). The moderating effect of social support and social integration on the relationship between involuntary job loss and health. *Journal of Applied Gerontology, 40*(10), 1272–1279. https://doi.org/10.1177/0733464820921082

Fredericksen, R. J., Gibbons, L. E., Fitzsimmons, E., Nance, R. M., Schafer, K. R., Batey, D. S., Loo, S., Dougherty, S., Mathews, W. C., Christopoulos, K., Mayer, K. H., Mugavero, M. J., Kitahata, M. M., Crane, P. K., & Crane, H. M. (2021). Impact and correlates of sub-optimal social support among patients in HIV care, *AIDS Care, 33*(9), 1178–1188. https://doi.org/10.1080/09540121.2020.1853660

Garza, V., Graf, N., Lerma, P., & Herold, M. (2021). Social support and companionship among people with end-stage renal disease. *Journal of Applied Rehabilitation Counseling, 52*(3), 176–193. https://doi.org/10.1891/JARC-D-20-00024

Gonzaga, I., Claumann, G. S., Scarabelot, K. S., Silva, D. A. S., & Pelegrini, A. (2021). Body image dissatisfaction in adolescents: Comparison with physical activity, teasing and social support. *Journal of Health Psychology, 26*(10), 1651–1660. https://doi.org/10.1177/1359105319887796

Lo, C. K., Ho, F. K., Yan, E., Lu, Y., Chan, K. L., & Ip, P. (2021). Associations between child maltreatment and adolescents' health-related quality of life and emotional and social problems in low-income families, and the moderating role of social support. *Journal of Interpersonal Violence, 36*(15–16), 7436–7455. https://doi.org/10.1177/0886260519835880

Koren, Y., Leveille, S., & You, T. (2021). Tai chi interventions promoting social support and interaction among older adults. *Research in Gerontological Nursing, 14*(3), 126–137. https://doi.org/10.3928/19404921-20210325-02

Ntontis, E., Drury, J., Amlôt, R., Rubin, G. J., Williams, R., & Saavedra, P. (2020). Collective resilience in the disaster recovery period: Emergent social identity and observed social support are associated with collective efficacy, well-being, and the provision of social support. *British Journal of Social Psychology, 60*, 1075–1095. https://doi.org/10.1111/bjso.12434

Orlas, C. P., Herrera-Escobar, J. P., Hau, K. M., Velmahos, A., Patel, N., Sanchez, S., Kaafarani, H. M. A., Salim, A., & Nehra, D. (2021). Perceived social support is strongly associated with recovery after injury. *Journal of Trauma and Acute Care Surgery, 91*(3), 552–558. https://doi.org/10.1097/TA.0000000000003230

Uhing, A., Williams, J. S., Garacci, E., & Egede, L. E. (2021). Gender differences in the relationship between social support and strain and mortality among a national sample of adults. *Journal of Behavioral Medicine, 44*, 673–681. https://doi.org/10.1007/s10865-021-00221-1

Spiritual Health   2001

Definition: Connectedness with self, others, higher power, all life, nature, and the universe that transcends and empowers the self

OUTCOME TARGET RATING: Maintain at _____ Increase to _____

		Severely Compromised	Substantially Compromised	Moderately Compromised	Mildly Compromised	Not Compromised	
OUTCOME OVERALL RATING		**1**	**2**	**3**	**4**	**5**	
Indicators:							
200101	Quality of faith	1	2	3	4	5	NA
200102	Quality of hope	1	2	3	4	5	NA
200103	Meaning and purpose in life	1	2	3	4	5	NA
200123	Joy in life	1	2	3	4	5	NA
200104	Achievement of spiritual world view	1	2	3	4	5	NA
200105	Feelings of peacefulness	1	2	3	4	5	NA
200106	Ability to love	1	2	3	4	5	NA
200107	Ability to forgive	1	2	3	4	5	NA
200109	Ability to pray	1	2	3	4	5	NA
200110	Ability to worship	1	2	3	4	5	NA
200108	Spiritual experiences	1	2	3	4	5	NA
200122	Spiritual contentment	1	2	3	4	5	NA
200111	Participation in spiritual rites and passages	1	2	3	4	5	NA
200113	Participation in meditation	1	2	3	4	5	NA
200115	Participation in spiritual reading	1	2	3	4	5	NA
200112	Interaction with spiritual leaders	1	2	3	4	5	NA
200114	Expression through music	1	2	3	4	5	NA
200119	Expression through art	1	2	3	4	5	NA
200120	Expression through writing	1	2	3	4	5	NA

S

Spiritual Health—cont'd

		Severely Compromised	Substantially Compromised	Moderately Compromised	Mildly Compromised	Not Compromised	
200116	Connectedness with inner self	1	2	3	4	5	NA
200117	Connectedness with others	1	2	3	4	5	NA
200124	Interaction with others to share thoughts and feelings	1	2	3	4	5	NA
200125	Interaction with others to share beliefs	1	2	3	4	5	NA

Domain-*Health & Life Quality (V)*   **Class**-*Perceived Health & Life Situation (U)*   *1st edition 1997; revised 2004, 2018*

OUTCOME CONTENT REFERENCES:

Burkhardt, M. A. (1989). Spirituality: An analysis of the concept. *Holistic Nursing Practice, 3*(3), 69–77. https://doi.org/10.1097/00004650-198905000-00011

Burkhart, L., & Solari-Twadell, P. A. (2001). Spirituality and religiousness: Differentiating the diagnoses through a review of the nursing literature. *Nursing Diagnosis: The International Journal of Nursing Language and Classification, 12*(2). 45–54. https://doi.org/10.1111/j.1744-618x.2001.tb00118.x

+Daaleman, T. P., & Frey, B. B. (2004). The Spirituality Index of Well-Being: A new instrument for health-related quality-of-life research. *Annals of Family Medicine, 2*(5), 499–503. https://doi.org/10.1370/afm.89

Ellison, C. W. (1983). Spiritual well-being: Conceptualization and measurement. *Journal of Psychology and Theology, 11*(4), 330–340. https://doi.org/10.1177/009164718301100406

Holt, N. (2016). What does the word spirituality really mean? In J. Mata-McMahon, T. Kovač, & G. Miller. (Eds.), *Spirituality: An interdisciplinary view* (pp. 79–97). Inter-Disciplinary Press.

Hungelmann, J., Kenkel-Rossi, E., Klassen, L., & Stollenwerk, R. (1996). Focus on spiritual well-being: Harmonious interconnectedness of mind-body-spirit: Use of the JAREL Spiritual Well-Being Scale. *Geriatric Nursing, 17*(6), 262–266. https://doi.org/10.1016/s0197-4572(96)80238-2

Munoz, A. R., Salsman. J., M., Stein, K. D., & Cella, D. (2015). Reference values of the functional assessment of chronic illness therapy-spiritual well-being: A report from American Cancer Society's studies of cancer survivors. *Cancer, 121*(11), 1838–1844. https://doi.org/10.1002/cncr.29286

+Peterman, A. H., Fitchett, G., Brady, M. J., Hernandez, L., & Cella, D. (2002). Measuring spiritual well-being in people with cancer: The Functional Assessment of Chronic Illness Therapy-Spiritual Well-Being Scale (FACIT-Sp). *Annals of Behavioral Medicine, 24*(1), 49–58. https://doi.org/10.1207/S15324796ABM2401_06

+Roberts, K. T., & Aspy, C. B. (1993). Development of the Serenity Scale. *Journal of Nursing Measurement, 1*(2), 145–164.

WHOQOL SRPB Group. (2006). A cross-cultural study of spirituality, religion, and personal beliefs as components of quality of life. *Social Science & Medicine, 62*(6), 1486–1497. https://doi.org/10.1016/j.socscimed.2005.08.001

Stress Level   1212

Definition: Severity of manifested physical or mental tension resulting from factors that alter an existing equilibrium

OUTCOME TARGET RATING: Maintain at _____ Increase to _____

		Severe	Substantial	Moderate	Mild	None	
OUTCOME OVERALL RATING		1	2	3	4	5	
Indicators:							
121201	Increased blood pressure	1	2	3	4	5	NA
121202	Increased radial pulse rate	1	2	3	4	5	NA
121203	Increased respiratory rate	1	2	3	4	5	NA
121204	Dilated pupils	1	2	3	4	5	NA
121205	Increased muscle tension in neck, shoulders, and back	1	2	3	4	5	NA
121206	Tension headache	1	2	3	4	5	NA
121207	Sweaty palms	1	2	3	4	5	NA
121208	Dry mouth and throat	1	2	3	4	5	NA
121209	Diarrhea	1	2	3	4	5	NA
121210	Urinary frequency	1	2	3	4	5	NA
121211	Change in food intake	1	2	3	4	5	NA
121212	Upset stomach	1	2	3	4	5	NA
121213	Restlessness	1	2	3	4	5	NA
121214	Sleep disturbance	1	2	3	4	5	NA
121235	Interruption of thought process	1	2	3	4	5	NA

S

Continued

Stress Level—cont'd

		Severe	Substantial	Moderate	Mild	None	
121215	Forgetfulness	1	2	3	4	5	NA
121216	Frequent cognitive mistakes	1	2	3	4	5	NA
121217	Diminished attention to detail	1	2	3	4	5	NA
121218	Inability to concentrate on tasks	1	2	3	4	5	NA
121219	Emotional outbursts	1	2	3	4	5	NA
121220	Irritability	1	2	3	4	5	NA
121221	Depression	1	2	3	4	5	NA
121222	Anxiety	1	2	3	4	5	NA
121223	Suspiciousness	1	2	3	4	5	NA
121224	Oppressive thoughts	1	2	3	4	5	NA
121225	Flashback episodes	1	2	3	4	5	NA
121226	Dissociation	1	2	3	4	5	NA
121227	Compulsive behavior	1	2	3	4	5	NA
121228	Increased alcohol use	1	2	3	4	5	NA
121229	Increased psychotropic medication use	1	2	3	4	5	NA
121230	Increased smoking	1	2	3	4	5	NA
121231	Absenteeism	1	2	3	4	5	NA
121232	Decreased productivity	1	2	3	4	5	NA
121233	Increased frequency of accidents	1	2	3	4	5	NA
121234	Change in libido	1	2	3	4	5	NA
121236	Hair loss	1	2	3	4	5	NA

Domain-Psychosocial Health (III)   **Class**-Psychological Well-Being (M)   3rd edition 2004; revised 2008, 2013

OUTCOME CONTENT REFERENCES:

American Psychiatric Association. (2000). *Diagnostic and statistical manual of mental disorders* (4th ed., text rev.).

Campbell, R. J. (1989). *Psychiatric dictionary* (6th ed.). Oxford University.

Curtis, R., Groarke, A., Coughlan, R., & Gsel, A. (2004). The influence of disease severity, perceived stress, social support and coping in patients with chronic illness: A 1 year follow up. *Psychology, Health & Medicine, 9*(4), 456–475. https://doi.org/10.1080/1354850042000267058

Lazarus, R. S., & Folkman, S. (1984). *Stress, appraisal, and coping.* Springer.

Richardson, C. G., & Ratner, P. A. (2005). Sense of coherence as a moderator of the effects of stressful life events of health. *Journal of Epidemiology & Community Health, 59*(11), 979–984. https://doi.org/10.1136/jech.2005.036756

Stanhope, M., & Lancaster, J. (1988). *Community health nursing: Process and practice for promoting health* (2nd ed.). Mosby.

Tasman, A., Kay, J., & Lieberman, J. A. (1997). *Psychiatry* (Vol. 2). Saunders.

Student Health Status

2005

Definition: Overall physical, psychological, and social functioning of a school-age child

OUTCOME TARGET RATING: Maintain at _____ Increase to _____

		Severely Compromised	Substantially Compromised	Moderately Compromised	Mildly Compromised	Not Compromised	
OUTCOME OVERALL RATING		1	2	3	4	5	
Indicators:							
200501	Physical health	1	2	3	4	5	NA
200502	Mental health	1	2	3	4	5	NA
200503	School attendance	1	2	3	4	5	NA
200504	Readiness to learn	1	2	3	4	5	NA
200505	Academic performance at grade level or higher	1	2	3	4	5	NA

Student Health Status—cont'd

		Severely Compromised	Substantially Compromised	Moderately Compromised	Mildly Compromised	Not Compromised	
200506	Standardized test performance at grade level or higher	1	2	3	4	5	NA
200507	Progression to graduation on expected schedule	1	2	3	4	5	NA
200508	Return to class after visit to health office	1	2	3	4	5	NA
200509	Physician office visits minimized	1	2	3	4	5	NA
200510	Emergency room visits minimized	1	2	3	4	5	NA
200511	Reports to the health office for medications at appropriate time	1	2	3	4	5	NA
200512	Participation in mandated screenings	1	2	3	4	5	NA
200513	Family follow-up of referrals	1	2	3	4	5	NA
200514	Participation in self-care activities	1	2	3	4	5	NA
200516	Financial resources for health care	1	2	3	4	5	NA
200517	Participation in curricular school activities	1	2	3	4	5	NA
200518	Participation in extracurricular school activities	1	2	3	4	5	NA
200519	Participation in physical activities	1	2	3	4	5	NA
200520	Growth	1	2	3	4	5	NA
200521	Development	1	2	3	4	5	NA
200522	Optimum weight	1	2	3	4	5	NA
200523	Healthy dietary habits	1	2	3	4	5	NA
200524	Postponement of sexual activity	1	2	3	4	5	NA

		Severe	Substantial	Moderate	Mild	None	
200527	Alcohol use	1	2	3	4	5	NA
200528	Recreational drug use	1	2	3	4	5	NA
200533	Performance enhancing drug use	1	2	3	4	5	NA
200529	Tobacco use	1	2	3	4	5	NA
200530	Occurrence of accidents	1	2	3	4	5	NA
200531	Disruptive behavior	1	2	3	4	5	NA
200534	Eating disorder	1	2	3	4	5	NA
200532	Occurrence of sexually transmitted disease	1	2	3	4	5	NA
200535	Risk for pregnancy	1	2	3	4	5	NA

Domain-Health & Life Quality (V)   **Class**-Health Status (JJ)   3rd edition 2004; revised 2008, 2013

OUTCOME CONTENT REFERENCES:

Council of Chief State School Officers. (1998). *Incorporating health-related indicators in education accountability systems.*

Howard, M. (1991). *How to help your teenager postpone sexual involvement.* Continuum.

Marx, E., & Wooley, S. F. (Eds). (1998). *Health is academic: A guide to coordinated school health programs.* Teachers College Columbia University.

Miller, B., Card, J., Paikoff, R. J., & Peterson, J. (1992). *Preventing adolescent pregnancy.*

Novello, A. C., DeGraw, C., & Kleinman, D. V. (1992). Healthy children ready to learn: An essential collaboration between health and education. *Public Health Reports, 107*(1), 3–10.

Tyson, H. (1999). A load off the teachers' backs: Coordinated school health programs. *Phi Delta Kappan, 80*(5), K1–K8.

Washington State Office of Superintendent of Public Instruction. (2001). *School nurse outcome measures.*

S

Substance Addiction Consequences

1407

Definition: Severity of change in health status, coping, and social functioning due to substance addiction

OUTCOME TARGET RATING: Maintain at _____ Increase to _____

		Severe	Substantial	Moderate	Mild	None	
OUTCOME OVERALL RATING		1	2	3	4	5	
Indicators:							
140724	Sense of isolation	1	2	3	4	5	NA
140725	Anxiety	1	2	3	4	5	NA
140726	Sadness	1	2	3	4	5	NA
140727	Concern about own health problems	1	2	3	4	5	NA
140701	Sustained decrease in physical activity	1	2	3	4	5	NA
140702	Chronic impaired motor function	1	2	3	4	5	NA
140704	Chronic fatigue	1	2	3	4	5	NA
140723	Chronic hygiene problems	1	2	3	4	5	NA
140705	Chronic impaired cognitive function	1	2	3	4	5	NA
140728	Difficulty making daily decisions	1	2	3	4	5	NA
140707	Prolonged recovery from illnesses	1	2	3	4	5	NA
140718	Absenteeism from work	1	2	3	4	5	NA
140719	Absenteeism from school	1	2	3	4	5	NA
140720	Difficulty maintaining role performance	1	2	3	4	5	NA
140729	Family relationship problems	1	2	3	4	5	NA
140709	Difficulty maintaining employment	1	2	3	4	5	NA
140710	Difficulty maintaining housing	1	2	3	4	5	NA
140711	Difficulty supporting self financially	1	2	3	4	5	NA
140721	Difficulty maintaining social interactions	1	2	3	4	5	NA
140722	Risk for infection from sharing needles	1	2	3	4	5	NA
140729	Frequency of hospitalizations	1	2	3	4	5	NA
140731	Frequency of emergency room visits	1	2	3	4	5	NA
140732	Participation in illegal activities	1	2	3	4	5	NA
140733	Concern about the future	1	2	3	4	5	NA

Domain-*Health & Life Quality (V)* **Class**-*Symptom Status (V)* *1st edition 1997; revised 2004, 2008, 2013, 2024*

OUTCOME CONTENT REFERENCES:

Ayalew, M., Tafere, M., & Asmare, Y. (2018). Prevalence, trends, and consequences of substance use among university students: Implication for intervention. *International Quarterly of Community Health Education, 38*(3), 169–173. https://doi.org/10.1177/0272684X17749570

de Andrade Boska, G., Carvalho Seabra, P. R., Ferreira de Oliveira, M. A., de Almeida Lopes Fernandes, I. F., Claro, H. G., & Russo Sequeira, R. M. (2021). Consequences of psychoactive substance use: A comparative study of two services in Brazil and Portugal. *Revista Da Escola de Enfermagem Da USP, 55*, 1–8. https://doi.org/10.1590/1980-220X-REEUSP-2021-0138

Manthey, J., Hassan, S. A., Carr, S., Kilian, C., Kuitunen-Paul, S., & Rehm, J. (2021). Estimating the economic consequences of substance use and substance use disorders. *Expert Review of Pharmacoeconomics & Outcomes Research, 21*(5), 869–876. https://doi.org/10.1080/14737167.2021.1916470

Seabra, P. R. C., Amendoeira, J. J. P., & Sá, L. O. (2018). Testing nursing sensitive outcomes in out-patient drug addicts, with "Nursing Role Effectiveness Model." *Issues in Mental Health Nursing, 39*(3), 200–207. https://doi.org/10.1080/01612840.2017.1378783

Seabra, P. R. C., Amendoeira, J. J. P., Sá, L. O., & Capelas, M. L. V. (2018). Clinical validation of the Portuguese version of "Substance Addiction Consequences" derived from the Nursing Outcomes Classification. *Issues in Mental Health Nursing, 39*(9), 779–785. https://doi.org/10.1080/01612840.2018.1462870

Seabra, P. R. C., Sa, L. O., & Amendoeira, J. (2013). Consequences of substance addiction: A contribution to the validation of NOC outcomes. *Reme: Revista Latina-Americana de Enfermagen, 17*(3), 673–679. https://doi.org/10.5935/1415-2762.20130049

S

Substance Withdrawal Severity   2108

Definition: Severity of signs and symptoms of withdrawal from addictive drugs, tobacco, or alcohol

OUTCOME TARGET RATING: Maintain at_____ Increase to_____

		Severe	Substantial	Moderate	Mild	None	
OUTCOME OVERALL RATING		1	2	3	4	5	
Indicators:							
210801	Substance seeking behavior	1	2	3	4	5	NA
210802	Substance cravings	1	2	3	4	5	NA
210843	Anxiety	1	2	3	4	5	NA
210844	Restlessness	1	2	3	4	5	NA
210845	Moodiness	1	2	3	4	5	NA
210803	Irritability	1	2	3	4	5	NA
210846	Psychomotor agitation	1	2	3	4	5	NA
210805	Emotional outbursts	1	2	3	4	5	NA
210806	Depression	1	2	3	4	5	NA
210832	Hallucinations	1	2	3	4	5	NA
210847	Paranoia	1	2	3	4	5	NA
210848	Mania	1	2	3	4	5	NA
210810	Muscle pain	1	2	3	4	5	NA
210807	Hyperreflexia	1	2	3	4	5	NA
210808	Myoclonus	1	2	3	4	5	NA
210809	Fasciculations	1	2	3	4	5	NA
210810	Muscle pain	1	2	3	4	5	NA
210849	Body aches	1	2	3	4	5	NA
210811	Tremors	1	2	3	4	5	NA
210850	Ataxia	1	2	3	4	5	NA
210851	Respiratory depression	1	2	3	4	5	NA
210852	Lightheadedness	1	2	3	4	5	NA
210853	Hypertension	1	2	3	4	5	NA
210854	Tachycardia	1	2	3	4	5	NA
210813	Dysrhythmia	1	2	3	4	5	NA
210814	Change in appetite	1	2	3	4	5	NA
210855	Anorexia	1	2	3	4	5	NA
210856	Weight change	1	2	3	4	5	NA
210815	Nausea	1	2	3	4	5	NA
210816	Vomiting	1	2	3	4	5	NA
210817	Abdominal pain	1	2	3	4	5	NA
210818	Diarrhea	1	2	3	4	5	NA
210819	Rhinorrhea	1	2	3	4	5	NA
210820	Lacrimation	1	2	3	4	5	NA
210857	Vertigo	1	2	3	4	5	NA
210858	Tinnitus	1	2	3	4	5	NA
210821	Pupil change	1	2	3	4	5	NA
210822	Goose bumps	1	2	3	4	5	NA
210859	Itching	1	2	3	4	5	NA
210823	Hot and cold flashes	1	2	3	4	5	NA
210824	Photophobia	1	2	3	4	5	NA

S

Continued

Substance Withdrawal Severity—cont'd

		Severe	Substantial	Moderate	Mild	None	
210825	Paresthesia	1	2	3	4	5	NA
210826	Abnormal sensitivity to sound	1	2	3	4	5	NA
210860	Pain sensitivity	1	2	3	4	5	NA
210827	Headaches	1	2	3	4	5	NA
210828	Yawning	1	2	3	4	5	NA
210829	Impaired concentration	1	2	3	4	5	NA
210830	Disorientation	1	2	3	4	5	NA
210861	Apathy	1	2	3	4	5	NA
210831	Difficulty sleeping	1	2	3	4	5	NA
210832	Hallucinations	1	2	3	4	5	NA
210862	Paranoia	1	2	3	4	5	NA
210833	Seizures	1	2	3	4	5	NA
210863	Dry mouth	1	2	3	4	5	NA
210834	Fever	1	2	3	4	5	NA
210835	Chills	1	2	3	4	5	NA
210836	Flushing	1	2	3	4	5	NA
210837	Diaphoresis	1	2	3	4	5	NA
210838	Fatigue	1	2	3	4	5	NA
210862	Lethargy	1	2	3	4	5	NA
210839	Weakness	1	2	3	4	5	NA

Identify substance(s)_____

Domain-Health & Life Quality (V)   **Class**-Symptom Status (V)   4th edition 2008; revised 2013, 2024

OUTCOME CONTENT REFERENCES:

American Society of Addiction Medicine. (2020). The ASAM national practice guideline for the treatment of opioid use disorder: 2020 focused update. *Journal of Addiction Medicine, 14*(2S), 1–91.

Bangert, M. K., & Aisenberg, G. M. (2020). Drug deprescription-withdrawal risk, prevention, and treatment. *Proceedings (Baylor. University Medical Center), 33*(2), 213–217. https://doi.org/10.1080/08998280.2019.1695510

Duong, T., Vytialingam, R., & O'Regan, R. (2018). *A brief guide to the management of alcohol and other drug withdrawal.* Mental Health Commission.

Hughes, J. R., Peters, E. N., Callas, P. W., Peasley-Miklus, C., Oga, E., Etter, J. F., & Morley, N. (2020). Withdrawal symptoms from E-cigarette abstinencea among former smokers: A pre-post clinical trial. *Nicotine & Tobacco Research, 22*(5), 734–739. https://doi.org/10.1093/ntr/ntz129

Knapp, A. A., Allan, N. P., Cloutier, R., Blumenthal, H., Moradi, S., Budney, A. J., & Lord, S. E. (2021). Effects of anxiety sensitivity on cannabis, alcohol, and nicotine use among adolescents: Evaluating pathways through anxiety, withdrawal symptoms, and coping motives. *Journal of Behavioral Medicine, 44*(2), 187–201. https://doi.org/10.1007/s10865-020-00182-x

Li, C., Li, Y., Ma, M., Zhang, Y., Bao, J., Ge, W., Liu, Y., Peng, C., & He, L. (2021). The impact of COVID-19 pandemic on headache symptoms and drug withdrawal among patients with medication overuse headache: A cross-sectional study. *The Journal of Headache and Pain, 22*(41), 1–11. https://doi.org/10.1186/s10194-021-01256-0

Manning, V., Arunogiri, S., Frei, M., Ridley, K., Mroz, K., Campbell, S., & Lubman, D. (2018). *Alcohol and other drug withdrawal: Practice guidelines* (3rd ed.). Turning Point.

Nguyen, T. A., & Lam, S. W. (2020). Phenobarbital and symptom-triggered lorazepam versus lorazepam alone for severe alcohol withdrawal in the intensive care unit. *Alcohol, 82*, 23–27. https://doi.org/10.1016/j.alcohol.2019.07.004

Pergolizzi, J. V., Raffa, R. B., & Rosenblatt, M. H. (2019). Opioid withdrawal symptoms, a consequence of chronic opioid use and opioid use disorder: Current understanding and approaches to management. *Journal of Clinical Pharmacy and Therapeutics, 45*, 892–903. https://doi.org/10.1111/jcpt.13114

Robinson, J. D., Li, L., Chen, M., Lerman, C., Tyndale, R. F., Schnoll, R. A., Hawk, L. W. Jr., George, T. P., Benowitz, N. L., & Cinciripini, P. M. (2019). Evaluating the temporal relationship between withdrawal symptoms and smoking relapse. *Psychology of Addictive Behaviors, 33*(2), 105–116. https://doi.org/10.1037/adb0000434

Srivastava, A. B., Mariani, J. J., & Levin, F. R. (2020). New directions in the treatment of opioid withdrawal. *Lancet, 395*(10241), 1938–1948. https://doi.org/10.1016/S0140-6736(20)30852-7

Tonkin, S. S., Williams, T. F., Simms, L. J., Tiffany, S. T., Mahoney, M. C., Schnoll, R. A., Cinciripini, P. M., & Hawk, L. W. Jr. (2020). Withdrawal symptom, treatment mechanism, and/or side effect? Developing an explicit measurement model for smoking cessation research. *Nicotine & Tobacco Research, 22*(4), 482–491. https://doi.org/10.1093/ntr/nty262

S

Successful Aging   **2016**

Definition: Personal actions to maintain a high state of physical, functional, psychological, and social functioning in old age

OUTCOME TARGET RATING: Maintain at _____ Increase to _____

		Never Demonstrated	Rarely Demonstrated	Sometimes Demonstrated	Often Demonstrated	Consistently Demonstrated	
OUTCOME OVERALL RATING		1	2	3	4	5	
Indicators:							
201601	Maintains purpose in life	1	2	3	4	5	NA
201602	Maintains independence	1	2	3	4	5	NA
201603	Positive expectations about aging	1	2	3	4	5	NA
201604	Maintains connections with family	1	2	3	4	5	NA
201605	Maintains connections with friends	1	2	3	4	5	NA
201606	Physiological resilience	1	2	3	4	5	NA
201607	Emotional resilience	1	2	3	4	5	NA
201608	Capacity to respond to stressful situations	1	2	3	4	5	NA
201609	Compensates for disabilities	1	2	3	4	5	NA
201610	High physical function	1	2	3	4	5	NA
201611	High cognitive function	1	2	3	4	5	NA
201612	Positive mood	1	2	3	4	5	NA
201613	Positive self-esteem	1	2	3	4	5	NA
201614	Influences others' lives in positive ways	1	2	3	4	5	NA
201615	Sustains engagement in social activities	1	2	3	4	5	NA
201616	Shows respect in social interactions	1	2	3	4	5	NA
201617	Sustains engagement in productive activities	1	2	3	4	5	NA
201618	Sustains engagement in community activities	1	2	3	4	5	NA
201619	Sustains engagement in spiritual activities	1	2	3	4	5	NA
201620	Financial security for needs and wants	1	2	3	4	5	NA

Domain-Health & Life Quality(V)   **Class**-Perceived Health & Life Situation (U)   7th edition 2024

OUTCOME CONTENT REFERENCES:

Borras, C., Ingles, M., Mas-Bargues, C., Dromant, M., Sanz-Ros, J., Román-Domínguez, A., Gimeno-Mallench, L., Gambini, J., & Viña, J. (2020). Centenarians: An excellent example of resilience for successful ageing. *Mechanisms of Ageing and Development, 186*, 111199. https://doi.org/10.1016/j.mad.2019.111199

Cotter, D. L., Walters, S. M., Fonseca, C., Wolf, A., Cobigo, Y., Fox, E. C., You, M. Y., Altendahl, M., Djukic, N., Staffaroni, A. M., Elahi, F. M., Kramer, J. H., Kaitlin B., & Casaletto, K. B. (2020). Aging and positive mood: Longitudinal neurobiological and cognitive correlates. *The American Journal of Geriatric Psychiatry, 28*(9), 946–956. https://doi.org/10.1016/j.jagp.2020.05.002

Gopinath, B., Gerald Liew, G., Burlutsky, G., McMahon, C. M., & Mitchell, P. (2020). Association between vision and hearing impairment and successful aging over five years. *Maturitas, 143*, 203–208. https//doi.org/10.1016/j.maturitas.2020.10.015

Lucena, A. F., Argenta, C., Luzia, M. F., Almeida, M. A., Barreto, L. N. M., & Swanson, E. (2020). Multidimensional Model of Successful Aging and nursing terminologies: Similarities for use in the clinical practice. *Revista Gaúcha de Enfermagem, 41*(spe), e20190148. https://doi.org/10.1590/1983-1447.2020.20190148

Maharani, A., Pendleton, N., & Iracema, L., I. (2019). Hearing impairment, loneliness, social isolation, and cognitive function: Longitudinal analysis using English Longitudinal Study on Ageing. *The American Journal of Geriatric Psychiatry, 27*(12), 1348–1356. https://doi.org/10.1016/j.jagp.2019.07.010

Moreno-Agostino, D., Daskalopoulou, C., Wu, Y.-T., Koukounari, A., Haro, J. M., Tyrovolas, S., Panagiotakos, D. B., Prince, M., & Prina, A. M. (2020). The impact of physical activity on healthy ageing trajectories: Evidence from eight cohort studies. *International Journal of Behavioral Nutrition & Physical Activity, 17*(1), 1–12. https://doi.org/10.1186/s12966-020-00995-8

Pietrzak, R. H., Levy, B. R., Tsai, J., & Southwick, S. M. (2021). Successful aging in older U.S. veterans: Results from the 2019–2020 National Health and Resilience in Veterans Study. *The American Journal of Geriatric Psychiatry, 29*(3), 251–256. https://doi.org/10.1016/j.jagp.2020.08.006

Reich, A. J., Claunch, K. D., Verdeja, M. A., Dung, M. T., Anderson, S., Clayton, C. K., Goates, M. C., & Thacker, E. L. (2020). What does "Successful Aging" mean to you? Systematic review and cross-cultural comparison of lay perspectives of older adults in 13 countries, 2010–2020. *Journal of Cross-Cultural Gerontology, 35*(4), 455–478. https://doi.org/10.1007/s10823-020-09416-6

S

Rowe, J. W., & Kahn, R. L. (1997). Successful aging. *The Gerontologist, 37*(4), 433–440, https://doi.org/10.1093/geront/37.4.433

Shrira, A., Carmel, S., Tovel, H., & Raveis, V. H. (2019). Reciprocal relationships between the will-to-live and successful aging. *Aging & Mental Health, 23*(10), 1350–1357. https://doi.org/10.1080/13607863.2018.1499011

Teater, B., & Chonody, J. M. (2020). How do older adults define successful aging? A scoping review. *The International Journal of Aging and Human Development, 91*(4), 599–625. https://doi.org/10.1177/0091415019871207

Teater, B., & Chonody, J. M. (2020). What attributes of successful aging are important to older adults? The development of a multidimensional definition of successful aging. *Social Work in Health Care, 59*(3), 161–179. https://doi.org/10.1080/00981389.2020.1731049

Urtamo, A., Jyväkorpi, S. K., & Strandberg, T. E. (2019). Definitions of successful ageing: A brief review of a multidimensional concept. *Acta Biomedical Atenei Parmensis, 90*(2), 359–363. https://doi.org/10.23750/abm.v90i2.8376

Suffering Severity

2003

Definition: Severity of signs and symptoms of long-term anguish due to a distressing event, injury, or loss

OUTCOME TARGET RATING: Maintain at _____ Increase to _____

OUTCOME OVERALL RATING	Severe	Substantial	Moderate	Mild	None	
	1	2	3	4	5	
Indicators:						
200301 Self-absorption	1	2	3	4	5	NA
200302 Depression	1	2	3	4	5	NA
200303 Sadness	1	2	3	4	5	NA
200304 Powerlessness	1	2	3	4	5	NA
200305 Grief	1	2	3	4	5	NA
200306 Guilt	1	2	3	4	5	NA
200307 Hopelessness	1	2	3	4	5	NA
200308 Helplessness	1	2	3	4	5	NA
200309 Worthlessness	1	2	3	4	5	NA
200314 Vulnerability	1	2	3	4	5	NA
200315 Spiritual distress	1	2	3	4	5	NA
200316 Despair	1	2	3	4	5	NA
200319 Loneliness	1	2	3	4	5	NA
200310 Fear of reoccurrence	1	2	3	4	5	NA
200311 Fear of unbearable pain	1	2	3	4	5	NA
200312 Fear of unknown circumstances	1	2	3	4	5	NA
200313 Fear of being alone	1	2	3	4	5	NA
200317 Bitterness toward others	1	2	3	4	5	NA

Domain-Health & Life Quality (V)   **Class**-Symptom Status (V)   *2nd edition 2000; revised 2004, 2013*

OUTCOME CONTENT REFERENCES:

Ankri, J., Adrieu, S., Beaufils, B., Grand, A., & Henrard, J. C. (2005). Beyond the global score of the Zarit Burden Interview: Useful dimensions for clinicians. *International Journal of Geriatric Psychiatry, 20*(3), 254–260. https://doi.org/10.1177/0272684X17749570

Cherny, N. I., Coyle, N., & Foley, K. M. (1994). The treatment of suffering when patients request elective death. *Journal of Palliative Care, 10*(2), 71–79.

Copp, L. A. (1974). The spectrum of suffering. *AJN, American Journal of Nursing, 74*(3), 491–495. https://doi.org/10.2307/3469642

Duffy, M. E. (1992). A theoretical and empirical review of the concept of suffering. In P. L. Starck & J. P. McGovern (Eds.), *The hidden dimension of illness: Human suffering* (Pub. No. 15-2451, pp. 291–303). National League for Nursing Press.

Fochtman, D. (2006). The concept of suffering in children and adolescents with cancer. *Journal of Pediatric Oncology Nursing, 23*(2), 92–102. https://doi.org/10.1177/1043454205285870

Hall, P. (2006). Mothers' experiences of postnatal depression: An interpretative phenomenological analysis. *Community Practitioner, 79*(8), 256–260.

Jacob, S. R., & Scandrett-Hobdon, S. (1994). Mothers grieving the death of a child: Case reports of maternal grief. *The Nurse Practitioner, 19*(7), 60–65. https://doi.org/10.1097/00006205-199407000-00011

Mako, C., Galek, K., & Poppito, S. R. (2006). Spiritual pain among patients with advanced cancer in palliative care. *Journal of Palliative Medicine, 9*(5), 1106–1113. https://doi.org/10.1089/jpm.2006.9.1106

Mount, B. M. (1984). Psychological and social aspects of cancer pain. In P. D. Wall & R. Melzack (Eds.), *Textbook of pain* (pp. 460–471). Churchill Livingstone.

Price, D. D., & Harkins, S. W. (1992). Psychophysical approaches to pain measurement and assessment. In D. C. Turk & R. Melzack (Eds.), *Handbook of pain assessment* (pp. 111–134). The Guilford Press.

Steeves, R. H., Kahn, D. L., & Benoliel, J. Q. (1990). Nurses' interpretation of the suffering of their patients. *Western Journal of Nursing Research, 12*(6), 714–731. https://doi.org/10.1177/019394599001200602

S

Suicide Self-Restraint   1408

Definition: Personal actions to refrain from gestures and attempts at killing self

OUTCOME TARGET RATING: Maintain at _____ Increase to _____

		Never Demonstrated	Rarely Demonstrated	Sometimes Demonstrated	Often Demonstrated	Consistently Demonstrated	
OUTCOME OVERALL RATING		1	2	3	4	5	
Indicators:							
140828	Maintains personal grooming and hygiene	1	2	3	4	5	NA
140801	Expresses feelings	1	2	3	4	5	NA
140815	Expresses sense of hope	1	2	3	4	5	NA
140802	Maintains connectedness in relationships	1	2	3	4	5	NA
140823	Obtains assistance as needed	1	2	3	4	5	NA
140804	Verbalizes suicidal ideas	1	2	3	4	5	NA
140805	Controls impulses	1	2	3	4	5	NA
140829	Engages in purposeful activities	1	2	3	4	5	NA
140830	Maintains consistent mood	1	2	3	4	5	NA
140831	Refrains from substance abuse	1	2	3	4	5	NA
140832	Maintains sleep pattern	1	2	3	4	5	NA
140806	Refrains from gathering means for suicide	1	2	3	4	5	NA
140807	Refrains from giving away possessions	1	2	3	4	5	NA
140816	Refrains from inflicting serious injury	1	2	3	4	5	NA
140833	Refrains from risk-taking behavior	1	2	3	4	5	NA
140809	Refrains from using non-prescribed mood-altering substances	1	2	3	4	5	NA
140810	Discloses plan for suicide if present	1	2	3	4	5	NA
140811	Upholds suicide contract	1	2	3	4	5	NA
140812	Maintains self-control without supervision	1	2	3	4	5	NA
140813	Refrains from attempting suicide	1	2	3	4	5	NA
140824	Obtains treatment for depression	1	2	3	4	5	NA
140825	Obtains treatment for substance abuse	1	2	3	4	5	NA
140834	Uses strategies to reduce stress	1	2	3	4	5	NA
140835	Obtains assistance for mental health issues	1	2	3	4	5	NA
140819	Reports adequate pain control for chronic pain	1	2	3	4	5	NA
140836	Uses crisis intervention hotline	1	2	3	4	5	NA
140826	Uses suicide prevention resources	1	2	3	4	5	NA
140827	Uses social support groups	1	2	3	4	5	NA
140821	Uses available mental health services	1	2	3	4	5	NA
140822	Plans for future	1	2	3	4	5	NA

Domain-Psychosocial Health (III)   *Class*-Self-Control (O)   *1st edition 1997; revised 2000, 2004, 2008, 2024*

OUTCOME CONTENT REFERENCES:
Bryan, C. J., May, A. M., Rozek, D. C., Williams, S. R., Clemans, T. A., Mintz, J., Leeson, B., & Burch, T. S. (2018). Use of crisis management interventions among suicidal patients: Results of a randomized clinical trial. *Depression and Anxiety, 35*(7), 619–628, https://doi.org/10.1002/da.22753

Choi, K. W., Na, E. J., Hong, J. P., Cho, M. J., Fava, M., Mischoulon, D., Cho, H., Jeon, H. J. (2018). Alcohol-induced disinhibition is associated with impulsivity, depression, and suicide attempt: A nationwide community sample of Korean adults. *Journal of Affective Disorders, 227*, 323–329. https://doi.org/10.1016/j.jad.2017.11.001

de Sousa, G. S., Perrelli, J. G. A., de Oliveira Mangueira, S., de Oliveira Lopes, M. V., & Sougey, E. B. (2020). Clinical validation of the nursing diagnosis risk for suicide in the older adults. *Archives of Psychiatric Nursing, 34*(2), 21–28. https://doi.org/10.1016/j.apnu.2020.01.003

Ji, Y. D., Robertson, F. C., Patel, N. A., Peacock, Z. S., & Resnick, C. M. (2020). Assessment of risk factors for suicide among U.S. health care professionals. *JAMA Surgery, 155*(8), 713–721, https://doi.org/10.1001/jamasurg.20201338

S

Kellerman, Q. D., Hartoonian, N., Beier, M. L., Leipertz, S. L., Maynard, C., Hostetter, T. A., Haselkorn, J. K., & Turner, A. P. (2020). Risk factors for suicide in a national sample of veterans with multiple sclerosis. *Archives of Physical Medicine and Rehabilitation, 101*, 1138–1143. https://doi.org/10.1016/j.apmr.2020.03.013

Nelson, P. A., & Adams, S. M. (2020). Role of primary care in suicide prevention during the COVID-19 pandemic. *The Journal of Nurse Practitioners, 16*, 654–659. https://doi.org/10.1016/j.nursra.2020.07.015

Nyberg, J., Gustavsson, S., Åberg, M. A., Kuhn, H. G., & Waern, M. (2020). Late-adolescent risk factors for suicide and self-harm in middle-aged men: Explorative prospective population-based study. *The British Journal of Psychiatry, 217*, 370–376. https://doi.org/10.1192/bjp.2019.243

Schmutte, T., Olfson, M., Xie, M., & Marcus, S. C. (2020). Self-harm, suicidal ideation, and attempted suicide in older adults: A national study of emergency department visits and follow-up care. *American Journal of Geriatric Psychiatry, 28*(6), 646–658. https://doi.org/10.1016/j.jagp.2019.12.003

Törnblom, A. W., Sorjonen, K., Runeson, B., & Rydelius, P.-A. (2020). Who is at risk of dying young from suicide and sudden violent death? Common and specific risk factors among children, adolescents, and young adults. *Suicide and Life-Threatening Behavior, 50*(4), 757–777. https://doi.org/10.1111/sltb.12614

Wilson, M. P., Moutier, C., Wolf, L., Nordstrom, K., Schulz, T., & Betz, M. E. (2020). ED recommendations for suicide prevention in adults: The ICAR2E mnemonic and a systematic review of the literature. *American Journal of Emergency Medicine, 38*, 571–581. https://doi.org/10.1016/j.ajem.2019.06.031

Surgical Recovery: Convalescence 2304

Definition: Extent of physiological, psychological, and role function following discharge from post-anesthesia care to the final post-operative clinic visit

OUTCOME TARGET RATING: Maintain at_____ Increase to_____

	Severe Deviation from Normal Range	Substantial Deviation from Normal Range	Moderate Deviation from Normal Range	Mild Deviation from Normal Range	No Deviation from Normal Range	
OUTCOME OVERALL RATING	1	2	3	4	5	
Indicators:						
230401 Systolic blood pressure	1	2	3	4	5	NA
230402 Diastolic blood pressure	1	2	3	4	5	NA
230403 Hemodynamic stability	1	2	3	4	5	NA
230404 Body temperature	1	2	3	4	5	NA
230405 Radial pulse rate	1	2	3	4	5	NA
230406 Radial pulse rhythm	1	2	3	4	5	NA
230407 Respiratory rate	1	2	3	4	5	NA
230408 Depth of inspiration	1	2	3	4	5	NA
230409 Urine output	1	2	3	4	5	NA
230410 Bowel sounds	1	2	3	4	5	NA
230411 Bowel elimination	1	2	3	4	5	NA
230412 Electrolyte balance	1	2	3	4	5	NA
230413 Fluid intake	1	2	3	4	5	NA
230414 Hydration	1	2	3	4	5	NA
230415 Food intake	1	2	3	4	5	NA
230416 Blood glucose level	1	2	3	4	5	NA
230417 Tissue integrity	1	2	3	4	5	NA
230418 Neurovascular integrity	1	2	3	4	5	NA
230419 Wound healing	1	2	3	4	5	NA
230420 Ambulation	1	2	3	4	5	NA
230421 Cognition	1	2	3	4	5	NA
230422 Concentration	1	2	3	4	5	NA
230423 Sleep	1	2	3	4	5	NA
230424 Performance of prescribed exercise	1	2	3	4	5	NA
230425 Performance of prescribed wound care	1	2	3	4	5	NA

S

Surgical Recovery: Convalescence—cont'd

		Severe Deviation from Normal Range	Substantial Deviation from Normal Range	Moderate Deviation from Normal Range	Mild Deviation from Normal Range	No Deviation from Normal Range	
230426	Adjustment to body changes due to surgery	1	2	3	4	5	NA
230427	Use of prescribed assistive devices	1	2	3	4	5	NA
230428	Performance of self-care activities	1	2	3	4	5	NA
230429	Resumption of normal activities	1	2	3	4	5	NA
230430	Resumption of normal role function	1	2	3	4	5	NA
		Severe	Substantial	Moderate	Mild	None	
230431	Atelectasis	1	2	3	4	5	NA
230432	Pneumonia	1	2	3	4	5	NA
230433	Pain	1	2	3	4	5	NA
230434	Drainage on dressing	1	2	3	4	5	NA
230435	Drainage from drains	1	2	3	4	5	NA
230436	Wound infection	1	2	3	4	5	NA
230437	Wound dehiscence	1	2	3	4	5	NA
230438	Thrombophlebitis	1	2	3	4	5	NA
230439	Pulmonary embolus	1	2	3	4	5	NA
230440	Nausea	1	2	3	4	5	NA
230441	Vomiting	1	2	3	4	5	NA
230442	Paralytic ileus	1	2	3	4	5	NA
230443	Constipation	1	2	3	4	5	NA
230444	Fatigue	1	2	3	4	5	NA
230445	Anxiety	1	2	3	4	5	NA
230446	Depression	1	2	3	4	5	NA

Domain-Physiologic Health (II)   **Class**-Therapeutic Response (AA)   5th edition 2013

OUTCOME CONTENT REFERENCES:

Capasso, V. A., Codner, C., Nuzzo-Meuller, G., Cox, E. M., & Bouvier, S. (2006). Peripheral arterial sheath removal program: A performance improvement initiative. *Journal of Vascular Nursing, 24*(4), 127–132. https://doi.org/10.1016/j.jvn.2006.09.001

Douglas, M., & Rowed, S. (2005). The implementation of a postoperative care process on a neurosurgical unit. *Journal of Neuroscience Nursing, 37*(6), 329–333. https://doi.org/10.1097/01376517-200512000-00006

Galli, B., Munver, R., Sawczuk, I., & Kochis, E. (2005). Laparoscopic radical nephrectomy in renal cell carcinoma. *Urologic Nursing, 25*(2), 83–86, 133.

Gilmartin, J. (2007). Contemporary day surgery: Patients' experience of discharge and recovery. *Journal of Clinical Nursing, 16*(6), 1109–1117. https://doi.org/10.1111/j.1365-2702.2007.01548.x

Hodgins, M. J., Ouellet, L. L., Pond, S., Knorr, S., & Geldart, G. (2008). Effect of telephone follow-up on surgical orthopedic recovery. *Applied Nursing Research, 21*(4), 218–226. https://doi.org/10.1016/j.apnr.2007.01.008

Montin, L., Leino-Kilpi, H., Suominen, T., & Lepisto, J. (2008). A systematic review of empirical studies between 1966 and 2005 of patient outcomes of total hip arthroplasty and related factors. *Journal of Clinical Nursing, 17*(1), 40–45. https://doi.org/10.1111/j.1365-2702.2007.01944.x

Oakes, C. L., Ellington, K. J., Oakes, K. J., Olson, R. L., Neill, K. M., & Vacchiano, C. A. (2002). Assessment of post anesthesia short-term quality of life: A pilot study. *AANA Journal, 70*(4), 27–273.

Pasero, C., & Belden, J. (2006). Evidence-based perianesthesia care: Accelerated postoperative recovery programs. *Journal of Peri Anesthesia Nursing 21*(3), 168–176. https://doi.org/10.1016/j.jopan.2006.03.010

Pop, R. S., Manworren, R. C., Guzzetta, C. E., & Hynan, L. S. (2007). Perianesthesia nurses' pain management after tonsillectomy and adenoidectomy: Pediatric patient outcomes. *Journal of PeriAnesthesia Nursing, 22*(2), 91–101. https://doi.org/10.1016/j.jopan.2007.01.003

Richards, N. M. (2007). Outcomes in special populations undergoing cardiac surgery: Octogenarians, women and adults with congenital heart disease. *Critical Care Nursing Clinics of North America, 19*(4), 467–485. https://doi.org/10.1016/j.ccell.2007.07.003

Slusarz, R., Beuth, W., & Ksiazkiewicz, B. (2009). Postsurgical examination of functional outcome of patients having undergone surgical treatment of intracranial aneurysm. *Scandinavian Journal of Caring Science, 23*(1), 130–139. https://doi.org/10.1111/j.1471-6712.2008.00599.x

S

Surgical Recovery: Immediate Post–Operative   2305

Definition: Extent to which an individual achieves physiological baseline function following major surgery requiring anesthesia

OUTCOME TARGET RATING: Maintain at_____ Increase to_____

		Severe Deviation from Normal Range	Substantial Deviation from Normal Range	Moderate Deviation from Normal Range	Mild Deviation from Normal Range	No Deviation from Normal Range	
OUTCOME OVERALL RATING		1	2	3	4	5	
Indicators:							
230501	Patent airway	1	2	3	4	5	NA
230502	Systolic blood pressure	1	2	3	4	5	NA
230503	Diastolic blood pressure	1	2	3	4	5	NA
230504	Pulse pressure	1	2	3	4	5	NA
230505	Body temperature	1	2	3	4	5	NA
230506	Apical heart rate	1	2	3	4	5	NA
230507	Apical heart rhythm	1	2	3	4	5	NA
230508	Radial pulse rate	1	2	3	4	5	NA
230509	Depth of inspiration	1	2	3	4	5	NA
230510	Respiratory rate	1	2	3	4	5	NA
230511	Respiratory rhythm	1	2	3	4	5	NA
230512	Oxygen saturation	1	2	3	4	5	NA
230513	Level of consciousness	1	2	3	4	5	NA
230514	Cognitive orientation	1	2	3	4	5	NA
230515	Urine output	1	2	3	4	5	NA
230516	Bowel sounds	1	2	3	4	5	NA
230517	Gag reflex	1	2	3	4	5	NA
230518	Tissue integrity	1	2	3	4	5	NA
230519	Peripheral sensation	1	2	3	4	5	NA
230520	Drainage from wound drains/ tubes	1	2	3	4	5	NA

		Severe	Substantial	Moderate	Mild	None	
230521	Bleeding	1	2	3	4	5	NA
230522	Pain	1	2	3	4	5	NA
230523	Drainage on dressing	1	2	3	4	5	NA
230524	Wound site swelling	1	2	3	4	5	NA
230525	Intracranial pressure	1	2	3	4	5	NA
230526	Nausea	1	2	3	4	5	NA
230527	Vomiting	1	2	3	4	5	NA
230528	Headache	1	2	3	4	5	NA
230529	Sore throat	1	2	3	4	5	NA
230530	Hyperglycemia	1	2	3	4	5	NA
230531	Hypoglycemia	1	2	3	4	5	NA

Domain-*Physiologic Health (II)*   **Class**-*Therapeutic Response (AA)*   *5th edition 2013*

OUTCOME CONTENT REFERENCES:

Capasso, V. A., Codner, C., Nuzzo-Meuller, G., Cox, E. M., & Bouvier, S. (2006). Peripheral arterial sheath removal program: A performance improvement initiative. *Journal of Vascular Nursing, 24*(4), 127–132. https://doi.org/10.1016/j.jvn.2006.09.001

Douglas, M., & Rowed, S. (2005). The implementation of a postoperative care process on a neurosurgical unit. *Journal of Neuroscience Nursing, 37*(6), 329–333. https://doi.org/10.1097/01376517-200512000-00006

Galli, B., Munver, R., Sawczuk, I., & Kochis, E. (2005). Laparoscopic radical nephrectomy in renal cell carcinoma. *Urologic Nursing, 25*(2), 83–86, 133.

Gilmartin, J. (2007). Contemporary day surgery: Patients' experience of discharge and recovery. *Journal of Clinical Nursing, 16*(6), 1109–1117. https://doi.org/10.1111/j.1365-2702.2007.01548.x

Hodgins, M. J., Ouellet, L. L., Pond, S., Knorr, S., & Geldart, G. (2008). Effect of telephone follow-up on surgical orthopedic recovery. *Applied Nursing Research, 21*(4), 218–226. https://doi.org/10.1016/j.apnr.2007.01.008

Montin, L., Leino-Kilpi, H., Suominen, T., & Lepisto, J. (2008). A systematic review of empirical studies between 1966 and 2005 of patient outcomes of total hip arthroplasty and related factors. *Journal of Clinical Nursing, 17*(1), 40–45. https://doi.org/10.1111/j.1365-2702.2007.01944.x

Oakes, C. L., Ellington, K. J., Oakes, K. J., Olson, R. L., Neill, K. M., & Vacchiano, C. A. (2002). Assessment of post anesthesia short-term quality of life: A pilot study. *AANA Journal, 70*(4), 27–273.

Pasero, C., & Belden, J. (2006). Evidence-based perianesthesia care: Accelerated postoperative recovery programs. *Journal of PeriAnesthesia Nursing 21*(3), 168–176. https://doi.org/10.1016/j.jopan.2006.03.010

Pop, R. S., Manworren, R. C., Guzzetta, C. E., & Hynan, L. S. (2007). Perianesthesia nurses' pain management after tonsillectomy and adenoidectomy: Pediatric patient outcomes. *Journal of PeriAnesthesia Nursing, 22*(2), 91–101. https://doi.org/10.1016/j.jopan.2007.01.003

Richards, N. M. (2007). Outcomes in special populations undergoing cardiac surgery: Octogenarians, women and adults with congenital heart disease. *Critical Care Nursing Clinics of North America, 19*(4), 467–485. https://doi.org/10.1016/j.ccell.2007.07.003

Slusarz, R., Beuth, W., & Ksiazkiewicz, B. (2009). Postsurgical examination of functional outcome of patients having undergone surgical treatment of intracranial aneurysm. *Scandinavian Journal of Caring Science, 23*(1), 130–139. https://doi.org/10.1111/j.1471-6712.2008.00599.x

Swallowing Status   1010

Definition: Ability to move fluids and/or solids safely from the mouth to the stomach

OUTCOME TARGET RATING: Maintain at _____ Increase to _____

		Severely Compromised	Substantially Compromised	Moderately Compromised	Mildly Compromised	Not Compromised	
OUTCOME OVERALL RATING		1	2	3	4	5	
Indicators:							
101001	Maintains food in mouth	1	2	3	4	5	NA
101002	Handles oral secretions	1	2	3	4	5	NA
101003	Saliva production	1	2	3	4	5	NA
101004	Chewing ability	1	2	3	4	5	NA
101005	Delivery of bolus to hypopharynx is timed with swallow reflex	1	2	3	4	5	NA
101006	Ability to clear oral cavity	1	2	3	4	5	NA
101007	Timely bolus formation	1	2	3	4	5	NA
101008	Number of swallows appropriate for bolus size/texture	1	2	3	4	5	NA
101009	Meal duration with respect to amount consumed	1	2	3	4	5	NA
101010	Timely swallow reflex	1	2	3	4	5	NA
101015	Maintains neutral head and trunk position	1	2	3	4	5	NA
101016	Food acceptance	1	2	3	4	5	NA
101018	Swallow study findings	1	2	3	4	5	NA
		Severe	**Substantial**	**Moderate**	**Mild**	**None**	
101011	Changes in voice quality	1	2	3	4	5	NA
101012	Choking	1	2	3	4	5	NA
101020	Coughing	1	2	3	4	5	NA
101021	Gagging	1	2	3	4	5	NA
101013	Increased swallow effort	1	2	3	4	5	NA
101014	Gastric reflux	1	2	3	4	5	NA
101017	Discomfort with swallowing	1	2	3	4	5	NA
101022	Maxillofacial trauma	1	2	3	4	5	NA

Domain-Physiologic Health (II)   *Class-Digestion & Nutrition (K)*   *2nd edition 2000; reviewed 2018; revised 2004, 2024*

S

OUTCOME CONTENT REFERENCES:

Arvedson, J., Brodsky, L., & Lefton-Greif, M. A. (Eds.). (2019). *Pediatric swallowing and feeding: Assessment and management* (3rd ed.). Plural.

Bahia, M. M., & Lowell, S. Y. (2020). A systematic review of the physiological effects of the effortful swallow maneuver in adults with normal and disordered swallowing. *American Journal of Speech-Language Pathology, 29*(3), 1655–1673. https://doi.org/10.1044/2020_AJSLP-19-00132

Belafsky, P. C., Mouadeb, D. A., Rees, C. J., Pryor, J. C., Postma, G. N., Allen, J., & Leonard, R. J. (2008). Validity and reliability of the Eating Assessment Tool (EAT-10). *Annals of Otology, Rhinology & Laryngology, 117*(12), 919–924. https://doi.org/10.1177/000348940811701210

Dharmarathna, I., Miles, A., & Allen, J. (2020). Twenty years of quantitative instrumental measures of swallowing in children: A systematic review. *European Journal of Pediatrics, 179*(2), 203–223. https://doi.org/10.1007/s00431-019-03546-x

Hida, Y., Nishida, T., Taniguchi, C., & Sakakibara, H. (2021). Association between swallowing function and oral bacterial flora in independent community-dwelling elderly. *Aging Clinical & Experimental Research, 33*(1), 157–163. https://doi.org/10.1007/s40520-020-01521-3

Kendall, K. A., Ellerston, J., Heller, A., Houtz, D. R., Zhang, C., & Presson, A. P. (2016). Objective measures of swallowing function applied to the dysphagia population: A one year experience. *Dysphagia, 31*(4), 538–546. https://doi.org/10.1007/s00455-016-9711-0

Oliveira-Kumakura, A. R. D. S., de Araujo, T. L., Costa, A. G. D. S., Cavalcante, T. F., Lopes, M. V. D. O., & Carvalho, E. C. (2017). Clinical validation of the nursing outcome "swallowing status" in people with stroke: Analysis according to the classical and item response theories. *International Journal of Nursing Knowledge, 29*(4), 234–241. https://doi.org/10.1111/2047-3095.12184

Oliveira-Kumakura, A. R. D. S., Alonso, J. B., & Campos de Carvalho, E. (2019). Psychometric assessment of the nursing outcome Swallowing Status: Rasch model approach. *International Journal of Nursing Knowledge, 30*(4), 197–202. https://doi.org/10.1111/2047-3095.12229

Pearson, W. G. Jr., Griffeth, J. V., & Ennis, A. M. (2019). Functional anatomy underlying pharyngeal swallowing mechanics and swallowing performance goals. *Perspectives of the ASHA Special Interest Groups, 4*(4), 648–655. https://doi.org/10.1044/2019_PERS-SIG13-2018-0014

Railka de Souza Oliveira, A., Leite de Araujo, T., Campos de Carvalho, E., Gabrielle de Sousa Costa, A., Frota Cavalcante, T., & Venícios de Oliveira Lopes, M. (2015). Construction and validation of indicators and respective definitions for the nursing outcome Swallowing Status. *Revista Latino–Americana de Enfermagem (RLAE), 23*(3), 450–457. https://doi.org/10.1590/0104-1169.0377.2575

Solomon, N. P., Dietsch, A. M., & Dietrich–Burns, K. (2020). Predictors of swallowing outcomes in patients with combat-injury related dysphagia. *Journal of Trauma & Acute Care Surgery, 89*(Suppl. 2), S192–S199. https://doi.org/10.1097/TA.0000000000002623

Warnecke, T., Dziewas, R., & Langmore, S. (2021). *Neurogenic dysphagia.* Springer.

Swallowing Status: Esophageal Phase   1011

Definition: Ability to move fluids and/or solids safely from the pharynx to the stomach

OUTCOME TARGET RATING: Maintain at _____ Increase to _____

		Severely Compromised	Substantially Compromised	Moderately Compromised	Mildly Compromised	Not Compromised	
OUTCOME OVERALL RATING		**1**	**2**	**3**	**4**	**5**	
Indicators:							
101106	Maintains neutral head and neck position	1	2	3	4	5	NA
101114	Food acceptance	1	2	3	4	5	NA
101115	Volume acceptance	1	2	3	4	5	NA
101116	Esophageal phase study findings	1	2	3	4	5	NA
		Severe	**Substantial**	**Moderate**	**Mild**	**None**	
101101	Choking with swallowing	1	2	3	4	5	NA
101118	Coughing with swallowing	1	2	3	4	5	NA
101102	Gastric reflux	1	2	3	4	5	NA
101103	Epigastric pain	1	2	3	4	5	NA
101104	Discomfort with swallowing	1	2	3	4	5	NA
101108	Nighttime coughing	1	2	3	4	5	NA
101109	Nighttime vomiting	1	2	3	4	5	NA
101119	Nighttime choking	1	2	3	4	5	NA
101110	Repetitive swallowing	1	2	3	4	5	NA
101111	Hematemesis	1	2	3	4	5	NA
101112	Acidic breath odor	1	2	3	4	5	NA
101113	Bruxism	1	2	3	4	5	NA

Domain-*Physiologic Health (II)*   **Class**-*Digestion & Nutrition (K)*   *2nd edition 2000; reviewed 2018; revised 2004, 2024*

S

OUTCOME CONTENT REFERENCES:

Arvedson, J., Brodsky, L., & Lefton-Greif, M. A. (Eds.). (2019). *Pediatric swallowing and feeding: Assessment and management* (3rd ed.). Plural.

Bahia, M. M., & Lowell, S. Y. (2020). A systematic review of the physiological effects of the effortful swallow maneuver in adults with normal and disordered swallowing. *American Journal of Speech-Language Pathology, 29*(3), 1655–1673. https://doi.org/10.1044/2020_AJSLP-19-00132

Belafsky, P. C., Mouadeb, D. A., Rees, C. J., Pryor, J. C., Postma, G. N., Allen, J., & Leonard, R. J. (2008). Validity and reliability of the Eating Assessment Tool (EAT-10). *Annals of Otology, Rhinology & Laryngology, 117*(12), 919–924. https://doi.org/10.1177/000348940811701210

Dharmarathna, I., Miles, A., & Allen, J. (2020). Twenty years of quantitative instrumental measures of swallowing in children: A systematic review. *European Journal of Pediatrics, 179*(2), 203–223. https://doi.org/10.1007/s00431-019-03546-x

Hida, Y., Nishida, T., Taniguchi, C., & Sakakibara, H. (2021). Association between swallowing function and oral bacterial flora in independent community-dwelling elderly. *Aging Clinical & Experimental Research, 33*(1), 157–163. https://doi.org/10.1007/s40520-020-01521-3

Kendall, K. A., Ellerston, J., Heller, A., Houtz, D. R., Zhang, C., & Presson, A. P. (2016). Objective measures of swallowing function applied to the dysphagia population: A one year experience. *Dysphagia, 31*(4), 538–546. https://doi.org/10.1007/s00455-016-9711-0

Oliveira-Kumakura, A. R. D. S., de Araujo, T. L., Costa, A. G. D. S., Cavalcante, T. F., Lopes, M. V. D. O., & Carvalho, E. C. (2017). Clinical validation of the nursing outcome "swallowing status" in people with stroke: Analysis according to the classical and item response theories. *International Journal of Nursing Knowledge, 29*(4), 234–241. https://doi.org/10.1111/2047-3095.12184

Pearson, W. G. Jr., Griffeth, J. V., & Ennis, A. M. (2019). Functional anatomy underlying pharyngeal swallowing mechanics and swallowing performance goals. *Perspectives of the ASHA Special Interest Groups, 4*(4), 648–655. https://doi.org/10.1044/2019_PERS-SIG13-2018-0014

Warnecke, T., Dziewas, R., & Langmore, S. (2021). *Neurogenic dysphagia.* Springer.

Swallowing Status: Oral Phase   1012

Definition: Ability to prepare and move fluids and/or solids to the posterior area of the mouth

OUTCOME TARGET RATING: Maintain at _____ Increase to _____

		Severely Compromised	Substantially Compromised	Moderately Compromised	Mildly Compromised	Not Compromised	
OUTCOME OVERALL RATING		1	2	3	4	5	
Indicators:							
101201	Maintains food in mouth	1	2	3	4	5	NA
101202	Handles oral secretions	1	2	3	4	5	NA
101203	Bolus formation	1	2	3	4	5	NA
101204	Timely bolus formation	1	2	3	4	5	NA
101205	Chewing ability	1	2	3	4	5	NA
101206	Delivery of bolus to hypopharynx timed with swallow reflex	1	2	3	4	5	NA
101207	Ability to clear oral cavity	1	2	3	4	5	NA
101209	Lip closure	1	2	3	4	5	NA
101210	Number of swallows appropriate for bolus size/texture	1	2	3	4	5	NA
101211	Nippling efficiency	1	2	3	4	5	NA
101212	Rate of food consumption	1	2	3	4	5	NA
101214	Gag reflex	1	2	3	4	5	NA
101215	Oral phase study findings	1	2	3	4	5	NA
		Severe	**Substantial**	**Moderate**	**Mild**	**None**	
101208	Coughing before swallowing	1	2	3	4	5	NA
101217	Choking before swallowing	1	2	3	4	5	NA
101218	Gagging before swallowing	1	2	3	4	5	NA
101213	Nasal reflux	1	2	3	4	5	NA
101219	Maxillofacial trauma	1	2	3	4	5	NA

Domain-Physiologic Health (II)   *Class*-Digestion & Nutrition (K)   *2nd edition 2000; reviewed 2018; revised 2004, 2024*

S

OUTCOME CONTENT REFERENCES:

Arvedson, J., Brodsky, L., & Lefton-Greif, M. A. (Eds.). (2019). *Pediatric swallowing and feeding: Assessment and management* (3rd ed.). Plural.

Bahia, M. M., & Lowell, S. Y. (2020). A systematic review of the physiological effects of the effortful swallow maneuver in adults with normal and disordered swallowing. *American Journal of Speech-Language Pathology, 29*(3), 1655–1673. https://doi.org/10.1044/2020_AJSLP-19-00132

Belafsky, P. C., Mouadeb, D. A., Rees, C. J., Pryor, J. C., Postma, G. N., Allen, J., & Leonard, R. J. (2008). Validity and reliability of the eating assessment tool (EAT-10). *Annals of Otology, Rhinology & Laryngology, 117*(12), 919–924. https://doi.org/10.1177/000348940811701210

Dharmarathna, I., Miles, A., & Allen, J. (2020). Twenty years of quantitative instrumental measures of swallowing in children: A systematic review. *European Journal of Pediatrics, 179*(2), 203–223. https://doi.org/10.1007/s00431-019-03546-x

Hida, Y., Nishida, T., Taniguchi, C., & Sakakibara, H. (2021). Association between swallowing function and oral bacterial flora in independent community–dwelling elderly. *Aging Clinical & Experimental Research, 33*(1), 157–163. https://doi.org/10.1007/s40520-020-01521-3

Kendall, K. A., Ellerston, J., Heller, A., Houtz, D. R., Zhang, C., & Presson, A. P. (2016). Objective measures of swallowing function applied to the dysphagia population: A one year experience. *Dysphagia, 31*(4), 538–546. https://doi.org/10.1007/s00455-016-9711-0

Oliveira-Kumakura, A. R. D. S., de Araujo, T. L., Costa, A. G. D. S., Cavalcante, T. F., Lopes, M. V. D. O., & Carvalho, E. C. (2017). Clinical validation of the nursing outcome "swallowing status" in people with stroke: Analysis according to the classical and item response theories. *International Journal of Nursing Knowledge, 29*(4), 234–241. https://doi.org/10.1111/2047-3095.12184

Pearson, W. G. Jr., Griffeth, J. V., & Ennis, A. M. (2019). Functional anatomy underlying pharyngeal swallowing mechanics and swallowing performance goals. *Perspectives of the ASHA Special Interest Groups, 4*(4), 648–655. https://doi.org/10.1044/2019_PERS-SIG13-2018-0014

Solomon, N. P., Dietsch, A. M., & Dietrich-Burns, K. (2020). Predictors of swallowing outcomes in patients with combat-injury related dysphagia. *Journal of Trauma & Acute Care Surgery, 89*, 192–199. https://doi.org/10.1097/TA.0000000000002623

Warnecke, T., Dziewas, R., & Langmore, S. (2021). *Neurogenic dysphagia.* Springer.

Swallowing Status: Pharyngeal Phase   1013

Definition: Ability to move fluids and/or solids safely from the mouth to the esophagus

OUTCOME TARGET RATING: Maintain at _____ Increase to _____

	Severely Compromised	Substantially Compromised	Moderately Compromised	Mildly Compromised	Not Compromised	
OUTCOME OVERALL RATING	1	2	3	4	5	
Indicators:						
101301 Timely swallow reflex	1	2	3	4	5	NA
101304 Number of swallows appropriate for bolus size/texture	1	2	3	4	5	NA
101305 Maintains neutral head and neck position	1	2	3	4	5	NA
101307 Laryngeal elevation	1	2	3	4	5	NA
101311 Food acceptance	1	2	3	4	5	NA
101312 Pharyngeal phase study findings	1	2	3	4	5	NA

	Severe	Substantial	Moderate	Mild	None	
101302 Changes in voice quality	1	2	3	4	5	NA
101303 Choking	1	2	3	4	5	NA
101314 Coughing	1	2	3	4	5	NA
101315 Gagging	1	2	3	4	5	NA
101306 Increased swallow effort	1	2	3	4	5	NA
101310 Nasal reflux	1	2	3	4	5	NA
101316 Aspirations	1	2	3	4	5	NA

Domain-*Physiologic Health (II)*   **Class**-*Digestion & Nutrition (K)*   *2nd edition 2000; reviewed 2018; revised 2004, 2024*

OUTCOME CONTENT REFERENCES:

Arvedson, J., Brodsky, L., & Lefton-Greif, M. A. (Eds.). (2019). *Pediatric swallowing and feeding: Assessment and management* (3rd ed.). Plural.

Bahia, M. M., & Lowell, S. Y. (2020). A systematic review of the physiological effects of the effortful swallow maneuver in adults with normal and disordered swallowing. *American Journal of Speech–Language Pathology, 29*(3), 1655–1673. https://doi.org/10.1044/2020_AJSLP-19-00132

Belafsky, P. C., Mouadeb, D. A., Rees, C. J., Pryor, J. C., Postma, G. N., Allen, J., & Leonard, R. J. (2008). Validity and reliability of the eating assessment tool (EAT-10). *Annals of Otology, Rhinology & Laryngology, 117*(12), 919–924. https://doi.org/10.1177/000348940811701210

Dharmarathna, I., Miles, A., & Allen, J. (2020). Twenty years of quantitative instrumental measures of swallowing in children: A systematic review. *European Journal of Pediatrics, 179*(2), 203–223. https://doi.org/10.1007/s00431-019-03546-x

Hida, Y., Nishida, T., Taniguchi, C., & Sakakibara, H. (2021). Association between swallowing function and oral bacterial flora in independent community–dwelling elderly. *Aging Clinical & Experimental Research, 33*(1), 157–163. https://doi.org/10.1007/s40520-020-01521-3

Kendall, K. A., Ellerston, J., Heller, A., Houtz, D. R., Zhang, C., & Presson, A. P. (2016). Objective measures of swallowing function applied to the dysphagia population: A one year experience. *Dysphagia, 31*(4), 538–546. https://doi.org/10.1007/s00455-016-9711-0

Oliveira-Kumakura, A. R. D. S., de Araujo, T. L., Costa, A. G. D. S., Cavalcante, T. F., Lopes, M. V. D. O., & Carvalho, E. C. (2017). Clinical validation of the nursing outcome "swallowing status" in people with stroke: Analysis according to the classical and item response theories. *International Journal of Nursing Knowledge, 29*(4), 234–241. https://doi.org/10.1111/2047-3095.12184

Pearson, W. G. Jr., Griffeth, J. V., & Ennis, A. M. (2019). Functional anatomy underlying pharyngeal swallowing mechanics and swallowing performance goals. *Perspectives of the ASHA Special Interest Groups, 4*(4), 648–655. https://doi.org/10.1044/2019_PERS-SIG13-2018-0014

Warnecke, T., Dziewas, R., & Langmore, S. (2021). *Neurogenic dysphagia.* Springer.

Symptom Control   1608

Definition: Personal actions to minimize perceived adverse physical and psychological manifestations or signs of illness

OUTCOME TARGET RATING: Maintain at _____ Increase to _____

		Never Demonstrated	Rarely Demonstrated	Sometimes Demonstrated	Often Demonstrated	Consistently Demonstrated	
OUTCOME OVERALL RATING		1	2	3	4	5	
Indicators:							
160801	Monitors symptom onset	1	2	3	4	5	NA
160814	Recognizing precipitating factors	1	2	3	4	5	NA
160802	Monitors symptom persistence	1	2	3	4	5	NA
160803	Monitors symptom severity	1	2	3	4	5	NA
160815	Monitors symptom distress	1	2	3	4	5	NA
160804	Monitors symptom frequency	1	2	3	4	5	NA
160805	Monitors symptom variation	1	2	3	4	5	NA
160816	Monitors physical functioning	1	2	3	4	5	NA
160817	Monitors psychological functioning	1	2	3	4	5	NA
160806	Uses preventive measures	1	2	3	4	5	NA
160807	Uses symptom relief measures	1	2	3	4	5	NA
160813	Obtains health care when warning signs occur	1	2	3	4	5	NA
160809	Uses available resources	1	2	3	4	5	NA
160818	Discusses symptoms with health professional	1	2	3	4	5	NA
160819	Follows recommendations from health professional	1	2	3	4	5	NA
160810	Uses diary or app to monitor symptoms over time	1	2	3	4	5	NA
160811	Reports symptoms controlled	1	2	3	4	5	NA

Domain-Health Knowledge & Behavior (IV)   **Class**-*Health Behavior (Q)*   *1st edition 1997; revised 2000, 2004, 2008, 2024*

OUTCOME CONTENT REFERENCES:

Alderman, B., Webber, K., & Davies, A. (2020). An audit of end-of-life symptom control in patients with corona virus disease 2019 (COVID-19) dying in a hospital in the United Kingdom. *Palliative Medicine, 34*(9), 1249–1255. https://doi.org/10.1177/0269216320947312

Ellershaw, J., Smith, C., Overill, S., Walker, S. E., & Aldridge, J. (2001). Care of the dying: Setting standards for symptom control in the last 48 hours of life. *Journal of Pain and Symptom Management, 21*(1), 12–17. https://doi.org/10.1016/s0885-3924(00)00240-2

Hegyvary, S. T. (1993). Patient care outcomes related to management of symptoms. In J. J. Fitzpatrick & J. S. Stevenson (Eds.), *Annual review of nursing research,* (Vol. 11, pp. 145–168). Springer.

Hyslop, S., Davis, H., Duong, N., Loves, R., Schechter, T., Tomlinson, D., Tomlinson, G. A., Dupuis, L. L., & Sung, L. (2019). Symptom documentation and intervention provision for symptom control in children receiving cancer treatments. *European Journal of Cancer, 109*, 120–128. https://doi.org/10.1016/j.ejca.2019.01.002

+McCorkle, R., & Benoliel, J. Q. (1983). Symptom distress, current concerns, and mood disturbances after diagnosis of life-threatening disease. *Social Science Medicine, 17*(7), 431–438. https://doi.org/10.1016/0277-9536(83)90348-9

+McCorkle, R., & Young, K. (1978). Development of a symptom distress scale. *Cancer Nursing, 1*(5), 373–378.

S

Quirino Afonso, B., da Costa Ferreira, N., & de Cassia Gengo Silva Butcher, R. (2020). Content validation of the symptom control outcome for heart failure patients in palliative care. *Revista Gaucha de Enfermagem, 41*, 1–8. https://doi.org/10.1590/1983-1447.2020.20190427

+ Rhodes, V. A., McDaniel, R. W., Homan, S. S., Johnson, M., & Madsen, R. (2000). An instrument to measure symptom experience. *Cancer Nursing, 23*(1), 49–54. https://doi.org/10.1097/00002820-200002000-00008

Symptom Severity 2103

Definition: Severity of adverse physical, emotional, and social responses

OUTCOME TARGET RATING: Maintain at _____ Increase to _____

		Severe	Substantial	Moderate	Mild	None	
OUTCOME OVERALL RATING		1	2	3	4	5	
Indicators:							
210301	Symptom intensity	1	2	3	4	5	NA
210302	Symptom frequency	1	2	3	4	5	NA
210303	Symptom persistence	1	2	3	4	5	NA
210304	Associated discomfort	1	2	3	4	5	NA
210305	Associated restlessness	1	2	3	4	5	NA
210306	Associated fear	1	2	3	4	5	NA
210307	Associated anxiety	1	2	3	4	5	NA
210317	Associated emotional stress	1	2	3	4	5	NA
210318	Impaired concentration	1	2	3	4	5	NA
210308	Impaired physical mobility	1	2	3	4	5	NA
210309	Impaired role performance	1	2	3	4	5	NA
210319	Impaired work performance	1	2	3	4	5	NA
210320	Impaired school performance	1	2	3	4	5	NA
210310	Impaired interpersonal relationships	1	2	3	4	5	NA
210311	Impaired mood	1	2	3	4	5	NA
210312	Impaired life enjoyment	1	2	3	4	5	NA
210313	Inadequate sleep	1	2	3	4	5	NA
210314	Loss of appetite	1	2	3	4	5	NA
210321	Respiratory distress	1	2	3	4	5	NA
210322	Fatigue	1	2	3	4	5	NA

Domain-Health & Life Quality(V)   **Class**-Symptom Status (V)   *1st edition 1997; revised 2004, 2013, 2024*

OUTCOME CONTENT REFERENCES:

Dhingra, L. K., Lam, K., Cheung, W., Shao, T., Li, Z., Van de Maele, S., Chang, V. T., Chen, J., Ye, H., Wong, R., Lam, W. L., Chan, S., Bookbinder, M., Dieckmann, N. F., & Portenoy, R. (2015). Variation in symptom distress in underserved Chinese American Cancer patients. *Cancer, 121*, 3352–3359. https://doi.org/10.1002/cncr.29497

Han, W., Peng, X., Qu, D., Yang, Y., & Li, K. (2020). Heavy shackles: The experience of symptom distress and coping behaviors of Chinese patients with chronic obstructive pulmonary disease. *Nursing & Health Science*, 22, 1177–1185. https://doi.org/10.1111/nhs.12790

Hegyvary, S. T. (1993). Patient care outcomes related to management of symptoms. In J. J. Fitzpatrick & J. S. Stevenson (Eds.), *Annual review of nursing research* (Vol. 11, pp. 145–168). Springer.

Hui, D., & Bruera, E. (2017). The Edmonton Symptom Assessment System 25 years later: Past, present, and future developments. *Journal of Pain and Symptom Management, 53*(3), 630–643. https://doi.org/10.1016/j.jpainsymman.2016.10.370

+McCorkle, R., & Benoliel, J. Q. (1983). Symptom distress, current concerns, and mood disturbances after diagnosis of life-threatening disease. *Social Science Medicine, 17*(7), 431–438. https://doi.org/10.1016/0277-9536(83)90348-9

+McCorkle, R., & Young, K. (1978). Development of a symptom distress scale. *Cancer Nursing, 1*(5), 373–378.

+ Rhodes, V. A., McDaniel, R. W., Homan, S. S., Johnson, M., & Madsen, R. (2000). An instrument to measure symptom experience. *Cancer Nursing, 23*(1), 49–54. https://doi.org/10.1097/00002820-200002000-00008

Rodgers, C., Highberger, M., Powers, K., Voigt, K., & Douglas, C. (2019). Symptom trajectories of adolescents during hematopoietic stem cell recovery. *Cancer Nursing, 42*(6), 468–474. https://doi.org/10.1097/NCC.0000000000000643

Vogt, J., Beyer, F., Sistermanns, J., Kuon, J., Kahl, C., Alt, E. B., Stevens, S., Ahlborn, M., George, C., Heider, A., Tienken, M., Loquai, C., Stahlhut, K., Ruellan, A., Kubin, T., Dietz, A., Oechsle, K., Mehnert, T. A., Oorschot, B., & Thomas, M. (2021). Symptom burden and palliative care needs of patients with incurable cancer at diagnosis and during the disease course. *Oncologist, 26*(6), e1058–e1065. https://doi.org/10.1002/onco.13751

S

Systemic Toxin Clearance: Dialysis 2302

Definition: Clearance of toxins from the body with peritoneal or hemodialysis

OUTCOME TARGET RATING: Maintain at _____ Increase to _____

		Severe Deviation from Normal Range	Substantial Deviation from Normal Range	Moderate Deviation from Normal Range	Mild Deviation from Normal Range	No Deviation from Normal Range	
OUTCOME OVERALL RATING		1	2	3	4	5	
Indicators:							
230212	Urea reduction ratio (URR) ≥ 65%	1	2	3	4	5	NA
230214	Serum potassium	1	2	3	4	5	NA
230217	Serum sodium	1	2	3	4	5	NA
230220	Serum creatinine	1	2	3	4	5	NA
230221	Serum calcium	1	2	3	4	5	NA
230224	Serum phosphorous	1	2	3	4	5	NA
230230	Serum inflammatory markers	1	2	3	4	5	NA
230225	Creatinine clearance	1	2	3	4	5	NA
230226	Blood urea nitrogen to creatinine ratio	1	2	3	4	5	NA

Domain-*Physiologic Health (II)* **Class**-*Therapeutic Response (AA)* *2nd edition 2000; revised 2004, 2008, 2024*

OUTCOME CONTENT REFERENCES:

Barzegar, H., Moosazadeh, M., Jafari, H., & Esmaeili, R. (2016). Evaluation of dialysis adequacy in hemodialysis patients: A systematic review. *Urology Journal*, *13*(4), 2744–2749.

National Kidney Foundation. (2015). KDOQI clinical practice guideline for hemodialysis adequacy: 2015 update. *American Journal of Kidney Diseases*, *66*(5), 884–930. https://doi.org/10.1053/j.ajkd.2015.07.015

Sangeetha Lakshmi, B., Harini Devi, N., Suchitra, M. M., Srinivasa Rao, P., & Siva Kumar, V. (2018). Changes in the inflammatory and oxidative stress markers during a single hemodialysis session in patients with chronic kidney disease. *Renal Failure*, *40*(1), 534–540. https://doi.org/10.1080/0886022X.2018.1487857

Sautenet, B., Tong, A., Williams, G., Hemmelgarn, B. R., Manns, B., Wheeler, D. C., Tugwell, P., van Biesen, W., Winkelmayer, W. C., Crowe, S., Harris, T., Evangelidis, N., Hawley, C. M., Pollock, C., Johnson, D. W., Polkinghorne, K. R., Howard, K., Gallagher, M. P., Kerr, P. G., McDonald, S. P., Ju, A., & Craig, J. C. (2018). Scope and consistency of outcomes reported in randomized trials conducted in adults receiving hemodialysis: A systematic review. *American Journal of Kidney Diseases*, *72*(1), 62–74. https://doi.org/10.1053/j.ajkd.2017.11.010

Steyaert, S., Holvoet, E., Nagler, E., Malfait, S., & Van Biesen, W. (2019). Reporting of "dialysis adequacy" as an outcome in randomised trials conducted in adults on haemodialysis. *PLOS One*, *14*(2), e0207045. https://doi.org/10.1371/journal.pone.0207045

Thermoregulation 0800

Definition: Balance among heat production, heat gain, and heat loss

OUTCOME TARGET RATING: Maintain at _____ Increase to _____

		Severely Compromised	Substantially Compromised	Moderately Compromised	Mildly Compromised	Not Compromised	
OUTCOME OVERALL RATING		1	2	3	4	5	
Indicators:							
080010	Sweating when hot	1	2	3	4	5	NA
080011	Shivering and goose bumps when cold	1	2	3	4	5	NA
080017	Apical heart rate	1	2	3	4	5	NA
080012	Radial pulse rate	1	2	3	4	5	NA
080013	Respiratory rate	1	2	3	4	5	NA
080024	Fever response	1	2	3	4	5	NA
080025	Muscle coordination	1	2	3	4	5	NA
080015	Reported thermal comfort	1	2	3	4	5	NA

T

Continued

Thermoregulation—cont'd

		Severe	Substantial	Moderate	Mild	None	
080001	Increased skin temperature	1	2	3	4	5	NA
080018	Decreased skin temperature	1	2	3	4	5	NA
080019	Hyperthermia	1	2	3	4	5	NA
080020	Hypothermia	1	2	3	4	5	NA
080003	Headache	1	2	3	4	5	NA
080004	Muscle aches	1	2	3	4	5	NA
080005	Irritability	1	2	3	4	5	NA
080006	Drowsiness	1	2	3	4	5	NA
080007	Skin color changes	1	2	3	4	5	NA
080008	Muscle twitching	1	2	3	4	5	NA
080014	Dehydration	1	2	3	4	5	NA
080026	Hypoglycemia	1	2	3	4	5	NA
080021	Heat cramps	1	2	3	4	5	NA
080027	Heat exhaustion	1	2	3	4	5	NA
080022	Heat stroke	1	2	3	4	5	NA
080023	Frost bite	1	2	3	4	5	NA
080028	Increased activity	1	2	3	4	5	NA
080029	Reduced activity	1	2	3	4	5	NA
080030	Increased appetite	1	2	3	4	5	NA
080031	Loss of appetite	1	2	3	4	5	NA
080032	Huddled body position	1	2	3	4	5	NA
080033	Stretched body position	1	2	3	4	5	NA
080034	Oliguria	1	2	3	4	5	NA
080035	Thirst	1	2	3	4	5	NA
080036	Nausea	1	2	3	4	5	NA
080037	Vomiting	1	2	3	4	5	NA
080038	Changes in mental status	1	2	3	4	5	NA

Domain-*Physiologic Health (II)*   **Class**-*Metabolic Regulation (I)*   *1st edition 1997; revised 2004, 2008, 2024*

OUTCOME CONTENT REFERENCES:

Ahima, R. S. (2020). Global warming threatens human thermoregulation and survival. *The Journal of Clinical Investigation, 130*(2), 559–561. https://doi.org/10.1172/JCI135006

Cheshire, W. P. Jr. (2016). Thermoregulatory disorders and illness related to heat and cold stress. *Autonomic Neuroscience: Basic & Clinical, 196*, 91–104. https://doi.org/10.1016/j.autneu.2016.01.001

Driscoll, R. L., McCarthy, D. G., Palmer, M. S., & Spriet, L. L. (2020). Mild dehydration impaired intermittent sprint performance and thermoregulation in females. *Applied Physiology, Nutrition, and Metabolism, 45*(9), 1045–1048. https://doi.org/10.1139/apnm-2020-0040

Giersch, G. E. W., Morrissey, M. C., Katch, R. K., Colburn, A. T., Sims, S. T., Stachenfeld, N. S., & Casa, D. J. (2020). Menstrual cycle and thermoregulation during exercise in the heat: A systematic review and meta-analysis. *Journal of Science and Medicine in Sport, 23*(12), 1134–1140. https://doi.org/10.1016/j.jsams.2020.05.014

Hockenberry, M. J., Rodgers, C. C., & Wilson, D. (2022). *Wong's essentials of pediatric nursing* (11th ed.). Elsevier.

Huether, S. E., McCance, K. L., & Brashers, V. L. (2020). *Understanding pathophysiology* (7th ed.). Elsevier.

Madden, C. J., & Morrison, S. F. (2019). Central nervous system circuits that control body temperature. *Neuroscience Letters, 696*, 225–232. https://doi.org/10.1016/j.neulet.2018.11.027

Tansey, E. A., & Johnson, C. D. (2015). Recent advances in thermoregulation. *Advances in Physiology Education, 39*(3), 139–148. https://doi.org/10.1152/advan.00126.2014

Watson, G., Casa, D. J., Fiala, K. A., Hile, A., Roti, M. W., Healey, J. C., Armstrong, L. E., & Maresh, C. M. (2006). Creatine use and exercise heat tolerance in dehydrated men. *Journal of Athletic Training, 41*(1), 18–29.

Williams, P. (2020). *Basic geriatric nursing* (7th ed.). Elsevier.

T

Thermoregulation: Newborn   **0801**

Definition: Balance among heat production, heat gain, and heat loss during the first 28 days of life

OUTCOME TARGET RATING: Maintain at _____ Increase to _____

		Severely Compromised	Substantially Compromised	Moderately Compromised	Mildly Compromised	Not Compromised	
OUTCOME OVERALL RATING		**1**	**2**	**3**	**4**	**5**	
Indicators:							
080106	Weight gain	1	2	3	4	5	NA
080107	Non-shivering thermogenesis	1	2	3	4	5	NA
080108	Assumes heat retention posture with hypothermia	1	2	3	4	5	NA
080109	Assumes heat dissipation posture with hyperthermia	1	2	3	4	5	NA
080110	Weaning from isolette to crib	1	2	3	4	5	NA
080113	Acid/base balance	1	2	3	4	5	NA
		Severe	**Substantial**	**Moderate**	**Mild**	**None**	
080116	Temperature instability	1	2	3	4	5	NA
080117	Hyperthermia	1	2	3	4	5	NA
080118	Hypothermia	1	2	3	4	5	NA
080119	Irregular respirations	1	2	3	4	5	NA
080120	Tachypnea	1	2	3	4	5	NA
080121	Bradycardia	1	2	3	4	5	NA
080103	Restlessness	1	2	3	4	5	NA
080122	Irritability	1	2	3	4	5	NA
080104	Lethargy	1	2	3	4	5	NA
080105	Skin color changes	1	2	3	4	5	NA
080123	Hypotonic	1	2	3	4	5	NA
080111	Dehydration	1	2	3	4	5	NA
080112	Blood glucose instability	1	2	3	4	5	NA
080114	Hyperbilirubinemia	1	2	3	4	5	NA

Domain-*Physiologic Health (II)*   **Class**-*Metabolic Regulation (I)*   *1st edition 1997; revised 2004, 2018*

OUTCOME CONTENT REFERENCES:
Bohnhorst, B., Heyne, T., Peter, C. S., & Poets, C. F. (2001). Skin-to-skin (kangaroo) care, respiratory control, and thermoregulation. *Journal of Pediatrics, 138*(2), 193–197. https://doi.org/10.1067/mpd.2001.110978
Hockenberry, M. J., & Wilson, D. (Eds.). (2015). *Wong's nursing care of infants and children* (10th ed.). Elsevier Mosby.
Mattson, S., & Smith, J. E. (Eds.). (2016). *Core curriculum for maternal-newborn nursing* (5th ed.). Elsevier.
Truman, P. (2006). Jaundice in the preterm infant. *Paediatric Nursing, 18*(5), 20–22. https://doi.org/10.7748/paed.18.5.20.s24
Verklan, M. T., & Walden, M. (Eds.). (2015). *Core curriculum for neonatal intensive care nursing* (5th ed.). Elsevier Saunders.

T

Tissue Injury Severity: Percutaneous Procedure   **1109**

Definition: Severity of complications from a needle-puncture access through the skin and into deeper tissues

OUTCOME TARGET RATING: Maintain at_____ Increase to_____

OUTCOME OVERALL RATING	Severe	Substantial	Moderate	Mild	None	
	1	2	3	4	5	
Indicators:						
110901 Pain at access site	1	2	3	4	5	NA
110902 Bruising at access site	1	2	3	4	5	NA
110903 Arteriovenous fistula at access site	1	2	3	4	5	NA
110904 Hematoma at access site	1	2	3	4	5	NA
110905 Retroperitoneal hematoma	1	2	3	4	5	NA
110906 Infection at access site	1	2	3	4	5	NA
110907 Ischemia of ipsilateral limb	1	2	3	4	5	NA
110908 Arterial occlusion at access site	1	2	3	4	5	NA
110909 Pseudoaneurysm at access site	1	2	3	4	5	NA
110910 Bleeding at access site	1	2	3	4	5	NA
110911 Ipsilateral limb compartment syndrome	1	2	3	4	5	NA

Domain- Physiologic Health (II)   *Class*-Tissue Integrity (L)   7th edition 2024

OUTCOME CONTENT REFERENCES:

Aziz, E. F., Pulimi, S., Coleman, C., Florita, C., Musat, D., Tormey, D., Fawzy, A., Lee, S., Herzog, E., Coven, D. L., Tamis-Holland, J., & Hong, M. K. (2010). Increased vascular access complications in patients with renal dysfunction undergoing percutaneous coronary procedures using arteriotomy closure devices. *Journal of Invasive Cardiology, 22*(1), 8–13.

Bertrand, O. F., De Larochellière, R., Rodés-Cabau, J., Proulx, G., Gleeton, O., Nguyen, C. M., Déry, J. P., Barbeau, G., Noël, B., Larose, E., Poirier, P., Roy, L., & Early Discharge After Transradial Stenting of Coronary Arteries Study Investigators. (2006). A randomized study comparing same day home discharge and abciximab bolus only to overnight hospitalization and abciximab bolus and infusion after transradial coronary stent implantation. *Circulation, 114*(24), 2636–2643. https://doi.org/10.1161/CIRCULATIONAHA.106.638627

Bhatty, S., Cooke, R., Shetty, R., & Jovin, I. S. (2011). Femoral vascular access site complications in the cardiac catheterization laboratory: Diagnosis and management. *Interventional Cardiology, 3*(4), 503–514.

Burzotta, F., Mariani, L., Trani, C., Coluccia, V., Brancati, M. F., Porto, I., Leone, A. M., Niccoli, G., Tommasino, A., Tinelli, G., Mazzari, M. A., Mongiardo, R., Snider, F., Schiavoni, G., & Crea, F. (2013). Management and timing of access-site vascular complications occurring after trans-radial percutaneous coronary procedures. *International Journal of Cardiology, 167*(5), 1973–1978. https://doi.org/10.1016/j.ijcard.2012.05.017

Chantal Magalhães da Silva, N., de Souza Oliveira, K. A. R., Moorhead, S., Pace, A. E., & Carvalho, E. (2017). Clinical validation of the indicators and definitions of the nursing outcome "Tissue Integrity: Skin and Mucous Membranes" in people with diabetes mellitus. *International Journal of Nursing Knowledge, 28*(4), 165–170. https://doi.org/10.1111/2047-3095.12150

Cheng, K. Y., Chair, S. Y., & Choi, K. C. (2013). Access site complications and puncture site pain following transradial coronary procedures: A correlational study. *International Journal of Nursing Studies, 50*(10), 1304–1313. https://doi.org/10.1016/j.ijnurstu.2012.12.023

Cosman, T. L., Arthur, H. M., & Natarajan, M. K. (2011). Prevalence of bruising at the vascular access site one week after elective cardiac catheterization or percutaneous coronary intervention. *Journal of Clinical Nursing, 20*(9-10), 1349–1356.

Kanei, Y., Kwan, T., Nakra, N. C., Liou, M., Huang, Y., Vales, L. L., Fox, J. T., Chen, J. P., & Saito, S. (2011). Transradial cardiac catheterization: A review of access site complications. *Catheterization and Cardiovascular Interventions, 78*(6), 840–846.

Kolluri, R., Fowler, B., & Nandish, S. (2013). Vascular access complications: Diagnosis and management. *Current Treatment Options in Cardiovascular Medicine, 15*(2), 173–187. https://doi.org/10.1007/s11936-013-0227-8

Lo, R. C., Fokkema, M. T. M., Curran, T., Darling, J., Hamdan, A. D., Martin, M. W. M., & Schermerhorn, M. L. (2015). Routine use of ultrasound-guided access reduces access site-related complications after lower extremity percutaneous revascularization. *Journal of Vascular Surgery, 61*(2), 405–412. https://doi.org/10.1016/j.jvs.2014.07.099

Mehran, R., Rao, S. V., Bhatt, D. L., Gibson, C. M., Caixeta, A., Eikelboom, J., Kaul, S., Wiviott, S. D., Menon, V., Nikolsky, E., Serebruany, V., Valgimigli, M., Vranckx, P., Taggart, D., Sabik, J. F., Cutlip, D. E., Krucoff, M. W., Ohman, E. M., Steg, P. G., & White, H. (2011). Standardized bleeding definitions for cardiovascular clinical trials: A consensus report from the Bleeding Academic Research Consortium. *Circulation, 123*(23), 2736–2747. https://doi.org/10.1161/CIRCULATIONAHA.110.009449

Merriweather, N., & Sulzbach-Hoke, L. M. (2012). Managing risk of complications at femoral vascular access sites in percutaneous coronary intervention. *Critical Care Nurse, 32*(5), 16–29. https://doi.org/10.4037/ccn2012123

Reich, R., Rabelo-Silva, E. R., Swanson, E., Moorhead, S., & Almeida, M. D. A. (2022). Development of a nursing outcome for a percutaneous procedure. *International Journal of Nursing Knowledge, 33*(2), 84–92. https://doi.org/10.1111/2047-3095.12329

Tavris, D. R., Wang, Y., Jacobs, S., Gallauresi, B., Curtis, J., Messenger, J., Resnic, F. S., & Fitzgerald, S. (2012). Bleeding and vascular complications at the femoral access site following percutaneous coronary intervention (PCI): An evaluation of hemostasis strategies. *Journal of Invasive Cardiology, 24*(7), 328–34.

Wong, H. F., Lee, C. W., Chen, Y. L., Wu, Y. M., Weng, H. H., Wang, Y. H., & Liu, H. M. (2013). Prospective comparison of angio-seal versus manual compression for hemostasis after neurointerventional procedures under systemic heparinization. *AJNR American Journal of Neuroradiology, 34*(2), 397–401.

Tissue Integrity: Skin & Mucous Membranes   1101

Definition: Structural intactness and normal physiological function of skin and mucous membranes

OUTCOME TARGET RATING: Maintain at _____ Increase to _____

		Severely Compromised	Substantially Compromised	Moderately Compromised	Mildly Compromised	Not Compromised	
OUTCOME OVERALL RATING		1	2	3	4	5	
Indicators:							
110101	Skin temperature	1	2	3	4	5	NA
110102	Sensation	1	2	3	4	5	NA
110103	Elasticity	1	2	3	4	5	NA
110104	Hydration	1	2	3	4	5	NA
110106	Perspiration	1	2	3	4	5	NA
110108	Texture	1	2	3	4	5	NA
110109	Thickness	1	2	3	4	5	NA
110111	Tissue perfusion	1	2	3	4	5	NA
110112	Hair growth on skin	1	2	3	4	5	NA
110113	Skin integrity	1	2	3	4	5	NA
		Severe	**Substantial**	**Moderate**	**Mild**	**None**	
110105	Abnormal pigmentation	1	2	3	4	5	NA
110115	Skin lesions	1	2	3	4	5	NA
110116	Mucous membrane lesions	1	2	3	4	5	NA
110126	Cellulitis	1	2	3	4	5	NA
110117	Scar tissue	1	2	3	4	5	NA
110118	Skin cancers	1	2	3	4	5	NA
110119	Skin flaking	1	2	3	4	5	NA
110120	Skin scaling	1	2	3	4	5	NA
110121	Erythema	1	2	3	4	5	NA
110122	Blanching	1	2	3	4	5	NA
110123	Necrosis	1	2	3	4	5	NA
110124	Induration	1	2	3	4	5	NA
110125	Corneal abrasion	1	2	3	4	5	NA
110127	Presence of foreign bodies	1	2	3	4	5	NA

Domain-*Physiologic Health (II)*   **Class**-*Tissue Integrity (L)*   *1st edition 1997; revised 2004, 2013, 2024*

OUTCOME CONTENT REFERENCES:

+Bergstrom, N., Braden, B. J., Laguzza, A., & Holman, V. (1987). The Braden Scale for predicting pressure sore risk. *Nursing Research, 36*(4), 205–210.

Campbell, J., Barakat-Johnson, M., Hogan, M., Maddison, K., McLean, J., Rando, T., Samolyk, M., Sage, S., Weger, K., & Dunk, A. M. (2020). A clinical guide to pelvic skin assessment. *Wounds International, 11*(1), 30–39.

Etcheverria, E. (2020). Recognizing and treating five common dermatologic conditions seen in primary care. *JAAPA: Journal of the American Academy of Physician Assistants, 33*(11), 33–37. https://doi.org/10.1097/01.JAA.0000718288.06130.dd

Hills, F. (2021). Connective tissue and dermatological conditions in pregnancy. *Obstetrics, Gynaecology & Reproductive Medicine, 31*(6), 162–169. https://doi.org/10.1016/j.ogrm.2021.04.004

Hogan-Quigley, B., Palm, M. L., & Bickley, L. (2021). *Bates nursing guide to physical examination and history taking* (3rd ed.). Wolters Kluwer.

Kim, K.-H. (2019). Sports-related skin conditions. *Journal of the Korean Medical Association/Taehan Uisa Hyophoe Chi, 62*(4), 202–208. https://doi.org/10.5124/jkma.2019.62.4.202

Oozageer Gunowa, N., Hutchinson, M., Brooke, J., & Jackson, D. (2018). Pressure injuries in people with darker skin tones: A literature review. *Journal of Clinical Nursing, 27*(17–18), 3266–3275. https://doi.org/10.1111/jocn.14062

Palmer, S. J. (2021). Dermatological conditions in older adults: Clinical overview. *Practice Nursing, 32*(Sup11), S8–S10. https://doi.org/10.12968/pnur.2021.32.Sup11.S8

Potter, P. A., Perry, A. G., Stockert, P. A., & Hall, A. (2021). *Fundamentals of nursing* (10th ed.). Elsevier.

Rupert, J., Honeycutt, J. D., & Odom, M. R. (2020). Foreign bodies in the skin: evaluation and management. *American Family Physician, 101*(12), 740–747.

Ud-Din, S., & Bayat, A. (2022). Noninvasive objective tools for quantitative assessment of skin scarring. *Advances in Wound Care* (2162-1918), *11*(3), 132–149. https://doi.org/10.1089/wound.2020.1387

T

Tissue Perfusion 0422

Definition: Adequacy of the blood flow through body organs to function at the cellular level

OUTCOME TARGET RATING: Maintain at_____ Increase to_____

		Severe Deviation from Normal Range	Substantial Deviation from Normal Range	Moderate Deviation from Normal Range	Mild Deviation from Normal Range	No Deviation from Normal Range	
OUTCOME OVERALL RATING		1	2	3	4	5	
Indicators:							
042201	Blood flow through the liver vasculature	1	2	3	4	5	NA
042202	Blood flow through the kidney vasculature	1	2	3	4	5	NA
042203	Blood flow through the gastrointestinal tract vasculature	1	2	3	4	5	NA
042204	Blood flow through the spleen vasculature	1	2	3	4	5	NA
042205	Blood flow through the pancreas vasculature	1	2	3	4	5	NA
042206	Blood flow through the coronary vasculature	1	2	3	4	5	NA
042207	Blood flow through the pulmonary vasculature	1	2	3	4	5	NA
042208	Blood flow through the cerebral vasculature	1	2	3	4	5	NA
042209	Blood flow through the peripheral vessels	1	2	3	4	5	NA
042210	Blood flow through the vasculature at the cellular level	1	2	3	4	5	NA

Domain-Physiologic Health (II)   **Class**-Cardiopulmonary (E)   5th edition 2013; reviewed 2024

OUTCOME CONTENT REFERENCES:

Abut, Y. C. (2019). Monitoring tissue perfusion in shock: From physiology to the bedside. *Anesthesia & Analgesia, 128*(6), e113. https://doi.org/10.1213/ANE.0000000000004122

Hinkle, J. L., Cheever, K. H., & Overbaugh, K. (2021). *Brunner & Suddarth's textbook of medical surgical nursing* (15th ed.). Wolters Kluwer.

Huether, S. E., McCance, K. L., & Brashers, V. L. (2020). *Understanding pathophysiology* (7th ed.). Elsevier.

Ignatavicius, D. D., Workman, M. L., Rebar, C. R., & Heimgartner, N. M. (2021). *Medical-surgical nursing: Concepts for interprofessional care* (10th ed.). Elsevier.

Lewis, S. M., Collier, I. C., Heitkermper, M. M., & Dirksen, S. R. (2019). *Medical-surgical nursing: Assessment and management of clinical problems* (11th ed.). Mosby.

Ma, K. F., Kleiss, S. F., Schuurmann, R., Bokkers, R., Ünlü, Ç., & De Vries, J. (2019). A systematic review of diagnostic techniques to determine tissue perfusion in patients with peripheral arterial disease. *Expert Review of Medical Devices, 16*(8), 697–710. https://doi.org/10.1080/17434440.2019.1644166

Rivers, E. P., Yataco, A. C., Jaehne, A. K., Gill, J., & Disselkamp, M. (2015). Oxygen extraction and perfusion markers in severe sepsis and septic shock: Diagnostic, therapeutic and outcome implications. *Current Opinion in Critical Care, 21*(5), 381–7. https://doi.org/10.1097/MCC.0000000000000241

Sánchez-Díaz, J. S., Peniche-Moguel, K. G., Rivera-Solís, G., Martínez-Rodríguez, E. A., Del-Carpio-Orantes, L., Pérez-Nieto, O. R., Zamarrón-López, E. I., Guerrero-Gutiérrez, M. A., & Monares-Zepeda, E. (2020). Hemodynamic monitoring with two blood gases: "A tool that does not go out of style". *Colombian Journal of Anesthesiology, 49*(1). https://doi.org/10.5554/22562087.e928

T

Tissue Perfusion: Abdominal Organs   0404

Definition: Adequacy of blood flow through the small vessels of the abdominal viscera to maintain organ function

OUTCOME TARGET RATING: Maintain at _____ Increase to _____

		Severe Deviation from Normal Range	Substantial Deviation from Normal Range	Moderate Deviation from Normal Range	Mild Deviation from Normal Range	No Deviation from Normal Range	
OUTCOME OVERALL RATING		1	2	3	4	5	
Indicators:							
040424	Diastolic blood pressure	1	2	3	4	5	NA
040425	Systolic blood pressure	1	2	3	4	5	NA
040426	Mean blood pressure	1	2	3	4	5	NA
040402	Urine output	1	2	3	4	5	NA
040403	Electrolyte and acid/base balance	1	2	3	4	5	NA
040405	Bowel sounds	1	2	3	4	5	NA
040419	Blood urea nitrogen	1	2	3	4	5	NA
040420	Plasma creatinine	1	2	3	4	5	NA
040421	Liver function test findings	1	2	3	4	5	NA
040421	Pancreatic enzymes	1	2	3	4	5	NA
040429	Intra-abdominal pressure	1	2	3	4	5	NA
		Severe	Substantial	Moderate	Mild	None	
040407	Abnormal thirst	1	2	3	4	5	NA
040408	Abdominal pain	1	2	3	4	5	NA
040409	Nausea	1	2	3	4	5	NA
040410	Vomiting	1	2	3	4	5	NA
040411	Malabsorption deficiencies	1	2	3	4	5	NA
040412	Chronic gastritis	1	2	3	4	5	NA
040413	Abdominal distention	1	2	3	4	5	NA
040414	Ascites	1	2	3	4	5	NA
040415	Gastrointestinal varices	1	2	3	4	5	NA
040416	Constipation	1	2	3	4	5	NA
040417	Diarrhea	1	2	3	4	5	NA
040427	Altered fluid balance	1	2	3	4	5	NA
040428	Loss of appetite	1	2	3	4	5	NA

Domain-*Physiologic Health (II)*   **Class**-*Cardiopulmonary (E)*   *1st edition 1997; revised 2004, 2008, 2024*

OUTCOME CONTENT REFERENCES:
Hinkle, J. L., Cheever, K. H., & Overbaugh, K. (2021). *Brunner & Suddarth's textbook of medical surgical nursing* (15th ed.). Wolters Kluwer.
Huether, S. E., McCance, K. L., & Brashers, V. L. (2020). *Understanding pathophysiology* (7th ed.). Elsevier.
Ignatavicius, D. D., Workman, M. L., Rebar, C. R., & Heimgartner, N. M. (2021). *Medical-surgical nursing: Concepts for interprofessional care* (10th ed.). Elsevier.
Pereira, B. M. (2021). Measurement protocols and intra-abdominal hypertension treatment. *Revista do Colégio Brasileiro de Cirurgiões, 48.*
    https://doi.org/10.1590/0100-6991e-20202838
Reintan, A., Parm, P., Kitus, R., Kern, H., & Starkopf, J. (2009). Gastrointestinal symptoms in intensive care patients. *Acta Anaesthesiologica Scandinavica*, 53(3), 318–324. https://doi.org/10.1111/j.1399-6576.2008.01860.x
Svorcan, P., Stojanovic, M., Stevanovic, P., Karamarkovic, A., Jankovic, R., & Ladjevic, N. (2017). The influence of intraabdominal pressure on the mortality rate of patients with acute pancreatitis. *Turkish Journal of Medical Sciences, 47*(3), 748–753. https://doi.org/10.3906/sag-1509-7

T

Tissue Perfusion: Cardiac

0405

Definition: Adequacy of blood flow through the coronary vasculature to maintain heart function

OUTCOME TARGET RATING: Maintain at _____ Increase to _____

		Severe Deviation from Normal Range	Substantial Deviation from Normal Range	Moderate Deviation from Normal Range	Mild Deviation from Normal Range	No Deviation from Normal Range	
OUTCOME OVERALL RATING		1	2	3	4	5	
Indicators:							
040515	Apical heart rate	1	2	3	4	5	NA
040523	Third heart sound	1	2	3	4	5	NA
040516	Radial pulse rate	1	2	3	4	5	NA
040517	Systolic blood pressure	1	2	3	4	5	NA
040518	Diastolic blood pressure	1	2	3	4	5	NA
040519	Mean blood pressure	1	2	3	4	5	NA
040501	Ejection fraction	1	2	3	4	5	NA
040502	Pulmonary wedge pressure	1	2	3	4	5	NA
040524	Oxygen saturation	1	2	3	4	5	NA
040503	Cardiac index	1	2	3	4	5	NA
040509	Electrocardiogram findings	1	2	3	4	5	NA
040510	Cardiac biomarkers	1	2	3	4	5	NA
040511	Coronary angiogram findings	1	2	3	4	5	NA
040525	Coronary tomography	1	2	3	4	5	NA
040512	Exercise stress test findings	1	2	3	4	5	NA
040513	Thallium scan findings	1	2	3	4	5	NA
040526	Color of mucus membranes	1	2	3	4	5	NA
040527	Skin color	1	2	3	4	5	NA
040528	Skin temperature	1	2	3	4	5	NA
040529	Peripheral pulses	1	2	3	4	5	NA
040530	Capillary refill	1	2	3	4	5	NA
		Severe	**Substantial**	**Moderate**	**Mild**	**None**	
040504	Unstable angina	1	2	3	4	5	NA
040520	Arrhythmia	1	2	3	4	5	NA
040521	Tachycardia	1	2	3	4	5	NA
040522	Bradycardia	1	2	3	4	5	NA
040505	Profuse diaphoresis	1	2	3	4	5	NA
040506	Nausea	1	2	3	4	5	NA
040507	Vomiting	1	2	3	4	5	NA
040531	Dizziness	1	2	3	4	5	NA
040532	Anxiety	1	2	3	4	5	NA
040533	Chest pain	1	2	3	4	5	NA
040534	Breathlessness	1	2	3	4	5	NA

Domain-Physiologic Health (II)   **Class**-Cardiopulmonary (E)   1st edition 1997; revised 2000, 2004, 2008, 2024

OUTCOME CONTENT REFERENCES:

Hinkle, J. L., Cheever, K. H., & Overbaugh, K. (2021). *Brunner & Suddarth's textbook of medical surgical nursing* (15th ed.). Wolters Kluwer.

Huether, S. E., McCance, K. L., & Brashers, V. L. (2020). *Understanding pathophysiology* (7th ed.). Elsevier.

Ibanez, B., James, S., Agewall, S., Antunes, M. J., Bucciarelli-Ducci, C., Bueno, H., Caforio, A., Crea, F., Goudevenos, J. A., Halvorsen, S., Hindricks, G., Kastrati, A., Lenzen, M. J., Prescott, E., Roffi, M., Valgimigli, M., Varenhorst, C., Vranckx, P., Widimský, P., & ESC Scientific Document Group (2018). 2017 ESC Guidelines for the management of acute myocardial infarction in patients presenting with ST-segment elevation: The Task Force for the Management of Acute Myocardial Infarction in Patients Presenting with ST-segment Elevation of the European Society of Cardiology (ESC). *European Heart Journal, 39*(2), 119–177. https://doi.org/10.1093/eurheartj/ehx393

Ignatavicius, D. D., Workman, M. L., Rebar, C. R., & Heimgartner, N. M. (2021). *Medical-surgical nursing: Concepts for interprofessional care* (10th ed.). Elsevier.

LeMone, P., Burke, K. M., Bauldoff, G., Gubrud-Howe, P., Levett-Jones, T., Hales, M., Berry, K., Dwyer, T., Knox, N., & Raymond, D. (2017). *Medical-surgical nursing: Critical thinking for person-centered care* (3rd ed.). Pearson.

Martinez, P. F., Oliveira-Junior, S. A., Polegato, B. F., Okoshi, K., & Okoshi, M. P. (2019). Biomarkers in acute myocardial infarction diagnosis and prognosis. *Arquivos Brasileiros de Cardiologia, 113*(1), 40–41. https://doi.org/10.5935/abc.20190131

Nicolau, J. C., Feitosa Filho, G. S., Petriz, J. L., Furtado, R. H. M., Précoma, D. B., Lemke, W., Timerman, A., Neto, J. A. M., Neto, L. B., Gomes, B. F. D. O., Santos, E. C. L., Piegas, L. S., Soeiro, A. D. M., Negri, A. J. D. A. Franci, Filho, B. M., Bccaro, B. M., Monenegro, C. E. L., Rochite, C. E., … Mathias, W. Jr. (2021). Brazilian Society of Cardiology Guidelines on Unstable Angina and Acute Myocardial Infarction without ST-Segment Elevation—2021. *Arquivos Brasileiros de Cardiologia, 117*(1), 181–264. https://doi.org/10.36660/abc.20210180

Santos, V. B., Atallah, Á. N., Lopes, C. T., Lopes, J. de L., & de Barros, A. L. B. L. (2015). Defining characteristics and related factors of Decreased Cardiac Tissue Perfusion: Proposal of a new nursing diagnosis. *International Journal of Nursing Knowledge, 27*(3), 175–180. https://doi.org/10.1111/2047-3095.12095

Tissue Perfusion: Cellular   0416

Definition: Adequacy of blood flow through the vasculature to maintain function at the cellular level

OUTCOME TARGET RATING: Maintain at_____ Increase to_____

	Severe Deviation from Normal Range	Substantial Deviation from Normal Range	Moderate Deviation from Normal Range	Mild Deviation from Normal Range	No Deviation from Normal Range	
OUTCOME OVERALL RATING	1	2	3	4	5	
Indicators:						
041601 Systolic blood pressure	1	2	3	4	5	NA
041602 Diastolic blood pressure	1	2	3	4	5	NA
041603 Mean arterial blood gases	1	2	3	4	5	NA
041604 Oxygen saturation	1	2	3	4	5	NA
041605 Fluid balance	1	2	3	4	5	NA
041606 Apical heart rate	1	2	3	4	5	NA
041607 Heart rhythm	1	2	3	4	5	NA
041608 Electrolyte and acid/base balance	1	2	3	4	5	NA
041609 Capillary refill	1	2	3	4	5	NA
041610 Urine output	1	2	3	4	5	NA
041611 Creatinine clearance	1	2	3	4	5	NA
041620 Lactate	1	2	3	4	5	NA
	Severe	Substantial	Moderate	Mild	None	
041612 Agitation	1	2	3	4	5	NA
041616 Pain	1	2	3	4	5	NA
041617 Decreased level of consciousness	1	2	3	4	5	NA
041621 Tissue hypoxia	1	2	3	4	5	NA
041618 Pale cool skin	1	2	3	4	5	NA
041619 Skin breakdown	1	2	3	4	5	NA
041613 Necrosis	1	2	3	4	5	NA
041622 Dry mouth	1	2	3	4	5	NA
041623 Fever	1	2	3	4	5	NA

Domain-*Physiologic Health (II)*   **Class**-*Cardiopulmonary (E)*   *4th edition 2008; revised 2024*

OUTCOME CONTENT REFERENCES:

Assuncao, M. S., Corrêa, T. D., Bravim, B., & Silva, E. (2015). How to choose the therapeutic goals to improve tissue perfusion in septic shock. *Einstein (Sao Paulo, Brazil), 13*(3), 441–447. https://doi.org/10.1590/S1679-45082015RW3148

Gauer, R., Forbes, D., & Boyer, N. (2020). Sepsis: Diagnosis and management. *American Family Physician, 101*(7), 409–418.

Guven, G., Hilty, M. P., & Ince, C. (2020). Microcirculation: Physiology, pathophysiology, and clinical application. *Blood Purification, 49*(1-2), 143–150. https://doi.org/10.1159/000503775

Huether, S. E., McCance, K. L., & Brashers, V. L. (2020). *Understanding pathophysiology* (7th ed.). Elsevier.

Ignatavicius, D. D., Workman, M. L., Rebar, C. R., & Heimgartner, N. M. (2021). *Medical-surgical nursing: Concepts for interprofessional care* (10th ed.). Elsevier.

T

Loiacono, L. A., & Shapiro, D. S. (2010). Detection of hypoxia at the cellular level. *Critical Care Clinics, 26*(2), 409–421. https://doi.org/10.1016/j.ccc.2009.12.001

Ramos Corrêa Pinto, L., Azzolin, K. d. O., Lucena, A. d. F., Moretti, M. M. S., Haas, J. S., Moraes, R. B., & Friedman, G. (2021), Septic shock: Clinical indicators and implications to critical patient care. *Journal of Clinical Nursing, 30*, 1607–1614. https://doi.org/10.1111/jocn.15713

Rivers, E. P., Yataco, A. C., Jaehne, A. K., Gill, J., & Disselkamp, M. (2015). Oxygen extraction and perfusion markers in severe sepsis and septic shock: Diagnostic, therapeutic and outcome implications. *Current Opinion in Critical Care, 21*(5), 381–387. https://doi.org/10.1097/MCC.0000000000000241

Sánchez-Díaz, J. S., Peniche-Moguel, K. G., Rivera-Solís, G., Martínez-Rodríguez, E. A., Del-Carpio-Orantes, L., Pérez-Nieto, O. R., Zamarrón-López, E. I., Guerrero-Gutiérrez, M. A., & Monares-Zepeda, E. (2020). Hemodynamic monitoring with two blood gases: "A tool that does not go out of style." *Colombian Journal of Anesthesiology, 49*(1). https://doi.org/10.5554/22562087.e928

Tissue Perfusion: Cerebral 0406

Definition: Adequacy of blood flow through the cerebral vasculature to maintain brain function

OUTCOME TARGET RATING: Maintain at _____ Increase to _____

	Severe Deviation from Normal Range	Substantial Deviation from Normal Range	Moderate Deviation from Normal Range	Mild Deviation from Normal Range	No Deviation from Normal Range	
OUTCOME OVERALL RATING	1	2	3	4	5	
Indicators:						
040602 Intracranial pressure	1	2	3	4	5	NA
040613 Systolic blood pressure	1	2	3	4	5	NA
040614 Diastolic blood pressure	1	2	3	4	5	NA
040617 Mean blood pressure	1	2	3	4	5	NA
040621 Cerebral perfusion pressure	1	2	3	4	5	NA
040615 Cerebral angiogram findings	1	2	3	4	5	NA
040622 Transcranial doppler findings	1	2	3	4	5	NA
040623 Near infrared spectrology findings	1	2	3	4	5	NA
040624 Bradycardia	1	2	3	4	5	NA
040625 Irregular respirations	1	2	3	4	5	NA
	Severe	Substantial	Moderate	Mild	None	
040603 Headache	1	2	3	4	5	NA
040604 Carotid bruit	1	2	3	4	5	NA
040605 Restlessness	1	2	3	4	5	NA
040606 Listlessness	1	2	3	4	5	NA
040607 Unexplained anxiety	1	2	3	4	5	NA
040608 Agitation	1	2	3	4	5	NA
040609 Vomiting	1	2	3	4	5	NA
040610 Hiccups	1	2	3	4	5	NA
040611 Syncope	1	2	3	4	5	NA
040616 Fever	1	2	3	4	5	NA
040618 Impaired cognition	1	2	3	4	5	NA
040619 Decreased level of consciousness	1	2	3	4	5	NA
040620 Impaired neurological reflexes	1	2	3	4	5	NA

Domain-Physiologic Health (II) **Class**-Cardiopulmonary (E) *1st edition 1997; revised 2004, 2008, 2024*

OUTCOME CONTENT REFERENCES:

Capizzi, A., Woo, J., & Verduzco-Gutierrez, M. (2020). Traumatic brain injury: An overview of epidemiology, pathophysiology, and medical management. *The Medical Clinics of North America, 104*(2), 213–238. https://doi.org/10.1016/j.mcna.2019.11.001

Donnelly, J., Budohoski, K. P., Smielewski, P., & Czosnyka, M. (2016). Regulation of the cerebral circulation: Bedside assessment and clinical implications. *Critical Care, 20*(1), 129. https://doi.org/10.1186/s13054-016-1293-6

Hinkle, J. L., Cheever, K. H., & Overbaugh, K. (2021). *Brunner & Suddarth's textbook of medical surgical nursing* (15th ed.). Wolters Kluwer.

Huether, S. E., McCance, K. L., & Brashers, V. L. (2020). *Understanding pathophysiology* (7th ed.). Elsevier.

Ignatavicius, D. D., Workman, M. L., Rebar, C. R., & Heimgartner, N. M. (2021). *Medical-surgical nursing: Concepts for interprofessional care* (10th ed.). Elsevier.

Kapoor, I., Prabhakar, H., & Mahajan, C. (2021). Impact of head-of-bed posture on brain oxygenation in patients with acute brain injury: A prospective cohort study. *Neurocritical Care, 35*(3), 919. https://doi.org/10.1007/s12028-021-01383-1

Nagata, K., Yamazaki, T., Takano, D., Maeda, T., Fujimaki, Y., Nakase, T., & Sato, Y. (2016). Cerebral circulation in aging. *Ageing Research Reviews, 30*, 49–60. https://doi.org/10.1016/j.arr.2016.06.001

Rohlwink, U. K., & Figaji, A. A. (2010). Methods of monitoring brain oxygenation. *Childs Nervous System, 26*, 453–464.

Skrifvars, M. B., Sekhon, M., & Åneman, E. A. (2021). Monitoring and modifying brain oxygenation in patients at risk of hypoxic ischaemic brain injury after cardiac arrest. *Critical Care, 25*(1), 1–8. https://doi.org/10.1186/s13054-021-03678-3

Tissue Perfusion: Peripheral   0407

Definition: Adequacy of blood flow through the small vessels of the extremities to maintain tissue function

OUTCOME TARGET RATING: Maintain at _____ Increase to _____

		Severe Deviation from Normal Range	Substantial Deviation from Normal Range	Moderate Deviation from Normal Range	Mild Deviation from Normal Range	No Deviation from Normal Range	
OUTCOME OVERALL RATING		1	2	3	4	5	
Indicators:							
040715	Capillary refill fingers	1	2	3	4	5	NA
040716	Capillary refill toes	1	2	3	4	5	NA
040710	Extremity skin temperature	1	2	3	4	5	NA
040730	Carotid pulse strength (right)	1	2	3	4	5	NA
040731	Carotid pulse strength (left)	1	2	3	4	5	NA
040732	Brachial pulse strength (right)	1	2	3	4	5	NA
040733	Brachial pulse strength (left)	1	2	3	4	5	NA
040734	Radial pulse strength (right)	1	2	3	4	5	NA
040735	Radial pulse strength (left)	1	2	3	4	5	NA
040736	Femoral pulse strength (right)	1	2	3	4	5	NA
040737	Femoral pulse strength (left)	1	2	3	4	5	NA
040738	Pedal pulse strength (right)	1	2	3	4	5	NA
040739	Pedal pulse strength (left)	1	2	3	4	5	NA
040727	Systolic blood pressure	1	2	3	4	5	NA
040728	Diastolic blood pressure	1	2	3	4	5	NA
040740	Mean blood pressure	1	2	3	4	5	NA
		Severe	Substantial	Moderate	Mild	None	
040711	Extremity bruits	1	2	3	4	5	NA
040712	Peripheral edema	1	2	3	4	5	NA
040713	Localized extremity pain	1	2	3	4	5	NA
040729	Necrosis	1	2	3	4	5	NA
040741	Numbness	1	2	3	4	5	NA
040742	Tingling	1	2	3	4	5	NA
040743	Pallor	1	2	3	4	5	NA
041449	Cyanosis	1	2	3	4	5	NA
040744	Muscle weakness	1	2	3	4	5	NA
040745	Muscle cramps	1	2	3	4	5	NA
040746	Skin breakdown	1	2	3	4	5	NA
040747	Rubor	1	2	3	4	5	NA
040748	Paresthesia	1	2	3	4	5	NA

Domain-*Physiologic Health (II)*   **Class**-*Cardiopulmonary (E)*   *1st edition 1997; revised 2004, 2008, 2024*

T

OUTCOME CONTENT REFERENCES:

Armstrong, D. W. J., Tobin, C., & Matangi, M. F. (2010). The accuracy of the physical examination for the detection of lower extremity peripheral arterial disease. *Canadian Journal of Cardiology, 26*(10), e346–e350. https://doi.org/10.1016/S0828-282X(10)70467-0

European Pressure Ulcer Advisory Panel| National Pressure Ulcer Advisory Panel| Pan Pacific Pressure Injury Alliance. (2019). *Prevention and treatment of pressure ulcers/injuries: Clinical practice guideline* (3rd ed.). https://www.internationalguideline.com/

García-Mayor, S., Morilla-Herrera, J. C., Lupiáñez-Pérez, I., Kaknani Uttumchandani, S., León Campos, Á., Aranda-Gallardo, M., Moya-Suárez, A. B., & Morales-Asencio, J. M. (2018). Peripheral perfusion and oxygenation in areas of risk of skin integrity impairment exposed to pressure patterns. A phase I trial (POTER Study). *Journal of Advanced Nursing, 74*(2), 465–471. https://doi.org/10.1111/jan.13414

Gómez-González, A. J., Morilla-Herrera, J. C., Lupiáñez-Pérez, I., Morales-Asencio, J. M., García-Mayor, S., León-Campos, Á., Marfil-Gómez, R., Aranda-Gallardo, M., Moya-Suárez, A. B., & Kaknani-Uttumchandani, S. (2020). Perfusion, tissue oxygenation and peripheral temperature in the skin of heels of healthy participants exposed to pressure: A quasi-experimental study. *Journal of Advanced Nursing. 76*(2), 654–663. https://doi.org/10.1111/jan.14250

Hariri, G., Joffre, J., Leblanc, G., Bonsey, M., Lavillegrand, J. R., Urbina, T., Guidet, B., Maury, E., Bakker, J., & Ait-Oufella, H. (2019). Narrative review: Clinical assessment of peripheral tissue perfusion in septic shock. *Annals of Intensive Care, 9*(1), 37. https://doi.org/10.1186/s13613-019-0511-1

Huether, S. E., McCance, K. L., & Brashers, V. L. (2020). *Understanding pathophysiology* (7th ed.). Elsevier.

Ignatavicius, D. D., Workman, M. L., Rebar, C. R., & Heimgartner, N. M. (2021). *Medical-surgical nursing: Concepts for interprofessional care* (10th ed.). Elsevier.

Lima, A., & Bakker, J. (2015). Clinical assessment of peripheral circulation. *Current Opinion in Critical Care, 21*(3), 226–231. https://doi.org/10.1097/MCC.0000000000000194

Santos, D. M., Quintans, J. S. S., Quintans-Junior L. J., Santana-Filho V. J., Cunha, C. L. P., Menezes, I. A. C., & Santos, M. R. V. (2019). Association between peripheral perfusion, microcirculation and mortality in sepsis: A systematic review. *Brazilian Journal of Anesthesiology, 69*(6), 605–621. https://doi.org/10.1016/j.bjane.2019.09.005

Tissue Perfusion: Pulmonary   0408

Definition: Adequacy of blood flow through pulmonary vasculature to perfuse alveoli/capillary unit

OUTCOME TARGET RATING: Maintain at _____ Increase to _____

		Severe Deviation from Normal Range	Substantial Deviation from Normal Range	Moderate Deviation from Normal Range	Mild Deviation from Normal Range	No Deviation from Normal Range	
OUTCOME OVERALL RATING		1	2	3	4	5	
Indicators:							
040810	Ventilation-perfusion scan	1	2	3	4	5	NA
040811	Pulmonary artery pressure (PAP)	1	2	3	4	5	NA
040814	Respiratory rhythm	1	2	3	4	5	NA
040815	Respiratory rate	1	2	3	4	5	NA
040816	Systolic blood pressure	1	2	3	4	5	NA
040817	Diastolic blood pressure	1	2	3	4	5	NA
040822	Mean blood pressure	1	2	3	4	5	NA
040818	Partial pressure of oxygen in arterial blood (PaO_2)	1	2	3	4	5	NA
040819	Partial pressure of carbon dioxide in arterial blood ($PaCO_2$)	1	2	3	4	5	NA
040820	Arterial pH	1	2	3	4	5	NA
040821	Oxygen saturation	1	2	3	4	5	NA
		Severe	Substantial	Moderate	Mild	None	
040805	Chest pain	1	2	3	4	5	NA
040806	Pleural friction rub	1	2	3	4	5	NA
040807	Hemoptysis	1	2	3	4	5	NA
040808	Unexplained anxiety	1	2	3	4	5	NA
040823	Shortness of breath	1	2	3	4	5	NA
040824	Impaired gas exchange	1	2	3	4	5	NA
040825	Dry cough	1	2	3	4	5	NA
040826	Use of accessory muscles	1	2	3	4	5	NA
040827	Fatigue	1	2	3	4	5	NA

Domain-Physiologic Health (II)   *Class*-Cardiopulmonary (E)   *1st edition 1997; revised 2004, 2008, 2024*

OUTCOME CONTENT REFERENCES:
Hinkle, J. L., Cheever, K. H., & Overbaugh, K. (2021). *Brunner & Suddarth's textbook of medical surgical nursing* (15th ed.). Wolters Kluwer.
Huether, S. E., McCance, K. L., & Brashers, V. L. (2020). *Understanding pathophysiology* (7th ed.). Elsevier.
Ignatavicius, D. D., Workman, M. L., Rebar, C. R., & Heimgartner, N. M. (2021). *Medical-surgical nursing: Concepts for interprofessional care* (10th ed.). Elsevier.
Lewis, S. M., Collier, I. C., Heitkermper, M. M., & Dirksen, S. R. (2019). *Lewis's medical-surgical nursing: Assessment & management of clinical problems* (11th ed.). Elsevier.
McCance, K. L., & Huether, S. E. (2018). *Pathophysiology: The biologic basis for disease in adults and children* (8th ed.). Elsevier.
Petersson J., & Glenny, R. W. (2014). Gas exchange and ventilation–perfusion relationships in the lung. *European Respiratory Journal, 44*, 1023–1041. https://doi.org/10.1183/09031936.00037014
Smeltzer, S. C., & Bare, B. G. (2020). *Brunner & Suddarth's textbook of medical surgical nursing* (14th ed.). Lippincott Williams & Wilkins.
So, M., Kabata, H., Fukunaga, K., Takagi, H., & Kuno, T. (2021). Radiological and functional lung sequelae of COVID-19: A systematic review and meta-analysis. *BMC Pulmonary Medicine, 21*(1), 97. https://doi.org/10.1186/s12890-021-01463-0
Ulrich, S., Schneider, S. R., & Bloch, K. E. (2017). Effect of hypoxia and hyperoxia on exercise performance in healthy individuals and in patients with pulmonary hypertension: A systematic review. *Journal of Applied Physiology, 123*(6), 1657–1670. https://doi.org/10.1152/japplphysiol.00186.2017
Wagner, P. D. (2015). The physiological basis of pulmonary gas exchange: Implications for clinical interpretation of arterial blood gases. *European Respiratory Journal, 45*(1), 227–243. https://doi.org/10.1183/09031936.00039214

Transfer Performance   0210

Definition: Ability to change body location independently with or without assistive device

OUTCOME TARGET RATING: Maintain at _____ Increase to _____

		Severely Compromised	Substantially Compromised	Moderately Compromised	Mildly Compromised	Not Compromised	
OUTCOME OVERALL RATING		1	2	3	4	5	
Indicators:							
021009	Transfers from one surface to another while lying	1	2	3	4	5	NA
021001	Transfers from bed to chair	1	2	3	4	5	NA
021002	Transfers from chair to bed	1	2	3	4	5	NA
021003	Transfers from chair to chair	1	2	3	4	5	NA
021010	Transfers from chair to wheelchair	1	2	3	4	5	NA
021011	Transfers from wheelchair to chair	1	2	3	4	5	NA
021004	Transfers from wheelchair to vehicle	1	2	3	4	5	NA
021005	Transfers from vehicle to wheelchair	1	2	3	4	5	NA
021007	Transfers from wheelchair to toilet	1	2	3	4	5	NA
021008	Transfers from toilet to wheelchair	1	2	3	4	5	NA

Domain-*Functional Health (I)*   **Class**-*Mobility (C)*   *1st edition 1997; revised 2004, 2008, 2024*

OUTCOME CONTENT REFERENCES:
Barbareschi, G., & Holloway, C. (2019). An investigation of factors affecting the performance of wheelchair transfers. *Disability and Rehabilitation: Assistive Technology, 14*(5), 479–488. https://doi.org/10.1080/17483107.2018.1463402
Ka, H. (2021). AI-empowered automatic evaluation of sitting-pivot-transfer performance based on 3D body motion tracking and ambient object recognition using a time-of-flight sensor. *Physical Medicine & Rehabilitation, 102*(4), e6. https://doi.org/10.1016/j.apmr.2021.01.020
Koontz, A. M., Bass, S., Kulich, H., & Cooper, R. A. (2018). Effects of grab bars and backrests on independent wheelchair transfer performance and technique. *Physiotherapy Research International, 24*(1), 1–8. https://doi.org/10.1002/pri.1758
Lee, S. J., Mehta-Desai, R., Oh, K., Sanford, J., & Prilutsky, B. I. (2019). Effects of bilateral swing-away grab bars on the biomechanics of stand-to-sit and sit-to-stand toilet transfers. *Disability and Rehabilitation: Assistive Technology, 14*(3), 292–300. https://doi.org/10.1080/17483107.2018.1447605
Witherspoon, J. W., Vuillerot, C., Vasavada, R. P., Waite, M. R., Shelton, M., Chrismer, I. C., Jain, M. S., & Meilleur, K. G. (2019). Motor function performance in individuals with RYR1-related myopathies. *Muscle & Nerve, 60*(10), 80–87. https://doi.org/10.1002/mus.26491

T

Urinary Continence   0502

Definition: Control of elimination of urine from the bladder

OUTCOME TARGET RATING: Maintain at _____ Increase to _____

	Never Demonstrated	Rarely Demonstrated	Sometimes Demonstrated	Often Demonstrated	Consistently Demonstrated	
OUTCOME OVERALL RATING	1	2	3	4	5	
Indicators:						
050201 Recognizes urge to void	1	2	3	4	5	NA
050202 Maintains predictable pattern of voiding	1	2	3	4	5	NA
050221 Uses bladder training strategies	1	2	3	4	5	NA
050224 Keeps bladder diary	1	2	3	4	5	NA
050203 Responds to urge in timely manner	1	2	3	4	5	NA
050204 Voids in appropriate receptacle	1	2	3	4	5	NA
050205 Gets to toilet between urge and passage of urine	1	2	3	4	5	NA
050218 Maintains barrier-free environment for independent toileting	1	2	3	4	5	NA
050225 Maintains privacy for voiding	1	2	3	4	5	NA
050206 Voids greater than150 milliliters each time	1	2	3	4	5	NA
050208 Starts and stops stream	1	2	3	4	5	NA
050209 Empties bladder completely	1	2	3	4	5	NA
050215 Drinks adequate amount of fluid	1	2	3	4	5	NA
050216 Manages clothing independently	1	2	3	4	5	NA
050217 Toilets independently	1	2	3	4	5	NA
050222 Keeps perineal area clean and dry	1	2	3	4	5	NA
050219 Identifies medication that interferes with urinary control	1	2	3	4	5	NA

	Consistently Demonstrated	Often Demonstrated	Sometimes Demonstrated	Rarely Demonstrated	Never Demonstrated	
050207 Urine leakage between voiding	1	2	3	4	5	NA
050210 Post-void residual >100–200 milliliters	1	2	3	4	5	NA
050223 Postpones voiding	1	2	3	4	5	NA
050211 Urine leakage with sneezing, laughing, or lifting	1	2	3	4	5	NA
050212 Wets clothing during day	1	2	3	4	5	NA
050213 Wets clothing or bedding during night	1	2	3	4	5	NA
050214 Urinary tract infection	1	2	3	4	5	NA

Domain-Physiologic Health (II)   **Class**-Elimination (F)   1st edition 1997; revised 2004, 2018, 2024

OUTCOME CONTENT REFERENCES:

+Góes, R. P., Pedreira, L. C., Valente, C. O., Mussi, F. C., Souza, M. L., & Amaral, J. B. (2020). Construction and validation of an instrument for the structural assessment of wards for urinary continence in older adults. *Revista Latino-Americana de Enfermagem, 28,* e3374. https://doi.org/10.1590/1518-8345.3361.3374

Kingan, M., & Martin, M. (2020). Getting ready for certification. *Journal of Wound, Ostomy and Continence Nursing, 47*(4), 407–408. https://doi.org/10.1097/WON.0000000000000682

Neves de Costa, J., de Oliveira Lopes, M. V., & Baena de Moraes Lopes, M. H. (2020). Simultaneous concept analysis of diagnoses related to urinary incontinence. *International Journal of Nursing Knowledge, 31*(2), 109–123. https://doi.org/10.1111/2047-3095.12254

Richards, D. A., Hilli, A., Pentecost, C., Goodwin, V. A., & Frost, J. (2017). Fundamental nursing care: A systematic review of the evidence on the effect of nursing care interventions for nutrition, elimination, mobility and hygiene. *Journal of Clinical Nursing, 27*(11-12), 2179–2188. https://doi.org/10.1111/jocn.14150

Saboia, D. M., Vasconcelos, C. T., Oriá, M. O. B., de C. Bezerra, K., Neto, J. A. V., & de M. Lopes, M. H. (2019). Continence app: Construction and validation of a mobile application for postnatal urinary incontinence prevention. *European Journal of Obstetrics & Gynecology and Reproductive Biology, 240,* 330–335.

Suzuki, M., Okochi, J., Iijima, K., Murata, T., & Kume, H. (2020). Nationwide survey of continence status among older adult residents living in long-term care facilities in Japan: The prevalence and associated risk factors of incontinence and effect of comprehensive care on continence status. *Geriatrics and Gerontology International, 20*(4), 285–290. https://doi.org/10.1111/ggi.13872

Yates, A. (2019). Basic continence assessment: What community nurses should know. *Journal of Community Nursing, 33*(3), 52–55.

U

Urinary Elimination   0503

Definition: Collection and discharge of urine

OUTCOME TARGET RATING: Maintain at _____ Increase to _____

		Severely Compromised	Substantially Compromised	Moderately Compromised	Mildly Compromised	Not Compromised	
OUTCOME OVERALL RATING		**1**	**2**	**3**	**4**	**5**	
Indicators:							
050301	Elimination pattern	1	2	3	4	5	NA
050302	Urine odor	1	2	3	4	5	NA
050303	Urine amount	1	2	3	4	5	NA
050304	Urine color	1	2	3	4	5	NA
050306	Urine clarity	1	2	3	4	5	NA
050307	Fluid intake	1	2	3	4	5	NA
050313	Empties bladder completely	1	2	3	4	5	NA
050314	Recognition of urge	1	2	3	4	5	NA
		Severe	**Substantial**	**Moderate**	**Mild**	**None**	
050305	Visible particles in urine	1	2	3	4	5	NA
050329	Visible blood in urine	1	2	3	4	5	NA
050309	Pain with urination	1	2	3	4	5	NA
050330	Burning with urination	1	2	3	4	5	NA
050310	Hesitancy with urination	1	2	3	4	5	NA
050331	Urinary frequency	1	2	3	4	5	NA
050311	Urgency with urination	1	2	3	4	5	NA
050332	Urinary retention	1	2	3	4	5	NA
050333	Nocturia	1	2	3	4	5	NA
050337	Overflow incontinence	1	2	3	4	5	NA
050334	Stress incontinence	1	2	3	4	5	NA
050335	Urge incontinence	1	2	3	4	5	NA
050336	Functional incontinence	1	2	3	4	5	NA

Domain-Physiologic Health (II)   **Class**-Elimination (F)   *1st edition 1997; reviewed 2018; revised 2004, 2024*

OUTCOME CONTENT REFERENCES:
Bitencourt, G. R., de Almeida Ferreira Alves, L., Ferreira Santana, R., & de Oliveira Lopes, M. V. (2016). Agreement between experts regarding assessment of postoperative urinary elimination nursing outcomes in elderly patients. *International Journal of Nursing Knowledge, 27*(3), 143–148. https://doi.org/10.1111/2047-095.12094
Davis, N. J., Wyman, J. F., Gubitosa, S., & Pretty, L. (2020). Urinary incontinence in older adults. *AJN, American Journal of Nursing, 120*(1), 57–62. https://doi.org/10.1097/01.NAJ.0000652124.58511.24
Góes, R. P., Pedreira, L. C., Valente, C. O., Mussi, F. C., Souza, M. L., & Amaral, J. B. (2020). Construction and validation of an instrument for the structural assessment of wards for urinary continence in older adults. *Revista Latino-Americana de Enfermagem, 28*, e3374. https://doi.org/10.1590/1518-8345.3361.3374
Hogan-Quigley, B., Palm, M. L., & Bickley, L. (2021). *Bates nursing guide to physical examination and history taking* (3rd ed.). Wolters Kluwer.
Kingan, M., & Martin, M. (2020). Getting ready for certification: Assessing principles of continence. *Journal of Wound, Ostomy, and Continence Nursing, 47*(4), 407–408. https://doi.org/10.1097/WON.0000000000000682
Neves de Costa, J., de Oliveira Lopes, M. V., & Baena de Moraes Lopes, M. H. (2020). Simultaneous concept analysis of diagnoses related to urinary incontinence. *International Journal of Nursing Knowledge, 31*(2), 109–123. https://doi.org/10.1111/2047-3095.12254
Richards, D. A., Hilli, A., Pentecost, C., Goodwin, V. A., & Frost, J. (2017). Fundamental nursing care: A systematic review of the evidence on the effect of nursing care interventions for nutrition, elimination, mobility and hygiene. *Journal of Clinical Nursing, 27*(11–12), 2179–2188. https://doi.org/10.1111/jocn.14150
Saboia, D. M., Vasconcelos, C. T., Oriá, M. O., de C. Bezerra, K., Neto, J. A. V., & de M. Lopes, M. H. (2019). Continence app: Construction and validation of a mobile application for postnatal urinary incontinence prevention. *European Journal of Obstetrics & Gynecology and Reproductive Biology, 240*, 330–335. https://doi.org/10.1016/j.ejogrb.2019.07.026
Yates, A. (2019). Basic continence assessment: What community nurses should know. *Journal of Community Nursing, 33*(3), 52–55.

V

Vision Compensation Behavior

1611

Definition: Personal actions to compensate for visual impairment

OUTCOME TARGET RATING: Maintain at _____ Increase to _____

	Never Demonstrated	Rarely Demonstrated	Sometimes Demonstrated	Often Demonstrated	Consistently Demonstrated	
OUTCOME OVERALL RATING	1	2	3	4	5	
Indicators:						
161101 Monitors symptoms of vision deterioration	1	2	3	4	5	NA
161114 Advocates for self	1	2	3	4	5	NA
161102 Positions self to advantage vision	1	2	3	4	5	NA
161103 Reminds others to use techniques that advantage vision	1	2	3	4	5	NA
161104 Uses adequate lighting for activity being performed	1	2	3	4	5	NA
161115 Adjusts schedule to natural light conditions	1	2	3	4	5	NA
161116 Uses fall prevention strategies	1	2	3	4	5	NA
161117 Uses other senses to support vision loss	1	2	3	4	5	NA
161118 Takes breaks from activity	1	2	3	4	5	NA
161105 Wears eyeglasses correctly	1	2	3	4	5	NA
161106 Wears contact lens correctly	1	2	3	4	5	NA
161107 Cares for eyewear correctly	1	2	3	4	5	NA
161108 Uses vision assistive devices	1	2	3	4	5	NA
161119 Uses large print materials	1	2	3	4	5	NA
161109 Uses computer assistive devices	1	2	3	4	5	NA
161113 Uses animal assistance	1	2	3	4	5	NA
161110 Uses support services for low vision	1	2	3	4	5	NA
161111 Uses Braille	1	2	3	4	5	NA
161120 Maintains social activities	1	2	3	4	5	NA

Domain-Health & Knowledge Behavior (IV) *Class*-Health Behavior (Q) 2nd edition 2000; revised 2004, 2018

OUTCOME CONTENT REFERENCES:

Costa, S. L., Pandey, K., Hrdina, J., Rondon, M., & Devos, H. (2020). Vision problems in multiple sclerosis. *Archives of Physical Medicine & Rehabilitation*, *101*(12), 2263–2265. https://doi.org/10.1016/j.apmr.2020.08.003

Hajek, A., Wolfram, C., Spitzer, M., & König, H.-H. (2021). Association of vision problems with psychosocial factors among middle-aged and older individuals: findings from a nationally representative study. *Aging & Mental Health*, *25*(5), 946–953. https://doi.org/10.1080/13607863.2020.1725806

Hinkle, J., & Cheever, K. (2014). *Brunner & Suddarth's textbook of medical-surgical nursing* (13th ed.). Wolters Kluwer Health/Lippincott Williams & Wilkins.

Magnus, E., & Vik, K. (2017). Older adults recently diagnosed with age-related vision loss: Readjusting to everyday life. *Activities, Adaption, & Aging, 40*(4), 296–319.

Schoessow, K. (2010). Shifting from compensation to participation: A model for occupational therapy in low vision. *British Journal of Occupational Therapy, 73*(4), 160–169.

Wettstein, M., Spuling, S. M., Hans-Werner-Wahl, & Heyl, V. (2021). Associations of self-reported vision problems with health and psychosocial functioning: A 9-year longitudinal perspective. *British Journal of Visual Impairment, 39*(1), 31–52. https://doi.org/10.1177/0264619620961803

V

Vital Signs   0802

Definition: Extent to which essential body functions are within normal ranges

OUTCOME TARGET RATING: Maintain at _____ Increase to _____

		Severe Deviation from Normal Range	Substantial Deviation from Normal Range	Moderate Deviation from Normal Range	Mild Deviation from Normal Range	No Deviation from Normal Range	
OUTCOME OVERALL RATING		1	2	3	4	5	
Indicators:							
080201	Body temperature	1	2	3	4	5	NA
080202	Apical heart rate	1	2	3	4	5	NA
080208	Apical heart rhythm	1	2	3	4	5	NA
080203	Radial pulse rate	1	2	3	4	5	NA
080204	Respiratory rate	1	2	3	4	5	NA
080210	Respiratory rhythm	1	2	3	4	5	NA
080212	Oxygen saturation	1	2	3	4	5	NA
080205	Systolic blood pressure	1	2	3	4	5	NA
080206	Diastolic blood pressure	1	2	3	4	5	NA
080209	Pulse pressure	1	2	3	4	5	NA
080211	Depth of inspiration	1	2	3	4	5	NA

Domain-*Physiologic Health (II)*   **Class**-*Metabolic Regulation (I)*   *1st edition 1997; revised 2004, 2008, 2024*

OUTCOME CONTENT REFERENCES:

Connor, N., McArthur, D., & Plazas, P. C. (2021). Reflections on vital sign measurement in nursing practice. *Nursing Philosophy, 22*, e12326. https://doi.org/10.1111/nup.12326

Dall'Ora, C., Griffiths, P., Hope, J., Barker, H., & Smith, G. B. (2020). What is the nursing time and workload involved in taking and recording patients' vital signs? A systematic review. *Journal of Clinical Nursing, 29*, 2053–2068. https://doi.org/10.1111/jocn.15202

Downey, C. L., Chapman, S., Randell, R., Brown, J. M., & Jayne, D. G. (2018). The impact of continuous versus intermittent vital signs monitoring in hospitals: A systematic review and narrative synthesis, *International Journal of Nursing Studies, 84*, 19–27. https://doi.org/10.1016/j.ijnurstu.2018.04.013

Potter, P. A., Perry, A. G., Stockert, P. A., & Hall, A. (2021). *Fundamentals of nursing* (10th ed.). Elsevier.

Schondelmeyer, A. C., Dewan, M. L., Brady, P. W., Timmons, K. M., Cable, R., Britto, M. T., & Bonafide, C. P. (2020). Cardiorespiratory and pulse oximetry monitoring in hospitalized children: A Delphi process. *Pediatrics, 146*(2), e20193336. https://doi.org/10.1542/peds.2019-3336

Scott, B. J., & Kaur, R. (2020). Monitoring breathing frequency, pattern, and effort. *Respiratory Care, 65*(6), 793–806. https://doi.org/10.4187/respcare.07439

Sorrentino, S. A., & Remmert, L. A. (2021). *Mosby's textbook for nursing assistants* (10th ed.). Elsevier.

Vocal Function   1110

Definition: Sounds made by individuals using the vocal tract to perform verbal interactions in daily living

OUTCOME TARGET RATING: Maintain at _____ Increase to _____

		Severely Compromised	Substantially Compromised	Moderately Compromised	Mildly Compromised	Not Compromised	
OUTCOME OVERALL RATING		1	2	3	4	5	
Indicators:							
111001	Vocal clarity	1	2	3	4	5	NA
111002	Voice pitch	1	2	3	4	5	NA
111003	Voice projection	1	2	3	4	5	NA
111004	Ability to clear throat	1	2	3	4	5	NA

V

Continued

Vocal Function—cont'd

		Severe	Substantial	Moderate	Mild	None	
111005	Breathiness	1	2	3	4	5	NA
111006	Mouth dryness	1	2	3	4	5	NA
111007	Hoarseness	1	2	3	4	5	NA
111008	Burning sensation	1	2	3	4	5	NA
111009	Choking	1	2	3	4	5	NA
111010	Voice breaks	1	2	3	4	5	NA
111011	Voice loss	1	2	3	4	5	NA
111012	Vocal fatigue	1	2	3	4	5	NA
111013	Throat irritation	1	2	3	4	5	NA
111014	Throat soreness	1	2	3	4	5	NA
111015	Vocal mucosal lesions	1	2	3	4	5	NA
111016	Vocal fold palsy	1	2	3	4	5	NA
111017	Polyps	1	2	3	4	5	NA
111018	Nodules	1	2	3	4	5	NA
111019	Laryngopharyngeal reflux	1	2	3	4	5	NA
111020	Allergens	1	2	3	4	5	NA

Domain-Physiologic Health (II) **Class**-Tissue Integrity (L) 7th edition 2024

OUTCOME CONTENT REFERENCES:

Buckley, K. L., O'Halloran, P. D., & Oates, J. M. (2014). Occupational vocal health of elite sports coaches: An exploratory pilot study of football coaches. *Journal of Voice, 29*(4), 476–483. https://doi.org/10.1016/j.jvoice.2014.09.017

de Lima Silva, C. R., da Silva Nunes, A. D., de Souza, L. B. R., Jerez-Roig, J., & Barbosa, I. R. (2021). Vocal and laryngeal symptoms and associated factors in wind instrumentalists: A systematic review. *Journal of Voice, 35*(2), 284–290. https://doi.org/10.1016/j.jvoice.2019.08.024

DeVore, E. K., Carroll, T. L., Rosner, B., & Shin, J. J. (2020). Can voice disorders matter as much as life-threatening comorbidities to patients' general health? *Laryngoscope, 130*(10), 2405–2411. https://doi.org/10.1002/lary.28417

Groll, M. D., Hablani, S., & Stepp, C. E. (2021). The relationship between voice onset time and increase in vocal effort and fundamental frequency. *Journal of Speech, Language, and Hearing Research, 64*(4), 1197–1209. https://doi.org/10.1044/2021_JSLHR-20-00505

Leonard, R. (2009). Voice therapy and vocal nodules in adults. *Current Opinion in Otolaryngology & Head and Neck Surgery, 17*(6), 453–457. https://doi.org/10.1097/MOO.0b013e3283317fd2

Manternach, J. N., & Schloneger, M. J. (2021). Vocal dose of preservice music therapists, preservice music teachers, and other undergraduate students. *Journal of Voice, 35*(2), 328.e1–328.e10. https://doi.org/10.1016/j.jvoice.2019.09.008

Menon, U. K., Raj, M., Antony, L., Soman, S., & Bhaskaran, R. (2019). Prevalence of voice disorders in school teachers in a district of South India. *Journal of Voice, 35*(1), 1–8. https://doi.org/10.1016/j.jvoice.2019.07.005

Won, S. J., Kim, R. B., Kim, J. P., Park, J. J., Kwon, M. S., & Woo, S. H. (2016). The prevalence and factors associated with vocal nodules in general population. Cross-sectional epidemiological study. *Medicine, 95*(39), 1–5. https://doi.org/10.1097/MD.0000000000004971

Weight: Body Mass   1006

Definition: Extent to which body weight, muscle, and fat are congruent to height, frame, gender, and age

OUTCOME TARGET RATING: Maintain at _____ Increase to _____

		Severe Deviation from Normal Range	Substantial Deviation from Normal Range	Moderate Deviation from Normal Range	Mild Deviation from Normal Range	No Deviation from Normal Range	
OUTCOME OVERALL RATING		1	2	3	4	5	
Indicators:							
100601	Weight	1	2	3	4	5	NA
100602	Triceps skinfold thickness	1	2	3	4	5	NA
100603	Subscapular skinfold thickness	1	2	3	4	5	NA
100604	Waist/hip circumference ratio (women)	1	2	3	4	5	NA

W

Weight: Body Mass—cont'd

		Severe Deviation from Normal Range	Substantial Deviation from Normal Range	Moderate Deviation from Normal Range	Mild Deviation from Normal Range	No Deviation from Normal Range	
100605	Neck/waist circumference ratio (men)	1	2	3	4	5	NA
100606	Body fat percentage	1	2	3	4	5	NA
100607	Head circumference percentile (child)	1	2	3	4	5	NA
100608	Height percentile (child)	1	2	3	4	5	NA
100609	Weight percentile (child)	1	2	3	4	5	NA

Domain-*Physiologic Health (II)*   **Class**-*Metabolic Regulation (I)*   *1st edition 1997; revised 2004; reviewed 2018*

OUTCOME CONTENT REFERENCES:

Aeberli, I., Gut-Knabenhans, M., Kusche-Ammann, R., Molinari, L., & Zimmermann, M. (2013). A composite score combining waist circumference and body mass index more accurately predicts body fat percentage in 6- to 13-year-old children. *European Journal of Nutrition, 52*(1), 247–253. https://doi.org/10.1007/s00394-012-0317-5

Flegal, K. M., Tabak, C. J., & Ogden, C. L. (2006). Overweight in children: Definitions and interpretation. *Health Education Research, 21*(6), 755–760.

Koo, W. W., & Hockman, E. M. (2006). Posthospital discharge feeding for preterm infants: Effects of standard compared with enriched milk formula on growth, bone mass, and body composition. *American Journal of Clinical Nutrition, 84*(6), 1357–1364. https://doi.org/10.1093/ajcn/84.6.1357

Power, B., Alfonso, H., Flicker, L., Hankey, G., Yeap, B., & Almeida, O. (2013). Changes in body mass in later life and incident dementia. *International Psychogeriatrics, 25*(3), 467–478. https://doi.org/10.1093/ajcn/84.6.1357

Rees, G., Porter, J., Bennett, S., Colleypriest, O., Ellis, L., & Stenhouse, E. (2012). The validity and reliability of weight and height measurements and body mass index calculations in early pregnancy. *Journal of Human Nutrition and Dietetics, 25*(2), 117–120. https://doi.org/10.1111/j.1365-277X.2011.01207.x

Reinders, I., Murphy, R., Martin, K., Brouwer, I., Visser, M., White, D., Newman, A. B., Houston, D. K., Kanaya, A. M., Nagin, D. S., Harris, T. B., & Health, Aging and Body Composition Study. (2015). Body mass index trajectories in relation to change in lean mass and physical function: The health, aging and body composition study. *Journal of the American Geriatrics Society, 63*(8), 1615–1621. https://doi.org/10.1111/jgs.13524

Yang, F., Lv, J.-H., Lei, S.-F., Chen, X.-D., Liu, M.-Y., Jian, W.-X., Xu, H., Tan, L.-J., Deng, F.-Y., Yang, Y.-J., Wang, Y.-B., Sun, X., Xiao, S.-M., Jiang, C., Guo, Y.-F., Guo, J.-J., Li, Y.-N., Zhu, X.-Z., Papasian, C.-J., & Deng, H.-W. (2006). Receiver-operating characteristic analyses of body mass index, waist circumference and waist-to-hip ratio for obesity: Screening in young adults in central south of China. *Clinical Nutrition, 25*(6), 1030–1039. https://doi.org/10.1016/j.clnu.2006.04.009

Yang, K., Turk, M., Allison, V., James, K., & Chasens, E. (2014). Body mass index self-perception and weight management behaviors during late adolescence. *Journal of School Health, 84*(10), 654–660. https://doi.org/10.1111/josh.12195

Weight Gain Behavior   1626

Definition: Personal actions to gain weight following voluntary or involuntary significant weight loss

OUTCOME TARGET RATING: Maintain at_____ Increase to_____

		Never Demonstrated	Rarely Demonstrated	Sometimes Demonstrated	Often Demonstrated	Consistently Demonstrated	
OUTCOME OVERALL RATING		**1**	**2**	**3**	**4**	**5**	
Indicators:							
162601	Obtains assistance from health professional	1	2	3	4	5	NA
162602	Identifies cause of weight loss	1	2	3	4	5	NA
162603	Receives proper dental care	1	2	3	4	5	NA
162604	Sets achievable weight gain goals	1	2	3	4	5	NA
162605	Selects a healthy target weight	1	2	3	4	5	NA
162606	Commits to a healthy eating plan	1	2	3	4	5	NA
162607	Identifies caloric intake requirements	1	2	3	4	5	NA
162608	Maintains an adequate supply of nutritious food and fluid	1	2	3	4	5	NA

W

Continued

Weight Gain Behavior—cont'd

		Never Demonstrated	Rarely Demonstrated	Sometimes Demonstrated	Often Demonstrated	Consistently Demonstrated	
162609	Obtains financial assistance for purchasing food	1	2	3	4	5	NA
162636	Uses community food pantries when needed	1	2	3	4	5	NA
162737	Refrains from skipping meals	1	2	3	4	5	NA
162610	Prepares food to enhance swallowing	1	2	3	4	5	NA
162738	Uses assistive devices	1	2	3	4	5	NA
162611	Uses flavor enhancers	1	2	3	4	5	NA
162612	Obtains assistance with food preparation	1	2	3	4	5	NA
162613	Identifies food and fluid preferences and dislikes	1	2	3	4	5	NA
162614	Identifies food allergies	1	2	3	4	5	NA
162615	Uses vitamin/mineral supplements	1	2	3	4	5	NA
162616	Drinks eight glasses of water daily	1	2	3	4	5	NA
162617	Recognizes signs and symptoms of electrolyte imbalance	1	2	3	4	5	NA
162618	Obtains treatment for electrolyte imbalance	1	2	3	4	5	NA
162619	Monitors appetite level	1	2	3	4	5	NA
162620	Uses prescribed medication to increase appetite	1	2	3	4	5	NA
162621	Uses prescribed medication to enhance weight gain	1	2	3	4	5	NA
162622	Uses nutrient supplements	1	2	3	4	5	NA
162623	Selects high protein, high caloric food and fluid	1	2	3	4	5	NA
162624	Eats nutritious food and drinks fluid between meals	1	2	3	4	5	NA
162625	Maintains fluid balance	1	2	3	4	5	NA
162626	Maintains adequate sleep	1	2	3	4	5	NA
162739	Monitors food and fluid intake using diary or mobile app	1	2	3	4	5	NA
162628	Administers enteral tube feedings as recommended	1	2	3	4	5	NA
162629	Administers parenteral nutrition as recommended	1	2	3	4	5	NA
162630	Monitors exercise for caloric requirements	1	2	3	4	5	NA
162631	Uses personal support system to enhance weight gain	1	2	3	4	5	NA
162632	Participates in support groups	1	2	3	4	5	NA
162633	Participates in nutritional monitoring	1	2	3	4	5	NA
162634	Monitors body mass index	1	2	3	4	5	NA
162635	Monitors body weight	1	2	3	4	5	NA
	Target weight _____ kg/lb						

Domain-Health Knowledge & Behavior (IV)   *Class*-Health Behavior (Q)   4th edition 2008; revised 2024

W

OUTCOME CONTENT REFERENCES:

Batchelor-Murphy, M. K., Steinberg, F. M., & Young, H. M. (2019). Dietary and feeding modifications for older adults. *AJN, American Journal of Nursing, 119*(12), 49–57. https://doi.org/10.1097/01.naj.0000615796.40279.9c

Caouette, S., Boss, L., & Lynn, M. (2020). The relationship between food insecurity and cost-related medication nonadherence in older adults: A systematic review. *AJN, American Journal of Nursing, 120*(6), 23–36. https://doi.org/10.1097/01.naj.0000668732.28490.c1

Clifton, M., Johnstone, W. M., & Kolasa, K. M. (2020). Feeding a person with advanced Alzheimer's disease: An update. *Nutrition Today, 55*(5), 202–210. https://doi.org/10.1097/NT.0000000000000430

Gelhorn, H. L., Gries, K. S., Speck, R. M., Duus, E. M., Bourne, R. K., Aggarwal, D., & Cella, D. (2019). Comprehensive validation of the Functional Assessment of Anorexia/ Cachexia Therapy (FAACT) Anorexia/Cachexia Subscale (A/CS) in lung cancer patients with involuntary weight loss. *Quality of Life Research,* *28*(6), 1641–1653. https://doi.org/10.1007/s11136-019-02135-7

Kamdar, N., Lester, H. F., Daundasekara, S. S., Greer, A. E., Hundt, N. E., Utech, A., & Hernandez, D. C. (2021). Food insecurity: Comparing odds between working-age veterans and nonveterans with children. *Nursing Outlook, 69*(2), 212–220. https://doi.org/10.1016/j.outlook.2020.08.011

U.S. Department of Health and Human Services and U.S. Department of Agriculture. (2020). *2020–2025 Dietary Guidelines for Americans* (9th ed.). https://www.dietaryguidelines.gov/

Weight Loss Behavior   1627

Definition: Personal actions to lose weight through diet, exercise, and behavior modification

OUTCOME TARGET RATING: Maintain at_____ Increase to_____

		Never Demonstrated	Rarely Demonstrated	Sometimes Demonstrated	Often Demonstrated	Consistently Demonstrated	
OUTCOME OVERALL RATING		1	2	3	4	5	
Indicators:							
162701	Obtains information on weight loss strategies from health professional	1	2	3	4	5	NA
162702	Selects a healthy target weight	1	2	3	4	5	NA
162703	Commits to a healthy eating plan	1	2	3	4	5	NA
162704	Selects nutritious food and fluid	1	2	3	4	5	NA
162705	Controls food portions	1	2	3	4	5	NA
162706	Establishes an exercise routine	1	2	3	4	5	NA
162728	Monitors time spent in sedentary activities	1	2	3	4	5	NA
162707	Caloric expenditure exceeds caloric intake	1	2	3	4	5	NA
162708	Controls preoccupation with food	1	2	3	4	5	NA
162709	Identifies emotional states that affect food and fluid intake	1	2	3	4	5	NA
162710	Identifies social situations that affect food and fluid intake	1	2	3	4	5	NA
162711	Plans for situations that affect food and fluid intake	1	2	3	4	5	NA
162712	Uses behavior modification strategies	1	2	3	4	5	NA
162713	Uses self-talk motivation	1	2	3	4	5	NA
162714	Avoids high caloric food and fluid	1	2	3	4	5	NA
162715	Drinks eight glasses of water daily	1	2	3	4	5	NA
162716	Includes vitamins in weight loss plan	1	2	3	4	5	NA
162717	Uses appetite suppressants as prescribed	1	2	3	4	5	NA
162718	Uses weight loss medication as prescribed	1	2	3	4	5	NA
162719	Uses personal support system to enhance weight loss	1	2	3	4	5	NA
162720	Participates in weight loss support group	1	2	3	4	5	NA
162721	Manages setbacks by resuming weight loss efforts	1	2	3	4	5	NA
162722	Monitors body weight	1	2	3	4	5	NA
162723	Monitors body mass index	1	2	3	4	5	NA
162729	Monitors waist circumference	1	2	3	4	5	NA
162730	Monitors food and fluid intake using diary or mobile app	1	2	3	4	5	NA

Continued

Weight Loss Behavior—cont'd

		Never Demonstrated	Rarely Demonstrated	Sometimes Demonstrated	Often Demonstrated	Consistently Demonstrated	
162731	Monitors exercise using diary or mobile app	1	2	3	4	5	NA
162726	Maintains progress toward target weight	1	2	3	4	5	NA
162727	Uses commercial diet products safely	1	2	3	4	5	NA
162732	Uses wearable technology to support weight loss efforts	1	2	3	4	5	NA
162733	Uses multiple strategies for weight loss	1	2	3	4	5	NA

Target weight _____ kg/lb

Domain-Health Knowledge & Behavior (IV)   **Class**-Health Behavior (Q)   4th edition 2008; revised 2024

OUTCOME CONTENT REFERENCES:

Aure, C. F., Kluge, A., & Moen, A. (2021), Older adults' engagement in technology-mediated self-monitoring of diet: A mixed-method study. *Journal of Nursing Scholarship, 53*(1), 25–34. https://doi.org/10.1111/jnu.12619

Batsis, J. A., & Zagaria, A. B. (2018). Addressing obesity in aging patients. *Medical Clinics of North America, 102*(1), 65–85. https://doi.org/10.1016/j.mcna.2017.08.007

Hall, K. D., & Kahan, S. (2018). Maintenance of lost weight and long-term management of obesity. *Medical Clinics of North America, 102*(1), 183–197. https://doi.org/10.1016/j.mcna.2017.08.012

Katz, A. (2019). CE: Obesity-related cancer in women: A clinical review. *AJN, American Journal of Nursing, 119*(8), 34–40. https://doi.org/10.1097/01.NAJ.0000577332.56265.51

Lee, M. K., Park, S. Y., & Choi, G. S. (2019). Facilitators and barriers to adoption of a healthy diet in survivors of colorectal cancer. *Journal of Nursing Scholarship, 51*(5), 509–517. https://doi.org/10.1111/jnu.12496

Marquez, B., & Murillo, R. (2017). Racial/ethnic differences in weight-loss strategies among U.S. adults: National health and nutrition examination survey 2007–2012. *Journal of the Academy of Nutrition and Dietetics, 117*(6), 923–928. https://doi.org/10.1016/j.jand.2017.01.025

Patel, M. L., Brooks, T. L., & Bennett, G. G. (2020). Consistent self-monitoring in a commercial app-based intervention for weight loss: Results from a randomized trial. *Journal of Behavioral Medicine, 43*(3), 391–401. https://doi.org/10.1007/s10865-019-00091-8

Tchang, B. G., Saunders, K. H., & Igel, L. I. (2021). Best practices in the management of overweight and obesity. *Medical Clinics of North America, 105*(1), 149–174. https://doi.org/10.1016/j.mcna.2020.08.018

Wang, E., Abrahamson, K., Liu, P. J., & Ahmed, A. (2020). Can mobile technology improve weight loss in overweight adults? A systematic review. *Western Journal of Nursing Research, 42*(9), 747–759. https://doi.org/10.1177/0193945919888224

Zhu, B., Chen, X., Park, C., Zhu, D., & Izci-Balserak, B. (2020). Fatigue and sleep quality predict eating behavior among people with type 2 diabetes. *Nursing Research, 69*(6), 419–426. https://doi.org/10.1097/NNR.0000000000000447

Weight Maintenance Behavior

1628

Definition: Personal actions to maintain optimum body weight

OUTCOME TARGET RATING: Maintain at _____ Increase to _____

		Never Demonstrated	Rarely Demonstrated	Sometimes Demonstrated	Often Demonstrated	Consistently Demonstrated	
OUTCOME OVERALL RATING		1	2	3	4	5	
Indicators:							
162801	Monitors body weight	1	2	3	4	5	NA
162822	Participates in exercise program	1	2	3	4	5	NA
162823	Monitors time spent in sedentary activities	1	2	3	4	5	NA
162802	Maintains optimal daily caloric intake	1	2	3	4	5	NA
162803	Balances exercise with caloric intake	1	2	3	4	5	NA
162804	Selects nutritious meals	1	2	3	4	5	NA
162805	Selects nutritious snacks	1	2	3	4	5	NA

W

Weight Maintenance Behavior—cont'd

		Never Demonstrated	Rarely Demonstrated	Sometimes Demonstrated	Often Demonstrated	Consistently Demonstrated	
162824	Controls food portions	1	2	3	4	5	NA
162806	Drinks eight glasses of water daily	1	2	3	4	5	NA
162807	Uses nutrient supplements as needed	1	2	3	4	5	NA
162808	Eats in response to hunger	1	2	3	4	5	NA
162809	Maintains recommended eating pattern	1	2	3	4	5	NA
162810	Retains ingested foods	1	2	3	4	5	NA
162811	Maintains fluid balance	1	2	3	4	5	NA
162812	Obtains assistance from health professional	1	2	3	4	5	NA
162813	Uses personal support systems	1	2	3	4	5	NA
162814	Identifies social situations that affect food and fluid intake	1	2	3	4	5	NA
162815	Identifies emotional states that affect food and fluid intake	1	2	3	4	5	NA
162816	Plans for situations that affect food and fluid intake	1	2	3	4	5	NA
162817	Controls preoccupation with food	1	2	3	4	5	NA
162818	Controls preoccupation with weight	1	2	3	4	5	NA
162825	Monitors food and fluid intake using diary or mobile app	1	2	3	4	5	NA
162819	Expresses realistic body image	1	2	3	4	5	NA
162820	Maintains adequate sleep	1	2	3	4	5	NA
162821	Maintains optimum weight	1	2	3	4	5	NA

Target weight _____ kg/lb

***Domain**-Health Knowledge & Behavior (IV)   **Class**-Health Behavior (Q)   4th edition 2008; revised 2024*

OUTCOME CONTENT REFERENCES:

Aure, C. F., Kluge, A., & Moen, A. (2021), Older adults' engagement in technology-mediated self-monitoring of diet: A mixed-method study. *Journal of Nursing Scholarship, 53*(1), 25–34. https://do.org/10.1111/jnu.12619

Dibb-Smith, A. E., Brindal, E., Chapman, J., & Noakes, M. (2019). A mixed-methods investigation of psychological factors relevant to weight maintenance. *Journal of Health Psychology, 24*(4), 440–452. https://doi.org/10.1177/1359105316678053

Hall, K. D., & Kahan, S. (2018). Maintenance of lost weight and long-term management of obesity. *Medical Clinics of North America, 102*(1), 183–197. https://doi.org/10.1016/j.mcna.2017.08.012

Soini, S., Mustajoki, P., Eriksson, J. G., & Lahti, J. (2018). Personality traits associated with weight maintenance among successful weight losers. *American Journal of Health Behaviors, 42*(6), 78–84. https://doi.org/10.5993/AJHB.42.6.8

U.S. Department of Health and Human Services and U.S. Department of Agriculture. (2020). *2020–2025 Dietary Guidelines for Americans* (9th ed.). https://www.dietaryguidelines.gov/

Varkevisser, R. D. M., van Stralen, M. M., Kroeze, W., Ket, J. C. F., & Steenhuis, I. H. M. (2019). Determinants of weight loss maintenance: A systematic review. *Obesity Reviews, 20*(4), 171–211. https://doi.org/10.1111/obr.12772

W

Will to Live

Definition: Desire, determination, and effort to survive by an individual facing adversity or a life challenge

OUTCOME TARGET RATING: Maintain at _____ Increase to _____

OUTCOME OVERALL RATING	Never Demonstrated	Rarely Demonstrated	Sometimes Demonstrated	Often Demonstrated	Consistently Demonstrated	
	1	2	3	4	5	
Indicators:						
120619 Reports a sense of well-being	1	2	3	4	5	NA
120620 Expresses determination to live	1	2	3	4	5	NA
120621 Expresses hope	1	2	3	4	5	NA
120622 Expresses connection to religious beliefs	1	2	3	4	5	NA
120623 Expresses optimism about the future	1	2	3	4	5	NA
120624 Expresses sense of control	1	2	3	4	5	NA
120625 Expresses feelings	1	2	3	4	5	NA
120626 Expresses interest in one's illness	1	2	3	4	5	NA
120627 Expresses interest in one's treatment	1	2	3	4	5	NA
120628 Uses strategies for problems associated with chronic disease	1	2	3	4	5	NA
120629 Uses strategies to cope with disabilities	1	2	3	4	5	NA
120630 Uses strategies to cope with life situation	1	2	3	4	5	NA
120631 Engages in treatments to lengthen life	1	2	3	4	5	NA
120632 Uses strategies to enhance health	1	2	3	4	5	NA
120633 Maintains relationships with others	1	2	3	4	5	NA

	Consistently Demonstrated	Often Demonstrated	Sometimes Demonstrated	Rarely Demonstrated	Never Demonstrated	
120634 Depression	1	2	3	4	5	NA
120635 Suicidal thoughts	1	2	3	4	5	NA
120636 Pessimistic thoughts	1	2	3	4	5	NA
120637 Loss of dignity	1	2	3	4	5	NA
120638 Pain	1	2	3	4	5	NA
120639 Social isolation	1	2	3	4	5	NA

Domain-Psychosocial Health (III)   **Class**-Psychological Well-Being (M)   *1st edition 1997; revised 2004, 2008, 2024*

OUTCOME CONTENT REFERENCES:

Bornet, M.-A., Bernard, M., Jaques, C., Rubli Truchard, E., Borasio, G. D., & Jox, R. J. (2021). Assessing the will to live: A scoping review. *Journal of Pain & Symptom Management*, *61*(4), 845. https://doi.org/10.1016/j.jpainsymman.2020.09.012

+Carmel, S. (2017). The Will-to-Live Scale: Development, validation, and significance for elderly people. *Aging & Mental Health*, *21*(3), 289–296. https://doi.org/10.1080/13607863.2015.1081149

+Cwik, J. C., Siegmann, P., Willutzki, U., Nyhuis, P., Wolter, M., Forkmann, T., Glaesmer, H., & Teismann, T. (2017). Brief Reasons for Living Inventory: A psychometric investigation. *BMC Psychiatry, 17*(4), 358. https://doi.org/10.1186/s12888-017-1521-x

+Ivanoff, A., Joon Jang, S., Smyth, N. J., & Linehan, M. M. (1994). Fewer reasons for staying alive when you are thinking of killing yourself: The Brief Reasons for Living Inventory. *Journal of Psychopathology and Behavioral Assessment, 16*(1), 1–13.

Julião, M., Antunes, B., Nunes, B., Sobral, M. A., Chaves, P., Runa, D., & Bruera, E. (2020). Measuring total suffering and will to live in an advanced cancer patient using a patient-centered outcome measure: A follow-up case study. *Journal of Palliative Medicine, 23*(5), 733–737. https://doi.org/10.1089/jpm.2019.0137

+Linehan, M. M., Goodstein, J. L., Nielsen, S. L., & Chiles, J. A. (1983). Reasons for staying alive when you are thinking of killing yourself: The Reasons for Living Inventory. *Journal of Consulting and Clinical Psychology, 51*(2), 276–286, 484–485.

Shrira, A., Carmel, S., Tovel, H., & Raveis, V. H. (2019). Reciprocal relationships between the will-to-live and successful aging. *Aging & Mental Health, 23*(10), 1350–1357. https://doi.org/10.1080/13607863.2018.1499011

Vatne, M., & Nåden, D. (2016). Crucial resources to strengthen the desire to live. *Nursing Ethics, 23*(3), 294–307. https://doi.org/10.1177/0969733014562990

Zamir, A., Granek, L., & Carmel, S. (2020). Factors affecting the will to live among elderly Jews living in Israel. *Aging & Mental Health, 24*(4), 550–556. https://doi.org/10.1080/13607863.2018.1537361

W

Wound Healing: Primary Intention   1102

Definition: Extent of regeneration of cells and tissues following intentional closure

OUTCOME TARGET RATING: Maintain at _____ Increase to _____

OUTCOME OVERALL RATING	None	Limited	Moderate	Substantial	Extensive	
	1	2	3	4	5	
Indicators:						
110201 Skin approximation	1	2	3	4	5	NA
110213 Wound edge approximation	1	2	3	4	5	NA
110214 Scar formation	1	2	3	4	5	NA
	Extensive	**Substantial**	**Moderate**	**Limited**	**None**	
110202 Purulent drainage	1	2	3	4	5	NA
110203 Serous drainage	1	2	3	4	5	NA
110204 Sanguineous drainage	1	2	3	4	5	NA
110205 Serosanguineous drainage	1	2	3	4	5	NA
110206 Sanguineous drainage from drain	1	2	3	4	5	NA
110207 Serosanguineous drainage from drain	1	2	3	4	5	NA
110208 Surrounding skin erythema	1	2	3	4	5	NA
110215 Surrounding skin bruising	1	2	3	4	5	NA
110209 Periwound edema	1	2	3	4	5	NA
110210 Increased skin temperature	1	2	3	4	5	NA
110211 Foul wound odor	1	2	3	4	5	NA

Location of wound (# from picture): _____

*Domain-Physiologic Health (II)   **Class**-Tissue Integrity (L)   1st edition 1997; revised 2004; reviewed 2018*

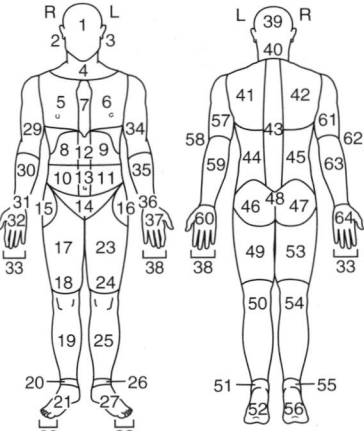

1. Front of head
2. Right ear
3. Left ear
4. Front of neck
5. Right chest
6. Left chest
7. Sternum
8. Right upper quadrant
9. Left upper quadrant
10. Right lower quadrant
11. Left lower quadrant
12. Abdominal midline
13. Navel
14. Pubic and perineal area
15. Right trochanter (hip)
16. Left trochanter (hip)
17. Right anterior thigh
18. Right knee
19. Right lower anterior leg
20. Right ankle (inner/outer)
21. Right foot
22. Right toes
23. Left anterior thigh
24. Left knee
25. Left lower anterior leg
26. Left ankle (inner/outer)
27. Left foot
28. Left toes
29. Right upper interior arm
30. Right interior forearm
31. Right wrist
32. Right palm
33. Right fingers _____ (specify)
34. Left upper interior arm
35. Left interior forearm
36. Left wrist
37. Left palm
38. Left fingers _____ (specify)
39. Back of head
40. Back of neck
41. Left scapula
42. Right scapula
43. Spine
44. Left back
45. Right back
46. Left buttock
47. Right buttock
48. Sacrum
49. Left posterior thigh
50. Left lower posterior leg
51. Left heel
52. Left bottom foot
53. Right posterior thigh
54. Right lower posterior leg
55. Right heel
56. Right bottom foot
57. Left upper posterior arm
58. Left elbow
59. Left posterior forearm
60. Left dorsal hand
61. Right upper posterior arm
62. Right elbow
63. Right posterior forearm
64. Right dorsal hand

W

OUTCOME CONTENT REFERENCES:

Cohen, I. K., Diegelmann, R. F., & Lindblad, W. L. (1992). *Wound healing: Biochemical and clinical aspects.* W.B. Saunders.

da Silva, M. B., de Almeida, M. A., Panato, B. P., de Siqueira, A. P. O., da Silva, M. P., & Reisderfer, L. (2015). Clinical applicability of nursing outcomes in the evolution of orthopedic patients with impaired physical mobility. *Revista Latino-Americana de Enfermagem, 23*, 51–58. https://doi.org/10.1111/2047-3095.12204

Flanagan, M. (Ed.). (2013). *Wound healing and skin integrity: Principles and practice.* John Wiley & Sons.

+Holden-Lund, C. (1988). Effects of relaxation with guided imagery on surgical stress and wound healing. *Research in Nursing & Health, 11*(4), 235–244.

Lazarus, G. S., Cooper, D. M., Knighton, D. R., Margohs, D. J., Pecoraro, R. E., Rodeheaver, G., & Robson, M. C. (1994). Definitions and guidelines for assessment of wounds and evaluation of healing. *Archives of Dermatology, 130*(4), 489–493.

McCulloch, J. M., & Kloth, L. C. (Eds.). (2010). *Wound healing: Evidence-based management.* F.A. Davis.

Potter, P. A., & Perry, A. G. (2001). *Fundamentals of nursing* (5th ed.). Mosby.

Scalise, A., Calamita, R., Tartaglione, C., Pierangeli, M., Bolletta, E., Gioacchini, M., Gesuita, R., & Di Benedetto, G. (2016). Improving wound healing and preventing surgical site complications of closed surgical incisions: A possible role of incisional negative pressure wound therapy. A systematic review of the literature. *International Wound Journal, 13*(6), 1260–1281. https://doi.org/10.1111/iwj.12492

Wound Healing: Secondary Intention   **1103**

Definition: Extent of regeneration of cells and tissues in an open wound

OUTCOME TARGET RATING: Maintain at _____ Increase to _____

		None	Limited	Moderate	Substantial	Extensive	
OUTCOME OVERALL RATING		**1**	**2**	**3**	**4**	**5**	
Indicators:							
110301	Granulation	1	2	3	4	5	NA
110320	Scar formation	1	2	3	4	5	NA
110321	Decreased wound size	1	2	3	4	5	NA
		Extensive	**Substantial**	**Moderate**	**Limited**	**None**	
110303	Purulent drainage	1	2	3	4	5	NA
110304	Serous drainage	1	2	3	4	5	NA
110305	Sanguineous drainage	1	2	3	4	5	NA
110306	Serosanguineous drainage	1	2	3	4	5	NA
110307	Surrounding skin erythema	1	2	3	4	5	NA
110322	Wound inflammation	1	2	3	4	5	NA
110308	Periwound edema	1	2	3	4	5	NA
110310	Blistered skin	1	2	3	4	5	NA
110311	Macerated skin	1	2	3	4	5	NA
110312	Necrosis	1	2	3	4	5	NA
110313	Sloughing	1	2	3	4	5	NA
110314	Tunneling	1	2	3	4	5	NA
110315	Undermining	1	2	3	4	5	NA
110316	Sinus tract formation	1	2	3	4	5	NA
110317	Foul wound odor	1	2	3	4	5	NA

Location of wound (# from picture) _____

Domain-Physiologic Health (II)   **Class**-Tissue Integrity (L)   *1st edition 1997; revised 2004; reviewed 2018*

W

1. Front of head
2. Right ear
3. Left ear
4. Front of neck
5. Right chest
6. Left chest
7. Sternum
8. Right upper quadrant
9. Left upper quadrant
10. Right lower quadrant
11. Left lower quadrant
12. Abdominal midline
13. Navel
14. Pubic and perineal area
15. Right trochanter (hip)
16. Left trochanter (hip)
17. Right anterior thigh
18. Right knee
19. Right lower anterior leg
20. Right ankle (inner/outer)
21. Right foot
22. Right toes
23. Left anterior thigh
24. Left knee
25. Left lower anterior leg
26. Left ankle (inner/outer)
27. Left foot
28. Left toes
29. Right upper interior arm
30. Right interior forearm
31. Right wrist
32. Right palm
33. Right fingers _____ (specify)
34. Left upper interior arm
35. Left interior forearm
36. Left wrist
37. Left palm
38. Left fingers _____ (specify)
39. Back of head
40. Back of neck
41. Left scapula
42. Right scapula
43. Spine
44. Left back
45. Right back
46. Left buttock
47. Right buttock
48. Sacrum
49. Left posterior thigh
50. Left lower posterior leg
51. Left heel
52. Left bottom foot
53. Right posterior thigh
54. Right lower posterior leg
55. Right heel
56. Right bottom foot
57. Left upper posterior arm
58. Left elbow
59. Left posterior forearm
60. Left dorsal hand
61. Right upper posterior arm
62. Right elbow
63. Right posterior forearm
64. Right dorsal hand

OUTCOME CONTENT REFERENCES:

Baranoski, S., LeBlanc, K., & Gloeckner, M. (2016). Preventing, assessing, and managing skin tears: A clinical review. *AJN, American Journal of Nursing, 116*(11), 24–31. https://doi.org/10.1097/01.NAJ.0000505581.01967.75

Flanagan, M. (Ed.). (2013). *Wound healing and skin integrity: Principles and practice.* John Wiley & Sons.

Frantz, R. A., & Gardner, S. (1994). Elderly skin care: Principles of chronic wound care. *Journal of Gerontological Nursing, 20*(9), 35–44.

Hadi, S. A., & Inwood, R. (2016). Current and emerging debridement options in wound care. *Podiatry Today, 29*(12), 44–49.

Lazarus, G. S., Cooper, D. M., Knighton, D. R., Margohs, D. J., Pecoraro, R. E., Rodeheaver, G., & Robson, M. C. (1994). Definitions and guidelines for assessment of wounds and evaluation of healing. *Archives of Dermatology, 130*(4), 489–493.

McCulloch, J. M., & Kloth, L. C. (Eds.). (2010). *Wound healing: Evidence-based management.* F.A. Davis.

Maklebust, J., & Sieggreen, M. (1996). *Pressure ulcers: Guidelines for prevention and nursing management* (2nd ed.). Springhouse.

Potter, P. A., & Perry, A. G. (2001). *Fundamentals of nursing* (5th ed.). Mosby.

+Thomas, D. R., Rodeheaver, G. T., Bartolucci, A. A., Frantz, R. A., Sussman, C., Ferrell, B. A., Cuddigan, J., Stotts, N. A., & Makleburt, J. (1997). Pressure ulcer scale for healing: Derivation and validation of the PUSH tool. *Advances in Wound Care, 10*(5), 96–101.

van Rijswijk, L. (1993). Full-thickness leg ulcers: Patient demographics and predictors of healing. *The Journal of Family Practice, 36*(6), 625–632.

W

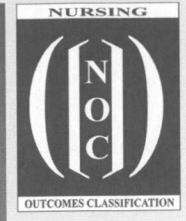

PART FOUR

NOC Performance Outcomes Related to NOC Knowledge Outcomes

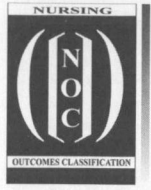

NOC Performance Outcomes Related to NOC Knowledge Outcomes

OVERVIEW

This section highlights the 82 knowledge outcomes in the current edition and links these to outcomes focused on behavior or performance. Nurses and other healthcare providers spend much of their time with patients, focusing on providing information about their health condition or disease. This is a critical step in helping patients to accept their diagnosis and initiate behavior changes in their daily routine. Nurses have always believed that knowledge leads to behavior. Today, patients and their families have access to an incredible amount of information through the internet. It is important that nurses and other healthcare providers guide patients to the best resources to learn about their clinical condition and the challenges they face. Many patients face multiple chronic health conditions that impact the complexity of their treatment regimen.

LINKAGE STRUCTURE

This section provides two tables to describe the linkages between knowledge and behavior outcomes. Table 4.1 contains the knowledge outcomes from the class, Knowledge Health Condition. There are a total of 45 outcomes in this class for this edition. Table 4.2 contains the 37 knowledge outcomes from the class Knowledge Health Promotion. The table has three columns with the knowledge outcomes listed in the left column. The middle column has primary behavioral outcomes that are considered the closest match to the knowledge outcome. The third column lists outcomes that support the primary outcomes and frequently include risk related outcomes. No status outcomes are included in these linkages. We find it useful to update this table each edition to make sure NOC includes behavioral outcomes for each of the knowledge outcomes. The linkages of knowledge and behaviors was first published in the NOC third edition. The tables provide a quick reference for care planning activities and can assist students and nurses learning how to use NOC to measure clinical outcomes regardless of their clinical practice setting or specialty.

Table 4.1	BEHAVIORAL NOCs TO CONSIDER FOR OUTCOMES IN THE KNOWLEDGE HEALTH CONDITION CLASS

CLASS: KNOWLEDGE HEALTH CONDITION

Definition: Outcomes that describe an individual's understanding in applying information to manage a health condition

Knowledge Outcomes	Primary Behavioral Outcomes	Secondary Behavioral Outcomes
Knowledge: Acute Illness Management	Participation in Health Care Decisions Self-Care Behavior Self-Care Behavior: Non-Parenteral Medication Self-Management: Acute Illness Self-Management: Treatment Regimen Sleep Enhancement Behavior	Health Seeking Behavior Nausea & Vomiting Control Personal Health Screening Behavior Risk Control: Infectious Process Symptom Control
Knowledge: Allergy Management	Adherence Behavior Adherence Behavior: Clinical Condition Adherence Behavior: Prescribed Diet Adherence Behavior: Prescribed Medication Self-Management: Known Allergy	Coping Participation in Health Care Decisions Personal Safety Behavior Psychosocial Adjustment: Life Change Risk Control: Environmental Hazards Risk Control: Infant Allergies Risk Control: Vocal Disorder Self-Care Behavior: Non-Parenteral Medication Self-Management: Asthma Symptom Control
Knowledge: Anticoagulation Therapy Management	Adherence Behavior: Clinical Condition Adherence Behavior: Prescribed Medication Risk Control: Thrombus Self-Management: Anticoagulation Therapy	Fall Prevention Behavior Personal Safety Behavior Psychosocial Adjustment: Life Change Risk Control: Stroke Self-Care Behavior: Non-Parenteral Medication Self-Care Behavior: Parenteral Medication Self-Management: Treatment Procedure Self-Management: Stroke Symptom Control
Knowledge: Anxiety Management	Adherence Behavior: Prescribed Medication Anxiety Self-Control Coping Lifestyle Balance Sleep Enhancement Behavior	Hoarding Cessation Behavior Psychosocial Adjustment: Life Change Self-Care Behavior: Non-Parenteral Medication Symptom Control
Knowledge: Arthritis Management	Adaptation to Physical Disability Adherence Behavior: Clinical Condition Adherence Behavior: Prescribed Activity Adherence Behavior: Prescribed Medication Ambulation Pain Control Self-Care Behavior: Activities of Daily Living: (ADL) Self-Management: Arthritis Sleep Enhancement Behavior	Coping Energy Conservation Exercise Participation Fall Prevention Behavior Lifestyle Balance Personal Resilience Psychosocial Adjustment: Life Change Self-Care Behavior: Instrumental Activities of Daily Living (IADL) Self-Care Behavior: Non-Parenteral Medication Symptom Control Weight Maintenance Behavior Weight Loss Behavior

Continued

Table 4.1	**BEHAVIORAL NOCS TO CONSIDER FOR OUTCOMES IN THE KNOWLEDGE HEALTH CONDITION CLASS—cont'd**

CLASS: KNOWLEDGE HEALTH CONDITION

Definition: Outcomes that describe an individual's understanding in applying information to manage a health condition

Knowledge Outcomes	Primary Behavioral Outcomes	Secondary Behavioral Outcomes
Knowledge: Asthma Management	Adherence Behavior: Clinical Condition Adherence Behavior: Prescribed Activity Adherence Behavior: Prescribed Medication Personal Safety Behavior Risk Control: Environmental Hazards Risk Control: Infectious Process Self-Management: Asthma	Coping Energy Conservation Family Participation in Professional Care Psychosocial Adjustment: Life Change Risk Control: Tobacco Use Self-Care Behavior: Non-Parenteral Medication Sleep Enhancement Behavior Smoking Cessation Behavior Symptom Control

Knowledge: Attention Deficit Hyperactivity Disorder (ADHD)	Abuse Protection
	Adherence Behavior: Prescribed Medication
	Family Participation in Professional Care
	Parenting Performance: Attention Deficit
	   Hyperactivity Disorder (ADHD)
		Family Coping
		Family Functioning
		Family Resilience
		Parenting Performance
		Parenting Performance: School Age Child
		   Psychosocial Safety
		Psychosocial Adjustment: Life Change
		Risk Control: Child Bullying
		Symptom Control

Knowledge: Autism Spectrum Disorder	Abuse Protection
	Adherence Behavior: Prescribed Medication
	Family Normalization: Autism Spectrum
	   Disorder
	Self-Management: Autism Spectrum
	   Disorder
	Sleep Enhancement Behavior
		Family Coping
		Family Functioning
		Family Participation in Professional Care
		Family Resilience
		Parenting Performance
		Psychosocial Adjustment: Life Change
		Risk Control: Child Bullying

Knowledge: Cancer Management	Adherence Behavior: Clinical Condition
	Adherence Behavior: Prescribed
	   Medication
	Coping
	Depression Self-Control
	Family Support During Treatment
	Hope
	Nausea & Vomiting Control
	Pain Control
	Participation in Health Care Decisions
	Patient Engagement Behavior
	Psychomotor Energy
	Psychosocial Adjustment: Life Change
	Self-Management: Cancer
	Sleep Enhancement Behavior
		Energy Conservation
		Family Resilience
		Personal Health Screening Behavior
		Personal Resilience
		Risk Control: Cancer
		Risk Control: Infectious Process
		Risk Control: Sun Exposure
		Self-Care Behavior
		Self-Care Behavior: Non-Parenteral
		   Medication
		Self-Care Behavior: Parenteral Medication
		Self-Management: Treatment Procedure
		Self-Management: Treatment Regimen
		Smoking Cessation Behavior
		Symptom Control

Table 4.1	BEHAVIORAL NOCs TO CONSIDER FOR OUTCOMES IN THE KNOWLEDGE HEALTH CONDITION CLASS—cont'd

CLASS: KNOWLEDGE HEALTH CONDITION

Definition: Outcomes that describe an individual's understanding in applying information to manage a health condition

Knowledge Outcomes	Primary Behavioral Outcomes	Secondary Behavioral Outcomes
Knowledge: Cardiac Disease Management	Adherence Behavior Adherence Behavior: Clinical Condition Adherence Behavior: Prescribed Activity Adherence Behavior: Prescribed Diet Adherence Behavior: Prescribed Medication Cardiac Rehabilitation Participation Pain Control Participation in Health Care Decisions Personal Health Screening Behavior Risk Control: Hypertension Risk Control: Lipid Disorder Self-Management: Cardiac Disease Self-Management: Coronary Artery Disease Self-Management: Heart Failure Self-Management: Treatment Regimen	Adaptation to Physical Disability Coping Energy Conservation Family Participation in Professional Care Family Support During Treatment Psychosocial Adjustment: Life Change Self-Care Behavior Self-Care Behavior: Non-Parenteral Medication Self-Care Behavior: Parenteral Medication Self-Management: Hypertension Self-Management: Treatment Procedure Smoking Cessation Behavior Symptom Control Weight Loss Behavior Weight Maintenance Behavior
Knowledge: Cardiac Rehabilitation	Adherence Behavior: Clinical Condition Cardiac Rehabilitation Participation Exercise Participation Fall Prevention Behavior Patient Engagement Behavior Self-Management: Cardiac Disease Self-Management: Coronary Artery Disease Self-Management: Heart Failure Smoking Cessation Behavior	Acceptance: Health Status Adherence Behavior: Prescribed Activity Adherence Behavior: Prescribed Diet Adherence Behavior: Prescribed Medication Coping Family Support During Treatment Motivation Risk Control: Hypertension Risk Control: Lipid Disorder Self-Care Behavior: Non-Parenteral Medication Symptom Control Weight Loss Behavior Weight Maintenance Behavior
Knowledge: Celiac Disease Management	Adherence Behavior: Clinical Condition Adherence Behavior: Prescribed Diet Pain Control Self-Management: Celiac Disease Symptom Control	Acceptance: Health Status Coping Psychosocial Adjustment: Life Change Self-Care Behavior: Non-Parenteral Medication Self-Management: Known Allergy Self-Management: Treatment Regimen Sleep Enhancement Behavior

Continued

Table 4.1	BEHAVIORAL NOCS TO CONSIDER FOR OUTCOMES IN THE KNOWLEDGE HEALTH CONDITION CLASS—cont'd

CLASS: KNOWLEDGE HEALTH CONDITION

Definition: Outcomes that describe an individual's understanding in applying information to manage a health condition

Knowledge Outcomes	Primary Behavioral Outcomes	Secondary Behavioral Outcomes
Knowledge: Chronic Anemia Management	Adherence Behavior: Clinical Condition Adherence Behavior: Prescribed Diet Adherence Behavior: Prescribed Medication Self-Management: Chronic Anemia	Adherence Behavior: Healthy Diet Energy Conservation Fall Prevention Behavior Psychosocial Adjustment: Life Change Self-Care Behavior: Non-Parenteral Medication Self-Management: Cancer Self-Management: Kidney Disease Self-Management: Kidney Failure Symptom Control
Knowledge: Chronic Disease Management	Adherence Behavior Clinical Condition Adherence Behavior: Healthy Diet Adherence Behavior: Prescribed Activity Adherence Behavior: Prescribed Diet Adherence Behavior: Prescribed Medication Exercise Participation Pain Control Psychosocial Adjustment: Life Change Self-Management: Chronic Disease Sleep Enhancement Behavior Symptom Control	Acceptance: Health Status Adaptation to Physical Disability Coping Family Support During Treatment Lifestyle Balance Risk Control: Infectious Process Self-Care Behavior Self-Care Behavior: Non-Parenteral Medication Self-Care Behavior: Parenteral Medication Self-Management: Treatment Procedure Self-Management: Treatment Regimen
Knowledge: Chronic Obstructive Pulmonary Disease Management	Adherence Behavior: Clinical Condition Adherence Behavior: Prescribed Activity Adherence Behavior: Prescribed Medication Energy Conservation Fall Prevention Behavior Pain Control Self-Management: Chronic Obstructive Pulmonary Disease Smoking Cessation Behavior Symptom Control	Acceptance: Health Status Adaptation to Physical Disability Coping Psychomotor Energy Psychosocial Adjustment: Life Change Risk Control: Cardiovascular Disease Risk Control: Infectious Process Risk Control: Tobacco Use Self-Care Behavior Self-Care Behavior: Non-Parenteral Medication Self-Care Behavior: Parenteral Medication Self-Management: Treatment Procedure Self-Management: Treatment Regimen Weight Loss Behavior Weight Maintenance Behavior
Knowledge: Coronary Artery Disease Management	Adherence Behavior: Clinical Condition Adherence Behavior: Prescribed Activity Adherence Behavior: Prescribed Diet Adherence Behavior: Prescribed Medication Cardiac Rehabilitation Participation Fall Prevention Behavior Self-Management: Coronary Artery Disease Smoking Cessation Behavior	Acceptance: Health Status Psychosocial Adjustment: Life Change Risk Control: Alcohol Use Risk Control: Cardiovascular Disease Risk Control: Tobacco Use Symptom Control Weight Loss Behavior Weight Maintenance Behavior

Table 4.1	BEHAVIORAL NOCs TO CONSIDER FOR OUTCOMES IN THE KNOWLEDGE HEALTH CONDITION CLASS—cont'd

CLASS: KNOWLEDGE HEALTH CONDITION

Definition: Outcomes that describe an individual's understanding in applying information to manage a health condition

Knowledge Outcomes	Primary Behavioral Outcomes	Secondary Behavioral Outcomes
Knowledge: Dementia Management	Family Coping Family Normalization: Dementia Family Participation in Professional Care Family Performance: Dementia Care Family Resilience Symptom Control	Caregiver Performance: Direct Care Caregiver Performance: Indirect Care Elopement Propensity Risk Family Risk Control: Elopement Fall Prevention Behavior Safe Wandering Self-Care Behavior
Knowledge: Depression Management	Acceptance: Health Status Adherence Behavior: Clinical Condition Adherence Behavior: Prescribed Medication Depression Self-Control Hope Mood Equilibrium Sleep Enhancement Behavior Psychomotor Energy Suicide Self-Restraint	Coping Family Support During Treatment Hoarding Cessation Behavior Lifestyle Balance Participation in Health Care Decisions Psychosocial Adjustment: Life Change Risk Control: Substance Use Self-Care Behavior Self-Harm Restraint Self-Management: Treatment Regimen Social Interaction Skills Social Involvement Weight Maintenance Behavior
Knowledge: Diabetes Management	Adherence Behavior: Clinical Condition Adherence Behavior: Prescribed Activity Adherence Behavior: Prescribed Diet Adherence Behavior: Prescribed Medication Exercise Participation Psychosocial Adjustment: Life Change Self-Management: Diabetes Self-Management: Treatment Regimen Sleep Enhancement Behavior Symptom Control	Acceptance: Health Status Coping Patient Engagement Behavior Risk Control: Hypertension Risk Control: Infectious Process Risk Control: Lipid Disorder Risk Control: Visual Impairment Self-Care Behavior: Feet Self-Care Behavior: Non-Parenteral Medication Self-Care Behavior: Parenteral Medication Self-Management: Hypertension Self-Management: Lipid Disorder Self-Management: Treatment Procedure Vision Compensation Behavior Weight Loss Behavior Weight Maintenance Behavior
Knowledge: Disease Management	Acceptance: Health Status Adherence Behavior: Clinical Condition Pain Control Self-Care Behavior Self-Management: Acute Illness Self-Management: Chronic Disease Symptom Control	Body Mechanics Performance Coping Energy Conservation Hearing Compensation Behavior Nausea & Vomiting Control Psychosocial Adjustment: Life Change Risk Control: Vocal Disorder Self-Care Behavior: Non-Parenteral Medication Self-Care Behavior: Parenteral Medication Vision Compensation Behavior

Continued

Table 4.1	BEHAVIORAL NOCS TO CONSIDER FOR OUTCOMES IN THE KNOWLEDGE HEALTH CONDITION CLASS—cont'd

CLASS: KNOWLEDGE HEALTH CONDITION

Definition: Outcomes that describe an individual's understanding in applying information to manage a health condition

Knowledge Outcomes	Primary Behavioral Outcomes	Secondary Behavioral Outcomes
Knowledge: Dysrhythmia Management	Adherence Behavior: Clinical Condition Adherence Behavior: Prescribed Activity Adherence Behavior: Prescribed Medication Pain Control Self-Management: Dysrhythmia Symptom Control	Acceptance: Health Status Anxiety Self-Control Coping Energy Conservation Psychosocial Adjustment: Life Change Risk Control: Cardiovascular Disease Risk Control: Stroke Risk Control: Thrombus Self-Care Behavior Self-Care Behavior: Non-Parenteral Medication Self-Care Behavior: Parenteral Medication Self-Management: Treatment Procedure Self-Management: Treatment Regimen
Knowledge: Eating Disorder Management	Adherence Behavior: Clinical Condition Adherence Behavior: Healthy Diet Adherence Behavior: Prescribed Activity Adherence Behavior: Prescribed Diet Coping Eating Disorder Self-Control Impulse Self-Control	Acceptance: Health Status Anxiety Self-Control Depression Self-Control Family Support During Treatment Psychosocial Adjustment: Life Change Risk Control: Cardiovascular Disease Risk Control: Dehydration Self-Care Behavior: Non-Parenteral Medication Weight Gain Behavior Weight Maintenance Behavior
Knowledge: Epilepsy Management	Adaptation to Physical Disability Adherence Behavior: Clinical Condition Adherence Behavior: Prescribed Medication Fall Prevention Behavior Seizure Self-Control	Acceptance: Health Status Coping Family Participation in Professional Care Personal Safety Behavior Psychosocial Adjustment: Life Change Risk Control: Falls Self-Management: Treatment Regimen Symptom Control

Table 4.1	BEHAVIORAL NOCS TO CONSIDER FOR OUTCOMES IN THE KNOWLEDGE HEALTH CONDITION CLASS—cont'd

CLASS: KNOWLEDGE HEALTH CONDITION

Definition: Outcomes that describe an individual's understanding in applying information to manage a health condition

Knowledge Outcomes	Primary Behavioral Outcomes	Secondary Behavioral Outcomes
Knowledge: Heart Failure Management	Adherence Behavior: Clinical Condition Adherence Behavior: Prescribed Activity Adherence Behavior: Prescribed Diet Adherence Behavior: Prescribed Medication Cardiac Rehabilitation Participation Energy Conservation Pain Control Psychomotor Energy Risk Control: Falls Self-Management: Heart Failure Self-Management: Hypertension	Acceptance: Health Status Adaptation to Physical Disability Alcohol Abuse Cessation Behavior Coping Depression Self-Control Family Participation in Professional Care Personal Resilience Psychosocial Adjustment: Life Change Self-Care Behavior Self-Care Behavior: Non-Parenteral Medication Self-Management: Lipid Disorder Self-Management: Treatment Procedure Self-Management: Treatment Regimen Smoking Cessation Behavior Symptom Control Weight Loss Behavior Weight Maintenance Behavior
Knowledge: Human Immunodeficiency Virus Management	Adherence Behavior: Clinical Condition Adherence Behavior: Prescribed Medication Coping Personal Safety Behavior Psychomotor Energy Self-Management: Human Immunodeficiency Virus Self-Care Behavior: Non-Parenteral Medication Self-Care Behavior: Parenteral Medication	Acceptance: Health Status Depression Self-Control Family Support During Treatment Guilt Resolution Psychosocial Adjustment: Life Change Risk Control: Infectious Process Risk Control: Sexually Transmitted Diseases (STD) Self-Management: Infection Self-Management: Treatment Procedure Self-Management: Treatment Regimen Symptom Control
Knowledge: Hypertension Management	Adherence Behavior: Clinical Condition Adherence Behavior: Prescribed Diet Adherence Behavior: Prescribed Medication Self-Management: Hypertension Weight Loss Behavior	Acceptance: Health Status Anxiety Self-Control Coping Exercise Participation Psychosocial Adjustment: Life Change Risk Control: Falls Risk Control: Lipid Disorder Risk Control: Prediabetes Self-Management: Cardiac Disease Self-Management: Treatment Procedure Self-Management: Treatment Regimen Smoking Cessation Behavior Symptom Control Weight Maintenance Behavior

Continued

Table 4.1	**BEHAVIORAL NOCS TO CONSIDER FOR OUTCOMES IN THE KNOWLEDGE HEALTH CONDITION CLASS—cont'd**

CLASS: KNOWLEDGE HEALTH CONDITION

Definition: Outcomes that describe an individual's understanding in applying information to manage a health condition

Knowledge Outcomes	Primary Behavioral Outcomes	Secondary Behavioral Outcomes
Knowledge: Infection Management	Adherence Behavior: Clinical Condition Adherence Behavior: Prescribed Medication Immunization Behavior Risk Control: Infectious Process Risk Control: Sexually Transmitted Diseases (STD) Self-Management: Infection Self-Management: Pneumonia Self-Management: Wound	Community Immune Status Community Risk Control: Communicable Disease Self-Care Behavior Self-Care Behavior: Hygiene Self-Care Behavior: Non-Parenteral Medication Self-Care Behavior: Parenteral Medication Self-Management: Human Immunodeficiency Virus Self-Management: Treatment Procedure
Knowledge: Inflammatory Bowel Disease Management	Adherence Behavior: Clinical Condition Adherence Behavior: Prescribed Activity Adherence Behavior: Prescribed Diet Adherence Behavior: Prescribed Medication Pain Control Self-Management: Inflammatory Bowel Disease Symptom Control	Acceptance: Health Status Coping Energy Conservation Psychosocial Adjustment: Life Change Risk Control: Dehydration Self-Care Behavior: Non-Parenteral Medication Self-Management: Treatment Procedure Self-Management: Treatment Regimen Smoking Cessation Behavior Weight Gain Behavior Weight Maintenance Behavior
Knowledge: Kidney Disease Management	Adherence Behavior: Clinical Condition Adherence Behavior: Prescribed Diet Adherence Behavior: Prescribed Medication Cardiac Rehabilitation Participation Musculoskeletal Rehabilitation Participation Risk Control: Hypertension Self-Management: Kidney Disease	Psychosocial Adjustment: Life Change Risk Control: Cardiovascular Disease Risk Control: Infectious Process Self-Care Behavior: Non-Parenteral Medication Self-Management: Diabetes Self-Management: Hypertension Self-Management: Lipid Disorder Self-Management: Treatment Procedure Self-Management: Treatment Regimen Symptom Control
Knowledge: Kidney Failure Management	Adherence Behavior: Clinical Condition Adherence Behavior: Prescribed Diet Adherence Behavior: Prescribed Medication Psychosocial Adjustment: Life Change Risk Control: Hypertension Self-Management: Kidney Failure Self-Management: Treatment Procedure Self-Management: Treatment Regimen Symptom Control	Acceptance: Health Status Adaptation to Physical Disability Coping Energy Conservation Risk Control: Cardiovascular Disease Risk Control: Hypotension Risk Control: Infectious Process Self-Care Behavior: Non-Parenteral Medication Self-Care Behavior: Parenteral Medication Self-Management: Anemia Self-Management: Diabetes Self-Management: Hypertension Self-Management: Lipid Disorder Self-Management: Treatment Procedure Self-Management: Treatment Regimen

Table 4.1	BEHAVIORAL NOCs TO CONSIDER FOR OUTCOMES IN THE KNOWLEDGE HEALTH CONDITION CLASS—cont'd

CLASS: KNOWLEDGE HEALTH CONDITION

Definition: Outcomes that describe an individual's understanding in applying information to manage a health condition

Knowledge Outcomes	Primary Behavioral Outcomes	Secondary Behavioral Outcomes
Knowledge: Lipid Disorder Management	Adherence Behavior: Clinical Condition Adherence Behavior: Prescribed Diet Adherence Behavior: Prescribed Medication Self-Management: Coronary Artery Disease Self-Management: Lipid Disorder	Acceptance: Health Status Risk Control: Cardiovascular Disease Risk Control: Hypertension Risk Control: Stroke Risk Control: Thrombus Self-Care Behavior: Non-Parenteral Medication Self-Management: Treatment Regimen Smoking Cessation Behavior Symptom Control Weight Loss Behavior Weight Maintenance Behavior
Knowledge: Liver Disease Management	Adherence Behavior: Clinical Condition Adherence Behavior: Prescribed Diet Adherence Behavior: Prescribed Medication Alcohol Abuse Cessation Behavior Self-Management: Liver Disease Symptom Control	Acceptance: Health Status Family Support During Treatment Psychosocial Adjustment: Life Change Risk Control: Alcohol Use Risk Control: Drug Use Self-Care Behavior: Non-Parenteral Medication Self-Care Behavior: Parenteral Medication Self-Management: Treatment Procedure Self-Management: Treatment Regimen
Knowledge: Lymphedema Management	Adaptation to Physical Disability Adherence Behavior: Clinical Condition Adherence Behavior: Prescribed Medication Self-Management: Lymphedema Self-Management: Treatment Procedure Sleep Enhancement Behavior Symptom Control	Adherence Behavior: Prescribed Medication Coping Family Support During Treatment Pain Control Psychosocial Adjustment: Life Change Self-Care Behavior Self-Care Behavior: Non-Parenteral Medication Self-Care Behavior: Parenteral Medication Self-Management: Cancer Self-Management: Treatment Procedure Self-Management: Treatment Regimen
Knowledge: Multiple Sclerosis Management	Adherence Behavior: Clinical Condition Adherence Behavior: Prescribed Diet Adherence Behavior: Prescribed Medication Fall Prevention Behavior Self-Management: Multiple Sclerosis Sleep Enhancement Behavior Symptom Control	Acceptance: Health Status Adherence Behavior: Prescribed Activity Coping Energy Conservation Psychosocial Adjustment: Life Change Risk Control: Falls Self-Care Behavior Self-Care Behavior: Non-Parenteral Medication Self-Care Behavior: Parenteral Medication Self-Management: Treatment Procedure Self-Management: Treatment Regimen

Continued

Table 4.1	BEHAVIORAL NOCs TO CONSIDER FOR OUTCOMES IN THE KNOWLEDGE HEALTH CONDITION CLASS—cont'd

CLASS: KNOWLEDGE HEALTH CONDITION

Definition: Outcomes that describe an individual's understanding in applying information to manage a health condition

Knowledge Outcomes	Primary Behavioral Outcomes	Secondary Behavioral Outcomes
Knowledge: Musculoskeletal Rehabilitation	Adherence Behavior: Clinical Condition Adherence Behavior: Prescribed Activity Body Mechanics Performance Fall Prevention Behavior Musculoskeletal Rehabilitation Participation Risk Control: Falls	Adaptation to Physical Disability Ambulation Exercise Participation Family Support During Treatment Motivation Pain Control Self-Care Behavior Self-Management: Treatment Regimen
Knowledge: Osteoporosis Management	Adherence Behavior: Prescribed Activity Adherence Behavior: Prescribed Diet Adherence Behavior: Prescribed Medication Psychosocial Adjustment: Life Change Self-Management: Osteoporosis	Acceptance: Health Status Adaptation to Physical Disability Ambulation Fall Prevention Behavior Pain Control Self-Care Behavior Self-Care Behavior: Non-Parenteral Medication Self-Management: Treatment Regimen Sleep Enhancement Behavior Smoking Cessation Behavior Symptom Control
Knowledge: Parkinson Disease Management	Adherence Behavior: Clinical Condition Adherence Behavior: Prescribed Activity Adherence Behavior: Prescribed Medication Fall Prevention Behavior Personal Safety Behavior Self-Management: Parkinson Disease	Acceptance: Health Status Adaptation to Physical Disability Exercise Participation Family Support During Treatment Participation in Health Care Decisions Psychosocial Adjustment: Life Change Self-Management: Treatment Regimen Symptom Control
Knowledge: Peripheral Artery Disease Management	Adherence Behavior: Clinical Condition Adherence Behavior: Prescribed Activity Adherence Behavior: Prescribed Diet Adherence Behavior: Prescribed Medication Pain Control Self-Management: Peripheral Artery Disease	Acceptance: Health Status Risk Control: Stroke Risk Control: Thrombus Risk Control: Tobacco Use Self-Care Behavior Self-Care Behavior: Non-Parenteral Medication Self-Management: Treatment Regimen Smoking Cessation Behavior Symptom Control
Knowledge: Pneumonia Management	Adherence Behavior: Clinical Condition Adherence Behavior: Prescribed Medication Pain Control Self-Management: Infection Self-Management: Pneumonia Sleep Enhancement Behavior Symptom Control	Energy Conservation Psychomotor Energy Risk Control: Tobacco Use Self-Care Behavior Self-Care Behavior: Non-Parenteral Medication Self-Management: Treatment Procedure

Table 4.1	BEHAVIORAL NOCs TO CONSIDER FOR OUTCOMES IN THE KNOWLEDGE HEALTH CONDITION CLASS—cont'd

CLASS: KNOWLEDGE HEALTH CONDITION

Definition: Outcomes that describe an individual's understanding in applying information to manage a health condition

Knowledge Outcomes	Primary Behavioral Outcomes	Secondary Behavioral Outcomes
Knowledge: Prescribed Activity	Adherence Behavior: Prescribed Activity Ambulation Exercise Participation Fall Prevention Behavior	Adaptation to Physical Disability Ambulation: Wheelchair Body Mechanics Performance Energy Conservation Personal Safety Behavior Risk Control: Falls Self-Management: Treatment Regimen
Knowledge: Prescribed Diet	Adherence Behavior: Prescribed Diet Weight Gain Behavior Weight Loss Behavior Weight Maintenance Behavior	Self-Care Behavior: Eating Prenatal Health Behavior
Knowledge: Stroke Management	Adaptation to Physical Disability Adherence Behavior: Clinical Condition Adherence Behavior: Prescribed Activity Adherence Behavior: Prescribed Diet Adherence Behavior: Prescribed Medication Fall Prevention Behavior Heedfulness of Affected Side Musculoskeletal Rehabilitation Participation Self-Management: Anticoagulation Therapy Self-Management: Stroke Symptom Control	Acceptance: Health Status Ambulation Exercise Participation Psychosocial Adjustment: Life Change Risk Control: Falls Risk Control: Stroke Risk Control: Thrombus Risk Control: Tobacco Use Risk Control: Vocal Disorder Self-Care Behavior Self-Care Behavior: Non-Parenteral Medication Self-Management: Treatment Procedure Self-Management: Treatment Regimen Sleep Enhancement Behavior
Knowledge: Treatment Procedure	Caregiver Performance: Direct Care Self-Direction of Care Self-Management: Treatment Procedure	Family Support During Treatment Motivation Risk Control: Infectious Process Self-Management: Ostomy Self-Management: Wound

Continued

Table 4.1	BEHAVIORAL NOCS TO CONSIDER FOR OUTCOMES IN THE KNOWLEDGE HEALTH CONDITION CLASS—cont'd

CLASS: KNOWLEDGE HEALTH CONDITION

Definition: Outcomes that describe an individual's understanding in applying information to manage a health condition

Knowledge Outcomes	Primary Behavioral Outcomes	Secondary Behavioral Outcomes
Knowledge: Treatment Regimen	Adherence Behavior Adherence Behavior: Clinical Condition Adherence Behavior: Prescribed Activity Adherence Behavior: Prescribed Diet Adherence Behavior: Prescribed Medication Caregiver Performance: Direct Care Pain Control Self-Care Behavior: Non-Parenteral Medication Self-Care Behavior: Parenteral Medication Self-Direction of Care Self-Management: Acute Illness Self-Management: Chronic Disease Self-Management: Treatment Regimen Symptom Control	Adaptation to Physical Disability Psychosocial Adjustment: Life Change Self-Management: Anticoagulation Therapy Self-Management: Arthritis Self-Management: Asthma Self-Management: Autism Spectrum Disorder Self-Management: Cancer Self-Management: Cardiac Disease Self-Management: Celiac Disease Self-Management: Chronic Anemia Self-Management: Chronic Obstructive Pulmonary Disease Self-Management: Coronary Artery Disease Self-Management: Diabetes Self-Management: Dysrhythmia Self-Management: Heart Failure Self-Management: Human Immunodeficiency Virus Self-Management: Hypertension Self-Management: Infection Self-Management: Inflammatory Bowel Disease Self-Management: Kidney Disease Self-Management: Kidney Failure Self-Management: Known Allergy Self-Management: Lipid Disorder Self-Management: Liver Disease Self-Management: Lymphedema Self-Management: Multiple Sclerosis Self-Management: Osteoporosis Self-Management: Ostomy Self-Management: Parkinson Disease Self-Management: Peripheral Artery Disease Self-Management: Pneumonia Self-Management: Stroke Self-Management: Wound
Knowledge: Wound Management	Self-Management: Treatment Procedure Self-Management: Wound	Pain Control Risk Control: Infectious Process Self-Management: Infection Self-Management: Treatment Regimen

Table 4.2	BEHAVIORAL NOCs TO CONSIDER FOR OUTCOMES IN THE KNOWLEDGE HEALTH PROMOTION CLASS

Class: Knowledge Health Promotion

Definition: Outcomes that describe an individual's understanding in applying information to optimize health

Knowledge Outcomes	Primary Behavioral Outcomes	Secondary Behavioral Outcomes
Knowledge: Body Mechanics	Body Mechanics Performance Fall Prevention Behavior Personal Safety Behavior	Ambulation Ambulation: Wheelchair Risk Control: Falls Transfer Performance
Knowledge: Bottle Feeding	Bottle Feeding Performance	Parenting Performance: Infant Risk Control: Aspiration Risk Control: Dehydration
Knowledge: Breastfeeding	Breastfeeding Establishment: Maternal Breastfeeding Maintenance Breastfeeding Weaning	Breastfeeding Establishment: Infant Pain Control Parent-Infant Attachment Risk Control: Dehydration
Knowledge: Cancer Threat Reduction	Personal Health Screening Behavior Risk Control: Cancer Risk Control: Tobacco Use	Risk Control: Environmental Hazards Risk Control: Sun Exposure Smoking Cessation Behavior
Knowledge: Child Physical Safety	Parenting Performance Parenting Performance: Adolescent Physical Safety Parenting Performance: Early Childhood Physical Safety Parenting Performance: Infant Physical Safety Parenting Performance: Toddler Physical Safety	Abuse Protection Alcohol Abuse Cessation Behavior Drug Abuse Cessation Behavior Family Risk Control: Violence Risk Control: Child Bullying Risk Control: Environmental Hazards Risk Control: Problematic Internet Use Smoking Cessation Behavior
Knowledge: Community Health Resources	Caregiver Performance: Indirect Care Financial Literacy Behavior Health Insurance Literacy Behavior	Digital Literacy Behavior
Knowledge: Conception Prevention	Risk Control: Unintended Pregnancy	Risk Control: Sexually Transmitted Diseases (STD)
Knowledge: Cup Feeding	Cup Feeding Performance	Parent-Infant Attachment Parenting Performance: Infant Risk Control: Aspiration Risk Control: Dehydration
Knowledge: Diagnostic & Therapeutic Procedures	Personal Health Screening Behavior Self-Management: Treatment Procedure	Participation in Health Care Decisions Personal Engagement Behavior Risk Control: Cancer Risk Control: Osteoporosis
Knowledge: Energy Conservation	Energy Conservation	Ambulation Body Mechanics Performance Risk Control: Falls Self-Care Behavior
Knowledge: Fall Prevention	Adherence Behavior: Prescribed Activity Fall Prevention Behavior Transfer Performance	Ambulation Ambulation: Wheelchair Heedfulness of Affected Side Hoarding Cessation Behavior Risk Control: Falls Safe Wandering Seizure Self-Control Self-Care Behavior Self-Care Behavior: Feet

Continued

Table 4.2	BEHAVIORAL NOCs TO CONSIDER FOR OUTCOMES IN THE KNOWLEDGE HEALTH PROMOTION CLASS—cont'd

Class: Knowledge Health Promotion

Definition: Outcomes that describe an individual's understanding in applying information to optimize health

Knowledge Outcomes	Primary Behavioral Outcomes	Secondary Behavioral Outcomes
Knowledge: Fertility Promotion	Prenatal Health Behavior Sexual Functioning	Coping Family Participation in Professional Care Risk Control: Sexually Transmitted Diseases (STD) Self-Care Behavior: Non-Parenteral Medication
Knowledge: Foot Care	Self-Care Behavior: Feet	Risk Control: Infectious Process Self-Care Behavior: Bathing Self-Care Behavior: Hygiene
Knowledge: Health Behavior	Adherence Behavior: Clinical Condition Pain Control Personal Safety Behavior Prenatal Health Behavior Risk Control: Alcohol Use Risk Control: Aspiration Risk Control: Cancer Risk Control: Cardiovascular Disease Risk Control: Child Bullying Risk Control: Dehydration Risk Control: Drug Use Risk Control: Dry Eye Risk Control: Environmental Hazards Risk Control: Falls Risk Control: Food Insecurity Risk Control: Hearing Impairment Risk Control: Housing Insecurity Risk Control: Hypertension Risk Control: Hyperthermia Risk Control: Hypotension Risk Control: Hypothermia Risk Control: Infant Allergies Risk Control: Infectious Process Risk Control: Lipid Disorder Risk Control: Obesity Risk Control: Osteoporosis Risk Control: Prediabetes Risk Control: Pressure Injury Risk Control: Problematic Internet Use Risk Control: Sexually Transmitted Diseases (STD) Risk Control: Stroke Risk Control: Sun Exposure Risk Control: Thrombus Risk Control: Tobacco Use Risk Control: Unintended Pregnancy Risk Control: Visual Impairment Risk Control: Vocal Disorder Risk Detection	Adaptation to Physical Disability Adherence Behavior Adherence Behavior: Healthy Diet Adherence Behavior: Prescribed Activity Adherence Behavior: Prescribed Diet Adherence Behavior: Prescribed Medication Alcohol Abuse Cessation Behavior Anxiety Self-Control Body Mechanics Performance Community Health Screening Effectiveness Community Program Effectiveness Community Risk Control: Bullying Community Risk Control: Chronic Disease Community Risk Control: Communicable Disease Community Risk Control: Environmental Hazards Community Risk Control: Lead Exposure Community Risk Control: Obesity Community Risk Control: Suicide Community Risk Control: Unhealthy Cultural Traditions Community Risk Control: Violence Coping Drug Abuse Cessation Behavior Energy Conservation Fall Prevention Behavior Family Risk Control: Bullying Family Risk Control: Obesity Family Risk Control: Violence Immunization Behavior Impulse Self-Control Leisure Participation Sleep Enhancement Behavior Smoking Cessation Behavior Weight Gain Behavior Weight Loss Behavior Weight Maintenance Behavior

Table 4.2	BEHAVIORAL NOCs TO CONSIDER FOR OUTCOMES IN THE KNOWLEDGE HEALTH PROMOTION CLASS—cont'd

Class: Knowledge Health Promotion

Definition: Outcomes that describe an individual's understanding in applying information to optimize health

Knowledge Outcomes	Primary Behavioral Outcomes	Secondary Behavioral Outcomes
Knowledge: Health Resources	Caregiver Performance: Indirect Care Digital Literacy Behavior Health Insurance Literacy Behavior Health Literacy Behavior	Family Participation in Professional Care Self-Direction of Care
Knowledge: Healthy Diet	Adherence Behavior: Healthy Diet	Health Promoting Behavior Health Seeking Behavior Motivation Risk Control: Dehydration Self-Care Behavior: Eating
Knowledge: Healthy Lifestyle	Adherence Behavior: Healthy Diet Exercise Participation Leisure Participation Lifestyle Balance Personal Safety Behavior Personal Time Management Risk Detection Sleep Enhancement Behavior Social Interaction Skills	Alcohol Abuse Cessation Behavior Coping Drug Abuse Cessation Behavior Eating Disorder Self-Control Motivation Personal Resilience Risk Control: Alcohol Use Risk Control: Drug Use Risk Control: Sun Exposure Risk Control: Tobacco Use Risk Control: Vocal Disorder Smoking Cessation Behavior Social Involvement Successful Aging Weight Loss Behavior Weight Maintenance Behavior
Knowledge: Infant Care	Abuse Prevention Parent-Infant Attachment Parenting Performance: Infant Parenting Performance: Infant Physical Safety Parenting Performance: Infant Psychosocial Safety	Abusive Behavior Self-Restraint Bottle Feeding Performance Cup Feeding Performance Family Functioning Immunization Behavior Parenting Performance Play Participation Risk Control: Dehydration Risk Control: Infant Allergies
Knowledge: Labor & Delivery	Family Participation in Professional Care Postpartum Maternal Health Behavior Symptom Control	Coping Energy Conservation Pain Control Risk Control: Hypertension Self-Direction of Care
Knowledge: Medication	Adherence Behavior: Prescribed Medication Caregiver Performance: Direct Care Self-Care Behavior: Non-Parenteral Medication Self-Care Behavior: Parenteral Medication	Personal Safety Behavior Self-Direction of Care Self-Management: Known Allergy

Continued

Table 4.2	BEHAVIORAL NOCS TO CONSIDER FOR OUTCOMES IN THE KNOWLEDGE HEALTH PROMOTION CLASS—cont'd

Class: Knowledge Health Promotion

Definition: Outcomes that describe an individual's understanding in applying information to optimize health

Knowledge Outcomes	Primary Behavioral Outcomes	Secondary Behavioral Outcomes
Knowledge: Ostomy Care	Psychosocial Adjustment: Life Change Risk Control: Dehydration Self-Management: Ostomy Symptom Control	Adherence Behavior: Healthy Diet Self-Care Behavior: Hygiene Self-Care Behavior: Non-Parenteral Medication Self-Management: Treatment Procedure
Knowledge: Pain Management	Adherence Behavior: Prescribed Medication Nausea & Vomiting Control Pain Control Sleep Enhancement Behavior Symptom Control	Coping Energy Conservation Personal Resilience Self-Care Behavior: Non-Parenteral Medication Self-Care Behavior: Parenteral Medication Self-Management: Treatment Procedure
Knowledge: Parenting	Abuse Protection Family Functioning Family Participation in Professional Care Immunization Behavior Parent-Infant Attachment Parenting Performance Parenting Performance: Adolescent Parenting Performance: Adolescent Physical Safety Parenting Performance: Early/Middle Childhood Physical Safety Parenting Performance: Infant Parenting Performance: Infant Physical Safety Parenting Performance: Middle Childhood Parenting Performance: Preschooler Parenting Performance: School Age Child Psychosocial Safety Parenting Performance: Toddler Physical Safety Play Participation	Bottle Feeding Performance Child Adaptation to Hospitalization Child Development: 1 Month Child Development: 2 Months Child Development: 4 Months Child Development: 6 Months Child Development: 9 Months Child Development: 12 Months Child Development: 18 Months Child Development: 2 Years Child Development: 3 Years Child Development: 4 Years Child Development: 5 Years Child Development: 6–7 Years Child Development: 8–10 Years Child Development: Early Adolescence Child Development: Late Adolescence Child Development: Middle Adolescence Cup Feeding Performance Family Coping Family Integrity Family Normalization: Autism Spectrum Disorder Family Resilience Family Risk Control: Bullying Family Risk Control: Household Food Insecurity Family Risk Control: Obesity Family Risk Control: Violence Family Social Climate Family Social Network Support Risk Control: Child Bullying Risk Control: Food Insecurity Risk Control: Housing Insecurity Risk Control: Infant Allergies Risk Control: Problematic Internet Use Risk Control: Vocal Disorder

Table 4.2	BEHAVIORAL NOCs TO CONSIDER FOR OUTCOMES IN THE KNOWLEDGE HEALTH PROMOTION CLASS—cont'd	
Class: Knowledge Health Promotion		
Definition: Outcomes that describe an individual's understanding in applying information to optimize health		
Knowledge Outcomes	**Primary Behavioral Outcomes**	**Secondary Behavioral Outcomes**
Knowledge: Personal Safety	Adherence Behavior: Prescribed Medication Fall Prevention Behavior Hearing Compensation Behavior Immunization Behavior Personal Safety Behavior Risk Detection Vision Compensation Behavior	Body Mechanics Performance Community Risk Control: Environmental Hazards Community Risk Control: Lead Exposure Impulse Self-Control Risk Control: Alcohol Use Risk Control: Aspiration Risk Control: Child Bullying Risk Control: Dehydration Risk Control: Drug Use Risk Control: Environmental Hazards Risk Control: Falls Risk Control: Food Insecurity Risk Control: Hearing Impairment Risk Control: Housing Insecurity Risk Control: Hyperthermia Risk Control: Hypothermia Risk Control: Pressure Injury Risk Control: Problematic Internet Use Risk Control: Sexually Transmitted Diseases (STD) Risk Control: Sun Exposure Risk Control: Tobacco Use Risk Control: Visual Impairment Risk Control: Vocal Disorder Safe Wandering Self-Management: Known Allergy
Knowledge: Postpartum Maternal Health	Breastfeeding Establishment: Maternal Pain Control Parent-Infant Attachment Postpartum Maternal Health Behavior Psychosocial Adjustment: Life Change Sleep Enhancement Behavior	Coping Depression Self-Control Energy Conservation Exercise Participation Family Participation in Professional Care Psychomotor Energy Personal Resilience Risk Control: Unintended Pregnancy Self-Care Behavior: Non-Parenteral Medication Self-Management: Wound

Continued

Table 4.2	**BEHAVIORAL NOCs TO CONSIDER FOR OUTCOMES IN THE KNOWLEDGE HEALTH PROMOTION CLASS—cont'd**	
Class: Knowledge Health Promotion		
Definition: Outcomes that describe an individual's understanding in applying information to optimize health		
Knowledge Outcomes	**Primary Behavioral Outcomes**	**Secondary Behavioral Outcomes**
Knowledge: Preconception Maternal Health	Adherence Behavior: Healthy Diet Immunization Behavior Prenatal Health Behavior Sexual Functioning	Adherence Behavior: Clinical Condition Alcohol Abuse Cessation Behavior Drug Abuse Cessation Behavior Personal Safety Behavior Risk Control: Alcohol Use Risk Control: Drug Use Risk Control: Environmental Hazards Risk Control: Sexually Transmitted Diseases (STD) Risk Control: Tobacco Use Risk Detection Smoking Cessation Behavior Weight Loss Behavior Weight Maintenance Behavior
Knowledge: Pregnancy	Adherence Behavior: Healthy Diet Alcohol Abuse Cessation Behavior Drug Abuse Cessation Behavior Nausea & Vomiting Control Prenatal Health Behavior Risk Control: Dehydration Smoking Cessation Behavior	Abuse Protection Adherence Behavior: Prescribed Diet Body Mechanics Performance Energy Conservation Exercise Participation Family Support During Treatment Personal Resilience Personal Safety Behavior Risk Control: Alcohol Use Risk Control: Drug Use Risk Control: Environmental Hazards Risk Control: Sexually Transmitted Diseases (STD) Risk Control: Tobacco Use Self-Care Behavior: Non-Parenteral Medication Sleep Enhancement Behavior Weight Maintenance Behavior
Knowledge: Pregnancy & Postpartum Sexual Function	Adherence Behavior: Healthy Diet Postpartum Maternal Health Behavior Risk Control: Unintended Pregnancy	Abuse Protection Coping Psychosocial Adjustment: Life Change Risk Control: Sexually Transmitted Diseases (STD) Sexual Functioning Symptom Severity
Knowledge: Preterm Infant Care	Child Development: 1 Month Coping Family Participation in Professional Care Parent Adaptation to Infant Hospitalization Parent-Infant Attachment Parenting Performance: Infant	Caregiver Home Care Readiness Caregiver Performance: Direct Care Caregiver Performance: Indirect Care Family Resilience Psychosocial Adjustment: Life Change

Table 4.2	BEHAVIORAL NOCS TO CONSIDER FOR OUTCOMES IN THE KNOWLEDGE HEALTH PROMOTION CLASS—cont'd	

Class: Knowledge Health Promotion

Definition: Outcomes that describe an individual's understanding in applying information to optimize health

Knowledge Outcomes	Primary Behavioral Outcomes	Secondary Behavioral Outcomes
Knowledge: School Age Child Psychosocial Safety	Abuse Protection Parenting Performance: Middle Childhood Parenting Performance: School Age Child Psychosocial Safety Play Participation	Family Risk Control: Violence Risk Control: Child Bullying Risk Control: Problematic Internet Use
Knowledge: Sexual Function	Sexual Functioning	Risk Control: Sexually Transmitted Diseases (STD) Risk Control: Unintended Pregnancy Symptom Control
Knowledge: Stress Management	Acceptance: Health Status Adherence Behavior: Clinical Condition Coping Lifestyle Balance Psychosocial Adjustment: Life Change	Adherence Behavior: Healthy Diet Exercise Participation Leisure Participation Personal Resilience Personal Time Management Self-Direction of Care Social Involvement
Knowledge: Stroke Threat Reduction	Adherence Behavior: Prescribed Diet Adherence Behavior: Prescribed Medication Risk Control: Hypertension Risk Control: Stroke Self-Management: Anticoagulation Therapy Self-Management: Coronary Artery Disease Smoking Cessation Behavior	Exercise Participation Risk Control: Alcohol Use Risk Control: Dehydration Risk Control: Hypertension Risk Control: Thrombus Risk Control: Tobacco Use Self-Management: Cardiac Disease Self-Management: Diabetes Self-Management: Hypertension Self-Management: Lipid Disorder
Knowledge: Substance Use Control	Alcohol Abuse Cessation Behavior Drug Abuse Cessation Behavior Smoking Cessation Behavior	Adherence Behavior: Healthy Diet Coping Family Coping Impulse Self-Control Personal Safety Behavior Risk Control: Alcohol Use Risk Control: Drug Use Risk Control: Tobacco Use Risk Control: Vocal Disorder Symptom Control
Knowledge: Thrombus Threat Reduction	Adherence Behavior: Clinical Condition Adherence Behavior: Prescribed Activity Adherence Behavior: Prescribed Diet Adherence Behavior: Prescribed Medication Self-Management: Anticoagulation Therapy	Ambulation Exercise Participation Risk Control: Dehydration Risk Control: Stroke Risk Control: Thrombus Self-Care Behavior: Non-Parenteral Medication

Continued

Table 4.2	BEHAVIORAL NOCs TO CONSIDER FOR OUTCOMES IN THE KNOWLEDGE HEALTH PROMOTION CLASS—cont'd

Class: Knowledge Health Promotion

Definition: Outcomes that describe an individual's understanding in applying information to optimize health

Knowledge Outcomes	Primary Behavioral Outcomes	Secondary Behavioral Outcomes
Knowledge: Time Management	Lifestyle Balance Personal Time Management Self-Direction of Care	Coping Leisure Participation Self-Direction of Instrumental Activities of Daily Living Sleep Enhancement Behavior
Knowledge: Weight Management	Adherence Behavior: Healthy Diet Adherence Behavior: Prescribed Activity Adherence Behavior: Prescribed Diet Exercise Participation Weight Gain Behavior Weight Loss Behavior Weight Maintenance Behavior	Adherence Behavior: Prescribed Medication Community Risk Control: Obesity Family Risk Control: Obesity Physical Fitness Risk Control: Obesity

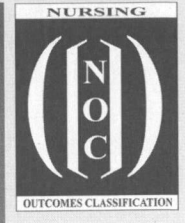

PART FIVE

Core Outcomes for Nursing Specialties

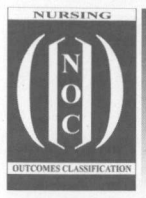

Core Outcomes for Nursing Specialties

This section provides an alphabetical list of core outcomes for 51 clinical nursing specialties used across a variety of care delivery settings. We have defined core outcomes as a set of outcomes that capture the essence of a specialty practice area. The outcomes reflect the content expertise of nurses practicing in the specialty and the needs of patients they treat. Specialties in nursing focus on specific populations of patients whom nurses care for on a day-to-day basis. The outcomes may also be used by other health care disciplines practicing in interdisciplinary teams. The specialty area outcome lists are not comprehensive of all outcomes used in the specialty but attempt to identify the key outcomes needed for practice. Specialty units in acute care organizations can use the core list of outcomes to identify outcomes for care planning activities and documentation of the nursing process in an electronic health record. In long-term care settings, the outcomes focused on gerontology and rehabilitation provide measurement options for care provided over an extended period of care. In today's health care environment, many of the treatments and surgeries previously provided in acute care hospitals are being done in surgical centers as outpatients. The nursing specialty content in this section can also be used to address short-term outcomes in these settings. The community nursing specialty provides outcomes used by nurses working in the public health arena and capture the health status at the community level. In addition, core outcomes can also be used to plan curriculum for nursing students and guide preparation of experienced nurses preparing for competency evaluations or seeking certification. NOC outcomes provide a means to measure the effectiveness of clinical practice and are one of the elements that direct the selection of interventions nurses use in the specialty.

EFFORTS TO IDENTIFY CORE OUTCOMES

Initial work to identify specialty core outcomes began after the second edition of NOC was published. Information to identify core outcomes was collected from surveys sent to 33 nursing specialty organizations and individual nurses. Only second edition NOC outcomes were used in the survey, and the survey methodology and results were summarized in the third edition of NOC. Since the survey work was completed, 76 new outcomes were added to the third edition, 58 new outcomes to the fourth edition, 107 new outcomes to the fifth edition, 52 new outcomes to the sixth edition, and 82 new outcomes to the current edition. This means that over 370 new outcomes have been published since the original survey work. A more detailed description of the development efforts

over the seven editions can be found in the overview of the taxonomy in Part 2. With each new publication of NOC core outcomes have been added to the specialty lists to reflect current practice. As we added outcomes to the lists, we used the higher conceptual level outcomes and did not list the more specific outcomes unless they were viewed as foundational to the specialty. For example, *Nutritional Status* was included rather than *Nutritional Status: Energy*. For this edition, we added five new specialty areas: Addiction, Burn Care, Chemical Dependency, Domestic Violence, Family Centered Care, and Men's Health and separated Women's Health and Obstetrics and Gynecology into two separate lists of outcomes.

CORE OUTCOMES THAT CROSS ALL SPECIALTIES

Some outcomes are not included in the core specialty outcome lists because they are viewed as a standard for all nursing practice specialties. This includes most of the client satisfaction outcomes, the discharge readiness outcomes, and *Safe Health Care Environment* and *Patient Engagement*

Box 5.1

Standards of Nursing Practice Across Specialties

Client Satisfaction
Client Satisfaction: Access to Care Resources
Client Satisfaction: Acute Care Transition Process
Client Satisfaction: Caring
Client Satisfaction: Case Management
Client Satisfaction: Communication
Client Satisfaction: Continuity of Care
Client Satisfaction: Cultural Needs Fulfillment
Client Satisfaction: Discharge Process
Client Satisfaction: Functional Assistance
Client Satisfaction: Pain Management
Client Satisfaction: Physical Care
Client Satisfaction: Physical Environment
Client Satisfaction: Protection of Rights
Client Satisfaction: Psychological Care
Client Satisfaction: Safety
Client Satisfaction: Symptom Control
Client Satisfaction: Teaching
Client Satisfaction: Technical Aspects of Care
Client Satisfaction: Telehealth Services
Discharge Readiness: Independent Living
Discharge Readiness: Supported Living
Patient Engagement Behavior
Safe Health Care Environment

Behavior. The 24 outcomes not included in the core specialties are found in Box 5.1.

NEXT STEPS

Further refinement of the core outcomes beyond expert opinion is an important next step. When actual data about specialty practice becomes more widely available, these core outcomes should be validated using clinical data. It is important to debate and analyze the following questions: What is a reasonable number of core outcomes for each specialty to address? How does the scope of a specialty impact the core? What methods can be used to maintain and refine current core outcomes for specialty practice? How can nursing specialty organizations be involved in the evolution and continued development of NOC outcomes for specialty practice? What impact do nurse practitioners have on the identification of core outcomes? Research to facilitate continued improvement in measuring the effectiveness of specialty practice using standardized terminologies and identifying new outcomes for development and inclusion in the taxonomy is essential.

Addiction

Abuse Cessation
Abuse: Disruptive Effects
Abuse Protection
Abuse Recovery
Abuse Recovery: Emotional
Abuse Recovery: Financial
Abuse Recovery: Physical
Abuse Recovery: Sexual
Adherence Behavior: Clinical Condition
Adherence Behavior: Prescribed Medication
Agitation Level
Alcohol Abuse Cessation Behavior
Anxiety Level
Anxiety Self-Control
Caregiver-Patient Relationship
Childhood Bullying Recovery
Comfort Status
Coping
Depression Level
Depression Self-Control
Distorted Thought Self-Control
Drug Abuse Cessation Behavior
Family Coping
Family Integrity
Family Normalization
Family Participation in Professional Care
Family Social Climate
Family Social Network Support
Family Support During Treatment
Financial Literacy Behavior
Group Therapy Participation
Health Beliefs: Perceived Control
Health Beliefs: Perceived Threat
Health Insurance Literacy Behavior
Health Literacy Behavior
Health Orientation
Health Seeking Behavior
Hoarding Behavior Severity
Hoarding Cessation Behavior
Impulse Self-Control
Infection Severity
Knowledge: Anxiety Management
Knowledge: Community Health Resources
Knowledge: Depression Management
Knowledge: Disease Management
Knowledge: Health Resources
Knowledge: Human Immunodeficiency Virus Management
Knowledge: Liver Disease Management

Knowledge: Medication
Knowledge: Pain Management
Knowledge: Personal Safety
Knowledge: Stress Management
Knowledge: Substance Use Control
Knowledge: Treatment Regimen
Liver Function
Medication Response
Metabolic Function
Neglect Cessation
Nutritional Status
Pain Control
Pain: Disruptive Effects
Pain Level
Panic Level
Panic Self-Control
Personal Autonomy
Personal Health Status
Personal Resilience
Personal Safety Behavior
Psychomotor Energy
Quality of Life
Risk Control: Alcohol Use
Risk Control: Drug Use
Risk Control: Food Insecurity
Risk Control: Housing Insecurity
Risk Control: Sexually Transmitted Diseases (STD)
Risk Control: Tobacco Use
Risk Control: Unintended Pregnancy
Role Performance
Seizure Self-Control
Seizure Severity
Self-Care: Non-Parenteral Medication Behavior
Self-Harm Restraint
Self-Management: Human Immunodeficiency Virus
Self-Management: Infection
Self-Management: Liver Disease
Self-Management: Treatment Regimen
Smoking Cessation Behavior
Spiritual Health
Stress Level
Substance Addiction Consequences
Substance Withdrawal Severity
Suffering Severity
Suicide Self-Restraint
Symptom Severity
Vital Signs

Air & Surface Transport

Abuse: Disruptive Effects
Acute Respiratory Acidosis Severity
Acute Respiratory Alkalosis Severity
Agitation Level
Allergic Response: Systemic
Blood Coagulation
Blood Glucose Control
Blood Loss Severity
Blood Product Transfusion Reaction
Burn Recovery
Cardiopulmonary Function
Circulation Status
Cognition
Cognitive Orientation
Communication
Community Disaster Readiness
Community Disaster Response
Dehydration Severity
Delirium Level
Discomfort Level
Electrolyte & Acid/Base Balance
Electrolyte Balance
Fatigue: Disruptive Effects
Fluid Balance
Fluid Overload Severity
Gastrointestinal Function
Hope
Hydration
Hypercalcemia Severity
Hyperchloremia Severity
Hyperglycemia Severity
Hyperkalemia Severity
Hypermagnesemia Severity
Hypernatremia Severity
Hyperphosphatemia Severity
Hypertension Severity
Hypoglycemia Severity
Hypokalemia Severity
Hypomagnesemia Severity
Hyponatremia Severity
Hypophosphatemia Severity
Hypotension Severity
Immune Hypersensitivity Response
Infection Severity
Infection Severity: Newborn
Joint Movement
Kidney Function
Knowledge: Allergy Management
Knowledge: Anticoagulation Management
Knowledge: Anxiety Management
Knowledge: Asthma Management
Knowledge: Cardiac Disease Management
Knowledge: Chronic Obstructive Pulmonary Disease
   Management
Knowledge: Diabetes Management
Knowledge: Dysrhythmia Management
Knowledge: Epilepsy Management
Knowledge: Heart Failure Management
Knowledge: Hypertension Management

Knowledge: Infection Management
Knowledge: Kidney Disease Management
Knowledge: Kidney Failure Management
Knowledge: Labor & Delivery
Knowledge: Medication
Knowledge: Pain Management
Knowledge: Pneumonia Management
Knowledge: Stroke Management
Knowledge: Wound Management
Liver Function
Maternal Status: Intrapartum
Mechanical Ventilation Response: Adult
Medication Response
Metabolic Acidosis Severity
Metabolic Alkalosis Severity
Metabolic Function
Nausea & Vomiting Severity
Neurological Function
Neurological Function: Central Motor Control
Neurological Function: Consciousness
Neurological Function: Cranial Sensory/Motor
Neurological Function: Peripheral
Neurological Function: Spinal Sensory/Motor
Newborn Adaptation
Pain: Adverse Psychological Response
Pain: Disruptive Effects
Pain Level
Panic Level
Physical Injury Severity
Respiratory Function
Respiratory Function: Airway Patency
Respiratory Function: Gas Exchange
Respiratory Function: Ventilation
Risk Control: Aspiration
Risk Control: Environmental Hazards
Risk Control: Vocal Disorder
Seizure Severity
Sensory Function
Shock Severity: Anaphylactic
Shock Severity: Cardiogenic
Shock Severity: Hypovolemic
Shock Severity: Neurogenic
Shock Severity: Septic
Stress Level
Substance Withdrawal Severity
Swallowing Status
Symptom Severity
Thermoregulation
Thermoregulation: Newborn
Tissue Integrity: Skin & Mucous Membranes
Tissue Perfusion
Tissue Perfusion: Abdominal Organs
Tissue Perfusion: Cardiac
Tissue Perfusion: Cellular
Tissue Perfusion: Cerebral
Tissue Perfusion: Peripheral
Tissue Perfusion: Pulmonary
Vital Signs
Will to Live

Ambulatory Care

Abuse Recovery
Acceptance: Health Status
Adaptation to Physical Disability
Adherence Behavior
Adherence Behavior: Healthy Diet
Adherence Behavior: Prescribed Activity
Adherence Behavior: Prescribed Diet
Adherence Behavior: Prescribed Medication
Alcohol Abuse Cessation Behavior
Blood Glucose Control
Cardiac Rehabilitation Participation
Chemotherapy: Disruptive Physical Effects
Digital Literacy Behavior
Drug Abuse Cessation Behavior
Exercise Participation
Family Coping
Fatigue: Disruptive Effects
Fatigue Level
Financial Literacy Behavior
Health Beliefs: Perceived Ability to Perform
Health Beliefs: Perceived Control
Health Beliefs: Perceived Resources
Health Beliefs: Perceived Threat
Health Literacy Behavior
Health Orientation
Health Promoting Behavior
Health Seeking Behavior
Hyperglycemia Severity
Hypertension Severity
Hypoglycemia Severity
Infection Severity
Infection Severity: Newborn
Knowledge: Acute Illness Management
Knowledge: Allergy Management
Knowledge: Chronic Disease Management
Knowledge: Diabetes Management
Knowledge: Diagnostic & Therapeutic Procedures
Knowledge: Disease Management
Knowledge: Health Behavior
Knowledge: Health Resources
Knowledge: Healthy Lifestyle
Knowledge: Infection Management

Knowledge: Medication
Knowledge: Sexual Function
Knowledge: Treatment Procedure
Knowledge: Treatment Regimen
Knowledge: Wound Management
Lifestyle Balance
Medication Response
Metabolic Function
Motivation
Musculoskeletal Rehabilitation Participation
Nutritional Status
Parenting Performance
Personal Health Screening Behavior
Personal Health Status
Physical Aging
Post-Procedure Recovery
Pre-Procedure Readiness
Respiratory Function
Risk Control: Obesity
Risk Control: Vocal Disorder
Risk Detection
Self-Care Behavior
Self-Care Behavior: Activities of Daily Living (ADL)
Self-Management: Acute Illness
Self-Management: Chronic Disease
Self-Management: Diabetes
Self-Management: Infection
Self-Management: Known Allergy
Self-Management: Treatment Procedure
Self-Management: Treatment Regimen
Self-Management: Wound
Smoking Cessation Behavior
Surgical Recovery: Convalescence
Surgical Recovery: Immediate Post-Operative
Vital Signs
Weight: Body Mass
Weight Gain Behavior
Weight Loss Behavior
Weight Maintenance Behavior
Wound Healing: Primary Intention
Wound Healing: Secondary Intention

Anesthesia

Acute Respiratory Acidosis Severity
Acute Respiratory Alkalosis Severity
Allergic Response: Systemic
Anxiety Level
Blood Coagulation
Blood Glucose Control
Blood Loss Severity
Blood Product Transfusion Reaction
Cardiac Pump Effectiveness
Cardiopulmonary Function
Circulation Status
Cognition
Cognitive Orientation
Comfort Status
Communication
Delirium Level
Electrolyte & Acid/Base Balance
Electrolyte Balance
Fear Level
Fear Level: Adolescent
Fear Level: Middle Childhood
Fear Level: Preschooler
Fetal Status: Intrapartum
Fluid Balance
Fluid Overload Severity
Hydration
Hypercalcemia Severity
Hyperchloremia Severity
Hyperglycemia Severity
Hyperkalemia Severity
Hypermagnesemia Severity
Hypernatremia Severity
Hyperphosphatemia Severity
Hypertension Severity
Hypocalcemia Severity
Hypochloremia Severity
Hypoglycemia Severity
Immune Hypersensitivity Response
Knowledge: Allergy Management
Knowledge: Asthma Management
Knowledge: Diabetes Management
Knowledge: Diagnostic & Therapeutic Procedures
Knowledge: Hypertension Management
Knowledge: Infection Management
Knowledge: Medication

Knowledge: Treatment Procedure
Lymphedema Severity
Mechanical Ventilation Response: Adult
Medication Response
Metabolic Acidosis Severity
Metabolic Alkalosis Severity
Metabolic Function
Nausea & Vomiting Severity
Neurological Function
Neurological Function: Autonomic
Neurological Function: Central Motor Control
Neurological Function: Consciousness
Neurological Function: Cranial Sensory/Motor
Neurological Function: Peripheral
Neurological Function: Spinal Sensory/Motor
Pain Level
Panic Level
Participation in Health Care Decisions
Post-Procedure Recovery
Pre-Procedure Readiness
Respiratory Function
Respiratory Function: Airway Patency
Respiratory Function: Gas Exchange
Respiratory Function: Ventilation
Risk Control: Vocal Disorder
Risk Detection
Seizure Severity
Shock Severity: Anaphylactic
Shock Severity: Cardiogenic
Shock Severity: Hypovolemic
Shock Severity: Neurogenic
Surgical Recovery: Immediate Post-Operative
Thermoregulation
Thermoregulation: Newborn
Tissue Injury Severity: Percutaneous Procedure
Tissue Integrity: Skin & Mucous Membranes
Tissue Perfusion
Tissue Perfusion: Abdominal Organs
Tissue Perfusion: Cardiac
Tissue Perfusion: Cellular
Tissue Perfusion: Cerebral
Tissue Perfusion: Peripheral
Tissue Perfusion: Pulmonary
Vital Signs
Vocal Function

Burn Care

Acute Respiratory Acidosis Severity
Acute Respiratory Alkalosis Severity
Adherence Behavior: Prescribed Medication
Allergic Response: Systemic
Anxiety Level
Blood Loss Severity
Blood Product Transfusion Reaction
Body Image
Burn Healing
Cardiopulmonary Function
Circulation Status
Comfort Status
Coping
Dehydration Severity
Discomfort Level
Electrolyte & Acid/Base Balance
Electrolyte Balance
Family Coping
Family Participation in Professional Care
Family Support During Treatment
Fear Level
Fear Level: Adolescent
Fear Level: Middle Childhood
Fear Level: Preschooler
Hydration
Hypercalcemia Severity
Hyperchloremia Severity
Hyperglycemia Severity
Hyperkalemia Severity
Hypermagnesemia Severity
Hypernatremia Severity
Hyperphosphatemia Severity
Hypertension Severity
Hypocalcemia Severity
Hypochloremia Severity
Hypoglycemia Severity
Hypokalemia Severity
Hypomagnesemia Severity
Hyponatremia Severity
Hypophosphatemia Severity
Hypotension Severity
Infection Severity
Knowledge: Anxiety Management
Knowledge: Diagnostic & Therapeutic Procedures
Knowledge: Dysrhythmia Management
Knowledge: Hypertension Management

Knowledge: Infection Management
Knowledge: Medication
Knowledge: Pain Management
Knowledge: Sexual Function
Knowledge: Treatment Procedure
Knowledge: Treatment Regimen
Knowledge: Wound Management
Medication Response
Metabolic Acidosis Severity
Metabolic Alkalosis Severity
Metabolic Function
Nutritional Status
Pain: Adverse Psychological Response
Pain Control
Pain: Disruptive Effects
Pain Level
Panic Level
Personal Resilience
Physical Injury Severity
Post-Procedure Recovery
Pre-Procedure Readiness
Psychological Adjustment: Life Change
Respiratory Function
Respiratory Function: Airway Patency
Respiratory Function: Gas Exchange
Respiratory Function: Ventilation
Risk Control: Infectious Process
Self-Esteem
Sexual Functioning
Shock Severity: Hypovolemic
Shock Severity: Septic
Sleep
Sleep Disruption Severity
Sleep Enhancement Behavior
Stress Level
Surgical Recovery: Immediate Post-Operative
Symptom Severity
Tissue Perfusion
Tissue Perfusion: Cardiac
Tissue Perfusion: Cellular
Tissue Perfusion: Cerebral
Tissue Perfusion: Pulmonary
Vital Signs
Will to Live
Wound Healing: Secondary Intention

Cardiac Rehabilitation

Acceptance: Health Status
Adherence Behavior
Adherence Behavior: Clinical Condition
Adherence Behavior: Prescribed Medication
Ambulation
Anxiety Level
Balance
Blood Glucose Control
Cardiac Pump Effectiveness
Cardiac Rehabilitation Participation
Cardiopulmonary Function
Circulation Status
Coping
Discomfort Level
Endurance
Energy Conservation
Exercise Participation
Fall Prevention Behavior
Family Support During Treatment
Fatigue: Disruptive Effects
Fatigue Level
Fluid Overload Severity
Gait
Health Beliefs
Health Beliefs: Perceived Ability to Perform
Health Beliefs: Perceived Control
Health Beliefs: Perceived Resources
Health Literacy Behavior
Health Orientation
Health Promoting Behavior
Health Seeking Behavior
Hope
Hypercalcemia Severity
Hyperkalemia Severity
Hypertension Severity
Hypocalcemia Severity
Hypokalemia Severity
Knowledge: Anticoagulation Therapy Management
Knowledge: Anxiety Management
Knowledge: Cardiac Disease Management
Knowledge: Cardiac Rehabilitation
Knowledge: Coronary Artery Disease Management
Knowledge: Diagnostic & Therapeutic Procedures
Knowledge: Disease Management
Knowledge: Dysrhythmia Management
Knowledge: Fall Prevention
Knowledge: Health Resources
Knowledge: Heart Failure Management
Knowledge: Hypertension Management
Knowledge: Lipid Disorder Management
Knowledge: Medication

Knowledge: Prescribed Activity
Knowledge: Prescribed Diet
Knowledge: Sexual Function
Knowledge: Stroke Management
Knowledge: Thrombus Threat Reduction
Knowledge: Treatment Procedure
Knowledge: Treatment Regimen
Knowledge: Weight Management
Lifestyle Balance
Medication Response
Pain Control
Pain: Disruptive Effects
Pain Level
Participation in Health Care Decisions
Personal Health Status
Personal Resilience
Personal Well-Being
Psychosocial Adjustment: Life Change
Quality of Life
Respiratory Function
Risk Control: Falls
Risk Control: Lipid Disorder
Risk Control: Obesity
Risk Control: Prediabetes
Risk Control: Thrombus
Risk Control: Vocal Disorder
Self-Care Behavior: Activities of Daily Living (ADL)
Self-Care Behavior: Non-Parenteral Medication
Self-Management: Anticoagulation Therapy
Self-Management: Cardiac Disease
Self-Management: Chronic Disease
Self-Management: Coronary Artery Disease
Self-Management: Dysrhythmia
Self-Management: Heart Failure
Self-Management: Stroke
Self-Management: Treatment Procedure
Self-Management: Treatment Regimen
Sexual Functioning
Sleep
Smoking Cessation Behavior
Stress Level
Tissue Perfusion
Tissue Perfusion: Cardiac
Tissue Perfusion: Peripheral
Tissue Perfusion: Pulmonary
Vital Signs
Vocal Function
Weight: Body Mass
Weight Loss Behavior
Weight Maintenance Behavior

Chemical Dependency

Abuse Cessation
Abuse: Disruptive Effects
Abuse Protection
Abuse Recovery
Abuse Recovery: Emotional
Abuse Recovery: Financial
Abuse Recovery: Physical
Abuse Recovery: Sexual
Adherence Behavior: Clinical Condition
Adherence Behavior: Prescribed Medication
Agitation Level
Alcohol Abuse Cessation Behavior
Anxiety Level
Anxiety Self-Control
Caregiver-Patient Relationship
Childhood Bullying Recovery
Comfort Status
Coping
Depression Level
Depression Self-Control
Distorted Thought Self-Control
Drug Abuse Cessation Behavior
Family Coping
Family Integrity
Family Normalization
Family Participation in Professional Care
Family Social Climate
Family Social Network Support
Family Support During Treatment
Financial Literacy Behavior
Group Therapy Participation
Health Beliefs: Perceived Control
Health Beliefs: Perceived Threat
Health Insurance Literacy Behavior
Health Literacy Behavior
Health Orientation
Health Seeking Behavior
Impulse Self-Control
Infection Severity
Knowledge: Anxiety Management
Knowledge: Community Health Resources
Knowledge: Depression Management
Knowledge: Health Resources
Knowledge: Human Immunodeficiency Virus Management
Knowledge: Liver Disease Management

Knowledge: Medication
Knowledge: Pain Management
Knowledge: Personal Safety
Knowledge: Sexual Function
Knowledge: Stress Management
Knowledge: Substance Use Control
Knowledge: Treatment Regimen
Liver Function
Medication Response
Metabolic Function
Nutritional Status
Pain: Disruptive Effects
Pain Level
Panic Level
Panic Self-Control
Personal Autonomy
Personal Health Status
Personal Resilience
Personal Safety Behavior
Psychomotor Energy
Quality of Life
Risk Control: Alcohol Use
Risk Control: Drug Use
Risk Control: Housing Insecurity
Risk Control: Sexually Transmitted Diseases (STD)
Risk Control: Tobacco Use
Risk Control: Unintended Pregnancy
Role Performance
Seizure Self-Control
Seizure Severity
Self-Harm Restraint
Self-Management: Infection
Self-Management: Treatment Regimen
Sexual Functioning
Sleep
Sleep Disruption Severity
Sleep Enhancement Behavior
Smoking Cessation Behavior
Spiritual Health
Stress Level
Substance Addiction Consequences
Substance Withdrawal Severity
Suffering Severity
Suicide Self-Restraint
Symptom Severity

Community & Public Health

Abuse Cessation
Abuse: Disruptive Effects
Abuse Protection
Abuse Recovery
Abuse Recovery: Emotional
Abuse Recovery: Financial
Abuse Recovery: Physical
Abuse Recovery: Sexual
Adherence Behavior
Alcohol Abuse Cessation Behavior
Comfort Status
Community Competence
Community Disaster Readiness
Community Disaster Response
Community Grief Recovery
Community Grief Response
Community Health Screening Effectiveness
Community Health Status
Community Immune Status
Community Immune Status: Adult
Community Immune Status: School Age Child
Community Immune Status: Young Child
Community Immunity Effectiveness
Community Pandemic Readiness
Community Pandemic Response
Community Program Effectiveness
Community Resilience
Community Risk Control: Bullying
Community Risk Control: Chronic Disease
Community Risk Control: Communicable Disease
Community Risk Control: Environmental Hazards
Community Risk Control: Lead Exposure
Community Risk Control: Obesity
Community Risk Control: Suicide
Community Risk Control: Unhealthy Cultural Traditions
Community Risk Control: Violence
Community Violence Level
Coping
Decision-Making
Digital Literacy Behavior
Drug Abuse Cessation Behavior
Family Coping
Family Functioning
Family Health Status

Family Integrity
Family Normalization
Family Participation in Professional Care
Family Resilience
Family Risk Control: Bullying
Family Risk Control: Household Food Insecurity
Family Risk Control: Obesity
Family Risk Control: Violence
Family Social Climate
Family Social Network Support
Family Support During Treatment
Financial Literacy Behavior
Health Beliefs
Health Literacy Behavior
Health Orientation
Health Promoting Behavior
Health Seeking Behavior
Hoarding Cessation Behavior
Immunization Behavior
Knowledge: Acute Illness Management
Knowledge: Chronic Disease Management
Knowledge: Community Health Resources
Knowledge: Health Behavior
Knowledge: Health Resources
Knowledge: Healthy Lifestyle
Knowledge: Parenting
Lifestyle Balance
Neglect Cessation
Neglect Recovery
Neglect: Disruptive Effects
Nutritional Status
Personal Resilience
Personal Well-Being
Physical Fitness
Quality of Life
Risk Control
Risk Control: Drug Use
Risk Control: Food Insecurity
Risk Control: Housing Insecurity
Risk Control: Prediabetes
Risk Control: Problematic Internet Use
Risk Control: Vocal Disorder
Risk Detection
Safe Home Environment
Smoking Cessation Behavior
Spiritual Health

Critical Care

Acute Respiratory Acidosis Severity
Acute Respiratory Alkalosis Severity
Allergic Response: Systemic
Anxiety Level
Blood Coagulation
Blood Glucose Control
Blood Loss Severity
Blood Product Transfusion Reaction
Burn Healing
Cardiopulmonary Function
Circulation Status
Cognitive Orientation
Comfort Status
Dehydration Severity
Delirium Level
Dignified Life Closure
Electrolyte & Acid/Base Balance
Electrolyte Balance
Family Coping
Family Participation in Professional Care
Family Support During Treatment
Fear Level
Fear Level: Adolescent
Fear Level: Middle Childhood
Fear Level: Preschooler
Fluid Overload Severity
Hemodialysis: Disruptive Effects
Hypercalcemia Severity
Hyperchloremia Severity
Hyperglycemia Severity
Hyperkalemia Severity
Hypermagnesemia Severity
Hypernatremia Severity
Hyperphosphatemia Severity
Hypertension Severity
Hypocalcemia Severity
Hypochloremia Severity
Hypoglycemia Severity
Hypokalemia Severity
Hypomagnesemia Severity
Hyponatremia Severity
Hypophosphatemia Severity
Hypotension Severity
Immune Hypersensitivity Response
Infection Severity
Infection Severity: Newborn
Kidney Function
Knowledge: Allergy Management
Knowledge: Anticoagulation Therapy Management
Knowledge: Anxiety Management
Knowledge: Asthma Management
Knowledge: Cardiac Disease Management
Knowledge: Coronary Artery Disease Management
Knowledge: Diagnostic & Therapeutic Procedures
Knowledge: Dysrhythmia Management
Knowledge: Epilepsy Management
Knowledge: Hypertension Management
Knowledge: Infection Management
Knowledge: Lipid Disorder Management
Knowledge: Medication
Knowledge: Ostomy Care

Knowledge: Pain Management
Knowledge: Pneumonia Management
Knowledge: Stroke Management
Knowledge: Stroke Threat Reduction
Knowledge: Thrombus Threat Reduction
Knowledge: Treatment Procedure
Knowledge: Treatment Regimen
Knowledge: Wound Management
Liver Function
Mechanical Ventilation Response: Adult
Mechanical Ventilation Weaning Response: Adult
Medication Response
Metabolic Acidosis Severity
Metabolic Alkalosis Severity
Metabolic Function
Nausea & Vomiting: Disruptive Effects
Nausea & Vomiting Severity
Neurological Function
Neurological Function: Autonomic
Neurological Function: Consciousness
Neurological Function: Cranial Sensory/Motor
Neurological Function: Peripheral
Neurological Function: Spinal Sensory/Motor
Newborn Adaptation
Nutritional Status
Pain: Adverse Psychological Response
Pain: Disruptive Effects
Pain Level
Panic Level
Peripheral Artery Disease Severity
Peritoneal Dialysis: Disruptive Effects
Physical Injury Severity
Post-Procedure Recovery
Pre-Procedure Readiness
Preterm Infant Organization
Respiratory Function
Respiratory Function: Airway Patency
Respiratory Function: Gas Exchange
Respiratory Function: Ventilation
Risk Control: Vocal Disorder
Seizure Severity
Shock Severity: Anaphylactic
Shock Severity: Cardiogenic
Shock Severity: Hypovolemic
Shock Severity: Neurogenic
Shock Severity: Septic
Stress Level
Surgical Recovery: Immediate Post-Operative
Swallowing Status
Symptom Severity
Systemic Toxin Clearance: Dialysis
Tissue Perfusion
Tissue Perfusion: Cardiac
Tissue Perfusion: Cellular
Tissue Perfusion: Cerebral
Tissue Perfusion: Pulmonary
Vital Signs
Vocal Function
Wound Healing: Primary Intention
Wound Healing: Secondary Intention

Dermatology

Adherence Behavior
Adherence Behavior: Clinical Condition
Adherence Behavior: Prescribed Medication
Allergic Response: Localized
Allergic Response: Systemic
Anxiety Level
Body Image
Burn Healing
Burn Recovery
Coping
Discomfort Level
Foot Health
Health Beliefs: Perceived Control
Health Promoting Behavior
Health Seeking Behavior
Infection Severity
Knowledge: Allergy Management
Knowledge: Cancer Management
Knowledge: Cancer Threat Reduction
Knowledge: Disease Management
Knowledge: Infection Management
Knowledge: Medication
Knowledge: Treatment Regimen
Knowledge: Wound Management
Medication Response
Pain Control
Pain Level
Personal Well-Being
Quality of Life
Risk Control: Infant Allergies
Risk Control: Sun Exposure
Self-Care Behavior: Non-Parenteral Medication
Self-Esteem
Self-Management: Known Allergy
Self-Management: Treatment Regimen
Self-Management: Wound
Social Anxiety Level
Suffering Severity
Symptom Severity
Tissue Integrity: Skin & Mucous Membranes
Wound Healing: Primary Intention
Wound Healing: Secondary Intention

Diabetes

Acceptance: Health Status
Adherence Behavior
Adherence Behavior: Clinical Condition
Adherence Behavior: Prescribed Activity
Adherence Behavior: Prescribed Diet
Adherence Behavior: Prescribed Medication
Anxiety Level
Blood Glucose Control
Cardiopulmonary Function
Cognition
Coping
Depression Level
Depression Self-Control
Exercise Participation
Family Participation in Professional Care
Fear Level
Fear Level: Adolescent
Fear Level: Middle Childhood
Fear Level: Preschooler
Financial Literacy Behavior
Foot Health
Gastrointestinal Function
Health Insurance Literacy Behavior
Health Literacy Behavior
Health Promoting Behavior
Hypertension Severity
Immunization Behavior
Kidney Function
Knowledge: Diabetes Management
Knowledge: Diagnostic & Therapeutic Procedures
Knowledge: Foot Care
Knowledge: Treatment Regimen
Knowledge: Weight Management
Knowledge: Wound Management
Medication Response
Metabolic Function
Neurological Function: Peripheral
Nutritional Status
Nutritional Status: Food & Fluid Intake
Nutritional Status: Nutrient Intake
Participation in Health Care Decisions
Personal Health Screening Behavior
Personal Health Status
Personal Resilience
Psychosocial Adjustment: Life Change
Risk Control: Falls
Risk Control: Hypertension
Risk Control: Lipid Disorder
Risk Control: Obesity
Risk Control: Pressure Injury
Risk Control: Stroke
Risk Control: Tobacco Use
Risk Control: Visual Impairment
Safe Home Environment
Self-Care Behavior: Feet
Self-Care Behavior: Parenteral Medication
Self-Management: Diabetes
Self-Management: Hypertension
Self-Management: Lipid Disorder
Self-Management: Stroke
Self-Management: Treatment Procedure
Self-Management: Treatment Regimen

Continued

Diabetes—cont'd

Knowledge: Hypertension Management
Knowledge: Kidney Disease Management
Knowledge: Lipid Disorder Management
Knowledge: Medication
Knowledge: Prescribed Activity
Knowledge: Sexual Function
Knowledge: Stress Management
Knowledge: Stroke Management
Knowledge: Treatment Procedure

Sensory Function: Proprioception
Sensory Function: Vision
Sexual Functioning
Sleep Disruption Severity
Sleep Enhancement Behavior
Social Support
Stress Level
Tissue Integrity: Skin & Mucous Membranes
Weight: Body Mass
Weight Loss Behavior

Domestic Violence

Abuse Cessation
Abuse: Disruptive Effects
Abuse Protection
Abuse Recovery
Abuse Recovery: Emotional
Abuse Recovery: Financial
Abuse Recovery: Physical
Abuse Recovery: Sexual
Abusive Behavior Self-Restraint
Adaptation to Physical Disability
Aggression Self-Restraint
Agitation Level
Anxiety Level
Anxiety Self-Control
Body Image
Comfort Status
Coping
Depression Level
Depression Self-Control
Discomfort Level
Family Risk Control: Violence
Family Social Support Network
Fatigue: Disruptive Effects
Fatigue Level
Fear Level
Fear Self-Control
Group Therapy Participation
Grief Resolution
Guilt Resolution
Hope
Impulse Self-Control
Knowledge: Anxiety Management
Knowledge: Depression Management
Knowledge: Healthy Lifestyle
Knowledge: Medication
Knowledge: Pain Management
Knowledge: Personal Safety
Knowledge: Sexual Function
Knowledge: Stress Management
Knowledge: Substance Use Control
Knowledge: Treatment Regimen

Loneliness Severity
Medication Response
Mood Equilibrium
Motivation
Neglect Cessation
Neglect: Disruptive Effects
Neglect Recovery
Nutritional Status
Pain: Adverse Psychological Response
Pain Control
Pain: Disruptive Effects
Pain Level
Panic Level
Personal Health Status
Personal Safety Behavior
Physical Injury Severity
Psychomotor Energy
Psychosocial Adjustment: Life Change
Quality of Life
Risk Control: Alcohol Use
Risk Control: Drug Use
Risk Control: Food Insecurity
Risk Control: Housing Insecurity
Risk Control: Tobacco Use
Self-Care Behavior
Self-Esteem
Sexual Functioning
Sleep
Sleep Disruption Severity
Sleep Enhancement Behavior
Smoking Cessation Behavior
Social Support
Stress Level
Suffering Severity
Suicide Self-Restraint
Symptom Control
Symptom Severity
Tissue Integrity: Skin & Mucous Membranes
Weight Maintenance Behavior
Will to Live

Emergency & Triage

Acute Respiratory Acidosis Severity
Acute Respiratory Alkalosis Severity
Adherence Behavior
Adherence Behavior: Prescribed Medication
Allergic Response: Systemic
Anxiety Level
Blood Glucose Control
Blood Loss Severity
Blood Product Transfusion Reaction
Cardiopulmonary Function
Cardiac Pump Effectiveness
Cognition
Community Disaster Readiness
Community Disaster Response
Community Pandemic Readiness
Community Pandemic Response
Community Risk Control: Communicable Disease
Dehydration Severity
Fear Level
Fear Level: Adolescent
Fear Level: Middle Childhood
Fear Level: Preschooler
Fluid Overload Severity
Gastrointestinal Function
Health Beliefs
Health Beliefs: Perceived Resources
Hydration
Hyperglycemia Severity
Hypertension Severity
Hypoglycemia Severity
Hypotension Severity
Infection Severity
Infection Severity: Newborn
Joint Movement
Kidney Function
Knowledge: Allergy Management
Knowledge: Asthma Management
Knowledge: Cardiac Disease Management
Knowledge: Diabetes Management
Knowledge: Diagnostic & Therapeutic Procedures
Knowledge: Hypertension Management

Knowledge: Kidney Disease Management
Knowledge: Medication
Knowledge: Pain Management
Knowledge: Stroke Management
Knowledge: Stroke Threat Reduction
Knowledge: Thrombus Threat Reduction
Knowledge: Treatment Procedure
Knowledge: Treatment Regimen
Knowledge: Wound Care
Liver Function
Metabolic Acidosis Severity
Metabolic Alkalosis Severity
Metabolic Function
Neurological Function
Neurological Function: Autonomic
Neurological Function: Central Motor Control
Neurological Function: Consciousness
Neurological Function: Cranial Sensory/Motor
Neurological Function: Peripheral
Neurological Function: Spinal Sensory/Motor
Pain Level
Panic Level
Participation in Health Care Decisions
Physical Injury Severity
Respiratory Function
Respiratory Function: Airway Patency
Respiratory Function: Gas Exchange
Respiratory Function: Ventilation
Risk Control: Vocal Disorder
Seizure Severity
Self-Harm Restraint
Sensory Function
Shock Severity: Anaphylactic
Shock Severity: Cardiogenic
Shock Severity: Hypovolemic
Shock Severity: Neurogenic
Shock Severity: Septic
Skeletal Function
Swallowing Status
Tissue Perfusion
Vital Signs
Vocal Function

Family Centered Care

Abuse Protection
Caregiver Emotional Health Status
Caregiver Lifestyle Disruption
Caregiver-Patient Relationship
Caregiver Performance: Direct Care
Caregiver Performance: Indirect Care
Caregiver Physical Health Status
Caregiver Role Endurance
Caregiver Stressors
Child Development: 1 Month
Child Development: 2 Months
Child Development: 4 Months
Child Development: 6 Months

Knowledge: Autism Spectrum Disorder
Knowledge: Child Physical Safety
Knowledge: Community Health Resources
Knowledge: Cup Feeding
Knowledge: Eating Disorder Management
Knowledge: Epilepsy Management
Knowledge: Health Behavior
Knowledge: Healthy Diet
Knowledge: Healthy Lifestyle
Knowledge: Infant Care
Knowledge: Infection Management
Knowledge: Medication
Knowledge: Parenting
Knowledge: Personal Safety

Continued

Family Centered Care—cont'd

Child Development: 9 Months
Child Development: 12 Months
Child Development: 18 Months
Child Development: 2 Years
Child Development: 3 Years
Child Development: 4 Years
Child Development: 5 Years
Child Development: 6–7 Years
Child Development: 8–10 Years
Child Development: Early Adolescence
Child Development: Late Adolescence
Child Development: Middle Adolescence
Digital Literacy Behavior
Family Coping
Family Functioning
Family Health Status
Family Integrity
Family Normalization
Family Normalization: Autism Spectrum Disorder
Family Performance: Dementia Care
Family Resilience
Family Risk Control: Bullying
Family Risk Control: Elopement
Family Risk Control: Household Food Insecurity
Family Risk Control: Obesity
Family Risk Control: Violence
Family Social Climate
Family Social Network Support
Family Support During Treatment
Financial Literacy Behavior
Grief Resolution
Health Insurance Literacy Behavior
Health Literacy Behavior
Parent Adaptation to Infant Hospitalization
Parent Adaptation to Toddler Hospitalization
Knowledge: Attention Deficit Hyperactivity Disorder (ADHD)

Knowledge: Preterm Infant Care
Knowledge: School Age Child Psychosocial Safety
Participation in Health Care Decisions
Parenting Performance
Parenting Performance: Adolescent
Parenting Performance: Adolescent Physical Safety
Parenting Performance: Attention Deficit Hyperactivity Disorder (ADHD)
Parenting Performance: Early Childhood Psychosocial Safety
Parenting Performance: Infant Physical Safety
Parenting Performance: Infant Psychosocial Safety
Parenting Performance: Middle Childhood
Parenting Performance: Preschooler
Parenting Performance: School Age Child Psychosocial Safety
Parenting Performance: Toddler
Parenting Performance: Toddler Physical Safety
Physical Fitness
Play Participation
Risk Control: Alcohol Use
Risk Control: Child Bullying
Risk Control: Drug Use
Risk Control: Infant Allergies
Risk Control: Infectious Process
Risk Control: Problematic Internet Use
Risk Control: Tobacco Use
Risk Control: Sun Exposure
Safe Home Environment
Safe Home Environment: Nursery
Self-Management: Autism Spectrum Disorder
Self-Management: Infection
Self-Management: Known Allergy
Spiritual Health

Gastroenterology

Acceptance: Health Status
Adherence Behavior: Clinical Condition
Adherence Behavior: Prescribed Diet
Adherence Behavior: Prescribed Medication
Anxiety Level
Appetite
Blood Loss Severity
Bowel Continence
Bowel Elimination
Discomfort Level
Electrolyte & Acid/Base Balance
Electrolyte Balance
Fatigue Level
Gastrointestinal Function
Health Literacy Behavior
Health Promoting Behavior
Health Seeking Behavior
Hydration
Infant Nutritional Status
Infection Severity

Liver Function
Medication Response
Metabolic Acidosis Severity
Metabolic Alkalosis Severity
Metabolic Function
Nausea & Vomiting Control
Nausea & Vomiting: Disruptive Effects
Nausea & Vomiting Severity
Nutritional Status
Nutritional Status: Biochemical Measures
Nutritional Status: Food & Fluid Intake
Nutritional Status: Nutrient Intake
Pain: Adverse Psychological Response
Pain Control
Pain: Disruptive Effects
Pain Level
Participation in Health Care Decisions
Risk Control: Aspiration
Risk Control: Vocal Disorder
Risk Detection

Continued

Gastroenterology—cont'd

Infection Severity: Newborn
Knowledge: Acute Illness Management
Knowledge: Allergy Management
Knowledge: Celiac Disease Management
Knowledge: Chronic Anemia Management
Knowledge: Diagnostic & Therapeutic Procedures
Knowledge: Disease Management
Knowledge: Eating Disorder Management
Knowledge: Healthy Lifestyle
Knowledge: Inflammatory Bowel Disease Management
Knowledge: Liver Disease Management
Knowledge: Medication
Knowledge: Ostomy Care
Knowledge: Pain Management
Knowledge: Prescribed Diet
Knowledge: Stress Management
Knowledge: Treatment Procedure
Knowledge: Treatment Regimen
Knowledge: Weight Management

Self-Care Behavior: Non-Parenteral Medication
Self-Care Behavior: Parenteral Medication
Self-Management: Celiac Disease
Self-Management: Chronic Anemia
Self-Management: Inflammatory Bowel Disease
Self-Management: Known Allergy
Self-Management: Liver Disease
Self-Management: Ostomy
Self-Management: Treatment Procedure
Self-Management: Treatment Regimen
Swallowing Status
Swallowing Status: Esophageal Phase
Swallowing Status: Oral Phase
Swallowing Status: Pharyngeal Phase
Symptom Control
Symptom Severity
Vital Signs
Vocal Function
Weight Body Mass
Weight Gain Behavior
Weight Loss Behavior

Genetics

Acceptance: Health Status
Anxiety Level
Anxiety Self-Control
Comfort Status: Psychospiritual
Comfort Status: Sociocultural
Coping
Decision-Making
Family Coping
Family Functioning
Family Integrity
Family Participation in Professional Care
Family Social Climate
Family Social Network Support
Fear Level
Fear Level: Adolescent
Financial Literacy Behavior
Health Beliefs
Health Beliefs: Perceived Control
Health Beliefs: Perceived Threat
Health Insurance Literacy Behavior
Health Literacy Behavior
Information Processing
Knowledge: Anxiety Management
Knowledge: Cancer Threat Reduction

Knowledge: Celiac Disease Management
Knowledge: Diagnostic & Therapeutic Procedures
Knowledge: Disease Management
Knowledge: Medication
Knowledge: Multiple Sclerosis Management
Knowledge: Stress Management
Knowledge: Stroke Threat Reduction
Participation in Health Care Decisions
Personal Autonomy
Personal Health Status
Personal Well-Being
Quality of Life
Risk Control: Cancer
Risk Control: Cardiovascular Disease
Risk Control: Infant Allergies
Risk Control: Obesity
Risk Control: Prediabetes
Risk Detection
Social Support
Spiritual Health
Stress Level
Will to Live

Gerontology

Acceptance: Health Status
Adaptation to Physical Disability
Adherence Behavior: Clinical Condition
Adherence Behavior: Healthy Diet
Adherence Behavior: Prescribed Activity
Adherence Behavior: Prescribed Diet
Adherence Behavior: Prescribed Medication
Appetite
Balance
Body Mechanics Performance
Bowel Continence
Bowel Elimination
Cardiac Rehabilitation Participation
Cardiopulmonary Function
Caregiver Emotional Health Status
Caregiver Physical Health Status
Caregiver-Patient Relationship
Caregiver Performance: Direct Care
Caregiver Performance: Indirect Care
Cognition
Comfort Status
Communication
Coordinated Movement
Dehydration Severity
Delirium Level
Dementia Level
Depression Level
Development: Late Adulthood
Digital Literacy Behavior
Discomfort Level
Dry Eye Severity
Elopement Occurrence
Elopement Propensity Risk
Endurance
Energy Conservation
Fall Prevention Behavior
Family Normalization: Dementia
Family Participation in Professional Care
Family Performance: Dementia Care
Family Social Network Support
Fatigue: Disruptive Effects
Fatigue Level
Financial Literacy Behavior
Foot Health
Gait
Health Insurance Literacy Behavior
Health Literacy Behavior
Hearing Compensation Behavior
Hoarding Behavior Severity
Hoarding Cessation Behavior
Hydration
Hyperglycemia Severity
Hypertension Severity
Hypoglycemia Severity
Knowledge: Acute Illness Management
Knowledge: Anticoagulation Therapy Management
Knowledge: Arthritis Management
Knowledge: Cardiac Rehabilitation
Knowledge: Chronic Anemia Management
Knowledge: Chronic Disease Management
Knowledge: Chronic Obstructive Pulmonary Disease Management

Knowledge: Stroke Management
Knowledge: Stroke Threat Reduction
Knowledge: Thrombus Threat Reduction
Knowledge: Weight Management
Lymphedema Severity
Memory
Musculoskeletal Rehabilitation Participation
Neurological Function
Nutritional Status
Nutritional Status: Food & Fluid Intake
Oral Health
Peripheral Artery Disease Severity
Personal Health Status
Personal Resilience
Quality of Life
Respiratory Function: Airway Patency
Respiratory Function: Gas Exchange
Respiratory Function: Ventilation
Rest
Risk Control: Aspiration
Risk Control: Falls
Risk Control: Hyperthermia
Risk Control: Obesity
Risk Control: Pressure Injury
Risk Control: Tobacco
Risk Control: Vocal Disorder
Risk Detection
Safe Home Environment
Safe Wandering
Self-Awareness
Self-Care Behavior
Self-Care Behavior: Activities of Daily Living (ADL)
Self-Care Behavior: Bathing
Self-Care Behavior: Dressing
Self-Care Behavior: Eating
Self-Care Behavior: Feet
Self-Care Behavior: Hygiene
Self-Care Behavior: Instrumental Activities of Daily Living (IADL)
Self-Care Behavior: Oral Hygiene
Self-Care Behavior: Parenteral Medication
Self-Care Behavior: Toileting
Self-Management: Acute Illness
Self-Management: Anticoagulation Therapy
Self-Management: Arthritis
Self-Management: Chronic Anemia
Self-Management: Chronic Disease
Self-Management: Chronic Obstructive Pulmonary Disease
Self-Management: Coronary Artery Disease
Self-Management: Dysrhythmia
Self-Management: Heart Failure
Self-Management: Hypertension
Self-Management: Kidney Disease
Self-Management: Lipid Disorder
Self-Management: Liver Disease
Self-Management: Lymphedema
Self-Management: Osteoporosis
Self-Management: Parkinson Disease
Self-Management: Peripheral Artery Disease
Self-Management: Pneumonia
Self-Management: Stroke

Continued

Gerontology—cont'd

Knowledge: Coronary Artery Disease Management
Knowledge: Dementia Management
Knowledge: Depression Management
Knowledge: Dysrhythmia Management
Knowledge: Fall Prevention
Knowledge: Foot Care
Knowledge: Health Behavior
Knowledge: Health Resources
Knowledge: Healthy Diet
Knowledge: Healthy Lifestyle
Knowledge: Hypertension Management
Knowledge: Inflammatory Bowel Disease Management
Knowledge: Infection Management
Knowledge: Kidney Disease Management
Knowledge: Lipid Disorder Management
Knowledge: Liver Disease Management
Knowledge: Lymphedema Management
Knowledge: Medication
Knowledge: Musculoskeletal Rehabilitation
Knowledge: Osteoporosis Management
Knowledge: Parkinson Disease Management
Knowledge: Peripheral Artery Disease Management
Knowledge: Pneumonia Management
Knowledge: Sexual Function
Knowledge: Stress Management

Self-Management: Treatment Procedure
Self-Management: Treatment Regimen
Sensory Function
Sensory Function: Hearing
Sensory Function: Proprioception
Sensory Function: Smell
Sensory Function: Taste
Sensory Function: Vision
Sexual Functioning
Sleep
Sleep Disruption Severity
Sleep Enhancement Behavior
Smoking Cessation
Social Involvement
Social Support
Successful Aging
Tissue Integrity: Skin & Mucous Membranes
Tissue Perfusion
Urinary Continence
Urinary Elimination
Vision Compensation Behavior
Vital Signs
Vocal Function
Weight: Body Mass

HIV/AIDS

Acceptance: Health Status
Activity Tolerance
Acute Respiratory Acidosis Severity
Acute Respiratory Alkalosis Severity
Adaptation to Physical Disability
Adherence Behavior
Adherence Behavior: Clinical Condition
Adherence Behavior: Prescribed Activity
Adherence Behavior: Prescribed Diet
Adherence Behavior: Prescribed Medication
Alcohol Abuse Cessation Behavior
Anxiety Level
Anxiety Self-Control
Appetite
Body Image
Bowel Continence
Caregiver Lifestyle Disruption
Caregiver Stressors
Circulation Status
Comfort Status
Comfort Status: Physical
Comfort Status: Psychospiritual
Coping
Decision-Making
Depression Level
Depression Self-Control
Dignified Life Closure
Discomfort Level
Electrolyte & Acid/Base Balance
Endurance

Memory
Metabolic Acidosis Severity
Metabolic Alkalosis Severity
Metabolic Function
Mood Equilibrium
Nausea & Vomiting: Disruptive Effects
Nausea & Vomiting Severity
Neurological Function: Consciousness
Nutritional Status
Oral Health
Pain: Adverse Psychological Response
Pain Control
Pain: Disruptive Effects
Pain Level
Panic Level
Panic Self-Control
Personal Resilience
Personal Well-Being
Psychosocial Adjustment: Life Change
Respiratory Function
Respiratory Function: Ventilation
Rest
Risk Control: Dehydration
Risk Control: Infectious Process
Risk Control: Pressure Injury
Risk Control: Sexually Transmitted Diseases (STD)
Risk Detection
Role Performance
Safe Home Environment
Self-Care Behavior

Continued

HIV/AIDS—cont'd

Energy Conservation
Family Coping
Family Normalization
Family Support During Treatment
Fatigue: Disruptive Effects
Fatigue Level
Fear Level
Fear Level: Adolescent
Fear Self-Control
Financial Literacy Behavior
Fluid Balance
Gastrointestinal Function
Grief Resolution
Guilt Resolution
Health Literacy Behavior
Hope
Hydration
Immunization Behavior
Infection Severity
Knowledge: Chronic Anemia Management
Knowledge: Depression Management
Knowledge: Diagnostic & Therapeutic Procedures
Knowledge: Energy Conservation
Knowledge: Healthy Diet
Knowledge: Human Immunodeficiency Virus Management
Knowledge: Infection Management
Knowledge: Medication
Knowledge: Pain Management
Knowledge: Sexual Function
Knowledge: Treatment Procedure
Knowledge: Treatment Regimen
Knowledge: Wound Management
Liver Function
Medication Response

Self-Care Behavior: Activities of Daily Living (ADL)
Self-Care Behavior: Instrumental Activities of Daily Living (IADL)
Self-Care Behavior: Non-Parenteral Medication
Self-Care Behavior: Parenteral Medication
Self-Esteem
Self-Management: Chronic Anemia
Self-Management: Depression
Self-Management: Human Immunodeficiency Virus
Self-Management: Pneumonia
Self-Management: Treatment Procedure
Self-Management: Treatment Regimen
Self-Management: Wound
Sensory Function
Sexual Functioning
Shock Severity: Septic
Sleep
Smoking Cessation Behavior
Social Support
Spiritual Health
Stress Level
Substance Withdrawal Severity
Suffering Severity
Symptom Severity
Thermoregulation
Tissue Integrity: Skin & Mucous Membranes
Tissue Perfusion
Urinary Elimination
Vital Signs
Weight Gain Behavior
Will to Live
Wound Healing: Primary Intention
Wound Healing: Secondary Intention

Home Health Care

Acceptance: Health Status
Activity Tolerance
Adaptation to Physical Disability
Adherence Behavior
Adherence Behavior: Clinical Condition
Adherence Behavior: Healthy Diet
Adherence Behavior: Prescribed Activity
Adherence Behavior: Prescribed Diet
Adherence Behavior: Prescribed Medication
Ambulation
Ambulation: Wheelchair
Balance
Blood Glucose Control
Body Mechanics Performance
Bone Healing
Bowel Elimination
Burn Recovery
Cardiac Rehabilitation Participation
Caregiver Emotional Health Status
Caregiver Physical Health Status
Caregiver Lifestyle Disruption
Caregiver Performance: Direct Care

Knowledge: Multiple Sclerosis Management
Knowledge: Musculoskeletal Rehabilitation
Knowledge: Osteoporosis Management
Knowledge: Ostomy Care
Knowledge: Pain Management
Knowledge: Parkinson Disease
Knowledge: Peripheral Artery Disease Management
Knowledge: Personal Safety
Knowledge: Pneumonia Management
Knowledge: Prescribed Activity
Knowledge: Stress Management
Knowledge: Stroke Management
Knowledge: Stroke Threat Reduction
Knowledge: Thrombus Threat Reduction
Knowledge: Treatment Procedure
Knowledge: Treatment Regimen
Knowledge: Weight Management
Knowledge: Wound Management
Lymphedema Severity
Medication Response
Metabolic Function
Mobility

Continued

Home Health Care—cont'd

Caregiver Performance: Indirect Care
Caregiver Physical Health Status
Caregiver Role Endurance
Caregiver Stressors
Caregiver-Patient Relationship
Chemotherapy: Disruptive Physical Effects
Childhood Bullying Recovery
Comfort Status
Dignified Life Closure
Discomfort Level
Endurance
Fall Prevention Behavior
Family Coping
Family Normalization
Family Normalization: Autism Spectrum Disorder
Family Normalization: Dementia
Family Participation in Professional Care
Family Performance: Dementia Care
Family Resilience
Family Risk Control: Bullying
Family Social Network Support
Family Support During Treatment
Fatigue: Disruptive Effects
Fatigue Level
Financial Literacy Behavior
Foot Health
Gait
Health Beliefs
Health Beliefs: Perceived Ability to Perform
Health Beliefs: Perceived Control
Health Beliefs: Perceived Resources
Health Beliefs: Perceived Threat
Health Literacy Behavior
Health Orientation
Hoarding Behavior Severity
Hoarding Cessation Behavior
Hyperglycemia Severity
Hypertension Severity
Hypotension Severity
Infection Severity
Joint Movement
Kidney Function
Knowledge: Acute Illness Management
Knowledge: Allergy Management
Knowledge: Anticoagulation Therapy Management
Knowledge: Arthritis Management
Knowledge: Asthma Management
Knowledge: Autism Spectrum Disorder
Knowledge: Cancer Management
Knowledge: Cancer Threat Reduction
Knowledge: Cardiac Disease Management
Knowledge: Cardiac Rehabilitation
Knowledge: Celiac Disease Management
Knowledge: Chronic Anemia Management
Knowledge: Chronic Disease Management
Knowledge: Chronic Obstructive Pulmonary Disease Management
Knowledge: Community Health Resources
Knowledge: Coronary Artery Disease Management
Knowledge: Dementia Management
Knowledge: Depression Management
Knowledge: Diabetes Management

Musculoskeletal Rehabilitation Participation
Nutritional Status
Parenting Performance
Peripheral Artery Disease Severity
Personal Health Screening Behavior
Personal Health Status
Personal Resilience
Psychomotor Energy
Risk Control: Aspiration
Risk Control: Child Bullying
Risk Control: Dehydration
Risk Control: Environmental Hazards
Risk Control: Falls
Risk Control: Infant Allergies
Risk Control: Infectious Process
Risk Control: Obesity
Risk Control: Prediabetes
Risk Control: Pressure Injury
Risk Control: Vocal Disorder
Risk Detection
Safe Home Environment
Safe Home Environment: Nursery
Self-Care Behavior
Self-Care Behavior: Activities of Daily Living (ADL)
Self-Care Behavior: Bathing
Self-Care Behavior: Dressing
Self-Care Behavior: Eating
Self-Care Behavior: Feet
Self-Care Behavior: Hygiene
Self-Care Behavior: Instrumental Activities of Daily Living (IADL)
Self-Care Behavior: Non-Parenteral Medication
Self-Care Behavior: Oral Hygiene
Self-Care Behavior: Parenteral Medication
Self-Care Behavior: Toileting
Self-Direction of Care
Self-Direction of Instrumental Activities of Daily Living
Self-Management: Acute Illness
Self-Management: Anticoagulation Therapy
Self-Management: Arthritis
Self-Management: Autism Spectrum Disorder
Self-Management: Cancer
Self-Management: Celiac Disease
Self-Management: Chronic Anemia
Self-Management: Chronic Disease
Self-Management: Chronic Obstructive Pulmonary Disease
Self-Management: Coronary Artery Disease
Self-Management: Dysrhythmia
Self-Management: Heart Failure
Self-Management: Human Immunodeficiency Virus
Self-Management: Hypertension
Self-Management: Inflammatory Bowel Disease
Self-Management: Kidney Disease
Self-Management: Kidney Failure
Self-Management: Known Allergy
Self-Management: Lipid Disorder
Self-Management: Liver Disease
Self-Management: Lymphedema
Self-Management: Osteoporosis
Self-Management: Ostomy
Self-Management: Parkinson Disease
Self-Management: Peripheral Artery Disease

Continued

Home Health Care—cont'd

Knowledge: Diagnostic & Therapeutic Procedures
Knowledge: Disease Management
Knowledge: Dysrhythmia Management
Knowledge: Eating Disorder Management
Knowledge: Epilepsy Management
Knowledge: Fall Prevention
Knowledge: Healthy Diet
Knowledge: Healthy Lifestyle
Knowledge: Heart Failure Management
Knowledge: Human Immunodeficiency Virus Management
Knowledge: Hypertension Management
Knowledge: Infection Management
Knowledge: Inflammatory Bowel Disease Management
Knowledge: Kidney Disease Management
Knowledge: Kidney Failure Management
Knowledge: Lipid Disorder Management
Knowledge: Liver Disease
Knowledge: Lymphedema Management
Knowledge: Medication

Self-Management: Pneumonia
Self-Management: Stroke
Self-Management: Treatment Procedure
Self-Management: Treatment Regimen
Self-Management: Wound
Sensory Function
Sleep
Sleep Disruption Severity
Sleep Enhancement Behavior
Smoking Cessation Behavior
Spiritual Health
Urinary Continence
Vital Signs
Vocal Function
Weight Maintenance Behavior
Wound Healing: Primary Intention
Wound Healing: Secondary Intention

Hospice & Palliative Care

Acceptance: Health Status
Caregiver Performance: Direct Care
Caregiver Performance: Indirect Care
Cognition
Comfort Status
Comfort Status: Environment
Comfort Status: Physical
Comfort Status: Psychospiritual
Comfort Status: Sociocultural
Communication
Coping
Delirium Level
Development: Late Adulthood
Dignified Life Closure
Discomfort Level
Fall Prevention Behavior
Falls Occurrence
Family Coping
Family Normalization
Family Participation in Professional Care
Family Social Climate
Family Social Network Support
Fatigue: Disruptive Effects
Fatigue Level
Fear Level
Financial Literacy Behavior
Grief Resolution
Guilt Resolution
Health Beliefs
Health Insurance Literacy Behavior
Hope
Hydration
Knowledge: Cancer Management
Knowledge: Chronic Anemia Management
Knowledge: Chronic Disease Management
Knowledge: Community Health Resources
Knowledge: Medication

Knowledge: Pain Management
Knowledge: Personal Safety
Knowledge: Treatment Procedure
Knowledge: Treatment Regimen
Medication Response
Nutritional Status
Nutritional Status: Food & Fluid Intake
Oral Health
Pain: Adverse Psychological Response
Pain Control
Pain: Disruptive Effects
Pain Level
Participation in Health Care Decisions
Personal Health Status
Personal Well-Being
Psychosocial Adjustment: Life Change
Quality of Life
Relocation Adaptation
Respiratory Function
Risk Control: Falls
Risk Control: Infectious Process
Risk Control: Pressure Injury
Safe Home Environment
Self-Awareness
Self-Care Behavior
Self-Direction of Care
Self-Esteem
Sleep
Sleep Disruption Severity
Sleep Enhancement Behavior
Social Support
Spiritual Health
Suffering Severity
Symptom Control
Symptom Severity
Will to Live
Vital Signs

Infection Control & Epidemiological

Acceptance: Health Status
Acute Respiratory Acidosis Severity
Acute Respiratory Alkalosis Severity
Adaptation to Physical Disability
Adherence Behavior: Prescribed Medication
Anxiety Level
Appetite
Blood Glucose Control
Blood Loss Severity
Bowel Elimination
Burn Healing
Burn Recovery
Cardiac Pump Effectiveness
Cardiopulmonary Function
Circulation Status
Comfort Status: Physical
Community Disaster Readiness
Community Disaster Response
Community Immune Status
Community Immune Status: Adult
Community Immunity Effectiveness
Community Pandemic Readiness
Community Pandemic Response
Community Program Effectiveness
Community Risk Control: Communicable Disease
Community Risk Control: Environmental Hazards
Coping
Discomfort Level
Electrolyte Balance
Endurance
Energy Conservation
Family Coping
Family Normalization
Family Support During Treatment
Fatigue: Disruptive Effects
Fatigue Level
Financial Literacy Behavior
Fluid Balance
Fluid Overload Severity
Gastrointestinal Function
Health Beliefs: Perceived Ability to Perform
Health Literacy Behavior
Health Orientation
Health Seeking Behavior
Hope
Hydration
Hypertension Severity
Hypotension Severity
Immobility Consequences: Physiological
Immobility Consequences: Psycho-Cognitive
Immune Status
Immunization Behavior
Infection Severity
Infection Severity: Newborn
Joint Movement
Knowledge: Chronic Anemia Management
Knowledge: Diagnostic & Therapeutic Procedures
Knowledge: Disease Management
Knowledge: Healthy Diet
Knowledge: Human Immunodeficiency Virus Management
Knowledge: Infection Management

Medication Response
Metabolic Acidosis Severity
Metabolic Alkalosis Severity
Metabolic Function
Nausea & Vomiting: Disruptive Effects
Nausea & Vomiting Severity
Neurological Function
Neurological Function: Consciousness
Nutritional Status
Nutritional Status: Nutrient Intake
Oral Health
Pain: Adverse Psychological Response
Pain Control
Pain: Disruptive Effects
Pain Level
Panic Level
Personal Health Status
Personal Well-Being
Prenatal Health Behavior
Psychosocial Adjustment: Life Change
Respiratory Function
Respiratory Function: Airway Patency
Respiratory Function: Gas Exchange
Respiratory Function: Ventilation
Rest
Risk Control: Environmental Hazards
Risk Control: Hyperthermia
Risk Control: Hypothermia
Risk Control: Infectious Process
Risk Control: Pressure Injury
Risk Control: Sexually Transmitted Diseases (STD)
Risk Control: Vocal Disorder
Risk Detection
Safe Home Environment
Self-Care Behavior
Self-Care Behavior: Oral Hygiene
Self-Management: Chronic Anemia
Self-Management: Human Immunodeficiency Virus
Self-Management: Infection
Self-Management: Pneumonia
Self-Management: Treatment Procedure
Self-Management: Treatment Regimen
Self-Management: Wound
Sensory Function
Shock Severity: Anaphylactic
Shock Severity: Cardiogenic
Shock Severity: Hypovolemic
Shock Severity: Neurogenic
Shock Severity: Septic
Sleep
Smoking Cessation Behavior
Social Support
Stress Level
Suffering Severity
Symptom Severity
Thermoregulation
Thermoregulation: Newborn
Tissue Injury Severity: Percutaneous Procedure
Tissue Integrity: Skin & Mucous Membranes
Tissue Perfusion: Abdominal Organs
Tissue Perfusion: Cardiac

Continued

Infection Control & Epidemiological—cont'd

Knowledge: Medication
Knowledge: Pain Management
Knowledge: Pneumonia Management
Knowledge: Treatment Procedure
Knowledge: Treatment Regimen
Knowledge: Wound Management
Mechanical Ventilation Response: Adult
Mechanical Ventilation Weaning Response: Adult

Tissue Perfusion: Peripheral
Tissue Perfusion: Pulmonary
Urinary Elimination
Vital Signs
Weight Gain Behavior
Weight Maintenance Behavior
Will to Live
Wound Healing: Primary Intention
Wound Healing: Secondary Intention

Infusion Therapy

Allergic Response: Localized
Allergic Response: Systemic
Anxiety Level
Blood Coagulation
Blood Product Transfusion Reaction
Chemotherapy: Disruptive Physical Effects
Circulation Status
Comfort Status
Dehydration Severity
Electrolyte & Acid/Base Balance
Family Participation in Professional Care
Financial Literacy Behavior
Fluid Balance
Fluid Overload Severity
Gastrointestinal Function
Health Insurance Literacy Behavior
Health Literacy Behavior
Hydration
Immobility Consequences: Physiological
Infant Nutritional Status
Infection Severity
Infection Severity: Newborn
Kidney Function
Knowledge: Acute Illness Management
Knowledge: Anxiety Management
Knowledge: Arthritis Management
Knowledge: Cancer Management
Knowledge: Celiac Disease Management
Knowledge: Chronic Illness Management
Knowledge: Diabetes Management
Knowledge: Diagnostic & Therapeutic Procedures
Knowledge: Heart Failure Management
Knowledge: Infection Management

Knowledge: Medication
Knowledge: Multiple Sclerosis Management
Knowledge: Prescribed Activity
Knowledge: Treatment Procedure
Knowledge: Treatment Regimen
Liver Function
Medication Response
Nutritional Status: Biochemical Measures
Pain: Adverse Psychological Response
Pain: Disruptive Effects
Pain Level
Pre-Procedure Readiness
Quality of Life
Respiratory Function
Risk Control: Infectious Process
Risk Control: Thrombus
Self-Care Behavior: Non-Parenteral Medication
Self-Care Behavior: Parenteral Medication
Self-Management: Arthritis
Self-Management: Cancer
Self-Management: Celiac Disease
Self-Management: Diabetes
Self-Management: Heart Failure
Self-Management: Infection
Self-Management: Treatment Procedure
Self-Management: Treatment Regimen
Shock Severity: Hypovolemic
Surgical Recovery: Immediate Post-Operative
Symptom Severity
Tissue Integrity: Skin & Mucous Membranes
Tissue Perfusion: Cellular
Tissue Perfusion: Peripheral
Urinary Elimination
Vital Signs

Medical-Surgical

Acceptance: Health Status
Acute Respiratory Acidosis Severity
Acute Respiratory Alkalosis Severity
Adaptation to Hospitalization: Adolescent
Adaptation to Hospitalization: Childhood
Adaptation to Hospitalization: Preschooler
Adaptation to Physical Disability
Adherence Behavior: Clinical Condition
Adherence Behavior: Prescribed Activity
Adherence Behavior: Prescribed Diet
Adherence Behavior: Prescribed Medication
Alcohol Abuse Cessation Behavior
Allergic Response: Localized
Allergic Response: Systemic
Ambulation
Ambulation: Wheelchair
Appetite
Balance
Blood Glucose Control
Body Positioning: Self-Initiated
Cardiac Rehabilitation Participation
Cardiopulmonary Function
Chemotherapy: Disruptive Physical Effects
Cognition
Cognitive Orientation
Comfort Status
Communication
Dehydration Severity
Delirium Level
Dementia Level
Development: Established Adulthood
Development: Late Adulthood
Development: Middle Adulthood
Development: Young Adulthood
Discomfort Level
Drug Abuse Cessation Behavior
Electrolyte Balance
Endurance
Family Support During Treatment
Fatigue: Disruptive Effects
Fatigue Level
Financial Literacy Behavior
Fluid Overload Severity
Gait
Gastrointestinal Function
Health Insurance Literacy Behavior
Health Literacy Behavior
Hemodialysis: Disruptive Effects
Hydration
Hypercalcemia Severity
Hyperchloremia Severity
Hyperglycemia Severity
Hyperkalemia Severity
Hypermagnesemia Severity
Hypernatremia Severity
Hyperphosphatemia Severity
Hypertension Severity
Hypocalcemia Severity
Hypochloremia Severity
Hypoglycemia Severity
Hypokalemia Severity

Knowledge: Ostomy Care
Knowledge: Pain Management
Knowledge: Parkinson Disease Management
Knowledge: Sexual Function
Knowledge: Treatment Procedure
Knowledge: Treatment Regimen
Knowledge: Weight Management
Knowledge: Wound Management
Liver Function
Medication Response
Metabolic Acidosis Severity
Metabolic Alkalosis Severity
Metabolic Function
Mobility
Nutritional Status: Food & Fluid Intake
Pain: Adverse Psychological Response
Pain Control
Pain Level
Parent Adaptation to Infant Hospitalization
Parent Adaptation to Toddler Hospitalization
Participation in Health Care Decisions
Peritoneal Dialysis: Disruptive Effects
Personal Safety Behavior
Physical Aging
Respiratory Function
Respiratory Function: Airway Patency
Respiratory Function: Gas Exchange
Respiratory Function: Ventilation
Rest
Risk Control: Aspiration
Risk Control: Dehydration
Risk Control: Falls
Risk Control: Hypertension
Risk Control: Lipid Disorder
Risk Control: Obesity
Risk Control: Osteoporosis
Risk Control: Prediabetes
Risk Control: Pressure Injury
Risk Control: Stroke
Risk Control: Thrombus
Risk Control: Vocal Disorder
Self-Care Behavior
Self-Care Behavior: Activities of Daily Living (ADL)
Self-Care Behavior: Feet
Self-Care Behavior: Instrumental Activities of Daily Living (IADL)
Self-Management: Anticoagulation Therapy
Self-Management: Arthritis
Self-Management: Asthma
Self-Management: Cancer
Self-Management: Cardiac Disease
Self-Management: Celiac Disease
Self-Management: Chronic Anemia
Self-Management: Chronic Obstructive Pulmonary Disease
Self-Management: Coronary Artery Disease
Self-Management: Diabetes
Self-Management: Dysrhythmia
Self-Management: Heart Failure
Self-Management: Human Immunodeficiency Virus
Self-Management: Hypertension
Self-Management: Infection

Continued

Medical-Surgical—cont'd

Hypomagnesemia Severity
Hyponatremia Severity
Hypophosphatemia Severity
Hypotension Severity
Immune Hypersensitivity Response
Infection Severity
Joint Movement
Kidney Function
Knowledge: Allergy Management
Knowledge: Arthritis Management
Knowledge: Cancer Management
Knowledge: Cancer Threat Reduction
Knowledge: Cardiac Disease Management
Knowledge: Cardiac Rehabilitation
Knowledge: Celiac Disease Management
Knowledge: Chronic Anemia Management
Knowledge: Chronic Obstructive Pulmonary Disease Management
Knowledge: Community Health Resources
Knowledge: Coronary Artery Disease Management
Knowledge: Diabetes Management
Knowledge: Diagnostic & Therapeutic Procedures
Knowledge: Disease Management
Knowledge: Dysrhythmia Management
Knowledge: Epilepsy Management
Knowledge: Heart Failure Management
Knowledge: Human Immunodeficiency Virus Management
Knowledge: Hypertension Management
Knowledge: Inflammatory Bowel Disease Management
Knowledge: Kidney Failure Management
Knowledge: Lipid Disorder Management
Knowledge: Liver Disease Management
Knowledge: Lymphedema Management
Knowledge: Medication
Knowledge: Multiple Sclerosis Management

Self-Management: Inflammatory Bowel Disease
Self-Management: Kidney Failure
Self-Management: Lipid Disorder
Self-Management: Liver Disease
Self-Management: Lymphedema
Self-Management: Multiple Sclerosis
Self-Management: Ostomy
Self-Management: Parkinson Disease
Self-Management: Pneumonia
Self-Management: Stroke
Self-Management: Treatment Procedure
Self-Management: Treatment Regimen
Self-Management: Wound
Shock Severity: Anaphylactic
Shock Severity: Cardiogenic
Shock Severity: Hypovolemic
Shock Severity: Neurogenic
Shock Severity: Septic
Sleep
Sleep Disruption Severity
Sleep Enhancement Behavior
Smoking Cessation Behavior
Surgical Recovery: Convalescence
Surgical Recovery: Immediate Post-Operative
Tissue Injury Severity: Percutaneous Procedure
Tissue Integrity: Skin & Mucous Membranes
Tissue Perfusion
Tissue Perfusion: Peripheral
Transfer Performance
Vital Signs
Vocal Function
Wound Healing: Primary Intention
Wound Healing: Secondary Intention

Men's Health

Abuse Recovery
Abuse Recovery: Emotional
Abuse Recovery: Financial
Abuse Recovery: Physical
Abuse Recovery: Sexual
Activity Tolerance
Adherence Behavior: Clinical Condition
Adherence Behavior: Healthy Diet
Adherence Behavior: Prescribed Activity
Adherence Behavior: Prescribed Diet
Adherence Behavior: Prescribed Medication
Alcohol Abuse Cessation Behavior
Blood Glucose Control
Body Image
Bowel Elimination
Cardiopulmonary Function
Circulation Status
Comfort Status
Coping
Depression Level
Depression Self-Control
Development: Established Adulthood
Development: Late Adulthood

Metabolic Function
Mobility
Neglect Recovery
Neurological Function
Nutritional Status
Pain: Adverse Psychological Effects
Pain Control
Pain: Disruptive Effects
Pain Level
Personal Autonomy
Personal Health Screening Behavior
Personal Health Status
Personal Resilience
Personal Time Management
Physical Fitness
Physical Maturation: Male
Quality of Life
Respiratory Function
Rest
Risk Control
Risk Control: Alcohol Use
Risk Control: Cancer

Continued

Men's Health—cont'd

Development: Middle Adulthood
Development: Young Adulthood
Discomfort Level
Drug Abuse Cessation Behavior
Eating Disorder Self-Control
Exercise Participation
Family Coping
Family Functioning
Family Participation in Professional Care
Family Risk Control: Violence
Family Social Climate
Fatigue Level
Financial Literacy Behavior
Gastrointestinal Function
Gender Identity
Grief Resolution
Health Insurance Literacy Behavior
Health Literacy Behavior
Health Seeking Behavior
Hypertension Severity
Immune Status
Infection Severity
Kidney Function
Knowledge: Acute Illness Management
Knowledge: Allergy Management
Knowledge: Arthritis Management
Knowledge: Cancer Threat Reduction
Knowledge: Cardiac Disease Management
Knowledge: Chronic Disease Management
Knowledge: Depression Management
Knowledge: Diabetes Management
Knowledge: Diagnostic & Therapeutic Procedures
Knowledge: Disease Management
Knowledge: Eating Disorder Management
Knowledge: Healthy Diet
Knowledge: Healthy Lifestyle
Knowledge: Human Immunodeficiency Virus Management
Knowledge: Hypertension Management
Knowledge: Infection Management
Knowledge: Medication
Knowledge: Osteoporosis Management
Knowledge: Sexual Function
Knowledge: Weight Management
Knowledge: Wound Management
Lifestyle Balance
Liver Function
Medication Response

Risk Control: Cardiovascular Disease
Risk Control: Dehydration
Risk Control: Drug Use
Risk Control: Hypertension
Risk Control: Obesity
Risk Control: Prediabetes
Risk Control: Sexually Transmitted Diseases (STD)
Risk Control: Sun Exposure
Risk Control: Tobacco Use
Risk Control: Vocal Disorder
Risk Detection
Safe Home Environment
Self-Awareness
Self-Care Behavior
Self-Esteem
Self-Management: Acute Illness
Self-Management: Arthritis
Self-Management: Chronic Disease
Self-Management: Diabetes
Self-Management: Human Immunodeficiency Virus
Self-Management: Hypertension
Self-Management: Infection
Self-Management: Known Allergy
Self-Management: Osteoporosis
Self-Management: Treatment Procedure
Self-Management: Treatment Regimen
Sexual Functioning
Sexual Identity
Skeletal Function
Sleep
Sleep Disruption Severity
Sleep Enhancement Behavior
Smoking Cessation Behavior
Successful Aging
Tissue Perfusion
Urinary Continence
Urinary Elimination
Vital Signs
Vocal Function
Weight: Body Mass
Weight Gain Behavior
Weight Loss Behavior
Weight Maintenance Behavior
Wound Healing: Primary Intention
Wound Healing: Secondary Intention

Neonatology

Blood Coagulation
Blood Glucose Control
Bottle Feeding Establishment: Infant
Bottle Feeding Performance
Bowel Elimination
Breastfeeding Establishment: Infant
Breastfeeding Maintenance
Cardiopulmonary Function
Child Development: 1 Month
Circulation Status
Cup Feeding Establishment: Infant
Cup Feeding Performance
Dehydration Severity
Electrolyte & Acid/Base Balance
Family Participation in Professional Care
Family Social Network Support
Family Support During Treatment
Fluid Balance
Growth
Hydration
Immune Status
Infant Nutritional Status
Infection Severity: Newborn
Knowledge: Bottle Feeding

Knowledge: Breastfeeding
Knowledge: Cup Feeding
Knowledge: Medication
Knowledge: Parenting
Knowledge: Preterm Infant Care
Medication Response
Newborn Adaptation
Parent Adaptation to Infant Hospitalization
Parent-Infant Attachment
Parenting Performance
Parenting Performance: Infant
Preterm Infant Organization
Respiratory Function: Airway Patency
Respiratory Function: Gas Exchange
Respiratory Function: Ventilation
Risk Control: Infant Allergies
Safe Home Environment: Nursery
Thermoregulation: Newborn
Tissue Integrity: Skin & Mucous Membranes
Tissue Perfusion
Urinary Elimination
Vital Signs
Weight: Body Mass

Nephrology

Activity Tolerance
Adherence Behavior
Adherence Behavior: Clinical Condition
Adherence Behavior: Prescribed Diet
Adherence Behavior: Prescribed Medication
Allergic Response: Systemic
Blood Glucose Control
Blood Product Transfusion Reaction
Body Image
Caregiver Performance: Direct Care
Caregiver-Patient Relationship
Comfort Status
Dehydration Severity
Delirium Level
Dementia Level
Electrolyte Balance
Fatigue: Disruptive Effects
Fatigue Level
Financial Literacy Behavior
Fluid Balance
Fluid Overload Severity
Health Beliefs
Health Beliefs: Perceived Control
Health Beliefs: Perceived Threat
Health Insurance Literacy Behavior
Health Literacy Behavior
Health Promoting Behavior
Health Seeking Behavior

Knowledge: Kidney Disease Management
Knowledge: Kidney Failure Management
Knowledge: Medication
Knowledge: Personal Safety
Knowledge: Prescribed Activity
Knowledge: Treatment Procedure
Knowledge: Treatment Regimen
Knowledge: Wound Management
Medication Response
Metabolic Function
Mood Equilibrium
Neurological Status
Nutritional Status
Nutritional Status: Biochemical Measures
Nutritional Status: Energy
Nutritional Status: Food & Fluid Intake
Nutritional Status: Nutrient Intake
Pain Control
Pain: Disruptive Effects
Pain Level
Participation in Health Care Decisions
Peritoneal Dialysis: Disruptive Effects
Personal Well-Being
Quality of Life
Risk Control: Cardiovascular Disease
Risk Control: Dehydration
Risk Control: Hypertension
Risk Control: Obesity

Continued

Nephrology—cont'd

Hemodialysis Access
Hemodialysis: Disruptive Effects
Hypercalcemia Severity
Hyperchloremia Severity
Hyperglycemia Severity
Hyperkalemia Severity
Hypernatremia Severity
Hypertension Severity
Hypotension Severity
Infection Severity
Kidney Function
Knowledge: Chronic Anemia Management
Knowledge: Diabetes Management
Knowledge: Diagnostic & Therapeutic Procedures
Knowledge: Disease Management
Knowledge: Energy Conservation
Knowledge: Health Resources
Knowledge: Healthy Diet
Knowledge: Hypertension Management
Knowledge: Infection Management

Self-Care Behavior: Non-Parenteral Medication
Self-Esteem
Self-Management: Chronic Anemia
Self-Management: Hypertension
Self-Management: Infection
Self-Management: Kidney Disease
Self-Management: Kidney Failure
Self-Management: Treatment Procedure
Self-Management: Treatment Regimen
Self-Management: Wound
Sensory Function: Tactile
Social Involvement
Spiritual Health
Suffering Severity
Symptom Control
Symptom Severity
Tissue Perfusion: Cellular
Vital Signs
Weight: Body Mass
Wound Healing: Primary Intention

Neuroscience

Abstract Reasoning
Activity Tolerance
Adaptation to Physical Disability
Adherence Behavior: Clinical Condition
Adherence Behavior: Prescribed Activity
Adherence Behavior: Prescribed Medication
Agitation Level
Ambulation
Ambulation: Wheelchair
Attention Deficit Level
Balance
Cognition
Cognitive Orientation
Comfort Status
Communication: Expressive
Communication: Receptive
Coordinated Movement
Coping
Delirium Level
Dementia Level
Elopement Occurrence
Elopement Propensity Risk
Family Coping
Family Normalization
Family Normalization: Dementia
Family Participation in Professional Care
Family Performance: Dementia Care
Family Resilience
Family Risk Control: Elopement
Family Social Network Support
Family Support During Treatment
Financial Literacy Behavior
Gait
Health Literacy Behavior
Heedfulness of Affected Side

Knowledge: Stroke Threat Reduction
Knowledge: Thrombus Threat Reduction
Knowledge: Treatment Regimen
Medication Response
Memory
Mobility
Musculoskeletal Rehabilitation Participation
Neurological Function
Neurological Function: Autonomic
Neurological Function: Central Motor Control
Neurological Function: Consciousness
Neurological Function: Cranial Sensory/Motor
Neurological Function: Peripheral
Neurological Function: Spinal Sensory/Motor
Oral Health
Pain: Adverse Psychological Response
Pain Control
Pain: Disruptive Effects
Pain Level
Personal Resilience
Physical Fitness
Psychomotor Energy
Rest
Risk Control: Aspiration
Risk Control: Falls
Risk Control: Pressure Injury
Risk Control: Stroke
Risk Control: Thrombus
Risk Control: Vocal Disorder
Safe Home Environment
Safe Wandering
Seizure Self-Control
Seizure Severity
Self-Management: Multiple Sclerosis
Self-Management: Stroke

Continued

Neuroscience—cont'd

Hope
Knowledge: Attention Deficit Hyperactivity Disorder (ADHD)
Knowledge: Dementia Management
Knowledge: Diagnostic & Therapeutic Procedures
Knowledge: Disease Management
Knowledge: Epilepsy Management
Knowledge: Healthy Lifestyle
Knowledge: Medication
Knowledge: Multiple Sclerosis Management
Knowledge: Musculoskeletal Rehabilitation
Knowledge: Sexual Function
Knowledge: Stroke Management

Self-Management: Treatment Procedure
Self-Management: Treatment Regimen
Sensory Function
Sexual Functioning
Shock Severity: Neurogenic
Sleep
Sleep Disruption Severity
Sleep Enhancement Behavior
Swallowing Status
Symptom Severity
Thermoregulation
Vital Signs
Vocal Function

Obstetrics & Gynecology

Activity Tolerance
Adherence Behavior: Healthy Diet
Adherence Behavior: Clinical Condition
Adherence Behavior: Prescribed Medication
Blood Glucose Control
Blood Loss Severity
Body Image
Bowel Elimination
Breastfeeding Establishment: Maternal
Breastfeeding Maintenance
Breastfeeding Weaning
Cardiopulmonary Function
Circulation Status
Client Satisfaction: Labor & Delivery
Comfort Status
Depression Level
Depression Self-Control
Development: Established Adulthood
Development: Late Adulthood
Development: Middle Adulthood
Development: Young Adulthood
Discomfort Level
Eating Disorder Self-Control
Exercise Participation
Family Coping
Family Functioning
Family Participation in Professional Care
Family Risk Control: Violence
Family Social Climate
Family Social Network Support
Fatigue Level
Fetal Status: Antepartum
Fetal Status: Intrapartum
Gastrointestinal Function
Grief Resolution
Health Insurance Literacy Behavior
Health Literacy Behavior
Health Seeking Behavior
Hypertension Severity

Knowledge: Wound Management
Lifestyle Balance
Liver Function
Medication Response
Metabolic Function
Mobility
Neurological Function
Nutritional Status
Pain Control
Pain Level
Parent-Infant Attachment
Perimenopause Symptom Severity
Perinatal Health Behavior
Personal Autonomy
Personal Health Screening Behavior
Personal Health Status
Personal Resilience
Personal Time Management
Physical Fitness
Physical Maturation: Female
Postpartum Maternal Health Behavior
Premenstrual Syndrome (PMS) Severity
Quality of Life
Respiratory Function
Rest
Risk Control
Risk Control: Alcohol Use
Risk Control: Cancer
Risk Control: Cardiovascular Disease
Risk Control: Dehydration
Risk Control: Drug Use
Risk Control: Hypertension
Risk Control: Obesity
Risk Control: Prediabetes
Risk Control: Sexually Transmitted Diseases (STD)
Risk Control: Sun Exposure
Risk Control: Tobacco Use
Risk Control: Unintended Pregnancy
Risk Detection

Continued

Obstetrics & Gynecology—cont'd

Immune Status
Infection Severity
Kidney Function
Knowledge: Acute Illness Management
Knowledge: Allergy Management
Knowledge: Breastfeeding
Knowledge: Cancer Threat Reduction
Knowledge: Cardiac Disease Management
Knowledge: Chronic Disease Management
Knowledge: Depression Management
Knowledge: Diabetes Management
Knowledge: Diagnostic & Therapeutic Procedures
Knowledge: Eating Disorder Management
Knowledge: Fertility Promotion
Knowledge: Healthy Diet
Knowledge: Healthy Lifestyle
Knowledge: Hypertension Management
Knowledge: Infection Management
Knowledge: Labor & Delivery
Knowledge: Postpartum Maternal Health
Knowledge: Preconception Maternal Health
Knowledge: Pregnancy
Knowledge: Pregnancy & Postpartum Sexual Function
Knowledge: Sexual Function
Knowledge: Weight Management

Safe Home Environment
Self-Esteem
Self-Management: Acute Illness
Self-Management: Chronic Disease
Self-Management: Diabetes
Self-Management: Hypertension
Self-Management: Infection
Self-Management: Known Allergy
Self-Management: Treatment Procedure
Self-Management: Treatment Regimen
Sexual Functioning
Skeletal Function
Sleep
Sleep Disruption Severity
Sleep Enhancement Behavior
Smoking Cessation Behavior
Tissue Perfusion
Urinary Continence
Urinary Elimination
Vital Signs
Weight: Body Mass
Weight Gain Behavior
Weight Loss Behavior
Weight Maintenance Behavior
Wound Healing: Primary Intention
Wound Healing: Secondary Intention

Occupational Health

Acceptance: Health Status
Adaptation to Physical Disability
Adherence Behavior
Adherence Behavior: Clinical Condition
Adherence Behavior: Prescribed Activity
Adherence Behavior: Prescribed Diet
Adherence Behavior: Prescribed Medication
Alcohol Abuse Cessation Behavior
Anger Self-Restraint
Anxiety Level
Anxiety Self-Control
Blood Glucose Control
Body Mechanics Performance
Burn Healing
Burn Recovery
Cardiac Rehabilitation Participation
Coping
Decision-Making
Depression Level
Depression Self-Control
Drug Abuse Cessation Behavior
Exercise Participation
Family Support During Treatment
Financial Literacy Behavior
Group Therapy Participation
Health Beliefs: Perceived Ability to Perform
Health Beliefs: Perceived Control
Health Beliefs: Perceived Resources
Health Beliefs: Perceived Threat
Health Insurance Literacy Behavior

Medication Response
Musculoskeletal Rehabilitation Participation
Nutritional Status
Oral Health
Pain: Adverse Psychological Response
Pain Control
Pain: Disruptive Effects
Pain Level
Personal Health Screening Behavior
Personal Safety Behavior
Personal Well-Being
Physical Injury Severity
Psychosocial Adjustment: Life Change
Risk Control
Risk Control: Alcohol Use
Risk Control: Cancer
Risk Control: Cardiovascular Disease
Risk Control: Drug Use
Risk Control: Environmental Hazards
Risk Control: Falls
Risk Control: Food Insecurity
Risk Control: Hearing Impairment
Risk Control: Housing Insecurity
Risk Control: Hypertension
Risk Control: Infectious Process
Risk Control: Lipid Disorder
Risk Control: Obesity
Risk Control: Prediabetes
Risk Control: Stroke
Risk Control: Sun Exposure

Continued

Occupational Health—cont'd

Health Literacy Behavior
Health Orientation
Health Promoting Behavior
Health Seeking Behavior
Hearing Compensation Behavior
Hypertension Severity
Hypoglycemia Severity
Immunization Behavior
Infection Severity
Knowledge: Acute Illness Management
Knowledge: Allergy Management
Knowledge: Anxiety Management
Knowledge: Asthma Management
Knowledge: Body Mechanics
Knowledge: Cancer Management
Knowledge: Cancer Threat Reduction
Knowledge: Cardiac Rehabilitation
Knowledge: Chronic Disease Management
Knowledge: Community Health Resources
Knowledge: Depression Management
Knowledge: Diabetes Management
Knowledge: Disease Management
Knowledge: Dysrhythmia Management
Knowledge: Epilepsy Management
Knowledge: Foot Care
Knowledge: Health Behavior
Knowledge: Health Resources
Knowledge: Healthy Diet
Knowledge: Healthy Lifestyle
Knowledge: Hypertension Management
Knowledge: Infection Management
Knowledge: Lipid Disorder Management
Knowledge: Liver Disease Management
Knowledge: Medication
Knowledge: Musculoskeletal Rehabilitation
Knowledge: Pain Management
Knowledge: Parkinson Disease Management
Knowledge: Personal Safety
Knowledge: Stroke Threat Reduction
Knowledge: Substance Use Control
Knowledge: Time Management
Knowledge: Treatment Procedure
Knowledge: Treatment Regimen
Knowledge: Weight Management
Knowledge: Wound Management
Lifestyle Balance

Risk Control: Tobacco Use
Risk Control: Visual Impairment
Risk Control: Vocal Disorder
Risk Detection
Role Performance
Safe Home Environment
Seizure Severity
Self-Care Behavior: Activities of Daily Living (ADL)
Self-Care Behavior: Feet
Self-Care Behavior: Instrumental Activities of Daily Living
Self-Management: Acute Illness
Self-Management: Asthma
Self-Management: Chronic Disease
Self-Management: Diabetes
Self-Management: Hypertension
Self-Management: Infection
Self-Management: Known Allergy
Self-Management: Lipid Disorder
Self-Management: Liver Disease
Self-Management: Lymphedema
Self-Management: Osteoporosis
Self-Management: Parkinson Disease
Self-Management: Pneumonia
Self-Management: Stroke
Self-Management: Treatment Procedure
Self-Management: Treatment Regimen
Self-Management: Wound
Sensory Function: Smell
Sleep
Sleep Disruption Severity
Sleep Enhancement Behavior
Smoking Cessation Behavior
Social Support
Stress Level
Substance Addiction Consequences
Substance Withdrawal Severity
Suffering Severity
Vision Compensation Behavior
Vocal Function
Weight: Body Mass
Weight Loss Behavior
Weight Maintenance Behavior
Wound Healing: Primary Intention

Oncology

Acceptance: Health Status
Activity Tolerance
Adaptation to Physical Disability
Adherence Behavior
Adherence Behavior: Clinical Condition
Adherence Behavior: Healthy Diet
Adherence Behavior: Prescribed Activity
Adherence Behavior: Prescribed Diet
Adherence Behavior: Prescribed Medication
Anxiety Level
Anxiety Self-Control
Appetite
Body Image
Chemotherapy: Disruptive Physical Effects
Comfort Status
Communication
Coping
Decision-Making
Dehydration Severity
Dignified Life Closure
Discomfort Level
Electrolyte & Acid/Base Balance
Electrolyte Balance
Endurance
Energy Conservation
Fall Prevention Behavior
Family Coping
Family Functioning
Family Participation in Professional Care
Family Resilience
Family Social Support Network
Family Support During Treatment
Fatigue: Disruptive Effects
Fatigue Level
Fear Level
Fear Level: Adolescent
Fear Level: Middle Childhood
Fear Level: Preschooler
Fear Self-Control
Fluid Balance
Grief Resolution
Health Insurance Literacy Behavior
Health Literacy Behavior
Hope
Hydration
Immobility Consequences: Physiological
Immobility Consequences: Psycho-Cognitive
Infection Severity
Knowledge: Anxiety Management
Knowledge: Cancer Management
Knowledge: Cancer Threat Reduction
Knowledge: Chronic Anemia Management
Knowledge: Diagnostic & Therapeutic Procedures
Knowledge: Energy Conservation
Knowledge: Health Behavior
Knowledge: Health Resources
Knowledge: Healthy Diet
Knowledge: Infection Management
Knowledge: Lymphedema Management
Knowledge: Medication
Knowledge: Ostomy Care

Lifestyle Balance
Lymphedema Severity
Medication Response
Memory
Nausea & Vomiting Control
Nausea & Vomiting: Disruptive Effects
Nausea & Vomiting Severity
Nutritional Status
Pain: Adverse Psychological Response
Pain Control
Pain: Disruptive Effects
Pain Level
Parent Adaptation to Infant Hospitalization
Parent Adaptation to Toddler Hospitalization
Participation in Health Care Decisions
Personal Autonomy
Personal Health Status
Personal Resilience
Personal Well-Being
Pre-Procedure Readiness
Psychomotor Energy
Psychosocial Adjustment: Life Change
Quality of Life
Risk Control: Cancer
Risk Control: Dehydration
Risk Control: Falls
Risk Control: Infectious Process
Risk Control: Pressure Injury
Safe Home Environment
Self-Awareness
Self-Care Behavior
Self-Care Behavior: Activities of Daily Living (ADL)
Self-Care Behavior: Instrumental Activities of Daily Living
Self-Care Behavior: Non-Parenteral Medication
Self-Care Behavior: Parenteral Medication
Self-Direction of Care
Self-Management: Cancer
Self-Management: Chronic Anemia
Self-Management: Infection
Self-Management: Lymphedema
Self-Management: Ostomy
Self-Management: Pneumonia
Self-Management: Treatment Procedure
Self-Management: Treatment Regimen
Self-Management: Wound
Sensory Function: Taste
Sexual Functioning
Sleep
Sleep Disruption Severity
Sleep Enhancement Behavior
Social Support
Spiritual Health
Stress Level
Suffering Severity
Surgical Recovery: Convalescence
Surgical Recovery: Immediate Post-Operative
Symptom Control
Symptom Severity
Vital Signs
Weight: Body Mass
Weight Gain Behavior

Continued

Oncology—cont'd

Knowledge: Pain Management
Knowledge: Prescribed Activity
Knowledge: Sexual Function
Knowledge: Treatment Procedure
Knowledge: Treatment Regimen
Knowledge: Wound Management

Weight Loss Behavior
Weight Maintenance Behavior
Will to Live
Wound Healing: Primary Intention
Wound Healing: Secondary Intention

Operating Room

Acute Respiratory Acidosis Severity
Acute Respiratory Alkalosis Severity
Allergic Response: Systemic
Anxiety Level
Blood Coagulation
Blood Glucose Control
Blood Loss Severity
Blood Product Transfusion Reaction
Cardiopulmonary Function
Circulation Status
Cognition
Delirium Level
Dehydration Severity
Discomfort Level
Dry Eye Severity
Electrolyte & Acid/Base Balance
Electrolyte Balance
Family Coping
Family Participation in Professional Care
Financial Literacy Behavior
Fluid Balance
Fluid Overload Severity
Health Beliefs: Perceived Control
Health Beliefs: Perceived Resources
Health Insurance Literacy Behavior
Health Literacy Behavior
Hydration
Hypercalcemia Severity
Hyperchloremia Severity
Hyperglycemia Severity
Hyperkalemia Severity
Hypermagnesemia Severity
Hypernatremia Severity
Hyperphosphatemia Severity
Hypertension Severity
Hypocalcemia Severity
Hypochloremia Severity
Hypoglycemia Severity
Hypokalemia Severity
Hypomagnesemia Severity
Hyponatremia Severity
Hypophosphatemia Severity
Hypotension Severity
Immobility Consequences: Physiological
Infection Severity
Infection Severity: Newborn
Joint Movement

Kidney Function
Knowledge: Anxiety Management
Knowledge: Diagnostic & Therapeutic Procedure
Knowledge: Infection Management
Knowledge: Medication
Knowledge: Treatment Procedure
Knowledge: Treatment Regimen
Liver Function
Medication Response
Metabolic Acidosis Severity
Metabolic Alkalosis Severity
Metabolic Function
Nausea & Vomiting Control
Nausea & Vomiting Severity
Pain Level
Panic Level
Participation in Health Care Decisions
Pre-Procedure Readiness
Respiratory Function
Respiratory Function: Airway Patency
Respiratory Function: Gas Exchange
Respiratory Function: Ventilation
Risk Control: Vocal Disorder
Seizure Severity
Shock Severity: Anaphylactic
Shock Severity: Cardiogenic
Shock Severity: Hypovolemic
Shock Severity: Neurogenic
Shock Severity: Septic
Surgical Recovery: Immediate Post-Operative
Swallowing Status
Symptom Severity
Thermoregulation
Thermoregulation: Newborn
Tissue Injury Severity: Percutaneous Procedure
Tissue Integrity: Skin & Mucous Membranes
Tissue Perfusion
Tissue Perfusion: Abdominal Organs
Tissue Perfusion: Cardiac
Tissue Perfusion: Cellular
Tissue Perfusion: Cerebral
Tissue Perfusion: Peripheral
Tissue Perfusion: Pulmonary
Vital Signs
Wound Healing: Primary Intention

Ophthalmology

Acceptance: Health Status
Adaptation to Physical Disability
Adherence Behavior: Prescribed Medication
Body Image
Decision-Making
Discomfort Level
Dry Eye Severity
Health Beliefs
Knowledge: Anticoagulation Therapy Management
Knowledge: Cardiac Disease Management
Knowledge: Child Physical Safety
Knowledge: Coronary Artery Disease Management
Knowledge: Diabetes Management
Knowledge: Diagnostic & Therapeutic Procedures
Knowledge: Disease Management
Knowledge: Dysthymia Management
Knowledge: Health Behavior
Knowledge: Health Resources
Knowledge: Healthy Lifestyle
Knowledge: Hypertension Management
Knowledge: Infection Management
Knowledge: Medication
Knowledge: Multiple Sclerosis Management
Knowledge: Personal Safety
Knowledge: Treatment Regimen
Knowledge: Treatment Procedure

Medication Response
Neurological Function
Neurological Function: Cranial Sensory/Motor
Pain Control
Pain Level
Parenting Performance: Infant Safety
Parenting Performance: Toddler Safety
Participation in Health Care Decisions
Personal Health Screening Behavior
Physical Aging
Physical Injury Severity
Post-Procedure Recovery
Pre-Procedure Readiness
Risk Control
Risk Control: Prediabetes
Risk Control: Visual Impairment
Self-Care Behavior: Non-Parenteral Medication
Self-Management: Cardiac Disease
Self-Management: Coronary Artery Disease
Self-Management: Dysrhythmia
Self-Management: Diabetes
Self-Management: Hypertension
Self-Management: Multiple Sclerosis
Self-Management: Treatment Regimen
Self-Management: Treatment Procedure
Sensory Function: Vision
Surgical Recovery: Immediate Post-Operative
Symptom Severity
Vision Compensation Behavior

Orthopedics

Activity Tolerance
Adaptation to Physical Disability
Adherence Behavior: Clinical Condition
Adherence Behavior: Prescribed Activity
Ambulation
Ambulation: Wheelchair
Balance
Blood Coagulation
Body Mechanics Performance
Body Image
Body Positioning: Self-Initiated
Bone Healing
Caregiver Home Care Readiness
Caregiver Performance: Direct Care
Caregiver Performance: Indirect Care
Communication
Coordinated Movement
Depression Level
Discharge Readiness: Independent Living
Discharge Readiness: Supported Living
Discomfort Level
Endurance
Exercise Participation
Fall Prevention Behavior
Family Support During Treatment
Fatigue Level
Foot Health

Knowledge: Pain Management
Knowledge: Prescribed Activity
Knowledge: Thrombus Threat Reduction
Knowledge: Treatment Procedure
Knowledge: Treatment Regimen
Knowledge: Wound Management
Medication Response
Mobility
Musculoskeletal Rehabilitation Participation
Neurological Function: Cranial Sensory/Motor
Neurological Function: Spinal Sensory/Motor
Nutritional Status: Biochemical Measures
Nutritional Status: Food & Fluid Intake
Pain: Adverse Psychological Response
Pain Control
Pain: Disruptive Effects
Pain Level
Participation in Health Care Decisions
Personal Well-Being
Physical Injury Severity
Post-Procedure Recovery
Pre-Procedure Readiness
Respiratory Function
Risk Control: Falls
Risk Control: Infectious Process
Risk Control: Osteoporosis
Risk Control: Pressure Injury

Continued

Orthopedics—cont'd

Gait
Health Insurance Literacy Behavior
Hypercalcemia Severity
Hypocalcemia Severity
Immobility Consequences: Physiological
Immobility Consequences: Psycho-Cognitive
Infection Severity
Joint Movement
Joint Movement: Ankle
Joint Movement: Elbow
Joint Movement: Fingers
Joint Movement: Hip
Joint Movement: Knee
Joint Movement: Neck
Joint Movement: Passive
Joint Movement: Shoulder
Joint Movement: Spine
Joint Movement: Wrist
Knowledge: Body Mechanics
Knowledge: Community Health Resources
Knowledge: Diagnostic & Therapeutic Procedures
Knowledge: Energy Conservation
Knowledge: Fall Prevention
Knowledge: Foot Care
Knowledge: Infection Management
Knowledge: Medication
Knowledge: Musculoskeletal Rehabilitation
Knowledge: Osteoporosis Management

Safe Home Environment
Self-Care Behavior: Activities of Daily Living (ADL)
Self-Care Behavior: Bathing
Self-Care Behavior: Dressing
Self-Care Behavior: Toileting
Self-Care Behavior: Feet
Self-Care Behavior: Instrumental Activities of Daily Living (IADL)
Self-Care Behavior: Non-Parenteral Medications
Self-Direction of Care
Self-Management: Infection
Self-Management: Osteoporosis
Self-Management: Pneumonia
Self-Management: Treatment Procedure
Self-Management: Treatment Regimen
Self-Management: Wound
Skeletal Function
Sleep
Sleep Disruption Severity
Sleep Enhancement Behavior
Surgical Recovery: Convalescence
Surgical Recovery: Immediate Post-Operative
Symptom Severity
Tissue Integrity: Skin & Mucous Membranes
Tissue Perfusion
Transfer Performance
Vital Signs
Wound Healing: Primary Intention
Wound Healing: Secondary Intention

Otorhinolaryngology & Head-Neck

Acceptance: Health Status
Activity Tolerance
Adaptation to Physical Disability
Adherence Behavior
Adherence Behavior: Clinical Condition
Adherence Behavior: Prescribed Medication
Ambulation
Anxiety Level
Appetite
Blood Loss Severity
Blood Product Transfusion Reaction
Body Image
Caregiver Emotional Health Status
Caregiver Home Readiness
Caregiver Lifestyle Disruption
Caregiver Performance: Direct Care
Caregiver Stressors
Communication
Coping
Dehydration Severity
Delirium Level
Depression Level
Discomfort Level
Electrolyte & Acid/Base Balance
Fluid Balance
Gait

Pain: Adverse Psychological Response
Pain Control
Pain: Disruptive Effects
Pain Level
Participation in Health Care Decisions
Personal Resiliency
Personal Well-Being
Post-Procedure Recovery
Pre-Procedure Readiness
Quality of Life
Respiratory Function: Airway Patency
Respiratory Function: Gas Exchange
Respiratory Function: Ventilation
Risk Control
Risk Control: Aspiration
Risk Control: Cancer
Risk Control: Falls
Risk Control: Infectious Process
Risk Control: Hearing Impairment
Risk Control: Pressure Injury
Risk Control: Tobacco Use
Risk Control: Vocal Disorder
Seizure Self-Control
Self-Care Behavior
Self-Care Behavior: Activities of Daily Living (ADL)
Self-Care Behavior: Oral Hygiene

Continued

Otorhinolaryngology & Head-Neck—cont'd

Health Insurance Literacy Behavior
Health Promoting Behavior
Health Seeking Behavior
Hearing Compensation Behavior
Hope
Hydration
Immobility Consequences: Physiological
Immobility Consequences: Psycho-Cognitive
Immune Status
Infection Severity
Knowledge: Allergy Management
Knowledge: Anxiety Management
Knowledge: Asthma Management
Knowledge: Depression Management
Knowledge: Diagnostic & Therapeutic Procedures
Knowledge: Health Resources
Knowledge: Healthy Lifestyle
Knowledge: Infection Management
Knowledge: Medication
Knowledge: Pneumonia Management
Knowledge: Treatment Procedure
Knowledge: Treatment Regimen
Knowledge: Wound Management
Medication Response
Mobility
Neurological Function: Cranial Sensory/Motor
Nutritional Status
Nutritional Status: Biochemical Measures
Nutritional Status: Nutrient Intake

Self-Esteem
Self-Management: Asthma
Self-Management: Infection
Self-Management: Known Allergy
Self-Management: Pneumonia
Self-Management: Treatment Procedure
Self-Management: Treatment Regimen
Self-Management: Wound
Sensory Function: Hearing
Sensory Function: Smell
Sensory Function: Taste
Sleep
Sleep Disruption Severity
Sleep Enhancement Behavior
Smoking Cessation Behavior
Social Support
Spiritual Health
Swallowing Status
Swallowing Status: Esophageal Phase
Swallowing Status: Oral Phase
Swallowing Status: Pharyngeal Phase
Symptom Control
Tissue Integrity: Skin & Mucous Membranes
Tissue Perfusion: Pulmonary
Vital Signs
Vocal Function
Will to Live
Wound Healing: Primary Intention
Wound Healing: Secondary Intention

Pain Management

Acceptance: Health Status
Agitation Level
Adherence Behavior: Prescribed Medication
Ambulation
Anxiety Level
Cognition
Cognitive Orientation
Comfort Status
Communication
Delirium Level
Dementia Level
Depression Level
Depression Self-Control
Dignified Life Closure
Discharge Readiness: Independent Living
Discharge Readiness: Supported Living
Discomfort Level
Electrolyte & Acid/Base Balance
Family Support During Treatment
Fluid Balance
Information Processing
Knowledge: Anxiety Management
Knowledge: Arthritis Management
Knowledge: Cancer Management
Knowledge: Diagnostic & Therapeutic Procedures
Knowledge: Medication

Pain Level
Personal Resilience
Post-Procedure Recovery
Pre-Procedure Readiness
Respiratory Function
Respiratory Function: Airway Patency
Respiratory Function: Gas Exchange
Respiratory Function: Ventilation
Risk Control: Falls
Safe Home Environment
Self-Care Behavior
Self-Care Behavior: Activities of Daily Living (ADL)
Self-Care Behavior: Bathing
Self-Care Behavior: Dressing
Self-Care Behavior: Instrumental Activities of Daily Living (IADL)
Self-Care Behavior: Non-Parenteral Medication
Self-Care Behavior: Parenteral Medication
Self-Management: Acute Illness
Self-Management: Arthritis
Self-Management: Cancer
Self-Management: Chronic Disease
Self-Management: Lymphedema
Self-Management: Osteoporosis
Self-Management: Treatment Procedure
Self-Management: Treatment Regimen
Sexual Functioning

Continued

Pain Management—cont'd

Knowledge: Musculoskeletal Rehabilitation
Knowledge: Pain Management
Knowledge: Sexual Function
Knowledge: Substance Use Control
Lymphedema Severity
Medication Response
Musculoskeletal Rehabilitation Participation
Nausea & Vomiting Severity
Pain: Adverse Psychological Response
Pain Control
Pain: Disruptive Effects

Skeletal Function
Sleep
Sleep Disruption Severity
Sleep Enhancement Behavior
Stress Level
Surgical Recovery: Convalescence
Surgical Recovery: Immediate Post-Operative
Symptom Control
Vital Signs

Parish Nursing

Abuse Cessation
Abuse: Disruptive Effects
Abuse Protection
Abuse Recovery
Adaptation to Physical Disability
Adherence Behavior
Adherence Behavior: Clinical Condition
Adherence Behavior: Healthy Diet
Adherence Behavior: Prescribed Activity
Adherence Behavior: Prescribed Diet
Adherence Behavior: Prescribed Medication
Anxiety Level
Anxiety Self-Control
Attention Deficient Level
Cardiac Rehabilitation Participation
Caregiver Adaptation to Patient Institutionalization
Caregiver Emotional Health Status
Caregiver Physical Health Status
Caregiver Stressors
Caregiver Well-Being
Caregiver-Patient Relationship
Chemotherapy: Disruptive Physical Effects
Childhood Bullying Recovery
Cognition
Comfort Status: Physical
Comfort Status: Psychospiritual
Community Disaster Recovery
Community Grief Recovery
Community Immune Status: Adult
Community Immune Status: School Age Child
Community Immune Status: Young Child
Community Immunity Effectiveness
Community Pandemic Readiness
Community Pandemic Recovery
Community Pandemic Response
Coping
Decision-Making
Dementia Level
Depression Level
Depression Self-Control
Dignified Life Closure
Family Coping
Family Functioning
Family Integrity

Knowledge: Hypertension Management
Knowledge: Kidney Disease Management
Knowledge: Liver Disease Management
Knowledge: Medication
Knowledge: Parenting
Knowledge: Parkinson Disease Management
Knowledge: Personal Safety
Knowledge: Preterm Infant Care
Knowledge: School Age Child Psychosocial Safety
Knowledge: Sexual Function
Knowledge: Time Management
Knowledge: Weight Management
Leisure Participation
Lifestyle Balance
Loneliness Severity
Lymphedema Severity
Medication Response
Mood Equilibrium
Neglect Cessation
Neglect: Disruptive Effects
Parenting Performance: Adolescent
Parenting Performance: Adolescent Physical Safety
Parenting Performance: Attention Deficit Hyperactivity Disorder (ADHD)
Parenting Performance: Early Childhood Psychosocial Safety
Parenting Performance: Infant Physical Safety
Parenting Performance: Infant Psychosocial Safety
Parenting Performance: School Age Child Psychosocial Safety
Parenting Performance: Toddler Physical Safety
Participation in Health Care Decisions
Personal Health Screening Behavior
Personal Resilience
Personal Time Management
Personal Well-Being
Physical Fitness
Psychomotor Energy
Quality of Life
Relocation Adaptation
Risk Control: Cancer
Risk Control: Cardiovascular Disease
Risk Control: Child Bullying
Risk Control: Food Insecurity
Risk Control: Housing Insecurity
Risk Control: Obesity

Continued

Parish Nursing—cont'd

Family Normalization
Family Normalization: Autism Spectrum Disorder
Family Normalization: Dementia
Family Performance: Dementia Care
Family Risk Control: Bullying
Family Risk Control: Household Food Insecurity
Family Risk Control: Obesity
Family Risk Control: Violence
Family Social Climate
Family Social Support Network
Fear Level
Gender Identity
Grief Resolution
Health Beliefs
Health Orientation
Health Promoting Behavior
Health Seeking Behavior
Hope
Knowledge: Acute Illness Management
Knowledge: Anxiety Management
Knowledge: Attention Deficit Hyperactivity Disorder (ADHD)
Knowledge: Autism Spectrum Disorder
Knowledge: Cancer Threat Reduction
Knowledge: Cardiac Rehabilitation
Knowledge: Chronic Disease Management
Knowledge: Community Resources
Knowledge: Diabetes Management
Knowledge: Fall Prevention
Knowledge: Health Behavior
Knowledge: Health Resources
Knowledge: Hypertension Management
Knowledge: Infection Management
Knowledge: Healthy Diet
Knowledge: Healthy Lifestyle
Knowledge: Heart Failure Management

Risk Control: Tobacco Use
Risk Control: Vocal Disorder
Risk Detection
Safe Home Environment
Self-Awareness
Self-Care Behavior: Activities of Daily Living (ADL)
Self-Care Behavior: Instrumental Activities of Daily Living (IADL)
Self-Care Behavior: Non-Parenteral Medication
Self-Esteem
Self-Harm Restraint
Self-Management: Autism Spectrum Disorder
Self-Management: Cancer
Self-Management: Cardiac Disease
Self-Management: Chronic Disease
Self-Management: Diabetes
Self-Management: Heart Failure
Self-Management: Hypertension
Self-Management: Infection
Smoking Cessation Behavior
Social Involvement
Social Support
Spiritual Health
Stress Level
Suffering Severity
Symptom Severity
Vital Signs
Vocal Function
Weight Loss Behavior
Weight Maintenance Behavior
Will to Live

Pediatrics

Abstract Reasoning
Abuse: Disruptive Effects
Abuse Protection
Abusive Behavior Self-Restraint
Abuse Recovery
Adaptation to Hospitalization: Adolescent
Adaptation to Hospitalization: Middle Childhood
Adaptation to Hospitalization: Preschooler
Agitation Level
Ambulation
Anxiety Level
Attention Deficient Level
Balance
Body Image
Bottle Feeding Establishment: Infant
Bottle Feeding Performance
Breastfeeding Maintenance
Breastfeeding Weaning
Cardiopulmonary Function
Caregiver Home Care Readiness
Caregiver Performance: Direct Care

Knowledge: Preterm Infant Care
Knowledge: School Age Child Psychosocial Safety
Knowledge: Sexual Function
Knowledge: Treatment Procedure
Knowledge: Treatment Regimen
Knowledge: Wound Management
Medication Response
Mobility
Neglect Cessation
Neglect: Disruptive Effects
Newborn Adaptation
Nutritional Status
Oral Health
Pain: Adverse Psychological Response
Pain Control
Pain: Disruptive Effects
Pain Level
Parent Adaptation to Infant Hospitalization
Parent Adaptation to Toddler Hospitalization
Parent-Infant Attachment
Parenting Performance

Continued

Pediatrics—cont'd

Child Development: 1 Month
Child Development: 2 Months
Child Development: 4 Months
Child Development: 6 Months
Child Development: 9 Months
Child Development: 12 Months
Child Development: 18 Months
Child Development: 2 Years
Child Development: 3 Years
Child Development: 4 Years
Child Development: 5 Years
Child Development: 6–7 Years
Child Development: 8–10 Years
Child Development: Early Adolescence
Child Development: Middle Adolescence
Child Development: Late Adolescence
Childhood Bullying Recovery
Coping
Cup Feeding Establishment: Infant
Cup Feeding Performance
Dehydration Severity
Digital Literacy Behavior
Dignified Life Closure
Discomfort Level
Eating Disorder Self-Control
Exercise Participation
Family Coping
Family Functioning
Family Health Status
Family Integrity
Family Normalization
Family Normalization: Autism Spectrum Disorder
Family Participation in Professional Care
Family Resilience
Family Risk Control: Bullying
Family Risk Control: Household Food Insecurity
Family Risk Control: Obesity
Family Risk Control: Violence
Family Social Climate
Family Social Network Support
Family Support During Treatment
Fear Level: Adolescent
Fear Level: Middle Childhood
Fear Level: Preschooler
Gender Identity
Grief Resolution
Growth
Health Promoting Behavior
Health Seeking Behavior
Hydration
Hyperactivity Level
Immobility Consequences: Physiological
Immobility Consequences: Psycho-Cognitive
Immunization Behavior
Infant Nutritional Status
Infection Severity
Infection Severity: Newborn
Joint Movement
Knowledge: Acute Illness Management
Knowledge: Allergy Management
Knowledge: Anxiety Management

Parenting Performance: Adolescent
Parenting Performance: Adolescent Physical Safety
Parenting Performance: Attention Deficit Hyperactivity Disorder (ADHD)
Parenting Performance: Early Childhood Psychosocial Safety
Parenting Performance: Infant Physical Safety
Parenting Performance: Infant Psychosocial Safety
Parenting Performance: Middle Childhood
Parenting Performance: Preschooler
Parenting Performance: School Age Child Psychosocial Safety
Parenting Performance: Toddler
Parenting Performance: Toddler Physical Safety
Physical Fitness
Physical Injury Severity
Physical Maturation: Female
Physical Maturation: Male
Play Participation
Preterm Infant Organization
Psychosocial Adjustment: Life Change
Respiratory Function
Respiratory Function: Airway Patency
Respiratory Function: Gas Exchange
Respiratory Function: Ventilation
Risk Control
Risk Control: Alcohol Use
Risk Control: Child Bullying
Risk Control: Dehydration
Risk Control: Drug Use
Risk Control: Food Insecurity
Risk Control: Housing Insecurity
Risk Control: Hyperthermia
Risk Control: Hypothermia
Risk Control: Infant Allergies
Risk Control: Infectious Process
Risk Control: Obesity
Risk Control: Prediabetes
Risk Control: Problematic Internet Use
Risk Control: Sexually Transmitted Diseases (STD)
Risk Control: Sun Exposure
Risk Control: Tobacco Use
Risk Control: Unintended Pregnancy
Risk Control: Vocal Disorder
Safe Home Environment
Safe Home Environment: Nursery
Seizure Severity
Self-Care Behavior: Activities of Daily Living (ADL)
Self-Esteem
Self-Management: Asthma
Self-Management: Autism Spectrum Disorder
Self-Management: Celiac Disease
Self-Management: Diabetes
Self-Management: Infection
Self-Management: Known Allergy
Self-Management: Treatment Procedure
Self-Management: Treatment Regimen
Sensory Function
Sexual Identity
Skeletal Function
Smoking Cessation Behavior
Social Interaction Skills

Continued

Pediatrics—cont'd

Knowledge: Asthma Management
Knowledge: Attention Deficit Hyperactivity Disorder (ADHD)
Knowledge: Autism Spectrum Disorder
Knowledge: Bottle Feeding
Knowledge: Celiac Disease Management
Knowledge: Child Physical Safety
Knowledge: Chronic Disease Management
Knowledge: Cup Feeding
Knowledge: Diabetes Management
Knowledge: Disease Management
Knowledge: Eating Disorder Management
Knowledge: Epilepsy Management
Knowledge: Health Behavior
Knowledge: Healthy Diet
Knowledge: Healthy Lifestyle
Knowledge: Infant Care
Knowledge: Infection Management
Knowledge: Medication
Knowledge: Parenting
Knowledge: Personal Safety

Social Support
Spiritual Health
Student Health Status
Symptom Severity
Thermoregulation
Thermoregulation: Newborn
Tissue Integrity: Skin & Mucous Membranes
Tissue Perfusion
Vital Signs
Weight: Body Mass
Weight Gain Behavior
Weight Loss Behavior
Wound Healing: Primary Intention
Wound Healing: Secondary Intention

Pediatric Oncology

Acceptance: Health Status
Activity Tolerance
Allergic Response: Systemic
Anxiety Level
Appetite
Blood Loss Severity
Blood Product Transfusion Reaction
Body Image
Caregiver Emotional Health Status
Caregiver Home Care Readiness
Caregiver Physical Health Status
Caregiver Performance: Direct Care
Caregiver Performance: Indirect Care
Chemotherapy: Disruptive Physical Effects
Comfort Status
Coping
Depression Level
Dehydration Severity
Dignified Life Closure
Discomfort Level
Family Coping
Family Functioning
Family Normalization
Family Participation in Professional Care
Family Resilience
Family Social Support Network
Family Support During Treatment
Fatigue: Disruptive Effects
Fatigue Level
Fear Level
Fear Level: Adolescent
Fear Level: Middle Childhood
Fear Level: Preschooler
Gastrointestinal Function
Hope
Immune Hypersensitivity Response

Knowledge: Treatment Regimen
Liver Function
Medication Response
Metabolic Function
Nausea & Vomiting Control
Nausea & Vomiting Severity
Nutritional Status
Pain: Adverse Psychological Response
Pain Control
Pain Level
Parent Adaptation to Infant Hospitalization
Parent Adaptation to Toddler Hospitalization
Parenting Performance
Parenting Performance: Adolescent
Parenting Performance: Adolescent Physical Safety
Parenting Performance: Early/Middle Childhood
    Physical Safety
Parenting Performance: Infant
Parenting Performance: Infant Physical Safety
Parenting Performance: Toddler Physical Safety
Parenting Performance: Middle Childhood
Parenting Performance: Preschooler
Parenting Performance: Toddler
Play Participation
Post-Procedure Recovery
Pre-Procedure Readiness
Psychomotor Energy
Risk Control: Aspiration
Risk Control: Child Bullying
Risk Control: Dehydration
Risk Control: Sun Exposure
Risk Control: Vocal Disorder
Safe Home Environment
Self-Esteem
Self-Management: Cancer
Self-Management: Chronic Anemia

Continued

Pediatric Oncology—cont'd

Immune Status
Infant Nutritional Status
Kidney Function
Knowledge: Cancer Management
Knowledge: Chronic Anemia Management
Knowledge: Diagnostic & Therapeutic Procedures
Knowledge: Disease Management
Knowledge: Healthy Diet
Knowledge: Healthy Lifestyle
Knowledge: Infection Management
Knowledge: Medication
Knowledge: Pain Management
Knowledge: Treatment Procedure

Self-Management: Treatment Procedures
Self-Management: Treatment Regimen
Sensory Function: Taste
Skeletal Function
Surgical Recovery: Convalescence
Surgical Recovery: Immediate Post-Operative
Swallowing Status
Swallowing Status: Esophageal Phase
Swallowing Status: Oral Phase
Swallowing Status: Pharyngeal Phase
Vital Signs
Will to Live

Peri-Anesthesia

Allergic Response: Systemic
Anxiety Level
Blood Coagulation
Blood Glucose Control
Blood Loss Severity
Blood Product Transfusion Reaction
Bowel Elimination
Cardiac Pump Effectiveness
Cardiopulmonary Function
Circulation Status
Comfort Status
Dehydration Severity
Delirium Level
Dementia Level
Discomfort Level
Electrolyte Balance
Fall Prevention Behavior
Fear Level
Fear Level: Adolescent
Fear Level: Middle Childhood
Fear Level: Preschooler
Fluid Balance
Fluid Overload Severity
Hydration
Hypertension Severity
Hypotension Severity
Immune Hypersensitivity Response
Immune Status
Infection Severity
Kidney Function
Knowledge: Allergy Management
Knowledge: Anxiety Management
Knowledge: Diagnostic & Therapeutic Procedures
Knowledge: Disease Management
Knowledge: Energy Conservation
Knowledge: Infection Management
Knowledge: Medication
Knowledge: Pain Management
Knowledge: Personal Safety
Knowledge: Treatment Procedure
Knowledge: Treatment Regimen
Knowledge: Wound Management

Liver Function
Medication Response
Nausea & Vomiting Severity
Neurological Function: Peripheral
Pain: Adverse Psychological Response
Pain Level
Panic Level
Parent Adaptation to Infant Hospitalization
Parent Adaptation to Toddler Hospitalization
Participation in Health Care Decisions
Personal Health Status
Post-Procedure Recovery
Pre-Procedure Readiness
Respiratory Function
Respiratory Function: Airway Patency
Respiratory Function: Gas Exchange
Respiratory Function: Ventilation
Risk Control: Vocal Disorder
Risk Detection
Seizure Severity
Self-Management: Infection
Self-Management: Known Allergy
Self-Management: Treatment Procedure
Self-Management: Treatment Regimen
Self-Management: Wound
Shock Severity: Anaphylactic
Shock Severity: Cardiogenic
Shock Severity: Hypovolemic
Shock Severity: Neurogenic
Shock Severity: Septic
Thermoregulation
Thermoregulation: Newborn
Tissue Perfusion
Tissue Perfusion: Abdominal Organs
Tissue Perfusion: Cardiac
Tissue Perfusion: Cellular
Tissue Perfusion: Cerebral
Tissue Perfusion: Pulmonary
Urinary Elimination
Vital Signs
Wound Healing: Primary Intention
Wound Healing: Secondary Intention

Peri-Operative Care

Allergic Response: Systemic
Anxiety Level
Blood Coagulation
Blood Glucose Control
Blood Loss Severity
Blood Product Transfusion Reaction
Cardiac Pump Effectiveness
Cardiopulmonary Function
Circulation Status
Communication
Coordinated Movement
Coping
Dehydration Severity
Delirium Level
Dementia Level
Discomfort Level
Electrolyte & Acid/Base Balance
Electrolyte Balance
Family Coping
Family Participation in Professional Care
Fluid Balance
Fluid Overload Severity
Gastrointestinal Function
Hemodialysis Access
Hydration
Hypertension Severity
Hypotension Severity
Immune Hypersensitivity Response
Infection Severity
Joint Movement
Joint Movement: Passive
Kidney Function
Knowledge: Anxiety Management
Knowledge: Diagnostic & Therapeutic Procedures
Knowledge: Infection Management
Knowledge: Medication
Knowledge: Treatment Procedure
Knowledge: Treatment Regimen
Mechanical Ventilation Response: Adult
Mechanical Ventilation Weaning Response: Adult
Medication Response
Nausea & Vomiting Severity
Neurological Function
Neurological Function: Autonomic

Neurological Function: Consciousness
Neurological Function: Cranial Sensory/Motor
Neurological Function: Peripheral
Neurological Function: Spinal Sensory/Motor
Nutritional Status: Food & Fluid Intake
Pain Level
Panic Level
Personal Resilience
Physical Injury Severity
Post-Procedure Recovery
Pre-Procedure Readiness
Respiratory Function
Respiratory Function: Airway Patency
Respiratory Function: Gas Exchange
Respiratory Function: Ventilation
Risk Control: Infectious Process
Risk Control: Vocal Disorder
Seizure Severity
Self-Management: Treatment Procedure
Self-Management: Treatment Regimen
Sensory Function: Tactile
Shock Severity: Anaphylactic
Shock Severity: Cardiogenic
Shock Severity: Hypovolemic
Shock Severity: Neurogenic
Shock Severity: Septic
Skeletal Function
Surgical Recovery: Convalescence
Surgical Recovery: Immediate Post-Operative
Symptom Severity
Thermoregulation
Thermoregulation: Newborn
Tissue Integrity: Skin & Mucous Membranes
Tissue Perfusion
Tissue Perfusion: Abdominal Organs
Tissue Perfusion: Cardiac
Tissue Perfusion: Cellular
Tissue Perfusion: Cerebral
Tissue Perfusion: Peripheral
Tissue Perfusion: Pulmonary
Urinary Elimination
Vital Signs
Weight: Body Mass
Wound Healing: Primary Intention
Wound Healing: Secondary Intention

Plastic Surgery

Anxiety Level
Anxiety Self-Control
Blood Glucose Control
Blood Loss Severity
Body Image
Burn Healing
Burn Recovery
Circulation Status
Comfort Status
Comfort Status: Physical
Coping
Dehydration Severity
Discomfort Level
Family Support During Treatment
Fear Level
Financial Literacy Behavior
Fluid Balance
Health Literacy Behavior
Hydration
Immune Status
Infection Severity
Knowledge: Anxiety Management
Knowledge: Diagnostic & Therapeutic Procedures
Knowledge: Infection Management
Knowledge: Medication
Knowledge: Pain Management
Knowledge: Treatment Procedure
Knowledge: Treatment Regimen
Knowledge: Wound Management
Nausea & Vomiting Severity

Neurological Function
Neurological Function: Consciousness
Pain: Adverse Psychological Response
Pain: Disruptive Effects
Pain Level
Personal Well-Being
Post-Procedure Recovery
Pre-Procedure Readiness
Psychosocial Adjustment: Life Change
Respiratory Function
Risk Control
Risk Control: Infectious Process
Risk Detection
Self-Care Behavior
Self-Care Behavior: Non-Parenteral Medication
Self-Esteem
Self-Management: Infection
Self-Management: Treatment Procedure
Self-Management: Treatment Regimen
Self-Management: Wound
Sensory Function
Shock Severity: Hypovolemic
Sleep
Social Support
Surgical Recovery: Convalescence
Surgical Recovery: Immediate Post-Operative
Tissue Integrity: Skin & Mucous Membranes
Tissue Perfusion
Vital Signs
Wound Healing: Primary Intention
Wound Healing: Secondary Intention

Psychiatric-Mental Health

Acceptance: Health Status
Abuse Cessation
Abuse: Disruptive Effects
Abuse Recovery
Abusive Behavior Self-Restraint
Acceptance: Health Status
Adherence Behavior: Prescribed Medication
Aggression Self-Restraint
Agitation Level
Alcohol Abuse Cessation Behavior
Anger Self-Restraint
Anxiety Level
Anxiety Self-Control
Body Image
Childhood Bullying Recovery
Cognition
Cognitive Orientation
Comfort Status: Psychospiritual
Communication
Concentration
Coping
Decision-Making
Delirium Level
Dementia Level
Depression Level

Knowledge: Stress Management
Knowledge: Time Management
Lifestyle Balance
Loneliness Severity
Medication Response
Memory
Mood Equilibrium
Motivation
Neglect Cessation
Neglect: Disruptive Effects
Nutritional Status
Nutritional Status: Food & Fluid Intake
Pain: Adverse Psychological Response
Pain Control
Pain: Disruptive Effects
Pain Level
Panic Level
Panic Self-Control
Participation in Health Care Decisions
Personal Autonomy
Personal Health Status
Personal Resilience
Personal Time Management
Psychomotor Energy
Psychosocial Adjustment: Life Change

Continued

Psychiatric-Mental Health—cont'd

Depression Self-Control
Digital Literacy Behavior
Distorted Thought Self-Control
Drug Abuse Cessation Behavior
Eating Disorder Self-Control
Elopement Occurrence
Elopement Propensity Risk
Family Coping
Family Functioning
Family Involvement in Professional Care
Family Risk Control: Bullying
Family Risk Control: Elopement
Family Risk Control: Violence
Family Social Climate
Fatigue Level
Fear Level
Fear Level: Adolescence
Fear Level: Middle Childhood
Fear Level: Preschooler
Fear Self-Control
Grief Resolution
Group Therapy Participation
Guilt Resolution
Health Insurance Literacy Behavior
Health Literacy Behavior
Hoarding Behavior Severity
Hoarding Cessation Behavior
Hope
Identity
Information Processing
Knowledge: Anxiety Management
Knowledge: Depression Management
Knowledge: Disease Management
Knowledge: Healthy Lifestyle
Knowledge: Medication
Knowledge: Sexual Function

Quality of Life
Relocation Adaptation
Rest
Risk Control: Alcohol Use
Risk Control: Child Bullying
Risk Control: Drug Use
Risk Control: Obesity
Risk Control: Problematic Internet Use
Risk Control: Tobacco Use
Safe Home Environment
Safe Wandering
Self-Awareness
Self-Care Behavior: Activities of Daily Living (ADL)
Self-Care Behavior: Bathing
Self-Care Behavior: Hygiene
Self-Esteem
Self-Harm Restraint
Self-Management: Treatment Procedure
Self-Management: Treatment Regimen
Sexual Functioning
Sleep
Sleep Enhancement Behavior
Smoking Cessation Behavior
Social Anxiety Level
Social Involvement
Social Support
Stress Level
Substance Withdrawal Severity
Suicide Self-Restraint
Symptom Control
Weight Gain Behavior
Weight Loss Behavior
Weight Maintenance Behavior
Will to Live

Radiology

Acceptance: Health Status
Agitation Level
Allergic Response: Systemic
Anxiety Level
Balance
Body Positioning: Self-Initiated
Cardiac Pump Effectiveness
Cardiopulmonary Function
Circulation Status
Coping
Dehydration Severity
Delirium Level
Dementia Level
Discomfort Level
Electrolyte & Acid/Base Balance
Family Support During Treatment
Fatigue Level
Fear Level
Fear Level: Adolescence
Fear Level: Middle Childhood
Fear Level: Preschooler
Fluid Balance
Health Insurance Literacy Behavior
Health Literacy Behavior
Hope
Hydration
Immune Hypersensitivity Response
Immune Status
Infection Severity
Joint Movement
Knowledge: Allergy Management
Knowledge: Anxiety Management
Knowledge: Cancer Management

Knowledge: Diagnostic & Therapeutic Procedures
Knowledge: Infection Management
Knowledge: Medication
Knowledge: Treatment Procedure
Medication Response
Mobility
Nausea & Vomiting Severity
Neurological Function
Nutritional Status
Nutritional Status: Biochemical Measures
Nutritional Status: Nutrient Intake
Pain: Adverse Psychological Response
Pain Control
Panic Level
Panic Self-Control
Post-Procedure Recovery
Pre-Procedure Readiness
Respiratory Function
Rest
Risk Control: Vocal Disorder
Self-Management: Cancer
Self-Management: Infection
Self-Management: Known Allergy
Self-Management: Treatment Procedure
Sleep
Swallowing Status
Thermoregulation
Thermoregulation: Newborn
Tissue Integrity: Skin & Mucous Membranes
Tissue Perfusion
Transfer Performance
Vital Signs
Vocal Function

Rehabilitation

Acceptance: Health Status
Activity Tolerance
Adaptation to Physical Disability
Adherence Behavior: Prescribed Activity
Adherence Behavior: Prescribed Medication
Ambulation
Ambulation: Wheelchair
Balance
Body Mechanics Performance
Body Positioning: Self-Initiated
Bowel Continence
Bowel Elimination
Burn Recovery
Cardiac Rehabilitation Participation
Communication
Concentration
Coordinated Movement
Decision-Making
Delirium Level
Dementia Level
Discharge Readiness: Independent Living
Discharge Readiness: Supported Living
Discomfort Level
Endurance
Exercise Participation
Fall Prevention Behavior
Fatigue: Disruptive Effects
Fatigue Level
Financial Literacy Behavior
Gait
Health Insurance Literacy Behavior
Health Literacy Behavior
Heedfulness of Affected Side
Immobility Consequences: Physiological
Immobility Consequences: Psycho-Cognitive
Joint Movement
Joint Movement: Ankle
Joint Movement: Elbow
Joint Movement: Fingers
Joint Movement: Hip
Joint Movement: Knee
Joint Movement: Neck
Joint Movement: Passive
Joint Movement: Shoulder
Joint Movement: Spine
Joint Movement: Wrist
Knowledge: Arthritis Management
Knowledge: Body Mechanics

Knowledge: Cardiac Rehabilitation
Knowledge: Fall Prevention
Knowledge: Foot Care
Knowledge: Musculoskeletal Rehabilitation
Knowledge: Osteoporosis Management
Knowledge: Pain Management
Knowledge: Prescribed Activity
Knowledge: Sexual Function
Knowledge: Treatment Procedure
Knowledge: Thrombus Threat Reduction
Knowledge: Weight Management
Memory
Mobility
Motivation
Musculoskeletal Rehabilitation Participation
Neurological Function
Pain Control
Pain Level
Participation in Health Care Decisions
Psychomotor Energy
Psychosocial Adjustment: Life Change
Relocation Adaptation
Risk Control: Falls
Risk Control: Pressure Injury
Safe Home Environment
Self-Care Behavior
Self-Care Behavior: Activities of Daily Living (ADL)
Self-Care Behavior: Feet
Self-Care Behavior: Hygiene
Self-Care Behavior: Instrumental Activities of Daily Living (IADL)
Self-Care Behavior: Non-Parenteral Medication
Self-Care Behavior: Oral Hygiene
Self-Care Behavior: Toileting
Self-Direction of Care
Self-Management: Arthritis
Self-Management: Osteoporosis
Self-Management: Treatment Procedure
Sexual Functioning
Sleep
Sleep Enhancement Behavior
Social Support
Swallowing Status
Transfer Performance
Urinary Continence
Urinary Elimination
Vital Signs

School Health

Abuse Cessation
Abuse: Disruptive Effects
Abuse Protection
Activity Tolerance
Adaptation to Physical Disability
Adherence Behavior: Clinical Condition
Adherence Behavior: Prescribed Activity
Adherence Behavior: Prescribed Diet
Adherence Behavior: Prescribed Medication
Aggression Self-Restraint
Alcohol Abuse Cessation Behavior
Ambulation
Anxiety Level
Anxiety Self-Control
Body Image
Cardiopulmonary Function
Child Development: 5 Years
Child Development: 6–7 Years
Child Development: 8–10 Years
Child Development: Early Adolescence
Child Development: Late Adolescence
Child Development: Middle Adolescence
Childhood Bullying Recovery
Communication
Communication: Expressive
Communication: Receptive
Concentration
Coordinated Movement
Digital Literacy Behavior
Drug Abuse Cessation Behavior
Eating Disorder Self-Control
Endurance
Family Normalization: Autism Spectrum Disorder
Family Risk Control: Bullying
Family Risk Control: Household Food Insecurity
Family Risk Control: Obesity
Family Risk Control: Violence
Fear Level: Adolescent
Fear Level: Middle Childhood
Fear Level: Preschooler
Gender Identity
Growth
Hope
Hyperactivity Level
Identity
Information Processing
Knowledge: Acute Illness Management
Knowledge: Allergy Management
Knowledge: Asthma Management
Knowledge: Attention Deficit Hyperactivity Disorder (ADHD)
Knowledge: Autism Spectrum Disorder
Knowledge: Celiac Disease Management
Knowledge: Chronic Disease Management
Knowledge: Diabetes Management
Knowledge: Eating Disorder Management
Knowledge: Epilepsy Management

Knowledge: Healthy Diet
Knowledge: Healthy Lifestyle
Knowledge: Medication
Knowledge: Sexual Function
Knowledge: Stress Management
Knowledge: Substance Use Control
Knowledge: Weight Management
Memory
Mood Equilibrium
Neglect Cessation
Neglect: Disruptive Effects
Neurological Function
Neurological Function: Central Motor Control
Nutritional Status
Oral Health
Personal Autonomy
Personal Health Screening Behavior
Personal Resilience
Personal Safety Behavior
Personal Time Management
Physical Fitness
Play Participation
Respiratory Function
Risk Control: Alcohol Use
Risk Control: Child Bullying
Risk Control: Drug Use
Risk Control: Food Insecurity
Risk Control: Housing Security
Risk Control: Obesity
Risk Control: Prediabetes
Risk Control: Problematic Internet Use
Risk Control: Sexually Transmitted Diseases (STD)
Risk Control: Sun Exposure
Risk Control: Tobacco Use
Risk Control: Unintended Pregnancy
Risk Detection
Safe Home Environment
Seizure Severity
Self-Awareness
Self-Esteem
Self-Management: Asthma
Self-Management: Autism Spectrum Disorder
Self-Management: Celiac Disease
Self-Management: Diabetes
Self-Management: Known Allergy
Sensory Function: Hearing
Sensory Function: Vision
Sleep
Sleep Disruption Severity
Sleep Enhancement Behavior
Smoking Cessation Behavior
Social Anxiety Level
Social Interaction Skills
Social Involvement
Student Health Status
Vital Signs

Spinal Cord Injury

Acceptance: Health Status
Abuse Protection
Activity Tolerance
Adaptation to Physical Disability
Adherence Behavior
Adherence Behavior: Prescribed Activity
Adherence Behavior: Prescribed Medication
Ambulation
Ambulation: Wheelchair
Anxiety Level
Bowel Continence
Bowel Elimination
Cardiopulmonary Function
Caregiver Emotional Health Status
Caregiver Home Care Readiness
Caregiver Lifestyle Disruption
Caregiver Physical Health Status
Caregiver Role Endurance
Comfort Status
Communication
Depression Level
Discharge Readiness: Independent Living
Discharge Readiness: Supported Living
Discomfort Level
Endurance
Energy Conservation
Fall Prevention Behavior
Family Coping
Family Functioning
Family Normalization
Family Participation in Professional Care
Family Resilience
Family Social Climate
Financial Literacy Behavior
Grief Resolution
Health Beliefs: Perceived Ability to Perform
Health Beliefs: Perceived Control
Health Insurance Literacy Behavior
Health Literacy Behavior
Heedfulness of Affected Side
Hope
Kidney Function
Knowledge: Anxiety Management
Knowledge: Depression Management
Knowledge: Diagnostic & Therapeutic Procedures
Knowledge: Health Resources
Knowledge: Healthy Lifestyle
Knowledge: Infection Management
Knowledge: Medication
Knowledge: Musculoskeletal Rehabilitation
Knowledge: Personal Safety
Knowledge: Sexual Function
Knowledge: Treatment Procedure

Knowledge: Treatment Regimen
Knowledge: Weight Management
Knowledge: Wound Management
Leisure Participation
Medication Response
Mobility
Mood Equilibrium
Musculoskeletal Rehabilitation Participation
Neurological Function
Pain Control
Pain Level
Personal Resilience
Physical Injury Severity
Psychomotor Energy
Psychosocial Adjustment: Life Change
Quality of Life
Respiratory Function
Risk Control: Aspiration
Risk Control: Falls
Risk Control: Hyperthermia
Risk Control: Infectious Process
Risk Control: Pressure Injury
Risk Control: Vocal Disorder
Safe Home Environment
Self-Care Behavior: Activities of Daily Living (ADL)
Self-Care Behavior: Feet
Self-Care Behavior: Instrumental Activities of Daily Living (IADL)
Self-Direction of Care
Self-Direction of Instrumental Activities of Daily Living
Self-Esteem
Self-Management: Infection
Self-Management: Non-Parenteral Medication
Self-Management: Pain
Self-Management: Pneumonia
Self-Management: Treatment Procedure
Self-Management: Treatment Regimen
Self-Management: Wound
Sexual Functioning
Shock Severity: Neurogenic
Skeletal Function
Surgical Recovery: Convalescence
Surgical Recovery: Immediate Post-Operative
Symptom Control
Tissue Integrity: Skin & Mucous Membranes
Transfer Performance
Urinary Continence
Urinary Elimination
Vital Signs
Vocal Function
Wound Healing: Primary Intention
Wound Healing: Secondary Intention

Transplant

Acceptance: Health Status
Activity Tolerance
Acute Respiratory Acidosis Severity
Acute Respiratory Alkalosis Severity
Adaptation to Physical Disability
Adherence Behavior
Adherence Behavior: Prescribed Activity
Adherence Behavior: Prescribed Diet
Adherence Behavior: Prescribed Medication
Alcohol Abuse Cessation Behavior
Anxiety Level
Anxiety Self-Control
Appetite
Blood Glucose Control
Blood Loss Severity
Blood Product Transfusion Reaction
Body Image
Bowel Elimination
Cardiac Pump Effectiveness
Cardiac Rehabilitation Participation
Cardiopulmonary Function
Circulation Status
Cognitive Orientation
Comfort Status
Comfort Status: Physical
Comfort Status: Psychospiritual
Coping
Decision-Making
Dehydration Severity
Depression Level
Depression Self-Control
Dignified Life Closure
Discharge Readiness: Independent Living
Discharge Readiness: Supported Living
Discomfort Level
Electrolyte & Acid/Base Balance
Endurance
Energy Conservation
Family Coping
Family Participation in Professional Care
Family Resilience
Family Social Network Support
Family Support During Treatment
Fatigue: Disruptive Effects
Fatigue Level
Fear Level
Fear Self-Control
Financial Literacy Behavior
Fluid Balance
Fluid Overload Severity
Gastrointestinal Function
Health Insurance Literacy Behavior
Health Literacy Behavior
Hope
Hydration
Hypertension Severity
Hypoglycemia Severity
Hypotension Severity
Immune Hypersensitivity Response
Immunization Behavior
Infection Severity

Knowledge: Treatment Regimen
Knowledge: Wound Management
Liver Function
Mechanical Ventilation Response: Adult
Mechanical Ventilation Weaning Response: Adult
Medication Response
Metabolic Acidosis Severity
Metabolic Alkalosis Severity
Metabolic Function
Mood Equilibrium
Nausea & Vomiting: Disruptive Effects
Nausea & Vomiting Severity
Neurological Function
Nutritional Status
Oral Health
Pain: Adverse Psychological Response
Pain Control
Pain: Disruptive Effects
Pain Level
Personal Health Status
Personal Resilience
Personal Well-Being
Post-Procedure Recovery
Pre-Procedure Readiness
Psychosocial Adjustment: Life Change
Respiratory Function
Respiratory Function: Gas Exchange
Respiratory Function: Ventilation
Rest
Risk Control: Aspiration
Risk Control: Cancer
Risk Control: Dehydration
Risk Control: Hypertension
Risk Control: Infectious Process
Risk Control: Lipid Disorder
Risk Control: Osteoporosis
Risk Control: Pressure Injury
Risk Control: Stroke
Risk Control: Vocal Disorder
Risk Detection
Role Performance
Safe Home Environment
Self-Care Behavior
Self-Care Behavior: Activities of Daily Living (ADL)
Self-Care Behavior: Instrumental Activities of Daily Living (IADL)
Self-Direction of Instrumental Activities of Daily Living
Self-Esteem
Self-Management: Chronic Anemia
Self-Management: Diabetes
Self-Management: Hypertension
Self-Management: Infection
Self-Management: Lipid Disorder
Self-Management: Osteoporosis
Self-Management: Pneumonia
Self-Management: Stroke
Self-Management: Treatment Procedure
Self-Management: Treatment Regimen
Self-Management: Wound
Sensory Function
Sexual Functioning
Shock Severity: Cardiogenic

Continued

Transplant—cont'd

Kidney Function
Knowledge: Anxiety Management
Knowledge: Cancer Threat Reduction
Knowledge: Cardiac Rehabilitation
Knowledge: Chronic Anemia Management
Knowledge: Chronic Disease Management
Knowledge: Conception Prevention
Knowledge: Depression Management
Knowledge: Diabetes Management
Knowledge: Diagnostic & Therapeutic Procedures
Knowledge: Disease Management
Knowledge: Energy Conservation
Knowledge: Healthy Diet
Knowledge: Hypertension Management
Knowledge: Infection Management
Knowledge: Kidney Failure Management
Knowledge: Lipid Disorder Management
Knowledge: Medication
Knowledge: Musculoskeletal Rehabilitation
Knowledge: Pain Management
Knowledge: Sexual Function
Knowledge: Stroke Threat Reduction
Knowledge: Treatment Procedure

Shock Severity: Hypovolemic
Shock Severity: Septic
Sleep
Sleep Disruption Severity
Sleep Enhancement Behavior
Smoking Cessation Behavior
Social Support
Spiritual Health
Stress Level
Suffering Severity
Surgical Recovery: Convalescence
Symptom Severity
Thermoregulation
Tissue Integrity: Skin & Mucous Membranes
Tissue Perfusion
Urinary Elimination
Vital Signs
Will to Live
Wound Healing: Primary Intention

Urology

Acceptance: Health Status
Activity Tolerance
Adherence Behavior: Clinical Condition
Adherence Behavior: Prescribed Activity
Adherence Behavior: Prescribed Diet
Adherence Behavior: Prescribed Medication
Dehydration Severity
Electrolyte & Acid/Base Balance
Electrolyte Balance
Fatigue Level
Financial Literacy Behavior
Fluid Balance
Health Insurance Literacy Behavior
Health Literacy Behavior
Health Promoting Behavior
Health Seeking Behavior
Hemodialysis: Disruptive Effects
Hydration
Hypertension Severity
Infection Severity
Kidney Function
Knowledge: Chronic Anemia Management
Knowledge: Diagnostic & Therapeutic Procedures
Knowledge: Hypertension Management
Knowledge: Infection Management
Knowledge: Kidney Disease Management
Knowledge: Kidney Failure Management
Knowledge: Medication
Knowledge: Prescribed Activity
Knowledge: Prescribed Diet
Knowledge: Sexual Function
Knowledge: Treatment Procedure
Knowledge: Treatment Regimen

Knowledge: Wound Management
Medication Response
Metabolic Function
Neurological Function: Central Motor Control
Pain Level
Peritoneal Dialysis: Disruptive Effects
Pre-Procedure Readiness
Psychomotor Energy
Psychosocial Adjustment: Life Change
Risk Control: Dehydration
Risk Control: Infectious Process
Self-Care Behavior: Non-Parenteral Medication
Self-Care Behavior: Toileting
Self-Management: Acute Illness
Self-Management: Chronic Anemia
Self-Management: Hypertension
Self-Management: Infection
Self-Management: Kidney Disease
Self-Management: Kidney Failure
Self-Management: Non-Parenteral Medication
Self-Management: Treatment Procedure
Self-Management: Treatment Regimen
Self-Management: Wound
Sexual Functioning
Sexual Identity
Sleep
Sleep Disruption Severity
Sleep Enhancement Behavior
Symptom Severity
Urinary Continence
Urinary Elimination
Vital Signs
Wound Healing: Primary Intention

Vascular

Acceptance: Health Status
Activity Tolerance
Adherence: Clinical Condition
Adherence: Prescribed Activity
Allergic Response: Systemic
Ambulation
Anxiety Level
Blood Glucose Control
Blood Product Transfusion Reaction
Cardiopulmonary Function
Cardiac Pump Effectiveness
Cardiac Rehabilitation Participation
Circulation Status
Cognition
Cognitive Orientation
Communication
Communication: Expressive
Communication: Receptive
Dehydration Severity
Delirium Level
Dignified Life Closure
Distorted Thought Self-Control
Electrolyte & Acid/Base Balance
Endurance
Exercise Participation
Fall Prevention Behavior
Fatigue Level
Fear Level
Fluid Balance
Foot Health
Grief Resolution
Health Insurance Literacy Behavior
Health Literacy Behavior
Health Seeking Behavior
Hope
Hydration
Immune Hypersensitivity Response
Infection Severity
Kidney Function
Knowledge: Cardiac Rehabilitation
Knowledge: Chronic Anemia Management
Knowledge: Diagnostic & Therapeutic Procedures
Knowledge: Foot Care
Knowledge: Infection Management
Knowledge: Lipid Disorder Management
Knowledge: Medication
Knowledge: Pain Management
Knowledge: Peripheral Artery Disease Management
Knowledge: Prescribed Activity
Knowledge: Stroke Threat Reduction
Knowledge: Thrombus Threat Reduction
Knowledge: Treatment Procedure

Knowledge: Treatment Regimen
Knowledge: Wound Management
Metabolic Function
Medication Response
Neurological Function
Neurological Function: Peripheral
Neurological Function: Spinal Sensory/Motor
Nutritional Status
Pain: Adverse Psychological Response
Pain Control
Pain Level
Participation in Health Care Decisions
Psychomotor Energy
Psychosocial Adjustment: Life Change
Quality of Life
Respiratory Function
Rest
Risk Control: Alcohol Use
Risk Control: Dehydration
Risk Control: Falls
Risk Control: Infectious Process
Risk Control: Pressure Injury
Risk Control: Stroke
Risk Control: Sun Exposure
Risk Control: Thrombus
Risk Control: Tobacco Use
Self-Care Behavior: Eating
Self-Care Behavior: Feet
Self-Management: Chronic Anemia
Self-Management: Coronary Artery Disease
Self-Management: Infection
Self-Management: Lipid Disorder
Self-Management: Peripheral Artery Disease
Self-Management: Stroke
Self-Management: Treatment Procedure
Self-Management: Treatment Regimen
Self-Management: Wound
Sensory Function
Sleep
Sleep Disruption Severity
Smoking Cessation Behavior
Spiritual Health
Suffering Severity
Symptom Severity
Thermoregulation
Tissue Integrity: Skin & Mucous Membranes
Tissue Perfusion
Tissue Perfusion: Peripheral
Urinary Elimination
Vital Signs
Weight: Body Mass
Wound Healing: Primary Intention
Wound Healing: Secondary Intention

Women's Health

Abuse Recovery
Abuse Recovery: Emotional
Abuse Recovery: Financial
Abuse Recovery: Physical
Abuse Recovery: Sexual
Activity Tolerance
Adherence Behavior: Healthy Diet
Adherence Behavior: Clinical Condition
Adherence Behavior: Prescribed Medication
Alcohol Abuse Cessation Behavior
Blood Coagulation
Blood Glucose Control
Blood Loss Severity
Body Image
Bowel Elimination
Breastfeeding Establishment: Maternal
Breastfeeding Maintenance
Breastfeeding Weaning
Cardiopulmonary Function
Circulation Status
Comfort Status
Depression Level
Depression Self-Control
Development: Established Adulthood
Development: Late Adulthood
Development: Middle Adulthood
Development: Young Adulthood
Discomfort Level
Drug Abuse Cessation Behavior
Eating Disorder Self-Control
Exercise Participation
Family Coping
Family Functioning
Family Participation in Professional Care
Family Risk Control: Violence
Family Social Climate
Fatigue Level
Fetal Status: Antepartum
Fetal Status: Intrapartum
Financial Literacy Behavior
Gastrointestinal Function
Gender Identity
Grief Resolution
Health Insurance Literacy Behavior
Health Literacy Behavior
Health Seeking Behavior
Hypertension Severity
Immune Status
Infection Severity
Kidney Function
Knowledge: Acute Illness Management
Knowledge: Allergy Management
Knowledge: Arthritis Management
Knowledge: Breastfeeding
Knowledge: Cancer Threat Reduction
Knowledge: Cardiac Disease Management
Knowledge: Chronic Disease Management
Knowledge: Depression Management
Knowledge: Diabetes Management
Knowledge: Diagnostic & Therapeutic Procedures
Knowledge: Disease Management

Knowledge: Weight Management
Knowledge: Wound Management
Lifestyle Balance
Liver Function
Medication Response
Metabolic Function
Mobility
Neglect Recovery
Neurological Function
Nutritional Status
Pain Control
Pain Level
Perinatal Health Behavior
Perimenopause Symptom Severity
Personal Autonomy
Personal Health Screening Behavior
Personal Health Status
Personal Resilience
Personal Safety Behavior
Personal Time Management
Physical Fitness
Physical Maturation: Female
Premenstrual Syndrome (PMS) Severity
Quality of Life
Respiratory Function
Rest
Risk Control
Risk Control: Alcohol Use
Risk Control: Cancer
Risk Control: Cardiovascular Disease
Risk Control: Dehydration
Risk Control: Drug Use
Risk Control: Hypertension
Risk Control: Obesity
Risk Control: Prediabetes
Risk Control: Sexually Transmitted Diseases (STD)
Risk Control: Sun Exposure
Risk Control: Tobacco Use
Risk Control: Unintended Pregnancy
Risk Detection
Safe Home Environment
Self-Awareness
Self-Care Behavior
Self-Esteem
Self-Management: Acute Illness
Self-Management: Arthritis
Self-Management: Chronic Disease
Self-Management: Diabetes
Self-Management: Human Immunodeficiency Virus
Self-Management: Hypertension
Self-Management: Infection
Self-Management: Known Allergy
Self-Management: Osteoporosis
Self-Management: Treatment Procedure
Self-Management: Treatment Regimen
Sexual Functioning
Sexual Identity
Skeletal Function
Sleep
Sleep Disruption Severity
Sleep Enhancement Behavior

Continued

Women's Health—cont'd

Knowledge: Eating Disorder Management
Knowledge: Healthy Diet
Knowledge: Healthy Lifestyle
Knowledge: Human Immunodeficiency Virus Management
Knowledge: Hypertension Management
Knowledge: Infection Management
Knowledge: Medication
Knowledge: Osteoporosis Management
Knowledge: Postpartum Maternal Health
Knowledge: Preconception Maternal Health
Knowledge: Pregnancy
Knowledge: Pregnancy & Postpartum Sexual Function
Knowledge: Sexual Function

Smoking Cessation Behavior
Successful Aging
Tissue Perfusion
Urinary Continence
Urinary Elimination
Vital Signs
Weight: Body Mass
Weight Gain Behavior
Weight Loss Behavior
Weight Maintenance Behavior
Wound Healing: Primary Intention
Wound Healing: Secondary Intention

Wound & Ostomy

Acceptance: Health Status
Adaptation to Physical Disability
Adherence Behavior: Healthy Diet
Adherence Behavior: Prescribed Medication
Body Image
Bowel Continence
Bowel Elimination
Burn Healing
Burn Recovery
Circulation Status
Coping
Dehydration Severity
Discomfort Level
Electrolyte & Acid/Base Balance
Electrolyte Balance
Gastrointestinal Function
Health Promoting Behavior
Hydration
Infection Severity
Knowledge: Disease Management
Knowledge: Infection Management
Knowledge: Inflammatory Bowel Disease Management
Knowledge: Medication
Knowledge: Ostomy Care
Knowledge: Sexual Function
Knowledge: Treatment Procedure

Knowledge: Treatment Regimen
Knowledge: Wound Management
Medication Response
Nutritional Status
Nutritional Status: Food & Fluids
Pain Control
Pain Level
Participation in Health Care Decisions
Post-Procedure Recovery
Pre-Procedure Readiness
Psychosocial Adjustment: Life Change
Risk Control: Dehydration
Risk Control: Infectious Process
Self-Esteem
Self-Management: Ostomy
Self-Management: Treatment Procedure
Self-Management: Treatment Regimen
Self-Management: Wound
Sexual Functioning
Surgical Recovery: Convalescence
Surgical Recovery: Immediate Post-Operative
Symptom Severity
Tissue Integrity: Skin & Mucous Membranes
Tissue Perfusion
Vital Signs
Wound Healing: Primary Intention
Wound Healing: Secondary Intention

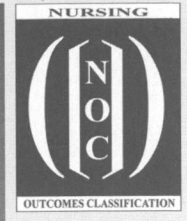

PART SIX

Appendices

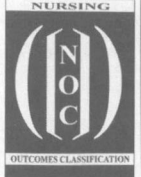

Outcomes: New, Revised, Reviewed, And Retired Since the Sixth Edition

Outcomes New to the Seventh Edition (n = 82)

2515 Abuse: Disruptive Effects
1315 Adaptation to Hospitalization: Adolescent
1314 Adaptation to Hospitalization: Middle Childhood
1313 Adaptation to Hospitalization: Preschooler
1640 Adherence Behavior: Clinical Condition
0921 Attention Deficit Level
0125 Child Development: 9 Months
0126 Child Development: 18 Months
0127 Child Development: 6–7 Years
0128 Child Development: 8–10 Years
0129 Child Development: Early Adolescence
0130 Child Development: Late Adolescence
0131 Child Development: Middle Adolescence
3017 Client Satisfaction: Acute Care Transition Process
3018 Client Satisfaction: Discharge Process
3019 Client Satisfaction: Labor & Delivery
3020 Client Satisfaction: Telehealth Services
2705 Community Disaster Recovery
2706 Community Grief Recovery
2796 Community Immune Status: Adult
2797 Community Immune Status: School Age Child
2798 Community Immune Status: Young Child
2799 Community Immunity Effectiveness
2707 Community Pandemic Readiness
2708 Community Pandemic Recovery
2709 Community Pandemic Response
0621 Dehydration Severity
0124 Development: Established Adulthood
2040 Digital Literacy Behavior
2614 Family Risk Control: Elopement
2620 Family Risk Control: Household Food Insecurity
2615 Family Risk Control: Violence
2630 Family Social Network Support
1218 Fear Level: Adolescent
1219 Fear Level: Middle Childhood
1220 Fear Level: Preschooler
1108 Foot Health
1221 Gender Identity
1641 Group Therapy Participation
2041 Health Insurance Literacy Behavior
2306 Hemodialysis: Disruptive Effects
1222 Hoarding Behavior Severity
1413 Hoarding Cessation Behavior
1868 Knowledge: Anxiety Management
1869 Knowledge: Attention Deficit Hyperactivity Disorder (ADHD)

1870 Knowledge: Community Health Resources
1871 Knowledge: Foot Care
1872 Knowledge: Kidney Failure Management
1873 Knowledge: Liver Disease Management
1874 Knowledge: Parkinson Disease Management
1875 Knowledge: School Age Child Psychosocial Safety
2516 Neglect: Disruptive Effects
1316 Parent Adaptation to Infant Hospitalization
1317 Parent Adaptation to Toddler Hospitalization
2908 Parenting Performance: Attention Deficit Hyperactivity Disorder (ADHD)
2909 Parenting Performance: Early Childhood Psychosocial Safety
2910 Parenting Performance: Infant Physical Safety
2911 Parenting Performance: Infant Psychosocial Safety
2912 Parenting Performance: School Age Child Psychosocial Safety
2913 Parenting Performance: Toddler Physical Safety
2307 Peritoneal Dialysis: Disruptive Effects
1943 Risk Control: Food Insecurity
1944 Risk Control: Housing Insecurity
1945 Risk Control: Prediabetes
1946 Risk Control: Problematic Internet Use
1948 Risk Control: Voice Disorder
1947 Safe Home Environment: Nursery
0314 Self-Care Behavior: Feet
1414 Self-Harm Restraint
3125 Self-Management: Kidney Failure
3126 Self-Management: Liver Disease
3127 Self-Management: Parkinson Disease
3128 Self-Management: Treatment Procedure
3129 Self-Management: Treatment Regimen
2406 Sensory Function: Smell
2407 Sensory Function: Taste
2119 Sleep Disruption Severity
1642 Sleep Enhancement Behavior
1223 Social Identity
2016 Successful Aging
1109 Tissue Injury Severity: Percutaneous Procedure
1110 Vocal Function

Outcomes Revised for the Seventh Edition

Label Name Changes (n = 37)

Outcomes in this category have minor label name changes

Sixth Edition Outcome	Label Change for Seventh Edition Outcome
2300 Blood Glucose Level	2300 Blood Glucose Control
0700 Blood Transfusion Reaction	0700 Blood Product Transfusion Reaction
0414 Cardiopulmonary Status	0414 Cardiopulmonary Function
2506 Caregiver Emotional Health	2506 Caregiver Emotional Health Status
2507 Caregiver Physical Health	2507 Caregiver Physical Health Status
1632 Compliance Behavior: Prescribed Activity	1632 Adherence Behavior: Prescribed Activity
1622 Compliance Behavior: Prescribed Diet	1622 Adherence Behavior: Prescribed Diet
1623 Compliance Behavior: Prescribed Medication	1623 Adherence Behavior: Prescribed Medication
2704 Community Resiliency	2704 Community Resilience
2608 Family Resiliency	2608 Family Resilience
1803 Knowledge: Disease Process	1803 Knowledge: Disease Management
1839 Knowledge: Pregnancy & Postpartum Sexual Functioning	1839 Knowledge: Pregnancy & Postpartum Sexual Function
1815 Knowledge: Sexual Functioning	1815 Knowledge: Sexual Function
0909 Neurological Status	0909 Neurological Function
0910 Neurological Status: Autonomic	0910 Neurological Function: Autonomic
0911 Neurological Status: Central Motor Control	0911 Neurological Function: Central Motor Control
0912 Neurological Status: Consciousness	0912 Neurological Function: Consciousness
0913 Neurological Status: Cranial Sensory/Motor Function	0913 Neurological Function: Cranial Sensory/Motor
0917 Neurological Status: Peripheral	0917 Neurological Function: Peripheral
0914 Neurological Status: Spinal Sensory/Motor Control	0914 Neurological Function: Spinal Sensory/Motor
1615 Ostomy Self-Care	1615 Self-Management: Ostomy
1309 Personal Resiliency	1309 Personal Resilience
0415 Respiratory Status	0415 Respiratory Function
0410 Respiratory Status: Airway Patency	0410 Respiratory Function: Airway Patency
0402 Respiratory Status: Gas Exchange	0402 Respiratory Function: Gas Exchange
0403 Respiratory Status: Ventilation	0403 Respiratory Function: Ventilation
0313 Self-Care Status	0313 Self-Care Behavior
0300 Self-Care: Activities of Daily Living (ADL)	0300 Self-Care Behavior: Activities of Daily Living (ADL)
0301 Self-Care: Bathing	0301 Self Care Behavior: Bathing
0302 Self-Care: Dressing	0302 Self-Care Behavior: Dressing
0303 Self-Care: Eating	0303 Self-Care Behavior: Eating
0305 Self-Care: Hygiene	0305 Self-Care Behavior: Hygiene
0306 Self-Care: Instrumental Activities of Daily Living (IADL)	0306 Self-Care Behavior: Instrumental Activities of Daily Living (IADL)
0307 Self-Care: Non-Parenteral Medication	0307 Self-Care Behavior: Non-Parenteral Medication
0308 Self-Care: Oral Hygiene	0308 Self-Care Behavior: Oral Hygiene
0309 Self-Care: Parenteral Medication	0309 Self-Care Behavior: Parenteral Medication
0310 Self-Care: Toileting	0310 Self-Care Behavior: Toileting

Definition Changes (n = 90)

Outcomes in this category have minor changes in definition that clarify the concept and improve definition consistency within each scale

2514 Abuse Recovery
2502 Abuse Recovery: Emotional
2503 Abuse Recovery: Financial
2504 Abuse Recovery: Physical
2505 Abuse Recovery: Sexual
1400 Abusive Behavior Self-Restraint
1308 Adaptation to Physical Disability
1600 Adherence Behavior
1621 Adherence Behavior: Healthy Diet
1623 Adherence Behavior: Prescribed Medication
0201 Ambulation: Wheelchair
0700 Blood Product Transfusion Reaction
1200 Body Image
1616 Body Mechanics Performance
1000 Breastfeeding Establishment: Infant
1001 Breastfeeding Establishment: Maternal
1003 Breastfeeding Weaning
1106 Burn Healing
1107 Burn Recovery
0400 Cardiac Pump Effectiveness
0414 Cardiopulmonary Function
2506 Caregiver Emotional Health Status
2202 Caregiver Home Care Readiness
2204 Caregiver-Patient Relationship
2507 Caregiver Physical Health Status
2210 Caregiver Role Endurance
2508 Caregiver Well-Being
0401 Circulation Status
3016 Client Satisfaction: Pain Management
3007 Client Satisfaction: Physical Environment
3013 Client Satisfaction: Technical Aspects of Care
0902 Communication
0903 Communication: Expressive
0904 Communication: Receptive
2700 Community Competence
2703 Community Grief Response
2704 Community Resilience
0121 Development: Late Adulthood
0122 Development: Middle Adulthood
0123 Development: Young Adulthood
1307 Dignified Life Closure
0311 Discharge Readiness: Independent Living
0312 Discharge Readiness: Supported Living
1919 Elopement Occurrence
0001 Endurance

2602 Family Functioning
0007 Fatigue Level
0915 Hyperactivity Level
0205 Immobility Consequences: Psycho-Cognitive
0707 Immune Hypersensitivity Response
1020 Infant Nutritional Status
1803 Knowledge: Disease Management
1806 Knowledge: Health Resources
1817 Knowledge: Labor & Delivery
1802 Knowledge: Prescribed Diet
1815 Knowledge: Sexual Function
1866 Knowledge: Time Management
1204 Mood Equilibrium
2513 Neglect Cessation
2512 Neglect Recovery
0912 Neurological Function: Consciousness
1004 Nutritional Status
1005 Nutritional Status: Biochemical Measures
1007 Nutritional Status: Energy
1008 Nutritional Status: Food & Fluid Intake
1009 Nutritional Status: Nutrient Intake
1306 Pain: Adverse Psychological Response
2102 Pain Level
1309 Personal Resilience
1635 Personal Time Management
1921 Pre-Procedure Readiness
0003 Rest
1501 Role Performance
1910 Safe Home Environment
1620 Seizure Self-Control
0305 Self-Care Behavior: Hygiene
0307 Self-Care Behavior: Non-Parenteral Medication
0309 Self-Care Behavior: Parenteral Medication
3105 Self-Management: Dysrhythmia
0119 Sexual Functioning
1207 Sexual Identity
0004 Sleep
1407 Substance Addiction Consequences
1010 Swallowing Status
1011 Swallowing Status: Esophageal Phase
1012 Swallowing Status: Oral Phase
1013 Swallowing Status: Pharyngeal Phase
1608 Symptom Control
0802 Vital Signs
1206 Will to Live

Scale Changes (n = 66)

0919 Abstract Thinking
2501 Abuse Protection
2514 Abuse Recovery
2502 Abuse Recovery: Emotional
2503 Abuse Recovery: Financial
2504 Abuse Recovery: Physical

2505 Abuse Recovery: Sexual
0200 Ambulation
0201 Ambulation: Wheelchair
1016 Bottle Feeding Establishment: Infant
1000 Breastfeeding Establishment: Infant
1001 Breastfeeding Establishment: Maternal

1002 Breastfeeding Maintenance
1003 Breastfeeding Weaning
0414 Cardiopulmonary Function
2202 Caregiver Home Care Readiness
2203 Caregiver Lifestyle Disruption
2204 Caregiver-Patient Relationship
2210 Caregiver Role Endurance
0900 Cognition
0901 Cognitive Orientation
2804 Community Disaster Readiness
2806 Community Disaster Response
2703 Community Grief Response
0905 Concentration
1018 Cup Feeding Establishment: Infant
0906 Decision-Making
0121 Development: Late Adulthood
0122 Development: Middle Adulthood
0123 Development: Young Adulthood
0311 Discharge Readiness: Independent Living
0007 Fatigue Level
0601 Fluid Balance
0602 Hydration
0204 Immobility Consequences: Physiological
0205 Immobility Consequences: Psycho-Cognitive
0707 Immune Hypersensitivity Response
0702 Immune Status
1020 Infant Nutritional Status

0907 Information Processing
0908 Memory
2512 Neglect Recovery
1008 Nutritional Status: Food & Fluid Intake
1009 Nutritional Status: Nutrient Intake
2102 Pain Level
1921 Pre-Procedure Readiness
1501 Role Performance
1934 Safe Health Care Environment
1910 Safe Home Environment
1926 Safe Wandering
0313 Self-Care Behavior
0300 Self-Care Behavior: Activities of Daily Living (ADL)
0301 Self-Care Behavior: Bathing
0302 Self-Care Behavior: Dressing
0303 Self-Care Behavior: Eating
0305 Self-Care Behavior: Hygiene
0306 Self-Care Behavior: Instrumental Activities of Daily Living (IADL)
0307 Self-Care Behavior: Non-Parenteral Medication
0308 Self-Care Behavior: Oral Hygiene
0309 Self-Care Behavior: Parenteral Medication
0310 Self-Care Behavior: Toileting
0004 Sleep
1504 Social Support
1407 Substance Addiction Consequences
2302 Systemic Toxin Clearance: Dialysis
1206 Will to Live

Revised Outcomes (n = 371)

Outcomes in this category have changes in label name, definition, or indicators

0919 Abstract Thinking
2501 Abuse Protection
2514 Abuse Recovery
2502 Abuse Recovery: Emotional
2503 Abuse Recovery: Financial
2504 Abuse Recovery: Physical
2505 Abuse Recovery: Sexual
1400 Abusive Behavior Self-Restraint
1300 Acceptance Health Status
0604 Acute Respiratory Acidosis Severity
0605 Acute Respiratory Alkalosis Severity
1308 Adaptation to Physical Disability
1600 Adherence Behavior
1621 Adherence Behavior: Healthy Diet
1632 Adherence Behavior: Prescribed Activity
1622 Adherence Behavior: Prescribed Diet

1623 Adherence Behavior: Prescribed Medication
1401 Aggression Self-Restraint
1629 Alcohol Abuse Cessation Behavior
0200 Ambulation
0201 Ambulation: Wheelchair
1211 Anxiety Level
0303 Balance
2300 Blood Glucose Control
0700 Blood Product Transfusion Reaction
1200 Body Image
1616 Body Mechanics Performance
0203 Body Positioning Self-Initiated
1016 Bottle Feeding Establishment: Infant
1017 Bottle Feeding Performance
0500 Bowel Continence
0501 Bowel Elimination

1000 Breastfeeding Establishment: Infant
1001 Breastfeeding Establishment: Maternal
1002 Breastfeeding Maintenance
1003 Breastfeeding Weaning
1106 Burn Healing
1107 Burn Recovery
0400 Cardiac Pump Effectiveness
0414 Cardiopulmonary Function
2200 Caregiver Adaptation to Patient Institutionalization
2506 Caregiver Emotional Health Status
2202 Caregiver Home Care Readiness
2203 Caregiver Lifestyle Disruption
2204 Caregiver Patient Relationship
2205 Caregiver Performance: Direct Care
2206 Caregiver Performance: Indirect Care
2507 Caregiver Physical Health Status
2210 Caregiver Role Endurance
2208 Caregiver Stressors
2508 Caregiver Well-Being
0120 Child Development: 1 Month
0100 Child Development: 2 Months
0101 Child Development: 4 Months
0102 Child Development: 6 Months
0103 Child Development: 12 Months
0104 Child Development: 2 Years
0105 Child Development: 3 Years
0106 Child Development: 4 Years
0107 Child Development: 5 Years
0401 Circulation Status
3014 Client Satisfaction
3000 Client Satisfaction: Access to Care Resources
3001 Client Satisfaction: Caring
3015 Client Satisfaction: Case Management
3002 Client Satisfaction: Communication
3003 Client Satisfaction: Continuity of Care
3004 Client Satisfaction: Cultural Needs Fulfillment
3005 Client Satisfaction: Functional Assistance
3016 Client Satisfaction: Pain Management
3006 Client Satisfaction: Physical Care
3007 Client Satisfaction: Physical Environment
3008 Client Satisfaction: Protection of Rights
3009 Client Satisfaction: Psychological Care
3010 Client Satisfaction: Safety
3011 Client Satisfaction: Symptom Control
3012 Client Satisfaction: Teaching
3013 Client Satisfaction: Technical Aspects of Care
0900 Cognition
0901 Cognitive Orientation
2008 Comfort Status
2009 Comfort Status: Environment
2010 Comfort Status: Physical
2011 Comfort Status: Psychospiritual
2012 Comfort Status: Sociocultural

0902 Communication
0903 Communication: Expressive
0904 Communication: Receptive
2700 Community Competence
2804 Community Disaster Readiness
2806 Community Disaster Response
2703 Community Grief Response
2701 Community Health Status
2800 Community Immune Status
2808 Community Program Effectiveness
2704 Community Resilience
2801 Community Risk Control: Chronic Disease
2802 Community Risk Control: Communicable Disease
0905 Concentration
1302 Coping
1018 Cup Feeding Establishment: Infant
1019 Cup Feeding Performance
0906 Decision-Making
0920 Dementia Level
1208 Depression Level
1409 Depression Self-Control
0121 Development: Late Adulthood
0122 Development: Middle Adulthood
0123 Development: Young Adulthood
1307 Dignified Life Closure
0311 Discharge Readiness: Independent Living
0312 Discharge Readiness: Supported Living
2109 Discomfort Level
1630 Drug Abuse Cessation Behavior
0600 Electrolyte & Acid/Base Balance
1919 Elopement Occurrence
1920 Elopement Propensity Risk
0001 Endurance
1909 Fall Prevention Behavior
1912 Falls Occurrence
2600 Family Coping
2602 Family Functioning
2606 Family Health Status
2603 Family Integrity
2604 Family Normalization
2605 Family Participation in Professional Care
2608 Family Resilience
0008 Fatigue: Disruptive Effects
0007 Fatigue Level
1210 Fear Level
0111 Fetal Status: Antepartum
0112 Fetal Status: Intrapartum
0601 Fluid Balance
0603 Fluid Overload Severity
1304 Grief Resolution
1700 Health Beliefs
1701 Health Beliefs: Perceived Ability to Perform
1703 Health Beliefs: Perceived Resources

1704 Health Beliefs: Perceived Threat
1602 Health Promoting Behavior
1610 Hearing Compensation Behavior
0602 Hydration
0915 Hyperactivity Level
2111 Hyperglycemia Severity
0610 Hypermagnesemia Severity
0611 Hypernatremia Severity
0612 Hyperphosphatemia Severity
0613 Hypocalcemia Severity
0614 Hypochloremia Severity
2113 Hypoglycemia Severity
0616 Hypomagnesemia Severity
0617 Hyponatremia Severity
0618 Hypophosphatemia Severity
0204 Immobility Consequences: Physiological
0205 Immobility Consequences: Psycho-Cognitive
0707 Immune Hypersensitivity Response
0702 Immune Status
1405 Impulse Self-Control
1020 Infant Nutritional Status
0907 Information Processing
1844 Knowledge: Acute Illness Management
1845 Knowledge: Anticoagulation Therapy Management
1831 Knowledge: Arthritis Management
1832 Knowledge: Asthma Management
1827 Knowledge: Body Mechanics
1846 Knowledge: Bottle Feeding
1800 Knowledge: Breastfeeding
1833 Knowledge: Cancer Management
1830 Knowledge: Cardiac Disease Management
1801 Knowledge: Child Physical Safety
3204 Knowledge: Chronic Anemia Management
1847 Knowledge: Chronic Disease Management
1848 Knowledge: Chronic Obstructive Pulmonary Management
1821 Knowledge: Conception Prevention
1849 Knowledge: Coronary Artery Disease Management
1850 Knowledge: Cup Feeding
1851 Knowledge: Dementia Management
1836 Knowledge: Depression Management
1820 Knowledge: Diabetes Management
1803 Knowledge: Disease Management
1852 Knowledge: Dysrhythmia Management
1853 Knowledge: Eating Disorder Management
1804 Knowledge: Energy Conservation
1828 Knowledge: Fall Prevention
1816 Knowledge: Fertility Promotion
1805 Knowledge: Health Behavior
1806 Knowledge: Health Resources
1855 Knowledge: Healthy Lifestyle

1835 Knowledge: Heart Failure Management
3206 Knowledge: Human Immunodeficiency Virus Management
1837 Knowledge: Hypertension Management
1819 Knowledge: Infant Care
1856 Knowledge: Inflammatory Bowel Disease Management
1857 Knowledge: Kidney Disease Management
1817 Knowledge: Labor & Delivery
1858 Knowledge: Lipid Disorder Management
3207 Knowledge: Lymphedema Management
1808 Knowledge: Medication
1838 Knowledge: Multiple Sclerosis Management
1859 Knowledge: Osteoporosis Management
1829 Knowledge: Ostomy Care
1843 Knowledge: Pain Management
1826 Knowledge: Parenting
1809 Knowledge: Personal Safety
1861 Knowledge: Pneumonia Management
1818 Knowledge: Postpartum Maternal Health
1822 Knowledge: Preconception Maternal Health
1810 Knowledge: Pregnancy
1839 Knowledge: Pregnancy & Postpartum Sexual Function
1811 Knowledge: Prescribed Activity
1802 Knowledge: Prescribed Diet
1840 Knowledge: Preterm Infant Care
1815 Knowledge: Sexual Function
1862 Knowledge: Stress Management
1864 Knowledge: Stroke Management
1812 Knowledge: Substance Use Control
1866 Knowledge: Time Management
1814 Knowledge: Treatment Procedure
1813 Knowledge: Treatment Regimen
1841 Knowledge: Weight Management
1604 Leisure Participation
1203 Loneliness Severity
2509 Maternal Status: Antepartum
2510 Maternal Status: Intrapartum
2511 Maternal Status: Postpartum
0411 Mechanical Ventilation Response: Adult
0412 Mechanical Ventilation Weaning Response: Adult
2301 Medication Response
0908 Memory
0619 Metabolic Acidosis Severity
0620 Metabolic Alkalosis Severity
0208 Mobility
1204 Mood Equilibrium
1209 Motivation
2106 Nausea & Vomiting: Disruptive Effects
1620 Nausea & Vomiting Severity
2513 Neglect Cessation

2512 Neglect Recovery
0909 Neurological Function
0910 Neurological Function: Autonomic
0911 Neurological Function: Central Motor Control
0912 Neurological Function: Consciousness
0913 Neurological Function: Cranial Sensory/Motor
0917 Neurological Function: Peripheral
0914 Neurological Function: Spinal Sensory/Motor
0118 Newborn Adaptation
1004 Nutritional Status
1005 Nutritional Status: Biochemical Measures
1007 Nutritional Status: Energy
1008 Nutritional Status: Food & Fluid Intake
1009 Nutritional Status: Nutrient Intake
1306 Pain: Adverse Psychological Response
1605 Pain Control
2101 Pain: Disruptive Effects
2102 Pain Level
1500 Parent-Infant Attachment
2211 Parenting Performance
2903 Parenting Performance: Adolescent
2902 Parenting Performance: Adolescent Physical Safety
2901 Parenting Performance: Early/Middle Childhood Physical Safety
2904 Parenting Performance: Infant
2905 Parenting Performance: Middle Childhood
2906 Parenting Performance: Preschooler
2907 Parenting Performance: Toddler
1606 Participation in Health Care Decisions
1638 Patient Engagement Behavior
2104 Perimenopause Symptom Severity
2006 Personal Health Status
1309 Personal Resilience
1911 Personal Safety Behavior
1635 Personal Time Management
2002 Personal Well-Being
0113 Physical Aging
0114 Physical Maturation: Female
0115 Physical Maturation: Male
1624 Postpartum Maternal Health Behavior
2303 Post-Procedure Recovery
2105 Premenstrual Syndrome (PMS) Severity
1921 Pre-Procedure Readiness
0006 Psychomotor Energy
2000 Quality of Life
1311 Relocation Adaptation
0415 Respiratory Function
0410 Respiratory Function: Airway Patency

0402 Respiratory Function: Gas Exchange
0403 Respiratory Function: Ventilation
0003 Rest
1903 Risk Control: Alcohol Use
1917 Risk Control: Cancer
1914 Risk Control: Cardiovascular Disease
1904 Risk Control: Drug Use
1915 Risk Control: Hearing Impairment
1923 Risk Control: Hypothermia
1924 Risk Control: Infectious Process
1905 Risk Control: Sexually Transmitted Diseases (STDs)
1925 Risk Control: Sun Exposure
1906 Risk Control: Tobacco Use
1916 Risk Control: Visual Impairment
1908 Risk Detection
1501 Role Performance
1934 Safe Health Care Environment
1910 Safe Home Environment
1926 Safe Wandering
1620 Seizure: Self Control
1215 Self-Awareness
0313 Self-Care Behavior
0300 Self-Care Behavior: Activities of Daily Living (ADL)
0301 Self-Care Behavior: Bathing
0302 Self-Care Behavior: Dressing
0303 Self-Care Behavior: Eating
0305 Self-Care Behavior: Hygiene
0306 Self-Care Behavior: Instrumental Activities of Daily Living (IADL)
0307 Self-Care Behavior: Non-Parenteral Medication
0308 Self-Care Behavior: Oral Hygiene
0309 Self-Care Behavior: Parenteral Medication
0310 Self-Care Behavior: Toileting
1613 Self-Direction of Care
1205 Self-Esteem
3100 Self-Management: Acute Illness
3101 Self-Management: Anticoagulation Therapy
0704 Self-Management: Asthma
1617 Self-Management: Cardiac Disease
3116 Self-Management: Chronic Anemia
3102 Self-Management: Chronic Disease
3103 Self-Management: Chronic Obstructive Pulmonary Disease
3104 Self-Management: Coronary Artery Disease
1619 Self-Management: Diabetes
3105 Self-Management: Dysrhythmia
3106 Self-Management: Heart Failure
3117 Self-Management: Human Immunodeficiency Virus

3107 Self-Management: Hypertension
3118 Self-Management: Infection
3119 Self-Management: Inflammatory Bowel Disease
1857 Self-Management: Kidney Disease
3109 Self-Management: Lipid Disease
3121 Self-Management: Lymphedema
1631 Self-Management: Multiple Sclerosis
1615 Self-Management: Ostomy
3122 Self-Management Pneumonia
3123 Self-Management Stroke
0119 Sexual Functioning
1207 Sexual Identity
0004 Sleep
1625 Smoking Cessation Behavior
1504 Social Support
1407 Substance Addiction Consequences
2108 Substance Withdrawal Severity
1408 Suicide Self-Restraint
1010 Swallowing Status
1011 Swallowing Status: Esophageal Phase

1012 Swallowing Status: Oral Phase
1013 Swallowing Status: Pharyngeal Phase
1608 Symptom Control
2103 Symptom Severity
2302 Systemic Toxin Clearance: Dialysis
0800 Thermoregulation
1101 Tissue Integrity: Skin & Mucous Membranes
0404 Tissue Perfusion: Abdominal Organs
0405 Tissue Perfusion: Cardiac
0416 Tissue Perfusion: Cellular
0406 Tissue Perfusion: Cerebral
0407 Tissue Perfusion: Peripheral
0408 Tissue Perfusion: Pulmonary
0210 Transfer Performance
0502 Urinary Continence
0503 Urinary Elimination
0802 Vital Signs
1626 Weight Gain Behavior
1627 Weight Loss Behavior
1628 Weight Maintenance Behavior
1206 Will to Live

Reviewed Outcomes (n = 28)

Outcomes in this category have been reviewed with updated literature but no changes to the outcome

0606 Electrolyte Balance
1702 Health Beliefs: Perceived Control
0607 Hypercalcemia Severity
0608 Hyperchloremia Severity
0609 Hyperkalemia Severity
0615 Hypokalemia Severity
1834 Knowledge: Cancer Threat Reduction
1854 Knowledge: Healthy Diet
1842 Knowledge: Infection Management
1860 Knowledge: Peripheral Artery Disease Management
0803 Liver Function
1100 Oral Health
2115 Peripheral Artery Disease Severity
1634 Personal Health Screening Behavior

1902 Risk Control
1927 Risk Control: Dry Eye
1939 Risk Control: Falls
1928 Risk Control: Hypertension
1922 Risk Control: Hyperthermia
1933 Risk Control: Hypotension
1940 Risk Control: Infant Allergies
1929 Risk Control: Lipid Disorder
1941 Risk Control: Obesity
1930 Risk Control: Osteoporosis
1931 Risk Control: Stroke
1907 Risk Control: Unintended Pregnancy
3124 Self-Management: Wound
0422 Tissue Perfusion

Outcomes in the Sixth Edition that were Retired for this Edition (n = 10)

1301 Child Adaptation to Hospitalization
0109 Child Development: Adolescence
0108 Child Development: Middle Childhood
2007 Comfortable Death
1601 Compliance Behavior

1213 Fear Level: Child
1406 Mutilation Self-Restraint
2900 Parenting Performance: Infant/Toddler Safety
1901 Parenting Performance: Psychosocial Safety
2403 Sensory Function: Taste & Smell

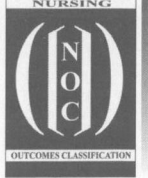

Previous Editions and Translations

Iowa Outcomes Project, Johnson, M., & Maas, M. (Eds.). (1997). *Nursing outcomes classification (NOC).* Mosby-Year Book. (190 outcomes)

    Translated into Dutch, 1999: Elsevier/Tijidstroom

    Translated into French, 1999: Masson

    Translated into Japanese, 1999: Igaku-Shoin MYW

    Translated into Korean, 1999: Hyun Moon Sa

Iowa Outcomes Project, Johnson, M., Maas, M., & Moorhead, S. (Eds.). (2000). *Nursing outcomes classification (NOC)* (2nd ed.). Mosby. (260 outcomes)

    Translated into German, 2005: Verlag Hans Huber

    Translated into Japanese, 2003: Igaku-Shoin MYW

    Translated into Portuguese, 2004: Artmed Editora

    Translated into Spanish, 2001: Ediciones Harcourt

Moorhead, S., Johnson, M., & Maas, M. (Eds.). (2004). *Nursing outcomes classification (NOC)* (3rd ed.). Mosby. (330 outcomes)

    Translated into Chinese (Simplified), 2005: Peking University Medical Press/ Elsevier (Singapore)

    Translated into Italian, 2007: Casa Editrice Ambrosiana

    Translated into Japanese, 2005: Igaku-Shoin MYW

    Translated into Norwegian, 2007: Akribe

    Translated into Portuguese, 2008: Artmed Editora

    Translated into Spanish, 2008: Elsevier España

Moorhead, S., Johnson, M., Maas, M. L., & Swanson, E. (Eds.). (2008). *Nursing outcomes classification (NOC)* (4th ed.). Mosby/Elsevier. (385 outcomes)

    Translated into Chinese (Traditional), 2011: Elsevier Taiwan

    Translated into Dutch, 2011: Reed Business

    Translated into German, 2013: Verlag Hans Huber

    Translated into Japanese, 2010: Igaku-Shoin

    Translated into Portuguese, 2010: Elsevier Editora

    Translated into Spanish, 2009: Elsevier España

Moorhead, S., Johnson, M., Maas, M. L., & Swanson, E. (Eds.). (2013). *Nursing outcomes classification (NOC): Measurement of health outcomes* (5th ed.). Elsevier Mosby. (490 outcomes)

    Translated into Dutch, 2016: Bohn Stafleu van Loghum

Translated into French, 2014: Elsevier Masson

Translated into Indonesian, 2016: CV. Mocomedia/Elsevier Singapore

Translated into Italian, 2013: Casa Editrice Ambrosiana

Translated into Japanese, 2015: Elsevier Japan

Translated into Portuguese, 2016: Elsevier Editora

Translated into Spanish, 2014: Elsevier España

Moorhead, S., Swanson, E., Johnson, M., & Maas, M., (Eds.). (2018). *Nursing outcomes classification (NOC): Measurement of health outcomes* (6th ed.). Elsevier Mosby. (540 outcomes)

    Translated into Dutch, 2020: Bohn Stafleu van Loghum

    Translated into Indonesian, 2018: CV. Mocomedia/Elsevier Singapore

    Translated into Italian, 2020: Casa Editrice Ambrosiana

    Translated into Japanese, 2018: Elsevier Japan

    Translated into Portuguese, 2020: GEN Guanabara Koogan

    Translated into Spanish, 2018: Elsevier Espanā

LINKAGE BOOKS

Johnson, M., Bulechek, G., Dochterman, J. M., Maas, M., & Moorhead, S. (Eds.). (2001). *Nursing diagnoses, outcomes, and interventions: NANDA, NOC, & NIC linkages.* Mosby.

    Translated into Chinese (Traditional), 2003: Tsan-Hai Book/Elsevier (Singapore)

    Translated into German, 2007: Verlog Hans Huber

    Translated into Italian, 2005: Casa Editrice Ambrosiana

    Translated into Japanese, 2002: Igaku-Shoin

    Translated into Portuguese, 2005: Artmed Editora

    Translated into Spanish, 2002: Ediciones Harcourt

Johnson, M., Bulechek, G., Butcher, H., Dochterman, J. M., Maas, M., Moorhead, S., & Swanson, E. (Eds.) (2006). *NANDA, NOC, & NIC linkages: Nursing diagnoses, outcomes, and interventions* (2nd ed.). Mosby.

    Translated into Chinese (Simplified), 2009: Peking University Medical Press/Elsevier (Singapore)

    Translated into Japanese, 2006: Igaku-Shoin

    Translated into Portuguese, 2009: Artmed Editora

    Translated into Spanish, 2007: Elsevier España

Johnson, M., Moorhead, S., Bulechek, G., Butcher, H., Maas, M., & Swanson, E. (2012). *NOC and NIC linkages to NANDA-I and clinical conditions: Supporting critical reasoning and quality care* (3rd ed.). Elsevier Mosby.

    Translated into Italian, 2014: Casa Editrice Ambrosiana
    Translated into Portuguese, 2013: Elsevier Editora
    Translated into Spanish, 2012: Elsevier España
    Translated into Spanish, 2012: Elsevier Espanã

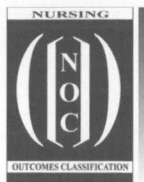

APPENDIX C

Breakdown of Outcomes for Each Measurement Scale in NOC

OUTCOMES WITH ONE MEASUREMENT SCALE

01 Compromised Scale		*n* = 24
Severely Compromised to Not Compromised		
Activity Tolerance	Communication: Expressive	Physical Fitness
Appetite	Communication: Receptive	Preterm Infant Organization
Body Positioning: Self-Initiated	Coordinated Movement	Rest
Caregiver Physical Health Status	Fluid Balance	Sensory Function
Comfort Status	Hydration	Skeletal Function
Comfort Status: Environment	Immune Status	Sleep
Comfort Status: Sociocultural	Mobility	Spiritual Health
Communication	Personal Health Status	Transfer Performance

02 Deviation Scale		*n* = 31
Severe Deviation to No Deviation from Normal Range		
Blood Glucose Control	Joint Movement: Knee	Nutritional Status: Food & Fluid
Electrolyte Balance	Joint Movement: Neck	Intake
Fetal Status: Antepartum	Joint Movement: Passive	Nutritional Status: Nutrient Intake
Fetal Status: Intrapartum	Joint Movement: Shoulder	Physical Aging
Growth	Joint Movement: Spine	Physical Maturation: Female
Infant Nutritional Status	Joint Movement: Wrist	Physical Maturation: Male
Joint Movement	Metabolic Function	Systemic Toxin Clearance:
Joint Movement: Ankle	Newborn Adaptation	Dialysis
Joint Movement: Elbow	Nutritional Status	Tissue Perfusion
Joint Movement: Fingers	Nutritional Status: Biochemical Measures	Vital Signs
Joint Movement: Hip	Nutritional Status: Energy	Weight: Body Mass

07 Occurrence Scale		*n* = 2
10 and Over to None		
Elopement Occurrence	Falls Occurrence	

09 Range Scale		*n* = 3
None to Extensive		
Abuse Cessation	Neglect Cessation	Social Support

11 Positive Scale		*n* = 2
Never Positive to Consistently Positive		
Body Image	Self-Esteem	

12 Strength Scale		*n* = 6
Very Weak to Very Strong		
Health Beliefs	Health Beliefs: Perceived Control	Health Beliefs: Perceived Threat
Health Beliefs: Perceived Ability to Perform	Health Beliefs: Perceived Resources	Health Orientation

13 Demonstrated Scale $n = 251$

Never Demonstrated to Consistently Demonstrated

Abstract Thinking
Abuse Protection
Abuse Recovery
Abuse Recovery: Emotional
Abuse Recovery: Financial
Abuse Recovery: Physical
Abuse Recovery: Sexual
Abusive Behavior Self-Restraint
Acceptance: Health Status
Adaptation to Physical Disability
Adherence Behavior
Adherence Behavior: Clinical Condition
Adherence Behavior: Healthy Diet
Adherence Behavior: Prescribed Activity
Adherence Behavior: Prescribed Diet
Adherence Behavior: Prescribed Medication
Aggression Self-Restraint
Alcohol Abuse Cessation Behavior
Ambulation
Ambulation: Wheelchair
Anger Self-Restraint
Anxiety Self-Control
Body Mechanics Performance
Bottle Feeding Establishment: Infant
Bottle Feeding Performance
Breastfeeding Establishment: Infant
Breastfeeding Establishment: Maternal
Breastfeeding Maintenance
Breastfeeding Weaning
Cardiac Rehabilitation Participation
Caregiver Adaptation to Patient
    Institutionalization
Caregiver Home Care Readiness
Caregiver-Patient Relationship
Caregiver Performance: Direct Care
Caregiver Performance: Indirect Care
Caregiver Role Endurance
Child Development: 1 Month
Child Development: 2 Months
Child Development: 4 Months
Child Development: 6 Months
Child Development: 9 Months
Child Development: 12 Months
Child Development: 18 Months
Child Development: 2 Years
Child Development: 3 Years
Child Development: 4 Years
Child Development: 5 Years

Child Development: 6–7 Years
Child Development: 8–10 Years
Child Development: Early
    Adolescence
Child Development: Late
    Adolescence
Child Development: Middle
    Adolescence
Childhood Bullying Recovery
Cognition
Cognitive Orientation
Concentration
Coping
Cup Feeding Establishment:
    Infant
Cup Feeding Performance
Decision-Making
Depression Self-Control
Development: Established
    Adulthood
Development: Late Adulthood
Development: Middle Adulthood
Development: Young Adulthood
Digital Literacy Behavior
Dignified Life Closure
Discharge Readiness: Independent
    Living
Discharge Readiness: Supported
    Living
Distorted Thought Self-Control
Drug Abuse Cessation Behavior
Elopement Propensity Risk
Energy Conservation
Exercise Participation
Fall Prevention Behavior
Family Coping
Family Functioning
Family Integrity
Family Normalization
Family Normalization: Autism
    Spectrum Disorder
Family Normalization: Dementia
Family Participation in
    Professional Care
Family Performance: Dementia Care
Family Resilience
Family Risk Control: Bullying
Family Risk Control: Elopement

Family Risk Control: Household
    Food Insecurity
Family Risk Control: Obesity
Family Risk Control: Violence
Family Social Climate
Family Social Network Support
Family Support During Treatment
Fear Self-Control
Financial Literacy Behavior
Gender Identity
Grief Resolution
Group Therapy Participation
Guilt Resolution
Health Insurance Literacy
    Behavior
Health Literacy Behavior
Health Promoting Behavior
Health Seeking Behavior
Hearing Compensation Behavior
Heedfulness of Affected Side
Hoarding Cessation Behavior
Hope
Immunization Behavior
Impulse Self-Control
Information Processing
Leisure Participation
Lifestyle Balance
Memory
Motivation
Musculoskeletal Rehabilitation
    Participation
Nausea & Vomiting Control
Neglect Recovery
Pain Control
Panic Self-Control
Parent Adaptation to Infant
    Hospitalization
Parent Adaptation to Toddler
    Hospitalization
Parent-Infant Attachment
Parenting Performance
Parenting Performance:
    Adolescent
Parenting Performance:
    Adolescent Physical Safety
Parenting Performance: Attention
    Deficit Hyperactivity Disorder
    (ADHD)

Parenting Performance: Early Childhood Psychosocial Safety
Parenting Performance: Early/Middle Childhood Physical Safety
Parenting Performance: Infant
Parenting Performance: Infant Physical Safety
Parenting Performance: Infant Psychosocial Safety
Parenting Performance: Middle Childhood
Parenting Performance: Preschooler
Parenting Performance: School Age Child Psychosocial Safety
Parenting Performance: Toddler
Parenting Performance: Toddler Physical Safety
Participation in Health Care Decisions
Patient Engagement Behavior
Personal Autonomy
Personal Health Screening Behavior
Personal Identity
Personal Resilience
Personal Safety Behavior
Personal Time Management
Play Participation
Postpartum Maternal Health Behavior
Prenatal Health Behavior
Pre-Procedure Readiness
Psychosocial Adjustment: Life Change
Risk Control
Risk Control: Alcohol Use
Risk Control: Aspiration
Risk Control: Cancer
Risk Control: Cardiovascular Disease
Risk Control: Child Bullying
Risk Control: Dehydration
Risk Control: Drug Use
Risk Control: Dry Eye
Risk Control: Environmental Hazards
Risk Control: Falls
Risk Control: Food Insecurity
Risk Control: Hearing Impairment
Risk Control: Housing Insecurity
Risk Control: Hypertension
Risk Control: Hyperthermia
Risk Control: Hypotension
Risk Control: Hypothermia
Risk Control: Infant Allergies
Risk Control: Infectious Process
Risk Control: Lipid Disorder
Risk Control: Obesity
Risk Control: Osteoporosis

Risk Control: Prediabetes
Risk Control: Pressure Injury
Risk Control: Problematic Internet Use
Risk Control: Sexually Transmitted Diseases (STD)
Risk Control: Stroke
Risk Control: Sun Exposure
Risk Control: Thrombus
Risk Control: Tobacco Use
Risk Control: Unintended Pregnancy
Risk Control: Visual Impairment
Risk Control: Voice Disorder
Risk Detection
Role Performance
Safe Wandering
Seizure Self-Control
Self-Awareness
Self-Care Behavior
Self-Care Behavior: Activities of Daily Living (ADL)
Self-Care Behavior: Bathing
Self-Care Behavior: Dressing
Self-Care Behavior: Eating
Self-Care Behavior: Feet
Self-Care Behavior: Hygiene
Self-Care Behavior: Instrumental Activities of Daily Living (IADL)
Self-Care Behavior Non-Parenteral Medication
Self-Care Behavior: Oral Hygiene
Self-Care Behavior: Parenteral Medication
Self-Care Behavior: Toileting
Self-Direction of Care
Self-Direction of Instrumental Activities of Daily Living
Self-Harm Restraint
Self-Management: Acute Illness
Self-Management: Anticoagulation Therapy
Self-Management: Arthritis
Self-Management: Asthma
Self-Management: Autism Spectrum Disorder
Self-Management: Cancer
Self-Management: Cardiac Disease
Self-Management: Celiac Disease
Self-Management: Chronic Anemia

Self-Management: Chronic Disease
Self-Management: Chronic Obstructive Pulmonary Disease
Self-Management: Coronary Artery Disease
Self-Management: Diabetes
Self-Management: Dysrhythmia
Self-Management: Heart Failure
Self-Management: Human Immunodeficiency Virus
Self-Management: Hypertension
Self-Management: Infection
Self-Management: Inflammatory Bowel Disease
Self-Management: Kidney Disease
Self-Management: Kidney Failure
Self-Management: Known Allergy
Self-Management: Lipid Disorder
Self-Management: Liver Disease
Self-Management: Lymphedema
Self-Management: Multiple Sclerosis
Self-Management: Osteoporosis
Self-Management: Ostomy
Self-Management: Parkinson Disease
Self-Management: Peripheral Artery Disease
Self-Management: Pneumonia
Self-Management: Stroke
Self-Management: Treatment Procedure
Self-Management: Treatment Regimen
Self-Management: Wound
Sexual Functioning
Sexual Identity
Sleep Enhancement Behavior
Smoking Cessation Behavior
Social Identity
Social Interaction Skills
Social Involvement
Successful Aging
Suicide Self-Restraint
Symptom Control
Vision Compensation Behavior
Weight Gain Behavior
Weight Loss Behavior
Weight Maintenance Behavior

14 Severity Scale   *n* = 80

Severe to None

Abuse: Disruptive Effects
Acute Respiratory Acidosis Severity
Acute Respiratory Alkalosis Severity
Agitation Level
Allergic Response: Localized
Allergic Response: Systemic
Anxiety Level
Attention Deficit Level
Blood Loss Severity
Blood Transfusion Product Reaction
Caregiver Lifestyle Disruption
Caregiver Stressors
Chemotherapy: Disruptive Physical Effects
Dehydration Severity
Delirium Level
Dementia Level
Depression Level
Discomfort Level
Dry Eye Severity
Fatigue: Disruptive Effects
Fatigue Level
Fear Level
Fear Level: Adolescent
Fear Level: Middle Childhood
Fear Level: Preschooler
Fluid Overload Severity
Hemodialysis: Disruptive Effects
Hoarding Behavior Severity
Hyperactivity Level

Hypercalcemia Severity
Hyperchloremia Severity
Hyperglycemia Severity
Hyperkalemia Severity
Hypermagnesemia Severity
Hypernatremia Severity
Hyperphosphatemia Severity
Hypertension Severity
Hypocalcemia Severity
Hypochloremia Severity
Hypoglycemia Severity
Hypokalemia Severity
Hypomagnesemia Severity
Hyponatremia Severity
Hypophosphatemia Severity
Hypotension Severity
Immobility Consequences: Physiological
Immobility Consequences: Psycho-Cognitive
Immune Hypersensitivity Response
Infection Severity
Infection Severity: Newborn
Loneliness Severity
Lymphedema Severity
Metabolic Acidosis Severity
Metabolic Alkalosis Severity
Nausea & Vomiting: Disruptive Effects

Nausea & Vomiting Severity
Neglect: Disruptive Effects
Pain: Adverse Psychological Response
Pain: Disruptive Effects
Pain Level
Panic Level
Perimenopause Symptom Severity
Peripheral Artery Disease Severity
Peritoneal Dialysis: Disruptive Effects
Physical Injury Severity
Premenstrual Syndrome (PMS) Severity
Seizure Severity
Shock Severity: Anaphylactic
Shock Severity: Cardiogenic
Shock Severity: Hypovolemic
Shock Severity: Neurogenic
Shock Severity: Septic
Sleep Disruption Severity
Social Anxiety Level
Stress Level
Substance Addiction Consequences
Substance Withdrawal Severity
Suffering Severity
Symptom Severity
Tissue Injury Severity: Percutaneous Procedure

17 Excellence Scale   *n* = 31

Poor to Excellent

Community Competence
Community Disaster Readiness
Community Disaster Recovery
Community Disaster Response
Community Grief Recovery
Community Grief Response
Community Health Screening Effectiveness
Community Health Status
Community Immune Status
Community Immune Status: Adult
Community Immune Status: School Age Child
Community Immune Status: Young Child

Community Immunity Effectiveness
Community Pandemic Readiness
Community Pandemic Recovery
Community Pandemic Response
Community Program Effectiveness
Community Resilience
Community Risk Control: Bullying
Community Risk Control: Chronic Disease
Community Risk Control: Communicable Disease
Community Risk Control: Environmental Hazards

Community Risk Control: Lead Exposure
Community Risk Control: Obesity
Community Risk Control: Suicide
Community Risk Control: Unhealthy Cultural Traditions
Community Risk Control: Violence
Community Violence Level
Safe Health Care Environment
Safe Home Environment
Safe Home Environment: Nursery

18 Satisfaction Scale $n = 24$

Not at all Satisfied to Completely Satisfied

Caregiver Well-Being
Client Satisfaction
Client Satisfaction: Access to Care
Resources
Client Satisfaction: Acute Care
Transition Process
Client Satisfaction: Caring
Client Satisfaction: Case Management
Client Satisfaction: Communication
Client Satisfaction: Continuity of Care

Client Satisfaction: Cultural Needs
Fulfillment
Client Satisfaction: Discharge Process
Client Satisfaction: Functional Assistance
Client Satisfaction: Labor & Delivery
Client Satisfaction: Pain Management
Client Satisfaction: Physical Care
Client Satisfaction: Physical Environment
Client Satisfaction: Protection of Rights
Client Satisfaction: Psychological Care

Client Satisfaction: Safety
Client Satisfaction: Symptom
Control
Client Satisfaction: Teaching
Client Satisfaction: Technical
Aspects of Care
Client Satisfaction: Telehealth
Services
Personal Well-Being
Quality of Life

20 Knowledge Scale $n = 82$

No Knowledge to Extensive Knowledge

Knowledge: Acute Illness Management
Knowledge: Allergy Management
Knowledge: Anticoagulation Therapy
Management
Knowledge: Anxiety Management
Knowledge: Arthritis Management
Knowledge: Asthma Management
Knowledge: Attention Deficit
Hyperactivity Disorder (ADHD)
Management
Knowledge: Autism Spectrum Disorder
Management
Knowledge: Body Mechanics
Knowledge: Bottle Feeding
Knowledge: Breastfeeding
Knowledge: Cancer Management
Knowledge: Cancer Threat Reduction
Knowledge: Cardiac Disease Management
Knowledge: Cardiac Rehabilitation
Knowledge: Celiac Disease
Management
Knowledge: Child Physical Safety
Knowledge: Chronic Anemia
Management
Knowledge: Chronic Disease
Management
Knowledge: Chronic Obstructive
Pulmonary Disease Management
Knowledge: Community Health Resources
Knowledge: Conception Prevention
Knowledge: Coronary Artery Disease
Management
Knowledge: Cup Feeding
Knowledge: Dementia Management
Knowledge: Depression Management
Knowledge: Diabetes Management

Knowledge: Diagnostic & Therapeutic
Procedures
Knowledge: Disease Management
Knowledge: Dysrhythmia Management
Knowledge: Eating Disorder Management
Knowledge: Energy Conservation
Knowledge: Epilepsy Management
Knowledge: Fall Prevention
Knowledge: Fertility Promotion
Knowledge: Foot Care
Knowledge: Health Behavior
Knowledge: Health Resources
Knowledge: Healthy Diet
Knowledge: Healthy Lifestyle
Knowledge: Heart Failure Management
Knowledge: Human Immunodeficiency
Virus Management
Knowledge: Hypertension Management
Knowledge: Infant Care
Knowledge: Infection Management
Knowledge: Inflammatory Bowel Disease
Management
Knowledge: Kidney Disease Management
Knowledge: Kidney Failure Management
Knowledge: Labor & Delivery
Knowledge: Lipid Disorder Management
Knowledge: Liver Disease Management
Knowledge: Lymphedema Management
Knowledge: Medication
Knowledge: Multiple Sclerosis
Management
Knowledge: Musculoskeletal
Rehabilitation

Knowledge: Osteoporosis
Management
Knowledge: Ostomy Care
Knowledge: Pain Management
Knowledge: Parenting
Knowledge: Parkinson Disease
Management
Knowledge: Peripheral Artery
Disease Management
Knowledge: Personal Safety
Knowledge: Pneumonia
Management
Knowledge: Postpartum Maternal
Health
Knowledge: Preconception Maternal
Health
Knowledge: Pregnancy
Knowledge: Pregnancy &
Postpartum Sexual Functioning
Knowledge: Prescribed Activity
Knowledge: Prescribed Diet
Knowledge: Preterm Infant Care
Knowledge: School Age Child
Psychosocial Safety
Knowledge: Sexual Function
Knowledge: Stress Management
Knowledge: Stroke Management
Knowledge: Stroke Threat Reduction
Knowledge: Substance Use Control
Knowledge: Thrombus Threat
Reduction
Knowledge: Time Management
Knowledge: Treatment Procedure
Knowledge: Treatment Regimen
Knowledge: Weight Management
Knowledge: Wound Management

OUTCOMES WITH COMBINATION MEASUREMENT SCALES

21 Compromised Scale & Severity Scale   *n* = 39

Severely Compromised to Not Compromised
Severe to None

Balance	Medication Response	Sensory Function: Smell
Bowel Elimination	Neurological Function	Sensory Function: Tactile
Cardiopulmonary Function	Neurological Function: Autonomic	Sensory Function: Taste
Caregiver Emotional Health Status	Neurological Function: Central	Sensory Function: Vision
Comfort Status: Physical	Motor Control	Student Health Status
Comfort Status: Psychospiritual	Neurological Function:	Swallowing Status
Endurance	Consciousness	Swallowing Status: Esophageal Phase
Family Health Status	Neurological Function: Cranial	Swallowing Status: Oral Phase
Foot Health	Sensory/Motor	Swallowing Status: Pharyngeal Phase
Gait	Neurological Function: Peripheral	Thermoregulation
Gastrointestinal Function	Neurological Function: Spinal	Thermoregulation: Newborn
Hemodialysis Access	Sensory/Motor	Tissue Integrity: Skin & Mucous
Kidney Function	Oral Health	Membranes
Liver Function	Sensory Function: Hearing	Urinary Elimination
	Sensory Function: Proprioception	Vocal Function

22 Deviation Scale & Severity Scale   *n* = 22

Severe to No Deviation from Normal Range
Severe to None

Blood Coagulation	Mechanical Ventilation Weaning	Surgical Recovery: Immediate Post-
Cardiac Pump Effectiveness	Response: Adult	Operative
Circulation Status	Post-Procedure Recovery	Tissue Perfusion: Abdominal Organs
Electrolyte & Acid/Base Balance	Respiratory Function	Tissue Perfusion: Cardiac
Maternal Status: Antepartum	Respiratory Function: Airway Patency	Tissue Perfusion: Cellular
Maternal Status: Intrapartum	Respiratory Function: Gas Exchange	Tissue Perfusion: Cerebral
Maternal Status: Postpartum	Respiratory Function: Ventilation	Tissue Perfusion: Peripheral
Mechanical Ventilation Response: Adult	Surgical Recovery: Convalescence	Tissue Perfusion: Pulmonary

23 Range & Reversed Range Scale   *n* = 5

None to Extensive
Extensive to None

Bone Healing	Burn Healing	Wound Healing: Primary Intention
	Burn Recovery	Wound Healing: Secondary Intention

24 Demonstrated & Reversed Demonstrated Scale   *n* = 10

Never Demonstrated to Consistently Demonstrated
Consistently Demonstrated to Never Demonstrated

Adaptation to Hospitalization: Adolescent	Bowel Continence	Psychomotor Energy
Adaptation to Hospitalization: Middle Childhood	Eating Disorder Self-Control	Relocation Adaptation
Adaptation to Hospitalization: Preschooler	Mood Equilibrium	Urinary Continence
		Will to Live

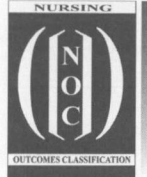

Timeline and Highlights of the Nursing Outcomes Classification

1991

Nursing Outcomes research team is established by Marion Johnson and Meridean Maas at the University of Iowa.

1992

Nursing Outcomes Classification (NOC) pilot work funded by Sigma Theta Tau International with Marion Johnson and Meridean Maas as the principal investigators.

1993

The first *Nursing Interventions Classification (NIC) Newsletter* published at the University of Iowa (later changed to *The NIC Letter* then to *The NIC/NOC Letter*).

NOC with Marion Johnson and Meridean Maas as the co-principal investigators is funded by Nursing Institute of Nursing Research (NINR) (Dec 1993–1997; extended to 1998).

1994

An institutional effectiveness grant for preparing pre- and post-doctoral students in effectiveness research with Joanne McCloskey and Meridean Maas, directors is funded at Iowa by NINR.

The Nursing Classifications Fund is established at the University of Iowa to provide ongoing financial support for the continued development and use of NIC and NOC.

The first publication about the *Nursing Outcomes Classification (*NOC) appears in print in *Current Issues in Nursing* (4th ed., pp. 136–142) published by Mosby.

1995

The Center for Nursing Classification (CNC) at the University of Iowa is approved (December 13) by the Iowa Board of Regents (without funding) to facilitate the ongoing research and implementation of NIC and NOC.

A fundraising advisory board for the Center is established and members appointed.

1996

The first journal article about the NOC appears in print in *Image–Journal of Nursing Scholarship*.

The first meeting of the Center's fundraising advisory board is held at the College of Nursing.

The first vendor (ERGO) signs licensing agreement for NIC and NOC.

1997

The first international NANDA, NIC, NOC Conference focused on facilitating use of the terminologies is held in St. Charles, Illinois, November 1–9.

The first edition of *Nursing Outcomes Classification (NOC)* is published by Mosby.

The *NIC Letter* becomes *the NIC/NOC Letter.*

1998

The second outcomes research grant funded by NINR (1998–2002) with 3 PIs: Marion Johnson, Meridean Maas, & Sue Moorhead.

NOC recognized by the American Nurses Association.

NOC is added to National Library of Medicine's Metathesaurus.

The Cumulative Index to Nursing and Health Care Literature (CINAHL) adds NOC to their index.

NIC and NOC submit information to American National Standards Institute Health Informatics Standards Board (ANSI HISB) for Inventory of Clinical Information Standards.

The NIC/NOC Letter is sponsored by Mosby Year Book.

The Center for Nursing Classification receives 3 years of support from the College of Nursing (1998–2001) and is allocated space on the fourth floor of the College of Nursing. Joanne McCloskey is appointed Director.

A monograph linking NIC interventions to NOC outcomes is published by the Center.

1999

The first Institute on Nursing Informatics and Classification is held at the University of Iowa, June 15–19.

NIC and NOC, along with other nursing language developers, give testimony about each classification to a subcommittee of the National Committee on Vital and Health Statistics (NCHVS). The goal is to include nursing terms in the standardized Patient Medical Record Information (PMRI).

NIC and NOC representatives participate in an invitational vocabulary conference at Vanderbilt University in Nashville, directed by Judy Osbolt with a goal toward developing a reference terminology for nursing.

NIC and NOC representatives attend an invitational meeting of the SNOMED (Systematized Nomenclature of Medicine) Convergent terminology group in Chicago, IL.

A second conference focused on NANDA, NIC, and NOC is held in New Orleans, Louisiana, April 14–17.

The first translations of the *Nursing Outcomes Classification* are published in Dutch, French, Japanese, and Korean.

2000

The *Nursing Interventions Classification, 3rd edition and the Nursing Outcomes Classification 2nd edition* are published by Mosby.

The NNN (Nursing Diagnoses, Nursing Interventions, and Nursing Outcomes) Alliance is created as a virtual organization, to foster a working relationship between NANDA, NIC, and NOC with Joanne McCloskey Dochterman and Dorothy Jones serving as co-chairs of the Alliance along with a governing board including members of the NANDA Board and Center for Classification Board at Iowa.

A monograph linking NIC and NOC with the long-term care minimum data set resident assessment instrument's (RAI) resident assessment protocols (RAPs) is published by the Center.

A monograph linking NIC and NOC with the Outcome and Assessment Information Set (OASIS) is published by the Center.

A monograph linking NOC with the Omaha Classification is published by the Center.

The second Institute on Nursing Informatics and Classification is held at the College of Nursing from June 11–14.

2001

The first edition, authored by the NIC and NOC PIs, of *Nursing Diagnoses, Outcomes, Interventions: NANDA, NOC, and NIC Linkages* is published by Mosby.

An NNN Invitational Common Structure Conference is funded by the National Library of Medicine (Joanne Dochterman and Dorothy Jones, PIs) and held in Utica, Illinois in August.

An effectiveness grant is funded Agency for Healthcare Research and Quality (AHRQ) & NINR for large data base research using NIC (Marita Titler and Joanne Dochterman). This is likely the first such grant to fund nursing effectiveness research using a clinical database with nursing standardized language.

NIC and NOC are registered in Health Level Seven (HL7).

The Center for Nursing Classification receives 3 years of support from University of Iowa central administrative offices.

The second edition of the *Nursing Outcomes Classification* is published in Spanish by Ediciones Harcourt.

The third Institute on Nursing Informatics and Classification is held at the College of Nursing in June.

Dr. Marion Johnson retires from the College of Nursing July 1.

2002

The NNN Alliance holds an international conference on nursing language, classification, and informatics in Chicago IL. NANDA's biennial conference becomes integrated into the NNN meeting. A White Paper on the Development of a Common Structure for NANDA, NIC, and NOC is presented to participants.

SNOMED licenses NIC and NOC for inclusion into their database.

The Center for Nursing Classification expands its name to Center for Nursing Classification and Clinical Effectiveness (CNC); its endowment reaches $600,000.

The fourth Institute on Nursing Informatics and Classification is held at the College of Nursing June 23–26.

A 4-hour web course, *NIC and NOC 101: The Basics,* is offered by the Center for Nursing Classification & Clinical Effectiveness at the University of Iowa.

A monograph, *Curriculum Guide for Implementation of NANDA, NIC, and NOC in an Undergraduate Nursing Curriculum*, authored by Cindy Finesilver and Debbie Metzler from Bellin College, is published by the Center.

A second institutional training grant for pre- and post-doctoral students in effectiveness research is funded at the University of Iowa by NINR, with Joanne Dochterman and Martha Craft-Rosenberg as Directors.

The position of Center Fellow is established (to assist in the ongoing development of NIC and NOC) and about 30 people are appointed for 3-year terms.

2003

ANA publishes the Common Taxonomy of Nursing Practice in a monograph, *Unifying Nursing Languages: The Harmonization of NANDA, NIC, and NOC* (edited by Joanne Dochterman and Dorothy Jones).

The first meeting of the CNC Fellows is held April 11th at the College of Nursing.

NANDA, NIC, NOC software program based on linkage book *Nursing Diagnoses, Outcomes, and Interventions: NANDA, NOC and NIC Linkages—CD-ROM* produced by Mosby.

The Center for Nursing Classification and Clinical Effectiveness receives the Sigma Theta Tau Board of Director's Award for in recognition of established excellence in integrating knowledge and clinical experience to achieve exemplary practice.

Fifth Institute on Nursing Informatics & Classification is held, June 9–12.

The second edition of the *Nursing Outcomes Classification* is translated into Japanese by Igaku-Shoin MYW.

Elizabeth Swanson and Howard Butcher join the CNC Executive Board.

A Spanish version of the web course, *NIC and NOC 101: The Basics,* translated by Patricia Levi is offered by the Center for Nursing Classification & Clinical Effectiveness at the University of Iowa.

Dr. Meridean Maas retires from the College of Nursing on July 1.

2004

The *Nursing Interventions Classification, 4th edition and the 3rd edition Nursing Outcomes Classification* are published by Mosby.

Dr. Renata Stemmer is sponsored by Sue Moorhead as a visiting scholar from Germany for 3 weeks in March.

The second meeting of the CNC Fellows is held in April.

The NNN Alliance holds the second International Conference on Nursing Language, Classification & Informatics in Chicago, Illinois.

The first Annette Scheffel Fundraising event was held in the fall.

Joanne McCloskey Dochterman retires as Director of the Center and Sue Moorhead is appointed Director effective July 1, 2004.

A monograph, *Guideline for Conducting Effectiveness Research in Nursing and Other Health Care Services,* authored by Marita Titler, Joanne Dochterman, and David Reed is published by the Center.

The Center for Nursing Classification and Clinical Effectiveness endowment reaches $700,000.

The second edition of the *Nursing Outcomes Classification* is published in Portuguese for the first time by Artmed Editora.

2005

NIC and NOC terms are incorporated into Geriatric Nursing Interventions Research Center (GNIRC) protocols.

Sixth Institute on Nursing Informatics & Classification is held June 13–15.

Center Fellows reappointed for 3-year term beginning July 1. Additional fellows were nominated and appointed.

The Center for Nursing Classification & Clinical Effectiveness celebrates its 10th anniversary in December.

The second Annette Scheffel fundraising event was held December 2nd with a reception and a live and silent auction.

The second edition of the *Nursing Outcomes Classification* is published in German for the first time by Verlag Hans Huber and the third edition of NOC into simplified Chinese by Peking University Medical Press/Elsevier (Singapore).

2006

The second edition *NANDA, NOC, and NIC Linkages: Nursing Diagnoses, Outcomes, Interventions* is published by Mosby.

The NNN Alliance holds the third International Conference on Nursing Language, Classification and Informatics in Philadelphia, Pennsylvania.

Five new fellows appointed at the Annual meeting in April.

American Nurses Association (ANA) recognition of NIC and NOC is renewed.

2007

The Seventh Institute on Nursing Informatics is held June 11–13.

The Center offers first research grant for $10,000.

The third edition of the *Nursing Outcomes Classification* is published for the first time in Italian by Casa Editrice Ambrosiana and Norwegian by Akribe.

2008

The fifth edition of the *Nursing Interventions Classification* and the fourth edition of the *Nursing Outcomes Classification* are published by Mosby Elsevier.

Joanne Dochterman retires from the CNC Executive Board.

The Eighth Institute of Nursing Informatics & Classification is held from June 9–11.

The Center becomes an affiliate member of the Alliance for Nursing Informatics (ANI).

2009

CNC submits materials to ANA for Biennial Recognition process.

Dr. Adenike Olagun is sponsored by Sue Moorhead as a visiting scholar from Nigeria through an International Network of Doctoral Education in Nursing (INDEN) Scholarship award.

CNC offers first postdoctoral fellowship for $10,000.

Dr. Gloria Bulechek retires from the College of Nursing July 1.

2010

The Center offers first real-time teleconference to Ile Ife, Nigeria, March 14–19.

The Ninth Institute on Nursing Informatics & Classification is held June 9–11.

Renata Pereira de Melo from Universidade Federal do Ceará, Brazil is sponsored by Sue Moorhead as a predoctoral student from Brazil.

A major renovation to the Center is completed with updated electronic equipment to facilitate conferencing and upkeep of the classifications.

2011

Cheryl Wagner accepts appointment as NIC editor.

Elsevier creates NIC/NOC Facebook site and supports quarterly newsletter.

Meridean Maas selected as a Living Legend of the American Academy of Nursing.

Dr. Prisca Adejurmo is sponsored by Sue Moorhead as a visiting scholar from Nigeria through an INDEN Scholarship award.

2012

The third edition of *NOC and NIC Linkages to NANDA-I and Clinical Conditions: Supporting Critical Reasoning and Quality Care* is published by Elsevier Mosby.

A celebration of the 20th anniversary of the *Nursing Interventions Classification* and the 15th anniversary of the *Nursing Outcomes Classification* is held at the NANDA International 40th anniversary conference in Houston, Texas.

Meridean Maas, Gloria Bulechek, and Sue Moorhead are inducted as Fellows of NANDA International (Inaugural Inductee) (FNI), NANDA.

Alice Gabrielle DeSousa Costa from Federal Universidade of Ceará, Fortalenza, Brazil is sponsored by Sue Moorhead as a visiting Fulbright Scholar as part of her PhD program.

2013

The sixth edition of the *Nursing Interventions Classification* and the fifth edition of the *Nursing Outcomes Classification* are published by Mosby Elsevier.

The Tenth Institute on Nursing Informatics and Classification is held June 13–14 at the College of Nursing, University of Iowa.

Sharon Sweeney completes 10 years of service to the Center as the Administrative Coordinator.

Sue Moorhead is inducted as a Fellow of the American Academy of Nursing.

2014

Camila Takao Lopez is sponsored as a pre-doctoral student from University Federal de Sao Paulo, Brazil by Sue Moorhead from 9/1/2014 to 11/30/2014.

Agueda Maria Ruiz Zimmer Calvacante is sponsored as a pre-doctoral student from University Federal de Sao Paulo, Brazil by Sue Moorhead from 9/1/2014 to 11/30/2014.

Dr. Hatis Bebis is sponsored by Sue Moorhead as a visiting scholar from Gulhane Military Medical Academy in Turkey from 9/17/14 to 9/30/15.

2015

Dr. Miriam de Abreu Almeida is sponsored by Sue Moorhead as a visiting scholar from University Federal do Rio Grande, Brazil from 9/1/2015 to 11/27/2015.

The Center celebrates 20 years as an Iowa Board of Regents Center focused on facilitating ongoing research and implementation of NIC and NOC.

2016

Stella Chinma Adereti is sponsored by Sue Moorhead as a pre-doctoral student from Obafemi Awolowo University, Nigeria funded by an INDEN Scholarship award from 3/16/2016 to 6/16/2016.

The fifth edition of the *Nursing Outcomes Classification* is published for the first time in Indonesian by CV Mocomedia/Elsevier (Singapore).

Noriko Abe is hired as a temporary part-time Administrative Service Coordinator.

Sue Moorhead receives the Founders Award for her service to NANDA International.

2017

Elsevier expands licensing process to other international offices.

Noriko Abe's Center position is changed to a part-time Research Support Coordinator.

Suellen Cristina Dias Emidio is sponsored by Sue Moorhead as a pre-doctoral student from University of Campinas (UNICAMP), Brazil from 8/14/2017 to 12/14/2017.

Natany da Costa Ferreira is sponsored by Sue Moorhead as a pre-doctoral student from University Federal de Sao Paulo, Brazil from 8/16/2017 to 12/16/2017.

Dr. Amalia de Fatima Lucena is sponsored by Sue Moorhead and Elizabeth Swanson as a visiting scholar from the Federal University Rio Grande do Sul, Brazil from 9/1/2017 to 11/30/2017.

Dr. Elenice Valentim Carmona is sponsored by Sue Moorhead as a visiting scholar from University of Campinas (UNICAMP), Brazil from 11/9/2017 to 11/23/2017.

2018

The seventh edition of the *Nursing Interventions Classification* and the sixth edition of the *Nursing Outcomes Classification* are published by Elsevier.

Noriko Abe hired as a full time CNC coordinator.

Vanessa M. Mantovani is sponsored by Sue Moorhead as a pre-doctoral student from Federal University Rio Grande do Sul, Brazil from 9/15/2018 to 02/22/2019.

Celebration of 120th anniversary of Nursing at Iowa.

2019

Elizabeth Swanson retires in July from the College of Nursing.

Karen Dunn Lopez is hired as Director of Research for the Center as part of her appointment as a tenured Associate Professor on August 1.

NIC & NOC terms updated in SNOMED Clinical Terms.

Cheryl Wagner is appointed as an Adjunct Assistant Professor at the College of Nursing for a 3-year term (9/1/2019–6/30/2022).

2020

A Strategic Planning Conference is held in February at the College of Nursing to establish a Strategic Plan for the next 5 years with external consultation support.

First Doctor of Nursing Practice (DNP) project using NIC and NOC completed by Erin Cullen.

Dr. Natany da Costa Ferreira is appointed as an Adjunct Associate for the College of Nursing and is funded for a 1-year post-doctoral experience.

Sue Moorhead steps down as Director of the Center and Karen Dunn Lopez becomes the Director on July 1.

Dr. Meridean Maas dies in November after a brief illness.

The Center celebrates 25 years as a Board of Regents approved Center in the College of Nursing.

2021

Sue Moorhead retires from the College of Nursing, January 1.

Three papers linking NANDA-I, NOC, and NIC to care of COVID-19 patients, families and communities are published in the *International Journal of Nursing Knowledge.*

Dr. Miriam de Abreu Almedia is appointed as an Adjunct Associate Professor at the College of Nursing for a 3-year term (7/1/2021–6/30/2024).

Dr. Vanessa Mantovani is appointed as an Adjunct Assistant Professor at the College of Nursing for a 3-year term (8/1/2021–6/30/2024).

Dr. Suellen Cristina Dias Emidio is appointed as an Adjunct Assistant Professor at the College of Nursing for a 3-year term (8/1/2021–6/30/2024).

Dr. Amalia de Fatima Lucena is appointed as an Adjunct Associate Professor at the College of Nursing for a 3-year term (9/1/2021–6/30/2024).

Elspeth Adriana McMullan is hired for a new position in the Center as a Center Administrator/Research Specialist in September.

Karen Dunn Lopez is inducted as a Fellow of the American Academy of Nursing.

Karen Dunn Lopez becomes the Center representative to the Alliance for Nursing Informatics.

Dr. Mary Clarke is appointed as an editor of NIC for the eighth edition.

The Center supports a full-time postdoctoral fellowship for Dr. Natany da Costa Ferreira Oberfrank.

2022

Dr. Natany da Costa Ferreira Oberfrank accepts a faculty position on the tenure track at the College of Nursing.

The University of Iowa celebrates its 175th anniversary in February.

Dr. Sena Chae accepts a faculty position on the tenure track at the College of Nursing.

CNC coordinator, Noriko Abe, receives the Iowa Women's Foundation award for her work with NIC and NOC editors.

The CNC celebrates the 30th anniversary of NIC and the 25th anniversary of NOC.

Dr. Howard K. Butcher is inducted as a fellow of the American Academy of Nursing.

CNC co-sponsors a virtual workshop, Honoring the Legacy of Virginia Saba Through Charting a Path Forward for Standardized Nursing Terminologies in Practice and Research, organized by the Friends of the National Library of Medicine (10/20-21/2022).

2023

Raisa Camilo Ferreira is sponsored as a pre-doctoral student from State University of Campinas, Sao Paulo, Brazil by Karen Dunn Lopez and Sue Moorhead from 1/17/2023 to 6/16/2023.

NANDA International celebrates 50-year anniversary at the international conference in June.

The eighth edition of the *Nursing Interventions Classification* and the seventh edition of the *Nursing Outcomes Classification* are published by Elsevier.

In addition to the aforementioned events, NOC has been presented over the years at numerous national and international conferences. Presentations in other countries include Australia, Austria, Brazil, Canada, Czech Republic, Columbia, Denmark, England, Estonia, France, Germany, Iceland, Italy, Ireland, Japan, Mexico, Netherlands, Nigeria, Portugal, Peru, Slovenia, Slovakia, Spain, South Korea, Sweden, Switzerland, Taiwan, Turkey, and Wales.

Guidelines for Submission of a New or Revised Outcome

The Nursing-Sensitive Outcomes Classification (NOC) editors are interested in feedback and submission of outcomes for review and potential addition to the NOC. Feedback may be organized in the following manner.

A. GENERAL COMMENTS ABOUT THE CLASSIFICATION

Comments about the classification in general are welcome as are suggestions for outcomes that need to be developed. The outcome suggestions for development can be at the individual, family, or community state, behavior, or perception to be measured along a continuum.

B. FEEDBACK ON AN OUTCOME

If the submission is a revision of an existing NOC outcome, provide a paragraph briefly describing the rationale for changes and note the changes on a copy of the existing outcome. Suggestions can include changes in the definition, indicators, or scale. Additional indicators and the most current references can be suggested.

C. FEEDBACK ON A MEASUREMENT SCALE(S)

Comments on a particular scale are encouraged. Please briefly explain your suggestions and provide background on your experience in using the scale. Identify the outcome and provide a brief description of the patient populations(s) you are using the outcome with.

D. GUIDELINES FOR OUTCOME SUBMISSION

Each submission of a proposed outcome must include a label, a definition, indicators, and a short list of up-to-date references that support the outcome and document the indicators selected. You also may suggest a scale(s) to use with the outcome. A brief paragraph describing the rationale for adding the outcome to the NOC should be included. The rationale should note how the proposed outcome is different from outcomes already included in the NOC.

General Principles for Developing Outcomes

1. Define the outcome as a variable patient or client state, behavior, or perception that is responsive to nursing intervention(s).
2. Labels should be concise, stated in five or fewer words.
3. Colons can be used to make broader concepts more specific.
4. Labels should describe concepts that can be measured along a continuum.
5. Labels should be neutral and not stated as goals.
6. A set of indicators, more specific than the outcome, must be identified
7. The definition should clearly define the concept and encompass the indicators and is consistent with definitions using the same scale.

E. FEEDBACK ON CORE OUTCOMES BY SPECIALTY

Comments on core specialty outcomes are welcome. Please send suggestions for additional outcomes as well as any deletions you think are needed.

Comments and suggestions can be sent to:
classification-center@uiowa.edu

or by mail to:

The University of Iowa
College of Nursing
Center for Nursing Classification and Clinical Effectiveness
CNB 407
50 Newton Road
Iowa City, Iowa 52242
USA
Phone: (319) 335-7051

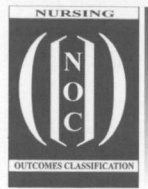

Index